Common haematology

Haemoglobin		
Mean cell volume, MCV		
Platelets		
White cells (total)		p322
neutrophils	$2.0\text{-}7.5 \times 10^9/\text{L}$	p322
lymphocytes	$1.0\text{-}4.5 \times 10^9/\text{L}$	p322
eosinophils	$0.04\text{-}0.4 \times 10^9/\text{L}$	p322

Blood gases

pH	7.35-7.45	p662
P_aO_2	>10.6kPa	p662
P_aCO_2	4.7-6kPa	p662
Base excess	± 2mmol/L	p662

U&Es (urea and electrolytes)

Sodium	135-145mmol/L	p664
Potassium	3.5-5.3mmol/L	p666
Creatinine	70-100μmol/L	p294-7
Urea	2.5-6.7mmol/L	p294-7
eGFR	$>60\text{mL/min/}1.73\text{m}^2$	p661

LFTs (liver function tests)

Bilirubin	3-17μmol/L	p268, p270
Alanine aminotransferase, ALT	5-35IU/L	p268, p270
Aspartate transaminase, AST	5-35IU/L	p268, p270
Alkaline phosphatase, ALP	30-130IU/L (*non-pregnant adults*)	p268, p270
Albumin	35-50g/L	p678

Cardiac enzymes

Troponin T	<99th percentile of upper reference limit: value depends on local assay	p115

Other biochemical values

Cholesterol	<5mmol/L	p682
Triglycerides	Fasting: 0.5-2.3mmol/L	p682
Amylase	0-180IU/dL	p628
C-reactive protein, CRP	<10mg/L	p678
Corrected calcium	2.12-2.60mmol/L	p668
Glucose, fasting	3.5-5.5mmol/L	p200
Thyroid-stimulating hormone, TSH	0.5-4.2mU/L	p210

For all other reference intervals, see p734-41

He moved

all the brightest gems

faster and faster towards the

ever-growing bucket of lost hopes;
had there been just one more year

of peace the battalion would have made
a floating system of perpetual drainage.

A silent fall of immense snow came near oily
remains of the recently eaten supper on the table.

We drove on in our old sunless walnut. Presently
classical eggs ticked in the new afternoon shadows.

We were instructed by my cousin Jasper not to exercise by country
house visiting unless accompanied by thirteen geese or gangsters.

The modern American did not prevail over the pair of redundant bronze puppies.
The worn-out principle is a bad omen which I am never glad to ransom in August.

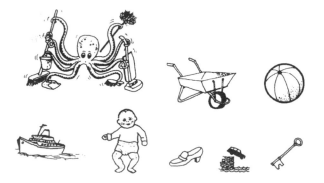

Reading tests Hold this chart (well-illuminated) 30cm away, and record the smallest type read (eg n12 left eye, n6 right eye, spectacles worn) or object named accurately.

OXFORD HANDBOOK OF
CLINICAL MEDICINE

ELEVENTH EDITION

Ian B. Wilkinson
Tim Raine
Kate Wiles
Peter Hateley
Dearbhla Kelly
Iain McGurgan

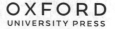

OXFORD
UNIVERSITY PRESS

Oxford University Press, Great Clarendon Street, Oxford OX2 6DP

Oxford University Press is a department of the University of Oxford. It furthers the University's objective of excellence in research, scholarship, and education by publishing worldwide. Oxford is a registered trade mark of Oxford University Press in the UK and in certain other countries.

Published in the United States by Oxford University Press Inc., New York

© Oxford University Press, 2024

The moral rights of the authors have been asserted

Database right Oxford University Press (maker)

First published 1985	Fifth edition 2001	Tenth edition 2017
(RA Hope & JM Longmore)	(JM Longmore & IB Wilkinson)	(IB Wilkinson, T Raine & K Wiles)
Second edition 1989	Sixth edition 2004	Eleventh edition 2024
Third edition 1993	Seventh edition 2007	
Fourth edition 1998	Eighth edition 2010	
	Ninth edition 2014	

Translations:

Chinese	French	Hungarian	Polish	Russian
Czech	German	Indonesian	Portuguese	Spanish
Estonian	Greek	Italian	Romanian	

British Library Cataloguing in Publication Data
Data available

Library of Congress Control Number: 2023944066

ISBN 978-0-19-884401-3

Printed in Italy by L.E.G.O. S.p.A. Lavis (TN)

Gender

Where guidelines apply to pregnancy and childbirth, the word 'women' should be assumed to cover all people who can get pregnant and would need access to healthcare services in this capacity. Their gender identity should be respected at the point of care.

Drugs

Except where otherwise stated, recommendations are for the **non-pregnant adult** who is **not breastfeeding** and who has reasonable **renal and hepatic function.**

We have made every effort to check this text, but it is still possible that drug or other errors have been missed. OUP makes no representation, express or implied, that doses are correct. Readers are urged to check with the most up to date product information, codes of conduct, and safety regulations. The authors and the publishers do not accept responsibility or legal liability for any errors in the text, or for the misuse or misapplication of material in this work.

For updates/corrections, see http://www.oup.co.uk/academic/series/oxhmed/updates/

Contents

Each chapter's contents are detailed on its first page

Preface to the eleventh edition

I must sincerely apologize for the delay in publishing the eleventh edition of the handbook, but to quote Harold MacMillan: 'Events, dear boy, events.' COVID hit midway through our programme of work on this edition, and we all devoted our time and effort to clinical duties, bringing work on the book to a complete halt. COVID has had a profound effect on all of us, both personally and professionally—who would have thought that we would be conducting consultations remotely, all know so much about a new virus, or have received our first mRNA vaccination. Pandemic over, we regrouped, doubled our efforts, and completed the book, aided in no small part by the endless patience and assistance of Kate and Elizabeth at OUP.

The formula is the same unique blend of fact, explanation, context-setting, and guidance that generations of medical students have enjoyed, but brought right up-to-date—including SARS viruses! We have tried to provide a greater emphasis on what really matters, whilst retaining a very personal perspective and creating a little more white space. Tim, Kate, and I have been joined by three new authors for this edition, providing a broad range of expertise including Clinical Pharmacology, Hepatology, Nephrology, Neurology, and General Practice as well as new ideas. As always, we greatly value the feedback from our junior and senior readers, and long may it continue.

I do hope that you will enjoy this edition of the *OHCM* as much as previous editions and that the twelfth edition is not as long in gestation as this one was.

IBW, 2024

Preface to the first edition

We wrote this book not because we know so much, but because we know we re-member so little ... the problem is not simply the quantity of information, but the diversity of places from which it is dispensed. Trailing eagerly behind the surgeon, the student is admonished never to forget alcohol withdrawal as a cause of post-operative confusion. The scrap of paper on which this is written spends a month in the pocket before being lost for ever in the laundry. At different times, and in in-convenient places, a number of other causes may be presented to the student. Not only are these causes and aphorisms never brought together, but when, as a sur-gical house officer, the former student faces a confused patient, none is to hand.

We aim to encourage the doctor to enjoy his patients: in doing so we believe he will prosper in the practice of medicine. For a long time now, house officers have been encouraged to adopt monstrous proportions in order to straddle the diverse pinnacles of clinical science and clinical experience. We hope that this book will make this endeavour a little easier by moving a cumulative memory burden from the mind into the pocket, and by removing some of the fears that are naturally felt when starting a career in medicine, thereby freely allowing the doctor's clinical acumen to grow by the slow accretion of many, many days and nights.

RA Hope and JM Longmore, 1985

Acknowledgements

Heart-felt thanks to our advisers on specific sections—each is acknowledged on the chapter's first page. Our thanks to our junior readers, Emma Flint, Adam Komorowski, Oliver Mowforth, Gemma Smith, Christina Taylor, and Tom Weatherby. We especially thank all our mentors and teachers, and patients who provide our inspiration and remind us that one never stops learning. We acknowledge the Department of Radiology at both the Leeds Teaching Hospitals NHS Trust and the Norfolk and Norwich University Hospital for their kind help in providing many images, particularly Dr Edmund Godfrey, whose tireless hunt for perfect images has improved so many chapters.

Readers' comments These have formed a vital part of our endeavour to provide an accurate, comprehensive, and up-to-date text. We sincerely thank the many students, doctors, and other health professionals who have found the time and the generosity to write to us on our Reader's Comments Cards, in editions past, or, in more recent times, via the web. These have now become so numerous for past editions that they cannot all be listed. See http://www.oup.com/uk/academic/series/oxhmed/links for a full list, and our very heart-felt tokens of thanks.

3rd-party web addresses We disclaim any responsibility for 3rd-party content.

Symbols and abbreviations

►	this fact or idea is important	CVS	cardiovascular system
►►	don't dawdle!—prompt action saves lives	CXR	chest x-ray
▲	warning	d	day(s); also expressed as /7; months are /12
!	reference	DC	direct current
♂:♀	male-to-female ratio. ♂:♀=2:1 means twice as common in males	DIC	disseminated intravascular coagulation
		DIP	distal interphalangeal
∴	therefore	dL	decilitre
∵	because of	DM	diabetes mellitus
~	approximately	DOAC	direct oral anticoagulant
≈	approximately equal to	DU	duodenal ulcer
–ve	negative	D&V	diarrhoea and vomiting
+ve	positive	DVT	deep venous thrombosis
>	greater than	EBV	Epstein–Barr virus
<	less than	ECG	electrocardiogram
↑↓	increased or decreased	Echo	echocardiogram
→	leading to	EDTA	ethylene diamine tetra-acetic acid (anticoagulant coating, eg in FBC bottles)
↔	normal (eg serum level)		
1°	primary	EEG	electroencephalogram
2°	secondary	eGFR	estimated glomerular filtration rate (in mL/min/1.73m²)
Δ	diagnosis		
ΔΔ	differential diagnosis	ELISA	enzyme-linked immunosorbent assay
A₂	aortic component of the 2nd heart sound	EM	electron microscope
Ab	antibody	EMG	electromyogram
ABC	airway, breathing, and circulation	ENT	ear, nose, and throat
ABG	arterial blood gas: P_aO_2, P_aCO_2, pH, HCO_3	ERCP	endoscopic retrograde cholangiopancreatography
ABPA	allergic bronchopulmonary aspergillosis		
ACE-i	angiotensin-converting enzyme inhibitor	ESR	erythrocyte sedimentation rate
ACR	albumin to creatinine ratio (mg/mmol)	ESRF	end-stage renal failure
ACS	acute coronary syndrome	EUA	examination under anaesthesia
ACTH	adrenocorticotropic hormone	FBC	full blood count
ADH	antidiuretic hormone	FDP	fibrin degradation products
AF	atrial fibrillation	FEV₁	forced expiratory volume in 1st second
AFB	acid-fast bacillus	F_iO_2	partial pressure of O_2 in inspired air
Ag	antigen	FFP	fresh frozen plasma
AIDS	acquired immunodeficiency syndrome	FSH	follicle-stimulating hormone
AKI	acute kidney injury	FVC	forced vital capacity
ALL	acute lymphoblastic leukaemia	g	gram
ALP	alkaline phosphatase	G6PD	glucose-6-phosphate dehydrogenase
AMA	antimitochondrial antibody	GA	general anaesthetic
AMP	adenosine monophosphate	GCS	Glasgow Coma Scale
ANA	antinuclear antibody	GFR	glomerular filtration rate
ANCA	antineutrophil cytoplasmic antibody	GGT	gamma-glutamyl transferase
APTT	activated partial thromboplastin time	GH	growth hormone
AR	aortic regurgitation	GI	gastrointestinal
ARA	angiotensin receptor antagonist (blocker)	GN	glomerulonephritis
ARDS	acute respiratory distress syndrome	GP	general practitioner
ART	antiretroviral therapy	GPA	granulomatosis with polyangiitis (formerly Wegener's granulomatosis)
AS	aortic stenosis		
ASD	atrial septal defect	GTN	glyceryl trinitrate
AST	aspartate transaminase	GTT	glucose tolerance test
ATN	acute tubular necrosis	GU(M)	genitourinary (medicine)
ATP	adenosine triphosphate	h	hour(s)
AV	atrioventricular	HAV	hepatitis A virus
AVM	arteriovenous malformation(s)	Hb	haemoglobin
AXR	abdominal x-ray (plain)	HbA1c	glycated haemoglobin
BAL	bronchoalveolar lavage	HBsAg	hepatitis B surface antigen
BD	*bis die* (Latin for twice a day)	HBV	hepatitis B virus
BNF	*British National Formulary*	HCC	hepatocellular cancer
BNP	brain natriuretic peptide	HCM	hypertrophic obstructive cardiomyopathy
BP	blood pressure	Hct	haematocrit
BPH	benign prostatic hyperplasia	HCV	hepatitis C virus
bpm	beats per minute	HDV	hepatitis D virus
ca	cancer	HDL	high-density lipoprotein
Ca²⁺	calcium	HHT	hereditary haemorrhagic telangiectasia
CABG	coronary artery bypass graft	HIV	human immunodeficiency virus
cAMP	cyclic adenosine monophosphate (AMP)	HLA	human leucocyte antigen
CAPD	continuous ambulatory peritoneal dialysis	HONK	hyperosmolar non-ketotic (coma)
CCF	congestive cardiac failure (ie left and right heart failure)	HPV	human papillomavirus
		HR	heart rate
CCU	coronary care unit	HRT	hormone replacement therapy
CDT	*Clostridium difficile* toxin	HSP	Henoch–Schönlein purpura
CHD	coronary heart disease	HSV	herpes simplex virus
CI	contraindication(s)	HUS	haemolytic uraemic syndrome
CK	creatine (phospho) kinase	IBD	inflammatory bowel disease
CKD	chronic kidney disease	IBW	ideal body weight
CLL	chronic lymphocytic leukaemia	ICD	implantable cardioverter defibrillator
CML	chronic myeloid leukaemia	ICP	intracranial pressure
CMV	cytomegalovirus	ICU	intensive care unit
CNS	central nervous system	IE	infective endocarditis
COPD	chronic obstructive pulmonary disease	Ig	immunoglobulin
CoV	coronavirus	IHD	ischaemic heart disease
COVID-19	coronavirus disease 2019	IM	intramuscular
CPAP	continuous positive airway pressure	INR	international normalized ratio
CPR	cardiopulmonary resuscitation	IP	interphalangeal
CRP	c-reactive protein	IPPV	intermittent positive pressure ventilation
CSF	cerebrospinal fluid	ITP	idiopathic thrombocytopenic purpura
CT	computed tomography	ITU	intensive therapy unit
CV	cardiovascular	IU	international unit
CVA	cerebrovascular accident	IV	intravenous
CVD	cardiovascular disease	IVC	inferior vena cava
CVP	central venous pressure	IVI	intravenous (infusion)

IVU	intravenous urography
JVP	jugular venous pressure
K⁺	potassium
kg	kilogram
kPa	kiloPascal
L	litre
LAD	left axis deviation on the ECG
LBBB	left bundle branch block
LDH	lactate dehydrogenase
LDL	low-density lipoprotein
LFT	liver function test
LH	luteinizing hormone
LIF	left iliac fossa
LMN	lower motor neuron
LMWH	low-molecular-weight heparin
LOC	loss of consciousness
LP	lumbar puncture
LUQ	left upper quadrant
LV	left ventricle of the heart
LVF	left ventricular failure
LVH	left ventricular hypertrophy
MALT	mucosa-associated lymphoid tissue
MAOI	monoamine oxidase inhibitor
MAP	mean arterial pressure
MC&S	microscopy, culture, and sensitivity
mcg	microgram(s)
MCP	metacarpophalangeal
MCV	mean cell volume
MDMA	3,4-methylenedioxymethamphetamine
ME	myalgic encephalomyelitis
mg	milligram(s)
Mg²⁺	magnesium
MI	myocardial infarction
min	minute(s)
mL	millilitre(s)
mmHg	millimetres of mercury
MND	motor neuron disease
MR	modified release or mitral regurgitation
MRA	magnetic resonance angiography
MRCP	magnetic resonance cholangiopancreatography
MRI	magnetic resonance imaging
MRSA	meticillin-resistant *Staphylococcus aureus*
MS	multiple sclerosis
MSM	men who have sex with men
MSU	midstream urine
mth(s)	month(s)
N&V	nausea and/or vomiting
Na⁺	sodium
NBM	nil by mouth
NEWS	National Early Warning Score
ng	nanogram(s)
NG	nasogastric
NHS	National Health Service (UK)
NICE	National Institute for Health and Care Excellence, http://www.nice.org.uk
NMDA	N-methyl-D-aspartate
NNT	number needed to treat
nocte	at night
NR	normal range (=reference interval)
NSAID	non-steroidal anti-inflammatory drug
OCP	oral contraceptive pill
OD	*omni die* (Latin for once daily)
OGD	oesophagogastroduodenoscopy
OGTT	oral glucose tolerance test
OHCS	*Oxford Handbook of Clinical Specialties*
OT	occupational therapist
P₂	pulmonary component of 2nd heart sound
P_aCO₂	partial pressure of CO₂ in arterial blood
PAN	polyarteritis nodosa
P_aO₂	partial pressure of O₂ in arterial blood
PBC	primary biliary cirrhosis
PCR	polymerase chain reaction or protein to creatinine ratio (mg/mmol)
PCV	packed cell volume
PE	pulmonary embolism
PEEP	positive end-expiratory pressure
PEF(R)	peak expiratory flow (rate)
PET	positron emission tomography
PID	pelvic inflammatory disease
PIP	proximal interphalangeal (joint)
PND	paroxysmal nocturnal dyspnoea
PO	*per os* (by mouth)

PPI	proton pump inhibitor, eg omeprazole
PR	*per rectum* (by the rectum)
PRL	prolactin
PRN	*pro re nata* (Latin for as required)
PRV	polycythaemia rubra vera
PSA	prostate-specific antigen
PTH	parathyroid hormone
PTT	prothrombin time
PUO	pyrexia of unknown origin
PVD	peripheral vascular disease
QDS	*quater die sumendus*; take 4 times daily
R	right
RA	rheumatoid arthritis
RAD	right axis deviation on the ECG
RBBB	right bundle branch block
RBC	red blood cell
RCT	randomized controlled trial
RDW	red cell distribution width
RFT	respiratory function tests
Rh	Rhesus status
RIF	right iliac fossa
RR	respiratory rate
RRT	renal replacement therapy
RUQ	right upper quadrant
RV	right ventricle of heart
RVF	right ventricular failure
RVH	right ventricular hypertrophy
℞	*recipe* (Latin for treat with)
s	second(s)
S₁, S₂	first and second heart sounds
SARS	severe acute respiratory syndrome
SBE	subacute bacterial endocarditis
SBP	systolic blood pressure
SC	subcutaneous
SD	standard deviation
SE	side effect(s)
SIADH	syndrome of inappropriate antidiuretic hormone secretion
SL	sublingual
SLE	systemic lupus erythematosus
SOB	short of breath
SPO₂	peripheral oxygen saturation (%)
SR	slow-release
Stat	*statim* (immediately; as initial dose)
STD/I	sexually transmitted disease/infection
SVC	superior vena cava
SVT	supraventricular tachycardia
T°	temperature
t½	biological half-life
T₃	tri-iodothyronine
T₄	thyroxine
TB	tuberculosis
TDS	*ter die sumendus* (take 3 times a day)
TFT	thyroid function test (eg TSH)
TIA	transient ischaemic attack
TIBC	total iron-binding capacity
TPN	total parenteral nutrition
TRH	thyrotropin-releasing hormone
TSH	thyroid-stimulating hormone
TTP	thrombotic thrombocytopenic purpura
U	unit(s)
UC	ulcerative colitis
U&E	urea and electrolytes (and creatinine)
UMN	upper motor neuron
URT(I)	upper respiratory tract (infection)
US(S)	ultrasound (scan)
UTI	urinary tract infection
VDRL	Venereal Diseases Research Laboratory
VE	ventricular extrasystole
VF	ventricular fibrillation
VHF	viral haemorrhagic fever
V/Q	ventilation/perfusion scan
VRE	vancomycin-resistant enterococci
VSD	ventricular septal defect
VT	ventricular tachycardia
VTE	venous thromboembolism
WBC	white blood cell
WCC	white blood cell count
WHO	World Health Organization
WPW	Wolff–Parkinson–White
wk(s)	week(s)
yr(s)	year(s)
ZN	Ziehl–Neelsen stain, eg for mycobacteria

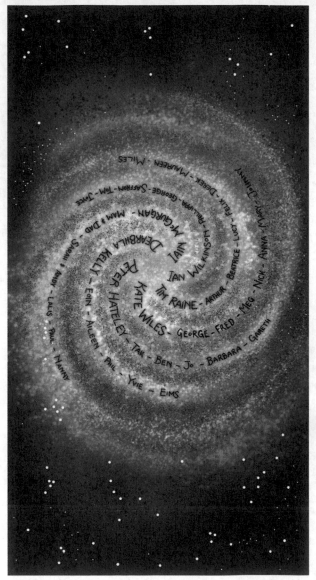

Artwork by Gillian Turner.

'He who studies medicine without books sails an uncharted sea, but he who studies medicine without patients does not go to sea at all'

William Osler 1849–1919

The word 'patient' occurs frequently throughout this book.
Do not skim over it lightly.
Rather pause and doff your metaphorical cap, offering due respect to those who by the opening up of their lives to you, become your true teachers.
Without your patients, you are a technician with a useless skill.
With them, you are a doctor.

1 Thinking about medicine

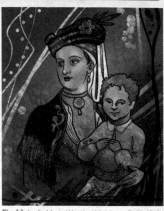

Fig 1.1 Lady Mary Wortley Montagu (1689–1762) was witty and affable, with the wisdom to reject her father's chosen match and marry the British ambassador to Turkey. There she witnessed older women attending parties, bringing with them 'a nut-shell full of the matter of the best sort of small-pox' to be injected into offered veins. Having had and been scarred by smallpox, she offered her son's vein, making him the first English person to receive inoculation against disease. She was 'patriot enough to take pains to bring this useful invention into fashion in England', inoculating her daughter before an audience at the court of George I. No harm occurred and her daughter would go on to marry the prime minister. But history respects the man who convinced the world, not the women who did it first. Inoculation became vaccination with Jenner's comparable use of cow- (*vacca*) pox more than 70 years after Montagu. Vaccination is one of our most powerful life-saving interventions and yet controversy has persisted since Montagu and Jenner.

The severe acute respiratory syndrome coronavirus 2 (SARS-CoV-2) pandemic changed lives, economies, education, politics, sport, and the arts, as well as medicine and our capacity to care for the sick. Change and uncertainty bred misinformation. Enforced lockdowns engendered revolt against establishment diktats. The disconnect between infection and serious illness for the majority distorted risk perception. Populism and non-scientific models of disease became the lifeblood of vaccine dissent.

Honesty, understanding, and communication have never been more important. The success of vaccination programmes is a test of community and cooperation. This remains our biggest challenge and one we cannot afford to fail.

Artwork by Gillian Turner.

We thank Josephine Fielding, our Specialist Reader for this chapter.

The Hippocratic oath

I swear by Apollo the physician and Asclepius and Hygieia and Panacea and all the gods and goddesses, making them my witnesses, that I will fulfil according to my ability and judgement this oath and this covenant.

To hold him who has taught me this art as equal to my parents and to live my life in partnership with him, and if he is in need of money to give him a share of mine, and to regard his offspring as equal to my own brethren and to teach them this art, if they desire to learn it, without fee and covenant. I will impart it by precept, by lecture and by all other manner of teaching, not only to my own sons but also to the sons of him who has taught me, and to disciples bound by covenant and oath according to the law of physicians, but to none other.

The regimen I shall adopt shall be to the benefit of the patients to the best of my power and judgement, not for their injury or any wrongful purpose.

I will not give a deadly drug to anyone though it be asked of me, nor will I lead the way in such counsel.[1] And likewise I will not give a woman a pessary to procure abortion.[2] But I will keep my life and my art in purity and holiness. I will not use the knife,[3] not even, verily, on sufferers of stone but I will give place to such as are craftsmen therein.

Whatsoever house I enter, I will enter for the benefit of the sick, refraining from all voluntary wrongdoing and corruption, especially seduction of male or female, bond or free.

Whatsoever things I see or hear concerning the life of men, in my attendance on the sick, or even apart from my attendance, which ought not to be blabbed abroad, I will keep silence on them, counting such things to be as religious secrets.

If I fulfil this oath and do not violate it, may it be granted to me to enjoy life and art alike, with good repute for all time to come; but may the contrary befall me if I transgress and violate my oath.

The human right to health

The constitution of the World Health Organization decrees that the highest attainable standard of health is a fundamental right of every human being.

But definitions of health are at best broad, and at worst nebulous. It is a limited view which focuses only on the prevention, treatment, and control of disease afforded by access to primary care, hospitals, and essential medicines. A wider discourse includes those factors that are equally, if not more, important for a healthy life including safe drinking water, sanitation, food, adequate housing, and pollution. The rapid progression of pharmaceutical and medical technologies means that social determinants of health including education, language, income, unemployment, housing, nutrition, inclusion, and discrimination are laid bare. Health should not be solely a product of a genetic and social lottery, but an essential resource that counters disadvantages when they occur.

The expectation that the flower of a universal health standard can grow and ripen from non-fertile ground is futile. A universal right to health can only flourish if fertilized in a rich soil of distributive justice with equal access to the essential resources required for human functioning including welfare, self-respect, liberty and opportunity, as well as health. This requires equity, not equality, with distribution according to need so that the worst off are taken care of.

The National Health Service (NHS) provides healthcare for all, based on clinical need and not capacity to pay. It is one of the best health services in the world.[1] Fight for it. Vote wisely, for its funding is a political choice. And remember, though the doors are always open, the road to them is paved with social determinants and may not be the same for all.

---

1 This is unlikely to be a commentary on euthanasia but to allude to the use of doctors as political assassins.

2 Abortion by oral methods was legal in ancient Greece. The oath cautions only against the use of pessaries as a potential source of lethal infection.

3 The oath does not disavow surgery, but merely asks the physician to cede to others with expertise.

Surviving life on the wards

Advice for doctors
- Do not blame the sick for being sick.
- Seek to discover your patient's wishes and adhere to them whenever possible.
- Ask for help.
- Learn.
- Work for your patients, not your consultant.
- Respect opinions.
- Treat a patient, not a disease.
- Admit a person, not a diagnosis.
- Spend time with the bereaved; help them to shed tears.
- Give the patient (and yourself) time: for questions, to reflect, and to allow healing.
- Be optimistic.
- Be kind to yourself: you are not an inexhaustible resource. Reflect on the emotional impact of your work (Schwartz round, Balint group).
- Question your conscience and tell the truth.
- Recognize that medicine may be finite, but kindness and empathy are limitless.

On being busy: Corrigan's secret door

Dr Corrigan of Dublin was:

'tall, erect, of commanding figure... He had the countenance of an intellectual... and his face "beamed with kindness"... In temperament his distinguishing traits were kindness and tenderness towards the sick, and the ability to make a bold decision.'

E. O'Brien, *Conscience and Conflict: A Biography of Sir Dominic Corrigan 1802–1880*, 1983.

Was Corrigan busy? At the start of his professional life he was advised that the best way to get business was to pretend to have it. It was suggested that a note marked 'Immediate and pressing' should be ostentatiously handed to him at the dinner table, but always at a suitable time so as not to miss the best food. Such advice was superfluous. Corrigan aspired to hard work and taught his students the value of 'never doing nothing'. The city in which he practised had a 'degree of filth, stench and darkness, inconceivable by those who have not experienced them', and yet 'not enough hospital beds to care for the great numbers in need'. And so the apocryphal tale of a secret door in his consulting room, to escape the ever-growing queue of eager patients.

In times of chaos—due to competing, urgent, simultaneous demands, excessive administration, not enough beds, effort–reward imbalance, and personal sacrifice—we need to take Corrigan by the hand, and walk with him through his secret door into a calm inner world. This metaphorical door reassures and guides:

1 However lonely you feel, you are not usually alone. Do not pride yourself on not asking for help. If a decision is a hard one, share it with a colleague.

2 Take any chance you get to sit down and rest. Have a cup of tea with other members of staff, or with a friendly patient (patients are sources of renewal, not just devourers of energies).

3 Do not miss meals. If there is no time to go to the canteen, ensure that food is put aside for you to eat when you can: hard work and sleeplessness are twice as miserable if you are hungry.

4 Avoid making work. It is too easy to become trapped by an expectation of excessive work, blackmailed by misplaced guilt, re-clerking patients, rewriting notes, or checking results at an hour when the priority should be self-care.

5 Look to the future. Timetable a good time within a bad rota.

The origins of the story of Corrigan's secret door are unknown and it may never have existed other than in these hallowed pages. But the study of mythology not only unlocks the treasure of tradition, it also offers a means to tackle the mightiest questions about the nature of humans (doctors) and the universe (medicine) when rationality falls short. Ask not, 'Why am I busy?', but, 'How can I be busy better?'

The ward round
- All entries on the patient record must have: date, time, the name of the clinician leading the interaction, the clinical findings and plan, your (electronic) signature, printed name, and contact details. If you work on paper, make sure the patient details are at the top of every side. Write legibly: it may save more than the patient.
- A problem list will help structure your thoughts and guide others.
- **BODEX: B**lood results, **O**bservations, **D**rug chart, **E**CG, **X**-rays. Look at these. If you think there is something of concern, make sure someone else looks at them too.
- Document what information has been given to the patient and relatives.

Handover
- Make sure you know when and where to attend.
- Make sure you understand what you need to do and why. 'Check blood results' or 'Review warning score' is not enough. Better to: 'Check potassium in 4 hours. Treat and discuss with a senior if it remains >6.0mmol/L'.

On call
- Write it down.
- The **ABCDE** approach (p763) to a sick patient is never wrong.
- Try and establish the clinical context of tasks you are asked to do. Prioritize and let staff know when you are likely to get to them.
- Use the national early warning score (**NEWS**) (p876, fig A1).
- Smile, even when talking by phone. Be polite.
- Eat and drink, preferably with your team.

Making a referral
- Have the clinical notes, observation chart, drug chart, and investigation results to hand. Read them before you call.
- Use **SBAR: S**ituation (who you are, who the patient is, the reason for the call), **B**ackground, **A**ssessment of the patient now, then outline your **R**equest.
- Anticipate: urine dip for the nephrologist, **PR** exam for the gastroenterologist.

Living with blood-spattered armour

With the going down of the sun we can momentarily cheer ourselves up by the thought that we are one day nearer to the end of life on earth and our responsibility for the unending tide of illness that floods into our wards and seeps into our consulting rooms. Of course, you may have many other satisfactions, but if not, wink with us as we hear some fool telling us that our aim should be the greatest health and happiness for the greatest number. When we hear this, we don't expect cheering from tattered ranks of doctors; rather, our ears detect a decimated groan, because these mere humans know that there is something at stake in doctoring far more elemental than health or happiness: namely survival.

Within weeks, however brightly your armour shone, it will be smeared and spattered, if not with blood, then with the fallout from decisions made without sufficient time and attention, due to deficiencies in the staff safety net that weakens without sufficient numbers to hold it up and check regularly for holes. *Force majeure* on the part of Nature and the exigencies of ward life have, we are stunned to realize, taught us to be second-rate; for to insist on being first-rate in all things is to toil as Sisyphus in a hopeless space, aiming for an absurd target that cannot be reached. Though unlike Sisyphus, such labour is not eternal, to strive like this is to accelerate our demise. So do not re-polish your armour, for perfectionism does not exist untarnished in our clinical world. Rather, furnish your mind and nourish your body in order to flourish. Food makes midnight groans less intrusive. Drink—doctors are more likely to be oliguric than their patients. Talk—it reduces the weight of the boulder you carry and the incline of the mountain you climb. And do not deny yourself the restorative power of sleep, for it is our natural state in which we were created, and we wake only to feed our dreams.

We cannot prepare you for finding out that you are not at ease with the person you are becoming, and neither would we dream of imposing a specific regimen of exercise, diet, and mental fitness. Finding out what can lead you through adversity is the art of living.

The Trust Equation attempts to quantify trustworthiness:

$$Trust = (Credibility + Reliability + Vulnerability)/Self$$

Credibility is the heart of medical education: the accumulation and application of knowledge. *Reliability* is the consistency and integrity with which the path to today's consultation was paved. But other aspects are harder, less familiar, and less taught. *Vulnerability* is the revealing of your humanity, shifting the weight of the medical relationship from paternalism (or maternalism) to interdependence. It is the mutuality of human weakness in both you and your patient. And as denominator, *Self* is the most powerful of all: too much of it reduces trust, no matter how credible and reliable you are. And so, the need for a vulnerable focus on another, revealed in your interactions, and communicated by you. A patient may not care how much you know, until they know how much you care. Without trust, there can be little healing.

Checklists for communication offer, at best, a guide:

Introduce yourself Every time you interact with a patient, give your name and your role. *Introductions are about making a human connection between one human being who is suffering and vulnerable, and another human being who wishes to help. They begin therapeutic relationships and can instantly build trust.* (Kate Granger, hellomynameis.org.uk, #hellomynameis)

Be friendly Smile. Sit down. Take an interest in the patient's world beyond this consultation. Ask an unscripted question. Use the patient's name more than once.

Listen Are you truly listening or are you contemplating the next question needed to realize your agenda? Be better than the average physician who interrupts after 20–30 seconds.

Look wise, say nothing, and grunt. Speech was given to conceal thought. (William Osler, 1849–1919)

Increase the wait-time Pause between listening and speaking. The patient may say more.

Pay attention to the non-verbal Observe gestures, body language, and eye contact. Be aware of your own.

Explain Consider written or drawn explanations. When appropriate, include relatives or other clinical team members to assist in understanding and recall.

Adapt your language An explanation in fluent medicalese may be meaningless.

Clarify understanding 'Acute', 'chronic', 'dizzy', 'jaundice', 'shock', 'malignant', 'remission': do these words have the same meaning for you and your patient?

Be polite
Rudeness is folly. To make enemies by being... unnecessarily rude is as crazy as setting one's house on fire. (Arthur Schopenhauer, 1788–1860). Being polite requires no talent.

Address silent fears Give patients a chance to raise their concerns: 'What are you worried this might be?', 'Some people worry about..., does that worry you?'

Consider the patient's disease model Patients may have their own explanations for their symptoms. Acknowledge their theories, try to understand what underpins their beliefs if you think them unlikely.

A physician is obligated to consider more than a diseased organ, more even than the whole man—he must view the man in his world. (Harvey Cushing, 1869–1939)

Keep the patient informed Explain your working diagnosis and relate this to the understanding, beliefs, and concerns of your patient. Let them know what will happen next, and the likely timing. 'Soon' may mean a month to a doctor, but a day to a patient. Apologize for any delay.

Summarize Is there anything you have missed?

Open questions 'How are you?', 'How does it feel?' The direction a patient chooses offers valuable information: 'Tell me about the vomit.' 'It was dark.' 'How dark?' 'Dark bits in it.' 'Like ...?' 'Like bits of soil in it.' This information is gold even though not cast in the form of coffee grounds.

Patient-centred questions Patients may have their own ideas about what is causing their symptoms, their impact, and what should be done. This is ever truer as patients are increasingly likely to have had a first consultation with Dr Google. Unless their ideas, concerns, and expectations are elucidated, your patient may never be fully satisfied or fully involved in their own care.

Considering the whole Humans are not self-sufficient units; we are complex relational beings, constantly reacting to events, environments, and each other. To understand your patient's concerns you must understand their context: home life, work, dreams, fears. Information from family and friends can be very helpful for identifying triggering and exacerbating factors, and elucidating the true underlying cause. A headache caused by anxiety is best treated not with analgesics, but by helping access support.

Silence and echoes Often the most valuable details are the most difficult to verbalize. Help your patients express such thoughts by giving them time: if you interrogate a robin, he will fly away; treelike silence may bring him to your hand. *Trade Secret: the best diagnosticians in medicine are not internists, but patients. If only the doctor would sit down, shut up, and listen, the patient will eventually tell him the diagnosis.* (Oscar London, *Kill as Few Patients as Possible*, 1987) Whilst powerful, silence should not be oppressive—try echoing the last words said to encourage your patient to continue vocalizing a particular thought.

Try to avoid
Closed questions: these permit no opportunity to deny assumptions. 'Have you had hip pain since your fall?' 'Yes, doctor.' Radiographs are performed even though the same hip pain was also present for many years before the fall.
Questions suggesting the answer: 'Was the vomit black—like coffee grounds?' 'Yes, like coffee grounds, doctor.' The doctor's expectations and hurry to get the evidence into a predefined format have so tarnished the story as to make it useless.

Shared decision-making: no decision about me, without me

Shared decision-making aims to place patients' needs, wishes, and preferences at the centre of clinical decision-making.
• *Inform* patients about their condition, treatment options, benefits, and risk.
• *Support* patients in understanding their condition.
• Make decisions based on *mutual understanding*.
Consider asking not, 'What is the matter?' but 'What matters to you?'

Consider your tendency towards libertarian paternalism or 'nudge'. This is when information is given in such a way as to encourage individuals to make a particular choice that is felt to be in their best interests, and to compensate for presumed 'reasoning failure' in the patient. This is done by *framing* the information in either a positive or negative light depending on your view and how you might wish to sway your audience. Consider the following correct statements made about a new drug which offers 96% survival compared to 94% with an older drug:
• More people survive if they take this drug.
• This new drug reduces mortality by a third.
• This new drug benefits only 2% of patients.
How do you choose? The equivalence in the above statements is transparent when they are presented together. But if you offer only one option, that may be all that is seen.

The diagnostic puzzle

How to formulate a diagnosis

Diagnosing by recognition For students, this is the most irritating method. You spend an hour asking all the wrong questions, and in waltzes a doctor who names the disease before you have even finished taking the pulse. This doctor has simply recognized the illness like they recognize an old friend (or enemy).

Diagnosing by probability Over our clinical lives we build up a personal database of diagnoses. We unconsciously run each new 'case' through this continuously developing probabilistic algorithm with increasing speed and effortlessness.

Diagnosing by reasoning Like Sherlock Holmes, we must exclude each differential, and the diagnosis is what remains. This is dependent on the quality of the differential and presupposes methods for *absolutely* excluding diseases. All tests are statistical rather than absolute (5% of the population lie outside the 'normal' range), which is why this method remains, like Sherlock Holmes, fictional at best.

Diagnosing by watching and waiting The dangers and expense of exhaustive tests may be obviated by the skilful use of time.

Diagnosing by selective doubting Diagnosis relies on clinical signs and investigative tests. Yet there are no hard signs or perfect tests. When diagnosis is difficult, try doubting the signs, then doubting the tests. But the game of medicine is unplayable if you doubt everything: so doubt selectively.

Diagnosis by iteration and reiteration A brief history suggests looking for a few signs, which leads to further questions and a few tests. As the process reiterates, various diagnostic possibilities crop up, leading to further questions and further tests. And so history taking and diagnosing never end.

A razor, a dictum, and a bludgeon

Consider three wise men:[2]

Occam's razor *Entia non sunt multiplicanda praeter necessitatem* translates as 'entities must not be multiplied unnecessarily'. The physician should therefore seek to achieve diagnostic parsimony and find a single disease to explain all symptoms, rather than proffer two or three unrelated diagnoses.

Hickam's dictum *Patients can have as many diagnoses as they damn well please.* Signs and symptoms may be due to more than one pathology. Indeed, a patient is statistically more likely to have two common diagnoses than one unifying rare condition.

Crabtree's bludgeon *No set of mutually inconsistent observations can exist for which some human intellect cannot conceive a coherent explanation however complicated.* This acts as a reminder that physicians prefer Occam to Hickam: a unifying diagnosis is a much more pleasing thing. Confirmation bias then ensues as we look for supporting information to fit with our unifying theory. Remember to test the validity of your diagnosis, no matter how pleasing it may seem.

Heuristic pitfalls

Heuristics are cognitive shortcuts which allow quick decision-making by focusing on predictors. Be vigilant of their traps. By making things simple, the answer may seem adequate, but it is unlikely to be the perfect solution to a difficult question.

Representativeness Diagnosis is driven by the 'classic case'. Do not forget the atypical variant.

Availability All heuristics are equal but availability is more equal than the others. The diseases we remember, or treated most recently, carry more weight in our diagnostic hierarchy. Yet, this readily available information may not be relevant now.

Overconfidence Are you overestimating how much you know and how well you know it? Probably.

Bias The hunt for, and recall of, clinical information that fits with our expectations. Can you disprove your own diagnostic hypothesis?

Illusory correlation Associated events are presumed to be causal. But was it treatment or time that cured the patient?

Clinical intuition

Do not aspire to clinical intuition, for it is nothing more than a cue to stored information. Though it is grounded in the expertise of experience, intuition alone is not enough. Remember that, like Pavlov, you can train a dog to intuit food from the sound of a bell and that this instinct will remain even when the food is gone.

Reliance on heuristic 'rules of thumb' is fraught with predictable biases and yet the beauty of people is that they are infinitely complex and wonderfully capricious. Intuition ignores heterogeneity. It inhibits the rare and atypical diagnosis. Clinical intuition may be nothing more than premonition. Or luck. Or magic.

But do not dismiss intuition entirely. It remains a hand to guide you through the unknown. Just do not follow blindly, for intuition reveals only an analogue version of the truth. Clarity of each clinical pixel is required to reveal the high-definition digital reality. And remember to zoom out so as not to make a decision based on a cropped image.

Hindsight is an unfair judge when it is revealed whether or not you were correct with your diagnoses last week, last year, and a decade ago. You can only try to ensure that it is not a cognitive illusion that you did your best at the time.

Duty of candour

In a world in which a 'mistake' can be redefined as a 'complication', it is easy to conceal error behind veils of technical language and superficial insight.

Duty of candour is statutory in England for incidents that cause death or significant harm (including psychological). As soon as practicable, communicate what happened, give details of further enquiries, and offer an apology.

Apology should be genuine, and freely and honestly given, for apology is not an admission of liability. Risks and imperfections are inherent to medicine. You have the freedom to be sorry whenever they occur. Human and system factors are innate to humans and systems. Focus not on legislation, but on transparency and learning. The ethics of forgiveness require a complete response in which the patient's voice is placed at the heart of the process.

The art of being wrong

Fallibility is a universal human phenomenon. The possibility that you are wrong is a perpetual state because you are blind to error while it is happening.[3] 'I *am* wrong' is a statement of impossibility. Once you are aware that you are wrong, you are no longer wrong, and can therefore only declare, 'I *was* wrong'.

Beware certainty. It is a comforting illusion that the world is knowable, and it is founded on our biases. It is introspective, and means other people's stories cease to matter. Certainty is lethal to empathy.

Error must be acknowledged and accepted. A focus on error does not diminish intelligence. Defensiveness is bad for progress. 'I was wrong, *but...*' rarely facilitates different and better. Only close scrutiny of mistakes reveals the possibility of change at the core of error. And yet, medicine is littered with examples of resistance to disclosure, and reward for concealment. This must change.[4] Presume error blindness and protect whistle-blowers. Listen. It is an act of humility that acknowledges the position of others, and the possibility of error in yourself.

Medicine desires a 'truth', but this is only ever transitory. Knowledge persists only until it is disproved by a better hypothesis or error. You may meet the exception to a rule today. Better to accept error and scrutinize it as a work of art. Look at it for long enough and the beauty within will be revealed. Art accepts the unknown, celebrating transience and subjectivity. By seeing the world through someone else's eyes, art teaches us empathy. It is at the point where art and medicine collide that doctors can re-attach themselves to the human race and feel the same emotions that motivate or terrify our patients. 'Unknowing' creates stories, music, and pictures. Though they are not 'right', they are the hallmark of our highest endeavours.

1 Thinking about medicine

►Consult the *BNF* or *BNF for Children* or similar before giving any drug with which you are not thoroughly familiar.

►Check the patient's allergy status and make all reasonable attempts to qualify the reaction (table 1.1). The burden of iatrogenic hospital admission and avoidable drug-related deaths is real. Equally, do not deny life-saving treatment based on a mild and predictable reaction.

►Check drug interactions meticulously.

Table 1.1 Drug reactions

Type of reaction	Examples
True allergy	Anaphylaxis: oedema, urticaria, wheeze (p776–7)
Side effect	All medications have side effects. The most common are rash, itch, nausea, diarrhoea, lethargy, and headache
Increased effect/ toxicity	Due to inter-individual variance. Dosage regimen normally corrects for this but beware states of altered drug clearance such as liver and kidney (p301) impairment
Drug interaction	Reaction due to drugs used in combination, eg azathioprine and allopurinol, erythromycin and warfarin

Remember *primum non nocere*: first do no harm. The more minor the illness, the more weight this carries. Overall, doctors have a tendency to prescribe too much rather than too little. Consider the following when prescribing any medication:

1 The *underlying pathology*. Do not let the amelioration of symptoms lead to failure of investigation and diagnosis.
2 Is this prescription according to *best evidence*?
3 *Side effects*. All medications come with risks, potential side effects, inconvenience to the patient, and expense.
4 Is the patient taking *other medications*?
5 *Alternatives to medication*. Does the patient really need or want medication? Are you giving medication out of a sense of needing to do something, or because you genuinely feel it will help the patient? Is it more appropriate to offer information, reassurance, or advise on lifestyle?
6 Is there a risk of *overdose or addiction*?
7 Can you *assist* the patient? Once per day is better than four times. How easy is it to open the bottle? Is there an intervention that can help with medicine management, eg a multicompartment compliance aid, patient counselling, an IT solution such as a smartphone app?
8 *Future planning*. How are you going to decide whether the medication has worked? What are the indications to continue, stop, or change?

Placebo and nocebo

The placebo effect is a phenomenon whereby a pharmacologically inactive substance is given in place of an active agent with benefit derived from suggestion and expectation. Benefit stems from provision of 'medicine', rather than pharmacodynamics. In contrast, the nocebo effect is a detrimental consequence due to negative psychosomaticity, eg disproportionate or improbable side effects.

Why evolution has bequeathed a degree of self-healing or harm in response to belief is unclear. Perhaps the modification of internal alarm systems by expectation confers a locus of control that improves outcome; improving symptoms during recovery whilst simultaneously preventing toxicity and ensuring that exit of the sick role remains the goal.

But placebos and nocebos have deceptive intent (unless consent for placebo is given in a clinical trial). They violate fiduciary duties of honesty and respect, and subvert self-truth. The patient may be disenfranchised and unable to participate in medical decision-making. Harm arises when placebos and nocebos dissuade patients from accessing medical help when it is available.

So do not use placebos and beware of nocebos. Rather, tell your patient a true story of how treatment may help. Provide an honest, realistic narrative of improvement, where it exists. In doing so, the patient, the treatment, and the doctor are bettered.

Compliance and concordance

Compliance embodies the imbalance of power between doctor and patient: the doctor knows best and it is the patient's responsibility to comply with that monopoly of knowledge. Devaluing of patients and ethically dubious, the term 'compliance' is now relegated from modern prescribing practice. In its place is 'concordance', a prescribing agreement that incorporates the beliefs and wishes of the patient.

Only 50-70% of patients take medicines as prescribed. This leads to concern over wasted resources and avoidable illness. Interventions that increase concordance are promoted using the mnemonic **E**very **P**atient, **E**qual **C**ontribution to **C**are:

• **E**xplanation: discuss the benefits and risks of taking and not-taking medication. Some patients will prefer not to be treated and, if the patient has capacity and understands the risks, such a decision should be respected.
• **P**roblems: talk through the patient's experience of treatment including side effects.
• **E**xpectations: this is important especially in the treatment of silent conditions and in preventative medicine where there may be no symptomatic benefit.
• **C**apability: talk through the medication regimen and consider ways to reduce complexity.
• **C**onsolidate: use visual aids/written information that detail the information they need to make their decision. Check how they are managing their medications when you next see them.

Patient education should not be presumed to increase concordance. There is little evidence for this. If the goal of 'education' is for the patient to subsume the views of the doctor then this is a reversion back to compliance and inequity in treatment decision-making. A shared agreement does not need to 'comply' or 'concord' with the prescriber. The capacity of every individual to consent to treatment or not, means that in some cases, concordance is also divergence. Provided it is informed, divergence needs to be accepted and respected.

QALYS and resource rationing

A QALY is a quality-adjusted life year. One year of healthy life expectancy = 1 QALY. One year of unhealthy life expectancy is worth <1 QALY, with the precise value falling with worsening quality of life. If an intervention means that you are likely to live for 8 years in perfect health then that intervention would have a QALY value of 8. If a new drug improves your quality of life from 0.5 to 0.7 for 25 years, then it has a QALY value of 5 $[(0.7 - 0.5) \times 25]$. The cost of 1 QALY is then calculated according to the price of an intervention. The National Institute for Health and Care Excellence (NICE) considers interventions cost-effective when 1 QALY costs less than £20 000–£30 000.

QALYS are both defended and criticized as a utilitarian approach: to provide the greatest health to the greatest number (table 1.2). How quantifiable are happiness, time spent with loved ones, a final holiday? Even time itself is ambiguous, for time experienced by patients may be more like literature than science: a minute might be a chapter, a year a single sentence. And what of egalitarianism: should individuals be abandoned because their treatment is considered an ineffective use of resources? And should the priority be equality or equity? What of distributive justice so that those who are worst off become better off? There is no perfect answer but your patients have the right to ask questions about decisions that affect their quality of life.

Table 1.2 The advantages and disadvantages of QALYs

Advantages	Disadvantages
Transparent societal decision-making	Focuses on slice (disease), not pie (health)
Allows cost-effectiveness analysis	Quality of life assessment comes from general public, not those with disease
Allows international comparison	Potentially ageist: older people will always have less life expectancy to gain
	Focus on outcomes and not process, ie care, compassion

1 Thinking about medicine

Race

It is unacceptable not to see race, for medicine is not immune to racial inequality. White privilege and structural racism do not sit outside the consultation room, waiting patiently to be invited in. This is about a system in which the positive affirmation of being white is so ubiquitous it has become part of the furniture. You must look for it. You will not change what you do not see.

Medicine continues to define disease according to race. Yet race is a dynamic and social construct, and physical traits are poor predictors of genetic and biological variability. Racial stereotypes of disease fail those on both sides of this tenuous division of peoples, though harm is more common to those who are not white. Racial correction in eGFR delays care and the assessment for kidney transplantation in those with black skin. The diagnosis of sarcoidosis is delayed for those with white skin. Race is presented as a risk factor for disease rather than a surrogate measure of inequality. It is frequently considered an independent variable for disease development and treatment response. Yet race is independent of nothing. It is entirely dependent. Dependent on socioeconomic status, deprivation, environmental exposure, entitlement to healthcare, language proficiency, and discrimination.

Racism has distorted the colour of your colleagues. Applicants from ethnic minority backgrounds are less likely to get into medical school. White doctors are more likely to pass postgraduate examinations. Ethnic minorities are underrepresented in consultant, clinical, and medical director roles, and those who get there earn less. There is racism in the smile and apology to those not appointed to hospital jobs in the UK, which are six times more likely to be offered to white compared to black candidates. The disadvantage of students and doctors through their careers due to race and ethnicity should be a source of embarrassment that drives systemic change.

See and include ethnicity to expose and address inequality and discrimination, but do not use it as a poor proxy for physiology or genetics. The validity of race-adjusted tools should be questioned. Consider whether the ubiquitous inclusion of race or ethnicity is needed in the traditional descriptor of a patient (eg a 50-year-old African Caribbean man) for it is more likely to reinforce subconscious bias than to provide useful clinical information. The onus is on all of us to move from a race-based profession, to a race-conscious one.[5] If the pages of this book fall short on this, then please point out our errors of omission to us. We are sorry that we did not look, and we did not see.

Sleep

It is a problem that we are physically, behaviourally, cognitively, socially, and emotionally dependent on sleep.[6] Think how much more we could achieve if we were awake for 6 or 7 more hours each day. Think how easy a night shift would be.

If only we could find our inner dolphin and adopt unihemispheric sleep. The two sides of our brain would uncouple; one side remaining awake whilst the other rests. Or let us evolve as a migrating bird that grabs seconds of sleep whilst in flight. Enough to avoid the effects of sleep deprivation and allow us to keep going.

Instead, the demands of our existence force us to compromise on the human requirement for sleep and we are destined to a permanent state of sleep bankruptcy. Unable to succumb to the evolutionary need for an afternoon nap, we soldier on until after dusk so that midnight is no longer mid-night. Adenosine accumulates like a cerebral egg timer counting the seconds since our last shuteye, driving an irresistible urge to sleep. But there is still more work to be done, so we suppress adenosine's signal with caffeine; another dose in the world's largest uncontrolled drug trial.

But it is better to sleep. And better still to rapid eye movement (REM) sleep for it is that which recalibrates our emotional circuits and allows intelligent decisions. Just as REM sleep distinguishes the emotional and social capabilities of mammals from other animals, perhaps it also distinguishes the good doctor from the bad.

Sex and gender

We should aspire to sexual equality for it is good for medicine. Females have a lower mortality from myocardial infarction when treated by female doctors, an effect attenuated when male doctors have more females as colleagues and patients. Yet scalar dichotomy persists. Females are underrepresented in clinical trials and largely excluded if pregnant. Pain is more commonly misdiagnosed in females. Females are less likely to receive bystander CPR. The majority of female doctors experience sexism,[7] which is a barrier to career progression. Gate-keeping restricts access to specialities for females. Even when corrected for working hours, there is a pay gap for females of 18.9% for hospital doctors, 15.3% for GPs, and 11.9% for clinical academics.[8]

Gender is distinct from sex, encompassing social and cultural aspects. Though physical characteristics define sex at birth, gender is not innate. Human lives cannot be described by categories of gender (or ethnicity or sexual orientation). Gender describes how a person identifies and it arises from an interplay between social and developmental influences, and environment. Gender develops over time and exists on a spectrum of behavioural, mental, and emotional traits. In the same way that computers are moving beyond binary code due to the limits of its capacity, gender identity is our comparably infinite new quantum code. It has moved beyond the confines of language and grammar, and the traditional mandate of a singular pronoun should no longer be the norm. But medicine needs to catch up. Equity in access to healthcare, cancer screening and mental health, and inclusivity in medical language are needed.

Equally, gender should not be restricted in the pages of this book. Where the words 'men' and 'women' occur, please read them as 'persons born male' or 'persons born female' only if biological categorization is important, and otherwise simply as 'persons'.

The environment

The earth is sick. Every biopsy yields a worrying result. Increasing numbers of variables are outside the reference range. Business as usual can no longer be prescribed. Yet, the environmental footprint is an often-unmeasured negative healthcare outcome. Healthcare produces greenhouse gas emissions, mountains of single-use plastic waste, and high levels of water consumption. One in every 20 road journeys in England relate to healthcare. Sustainable solutions include car shares, electric car charging points, safe cycle stores, local seasonal food for patients and staff, and changes in procurement. A cut in greenhouse gases includes anaesthetic agents and inhaler propellants. Energy-efficient building design should be prioritized as old hospitals crumble. Use your voice. People may listen.

Compassion

The importance of compassion[4] in medicine is undisputed but it is poorly described and impossible to teach. It is an emotional response to suffering that motivates a desire to help. It is more than pity, which has connotations of inferiority; and different from empathy, which is a vicarious experience of the emotional state of another. It requires imaginative indwelling into another's condition. The compassionate, though fictional, Jules Henri loses his sense of self; another person's despair alters his perception so that they are '*connected in some universal, though unseen, pattern of humanity*'.[4] With compassion, the pain of another is '*intensified by the imagination and prolonged by a hundred echoes*'.[5] Compassion has been valued by patients for at least the last 2000 years: '*For I could never even have prayed for this: that you would... endure my agonies and stay with me and help me*'.[6] Compassion requires engagement with suffering, cultural understanding, and mutuality, rather than paternalism. Fatigue, overwork, excess demands, and technical and efficiency targets inhibit its expression. When compassion (what is felt) is too hard, etiquette (what is done) must not fail: empathy, respectfulness, attention, and manners may offer partial compensation.

4 Sebastian Faulkes, *Human Traces*, 2005.

5 Milan Kundera, *The Unbearable Lightness of Being*, 1984.

6 *Philoctetes* by Sophocles 409 BC (translation Phillips and Clay, 2003).

1 Thinking about medicine

Diagnosing dying

Would you be surprised if your patient were to die in the next few days, weeks, or months? If the answer is 'no' then end of life choices, decisions, and care should be addressed. The following can aid in the diagnosis of dying:

• Decline in functional performance, eg in bed or chair >50% of day.
• Increasing dependence or sentinel event, eg fall, transfer to nursing home.
• Number and severity of comorbidities.
• Unstable or deteriorating symptoms, crisis admissions.
• Decreasing treatment response.
• Weight loss >10% in 6 months, serum albumin <25g/L.

Managing life-in-death

Death is an inevitable consequence of life but it is not inevitable that it is due to medical failure. Where failure does exist is in the narrow focus of medicine, concerned more with the repair of health rather than the sustenance of the soul: a failure to make life-in-death better. But when medical treatments can no longer offer a cure, and a patient enters the end of life, active management of dying is vital. Though priorities at the end of life are different, they still need to be met: freedom from pain, achieving a sense of completeness, being treated as a whole person, finding peace.

Swift death due to a catastrophic event is rare. Most death is the end product of a struggle with chronic, progressive disease: cancer, COPD, vascular disease, neurological disease, dementia, or frailty. Although death is inevitable, prognostication is difficult and inaccurate with remarkable variation in time to death. The patient in front of you may be the median, mean, or on the 99th centile. Preparation for death is an uncomfortable but necessary bedfellow for hope.

Prioritize preferences and aim to meet individual needs.[9]
• Seek help from experienced members of staff including palliative care teams.
• Elicit needs: physiological, psychological, social, and spiritual. Discuss fears.
• Establish the wishes of the patient. What trade-offs are they willing to accept, eg treatment toxicity for potential time gained? What is unacceptable to them?
• Consider the views of persons important to the patient.
• Hydration: give support to allow the dying to drink, offer mouth care. Consider clinically assisted hydration (parenteral, enteral, IV) according to wishes and if distressing signs/symptoms of dehydration are possible. Stop according to wishes and harm.
• Manage pain promptly and effectively. Treat any reversible causes of pain.
• Consider a syringe pump if symptom-control medications are needed more than twice in 24h (p533).
• Anticipate symptoms: the PRN drug chart should cover all possibilities (p532).
• Death may or may not come with peace and acceptance. Patients may rage mightily against the dying of the light. Listen and bear witness.

The wisdom of death

Death is nature's cruel master stroke, allowing genotypes space to try new phenotypes. The time comes in the life of every organism when it is better to start from scratch, rather than carry on with the weight and muddle of endless accretions. Our bodies and minds are the perishable phenotypes on the wave of our genes. But our genes are not really *our* genes. It is we who belong to them for a few decades. And death is nature's great insult, that she should prefer to put all her eggs in the basket of a defenceless, incompetent neonate; rather than in the tried and tested custody of our own superb minds. But as our neurofibrils begin to tangle, and that neonate walks to a wisdom that eludes us, we are forced to give nature credit for her daring idea. Of course, nature, in her careless way, can get it wrong; people often die in the wrong order and one of our chief roles is to prevent this misordering of deaths, not the phenomenon of death itself. With that exception, we must admit that dying is a brilliant idea, and one that it is most unlikely we would ever have devised ourselves.

Diagnosing death

Death[10] is the irreversible loss of the essential characteristics which are necessary for the existence of a human being.

Death following cessation of cardiorespiratory function
▶Simultaneous and irreversible onset of apnoea, absence of circulation, and unconsciousness.

Cardiorespiratory arrest is confirmed by observation of the following:
• Absence of central pulse on palpation.
• Absence of heart sounds on auscultation.

After 5 minutes of cardiorespiratory arrest, absence of brainstem activity is confirmed by the absence of pupillary responses to light, an absent corneal reflex, and no motor response to supra-orbital pressure.

The time of death is the time at which these criteria are fulfilled.

Brainstem death
▶Brainstem pathology causing irreversible damage to its integrative functions including neural control of cardiorespiratory function and consciousness.
Diagnosed by an absence of brainstem reflexes:
• No pupil light response.
• No corneal reflex (blink to touch).
• Absent oculovestibular reflexes (no eye movements seen with injection of ice-cold water into each external auditory meatus, tympanic membranes visualized).
• No motor response to stimulation within the cranial nerve distribution (supra-orbital pressure).
• No cough/gag reflex.
• No respiratory response to hypercarbia: oxygenation is maintained (SpO_2>85%) but ventilation is reduced to achieve $P_aCO_2 \geq 6.0$kPa with pH ≤ 7.40. No respiratory response is seen within 5 minutes and P_aCO_2 rises by >0.5kPa.

Diagnosis is made by two competent doctors registered for >5 years testing together completely and successfully on two separate occasions.

Organ donation

Around 7000 people are waiting for an organ transplant in the UK and approximately 500 people in need of a transplant will die each year (see p304).

Any patient who is a potential donor can be referred to a specialist organ donation service for advice as to suitability for transplantation and to coordinate approach to families. They are contactable 24h/d and their details will be held in your A&E and/or ITU departments.

Organs can be retrieved from:
• *Donor after brainstem death* or heart-beating donor.
• *Donor after cardiac death* or non-heart-beating donor. Includes death following unsuccessful CPR and patients for whom death is inevitable but do not meet the criteria for brainstem death.

There are two legislative frameworks for organ donation:
• *Opt-in*—donors give their explicit consent.
• *Opt-out*—anyone who has not refused consent is a donor (deemed consent).

The UK has an opt-out system of donation. The association between an opt-out system and higher organ donation rates is complicated by the presence of cofounding factors. National coordination, support and training of clinicians, routine discussion as part of end of life care, and efficient organ retrieval also increase donation rates. The ethics of presumed consent should not be forgotten: the absence of an objection is not an acceptable substitute for informed consent in other areas of clinical practice.

In the UK, regardless of legislation, if the patient's family or representative cannot support donation then it will not go ahead. Register your decision on the NHS Organ Donor Register (https://www.organdonation.nhs.uk/register-to-donate/register-your-details/) and, more importantly, let your family know your wishes.

Medical ethics

Our clinical practice is steered by ethical principles. They guide the decisions we make in our clinics and ward rounds, what we tell our patients, and what we omit to tell them. Tony Lopez, Journal of Royal Society of Medicine 2001;94:603-4.

In the silences of our consultations it is we who are under the microscope, unable to escape scrutiny in the sphere of ethics. To give us courage, we recall the law of the aviator and seagull: it is only by facing the prevailing wind that we can become airborne, and achieve a new vantage point. We hope for moral perception: to be able to visualize the salient features of a situation. For without this, ethical issues may float past never to be resolved. Be alert to words which may carry hidden assumptions: 'futility', 'consent', 'best interests'.

Consider **WIGWAM** in routine patient reviews:
• **W**ishes of the patient: are they known or unknown?
• **I**ssues of confidentiality/disclosure.
• **G**oals of care: are they clear? Whose are they: yours or the patient's?
• **W**ants: to decline treatment or discharge against advice.
• **A**rguments between family/friends/doctors.
• **M**oney: concerns of the patient, concerns of the healthcare provider.

Ethical frameworks
Offer structure, comprehensiveness, and transparency in deliberation.[11]

Four principles
• *Autonomy:* self-governance, the ability of a patient to make a choice based on their values and beliefs.
• *Beneficence:* the obligation to benefit patients. Links with autonomy as benefit is dependent upon the view of the patient.
• *Non-maleficence:* do no harm. Or more appropriately, do no overall harm: you can stick a needle into someone when they need dialysis.
• *Justice:* a collection of obligations including legality, human rights, fairness, and resource distribution.

Four quadrants method
• *Medical indications:* treatment options, goals, and likelihood of success.
• *Patient preferences:* what is the patient's autonomous decision? If capacity is lost, look for previously expressed wishes: advance directives, family, friends, GP.
• *Quality of life:* this is subjective: recognize your biases and accommodate those of the patient.
• *Contextual factors:* the wider context—legal, cultural, religious, familial.

These frameworks describe individual voices within the ethics choir. Sometimes there is harmony. But how is discordance managed? There is no hierarchy of principles. Each is binding unless it is trumped by a stronger principle. How you weigh and balance the ethical components of a situation is not easy, but it should be clear and justified. Know your patient and learn from those who know them. Consult others, especially those who hold different opinions. Talk to your local ethics committee. Can you explain your decision to the patient? Their family? A lawyer? If an investigative journalist were to sit on a sulcus of yours, having full knowledge of all thoughts and actions, would they be composing vitriol for tomorrow's newspapers? If so, can you answer them, point for point?

Beyond the ethical framework

To force an ethical problem to fit a framework may be inadequate and reductionistic. It is potentially biased towards Western culture, discounts the non-autonomous, and is vulnerable to poorly considered emphasis and error. 'Doing' ethics can become a checklist exercise where thinking is lost. But doctors are not moral philosophers. They are clinicians. A framework therefore provides a starting point from which to work. It is the toe which tests the water of moral deliberation. Be aware of the cultural setting of your dilemma and consider carefully the weight of synthesis. Be prepared to wade deeper if needed. But acknowledge that moral wisdom may well be out of your depth.

Body and soul cannot be separated for purposes of treatment, for they are one and indivisible. Sick minds must be healed as well as sick bodies. C Jeff Miller, 1931.

Mental state examination: ASEPTIC
• **A**ppearance and behaviour: dress, hygiene, eye contact, rapport.
• **S**peech: volume, rate, tone.
• **E**motion: mood (subjective and objective), affect (how mood is expressed with behaviour—appropriate or incongruent?).
• **P**erception: hallucinations—auditory (in the second or third person)? Visual?
• **T**hought:
  • Form: block, insertion, broadcast, flight of ideas, knight's move.
  • Content: delusions, obsessions, phobias, preoccupations, *self-harm*, *suicide*.
• **I**nsight: ask the patient why they have presented today.
• **C**ognition: orientation, registration, recall, concentration, knowledge.
►Ask about suicidal thoughts and plans.
►Remove yourself from the situation if you feel threatened.

Depression
Two questions can be used to identify depression:[12]
  1 *During the last month, have you been feeling down, depressed, or hopeless?*
  2 *During the last month, have you often been bothered by having little interest or pleasure in doing things?*

If a person answers 'yes' to either question they should undergo mental health assessment including a risk assessment of self-harm and suicide. Appropriate treatments include psychosocial intervention (guided self-help, cognitive behavioural therapy, structured physical activity) and medication. Treatment choice depends on disease severity, previous psychiatric history, response to treatment, and patient preference. If medication is indicated, a generic SSRI should be considered first line after consideration of GI bleeding risk, drug interactions, toxicity, overdose, and discontinuation symptoms. The full effect of medication is gradual, over 4–6 weeks.

Capacity
The Mental Capacity Act (MCA) 2005 has a two-stage test for lack of capacity:
  1 There is an impairment or disturbed functioning of the mind (due to physical illness or a mental health disorder).
  2 The patient is unable to make a decision.

Decision-making is impaired if the patient is unable to: *understand* relevant information, *retain* it for long enough to make a decision, *weigh up* information, *communicate* their decision. Capacity is decision-specific, not patient-specific. A capacity advocate should be provided for those who lack capacity. Even patients without capacity should be as involved as possible in decision-making.

Mental Health Act (MHA) and common law
A patient can be detained under common law (subject to a test of reasonableness) or under the MHA (for assessment/treatment for a mental health disorder) if they lack capacity to remain informally and are a danger to themselves or others. You will have more experience in verbal and non-verbal communication than in detention under the MHA, so use these skills first to try and de-escalate. If rapid tranquillization is needed, be familiar with dosage, side effects, and ongoing observation. If there is no history to guide choice of medication, intramuscular lorazepam can be used.[13]

Doctors and mental health
Suicide rates are three times higher in doctors compared to the general population. Up to 7% of doctors will have a substance abuse problem within their lifetime. Do not ignore feeling low, poor concentration, and reduced energy levels. Do not self-diagnose and manage. Avoid 'corridor consultations'. Trust your GP and seek support:
• British Medical Association: https://www.bma.org.uk/advice-and-support/your-wellbeing
• Support for doctors: https://doctors-in-distress.org.uk/ and https://www.dsn.org.uk/
• NHS mental health support: https://www.nhs.uk/mental-health/ and
  https://www.practitionerhealth.nhs.uk/

Medicalization

In *Illness as a Metaphor*,[7] Susan Sontag describes two kingdoms: that of the well, and that of the sick. She describes our dual citizenship, and the use of a passport to travel from one kingdom to the other. But medicalization blurs this distinction and the boundary between the 'Kingdom of the Sick' and the 'Kingdom of the Well' is lost. There is an anschluss of healthy people annexed into the potentially predatory and frightening kingdom of the sick from which there may well be no escape.

'Too much medicine' occurs as a result of:
- *Overdiagnosis:* labelling an (asymptomatic) person as 'sick' despite the fact that subsequent treatment, lifestyle advice, or monitoring provides no benefit to their outcome (and potentially causes harm), eg localized prostate cancer.
- *Overdetection:* increasingly sensitive tests identify pathology that is indolent or non-progressive, eg subsegmental pulmonary emboli on CT angiography.
- *Overdefinition:* expansion of disease definitions or lowering of disease thresholds, eg an eGFR diagnosis of chronic kidney disease means that 1 in 10 adults are labelled with the disease, many of whom will never progress to symptomatic kidney failure.
- *Disease mongering:* the creation of pseudo-diseases which pose no threat to health, eg restless legs, multiple chemical sensitivity.
- *Overutilization:* healthcare practice that provides no net benefit, eg routine MRI for lower back pain.
- *Overtreatment:* treatment that is of no benefit (and may cause harm), eg antibiotics for viral infections, polypill for the population.

Too much medicine arises from the fear of missing a diagnosis, and concern about avoidable morbidity or mortality. A punitive society means there is a perceived need for more tests, to seek more certainty. But certainty is a holy grail and the stuff of myth and legend. The individual patient is a unique set of symptoms, stoicism, experience, and need. And by the nature of life, cure can only ever be temporary.

Choosing wisely

'Too Much Medicine' (www.bmj.com/too-much-medicine) and 'Choosing Wisely' (www.choosingwisely.org) are initiatives which highlight the danger to human health and the waste of resources that comes from interventions which are not:
- Supported by evidence.
- Free from harm.
- Necessary (including duplicative tests).

Evidence, judgement, context, resources, ethics, and the perspective of the service user are all needed.

Screening

Consider medicalization when screening for disease. Remember all screening programmes do harm, some do good. The Wilson criteria for screening list the important features necessary for a screening programme and the mnemonic **IATROGENIC** reminds of our pressing duty to do no harm:
1 The condition screened for should be an **I**mportant one.
2 There should be an **A**cceptable treatment for the disease.
3 Diagnostic and **T**reatment facilities should be available.
4 A **R**ecognizable latent or early symptomatic stage is required.
5 **O**pinions on who to treat must be agreed.
6 The test must be **G**ood: high discriminatory power, valid, and reproducible with safety **G**uaranteed.
7 The **E**xamination must be acceptable to the patient.
8 The untreated **N**atural history of the disease must be known.
9 It should be **I**nexpensive.
10 Screening must be **C**ontinuous (ie not a 'one-off' affair).

7 Susan Sontag, *Illness as a Metaphor*, 1978.

The work of epidemiology is related to unanswered questions, but also to unquestioned answers.   Patricia Buffler, North American Congress of Epidemiology, 2011.

▶Who, what, when, where, why, and how?

Epidemiology is the study of the distribution of clinical phenomena in populations. It analyses disease in terms of host, agent, and environment (the 'epidemiologist's triad'). It elucidates risks and mechanisms for the development of disease. It reveals potential targets for disease prevention and treatment. Epidemiology does not look at the individual patient, but examines a defined population. How applicable its findings are depend upon how well the *sample* population mirrors the *study* population, which must, in turn, mirror the *target* population. Does your patient fit in this 'target'? If 'yes', then the epidemiological findings may be applicable.

Measures of disease frequency

- *Incidence proportion* is the number of new cases of disease as a proportion of the population. Synonyms include probability of disease, cumulative incidence, risk.
- *Incidence rate* is the number of new cases per unit of person-time, ie one person observed for 5 years contributes 5 person-years of follow-up.
- *Prevalence* is the number of cases that exist at a given time (point prevalence) or time frame (period prevalence), divided by the total population being studied. For example, the lifetime prevalence of hiccups is ~100% and incidence is millions/year. However, the point prevalence at 3am may be 0 if no one is actually having hiccups.

Comparisons of outcome frequency

Differences in outcome rates between populations point to an *association* between the outcome and factors distinguishing the populations (eg a smoking population compared to a non-smoking population). Challenges arise as populations tend to differ from each other in many ways, so it may not be clear which factors affect outcome frequency. This leads to *confounding*. For example, we might find that heart disease is more common in those who use walking sticks. But we cannot conclude that walking sticks cause heart disease as age is a confounding factor: age is causal, not walking sticks.

Ways of accounting for associations A may cause B (cycling leads to a lower BMI), B may cause A (thinner people are more likely to cycle), a 3rd unknown agent X may cause A and B (living further from the shops leads to cycling and a lower BMI), or the association may be a chance finding. When considering the options, it is useful to bear in mind the Bradford Hill 'criteria' for causation (NB none are essential):

1 Consistency of findings: among different populations, studies, time periods.
2 Temporality: the effect must occur after the cause.
3 Biological gradient: a dose response whereby more exposure = more effect.
4 Specificity: exposure causes a single outcome (smoking does not conform!).
5 Strength of association: strong associations are more likely to be causal.
6 Biological plausibility: there is a mechanism linking cause and effect.
7 Coherence: the relationship is supported by current disease knowledge.
8 Experiment: does removal of exposure reduce outcome frequency?

Epidemiological studies

Studies should be designed to give an adequate answer to a specific research question. Samples need to be representative and of sufficient size to answer the question.

Ecological studies Outcome rates are examined in different populations, eg trend over time, geographically distinct groups, social class. Populations rather than individuals are the unit of study.

Longitudinal (cohort) studies Subjects are followed over time with measurement of exposure and outcome.

Case–control studies Patients with the outcome of interest are identified and past exposure is assessed in comparison to 'controls' who did not develop the outcome. Cases and controls should be adequately matched for other factors that may affect outcome, or these differences should be corrected for (mathematical assumption).

Experimental studies Exposure is allocated to a study group and compared to those who are not exposed, eg randomized controlled trials (p21).

Medical mathematics

When you can measure what you are speaking about, and express it in numbers, you know something about it; but when you cannot measure it, when you cannot express it in numbers, your knowledge is of a meagre and unsatisfactory kind. Lord Kelvin, 1883.

Comparison measures

Comparisons between 'exposed' and 'unexposed' populations are made in terms of the risk or likelihood of an outcome This can be appreciated by plotting a 2×2 table (table 1.3).

Table 1.3 2×2 table analysis

Exposure	Outcome		
	Event	No event	Total
Yes	70	20	90
No	120	450	570
Total	190	470	

- **Absolute risk difference (attributable risk)** = disease frequency in exposed minus the disease frequency in unexposed. Example (table 1.3): (70/90) − (120/570) = 0.57 ∴ exposure increases risk by 57%.
- **Relative risk** = ratio of outcome in exposed population compared to unexposed. Relative risk of 1 means risk is same in both populations. Relative risk >1 means exposure increases risk. Relative risk <1 means exposure lessens risk. Example (table 1.3): (70/90) ÷ (120/570) = 3.69 ∴ risk is 3.69×higher with exposure.
- **Odds ratio** = ratio of the probability of an outcome occurring compared to the probability of an outcome not occurring. Example (table 1.3): (70/20) ÷ (120/450) = 13.13 ∴ odds of outcome are 13.13×higher with exposure.

Relative risk is easier to interpret than odds ratio but relies on a meaningful prevalence/incidence. For the individual, absolute risk difference may be most relevant.

P-values and confidence intervals

In a study of two groups (eg new treatment versus placebo), it is possible that there is no difference (ie new treatment has no benefit). This is the *null hypothesis*. A p-value measures the strength of evidence in relation to the null hypothesis:
- Low p-value: result is unlikely if null hypothesis is true. Null hypothesis is rejected.
- High p-value: result is likely if null hypothesis is true. Null hypothesis is accepted.

A p-value is not the probability that your results occurred by chance, and it cannot tell you how good a study is. There will be many assumptions in the statistical model. Look at the details: has confounding or bias affected the result? *Do not consider $p < 0.05$ as 'statistically significant'*: a small p-value just flags the data as unusual.[14] You need to question why and decide if this is clinically important.

Confidence intervals give a guide as to the effect size and direction (eg benefit/harm). They give a margin of error that indicates the amount of uncertainty in the statistical analysis.

Assessing validity

The validity of a test which dichotomizes study participants can be assessed by examining the results from the test against a standard reference or outcome: did the participant actually have the disease? (table 1.4).

Table 1.4 Table of possible test results

Test result	Patient has condition	Patient does not have condition
Positive	True positive (TP)	False positive (FP)
Negative	False negative (FN)	True negative (TN)

Sensitivity TP/(TP + FN) = of those with the condition, how many test positive? A sensitive test is able to correctly identify those with the disease.

Specificity TN/(TN + FP) = of those who do not have the condition, how many test negative? A specific test is able to correctly identify those without a disease. 'Do they have abdominal pain?' as a test for appendicitis will have ↑sensitivity (most cases have pain), but ↓specificity (many patients with pain do not have appendicitis).

Positive predictive value TP/(TP + FP) indicates how likely it is that someone with a positive test result has the condition.

Negative predictive value TN/(TN + FN) indicates how likely it is that someone with a negative test result does not have the condition. When you receive a test result, you need to know how likely it is to be correct.

Number needed to treat (NNT)

NNT is a useful way of reporting the results of randomized clinical trials. It is the reciprocal of the absolute risk difference: 1 ÷ ARR.

A large treatment effect means that fewer patients need to receive treatment in order for one to benefit. It is specific to the chosen comparator (eg placebo or usual care), the measured outcome (eg death, blood pressure fall), and the duration of treatment follow-up used in the study. Look carefully at the details of the question that the NNT is attempting to quantify.

- Advantages: easily calculated, single numerical value for efficacy, can be used to examine harm (becomes the number needed to harm).
- Disadvantages: confidence intervals are difficult when the differences between treatments are not significant.

The doctor as a gambler

Yes or No? Your tutor asks whether Gobble's disease is more common in the north or the south. You have no idea, and make a guess. What is the chance of getting it right? Common sense decrees that you have a 50:50 chance. Sod's law predicts that whatever you guess, you will always be wrong. Somewhere between the two is Damon Runyon's view that 'all life is 6 to 5 against': Will you pick the right answer? Perhaps, but don't bet on it!

New or existing disease? Suppose singultus is a rare symptom of the common Gobble's disease (5% of patients) but a common symptom of the rarer Kobble's disease (90% of patients). If a patient already known to have Gobble's disease develops singulitis, is it more likely to be due to new Kobble's disease or known Gobble's disease? The answer is usually no: it is generally the case that most symptoms are due to a disease that is already known, and do not imply a new disease (Occam's razor, p6). The 'odds ratio' makes this clearer, ie the ratio of [the probability of the symptom, given the known disease] to [the probability of the symptom due to new disease ≈ the probability of developing the new disease]. Usually this is vastly in favour of the symptom being due to the known disease, because of the prior odds of the two diseases. This will work until Kobble's disease increases in prevalence so as to increase the odds of a second disease (then Hickam trumps Occam, p6).

How to play the odds It is distasteful to think that doctors gamble with patients' lives. It is also distasteful to think of serious diseases being 'missed', and invasive procedures being done unnecessarily. Yet we do not have an evidence base or an experience base which can tell us definitively which cough or lethargy or sore toe is just 'one of those things', and which is the result of undiagnosed cancer or HIV or osteomyelitis. And so we gamble.

Medicine is not for pessimists—almost anything can be made to seem fatal, so that a pessimistic doctor would never get any sleep at night due to worry about the meaning of their patients' symptoms. Medicine is not for blind optimists either, who too easily embrace a fool's paradise of false reassurance. Rather, medicine is for informed gamblers: gamblers who are happy to use subtle clues to change their outlook from pessimism to optimism and vice versa. Sometimes the gambling is scientific, rational, methodical, and reproducible (odds ratio); sometimes it is based on the vital but ill-defined framework of experience ('Clinical intuition', p7).

Of course, gambling inevitably results in losses, and in medicine the chips are not just financial. They betoken the health of your patient, the wellbeing of families, your reputation, and your confidence. Perhaps the hardest part of medicine is the inevitability of making mistakes whilst attempting to help ('Being wrong', p7). But do not worry about gambling: gambling is your job. If you cannot gamble, you cannot walk the thin line between successfully addressing health needs, and causing over-medicalization (p16). But try hard to assemble sufficient evidence to maximize the chance of being lucky. Lucky gambling is a requisite for successful doctoring and the casino of medical practice celebrates the card counter. But the cardinal clinical virtue is courage: without it we would not follow our hunches and take justified risks.

EBM is the conscientious and judicious use of current, best research evidence to optimize management plans and integrate them with patients' values by:

1 Asking answerable questions.
2 Finding the best information.
3 Appraising the information for quality, validity, and relevance.
4 Dialogue to find out what the patient wants.
5 Applying data to patient care.
6 Evaluation.

The amount of evidence

More than 2 million new biomedical papers are published each year including >20 000 new randomized trials. Patients benefit directly from a tiny fraction of these papers. How do we find them?

• A hierarchy of evidence (fig 12) is used to identify the best research available to answer our question.

• Specialist journals, eg *Evidence-based Medicine*, appraise published information for quality, relevance, and interest on our behalf.

• Cochrane gathers and summarizes best evidence, free from commercial sponsorship and conflicts of interest. >37 000 researchers from 130 countries contribute.

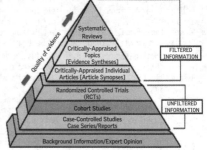

Fig 1.2 Hierarchy of evidence.
EBM Pyramid and EBM Page Generator, copyright 2006 Trustees of Dartmouth College and Yale University.

Problems

• The concept of scientific rigour is opaque. What do we want? The science, the rigour, the truth, or what will be most useful to patients? These may overlap, but they are not the same. Can average cohort results inform clinical decisions on an individual level (especially in the context of comorbidity)?

• Can we really appraise *all* the evidence? We are hindered by publication bias. Around half of all clinical trials remain unpublished. See www.alltrials.net for the campaign to register all trials, and ensure methods and summary results are available.

• Evidence can be expensive. Who paid the bill and what is their vested interest?

• Is the result clinically significant? What is the level of benefit to the individual, as opposed to the population? Is the EBM tail wagging the clinical dog?

• How is our innate hierarchy of evidence constructed? Do we maintain the same standard of evidence for all changes to our practice?

• Have you checked the correspondence columns in journals from which winning papers are extracted? It may take years for unforeseen flaws to surface.

• There is a danger that by always asking, 'What is the evidence?', we will divert resources from hard-to-prove areas (eg psychosocial interventions).

• EBM is never 100% up to date and reworking meta-analyses takes time and money. Specialists may ostensibly reject a new trial due to a tiny flaw, when the real dread is that it might flip their once-perfect formulation.

• EBM sits uncomfortably in a world of intuition and instinctual premonition, yet these instincts may be vital.

• If EBM is prescriptive, patient choice declines. Does our zeal for EBM make us arrogant, mechanical, and defensive? Where is the shared decision-making (p5)?

• By focusing on answerable questions, EBM can distract us from our patients' unanswerable questions—questions that require time and acknowledgement.

▶EBM must be informed by clinical judgement and compassion.

Randomized controlled trials (RCTs)

In a RCT, participants are allocated to an intervention/exposure (eg new drug treatment) or no intervention (eg placebo, standard care) by a process which equates to the flip of a coin, ie all participants have an equal chance of being in either arm of the study. The aim is to minimize bias and attempt to get at the truth as to whether the intervention is good or not. Both groups are followed up and analysed against predefined end-points.

Randomizing Done with the aim of eliminating the effects of non-studied factors. With randomization (and sufficient study size) the two arms of the study will be identical (on average), with the exception of the intervention of interest.

Blinding There is a risk that factors during the trial may affect the outcome, eg participant or clinician optimism if they know the patient is on active treatment, or an unwillingness to expose more severe disease to placebo. If the subject does not know which intervention they are having, the trial is single-blind. Ideally, the experimenter should not know either, and the study is double-blind.

▶In a good trial, the blind lead the blind.

When a RCT might not be the best method

* Generating new ideas beyond current paradigms (case reports).
* Researching causes of illnesses and prognoses (cohort studies).
* Evaluating diagnostic tests (cohort study and decision model).
* Where the researcher has no idea of the effective dose of a drug (dose-ranging design).
* When recruiting of patients would be impossible or unethical.
* When personalized medicine is the aim, eg treatments matched to patients' biomarker profiles (adaptive design, cohort study).

▶In the end, all randomized trials have to submit to the ultimate test when the statistical collides with the personal: 'Will this treatment/procedure benefit me?'

No randomized trial is complete until real-life decisions taken in the light of its findings are scrutinized.

Remember Osler: '*no two individuals react alike and behave alike under the abnormal conditions which we know as disease. This is the fundamental difficulty of the physician*'. Do not ask for definitive trials: everything is provisional.

▶Involve service users in all research to improve quality, relevance, accountability, and transparency.

Journal club: how good is this RCT?

Consider the following:[15]
* Does the study answer a useful question? Does it add to current literature: bigger, better, different target population?
* Does the target population in the study include your patient(s)? Check the inclusion and exclusion criteria including age and comorbidity.
* Is the intervention well described so it can be replicated in clinical practice?
* Was the sample size big enough to detect an effect? Can you find a sample size calculation? Watch out for sub-group analyses without a sample size calculation.
* Were outcome measures predefined?
* Is randomization adequate? Look at the baseline data for each group—are there significant differences? Are any parameters of interest (that might affect outcome) not included?
* Who was blinded and how blind were they?
* Are statistical methods reported and appropriate? There should be a measure of the effect size and its precision (confidence interval; p18).
* Is the effect clinically significant? Watch out for surrogate end-points which do not directly measure benefit, harm, or the treatment response of interest.
* How long was the follow-up? Was it long enough to determine outcome?
* How complete was the follow-up? How many patients were left at the end of the follow-up period? Were those who left the study included in the analysis (intention-to-treat)?

Special populations: the older person

To know how to grow old is the master-work of wisdom, and one of the most difficult chapters in the great art of living.   Henri Amiel, *Journal Intime*, 21 Sept 1874.

Ageing is the inevitable and irreversible decline in organ function with time, in the absence of injury or illness, and despite physiological pathways of repair.

Healthy ageing is the maintenance of physical and mental abilities that enable wellbeing and independence in older age.

►Do not presume ageing. Look for preventable and reversible pathology. Old age does not cause disease (although it can increase vulnerability and recovery time).

►Look for ways to reduce disability and support older people in their own homes.

Differences in the evaluation of the older person

1 **Multiple pathologies** Older patients have, on average, six diagnosable disorders. Effects may be multiplicative. Treatment must be integrated.

2 **Multiple aetiologies** One problem may have several causes, eg falls. Treating each alone may do little good, treating all may be of great benefit.

3 **Non-specific/atypical presentation** Delirium, dizziness, falls, mobility problems, weight loss, and incontinence can be due to disorders in more than one organ system. Typical signs and symptoms may be absent. Ask about functional decline in activities of daily living—this may be the only symptom.

4 **Missed or delayed diagnosis** The older person may decline quickly if treatment is delayed. Complications are common. Use a collateral history: what is the patient usually like?

5 **Pharmacy and polypharmacy** NSAIDs, anticoagulants, anti-parkinson drugs, hypoglycaemic drugs, and psychoactive drugs can pose particular risks in the older patient. Double check for interactions. Consider body weight, liver and kidney function—drug doses may need to be modified. The STOPP/START criteria detail more than 100 potentially inappropriate prescriptions and prescribing omissions relevant to the older patient.[16]

6 **Prolonged recovery time** Anticipate and plan for this. Don't forget nutrition.

7 **Rehabilitation and social factors** Essential for healthy ageing.

A quick ward assessment of the older person

History

In addition to routine elements, include function in activities of daily living, continence, and social support. Ask if there is an advanced care directive and nominated proxy healthcare decision-maker.

Examination
- Appearance and affect: hygiene, nutrition, hydration. Briefly assess mood.
- Senses: vision, hearing, assess swallowing with 20mL of water.
- Cognition: brief screening test, eg AMTS (p61), 2-step command.
- Pulse and blood pressure: lying/sitting *and* standing.
- Peripheral neurological exam: tone, power, wasting, active range of movement.
- Other periphery: pulses, oedema, skin integrity, pressure areas.
- Walking: stand patient, balance, transfers, observe gait (be ready to assist).
- Other systems: CV, respiratory, abdomen (don't forget to palpate for a bladder).

Falls

50% aged >80 will fall at least once per year leading to pain, distress, loss of confidence and independence, and mortality.[17] Fragility fractures cost the NHS £4.4bn/year.
- History: frequency, context and circumstances, severity, injuries.
- Multifactorial risk assessment: gait, balance, muscle strength, osteoporosis risk, perceived functional ability, fear of falls, vision, cognition, neurological examination, continence, home and hazards, cardiovascular examination, medications.
- Interventions: strength and balance training, home hazard intervention, correct vision, modification/withdrawal of medication (cardiovascular, psychotropic), integrated management of contributing morbidities. Consider barriers to change, eg fear, patient preference.

►Pre-existing conditions and non-obstetric disease cause more maternal deaths in the UK than obstetric complications.[18]

►Pregnant patients should receive the same investigations and treatment as non-pregnant patients, with avoidance of harm to the fetus whenever possible.

►Most deficiencies in the management of medical conditions in pregnancy are due to omission caused by inappropriate weighting of risk and benefit.

Physiological changes in pregnancy

Clinical assessment in pregnancy requires knowledge of the physiological changes associated with the gravid state. Expected changes and guidance on when to investigate for possible underlying pathology are given in table 1.5.

Table 1.5 Physiology and pathology in pregnancy

System	Normal pregnancy	Consider pathology
Cardiovascular	Vasodilatation	BP ≥140/90, systolic BP <90mmHg
	↑Heart rate	Sustained tachycardia >110/min
Respiratory	Respiratory alkalosis	Serum bicarbonate <18mmol/L
	No change in PEFR	Decrease in PEFR
	No change in respiratory rate	Respiratory rate >20/min
Kidney	↑Creatinine clearance	Creatinine >77μmol/L (eGFR not valid)
	↑Urinary protein excretion	uPCR >30mg/mmol, uACR >8mg/mmol
Endocrine	Altered glucose handling	Fasting glucose >5.0mmol/L
Haematology	Haemodilution	Hb <10.5g/dL, platelets <100×10⁹/L

Radiology

Image wisely and when required. History and examination will guide. If the uterus is positioned outside the field of view, the radiation dose to the conceptus is minimal. Exposure is well below the threshold of risk to the fetus in:

• Plain radiographs: chest, extremities, spine.

• CT: head, chest (negligible maternal breast cancer risk with modern CTPA techniques).

For most imaging, diagnostic benefit is greater than risk.

Ultrasound and MRI are used preferentially when imaging the abdomen.

►Reassure. Exposure from a chest radiograph is equivalent to 3 days of background radiation and less than a transatlantic flight. Do not presume it is not required: how else will you find the widened mediastinum in chest pain?

Medication

For all drugs prescribed in pregnancy, benefit is balanced against risk (table 1.6). For information on drugs in lactation see: https://www.ncbi.nlm.nih.gov/books/NBK501922/

Table 1.6 Common drugs used in pregnancy (T1 = 1st trimester, T3 = 3rd trimester)

Class	Considered safe	Considered unsafe
Antibiotics	Penicillins, cephalosporins, macrolides, metronidazole	Tetracyclines, ciprofloxacin, trimethoprim in T1
Antiemetics	Cyclizine, metoclopramide	
BP	Labetalol, nifedipine, methyldopa	ACE-i, ARB
Analgesia	Paracetamol	NSAIDs in T3
Anticoagulation	LMWH	Warfarin, DOAC
Endocrine	Insulin, metformin, thyroxine	
Cardiovascular	Aspirin, bisoprolol, adenosine	Amiodarone
Respiratory	Salbutamol, ipratropium, aminophylline, leukotriene antagonists	
Immune system	Prednisolone, azathioprine, CNI, hydroxychloroquine	Mycophenolate, methotrexate
Vaccination	Non-live, eg influenza and SARS-COV-2	Live: MMR, BCG, varicella

►►Do not underestimate sepsis in pregnancy. *Do not ignore tachypnoea.*

►►Counsel all about the increased risks of influenza and SARS-COV-2 (COVID-19) infection, and offer influenza and SARS-COV-2 (COVID-19) vaccinations.

2　History and examination

Contents

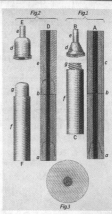

Fig 2.1 Laennec stethoscope of 1819. In an era when the blanket diagnosis of 'hysteria' could be given to women presenting with almost any symptom, it was to Laennec's credit that he sought a more sophisticated method of examination. He was unable to elicit physical signs in the female chest by percussion and application of the hand due to breast tissue and subcutaneous fat. Direct auscultation using the ear was 'as uncomfortable for the doctor as it was for the patient' and unacceptable to a Catholic bachelor. And so an improvised rolled-up piece of paper was honed and perfected to become a 'pectrolique', a 'medical cornet', and a 'thoraciscope' before finally being named the stethoscope. Despite unfavourable peer review, 'there is something even ludicrous in a grave physician formally listening through a long tube applied to the patient's thorax, as if the disease within were a living being that could communicate its condition to the sense without', its utility meant that the stethoscope became the hallmark of the medical phenotype, slung conventionally around the neck. Perhaps Laennec used one himself to 'scope' his 'stethos' (chest) before dying of tuberculosis.

Symptoms and signs

Symptoms are reported and described by patients.

Signs are elicited on inspection and by physical examination.

Together, they produce a picture of health or disease. Signs and symptoms evolve over time according to the natural history of disease or due to a response to treatment.

Throughout this chapter, we discuss symptoms and signs according to organ systems, or describe them as 'non-specific' when they do not conform to this classification. This is unnatural but it is a good first step in learning how to diagnose.

All doctors have to know about symptoms and their relief. Part of becoming a good doctor is learning to link symptoms together, to distinguish those that may be normal from those that are caused by disease. There is no way to distinguish what is worrying from what is not: all symptoms may be worrying (to the patient) and some diseases are self-limiting and not worrying (to the doctor).

There are many books and online resources that can help with learning clinical history taking and physical examination, but there is no substitute for experience. If you aren't sure, ask for help from someone with more experience.

Remember:
* We ask questions to get information to help with our differential diagnosis. But we should also ask questions to find out about the lives our patients live. Rapport and respect will help you to diagnose and to understand what disease means to the patient in front of you. Only with this understanding can you work with your patient to select the right treatment for them.
* Patients (and diseases) rarely read textbooks, so don't be surprised if some symptoms are ambiguous, and others are meaningless. Learn to recognize patterns, but do not be so presumptuous as to create them when none exist.
* Signs can be easy to detect, or subtle. Some will be found by medical students, others require experienced ears or eyes. *You can be a fine doctor without being able to elicit every sign*—listen and look, listen better and look again (later).
* Finding signs and putting together the clues they offer is to become a doctor. It is essential that we learn the signs of diseases that we should never miss.
* Learning is a lifelong process

Finding your way

On paper, history taking seems deceptively easy as if the patient knows the facts and the only problem is extracting them; but what a patient says may include hearsay ('She said I looked pale'), innuendo ('You know, doctor, down below'), legend ('I suppose I must have bitten my tongue; it was a real fit, you know'), exaggeration ('I didn't sleep a wink'), and improbability ('The Pope put a transmitter in my brain').

The great skill (and pleasure) in taking a history lies not in ignoring these garbled messages but in understanding those who voice them, making sense of them, and using them to direct clinical examination. No two doctors will have identical examination techniques. Relish this variation and craft your own routine.

Taking a good history is an art and an essential skill: 80% of diagnoses should be made on history alone, with the signs you elicit adding an extra 10%. A good history may negate the need for invasive tests and irradiation. Do not rely on signs or investigations for your diagnosis, but use them to confirm what you suspect.
A general approach:
• Introduce yourself and check whether the patient is comfortable.
• Seek consent for everything: to talk, to examine, to perform tests.
• Put the patient at ease: a good rapport may relieve distress.
• Be conversational rather than interrogative.
• Start with open questions and allow the patient to tell their story. Steer them back towards important diagnostic points later if necessary.

Presenting problem
Use open questions: 'Why have you come to see me today?' Record the patient's own words rather than medical terms.

History of the presenting problem
When did it start? How did it start: what was the first thing you noticed? How have things changed since then? Have you ever had it before? For pain use SOCRATES:
• **S**ite.
• **O**nset: gradual, sudden.
• **C**haracter: what does it feel like?
• **R**adiation: where does it move to?
• **A**ssociations, eg nausea, sweating.
• **T**iming: constant, intermittent.
• **E**xacerbating and alleviating factors: exercise, food, time of day.
• **S**everity: eg scale of 1–10, compared with worst ever previous pain.

Direct questioning narrows the list of possible diagnoses. Use specific or 'closed' questions about the differential diagnoses you have in mind. Review relevant systems (p28). Don't forget risk factors: travel, occupation, sexual contact.

Past medical history
Ever in hospital? Illnesses? Operations? Anaesthetic problems? Previous investigations even if a diagnosis was not made?

Drug history
Tablets, injections, 'over-the-counter' drugs, herbal remedies, and contraceptives. Ask about *allergies* and what the patient experienced: distinguish side effects (nausea, diarrhoea) from sensitization (rash, wheeze, anaphylaxis).

Social history
Probe without prying. 'Who else is there at home?' Daily life: job, meals, self-care, exercise, mobility (walking aids, stairs). Quality of life is subjective, not objective: What does the patient enjoy? What can they not do because of illness? Utilize the valuable and unique perspective of the GP—they may have known them and their family for decades. Do they have an advance directive? Consider smoking (1 pack-year =20 cigarettes/day for 1 year), alcohol (CAGE questionnaire, p276), illicit drug use.

Family history
Ask about health and cause of death in 1st- and 2nd-degree relatives. Include diseases of relevance to the presenting problem, eg kidney disease, liver disease. Consider cardiovascular risk factors/disease and cancer. Draw a family tree (see BOX). Systemic enquiry (p28) helps to uncover undeclared symptoms although some will already have been covered in a good history of the presenting problem.

►Ask if your patient has any *ideas* or *concerns* about what the problem might be. You may be able to reassure. Or you might agree: 'I am also worried that this might be cancer. I want to find out as soon as possible so we can make a plan for treatment together.'

►Recap with your patient. Ask them to tell you anything you have missed.

►Do not hesitate to review the history later: recollections change (often on the post-take ward round when your consultant asks the same questions).

Drawing a pedigree of inherited disease

Advances in genetics are touching all branches of medicine. It is increasingly important for doctors to identify patients at high risk of genetic disease, and to make appropriate referrals. A key skill is drawing a family tree (fig 2.2) to help you structure a family history:

1 Start with your patient. Draw a square for ♂ and a circle for ♀. Add a small arrow to show that this person is the *propositus/proband* (the person through whom the family tree is ascertained).

2 Add your patient's parents, brothers, and sisters. Record basic information only, eg age and if alive and well (a&w, fig 2.2). If dead, note age and cause of death, and pass an oblique stroke through that person's symbol.

3 Ask the key question, 'Has anybody else in your family had a similar problem as yourself, eg heart attack/angina/stroke/cancer?' Ask about diseases (or possible symptoms of disease) that relate to your patient's main problem.

4 Extend the family tree upwards to include grandparents. If good information about grandparents is not available extend to maternal and paternal uncles and aunts and their children (proband's cousins). If you haven't revealed a problem by now, *go no further*—you are unlikely to have missed important dominantly inherited disease. The pedigree may need to be extended further for recessive and sex-linked disease.

5 Ask about consanguinity (shown using a double line) which increases the risk of recessive disease.

6 Shade those in the family tree affected by the disease. • = an affected female; ■ = an affected male. This will help demonstrate the pattern of inheritance.

7 If you have identified a familial susceptibility, or your patient has a known genetic condition, extend the family tree down and across (children, nieces, nephews) to identify others who may be at risk and may benefit from screening. Refer to a genetics specialist for advice and counselling (*оหсs* p274).

The family tree (fig 2.2) shows these ideas at work and indicates that there is evidence for a genetic risk of colon cancer.

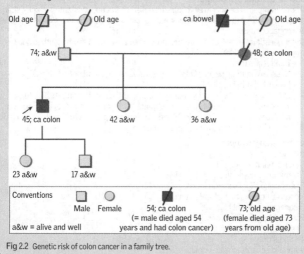

Fig 2.2 Genetic risk of colon cancer in a family tree.

Acknowledgement
Thank you to Dr Helen Firth for her contribution to this topic.

2 History and examination

Just as skilled acrobats are happy to work without safety nets, so experienced clinicians may operate without an enquiry covering the spectrum of symptoms that can arise in disease. To do this you must be skilled enough to understand all the nuances of the presenting complaint. Until you are sure that you have included all the symptoms that will help you to achieve/refine a diagnosis, or when the constellation of symptoms given fails to guide you, try systems enquiry.

General questions
May be the most significant.
- Weight loss (p35).
- Fever/night sweats (p30).
- Lump (p586).
- Fatigue (p30)/malaise/lethargy.
- Sleep (p31).
- Appetite (p35).
- Itch (p31)/rash.
- Mood (p72).

Cardiorespiratory symptoms
- Chest pain (p86).
- Breathlessness: quantify exercise tolerance (before needing to stop due to breathlessness) and how it has changed, eg stairs climbed, distance/speed walked.
- *Paroxysmal nocturnal dyspnoea* (PND) due to *orthopnoea* (breathlessness on lying flat, a symptom of left ventricular dysfunction). Quantify by number of pillows needed for sleep.
- Oedema: ask about dependent areas—ankles, legs, lower back if sitting.
- Palpitations (awareness of heartbeat): can they tap out the rhythm?
- Syncope/pre-syncope.
- Cough: sputum, *haemoptysis* (coughing up blood).

Gastrointestinal symptoms
- Abdominal pain. Use SOCRATES (p26): site; onset; character: constant or colicky, sharp or dull; radiation; associated factors: eating, bowel motion; timing; exacerbating/relieving factors; severity.
- Other questions—think of symptoms throughout the GI tract, from mouth to anus:
  - Swallowing (p246).
  - Indigestion (p248).
  - Nausea/vomiting (p246). *Haematemesis* is vomiting blood.
  - Bowel habit (p254, p256).
  - Stool: colour, consistency, blood, mucus, difficulty flushing (p262), urgency. *Tenesmus* is the feeling of incomplete evacuation (eg due to a tumour). *Melaena* is altered (black) blood passed PR (p252), with a characteristic offensive smell and tar-like appearance.

Genitourinary symptoms
- Incontinence: stress or urge (p640).
- Dysuria: painful micturition.
- Haematuria: visible blood or pink urine.
- Frothy urine suggests proteinuria.
- Nocturia: needing to micturate at night.
- Frequency: frequent micturition.
- Polyuria: large volumes of urine.
- Hesitancy: difficulty starting micturition.
- Terminal dribbling.
- Vaginal discharge: colour, odour.
- Dyspareunia: pain on intercourse (p408).
- Menses: frequency, regularity, duration, pain, clots. First day of last menstrual period (LMP). Number of pregnancies and births. Menarche. Menopause. Any chance of pregnancy now?

Neurological symptoms
• *Special senses*: sight, hearing, smell, and taste.
• Seizures, faints, 'funny turns'.
• Headache.
• Paraesthesiae ('pins and needles').
• Numbness.
• Limb weakness.
• Poor balance.
• Speech problems (p70).
• Sphincter disturbance: urinary retention, incontinence.
• Higher mental function and psychiatric symptoms (pp70–3).

▶Neurological symptoms always warrant functional assessment: what the patient can and cannot do at home, work, etc.

▶Does (and should) the patient drive, and special licence, eg HGV

Musculoskeletal symptoms
• Pain, stiffness, swelling of joints.
• Diurnal variation in symptoms (eg worse in mornings).
• Functional deficit.
• Symptoms of systemic disease: rashes, mouth ulcers, hair loss, nasal stuffiness, malaise. Ask, 'When did you last feel well?'

Thyroid symptoms
Hyperthyroidism
• Heat intolerance/sweating.
• Anxiety.
• Diarrhoea.
• Oligomenorrhoea.
• ↑Appetite, weight loss.
• Tremor.
• Palpitations.
• Visual symptoms due to thyroid eye disease (p78).

Hypothyroidism
• Cold intolerance.
• Low mood.
• Fatigue.
• Thin hair.
• Change in voice.
• Constipation.
• Dry skin.
• Weight gain.

Non-specific symptoms can be caused by a wide range of conditions, and do not conveniently direct the physician to a diagnosis.

Fatigue

So common that it is a variant of normality. Only 1 in 400 episodes of fatigue present to a doctor.

►Do not miss depression (p72).

►Exclude orthopnoea.

►Look for common treatable causes: anaemia, hypothyroidism, diabetes.

Ask: when it started and progression over time, length of sleep, difficulties going to sleep or staying asleep, nocturia, sleep during the day, exacerbating/relieving factors (eg exercise, pain), effect on daily life, life stressors, medications (and when they are taken), alcohol, illicit drug use.

Consider: FBC, ESR, U&E, plasma glucose, TFT.

Sweating

While some night sweating is common, drenching sweats requiring changes of clothes/bedding are a more ominous symptom associated with infection (eg TB, brucellosis), lymphoproliferative disease, and other malignancies. Patterns of fever may be relevant (p438).

Hyperhidrosis = excessive sweating

• Primary, eg hidradenitis suppurativa. Treatment: antiperspirants (aluminium chloride 20% = Driclor®), sympathectomy, iontophoresis.

• Secondary to another cause (table 2.1).

Table 2.1 Secondary causes of sweating

Category	Examples
Infection	Any—bacterial, viral, fungal. Typical and atypical
Acute trigger	Pain, anxiety
Endocrine	Hyperthyroidism, acromegaly, phaeochromocytoma, menopause
Infiltrative	Malignancy, amyloidosis
Medication	Mental health: SSRIs, amitriptyline, haloperidol, clozapine
	Parkinson's: anticholinesterase inhibitors, eg donepezil
	Analgesia: opioids, NSAIDs
	Antimicrobials: cephalosporins, quinolones, aciclovir, ribavirin
	Endocrine: steroids, levothyroxine, sulfonylureas, insulin
Withdrawal	Opioids, gabapentin, alcohol, caffeine

Ask about medications. Consider infection. Examine for lymphadenopathy and splenomegaly. Any signs of hyperthyroidism?

Check: T°, ESR, TFT, FBC, culture—blood, urine, other as indicated.

Falls

Lead to hospital admission, loss of confidence, and dependence.

• MSK: osteo/rheumatoid arthritis, (missed) fracture, eg neck of femur.

• CNS: ↓vision, cognitive impairment, depression, peripheral neuropathy, Parkinsonism, myopathy, malignancy, cord lesion/compression (p462).

• Infection: UTI, pneumonia.

• Endocrine: hypothyroidism.

• CV: postural hypotension (p37), arrhythmia.

• Medication: benzodiazepines, sleeping tablets (the 'Z's), tricyclics, MAOI, antipsychotics, opioids, anti-epileptics, antihypertensives, antianginals, alcohol.

• Environment: lighting, walking surface.

Treatment includes addressing injuries, reducing risk factors, and reducing the risk of injury, eg osteoporosis (p674).

An MDT approach is best including occupational therapists and physiotherapists as most falls are multifactorial.

Insomnia

This is trivial—until we ourselves have a few sleepless nights. Then sleep becomes the most desirable thing imaginable, and bestowing it the best thing we can do, like relieving pain. But don't give drugs without looking for a cause.
* *Self-limiting:* jet lag, stress, shift work, hospital admission.
* *Mental health:* depression, anxiety, mania, psychomotor agitation/psychosis.
* *Organic:*
   * Sensory disturbance: pain, tinnitus, itch.
   * Breathlessness: asthma, orthopnoea, obstructive sleep apnoea (p188).
   * Movement: dystonia, restless legs (p688, check ferritin).
   * Dementia.
* *Drugs:* eg diuretics, steroids, dopamine agonists, cocaine, alcohol.
* *Rare:* encephalitis (West Nile virus), encephalopathy (Whipple's, pellagra, HIV), fatal familial insomnia.

Sleep hygiene No daytime naps, regular bedtime routine. Stop caffeine and nicotine. Avoid late exercise, screen time, and alcohol. Look for patterns and possible modification in a sleep diary. Music and relaxation may make sleep more restorative and augment personal resources.

Hypnotic drugs Do not induce natural sleep. SE: daytime somnolence, rebound insomnia, addiction. Warn about driving/machine use. CBT is better.

Parasomnias, OHCS p739; narcolepsy, p688.

Pruritis (itch)

Ask What provokes it? eg after a bath ≈ polycythaemia rubra vera (p362). Exposure, eg to animals (atopy) or contact (irritant eczema). Are any others affected? eg scabies. Causes are shown in table 2.2.
Examine
* *Skin:* scabies burrows in finger webs, lice on hair shafts, knee and elbow blisters (dermatitis herpetiformis), wheals (urticaria).
* *Systemic:* jaundice, splenomegaly (p54, p59), lymphadenopathy, thyroid (p78)?

Investigate FBC, ESR, glucose, LFT, kidney function, ferritin, TFT.

Table 2.2 Aetiology of pruritus

Primary skin disease	Secondary causes	
Eczema, atopy, urticaria	Liver disease (bile salts, eg PBC)	HIV seroconversion
Scabies	Uraemia (eg CKD)	Drugs (eg opioids)
Lichen planus	Malignancy (eg lymphoma)	Diabetes mellitus
Dermatitis herpetiformis	Polycythaemia rubra vera	Thyroid disease
Dry skin	Iron deficiency anaemia	

Treat Cause, emollients, emollient bath oils, antihistamine (for sleep if not for itch).

Non-specific symptom pathways

A concern for both patients and physicians is that non-specific symptoms herald an underlying malignancy. Although non-specific symptoms have a low predictive value for individual cancers, the overall risk of harbouring cancer of any type is higher, and non-specific symptoms (including unexplained weight loss, fatigue, atypical abdominal pain, and persistent nausea) are present in a significant proportion of cancer diagnoses.

As non-specific symptoms can be caused by a range of conditions of which cancer is only one possible diagnosis amongst many, identifying the appropriate diagnostic tests and referral route for non-specific symptoms is challenging. There are emerging data to support dedicated referral pathways for patients presenting with non-specific *and concerning* symptoms, who do not qualify for an appropriate tumour-specific urgent referral pathway (p517).

Method and order for physical examination

The aim of physical examination is to confirm, exclude, or define the diagnosis revealed in the history. Conventional examination starts with a visual survey of the patient and the patient's environment. It then moves from the hand, up the arm, to the face and neck, and then down the body to include cardiac, respiratory, and abdominal examinations. The whole body is then revisited with central and peripheral neurological examinations. With experience, physical examination gets quicker as the patient's story directs your approach.

► Practice is key.

1 Visual survey

- General wellbeing: are they well or sick? Could they be sicker than they look?
- Appearance: does this suggest a diagnosis, eg acromegaly, Cushing's syndrome, hypopituitarism (p226), hyper/hypothyroidism (p212, 214), Marfan's, systemic sclerosis (p548), Turner's (p143), neurofibromatosis (p510), Parkinsonism (p490), svc syndrome (p524). Cachexia? Obesity?
- Pain: does this make them lie still (peritonitis) or writhe about (colic)?
- Breathing: laboured, rapid, shallow, irregular?
- Mood/affect? Appropriate or not (p72)?
- Look for clues: oxygen, GTN spray, asthma inhaler, glucose monitor, walking aid.

2 Hands

- *Signs of systemic disease in the hands*, see p74.
- Nails: clubbing, koilonychia (iron deficiency), onycholysis (psoriasis), nail fold infarcts (small vessel vasculitis), splinter haemorrhage (trauma, endocarditis).
- Joints: swelling, deformity, Heberden's/Bouchard's nodes (osteoarthritis).
- Skin: jaundice, palmar erythema, scleroderma, lesions (psoriasis, vasculitic changes, xanthomata, telangiectasia, tophi, neurofibromatosis).
- Muscle: wasting, fasciculation.
- Palpation: Dupuytren's contracture (fig 2.24, p58), calcinosis (connective tissue disease, hypercalcaemia).
- Capillary refill: if well perfused <2s.

3 Arm

- Radial and brachial pulses, see p40.
- Blood pressure: trend may be more important than a single value, see p108.
- Arteriovenous fistulae (p302), venous access (chronic/recurrent IV treatment).

4 Face

- Appearance: Bell's palsy (p498), exophthalmos (p79).
- Colour:
  - Blue/purple: cyanosis (p48, fig 2.15).
  - Yellow: jaundice, uraemia, pernicious anaemia, carotenaemia. If the sclera are also yellow it is jaundice.
  - Pallor: non-specific. Anaemia may be better assessed from palmar skin creases (when spread) and conjunctivae (fig 8.18, p325).
  - Hyperpigmentation: haemochromatosis (slate-grey), amiodarone, minocycline.
- Rash: malar flush (mitral valve disease), butterfly rash (SLE).
- Eyes: ptosis (fig 2.18, p48, and p69), myasthenia gravis, heliotrope rash, arcus senilis, cataract (myotonic dystrophy, DM), xanthelasma.
- Mouth: systemic sclerosis (p548), telangiectasia (Osler–Weber–Rendu, p694), cyanosis, pigmentation (Addison's, p220), IX, X, XII nerve lesions (p66), candida.
- Smell: hepatic fetor (p270), ketosis, alcohol, cannabis.

5 Neck
- Carotid pulse, see p40.
- Jugular venous pressure (JVP), see p41. Ensure patient is at 45°.
- Trachea: tug, position.
- Scars: tracheostomy, central venous access (critical illness, dialysis).
- Goitre (p78): palpate from behind. Moves with swallowing. Auscultate for bruit.
- Lymphadenopathy: supraclavicular (Virchow's node), submandibular, post-auricular.

6 Chest
- *Cardiovascular examination*, see p38.
- *Respiratory examination*, see p48.
- Breast examination (p80) if indicated (chaperone for all intimate examinations, and whenever requested).
- Check for axillary lymphadenopathy.

7 Abdomen
- *Abdominal examination*, see p58. Lie patient flat (one pillow).
- Check for inguinal lymphadenopathy.
- Consider rectal examination and urine output.
- Gynaecological examination if indicated.

8 Legs
- Vascular disease (p82): absence of hair, shiny skin, pulseless feet, varicosities (p83), ulcers, gangrene.
- Skin disease: erythema nodosum.
- Other: musculoskeletal, eg tibial bowing (Paget's disease, check also for enlargement of the skull), Charcot's (neuropathic) joint.

9 Neurological examination
- *Examination of the central nervous system*, see p66.
- *Examination of the peripheral nervous system*, see p62, p64.

10 Other
- Mental state examination, see p72.
- Musculoskeletal examination of the hand, see p76.

Temperature
- Strictly speaking not 'observation', but traditionally included with examination.
- Varies during the day with a 95% reference range of 35.7–37.3°C.
- Rectal temperatures are approximately 0.6°C above oral temperatures.
- Temperature falls by –0.021°C for every decade, so fever may not be so pronounced with age.
- Core temperature <35°C = hypothermia. Specific low-reading thermometers may be required.

Non-specific signs can be caused by a range of conditions, and do not conveniently direct the physician to a diagnosis.

Changes in colour

Cyanosis
Peripheral: dusky blue skin, usually fingers. Will occur with central cyanosis but can also be due to peripheral changes, eg cold, hypovolaemia, arterial disease.

Central: blue discolouration of the mucous membranes (check the tongue). Requires 50g/L of deoxyHb. Central cyanosis therefore indicates hypoxaemia, but do not assume that absence of cyanosis means adequate oxygenation.

▶▶ Acute cyanosis is an emergency.

Causes
• *Lung disease:* luminal obstruction, asthma, COPD, pneumonia, PE, pulmonary oedema, pneumothorax. May be corrected by ↑inspired O_2.
• *Congenital cyanotic heart disease:* a right-to-left shunt allows deoxygenated blood to reach the systemic circulation, eg transposition of the great arteries, VSD with Eisenmenger's syndrome (p148). Will not be reversed by ↑inspired O_2.
• *Rare:* methaemoglobinaemia, globin gene mutations.

Pallor
May not be pathological. Possible pathologies: anaemia, hypotension, Stokes–Adams (p456, pale first, then flushing), hypothyroidism, hypopituitarism, albinism.

Anaemia is haemoglobin concentration <130g/L in men and <120g/L in non-pregnant women (p324). It may be assessed from the conjunctivae and skin creases. Koilonychia and stomatitis (p58) suggest iron deficiency. Anaemia with jaundice suggests haemolysis. If pallor in just one limb/digit, consider emboli.

Other colour changes
• Genetic.
• Irradiation, scarring.
• ↑ACTH which cross-reacts with melanin receptors: Addison's (p220), Nelson's syndrome after adrenalectomy for Cushing's (p75), ectopic ACTH secretion.
• Sallow colouration in chronic kidney disease with uraemia (p298).
• Melasma due to increase in melanin and melanocytes. Can be triggered by OCP and pregnancy. No longer called chloasma (= green), which is a misnomer.
• Biliary cirrhosis, malabsorption.
• Haemochromatosis ('bronzed diabetes').
• Carotenaemia.
• Drugs: chlorpromazine, busulfan, amiodarone, gold.

Lymphadenopathy
Can be reactive or infiltrative:

Reactive
Infective:
• Bacterial: eg pyogenic, TB, brucella, syphilis.
• Viral: EBV, HIV, CMV, infectious hepatitis.
• Others: toxoplasmosis, trypanosomiasis.

Non-infective:
Sarcoidosis, berylliosis, connective tissue disease (eg rheumatoid, SLE), dermatopathic lymphadenitis, drugs (eg phenytoin).

Infiltrative
• Amyloidosis.
• Histiocytosis (*OHCS* p848).
• Lipoidoses.
• Cancer:
    • Haematological: lymphoma, leukaemias (ALL, CLL, AML, p354).
    • Metastatic: breast, lung, bowel, prostate, kidney, head and neck cancers.

Oedema

Pitting oedema

Due to increased hydrostatic pressure (eg DVT, right heart failure) or reduced oncotic pressure due to low concentrations of plasma proteins (eg cirrhosis, nephrotic syndrome, protein-losing enteropathy). Though the pathophysiology of oedema is not completely understood.

Periorbital oedema

Eyelid skin is very thin and susceptible to small fluid shifts. Causes include:
- Contact dermatitis: eye make-up.
- Angioedema: hereditary or acquired.
- Infection: ►orbital cellulitis can be life-threatening and needs urgent treatment. Also EBV.
- If there is proptosis, think Graves' disease (p78).
- Connective tissue disease: dermatomyositis, SLE, sarcoid, amyloid.
- Always dip the urine to exclude nephrotic syndrome.

Non-pitting oedema

Lymphoedema due to poor lymphatic drainage is non-indentable. Causes include radiotherapy, malignant infiltration, infection, filariasis, or rarely primary lymphoedema (Milroy disease, p692).

Weight

Weight loss

A symptom (reported by the patient) and a sign (identified by physician).
Causes include:
- Malnutrition/malabsorption.
- Chronic infection, eg TB.
- Depression.
- Cancer.
- Endocrine disorders: diabetes mellitus, hyperthyroidism.
- Degenerative neurological disease.
- Cardiac failure (cardiac cachexia), though right heart failure may mask weight loss by the scales.
- Anorexia nervosa (OHCS p746).
- Advanced chronic kidney disease.

Unintentional weight loss should ring alarm bells—assess patients carefully. Investigations: blood glucose, TFT, CXR, and as directed by history/examination.

Cachexia

General muscle wasting from ↓*eating* (neurological disease: stroke, dementia; anorexia nervosa), *malabsorption* (enteropathic AIDS, slim disease, *Cryptosporidium*, Whipple's), ↑*catabolism* (neoplasia, TB). Also poverty/famine.

Obesity

= BMI >30kg/m². Most not due to metabolic disease.
Associated health risks:
- Type 2 diabetes mellitus (p200).
- IHD.
- Dyslipidaemia.
- ↑BP.
- Osteoarthritis.
- Cancer.
- Non-alcoholic fatty liver disease.
- Infection, eg SARS-COV-2.

Treatment: lifestyle change is key—increase energy expenditure and reduce intake (p238). Medication ± surgery is considered if BMI >40 kg/m², or >35 kg/m² with significant disease that could improve with weight loss. Non-surgical measures should be tried first. Surgical and anaesthetic risks should be considered.

Rare secondary causes of obesity include genetic conditions (Prader–Willi, Lawrence–Moon) and endocrine conditions (hypothyroidism, Cushing's, hypothalamic damage, eg tumour or trauma → damage to satiety regions).

Table 2.3 Presenting symptoms and questions to ask

Presenting symptoms	Direct questions
Chest pain (see pp86–7 and p764)	**S**ite: eg central
	Onset: what was the patient doing when it started?
	Character: ask patient to describe pain (crushing? heavy?)
	Radiation: ask specifically if moves to arm, neck, or jaw
	Associations: ask specifically about shortness of breath, nausea, sweating
	Timing: will help interpret investigations, eg troponin
	Exacerbating and alleviating factors: ischaemic pain may be relieved by GTN. Worse on inspiration and better if sitting forwards suggests pericarditis. Worse with respiration or movement is less likely to be angina
	Severity: out of 10
	Is patient known to have angina or chest pain? Better/worse/same as usual pain? More frequent? Decreasing exercise tolerance?
	NB: GI cause more likely if 'burning', onset after eating/drinking, worse lying flat, or associated with dysphagia
Palpitations	'Are you aware of your own heartbeat?' When and how did it start/stop? Sudden/gradual onset? Duration? Associated with pre-syncope/syncope/chest pain/dyspnoea? Lifestyle trigger, eg caffeine?
	Regular fast palpitations may be paroxysmal supraventricular tachycardia (SVT) or ventricular tachycardia (VT)
	Irregular fast palpitations may be paroxysmal AF, or atrial flutter with variable block
	Dropped or missed beats related to rest, recumbency, or eating may be atrial or ventricular ectopics
	Regular pounding may be normal or due to anxiety
	Slow palpitations may be due to rate-controlling drugs, eg β-blockers. Also bigeminy (fig 3.39, p125)
	Check TSH. Consider a 24h ECG (Holter monitor, p121). An event recorder, if available, may be better than a 24h ECG
Dyspnoea (see p48 and p765)	Duration? On exertion or at rest? Determine exercise tolerance (and any other reason for limitation, eg arthritis). NYHA classification (p135)? Worse when lying flat (orthopnoea, ask how many pillows the patient sleeps with)? Does the patient ever wake up in the night gasping for breath (paroxysmal nocturnal dyspnoea), and how often? Any ankle swelling?
Dizziness/ blackouts (see pp456–8)	*Dizziness:* a loose term, try to clarify what your patient means
	Syncope: did they lose consciousness, and for how long (short duration suggests cardiovascular cause may be more likely than epilepsy)? Any warning (*pre-syncope*)? What was patient doing at the time? Sudden/gradual? Associated symptoms? Tongue biting (pp456–7) and incontinence suggest seizure. Any residual symptoms, eg confusion? How long did it take to feel 'normal'? Witnessed?
	Vertigo: the illusion of rotation of either the patient or their surroundings ± difficulty walking/standing (p458)
	Imbalance: difficulty in walking, without vertigo. Causes include neurological (peripheral nerve, posterior column, cerebellar or other central nerve disorder) and musculoskeletal disease
	Faintness: 'light-headedness'. Seen in anaemia, ↓BP, postural hypotension, hypoglycaemia, carotid sinus hypersensitivity, epilepsy
Claudication	SOCRATES? Foot/calf/thigh/buttock? 'Claudication distance', ie how long can patient walk before onset of pain? Is there rest pain?

Presenting problem
Presenting symptoms and useful questions to ask are shown in **table 2.3**.

Past history
Ask specifically about:
- History of cardiovascular disease: angina, heart attack, stroke.
- Cardiovascular risk factors (see BOX 'Ischaemic heart disease risk factors').
- Rheumatic fever.
- Previous tests/procedures: ECG, angiogram, angioplasty/stents, echocardiogram, cardiac scintigraphy, coronary artery bypass grafts (CABGs).

Drug history
Particularly note cardiovascular medications: aspirin/anti-platelet, GTN, β-blocker, ACE-i/ARB, diuretics, statin, SGLT2 inhibitor, anticoagulant, anti-arrhythmic.

Family history
Enquire specifically if any 1st-degree relatives have cardiovascular disease/events. Any sudden/unexplained death?

Social history
Smoking, impact of symptoms on daily life, alcohol (clarify number of units), exercise.

Ischaemic heart disease risk factors
- Hypertension.
- Smoking.
- Diabetes mellitus.
- Family history of premature CVD (age ≤60).
- Hyperlipidaemia.
- Pregnancy-induced hypertension, pre-eclampsia/eclampsia.

Postural hypotension

This is an important cause of falls and faints, particularly in the elderly. It is defined as a drop in systolic BP >20mmHg or diastolic >10mmHg after standing for 3min vs lying.

Causes Hypovolaemia (early sign). Drugs: antihypertensives, nitrates, diuretics, antipsychotics. Hypocortisolaemia: Addison's (p??0), hypopituitarism (↓ACTH). Autonomic disease: neuropathy (p501), multisystem atrophy (p490). Idiopathic. After a marathon run, peripheral resistance is low for some hours!

Treatment
- Postural hypotension is not a diagnosis, merely a description of a physical sign. Search for the underlying diagnosis to determine the best management.
- Consider referral to a 'falls clinic', where special equipment is available for assessment under various tilts.
- Generic management:
  - Lie down if feeling faint.
  - Stand slowly (with escape route: don't move away from the chair too soon).
  - ↑Water and salt ingestion, eg 9g salt (3.6g/150mmol sodium) per day (but salt has its problems).
  - Physical measures: leg crossing, squatting, elastic compression stockings (check dorsalis pedis pulse is present), and careful exercise may help.
  - If post-prandial dizziness, eat little and often: ↓carbohydrate and alcohol intake.
  - Head-up tilt of the bed at night (10°) ↑renin release, so may ↑standing BP.
- Drug options:
  - Fludrocortisone: 50–100mcg/day PO, then up to 300mcg/day if tolerated. Monitor weight, beware in heart failure, kidney impairment, or ↓albumin as fludrocortisone worsens oedema.
  - Other: sympathomimetics, eg midodrine; pyridostigmine (if underactive bladder too).

The cardiovascular system: examination

Introduce yourself, obtain consent to examine, and position sitting up at 45°. Expose to the waist (for female patients delay until examining the praecordium). Explain throughout.

1 Inspection

- **General** Ill or well? In pain?
- **Breathing pattern** Short of breath?
- **Colour** Pale, cyanosed, flushed?
- **Scars** Median sternotomy (fig 2.3)—CABG, valve replacement, congenital heart disease. Pacemaker/internal cardiac defibrillator.
- **Listen** Audible prosthetic valve click.
- **Clues** Oxygen, GTN spray.

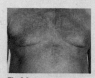

Fig 2.3 Sternotomy scar.

2 Hands

- **Colour** Cyanosis (fig 2.4), tobacco staining.
- **Perfusion** Temperature, capillary refill time.
- **Fingers** Arachnodactyly (Marfan's), polydactyly (ASD).
- **Nails** Clubbing (p74, cyanotic heart disease, endocarditis), splinter haemorrhages (endocarditis).
- **Nail bed** Nail fold infarcts (vasculitis), nail bed pulsations (Quincke's sign of aortic regurgitation).
- **Other** Osler's nodes (tender nodules, eg in finger pulps, endocarditis), Janeway lesions (red macules, endocarditis), tendon xanthomata (hyperlipidaemia).

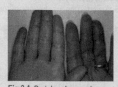

Fig 2.4 Peripheral cyanosis.
Reproduced from Ball G, et al. (eds). *Oxford Textbook of Vasculitis* (2014), with permission from Oxford University Press.

3 Pulse (pp40–1)

- **Radial** (fig 2.5) Rate, rhythm (AF, p126); radio-radial delay (palpate radial pulses simultaneously bilaterally, aortic arch aneurysm), radio-femoral delay (palpate ipsilateral pulses simultaneously, coarctation).
- **Collapsing pulse**
  1 Identify radial pulse then wrap your fingers around wrist.
  2 Before elevating arm check for pain.
  3 Lift arm straight up, collapsing pulse is felt as 'waterhammer' pulsation.
- **Brachial** Waveform character.

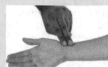

Fig 2.5 Radial pulse.
Reproduced from Thomas J, et al. (eds). *Oxford Handbook of Clinical Examination and Practical Skills* (2014), with permission from Oxford University Press.

4 Blood pressure

- **Systolic** (1st Korotkoff sound) and **diastolic** (5th Korotkoff sound = silence) Hypertension (p108), postural hypotension (p37).
- **Pulse pressure** Difference between systolic and diastolic pressures. Narrow in aortic stenosis, volume depletion; wide in aortic regurgitation, arteriosclerosis.

Top tip

The hand can be used as a manometer to estimate JVP/CVP if you cannot see the neck properly (eg central line *in situ*). Hold the hand palm down below the level of the heart until the veins dilate (patient must be warm!), then lift slowly, keeping the arm horizontal. The veins should empty as the hand is raised. Empty veins below the level of the heart suggest a low CVP, if they remain full it suggests a normal/high CVP.

5 Neck

- **JVP** (p41) Height above manubriosternal angle (not sternal notch) at 45° (fig 2.6). Waveform. Hepatojugular reflux: venous distension with pressure on liver (right heart incompetence).
- **Carotid pulse** Inspect: *Corrigan's sign* (excess pulsations due to aortic regurgitation). Palpate: volume and character on one side, then the other.

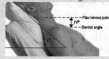

Fig 2.6 The JVP. Reproduced from Thomas J, *et al.* (eds). *Oxford Handbook of Clinical Examination and Practical Skills* (2014), with permission from Oxford University Press.

6 Face

- **Colour** Malar flush (mitral stenosis), central cyanosis.
- **Eyes** Corneal arcus (may suggest hyperlipidaemia, fig 2.7), xanthelasma (eyelid xanthomata), exophthalmos (arrhythmia due to Graves' disease, p78), conjunctival pallor (anaemia).
- **Dysmorphia** Marfan's (aortic dissection), Down's (ASD, VSD, MR), Turner's (coarctation), Williams' (AS, p143).

Fig 2.7 Corneal arcus.

7 The praecordium

- **'Heaves' and 'thrills'** Place heel of hand flat on chest to left then right of sternum. *Heave:* sustained thrusting usually felt at left sternal edge (= RV enlargement, eg pulmonary stenosis, cor pulmonale, ASD). *Thrill:* palpable murmur felt as vibration.
- **Apex beat** Lowermost lateral pulsation normally felt in 5th intercostal space, mid-clavicular line (sternal notch = 2nd intercostal space). Lateral displacement (cardiomegaly), impalpable (dextrocardia/COPD), tapping (palpable s_1 in mitral stenosis), thrusting (volume overload), double impulse (hypertrophic cardiomyopathy).
- **Auscultation** Palpate the carotid pulse simultaneously. Identify *1st* and *2nd heart sounds*. Are they normal? Listen for *added sounds* (p42) and *murmurs* (p44) in all valve areas (fig 2.8):
  1 *Mitral area* (apex). Listen with diaphragm for *mitral regurgitation*, a *pansystolic murmur* radiating to the axilla. Ask patient to, 'Roll to your left side, breathe out, and hold' then listen with the bell for *mitral stenosis*, a *rumbling mid-diastolic murmur*.
  2 *Tricuspid area* (lower left sternal edge) and
  3 *Pulmonary area* (left of manubrium in the 2nd intercostal space). If you suspect a right-sided murmur, listen with the patient's breath held in inspiration.
  4 *Aortic area* (right of manubrium in 2nd intercostal space). Listen for *aortic stenosis*, an *ejection systolic murmur* radiating to the carotids.
  5 Finally, sit the patient forwards and listen at the lower left sternal edge in expiration for *aortic regurgitation*, an *early diastolic murmur*.

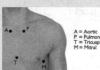

A = Aortic
P = Pulmonary
T = Tricuspid
M = Mitral

Fig 2.8 Valve areas. Reproduced from Thomas J, *et al.* (eds). *Oxford Handbook of Clinical Examination and Practical Skills* (2014), with permission from Oxford University Press.

8 Complete the examination

- Palpate for *sacral/ankle oedema* (fig 2.9).
- *Lung bases:* inspiratory crepitations, pleural effusions.
- Abdomen: *pulsatile liver, ascites* (right-sided heart failure), *splenomegaly* (endocarditis), *aortic aneurysm.*
- Fundoscopy for *Roth's spots* (infective endocarditis).
- Peripheral pulses and bruits (p82), urinalysis, BP, temperature, oxygen saturation, urinalysis.

Fig 2.9 Oedema 'pits' after firm pressure for a few seconds.

The radial pulse is used to determine rate and rhythm. A *collapsing pulse* is felt at the radial (or brachial) artery when the patient's arm is elevated above their head (fig 2.10). Other *character and volume* changes are assessed at the carotid (or brachial) arteries.

Rate Is the pulse fast (≥100bpm, p122) or slow (≤60bpm, p120)?

Rhythm An irregularly irregular pulse occurs in AF and with ectopics. A regularly irregular pulse occurs in 2° heart block and ventricular bigeminy.

Character (waveform) and volume
• *Bounding pulse:* CO_2 retention, liver failure, sepsis.
• *Small volume pulse:* aortic stenosis, shock, pericardial effusion.
• *Collapsing ('waterhammer') pulse:* aortic regurgitation, AV malformation, patent ductus arteriosus.
• *Anacrotic (slow-rising) pulse:* aortic stenosis.
• *Bisferiens pulse:* combined aortic stenosis and regurgitation.
• *Pulsus alternans:* alternating strong and weak beats. LVF, cardiomyopathy, aortic stenosis.
• *Jerky pulse:* H(O)CM.
• *Pulsus paradoxus:* (>10mmHg) fall in systolic pressure with inspiration. Cardiac tamponade, pericardial constriction, severe asthma, tension pneumothorax.

Other pulses: see peripheral vascular examination, p82.

Waterhammer pulse

The waterhammer was a vacuum tube toy half-filled with water. On inversion, the whoosh of water produced a hammer-blow as it rushed from end to end. This is the alternative name for Corrigan's collapsing pulse: the upstroke is abrupt and steep, reaching an early peak (felt as a flick), before a rapid downstroke (felt across all four fingers placed on the patient's pulse) as blood whooshes back into the left ventricle through an incompetent aortic valve.

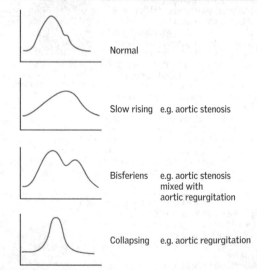

Normal

Slow rising   e.g. aortic stenosis

Bisferiens   e.g. aortic stenosis
mixed with
aortic regurgitation

Collapsing   e.g. aortic regurgitation

Fig 2.10 Arterial pulse waveforms.
Reproduced from Thomas J, *et al.* (eds). *Oxford Handbook of Clinical Examination and Practical Skills* (2014), with permission from Oxford University Press.

The internal jugular vein acts as a capricious manometer of right atrial pressure. JVP examination is difficult so do not be downhearted when the skill eludes you. Observe the *height* and the *waveform* of the pulse. Concomitantly palpate the arterial pulse to help decipher patterns.

Distinguishing the venous pulse
• Usually impalpable and obliterated by finger pressure on the vessel.
• Rises transiently with pressure on abdomen (*abdominojugular reflux*)[1] or liver (*hepatojugular reflux*).
• Changes with posture and respiration: disappears/falls when patient sits upright.
• Usually has a double pulse for every arterial pulse (fig 2.11).

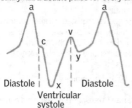

• a wave: atrial systole
• c wave: closure of tricuspid valve, not normally visible
• x descent: fall in atrial pressure during ventricular systole
• v wave: atrial filling against a closed tricuspid valve
• y descent: opening of tricuspid valve

Fig 2.11 The jugular venous pressure wave. The JVP drops (x descent) during ventricular systole because the right atrium is no longer contracting. This means that the pressure in the right atrium is dropping and this is reflected by the JVP.

After *Clinical Examination*, Macleod, Churchill and *Aids to Undergraduate Medicine*, J Burton, Churchill.

Height
Observe the patient at 45° with their head turned slightly to the left and neck relaxed. Good lighting and correct positioning are key. Look for the right internal jugular vein as it passes just medial to the clavicular head of the sternocleidomastoid, behind the angle of the jaw (fig 2.12). The JVP is assessed by measuring the vertical height of the top of the pulse above the manubriosternal

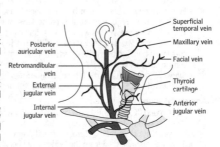

Fig 2.12 The jugular venous system.

angle (*not* the sternal notch). Pressure at zero (the sternal angle) is 5cm, so add 5 to the height of the JVP to obtain the right heart filling pressure in cm of water. A pressure above 9cm (4cm above the manubriosternal angle at 45°) is elevated.

Abnormalities of the JVP
• *Raised JVP with normal waveform:* fluid overload, right heart failure.
• *Fixed raised JVP with absent pulsation:* SVC obstruction (p524).
• *Large a wave:* pulmonary hypertension, pulmonary stenosis.
• *Cannon a wave:* when the right atrium contracts against a closed tricuspid valve, large 'cannon' a waves result. Seen in complete heart block, single chamber ventricular pacing, ventricular arrhythmias/ectopics.
• *Absent a wave:* atrial fibrillation.
• *Large v waves:* tricuspid regurgitation, look for earlobe movement.
• *Constrictive pericarditis:* high plateau JVP which rises on inspiration (*Kussmaul's sign*) with deep x and y descents.
• *Absent JVP:* when lying flat, the jugular vein should be filled. If there is reduced circulatory volume (eg volume depletion, haemorrhage) the JVP may be absent.

1 This sign was first described by Pasteur in 1885 in the context of tricuspid incompetence.

▶Listen systematically: heart sounds then murmurs. While listening, palpate the carotid artery: the carotid upstroke corresponds to systole (**fig 2.13**).

Heart sounds The 1st and 2nd sounds are usually clear. Confident pronouncements about other sounds and soft murmurs may be difficult. Even senior colleagues may disagree with one another, before deferring to an echocardiogram.

The 1st heart sound (S_1) represents mitral (M_1) and tricuspid (T_1) valve closure.
- *Loud S_1* occurs in mitral stenosis. The narrowed valve orifice limits ventricular filling so there is no gradual decrease in flow towards the end of diastole. The valves are, therefore, at their maximum excursion at the end of diastole, and so shut rapidly leading to a loud and palpable (the 'tapping' apex) S_1. S_1 is also loud if diastolic filling time is shortened, eg if the PR interval is short, and in tachycardia.
- *Soft S_1* occurs if the diastolic filling time is prolonged, eg prolonged PR interval, or when the mitral valve leaflets fail to close properly in mitral incompetence.
- *Variable intensity S_1* in AV block, AF, and nodal and ventricular tachycardias.
- *Splitting of S_1* may be heard in inspiration. It is normal and due to physiological asynchrony in the closure of mitral and tricuspid valves.

The 2nd heart sound (S_2) represents aortic (A_2) and pulmonary valve (P_2) closure.
- *Soft A_2* occurs in aortic stenosis.
- *Loud A_2* can occur in tachycardia, hypertension, and transposition, though diagnostic discrimination is limited in clinical practice.
- *P_2* is *loud* in pulmonary hypertension and *soft* in pulmonary stenosis.
- *Splitting of S_2* is best heard in the pulmonary area:
  - *Normal splitting in inspiration* due to the variation of right heart venous return with respiration, delaying the pulmonary component.
  - *Wide splitting* occurs in right bundle branch block, pulmonary stenosis, deep inspiration, mitral regurgitation, and ventricular septal defects (VSDs).
  - *Wide fixed splitting* occurs with atrial septal defects.
  - *Reversed splitting* (ie A_2 following P_2, with splitting increasing on expiration) occurs in left bundle branch block, aortic stenosis, patent ductus arteriosus, and right ventricular pacing.
  - *Single S_2* occurs in Fallot's tetralogy, severe aortic or pulmonary stenosis, pulmonary atresia, Eisenmenger's syndrome (p148), and with a large VSD.

Additional sounds
- *3rd heart sound* (S_3) occurs just after S_2, due to rapid ventricular filling. This can be due to increased volume load (mitral regurgitation, VSD), ventricular dysfunction (dilated cardiomyopathy), or physiology (pregnancy). It is low pitched and best heard with the bell. It can be distinguished from the 'pericardial knock' of constrictive pericarditis or restrictive cardiomyopathy as this is higher pitched and associated with constrictive changes in the JVP (p41).
- *4th heart sound* (S_4) occurs just before S_1. Always abnormal, it represents atrial contraction against a ventricle made stiff by any cause, eg aortic stenosis or hypertensive heart disease.
- *Triple and gallop rhythms:* a 3rd or 4th heart sound occurring with a sinus tachycardia may give the impression of galloping hooves. An S_3 gallop has the same rhythm as '*Ken*-tucky', whereas an S_4 gallop has the same rhythm as 'Tenne-*ssee*'. When S_3 and S_4 occur in a tachycardia, eg with pulmonary embolism, they may summate and appear as a single sound, a summation gallop.
- *An ejection systolic click* is heard early in systole with a bicuspid aortic valve, and in hypertension. Equivalent lesions in the right heart may also cause clicks.
- *Mid-systolic clicks* occur in mitral valve prolapse (p138).
- *An opening snap* precedes the mid-diastolic murmur of mitral (and tricuspid) stenosis. It indicates a pliable (non-calcified) valve.
- *Prosthetic sounds* are caused by non-biological valves opening and closing: *rumbling sounds* ≈ ball and cage valves, eg Starr–Edwards; *single clicks* ≈ tilting disc valves, eg single disc (Bjork-Shiley), bileaflet (St. Jude—often quieter). Prosthetic mitral valve clicks occur with S_1 and aortic valves click in time with S_2.

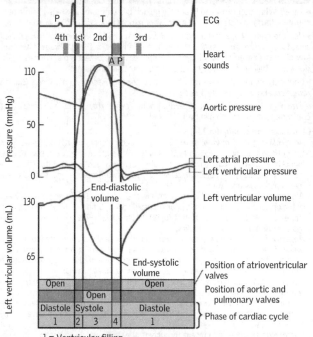

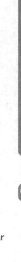

1 = Ventricular filling
2 = Isovolumetric ventricular contraction
3 = Ventricular ejection
4 = Isovolumetric ventricular relaxation

Fig 2.13 The cardiac cycle.

▶Think: 'What do I expect to hear?' Be guided by symptoms and signs before auscultation (but not dictated to: don't let your expectations determine auscultation).

▶Use the stethoscope correctly: remember that the bell is good for low-pitched sounds (eg mitral stenosis) and should be applied *gently*. The diaphragm filters out low pitches, making higher-pitched murmurs easier to detect (eg aortic regurgitation). NB: a bell applied tightly to the skin becomes a diaphragm.

▶Consider any murmur in terms of *character, timing, intensity, area where loudest, radiation,* and *accentuating manoeuvres.*

▶When in doubt, rely on echocardiography rather than disputed sounds (but continue to enjoy the challenge!).

Character and timing (fig 2.14)

• *An ejection-systolic murmur* (*ESM*, crescendo–decrescendo) usually originates from the outflow tract and waxes and wanes with intraventricular pressure. ESMs may be innocent in children and are not due to valve disease in high-output states (eg tachycardia, pregnancy). Pathological causes include aortic stenosis and sclerosis, pulmonary stenosis, and H(O)CM.

• *A pansystolic murmur* (*PSM*) is of uniform intensity and merges with S_2. It is usually pathological and heard with mitral or tricuspid regurgitation (S_1 may also be soft in these), or a ventricular septal defect (p148). Mitral valve prolapse may produce a late systolic murmur ± mid-systolic click.

• *An early diastolic murmur* (*EDM*) is high pitched and easily missed: listen for the 'absence of silence' in early diastole. An EDM occurs in aortic and pulmonary (rare) regurgitation. If pulmonary regurgitation is secondary to pulmonary hypertension resulting from mitral stenosis, then the EDM is called a *Graham Steell* murmur.

• *A mid-diastolic murmur* (*MDM*) is low pitched and rumbling. They occur in mitral stenosis (accentuated presystolically if in sinus rhythm). If due to rheumatic thickening of the mitral valve = *Carey Coombs' murmur*. An *Austin Flint murmur* is an MDM in the context of aortic regurgitation due to the fluttering of the anterior mitral valve cusp by the regurgitant stream.

• *Continuous murmurs* are present throughout the cardiac cycle and occur with a patent ductus arteriosus, arteriovenous fistula, or ruptured sinus of Valsalva.

Intensity All murmurs are graded on a scale of 1–6 (table 2.4), though in practice diastolic murmurs, being less loud, are only graded 1–4. Intensity is a poor guide to the severity of a lesion: an ESM may be inaudible in severe aortic stenosis.

Area where loudest Though there are no guarantees, mitral murmurs tend to be loudest over the apex, aortic murmurs over the right 2nd intercostal space, pulmonary over the left 2nd intercostal space, and tricuspid murmurs at the lower left sternal edge (fig 2.8, p39).

Radiation The ESM of aortic stenosis classically radiates to the carotids. The PSM of mitral regurgitation radiates to the axilla.

Accentuating manoeuvres

• Movements that bring the relevant part of the *heart closer to the stethoscope* accentuate murmurs: lean forward for aortic regurgitation, left lateral position for mitral stenosis.

• *Expiration* increases blood flow to the left side of the heart and therefore accentuates left-sided murmurs. *Inspiration* accentuates right-sided murmurs.

• *Valsalva manoeuvre* (forced expiration against a closed glottis) decreases systemic venous return, accentuating mitral valve prolapse and H(O)CM, but softening mitral regurgitation and aortic stenosis. *Squatting* has the opposite effect. *Exercise* accentuates the murmur of mitral stenosis.

Non-valvular added sounds

A *pericardial friction rub* may be heard in pericarditis. It is a superficial scratching sound, not confined to systole or diastole.

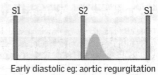

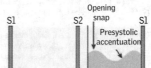

Fig 2.14 Typical waveforms of common heart murmurs.

S1   S2   S1

Ejection-systolic eg: aortic stenosis

S1   S2   S1

Early diastolic eg: aortic regurgitation

S1   S2   S1

Pansystolic eg: mitral regurgitation

S1   S2   S1

Opening snap

Presystolic accentuation

Mid-diastolic eg: mitral

Grading intensity of heart murmurs

▶The following grading is commonly used for murmurs: systolic murmurs from 1 to 6 and diastolic murmurs from 1 to 4 (as they cannot reach grading 5 or 6).

Table 2.4 Grading of heart murmurs.

Grade	Description
1/6	Very soft, only heard after listening for a while
2/6	Soft, but detectable immediately
3/6	Clearly audible, but no thrill palpable
4/6	Clearly audible, palpable thrill
5/6	Audible with stethoscope only partially touching chest
6/6	Can be heard without placing stethoscope on chest

Prosthetic valve murmurs

Prosthetic valves Created either from synthetic material (mechanical prosthesis, see prosthetic sounds, p42) or from biological tissue (bioprosthesis). The choice of prosthesis is determined by the anticipated lifespans of the patient and the graft, and the risks of anticoagulation (including plans for pregnancy). Three mechanical valve designs exist: the caged ball valve, the tilting disc single leaflet valve, and the bileaflet valve. Tissue valves are made from porcine valves or bovine pericardium.

Prosthetic aortic valves All produce a degree of outflow obstruction and thus have an ESM. The intensity of this murmur increases as the valve fails. Ball and cage valves (eg Starr–Edwards) and tissue valves *do* close completely in diastole and so a diastolic murmur warrants assessment for valve failure.

Prosthetic mitral valves Ball and cage valves project into the left ventricle and can cause a low-intensity ESM as they interfere with the ejected stream. Tissue valves and bileaflet valves can also have a low-intensity diastolic murmur. Consider any systolic murmur of loud intensity to be a sign of regurgitation and ∴ failure.

Eponymous signs of aortic regurgitation

- *de Musset's sign:* head nodding in time with the pulse.
- *Müller's sign:* systolic pulsations of the uvula.
- *Corrigan's sign:* visible carotid pulsations due to a rapid systolic rise and a rapid diastolic collapse.
- *Quincke's sign:* capillary nailbed pulsation in the fingers.
- *Traube's sign:* 'pistol shot' femorals, a booming sound heard over the femorals.
- *Duroziez's sign:* to-and-fro diastolic murmur heard when compressing the femorals proximally with the stethoscope.

The respiratory system: history

Table 2.5 Presenting symptoms and questions to ask

Presenting symptoms	Direct questions and possible causes
Dyspnoea (table 2.6 and p765)	Duration? Exercise tolerance: steps climbed/distance walked? NYHA classification (p135)? Diurnal variation (≈ asthma)? Ask specifically about circumstances in which dyspnoea occurs (eg occupational allergen exposure)
Cough (p47)	Duration? Character (eg barking/dry)? Nocturnal (≈ asthma, ask about other atopic symptoms, eg eczema, hay fever)? Exacerbating factors? Sputum (colour? how much?). Haemoptysis?
Haemoptysis (table 2.7)	Always consider risk factors for TB and malignancy (weight loss, night sweats (p30), smoking). Blood not mixed with sputum may suggest pulmonary embolism, trauma, or bleeding into a lung cavity. Melaena can occur if enough blood is swallowed
Hoarseness (OHCS p418)	Laryngitis, recurrent laryngeal nerve palsy, Singer's nodules, or laryngeal tumour
Wheeze (p51)/ stridor(p47)	Wheeze is common in asthma but also foreign body, congestive heart failure, malignancy, and any lesion causing airway narrowing
Chest pain (p86, p764)	SOCRATES (see p36), 'pleuritic' (worse on inspiration) suggests pleural involvement

History Ask about current symptoms (table 2.5) and past history: pneumonia/ bronchitis, TB, atopy (asthma/eczema/hay fever), previous CXR abnormalities, lung surgery, myopathy/neurological disorders, connective tissue disorders/symptoms, eg rheumatoid, SLE.

Drug history Respiratory medications: bronchodilators, corticosteroids? Any medications with respiratory side effects, eg ACE-i, cytotoxics, β-blockers, amiodarone?

Family history Atopy? Emphysema? TB?

Social history Quantify smoking in 'pack-years' (20 cigarettes/day for 1 year = 1 pack-year). Occupation: farming, mining, asbestos. Pets? Recent travel/TB contacts?

Dyspnoea

Subjective sensation of shortness of breath, often exacerbated by exertion. Speed of onset may aid diagnosis (table 2.6). Causes include:
- *Lung disease:* airway and interstitial disease. May be hard to differentiate from cardiac causes. Asthma: nocturnal cough, early morning dyspnoea & wheeze.
- *Cardiac disease:* left ventricular failure of any cause. Orthopnoea (dyspnoea worse on lying down; 'How many pillows?') and paroxysmal nocturnal dyspnoea (PND; dyspnoea waking one up). Also peripheral oedema, ↑JVP, crepitations (p51).
- *Anatomical:* diseases of the chest wall (p50), muscles, pleura. Ascites can cause breathlessness by splinting the diaphragm and restricting its movement.
- *Other:* ▶shock—dyspnoea may be shock's presenting feature (p599, p770). Anaemia. Metabolic acidosis with respiratory compensation, eg ketoacidosis, salicylate poisoning. Dyspnoea at rest *unassociated with exertion* may be psychogenic. Prolonged hyperventilation causes respiratory alkalosis, and a fall in ionized calcium leading to peripheral/perioral paraesthesiae ± carpopedal spasm. Physiological breathlessness of pregnancy (breathe deeper, not faster).

Table 2.6 Aetiology of dyspnoea by timing of onset

Acute	Subacute	Chronic
Foreign body	Asthma	COPD
Pneumothorax (p733, fig 16.44)	Pneumonia	Interstitial lung disease
Pulmonary embolus	Effusion	LV dysfunction
Acute pulmonary oedema		Anaemia

Haemoptysis is blood that is *coughed* up: frothy, *alkaline*, and bright red, often in a context of known lung disease (table 2.7). (NB: *Vomited* blood is acidic and dark.)

Table 2.7 Causes of haemoptysis

Infective	Pneumonia, pneumonitis, bronchiectasis, bronchitis, abscess. Can be bacterial (pneumococcus, TB), fungal (aspergillosis), viral (influenza, SARS-COV-2), and helminths (schistosomiasis)
Neoplastic	Primary or secondary
Vascular	Lung infarction (PE), vasculitis (ANCA-associated, anti-GBM disease, SLE), hereditary haemorrhagic telangiectasia, arteriovenous malformation
Parenchymal	Interstitial lung disease, sarcoidosis, haemosiderosis, cystic fibrosis
Pulmonary hypertension	Idiopathic, thromboembolic, congenital cyanotic heart disease (p148)
Coagulopathy	Any, eg thrombocytopenia (p342), DIC, warfarin toxicity. Always exclude underlying pathology.
Trauma/foreign body	Includes following intubation
Pseudo-haemoptysis	Oropharyngeal bleeding, aspirated haematemesis. Red pigment (prodigiosin) from *Serratia marcescens*. Munchausen's (p694)

Rare causes refuse to be classified neatly: vascular causes may have infective origins, eg hydatid cyst may count as a foreign body *and* infection *and* vascular if it fistulates with the aorta; ditto for infected (mycotic) aneurysm rupture, or TB aortitis. Infective causes may cause coagulopathy: dengue; leptospirosis. If monthly haemoptysis, consider lung endometriosis.

Treatment If massive (eg trauma, TB, hydatid cyst, cancer, AV malformation): prepare (IV access, blood gas, FBC, INR/APTT, crossmatch) for embolization by interventional radiology, bronchoscopic (stent/balloon) tamponade, or cardiothoracic surgery (lobe resection). IV morphine if distressed by symptoms, eg inoperable malignancy.

Cough
Coughing is relatively non-specific, resulting from irritation anywhere from the pharynx to the lungs. The character of a cough may, however, give clues as to the underlying cause:
• *Loud, brassy:* pressure on the trachea, eg tumour.
• *Hollow, 'bovine':* recurrent laryngeal nerve palsy.
• *Barking:* laryngotracheobronchitis (croup).
• *Chronic:* TB, foreign body, asthma (nocturnal), pertussis.
• *Dry, chronic:* oesophageal reflux, side effect of ACE-i.

►Do not ignore a change in character of a chronic cough; it may signify a new problem, eg infection, malignancy.

Stridor
Inspiratory sound due to partial obstruction of upper airways. Obstruction may be:
• Within the lumen: foreign body, tumour, bilateral vocal cord palsy.
• Within the airway wall: oedema (eg anaphylaxis), laryngospasm, epiglottitis, laryngotracheobronchitis (croup), amyloidosis.
• Extrinsic to the airway: goitre (p78), oesophagus, lymphadenopathy.

►If gas exchange is impaired, manage as an emergency (p756).

Introduce yourself, obtain consent to examine, and position sitting up at 45°. Expose to the waist (for female patients delay until examining the chest). Explain throughout.

1 Inspection

- **General** Ill or well? Respiratory distress (p49)? Stridor (p47)? Short of breath (p46)? Accessory muscle use? Cachexia (p35)?
- **Chest wall** Movement: ask patient to take a deep breath (pathology is on the restricted side). Deformities of chest wall (p50). Scars: skin thickening/

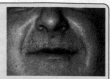

Fig 2.15 Cyanosis.

tattoos from radiotherapy, chest drain insertion.
- **Respiratory rate and breathing pattern** See p50. Paradoxical respiration: abdomen sucked in with inspiration in diaphragmatic paralysis (p496).
- **Colour** Pale, cyanosed (fig 2.15), flushed.
- **Clues** Oxygen, inhaler, peak flow meter, nebulizer.

2 Hands

- **Inspect** Peripheral cyanosis, clubbing (p74), systemic disease (sclerosis, rheumatoid arthritis), tremor (β-agonist use), tobacco staining (fig 2.16), muscle wasting (T1 lesions, eg Pancoast's tumour, p694), tender wrists (hypertrophic pulmonary osteoarthropathy in cancer).

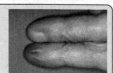

Fig 2.16 Tar stains.

- **Asterixis** Ask the patient to hold their hands out and cock their wrists back: CO_2 retention.
- **Pulse** Pulsus paradoxus (respiratory distress, p40), bounding (CO_2 retention).

3 Neck

- **Trachea** Sternal notch (fig 2.17)—is trachea deviated towards collapse or away from pleural effusion/tension pneumothorax? (A slight deviation to right is normal.) Assess cricosternal distance: <3cm is hyperexpansion. Feel for tracheal tug: descent of trachea with inspiration due to severe airflow limitation.
- **Lymphadenopathy** Sit patient forward and examine from behind (TB, malignancy, sarcoid).
- **JVP** See p41. Raised in cor pulmonale, fixed and raised in superior vena cava obstruction.

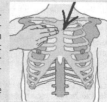

Fig 2.17 Sternal notch.

4 Face

- **Eyes** Horner's syndrome: ptosis, miosis, anhidrosis, enophthalmos (fig 2.18, and p69). Conjunctival pallor.
- **Mouth** Central cyanosis (ask patient to stick out tongue), pursed lip breathing.

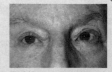

Fig 2.18 Horner's syndrome.

Top tips

- Whispering pectoriloquy is a classic and specific sign of consolidation.
- Expose the chest so not to miss small scars, eg from video thoracoscopy.
- If you see Horner's syndrome (fig 2.18), check for wasting of the small muscles of the hand.

5 Chest

• **Apex beat** Impalpable due to COPD/pleural effusion/dextrocardia?

Complete the next steps on the front of the chest before sitting the patient forward to perform again on the back of the chest.

1 **Expansion** Horizontal: place hands as positioned in fig 2.19 in expiration ('Breathe all the way out'), note movement of thumbs from midline. Vertical: place finger tips on clavicles in expiration and note symmetry of movement in inspiration.

2 **Tactile vocal fremitus** Palpate the chest with the lateral surface of your hand asking the patient to say '99' each time they feel your hand. Compare right to left. Often omitted (in clinical practice, but not in exams) in preference for vocal resonance.

3 **Percussion** Percuss all respiratory segments, comparing right and left (fig 2.20). *Dull*: collapse, consolidation, pleural thickening, effusion (*'stony dull'*). *Cardiac dullness* detectable on the left side. *Liver dullness* usually extends to 5th rib, right mid-clavicular line; hyperinflation (eg asthma, COPD) may push liver down. *Hyperresonance*: pneumothorax or hyperinflation (COPD).

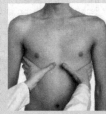
Fig 2.19 Hand placement for testing expansion: anchor fingers with thumbs free-floating.
Reproduced from Thomas J, et al. (eds). Oxford Handbook of Clinical Examination and Practical Skills (2007), with permission from Oxford University Press.

4 **Auscultation** With diaphragm, from apices to bases, comparing right and left (fig 2.23, table 2.8, p51).

5 **Vocal resonance** Repeat auscultation, asking patient to say (whisper) '99' each time they feel the stethoscope. ↑Resonance with whispering ('whispering pectoriloquy') is a sensitive sign for consolidation.

6 Complete the examination

• Palpate for *sacral and ankle oedema* (fig 29, p39).
• Observation chart for temperature and O_2 saturation.
• Examine the sputum pot (p50) and check peak flow.

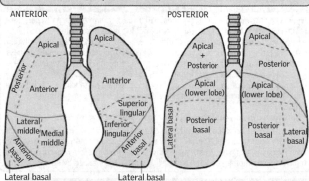
Fig 2.20 The respiratory segments supplied by the segmental bronchi.

ANTERIOR — Apical, Posterior, Anterior, Lateral middle, Medial middle, Anterior basal, Lateral basal; Apical, Anterior, Superior lingular, Inferior lingular, Anterior basal, Lateral basal

POSTERIOR — Apical, Apical + Posterior, Apical (lower lobe), Lateral basal, Posterior basal; Apical, Posterior, Apical (lower lobe), Posterior basal, Lateral basal

⚠ Signs of respiratory distress

• Tachypnoea.
• Nasal flaring.
• Tracheal tug: pulling of thyroid cartilage towards sternal notch in inspiration.
• Accessory muscle use: sternocleidomastoid, platysma, and infrahyoid.
• Recession: intercostal, subcostal, and sternal.
• Pulsus paradoxus (p40).

2 History and examination

Chest deformities
- **Barrel chest** ↑Diameter, ↓chest expansion. Seen in hyperinflation (asthma/COPD).
- **Pectus carinatum (pigeon chest)** Prominent sternum (fig 2.21).
- **Pectus excavatum (funnel chest)** Depression of sternum (fig 2.22).
- **Kyphosis** ↑AP thoracic spine curvature.
- **Scoliosis** Lateral curvature (*OHCS* p480).

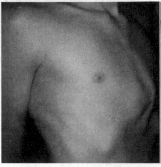 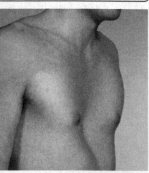

Fig 2.21 Pectus carinatum. Prominent sternum from lung hyperinflation while bony thorax develops, eg chronic childhood asthma. Often seen with *Harrison's sulcus*: groove deformity due to indrawing of lower ribs at diaphragm attachment. Usually no significance for function, may have psychological effects.

Image courtesy of Prof Eric Fonkalsrud.

Fig 2.22 Pectus excavatum. Often asymptomatic, but may cause displacement of the heart to the left, and restricted ventilatory capacity ± mild air-trapping. Associations: scoliosis; Marfan's; Ehlers–Danlos.

Image courtesy of Prof Eric Fonkalsrud.

Breathing patterns

Hyperventilation Rapid (tachypnoea >20 breaths/min) or deep (hyperpnoea (↑tidal volume)) breathing. In the absence of lung disease consider:
- *Hyperventilation syndrome:* a panic attack associated with hyperventilation. Associated symptoms include: palpitations, dizziness, tinnitus, chest pain/tightness, perioral/limb paraesthesiae (plasma ↓Ca^{2+}). Treatment: relaxation techniques and breathing into a paper bag (↑inspired CO_2 corrects the alkalosis).
- *Kussmaul respiration:* deep, sighing breaths in severe metabolic acidosis (blowing off CO_2), eg diabetic or alcoholic ketoacidosis, kidney failure, aspirin overdose (p825).
- *Neurogenic hyperventilation* is produced by pontine lesions.

Cheyne–Stokes breathing Breaths get deeper and deeper, then shallower (± episodic apnoea) in cycles. Caused by brainstem lesions/compression, eg stroke, ↑ICP). If cycle is long (eg 3min), there may be a long lung-to-brain circulation time (eg chronic pulmonary oedema or ↓cardiac output). Enhanced by opioids.

Sputum examination

Inspect sputum as part of routine respiratory examination. Send for culture, Gram stain (auramine/ZN stain if indicated), and cytology.
- *Black carbon specks* suggest smoking: commonest cause of increased sputum.
- *Yellow/green sputum* suggests infection, eg bronchiectasis, pneumonia.
- *Pink frothy sputum* suggests pulmonary oedema.
- *Bloody sputum (haemoptysis)* may be due to malignancy, TB, infection, trauma, pulmonary vasculitis. Always requires investigation (p47).
- *Clear sputum* is probably saliva.

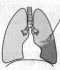

(There may be bronchial breathing at the top of an effusion)

Expansion: ↓
Percussion: ↓ (stony dull)
Air entry: ↓
Vocal resonance: ↓
Trachea + mediastinum central (shift away from affected side only with massive effusions ≥1000mL)

PLEURAL EFFUSION

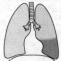

Expansion ↓
Percussion note ↓
Vocal resonance ↑
Bronchial breathing ± coarse crackles (with whispering pectoriloquy)
Trachea + mediastinum central

CONSOLIDATION

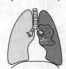

Expansion ↓
Percussion note ↑
Breath sounds ↓
Trachea + mediastinum shift towards the affected side

SPONTANEOUS PNEUMOTHORAX/ EXTENSIVE COLLAPSE (∆∆ LOBECTOMY/ PNEUMONECTOMY)

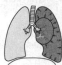

Expansion ↓
Percussion note ↑
Breath sounds ↓
Trachea + mediastinum shift away from the affected side

TENSION PNEUMOTHORAX (See fig 16.44, p733 for chest x-ray image)

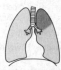

Expansion ↓
Percussion note ↓
Breath sounds bronchial ± crackles
Trachea + mediastinum central or pulled towards the area of fibrosis

FIBROSIS

Fig 2.23 Physical signs on respiratory examination.

Table 2.8 Auscultation

Breath sounds	Description	Pathology
Vesicular	Soft, low-pitched blowing/rustling	Normal
Bronchial breathing	Harsh. Expiration and inspiration of equal volume and length with a gap between inspiration and expiration	Consolidation, localized fibrosis, above pleural/percardial effusion (Ewart's sign, p132)
Reduced breath sounds	Quiet, difficult to hear	Pleural effusion/thickening, pneumothorax, occlusion
Silent	Inaudible breath sounds	Life-threatening asthma
Wheeze (rhonchi)	• Monophonic: single note, partial obstruction of one airway	• Airway occlusion: tumour, foreign body
	• Polyphonic: multiple notes, wide-spread airway narrowing	• Asthma, 'cardiac' wheeze from pulmonary oedema
Crepitations	Crackles: small airways reopen in inspiration:	
	• Fine and late in inspiration	• Pulmonary oedema
	• Coarse and mid inspiratory	• Bronchiectasis
	• Early inspiratory	• Small airway disease
	• Late/pan inspiratory	• Alveolar disease
Pleural rub	Creak like foot in snow. Due to movement of visceral over parietal pleura when both are inflamed	Pneumonia, pulmonary infarction
Pneumothorax click	Click during cardiac systole	Shallow left pneumothorax overlying heart

The gastrointestinal system: history

Gastrointestinal symptoms are detailed in table 2.9

Table 2.9 Presenting symptoms and questions to ask

Presenting symptom	Questions
Abdominal pain (p53, p598)	SOCRATES (p26)
Nausea, vomiting (table 2.10)	Timing? Relation to meals? Amount? Content: liquid, solid, bile, blood? Frequency?
Haematemesis (pp252–3)	Fresh (bright red)? Dark or 'coffee grounds'? Consider cancer: weight loss, dysphagia, pain, melaena? Medications: NSAIDs, anticoagulants?
Dysphagia (p246)	Level? Onset? Progressive? Painful swallow (odynophagia)?
Indigestion/dyspepsia/reflux (p248)	Timing (relation to meals)? NSAIDs?
Change in bowel habit: diarrhoea (p254), constipation (p256)	Symptoms of malignancy: weight loss, anaemia, melaena? Pale stools/steatorrhoea (p55)? Pain on defecation? Mucus? Polyuria/kidney stones (↑Ca²⁺). Antibiotics? Thyroid symptoms (p29)
Rectal bleeding (p621), melaena (p252)	Fresh/dark/black? Pain on defecation? Perianal pain? Mucus? Mixed with stool/on surface/on paper/in the pan?
Appetite, weight change	Quantify. Intentional? Dysphagia? Pain? See p35
Distension (p54)	Timing? Alcohol use? Pain? Itch? Jaundice? LMP?
Jaundice (p268)	Pruritus? Dark urine? Pale stools?

Past history Peptic ulcer disease, cancer, jaundice, hepatitis, blood transfusion, tattoos, surgery, last menstrual period, dietary changes, surgery/dialysis abroad.

Drug history Especially steroids, NSAIDs, antibiotics, anticoagulants.

Family history Irritable bowel syndrome (IBS), inflammatory bowel disease (IBD), polyps, cancer, jaundice.

Social history Smoking, alcohol (quantify units/week), recreational drug use, travel history, contact with jaundiced persons, occupational exposure, sexual history.

Vomiting History is vital. Associated symptoms and medical history may indicate cause (table 2.10). Examine for dehydration, distension, tenderness, mass, succussion splash in children (pyloric stenosis), tinkling bowel sounds (intestinal obstruction).

Table 2.10 Causes of vomiting

Gastrointestinal	CNS	Metabolic/endocrine
• Gastroenteritis	• Meningitis/encephalitis	Uraemia
• Peptic ulceration	• Migraine	Hypercalcaemia
• Pyloric stenosis	• ↑Intracranial pressure	Hyponatraemia
• Intestinal obstruction	• Brainstem lesion	Pregnancy
• Paralytic ileus	• Motion sickness	Diabetic ketoacidosis
• Acute cholecystitis	• Ménière's disease	Addison's disease
• Acute pancreatitis	• Labyrinthitis	
Alcohol and drugs	**Psychiatric**	**Other**
• Antibiotics	• Psychogenic	• Myocardial infarction
• Opioids	• Bulimia nervosa	• Autonomic neuropathy
• Cytotoxics		• Sepsis

Non-gastrointestinal causes of vomiting? Try ABCDEFGHI:

Addison's disease.

Brain (eg ↑ICP).

Cardiac (myocardial infarct).

Diabetic ketoacidosis.

Ears (labyrinthitis, Ménière's disease).

Foreign substances (alcohol, drugs).

Gravidity (hyperemesis).

Hypercalcaemia/Hyponatraemia.

Infection.

Abdominal pain Occurs due to a number of possible pathological mechanisms: irritation of the mucosa (acute gastritis), smooth muscle spasm (enterocolitis), capsular stretch (liver lesion/bleed), peritoneal inflammation (acute appendicitis), direct splanchnic nerve stimulation (retroperitoneal extension of tumour).

Character Constant or colicky, sharp or dull?

Duration and frequency Depend on the mechanism of production. Colic is an intermittent pain with sudden onset and cessation. It is due to the contraction of muscles around a partial or complete blockage in a luminal organ: small intestine, large intestine, rectum, gallbladder, ureter.

Location and distribution May help determine aetiology:
  - *Epigastric:* gastritis/duodenitis, peptic ulcer, gallbladder disease, pancreatitis, aortic aneurysm.
  - *Left upper quadrant:* peptic ulcer, gastric or colonic (splenic flexure) disease, splenic rupture, subphrenic abscess, renal colic, pyelonephritis.
  - *Right upper quadrant:* cholecystitis, biliary colic, hepatitis, peptic ulcer, colonic (hepatic flexure) disease, renal colic, pyelonephritis, subphrenic abscess.
  - *Loin* (lateral ⅓ of back between thorax and pelvis), merges with *flank* (side between ribs and pelvis, p563): renal colic, pyelonephritis, renal tumour, referred pain from spine.
  - *Left iliac fossa:* diverticulitis, volvulus, colon cancer, inflammatory bowel disease, hip pathology, renal colic, UTI (p292), pelvic abscess, ovarian cyst torsion, salpingitis, ectopic pregnancy.
  - *Right iliac fossa:* all causes of left iliac fossa pain plus appendicitis and Crohn's ileitis, and usually excluding diverticulitis.
  - *Pelvic:* UTI, urinary retention, menstruation, ectopic pregnancy, endometriosis (*OHCS* p140), endometritis (*OHCS* p136), salpingitis, ovarian cyst torsion.
  - *Generalized:* gastroenteritis, irritable bowel syndrome, peritonitis, constipation.
  - *Central:* mesenteric ischaemia, abdominal aneurysm, pancreatitis.
  - *Referred pain:* myocardial infarct, pleural pathology, hip disease, herpes zoster.

Time of occurrence Meals, defecation, sleep.

Aggravating/relieving factors Food, defecation, urinary symptoms, movement.

Abdominal distension

* Resonant: flatus.
* Dull: solid lesion, eg colon, stomach, pancreas, liver, or kidney tumour. Fluid, eg ascites (shifting dullness) due to malignancy or cirrhosis; distended bladder (cannot get below it).
* Expansile: aneurysm.
* Pelvic: uterine fibroids, ovarian cyst/tumour.

See also *ascites with portal hypertension* (p596), *other abdominal masses* (p596).

Hepatomegaly and splenomegaly

Hepatomegaly

* *Malignancy:* primary or metastatic. Usually craggy, irregular edge.
* *Congestion:* right heart failure (pulsatile hepatomegaly if severe tricuspid regurgitation), hepatic vein thrombosis (Budd–Chiari syndrome, p686).
* *Anatomical:* Riedel's lobe—a normal variant.
* *Infection:* infectious mononucleosis, viral hepatitis, malaria, schistosomiasis, amoebic abscess, hydatid cyst.
* *Haematological:* leukaemia, lymphoma, myeloproliferative disease, sickle cell disease, haemolytic anaemia.
* *Other:* fatty liver, porphyria, amyloidosis, glycogen storage disorder.

Splenomegaly (p596). If **M**assive, think of the '**M**'s: chronic **M**yeloid leukaemia, **M**yelofibrosis, **M**alaria, leish**M**aniasis.

Hepatosplenomegaly See p596.

Spleen or enlarged kidney?

* Cannot get above a spleen (ribs overlie the upper border of the spleen).
* Spleen is dull to percussion (kidney usually resonant because of overlying bowel).
* Spleen moves towards RIF with inspiration (kidney tends to move downwards).
* Spleen may have palpable notch on its medial side.

Faecal incontinence

Affects daily activity in 1–2% of adults. Continence depends on mental function, stool volume/consistency, sphincter function, rectal distensibility, anorectal sensation, and reflexes. Defects in any can cause incontinence. Distinguish from faecal soiling.

Causes

▶▶ Consider cord compression if acute faecal incontinence.
* *Sphincter dysfunction:* sphincter tears or pudendal nerve damage, eg at vaginal delivery, surgical trauma, fissure.
* *Impaired sensation:* diabetes, MS, dementia, spinal cord lesions.
* *Faecal impaction:* overflow diarrhoea is common and treatable.
* *Idiopathic:* no clear cause found, may be multifactorial, eg poor sphincter tone plus pudendal damage.

Assessment

▶ Rectal examination: overflow incontinence? Poor tone?
▶ Neurological examination of legs, particularly checking sensation.
▶ Consider anorectal manometry, pelvic ultrasound/MRI, pudendal nerve testing.

Treat according to cause, and to promote dignity

▶▶ Urgent referral if possible cord compression.
* Find and use specialist continence services. Skin care.
* Ensure toilet is in easy reach. Plan trips in the knowledge of toilet location.
* Obey call-to-stool impulses (especially after meal: the gastro-colic reflex).
* Ensure access to continence aids and individualized advice on their use: an anal cotton plug may help isolated internal sphincter weakness.
* Pelvic floor rehabilitation can improve squeeze pressure and tolerated volume.
* There is limited evidence that drug treatments including antidiarrhoeal agents (loperamide, diphenoxylate plus atropine, codeine) and drugs to enhance anal sphincter function (phenylephrine gel, sodium valproate) work.

Dyspepsia

Dyspepsia and indigestion (p248) are broad terms. Dyspepsia is defined as one or more of: post-prandial fullness, early satiety, epigastric/retrosternal pain or burning. 'Indigestion' reported by the patient can refer to dyspepsia, bloating, nausea, or vomiting. Try to find out exactly what your patient means and when these symptoms occur in relation to meals, eg classic symptoms of peptic ulceration 2–5 hours after a meal. Check for red flag symptoms (p245). If all patients with dyspepsia undergo endoscopy, <33% have clinically significant findings. Myocardial infarction may present as 'indigestion'.

Regurgitation

Gastric and oesophageal contents are regurgitated effortlessly into the mouth without contraction of abdominal muscles and diaphragm (so distinguishing it from true vomiting). It may be worse on lying flat, and can cause cough and nocturnal asthma. Commonly associated with dyspepsia. Consider other causes if associated with nausea. Contributing pathologies: oesophageal pouch, high upper GI obstruction.

Flatulence

Normally 400–1300mL of gas is expelled PR in 8–20 discrete (or indiscrete) episodes per day. If this, with any eructation (belching) or distension, seems excessive to the patient, they may complain of flatulence. Eructation occurs in hiatus hernia, but most patients with 'flatulence' have no GI pathology. Knowledge of the chief gas may be useful: N_2 in air swallowing (aerophagy), methane if fermentation by bowel bacteria (and reducing carbohydrate intake may help).

Tenesmus

A sensation in the rectum of incomplete emptying *after* defecation. ▸▸Malignancy needs exclusion before it can be attributed to irritable bowel syndrome (p264).

Steatorrhoea

Pale stools that are difficult to flush, and are caused by malabsorption of fat in the small intestine and hence greater fat content in the stool. **Causes** Ileal disease (eg Crohn's, ileal resection), pancreatic disease, obstructive jaundice (↓excretion of bile salts from the gallbladder). **Treatment** According to cause. May be deficient in fat-soluble vitamins (A, D, E, K).

Halitosis

Halitosis (fetor oris, oral malodour) results from gingivitis (rarely severe enough to cause Vincent's angina, p698), metabolic activity of bacteria in plaque, or sulfur compound-producing bacteria (locally retained bacteria on tongue metabolize sulfur-containing amino acids to yield volatile (∴ smelly) hydrogen sulfide and methyl mercaptan). Patients can be anxious and convinced of halitosis when it is not present (and vice versa!). **Contributory factors** Smoking, drugs (disulfiram, isosorbide), lung disease, dry mouth (so eat/drink regularly). **Treatment** Dental hygiene (floss, tongue scraping), mouthwash (0.2% aqueous chlorhexidine gluconate mouthwash), or products containing metal ions (eg Zn) to inhibit odour via affinity of metal ion to sulfur.

The Famous Five

Enid Blyton's Famous Five characters can solve any crime or diagnostic problem using 1950s methodologies steeped in endless school holidays, copious confection-laden midnight feasts, and lashings of ginger beer. Let us give them the problem of abdominal distension. The sweets and drinks used by the Famous Five actually contribute to the causes of abdominal distension:

Fat   **F**luid   **F**aeces   **F**latus   **F**etus

If you think it is far-fetched to implicate ginger beer in the genesis of fetuses, note that it was home-made. Like fun, there is no limit to the intoxicating power of a home-made remedy in a long-ago vintage summer. So do not forget to ask, 'When was your last period?' in all those born female.

Symptoms
• Fever.
• Dysuria (see BOX).
• Loin pain.
• Scrotal/testicular pain: must rule out testicular torsion (p644).
• Haematuria (p289, p639).
• Urethral/vaginal discharge (p409).
• Dyspareunia (*OHCS* p137).

Past history Renal colic, UTI, diabetes, ↑BP, gout, analgesic use (p314), surgery.

Menstrual history Menarche, last menstrual period, timing of cycle, menopause, bleeding pattern, additional bleeding (intermenstrual/postcoital/postmenopausal).

Sexual history 5Ps: **P**artners, **P**ractices, **P**rotection from STI, **P**revious STI, **P**regnancy.

Drug history Anticholinergics, antibiotics.

Family history Prostate carcinoma? Kidney disease?

Dysuria

Be sure you mean the same as your patient and your colleagues.

Dysuria Typically pain derived from urethra or bladder. Consider UTI prostatitis, STI/urethritis (p409), spermicides, urethral syndrome (p292). If postmenopausal, look for a urethral caruncle: fleshy outgrowth of distal urethral mucosa, ≤1cm, typically originating from the posterior urethral lip. It may be difficult to distinguish from vaginal pain (consider vaginitis, vulvitis, or vaginal inflammation, eg from spermicides, perfumed bath products). *Rare causes*: stones, urethral lesions (eg carcinoma, lymphoma, papilloma), postpartum trauma.

Strangury Urethral pain, usually referred from the bladder base, causing a constant distressing desire to urinate even if there is little urine to void. *Causes:* bladder stone, catheter, cystitis, prostatitis, bladder neoplasia, bladder endometriosis, schistosomiasis.

Voiding difficulty A sign of obstruction to normal urine outflow. Features include poor flow, straining to void, hesitancy, intermittent stream, incontinence (overflow), urinary retention (acute or chronic), incomplete emptying (± UTI in residual urine). Ask about lower urinary tract symptoms: pain, frequency, urgency, nocturia, obstructive symptoms:
• On trying to pass water, is there delay before you start? (*Hesitancy*.)
• Do you go on dribbling after you have tried to stop? (*Terminal dribbling*.)
• Is your stream getting weaker? (*Poor stream*.)
• Is your stream painful/slow/'drop-by-drop'? (Eg from bladder stone.)
• Do you feel the bladder is not empty after passing urine?
• Do you ever pass urine when you do not want to? (*Incontinence*, p640.)
• On feeling the need to pass urine, do you have to go straight away? (*Urgency*.)
• Do you urinate often during the day? (*Frequency*.). How often?
• Do you urinate often at night? (*Nocturia*.).[2] How often?

Causes
Obstructive: prostatic hyperplasia, uterine prolapse, retroverted gravid uterus, fibroids, ovarian cyst, urethral foreign body, ectopic ureterocele, bladder polyp, bladder cancer, oedema after surgery/catheter.
Bladder overdistension: eg after epidural.
Detrusor weakness/myopathy: incomplete emptying + overflow incontinence secondary to neurological disease, eg suprapontine stroke, cord lesion, multiple sclerosis, neuropathy (spinal cord compression, diabetic neuropathy).
Drugs: epidural anaesthesia, tricyclics, anticholinergics.
Other: reflex due to pain (eg herpes infection), interstitial cystitis (*OHCS* p158).

▶Remember faecal impaction as a cause of urinary retention.

2 With advanced age, nocturia (1–2/night) may be 'normal' because of: i) loss of ability to concentrate urine; ii) peripheral oedema returns to the circulation at night; iii) circadian rhythm may be lost; iv) less sleep is needed and waking may be interpreted as a need to void (a conditioned Pavlovian response).

Irritative or obstructive bladder symptoms

Symptoms of prostate enlargement are miscalled 'prostatism' (thereby excluding other pathologies, eg bladder neck obstruction, stricture (p634)). It is better to define *irritative* or *obstructive bladder* symptoms:
• **Irritative bladder symptoms** Urgency, dysuria, frequency, nocturia.
• **Obstructive symptoms** Reduced size and force of urinary stream, hesitancy, interruption of stream during voiding, terminal dribbling. The most common cause in men is enlargement of the prostate (prostatic hyperplasia). Also urethral stricture, tumour, urethral valves, bladder neck contracture.

Polyuria and urinary frequency

Polyuria = ↑urine volume, eg >3L/24h (but consider body mass).

Causes Over-enthusiastic IV fluid therapy, diabetes mellitus & insipidus (diabetes is Greek for fountain), ↑Ca^{2+}, psychogenic polydipsia/PIP syndrome (p234), polyuric phase of recovery after acute tubular necrosis, diuretics, alcohol, renal tubular disease, adrenal insufficiency.

Differentiate polyuria from frequent passage of small amounts of urine (eg cystitis, urethritis, neurogenic bladder, bladder compression).

Oliguria/anuria
• *Oliguria* is defined as a urine output of <0.5mL/kg/h and can be a sign of reduced circulating volume, acute kidney injury, or advanced chronic kidney disease.
• *Anuria* is defined as <50mL/24h. A catheterized patient with sudden anuria has a blocked catheter until proven otherwise. Slower progression from oliguria to anuria is more likely due to kidney disease.

Urinary changes
• *Cloudy urine* can be pus (UTI) but is often normal phosphate precipitation in an alkaline urine.
• *Pneumaturia* (bubbles in urine as it is passed) occurs with UTI due to gas-forming organisms or may signal an enterovesical (bowel–bladder) fistula from diverticulitis, Crohn's disease, or neoplastic disease of the bowel.
• *Nocturia* occurs with 'irritative bladder', diabetes mellitus, UTI, and reversed diurnal rhythm (seen in renal and cardiac failure).
• Once UTI is excluded, *haematuria* is due to neoplasia or glomerulonephritis (p306) until proven otherwise.

Examination of the abdomen

Introduce yourself, obtain consent to examine, and position lying down as flat as possible, conventionally exposing from 'nipples to knees'. (In female patients delay until examining the abdomen. In practice, maximize dignity: minimize intimate exposure time needed for examination.)

1 Inspection
- General: ill/well/cachexic/in pain?
- Colour: pale, jaundiced, uraemic, tattoos, acanthosis nigricans (axilla, groin).
- The '**S**'s: **S**hape, **S**cars, **S**toma, **S**teroids (striae, Cushingoid, eg transplant/IBD).
- Ask the patient to lift their head or *cough test:* look for bulges, distension. If this causes pain, suspect peritonitis.
- Targeted inspection for:
  - *Liver disease:* jaundice, purpura, spider naevi, gynaecomastia, hair loss.
  - *Malignancy:* cachexia, mass, anaemia, jaundice.

2 Hands
- **Inspect** Clubbing (p74), *palmar erythema* (fig 2.38, p75), *Dupuytren's contracture* (fig 2.24), crease pigmentation.
- **Nails** See p75. *Leuconychia* in hypoalbuminaemia, *koilonychia* in iron/B₁₂/folate deficiency, *Muehrcke's lines* in hypoalbuminaemia, *blue lunulae* in Wilson's disease.
- **Asterixis** Negative myoclonus characterized by irregular lapse of hand posture, due to metabolic (hepatic/renal) encephalopathy (may not be a useful test in a well patient).

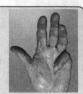
Fig 2.24 Dupuytren's contracture.

3 Arms
- Pulse (p40) and blood pressure.
- **Forearm** AV fistulae (haemodialysis access in kidney failure, p299), track marks, bruising, pigmentation, scratch marks.
- Inspect the *distribution of the SVC* (arms, upper chest, upper back) for spider naevi (fig 2.25).

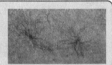
Fig 2.25 Spider naevi.

4 Neck
- Examine cervical and supraclavicular lymph nodes (fig 2.26) (*Virchow's node/Troisier's sign* = enlarged left supraclavicular node in gastric cancer).
- **JVP:** see p41. Raised in volume overload, tricuspid regurgitation (examine for pulsatile hepatomegaly).
- Scars from tunnelled haemodialysis lines (p299) or other central venous access.

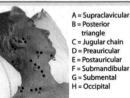

A = Supraclavicular
B = Posterior triangle
C = Jugular chain
D = Preauricular
E = Postauricular
F = Submandibular
G = Submental
H = Occipital

Fig 2.26 Cervical and supraclavicular nodes.
Reproduced from Thomas J, *et al.* (eds). *Oxford Handbook of Clinical Examination and Practical Skills* (2014), with permission from Oxford University Press.

5 Face
- **Eyes** Jaundice, conjunctival pallor, xanthelasma (PBC, chronic obstruction). *Kayser–Fleisher rings* = green-yellow ring at corneal margin in Wilson's disease.
- **Mouth** Angular stomatitis (thiamine/B₁₂/iron deficiency), pigmentation (Peutz–Jeghers syndrome, p695, fig 15.9), telangiectasia (Osler–Weber–Rendu syndrome/hereditary haemorrhagic telangiectasia, p695, fig 15.7), ulcers, glossitis, hepatic fetor.

6 Abdomen

Inspection

Scars: previous surgery, transplant, stoma. Check flanks for nephrectomy scars. *Masses:* hernias, pulsatile/expansile AAA. *Veins:* assess *direction of flow*:
• IVC obstruction = blood flows up below umbilicus.
• Portal hypertension (*caput medusae*) = flow radiates out from umbilicus.

Palpation (p563)

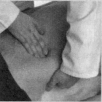

Fig 2.27 Ballottement of kidneys.
Reproduced from Thomas J, *et al.* (eds). *Oxford Handbook of Clinical Examination and Practical Skills* (2014), with permission from Oxford University Press.

Squat so patient's abdomen is at your eye level. Ask if there is pain and examine painful area last. Watch the patient's face for discomfort.

Light palpation: if pain, check for *rebound tenderness* (increased pain on removing hand = peritoneal inflammation). Any *guarding* (involuntary tensing of abdominal muscles, p598)? Rovsing's sign (appendicitis, p600), Murphy's sign (cholecystitis, p626). *Deep palpation:* to detect masses. *Liver:* starting in RIF, using radial border of index finger aligned with costal margin. Press down and ask patient to take a deep breath feeling for a liver edge. Repeat, working towards the right costal margin. Assess size (p54), texture, tenderness, pulsatility. *Scratch test:* place diaphragm of stethoscope at right costal margin, gently scratch abdominal wall, starting in RIF working towards RUQ—an increase in scratch transmission is audible at the liver border. *Spleen:* start in RIF. Press down and ask patient to take a deep breath feeling for edge of spleen. Repeat working towards the left costal margin. To help: roll the patient onto their right side to tip the spleen forward while pressing from behind. *Kidneys:* place one hand in patient's loin, pressing down on the abdomen from above and 'ballot' the kidney up with your lower hand against your upper hand (fig 2.27). *Aorta:* palpate midline above umbilicus, is it expansile (fig 2.49, p82)?

Percussion (Some percuss first, before palpation to fully exclude pain.)
• *Liver:* percuss and map upper & lower borders of liver.
• *Spleen:* percuss from border of spleen as palpated, to mid-axillary line.
• *Bladder:* if enlarged, suprapubic region will be dull.
• *Ascites:* *shifting dullness* (p596)—percuss from centre to flanks until dull, keep your finger at the dull spot and ask patient to lean onto opposite side. If the dullness is fluid, this will move with gravity and the dull area will become resonant.

Auscultation
• *Bowel sounds:* listen just below umbilicus. Absence = ileus. Enhanced and tinkling = bowel obstruction.
• *Bruits:* aorta, femoral and renal arteries (posteriorly, either side of midline, p82).

7 Complete the examination

Peripheral oedema, external genitalia, and *hernial orifices* (p604), dip *urine*.
Rectum and anus ►Have a chaperone present. Explain. Use gloves and lubricant. Ask the patient to lie on their left side, with knees up towards the chest.
Inspect: haemorrhoids, subanodermal clot, prolapsed rectum (= descent of >3cm when asked to strain), anodermatitis from soiling, gaping anus (= neuropathy/megarectum), asymmetry/tender unilateral bulge (= abscess).
Anocutaneous reflex: tests sensory and motor innervation. On lightly stroking the anal skin, does the external sphincter briefly contract?
Palpate: press index finger against the side of anus. Ask the patient to breathe in and insert finger slowly. Feel for masses (haemorrhoids are not palpable), and impacted stool. Then twist your arm so the pad of your finger is feeling anteriorly for cervix/prostate. Note consistency, size, and symmetry of prostate. Ask the patient to squeeze your finger and note the tone (best done with finger pad facing posteriorly). Note stool/blood on glove. Consider proctoscopy (anus) or sigmoidoscopy (rectum). Test for occult blood in faeces.

History From the patient, and whenever possible get a collateral history from another observer of the neurological symptoms. The patient's memory, perception, or speech may be affected by the disorder. Note the progression of symptoms and signs: gradual deterioration (eg slow-growing tumour) or intermittent exacerbations (eg multiple sclerosis) or rapid onset (eg stroke). Note if right- or left-hand dominant.

Presenting symptoms

- **Headache** See p452. Different to usual headaches? Acute/chronic? Speed of onset? Single/recurrent? Unilateral/bilateral? Associated symptoms (eg aura with migraine, p454)? Meningism (p806)? Worse on waking (may suggest ↑ICP)? Conscious level? ▶ Take a 'worst-ever' headache very seriously (p733).
- **Muscle weakness** See p462. Speed of onset? Muscle groups affected? Sensory loss? Any sphincter disturbance? Loss of balance? Associated spinal/root pain?
- **Visual disturbance** Includes blurring, double vision (diplopia), photophobia, visual loss. Speed of onset? Any preceding symptoms? Eye pain? See *oHcs* p323.
- **Other senses** Hearing (p459), smell, taste? May not be due to neurological disease: consider also ENT disease.
- **Dizziness** See p458. Illusion of surroundings moving (vertigo)? Associated hearing loss/tinnitus? Any syncope (consider cardiac disease)? Positional?
- **Speech disturbance** See p71. Difficulty in expression (expressive dysphasia), articulation (dysarthria), or comprehension (receptive dysphasia)? Sudden or gradual?
- **Dysphagia** See p246. To solids, liquids, or both? Intermittent or constant? Any associated pain (odynophagia)?
- **Fits/faints/'funny turns'/involuntary movements** See p464. A collateral history is helpful. Frequency? Duration? Mode of onset? Preceding symptoms/aura? Loss of consciousness? Tongue biting? Incontinence? Any residual weakness/confusion? Family history?
- **Abnormal sensation** Eg numbness, 'pins & needles' (paraesthesiae), pain. Distribution? Speed of onset? Associated weakness?
- **Tremor** Rapid or slow? Present at rest? Worse with deliberate movement? β-agonist use? Thyroid disease/symptoms (p29)? Fasciculation (spontaneous and involuntary muscle contraction)? Any family history?

Past medical history Meningitis/encephalitis, head/spine trauma, seizures, operations, risk factors for vascular disease (p466, AF, hypertension, hyperlipidaemia, diabetes, smoking), travel. Is there any possibility of pregnancy (eclampsia, *oHcs* p90)?

Drug history Anticonvulsant/antipsychotic/antidepressant medication? Any psychotropic/illicit drugs? Medications with known neurological side effects (eg isoniazid can cause a peripheral neuropathy)?

Social and family history What can the patient do/not do, ie activities of daily living (ADLs) and Barthel Index score? Any family history of neurological or psychiatric disease? Consanguinity? Consider sexual history, eg syphilis.

Tremor

Tremor is rhythmic oscillation of limbs, trunk, head, or tongue. Classified as:
1 **Resting tremor** Worst at rest, usually a slow tremor (frequency 3–5Hz), typically 'pill-rolling' of the thumb over a finger, eg Parkinsonism (± bradykinesia and rigidity, tremor is more resistant to treatment than other symptoms).
2 **Postural tremor** Worst if arms are outstretched. Typically rapid (8–12Hz). Includes *exaggerated physiological tremor* (eg anxiety, hyperthyroidism, alcohol, drugs), *cns pathology* (eg Wilson's disease, syphilis), *essential tremor* (autosomal dominant tremor of arms and head, cogwheeling but no bradykinesia, suppressed by alcohol, rarely progressive unless onset is unilateral. Propranolol (40–80mg/8–12h PO) may help, but not in all).
3 **Intention tremor** Worst on movement, seen in cerebellar disease, with pastpointing and dysdiadochokinesis (p495).

Cognition

If there is any concern about cognition, cognitive testing should be undertaken. The *Abbreviated Mental Test Score* (AMTS) is a commonly used screening tool based on 10 questions:

1 If the patient is able to repeat an address (eg 42 West Street), then test recall after the other questions have been completed.
2 Age?
3 Time (to nearest hour)?
4 Year?
5 Can they recognize 2 people by role (eg doctor, nurse, hospital visitor)?
6 Date of birth?
7 Dates of Second World War?[3]
8 Name of current monarch/prime minister?
9 Where are you now (which hospital)?
10 Count backwards from 20 to 1.

Score of 6 or less suggests dementia (chronic) or delirium (acute). AMTS correlates with the more detailed Mini-Mental State Examination (MMSE™, subject to strict copyright). Impaired hearing/deafness, mood disorders, and language barriers may lead to a falsely positive screen result. Other tools include the General Practitioner Assessment of Cognition (GPCOG), the Test Your Memory Test (TYM), and Six Item Cognitive Impairment Test (6-CIT).

Cramp

Painful muscle spasm. Common at night or after heavy exercise, and in patients with advanced kidney failure, including dialysis. Other possible causes include dystonia (writer's cramp, p465), salt depletion, muscle ischaemia (claudication, DM), myopathy (McArdle's, p692). Quinine bisulfate 200–300mg PO at night may be moderately effective for nocturnal cramps.

Drugs with possible causative role in cramp include diuretics (?related to ↓K⁺), domperidone, salbutamol/terbutaline IVI, ACE-i/ARB, celecoxib, lacidipine, ergot alkaloids, levothyroxine.

Paraesthesiae

'Pins and needles', numbness/tingling. Can be painful/'burn' (dysaesthesia).

Causes
• *Metabolic:* ↓Ca²⁺ (perioral), ↑P_aCO_2, hypothyroidism, neurotoxins (ask about bite/sting).
• *Vascular:* ▸▸ arterial emboli, Raynaud's, DVT, high plasma viscosity.
• *Antibody mediated:* paraneoplastic, SLE.
• *Infection:* Lyme disease, rabies.
• *Brain:* thalamic/parietal lesions.
• *Neuropathy:* MS, myelitis/HIV, ↓B₁₂, ▸▸ lumbar fracture, peripheral neuropathy (glove & stocking, eg DM, CKD, p500), cervical rib, carpal tunnel, sciatica, plexopathy/ mononeuropathy (p496). If *paroxysmal* consider migraine, epilepsy, phaeochromocytoma. If *wandering* consider infection (take travel history), eg *Strongyloides*.

Facial pain

CNS causes Migraine, trigeminal, glossopharyngeal neuralgia (p453), or from any other pain-sensitive structure in head/neck. *Post-herpetic neuralgia:* classically a burning/stabbing pain, involves dermatomal areas affected by shingles (p400), may become chronic/intractable with hyperalgesia/allodynia of affected skin.

Vascular and non-neurological causes
• Neck—cervical disc pathology.
• Bone/sinuses—sinusitis, malignancy.
• Eye—glaucoma, iritis, orbital cellulitis, eye strain, AVM.
• Temporomandibular joint—arthritis, idiopathic dysfunction (common).
• Teeth/gums—caries, broken teeth, abscess, malocclusion.
• Ear—otitis media, otitis externa.
• Vascular/vasculitis—aneurysm, AVM, giant cell arteritis, SLE.

3 The AMTS was established in 1972. A contemporary update of this question to an event within the life of patients questioned today should be considered. It needs to be a fair and multicultural test of long-term memory, not knowledge of taught history.

Neurological examination of the upper limbs

The neurological system can be daunting. Learn at the bedside. Practise. Signs may be equivocal or contrary to expectation. Always consider signs in the context of the history. Try re-examining as signs may evolve over time. An essential point is to distinguish whether a lesion is *upper (UMN)* or *lower motor neuron (LMN)* (p442).

Infection control means that the handshake is fast becoming a historical method of greeting. This is a shame, as it may have given vital diagnostic clues: unable to see hand in neglect/blindness; unable to lift hand due to weakness; difficulty reaching hand due to tremor or impaired coordination; unable to release hand in myotonia.

Position the patient comfortably, sitting up at 45° and with arms exposed.

---

1 Inspection

- Muscle wasting/atrophy: especially small muscles of the hand. Is this symmetrical/asymmetrical? Is there compensatory hypertrophy?
- Abnormal posturing/movement: fasciculation (if suspicion, try gently tapping), tremor, dystonia, athetosis. Is this localized or general?

---

2 Tone

Assesses resistance to stretch. Exclude pain in hands/arm/shoulder prior.

Ask patient to, 'Relax/go floppy like a rag-doll/let me take the weight of your arm/try not to help me'. Passively flex and extend elbow/wrist while also pronating and supinating.

Hypertonia is an increase in resistance to passive movement independent of velocity. Includes *rigidity:* resistance throughout stretch ('lead-pipe'). Rigidity plus tremor = *'cog-wheel'. Spasticity:* velocity-dependent resistance to sudden, passive movement, faster movement = stronger resistance.

---

3 Power

Direct patient to follow commands while you stabilize the joint above and resist movements in order to grade power (see BOX 'Muscle weakness grading', p443). Test left then right before moving to the next position. For myotomes, see pp448–9.

- **Shoulder abduction** 'Hold your arms out' (chicken-wing position). 'Don't let me push down' (at the elbow).
- **Elbow flexion/extension** 'Bend your arms up in front of you' (boxer-position, fist facing in). 'Stop me from pulling your arm out. Now push me away.'
- **Wrist flexion/extension** 'Make a fist, arms out straight.' Stabilize the forearm with one hand and put your other hand under their fist ('Push my hand to the ground'), then above ('Cock wrist up/stop me pushing your hand down').
- **Hand** Offer the patient two fingers and ask them to squeeze.
- **Finger abduction** 'Spread your fingers out. Stop me pushing them together.' Test like with like: your thumb versus theirs, your little finger versus theirs. 'Grip a piece of paper between two fingers.' Try to pull the paper away using the same grip.
- **Thumb abduction** 'Point your thumb (at 90°) towards the ceiling' (palm facing up). 'Don't let me push down' (with thumb, towards palm).

---

4 Reflexes

- **Biceps** c5/6. Strike your finger placed over biceps tendon in antecubital fossa.
- **Supinator** c6. Strike your fingers placed on distal radius.
- **Triceps** c7. Hold wrist on abdomen with elbow at 90°. Strike above the olecranon.

Test right, then left to compare. If absent, use 'reinforcement': ask patient to clench teeth on a count of three, at which time you strike (Jendrassik manoeuvre). Describe as absent, hyporeflexia (present only with reinforcement), normal, or brisk/hyperreflexia.

5 Coordination

- **Pronator drift** With arms outstretched (palms up), ask patient to close their eyes and watch for maintained supination.
- **Finger–nose test** Hold your finger an arm's length in front of patient. 'Touch your nose, then my finger. As fast as you can.' Look for *intention tremor* and *past pointing*.
- **Dysdiadochokinesis** Ask patient to touch palms together (pronation of forearm), then turn hand so dorsal side contacts palm (supination of forearm). Ask them to repeatedly pronate and supinate forearm. Failure to perform rapidly alternating movements is dysdiadochokinesis.

6 Sensation

Ask the patient to close their eyes while stimuli are applied. Test in all dermatomes (**fig 2.28** and p450), comparing left with right. Alter the rate of touch so it is not predictable.

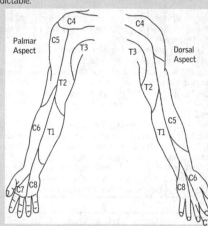

Fig 2.28 Sensory dermatomes of upper limb.
Reproduced from Harrison (ed) *Revision Notes for MCEM Part A*
(2011), with permission from Oxford University Press.

- **Light touch** Use cotton wool. Touch/dab (don't stroke or tickle) manubrium first. 'This is what it should feel like. Say, "Yes" if you feel it again on your arm. Does it feel the same or different?'
- **Pain (pin-prick)** Repeat using a neurological pin (not hypodermic needle), asking patient to tell you if it feels sharp. Allow pin to slide between your fingers—do not apply pressure.
- **Temperature** Repeat using alternating hot and cold probes (a tuning fork or testtube are also cold). Can the patient tell hot from cold?
- **Vibration** Use a 128Hz tuning fork. Confirm the patient can feel buzzing at a reference point (vertex of head/manubrium). Test for the start and end of vibration sensation (to distinguish from pressure, stop it with your fingers) at most distal bony prominence. Move proximally to next most distal bony prominence until vibration is correctly identified.
- **Proprioception** With the patient's eyes closed, hold the distal phalanx of the big finger at the sides, not on top/below. Flex and extend the joint explaining, 'This is up', and, 'This is down'. Repeat movements stopping at intervals to ask whether the fingertip is up or down. If impaired, test at the next most distal joint.

Top tips

- Use the tendon hammer like a pendulum, let it drop, don't grip it too tightly.
- Ensure you are testing light touch, not stroke sensation.

If the patient is able, begin your examination with gait analysis. Gait analysis (p463) may give more clinical information than any other test. If they aren't able to walk, start with them lying down, legs fully exposed.

1 Gait and inspection

Gait Ask patient to walk a few metres, turn, and walk back to you. Note walking aids, symmetry, size of paces, arm swing. Look for abnormalities of gait cycle (eg abnormalities in toe-off or heel-strike). Ask patient to 'walk heel-to-toe as if on a tightrope' to exaggerate instability. Ask patient to walk on tiptoes (s1 or gastrocnemius lesion), then on heels (L4,5 lesion, foot drop). Range of movement may be reduced by joint pathology. Exclude pain (*antalgic gait*) before you diagnose weakness. Unequal wear on the sole of the shoe may suggest an abnormal gait.

* *Trendelenburg gait:* unilateral weakness of hip abductor, eg superior gluteal nerve/L5 lesion.
* *Waddling/myopathic gait:* inability to stabilize pelvis due to bilateral hip abductor weakness (eg muscular dystrophy). Pelvis tilts to non-weight-bearing leg with each step leading to a waddle.
* *Hemiplegic (diplegic) gait:* foot (feet) in extension (UMN lesion) need to be circumverted/swung round to move forward.
* *Neuropathic gait:* weak foot dorsiflexion leads to a high step to avoid toe drag.
* *Parkinsonian gait:* slow initiation, stooped posture, small and shuffling steps, turning 'en bloc' (head, trunk, and pelvis turn together like a statue).
* *Choreiform gait:* irregular, jerky, involuntary movements in arms and legs (eg basal ganglia disorder).
* *Ataxic gait:* wide-based irregular steps, lateral veering/falling, truncal instability.

Romberg's test Ask patient to stand unaided with arms by sides and close their eyes (be ready to support). If they sway/lose balance the test is positive and indicates posterior column disease (proprioception-related disease).

Inspect Abnormal posturing, muscle wasting, fasciculation, deformities of the foot, eg pes cavus (Friedreich's ataxia, Charcot–Marie–Tooth disease). Is one leg smaller than the other (old polio, infantile hemiplegia)?

2 Tone

Assesses resistance to stretch. Exclude pain prior. Ask patient to, 'Relax/go floppy like a rag-doll/let me take the weight of your leg/try not to help me'. Roll knee from side to side to passively internally/externally rotate leg. Put your hand behind the knee and raise it quickly. If the heel lifts away from the bed, tone is increased.

Clonus Plantar-flex foot then quickly dorsiflex and hold. More than 3 'beats' of plantar flexion is abnormal. Rapid downward movement of patella may elicit patella clonus. Hypertonia and clonus suggest an UMN lesion.

3 Power

Direct patient to follow commands while you resist movements in order to grade power (see box 'Muscle weakness grading', p443). Test left then right before moving to the next position. For myotomes see pp450–1.

* **Hip flexion/extension** 'Keep your leg straight and lift it up. Don't let me push it down.' Then position hand under thigh. 'Now push my hand into the bed.'
* **Hip abduction** Position hands on outer thigh: 'Push your leg out to the side.'
* **Hip adduction** Position hand on inner thighs: 'Push your legs together.'
* **Knee flexion/extension** 'Bend your knee and bring your heel to your bottom. Don't let me pull it away.' 'Now kick out/push me away.'
* **Ankle plantar flexion** Position hand on sole of foot. 'Push your foot down/push my hand.'
* **Ankle dorsiflexion** Position hand on dorsum of foot. 'Lift your foot so your toes point to the ceiling. Don't let me push your foot down.'

4 Reflexes

Test right, then left to compare.
- **Knee** L3,4. Bend knee, take weight of leg. Strike patella tendon, just below patella.
- **Ankle** L5, s1. Bend knee, then move it laterally. Hold and dorsiflex the foot, then strike the Achilles tendon. If hip pain or limited mobility, dorsiflex the foot with a straight leg and position hand on sole. Strike your hand, feeling for an ankle jerk.
- **Plantar reflexes** L5, s1, s2. Run an orange stick up the lateral sole of the foot in the direction of the big toe. As you approach the base of the toes move medially. Plantar flexion of the great toe is normal. Dorsiflexion (positive *Babinski sign*) is abnormal (in adults).

5 Coordination

Heel–shin test Using your finger on the patient's shin to demonstrate, instruct patient to, 'Put your (left/right) heel just below your (right/left) knee. Run your heel smoothly down your shin. Lift it up and place it back on your knee. Now run it down again.'
Foot tap test Place your palms just below the patient's feet. Ask them to tap your palms with their left foot only, right foot only, both feet together, and both feet interchangeably.

6 Sensation

Ask the patient to close their eyes while stimuli are applied. Test in all dermatomes (**fig 2.29** and **p450**), comparing left with right. Alter the rate of touch so it is not predictable.

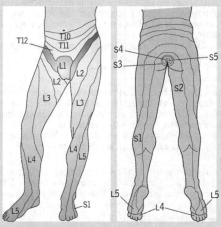

Fig 2.29 Sensory dermatomes of lower limb.
Reproduced from Harrison (ed) *Revision Notes for MCEM Part A* (2011), with permission from Oxford University Press.

- **Light touch** As upper limbs (**p63**).
- **Pain (pin-prick)** As upper limbs (**p63**).
- **Temperature** As upper limbs (**p63**).
- **Vibration** As upper limbs (**p63**).
- **Joint position sense** With the patient's eyes closed, hold the distal phalanx of the big toe at the sides, not on top/below. Flex and extend the joint explaining, 'This is up', and, 'This is down'. Repeat movements stopping at intervals to ask whether the toe tip is up or down. If impaired, test at the next most distal joint.

Top tips
- If you are limited for time, gait is the most useful test to start with.
- Make sure you test each muscle group individually by stabilizing above the joint you are testing.

2 History and examination

I Olfactory nerve
Ask if they have noticed a change in sense of taste/smell. Test familiar smells, eg coffee at each nostril (test nostrils separately, exclude occlusion of the nostril).

II Optic nerve
- **Acuity** Test each eye separately. Correction with glasses/pin-hole. Use Snellen chart (inside front cover).
- **Visual fields** Compare with yours (confrontation): ask the patient to look at your eye/nose and ask them to indicate when they see finger movement (or count your fingers) in each outer quadrant of the visual field. Or test formally via perimetry.
- **Pupils** Size, shape, symmetry. Reaction to light (fig 2.30) should be direct (pupil responds to light) and consensual (opposite pupil responds). Swinging light test for *relative afferent pupillary defect* detects asymmetrical disease: light shone into the normal eye causes bilateral pupillary constriction. When light is moved to the abnormal eye, both pupils paradoxically dilate as consensual pupillary relaxation in the normal eye dominates. *Accommodation:* ask the patient to focus on your finger/pen at arm's length, then move it towards their nose. Pupils constrict on near gaze.
- **Ophthalmoscopy** Darken the room. Warn the patient you need to get close to their face. Optic disc (pale? swollen?). Follow vessels from disc to view each quadrant. If the view is obscured, look for a cataract. View the fovea by asking the patient to look directly at the light. See *OHCS* p327. ►Slit lamp examination is superior.

III Oculomotor nerve, IV Trochlear nerve, VI Abducens nerve
Gently stabilize the patient's head. Ask them to look at your finger as you trace a 'H-shape'. *Nystagmus* is an involuntary, repetitive, to–fro movement of the eyes. A few beats of nystagmus may be physiological, especially at extremes of gaze.
- **III*rd nerve palsy:*** eye looks down and out. Ptosis, large pupil if external parasympathetic fibres compressed/damaged.
- **IV*th nerve palsy:*** diplopia on looking down and in (often noticed on descending stairs), head tilt (ocular torticollis) compensates.
- **VI*th nerve palsy:*** impaired lateral movement/lateral diplopia.

V Trigeminal nerve
- **Sensory** Check sensation (usually light touch) in all three divisions of the nerve (ophthalmic = forehead, mandibular = cheek, mandibular = jaw). Corneal reflex may be lost first: approach the eye from the side (outside line of vision) and lightly touch a thin strand of clean cotton to the cornea. Observe for blinking and tearing.
- **Motor** 'Open your mouth' and jaw deviates to the side of lesion. Palpate muscles of mastication (temporalis, masseter, pterygoids) as patient clenches teeth.

VII Facial nerve
'Raise your eyebrows', 'Close your eyes tightly', 'Show me your teeth', 'Puff out your cheeks'. Weakness leads to facial droop. UMN lesions affect the lower two-thirds of the face (cortical innervation to upper face is bilateral). LMN lesions affect all of one side of face. Test taste (anterior two-thirds of tongue) with salt/sweet solutions.

VIII Vestibulocochlear nerve
Test hearing: ask to repeat a number whispered in each ear while you block the other. *Balance/vertigo* (p458). Weber's and Rinne's tests (p459).

IX Glossopharyngeal nerve, X Vagus nerve
The palate should move symmetrically on saying 'Ah'. 10th nerve lesions cause paralysis of the palate. The asymmetric lift of the uvula means that it will point away from the lesion, towards the normal side. *Gag reflex:* gently touch the back of the soft palate with an orange stick. The afferent arm of the reflex involves IX; the efferent arm involves X.

XI Accessory nerve
'Shrug your shoulders' against resistance. 'Turn your head' against resistance.

XII Hypoglossal nerve
'Stick out your tongue.' The tongue deviates to the side of the lesion.

Causes of cranial nerve lesions

Where is the lesion? Think systematically: in brainstem (eg MS), pressing on the brainstem (eg tumour), at the neuromuscular junction (eg myasthenia), or in the muscles (eg a dystrophy)? Cranial nerves may be affected singly or in groups. Any cranial nerve may be affected by DM, stroke, MS, cancer, sarcoidosis, vasculitis (p552), SLE (p552), syphilis. Chronic meningitis (malignant, TB, or fungal) can pick off the lower cranial nerves one by one. Causes of cranial nerve lesions include:

- *I* Trauma, respiratory tract infection, meningitis, frontal lobe tumour.
- *II* (Also see p66.) *Monocular blindness:* lesions of one eye/optic nerve, eg MS, giant cell arteritis. *Bilateral blindness:* any cause of multifocal neuropathy/mononeuritis multiplex, eg DM, MS, neurosyphilis, rarely methanol. *Bitemporal hemianopia:* compression of optic chiasm, eg pituitary adenoma, craniopharyngioma, internal carotid artery aneurysm (fig 10.3, p447). *Homonymous hemianopia* (affects half the visual field, contralateral to the lesion) due to lesions beyond the chiasm, eg stroke, abscess, tumour. *Optic neuritis* causes pain on moving eye, loss of central vision, relative afferent papillary defect, disc swelling (papillitis) due to, eg MS, syphilis, collagen vascular disorders. *Ischaemic papillopathy:* (swelling of optic disc due to stenosis of the posterior ciliary artery) due to, eg giant cell arteritis. *Papilloedema* (fig 12.21, p558) most commonly due to ↑ICP (tumour, abscess, encephalitis, hydrocephalus, idiopathic intracranial hypertension); rarer is a retro-orbital lesion (eg cavernous sinus thrombosis, p478). *Optic atrophy:* MS, frontal tumours, Friedreich's ataxia, retinitis pigmentosa, syphilis, glaucoma, Leber's optic atrophy, chronic optic nerve compression. *Nystagmus:* horizontal nystagmus often vestibular (acute = nystagmus away from lesion, chronic = towards lesion), or cerebellar (nystagmus towards the affected side). Nystagmus in abduction: consider internuclear ophthalmoplegia (p69, fig 2.31). Nystagmus plus deafness/tinnitus: VIIIth nerve lesion, barotrauma, Ménière's (p458). Variable nystagmus with head position: benign positional vertigo (p458). Upbeat nystagmus: lesion in midbrain/base of the 4th ventricle. Downbeat nystagmus: foramen magnum lesion. *Pupil abnormalities:* see p68.
- *III* Pupil sparing = parasympathetic fibres unaffected ('medical'), eg DM, giant cell arteritis, syphilis. With dilated pupil = external compression of parasympathetic fibres ('surgical'): ↑ICP (uncal herniation through the tentorium), eg space-occupying lesion, posterior communicating artery aneurysm (p814).
- *IV* Usually due to trauma when occurs in isolation.
- *V* Trigeminal neuralgia (p453), herpes zoster, nasopharyngeal cancer, acoustic neuroma (p459).
- *VI* MS, Wernicke's encephalopathy, false localizing sign in ↑ICP, pontine stroke (fixed small pupils ± quadriparesis).
- *VII LMN* Bell's palsy (p498), Ramsay Hunt syndrome (p499, OHCS p856), polio, otitis media, skull fracture, cerebellopontine angle tumour, eg acoustic neuroma, malignant parotid tumour. *UMN* CVA, tumour.
- *VIII* (p458, p459) Noise damage, Paget's disease, Ménière's disease, herpes zoster, acoustic neuroma, brainstem CVA, drugs (eg aminoglycosides).
- *IX, X, XI* Trauma, brainstem lesions, neck tumours.
- *XII* Syringomyelia, tumour, stroke, bulbar palsy, trauma, TB, polio.

Groups of cranial nerves

- *VIII, then V, VI, IX, and X:* cerebellopontine angle pathology, eg acoustic neuroma.
- *III, IV, V (ophthalmic division), VI:* cavernous sinus pathology, eg thrombosis, superior orbital fissure lesion (Tolosa–Hunt syndrome, OHCS p858).
- *IX, X, XI:* jugular foramen lesion.
- *ΔΔ:* myasthenia gravis, muscular dystrophy, myotonic dystrophy, mononeuritis multiplex (p496).

Top tips

- Partial visual field loss is due to neurological disease. Monocular/binocular blindness is most commonly a disease of the eye, eg cataracts, retinopathy.
- Papillitis = unilateral optic disc swelling. Papilloedema = bilateral. Check both eyes!

Pupillary abnormalities
• Symmetry: equal and circular?
• Dilated or constricted?
• React to light, directly and consensually?
• Constrict normally on convergence/accommodation?

Irregular pupils
Anterior uveitis (iritis), trauma, syphilis.

Dilated pupils
Confirm pathological dilatation (not pathological constriction in the other eye). Dilated pupil occurs with external compression of CNIII (parasympathetic fibres) due to: ↑ICP (p814) (uncal herniation through the tentorium), space-occupying lesion, posterior communicating artery aneurysm. Also mydriatic drugs.

Constricted pupils
Sympathetic nerve damage (Horner's, p48, and ptosis, p69), opiates, miotics (pilocarpine drops for glaucoma), pontine damage.

Unequal pupils (anisocoria)
Unilateral lesion, mydriatic/miotic medication, eye surgery, syphilis, Holmes–Adie pupil. Some inequality may be normal.

Light reaction
Both pupils should constrict, one by a direct and the other by a consensual light reflex (fig 2.30). The lesion site is deduced by knowing the pathway: from the retina the message passes up the optic nerve (CNII) to the superior colliculus (midbrain) and thence to the CNIII nuclei on both sides producing pupillary constriction. If a light in one eye causes only contralateral constriction, the defect is 'efferent', as the afferent pathways from the retina being stimulated must be intact = *Marcus Gunn sign.*

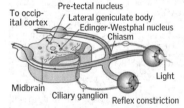

Fig 2.30 Light reflex. Action potentials go along the optic nerve (red), traverse the optic chiasm, pass synapses at the pre-tectal nucleus, en route to Edinger–Westphal nuclei of CNIII. These send fibres to *both* irises' ciliary muscles (so *both* pupils constrict) via *ciliary ganglion* (also relays accommodation and corneal sensation, and gets sympathetic roots from C8–T2, carrying fibres to dilate pupil).

Holmes–Adie (myotonic) pupil
The affected pupil is moderately dilated and poorly/non-reactive to light. It is slowly reactive to accommodation; wait and watch: it may eventually constrict more than a normal pupil. It is often associated with diminished or absent ankle and knee reflexes, in which case the *Holmes–Adie syndrome* is present. Usually a benign incidental finding. Rare causes: Lyme disease, syphilis, parvovirus B19, HSV, autoimmunity.

Argyll Robertson pupil
The pupil is constricted and unreactive to light, but reacts to accommodation. Occurs in late neurosyphilis. Hypothesized due to rostral midbrain pathology affecting efferent pupillary fibres on the dorsal aspect of the Edinger–Westphal nucleus (part of the light reflex) while sparing more ventral fibres associated with the accommodation. Mimicked (pseudo-Argyll Robertson pupil) by: Lyme disease, HIV, zoster, DM, sarcoidosis, MS, paraneoplastic, ↓B12, Parinaud's syndrome (pupillary hyporeflexia, impaired upward gaze, convergence retraction nystagmus, p694).

Hutchinson pupil
This is the sequence of events resulting from rapidly rising unilateral intracranial pressure (eg intracerebral haemorrhage). The pupil on the side of the lesion first constricts then widely dilates. The other pupil then goes through the same sequence ►See p814.

Ptosis

Drooping of the upper eyelid. Best observed with patient sitting up. **Causes**

1 CNIII lesions. Oculomotor nerve (CNIII) innervates main muscle concerned (levator palpebrae). Lesions therefore cause *unilateral complete* ptosis. Look for other evidence of a CNIII lesion: ophthalmoplegia with 'down and out' deviation of the eye, dilated pupil unreactive to light or accommodation. If eye pain, suspect infiltration (eg lymphoma, sarcoidosis). If ↑T° or ↓consciousness, suspect infection (tick bite?).

2 Sympathetic lesions. Nerves from the cervical sympathetic chain innervate the superior tarsal muscle with lesions leading to a milder ptosis. Usually *unilateral partial* ptosis, which may be overcome by looking up. *Horner's syndrome* (fig 2.18, p48) = ptosis + miosis (constricted pupil), + anhidrosis (lack of sweating), + enophthalmos (sinking of eye). Causes: usually malignancy/trauma along nerve path, ie midbrain, brainstem, upper spinal cord, neck, lung apex (Pancoast's tumour), orbit.

3 Myopathy, eg dystrophia myotonica, myasthenia gravis. Usually *bilateral partial* ptosis.

4 Congenital. Usually partial and without other CNS signs.

Internuclear ophthalmoplegia

To produce synchronous eye movements, cranial nerves III, IV, and VI communicate through the medial longitudinal fasciculus in midbrain (fig 2.31). In internuclear ophthalmoplegia a lesion disrupts communication causing:

• Weakness of the ipsilateral eye in adduction.

• Nystagmus of the contralateral eye in abduction.

There may be incomplete or slow abduction of the ipsilateral eye during lateral gaze. Convergence is preserved.

Causes MS, vascular. Rare: HIV, syphilis, Lyme disease, brainstem tumour, phenothiazine toxicity.

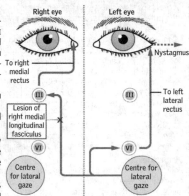

Fig 2.31 Internuclear ophthalmoplegia.

Visual loss

▶Get ophthalmology help. See *OHCS* pp344–63.

Consider:

• Red eye: *glaucoma, uveitis* (p559).

• Pain: *giant cell arteritis*—temporal headache, jaw claudication, scalp tenderness, ↑ESR ▶urgent steroids (p554). Also *optic neuritis*, eg MS.

• Cloudy cornea: *corneal ulcer* (*OHCS* p334), *glaucoma* (*OHCS* p331).

• Flashes/floaters: *TIA, migraine, retinal detachment*.

• Visual field defect: *cerebrovascular disease, space-occupying lesion, glaucoma, emboli* (examine for valvular heart disease/carotid bruit).

• Relevant history: *trauma, migraine, hypertension, MS, diabetes, connective tissue disease, hyperlipidaemia.*

• Systemic disease: *HIV retinitis, SLE, sarcoidosis.*

Sudden Acute glaucoma, retinal detachment, vitreous haemorrhage (eg proliferative DM retinopathy), central retinal artery/vein occlusion, optic neuritis (eg MS), migraine, CNS lesions (eg TIA (amaurosis fugax), stroke, space-occupying lesion), temporal arteritis, drugs (eg quinine/methanol), pituitary apoplexy.

Gradual Optic atrophy, chronic glaucoma, cataracts, macular degeneration, toxic amblyopia.

Higher mental functions include language, memory, thinking, attention, abstraction, and perception. In order to assess:
- Reassure: 'I know this may be difficult...'
- Engage in conversation. Ask open questions that require more than yes or no to answer. This tests fluency, reception, understanding, and allows assessment of articulation.
- Assess for dysphasia: 'What is this?' while pointing to, eg pen (nominal dysphasia).
- Test for conduction dysphasia and dysarthria: Ask patient to repeat complex words, eg 'British constitution', 'baby hippopotamus'.
- Assess movement (and comprehension) using complex instructions that require movement across the midline, eg 'Make a fist with your right hand, then extend your right index finger, then touch your left ear'.

Assessment will be affected by hearing loss, visual loss, and cognitive impairment.

Movement

Movement disorders
- ***Athetosis:*** slow sinuous writhing movements, present at rest. Due to a lesion in the putamen. ***Pseudoathetosis:*** athetoid movements due to severe proprioceptive loss.
- ***Chorea:*** a flow of jerky movements, flitting from one limb to another (each seemingly a fragment of a normal movement). Meaning = *dance* (hence 'choreography'). The early stages of chorea may be detected by feeling fluctuations in muscle tension while the patient grips your finger. Causes: basal ganglia lesion (stroke, Huntington's p464); Sydenham's chorea (St Vitus' dance) (p146); SLE (p552); Wilson's disease (p281); neonatal kernicterus; polycythaemia (p362); neuroacanthocytosis (acanthocytes in peripheral blood, chorea, orofacial dyskinesia, axonal neuropathy); hyperthyroidism (p212); drugs (levodopa, oral contraceptives/HRT, chlorpromazine, cocaine—'*crack dancing*'). See p464.
- ***Hemiballismus:*** uncontrolled unilateral flailing movements of proximal limb joints. Due to contralateral subthalamic lesions (p464).

Dyspraxia
Poor performance of complex movements despite ability to do each individual component. Test by asking the patient to copy unfamiliar hand positions, or mime an object's use, eg a comb.
- ***Dressing dyspraxia:*** the patient is unsure of the orientation of clothes. Test by pulling the sleeve of a sweater inside-out before asking the patient to put it on (mostly non-dominant hemisphere lesions).
- ***Constructional dyspraxia:*** difficulty in assembling or drawing objects, eg a five-pointed star (non-dominant hemisphere lesions, hepatic encephalopathy).
- ***Gait dyspraxia:*** difficulty performing the complex movement of walking (bilateral frontal lesions, posterior temporal region lesions, and hydrocephalus).

Cerebellar disease
Think **DASHING**:

Dysdiadochokinesis	**A**taxia	**S**lurred speech
Hypotonia and reduced power	**I**ntention tremor	**N**ystagmus
Gait: broad based		

Examination:
Speech: slurred/ataxic/staccato.
Eye movements: nystagmus.
Tone and power: hypotonia and reduced power.
Coordination: coordination tests for dysdiadochokinesis (p63, p65, p495).
Gait: broad based, patients fall to the side of the lesion. Romberg's test is negative.

Dysphasia

A disorder that affects the ability to produce and understand spoken language.
►It is one of the most debilitating neurological conditions, especially when cognitive function is intact.

Assessment

Dysphasia is unlikely when speech is fluent, grammatically correct, and meaningful.
1 *Comprehension:* test capacity to follow one-, two-, and several-step commands, eg 'Touch your ear, stand up, then close the door'.
2 *Articulation:* test repetition of complex words/phrases, eg 'British constitution', 'No ifs, ands, or buts', 'baby hippopotamus'.
3 *Naming:* test ability to name common and uncommon things, eg parts of a watch/clock/pen.
4 *Reading and writing:* usually affected like speech in dysphasia. If normal, consider other pathology, eg psychogenic, developmental. Remember to check hearing.

Classification (See box 'Problems with classifying dysphasias'.)

* *Broca's (expressive) anterior dysphasia:* non-fluent speech, effort and frustration with malformed words (eg 'spoot' for 'spoon'), or impaired recall of words (eg 'That thing'). Comprehension is relatively intact: patients understand questions and attempt to convey meaningful answers. *Site of lesion:* inferolateral dominant frontal lobe.
* *Wernicke's (receptive) posterior dysphasia:* empty, fluent speech with phonemic ('flush' for 'brush') and semantic ('comb' for 'brush') paraphasias/neologisms. May be mistaken for psychotic speech. The patient is unaware of errors. Comprehension may be impaired. *Site of lesion:* posterior superior dominant temporal lobe.
* *Conduction aphasia:* repetition is impaired, comprehension and fluency less so. *Site of lesion:* communication between Broca's and Wernicke's areas.
* *Nominal dysphasia:* objects cannot be named but other aspects of speech are normal. *Site of lesion:* posterior dominant temporoparietal lesions.

►Mixed dysphasia is common. Discriminating features may take time to emerge after acute brain injury. Speech therapy is offered, though it may not help.

Problems with classifying dysphasias

The classical model of language comprehension occurring in Wernicke's area and language expression in Broca's area is too simple. Functional MRI studies defy simplistic teaching that the processing of abstract words is confined to the left hemisphere and concrete words are processed on the right. Consider instead a mosaic of language centres in the brain with more and less specialized functions. There is evidence that tool-naming is handled differently and in a different area to fruit-naming. There is also inter-individual variation in the anatomy of these mosaics. This is depressing for those who want a rigid classification of dysphasia, but a source of hope to those who have had a stroke: recovery may be better than teaching and non-functional imaging lead us to believe.

Dysarthria

Difficulty with articulation due to incoordination/weakness of muscles needed for speech. Language is normal. Detected with assessment of articulation. Causes:
* **Cerebellar disease** Ataxic speech muscles lead to slurring (as if drunk). Speech may be irregular in volume and staccato in quality.
* **Extrapyramidal disease** Soft, indistinct, monotonous speech.
* **Bulbar palsy** LMN lesion causing palatal weakness (eg CNIX/X lesion; Guillain–Barré; MND, p502). Speech may have a nasal character.
* **Pseudobulbar palsy** UMN lesion causes spastic dysarthria: slow, indistinct, nasal, effortful speech (eg MND, p502; MS). A 'hot potato voice' occurs with bilateral lesions.

Dysphonia

Weakness of respiratory muscles and/or vocal cords (eg myasthenia, p508; Guillain–Barré, p500) leads to abnormal voice/volume. It may be precipitated in myasthenia by counting to 100. Parkinson's disease can produce a mix of dysarthria and dysphonia.

▶Psychiatric symptoms reflect dysfunction of the brain.
▶Just because a presentation is odd does not mean it is psychiatric.
▶Physical, neurological, and cognitive examination are needed before a psychiatric diagnosis is made.
▶If psychiatric symptoms are due to medical/neurological conditions there may be other evidence of nervous system dysfunction, eg dysarthria (p71), language disturbance (p71), altered gait (p64), sensory deficit.
▶If rapid onset, altered conscious level and/or fluctuating presentation consider delirium.

Psychiatric symptoms
▶Consider all symptoms in their cultural and religious context.
• *Negative symptoms:* the absence of a behaviour, thought, feeling, or sensation, eg lack of appetite, apathy, blunted emotion.
• *Positive symptoms:* the presence of symptoms that are not normally expected, eg hallucinations.

Mood
• Lost of interest/pleasure (*anhedonia*) in usual activities, feeling sad, hopeless, decreased energy, social withdrawal.
• *Anxiety*.
• *Mania:* non-contextualized elevated mood and/or disinhibition. Hypomania: milder than mania.
▶Always ask, 'Have you ever felt so low that you thought of harming yourself?'

Sensory
• *Hallucinations:* 'Have you ever heard voices or seen things when there hasn't been anyone or anything there?'

Thoughts
• *Delusion:* a fixed, false, idiosyncratic belief. 'What thoughts have you had?', 'Have you ever had any thoughts or beliefs that have struck you afterwards as strange?'
• *Thought insertion:* delusion that thoughts belong to someone else and have been inserted.
• *Thought broadcasting:* delusion that thoughts are heard or known by others.
• *Obsessions:* repeated unwanted/unpleasant thoughts that cause anxiety, disgust, or unease.
• *Flight of ideas:* speech races through themes, switching whimsically or through associations, eg 'clang' association: 'Yesterday I went to the shop. I didn't hop (*clang*), but I walked. Kangaroos hop, don't they? My friend Joey wasn't there.'
• *Knight's move:* an unexpected change in the direction of thinking (akin to the lateral component of the move of the knight's piece in chess).

Language
• *Pressure of speech:* rapid and frenzied speech, inappropriate to the situation.
• *Neologism* (new words), *echolalia* (repeating others' words), *paralalia* (repetition of own words).

Behaviour
• Avoidance: due to anxiety/phobia.
• Compulsions: performing an action persistently and repetitively.
• Eating disorders.
• Altered sleep.
• Distractibility.
• Increased goal-directed activity.
• Excessive involvement in risky activity. Alcohol/drug misuse (p276).

Somatic
Physical symptoms for which no physiological basis can be found. Include: fatigue, dizziness, insomnia, reduced appetite, weight loss, breathlessness, chest pain, headache, nausea, abdominal/muscular pain.

Mental state examination

Tips
- Explain the reason for meeting. Help to make the patient feel comfortable.
- Respect concerns and distress.
- Take into account culture, ethnicity, language, and comprehension.
- Consider whether physical health is impacting mental health, particularly pain and cognition.
- Write down the patient's exact words including the order in which they are expressed. This may be important for diagnosis.

Aims
- To achieve a snapshot of thoughts and behaviour at the time of examination.
- Identify the presence and severity of mental health conditions.
- Identify risk to self and to others.

Appearance
- Is dress appropriate for the setting?
- Do clothes reflect mood, ie bright/dark?
- Is personal hygiene maintained?
- Signs of possible withdrawal: tremor, agitation, perspiration.
- Signs of neurological disease: ataxia, dysarthria, motor asymmetry.

Behaviour
An examination of non-verbal communication. Avoid stigmatization and pejorative terminology.
- *Attitude:* cooperative, defensive, hostile, apathetic, distracted, agitated, anxious.
- *Eye contact:* able to maintain or not? Appropriate?
- *Facial expression:* expressive, relaxed, smiling/laughing, sad, distrustful, slow.
- *Mannerisms:* repetition, compulsions, rituals.
- *Psychomotor activity:* pacing, tremors, foot tapping, psychomotor slowing, pauses. If taking antipsychotic medication, observe for possible *extrapyramidal side effects:* oro-buccal dyskinesia, tremor, choreiform movements, dystonia.
- *Arousal:* level of attention/distraction. Signs of hyperarousal, delirium?
- *Disinhibited behaviour:* a disregard of social conventions affecting emotion, cognition, or motor function/response.
- *Engagement and rapport:* a key component of the examination. Note if rapport established, if easy, easier over time, tenuous, poor, or difficult.

Speech
- *Quantity:* spontaneous, talkative, expansive, paucity/poverty.
- *Rate:* rapid/pressure (mania), slow (depression, negative symptom in psychosis).
- *Flow and route:* tangential (mania), circumstantial (anxiety/obsession).
- *Specific pathology:* neologism, echolalia, paralalia (p72).

Mood (Sustained emotional state.); Affect (Expression of emotion, may fluctuate.)
- Assess subjective and objective: elated, euthymic, dysthymic, depressed, anxious. Fluctuation, range, and congruence.

Thoughts
- *Stream:* pressure/poverty, blocking of thoughts.
- *Form:* logical? Linked or tangential?
- *Possession:* insertion/withdrawal/broadcasting (p72).
- *Content:* delusions (eg persecutory, grandiose), obsession, phobia.
- ▶Suicidal ideation, self-harm, plans to violence/harm/abscond.

Perception
- Hallucination (visual/auditory).
- *Phenomenology:* the patient's perception and understanding of thoughts/phenomena.

Cognition
- Attention, memory, alertness, functioning (p61).

Insight
- Do they recognize their symptoms?
- Are they willing to work with healthcare professionals on treatment/recovery?

2 History and examination

The hands can give you a wealth of diagnostic information:
• Thyroid disease: warm, sweaty, tremor.
• Heart/lung disease: cold, cyanosis.
• Neurological disease: difficulty relaxing grip in myotonia, weak grip in myopathy/peripheral neuropathy.

Clubbing

Clubbed fingernails (± toenails) have:
• Soft tissue swelling of the terminal phalanx.
• Increased curvature in all directions.
• Loss of angle between nail and nail fold (figs 2.32, 2.33).

Hypothesized pathogenesis:
1 Disruption to normal pulmonary circulation means that megakaryocytes, which are usually fragmented in the lung, enter the systemic circulation.
2 Megakaryocytes become lodged in the capillaries of the fingers and toes, releasing platelet-derived growth factor (PDGF) and vascular endothelial growth factor (VEGF). Release of PDGF and VEGF may also be enhanced by hypoxia.
3 Other hypothesized pathogenic signalling proteins include prostaglandins, bradykinin, ferritin, adenosine nucleotides, interleukin-6, von Willebrand factor, serum transforming growth factor-β1, tumour necrosis factor, and epidermal growth factor. These are altered by disruption to production/metabolism, eg in the liver/bowel.
4 An altered growth factor/signalling profile leads to increased vascularity, permeability, and connective tissue damage.

Unilateral clubbing remains unexplained.

Causes

Respiratory
• Bronchial cancer (women>men), usually *not* small cell cancer.
• Chronic lung suppuration: empyema, abscess, bronchiectasis, cystic fibrosis.
• Fibrosing alveolitis.
• Mesothelioma.
• TB.

Gastrointestinal
• Inflammatory bowel disease.
• Cirrhosis.
• GI lymphoma.
• Malabsorption, eg coeliac disease.

Cardiovascular
• Cyanotic congenital heart disease.
• Endocarditis.
• Atrial myxoma.
• Aneurysms.
• Infected grafts.

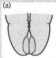

Fig 2.32 Finger clubbing.

Rare
• Familial.
• Thyroid acropachy (p560).

Unilateral clubbing
• Hemiplegia.
• Vascular lesions:
    • Upper limb artery aneurysm.
    • Takayasu's arteritis.
    • Brachial arteriovenous malformations (including iatrogenic: haemodialysis fistulas).

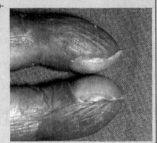

(a)

The dorsal aspect of 2 fingers, side by side with the nails touching. Normally, you should see a kite-shaped gap. If not, there is clubbing.

(b)   (c)

No dip therefore clubbing

Fig 2.33 Testing for finger clubbing.

Nail abnormalities

- *Koilonychia:* spoon-shaped nails (fig 2.34): iron deficiency, haemochromatosis, infection (eg fungal), endocrine disorders (eg acromegaly, hypothyroidism), malnutrition.
- *Leuconychia:* whitening of nails (fig 2.42, p76): punctate due to trauma, alopecia, psoriasis, fungal infection. See also Beau's lines and Terry's nails below.
- *Onycholysis:* detachment of the nail from the nailbed: hyperthyroidism, fungal infection, psoriasis.
- *Beau's lines:* transverse furrows from temporary arrest of nail growth (fig 2.35). Corresponds to times of physiological stress, eg severe infection, chemotherapy. The furrow's distance from the cuticle allows dating of the stress: ~0.1mm/day.
- *Mees' lines:* single white transverse bands: arsenic poisoning, chronic kidney disease, carbon monoxide poisoning.
- *Muehrcke's lines:* paired white parallel transverse bands (without furrowing of the nail itself, distinguishing them from Beau's lines) seen in chronic hypoalbuminaemia, Hodgkin's disease, pellagra (p240), chronic kidney disease.
- *Terry's nails:* proximal portion of nail is white/pink, nail tip is red/brown. Causes include cirrhosis, chronic kidney disease, congestive cardiac failure.
- *Pitting:* seen in psoriasis, alopecia areata.
- *Splinter haemorrhages:* fine longitudinal haemorrhagic streaks under the nails (fig 2.36). Due to microemboli or trauma. In the febrile patient, look for infective endocarditis. In the well gardener, look no further.
- *Nail-fold infarcts:* vasculitis, connective tissue (CT) disease, eg scleroderma, mixed CT disease.
- *Chronic paronychia:* chronic infection of the nail fold (fig 2.37). Presents as a painful swollen nail with intermittent discharge.

Skin changes

- *Palmar erythema* (fig 2.38): associated with pregnancy, hyperthyroidism, rheumatoid arthritis, polycythaemia, chemotherapy-induced palmar/plantar erythrodysaesthesia. Also chronic liver disease/cirrhosis via ↓inactivation of vasoactive endotoxins.
- *Pallor* of the palmar creases suggests anaemia.
- *Pigmentation:* normal pigmentation in dark skin. Also Addison's disease and Nelson's syndrome (↑ACTH after removal of the adrenal glands in Cushing's disease).

Nodules and contractures

- *Dupuytren's contracture:* fibrosis and contracture of palmar fascia (fig 2.24, p58): liver disease, trauma, ageing.
- *Heberden's* (distal interphalangeal joint, fig 2.39) and *Bouchard's* (fig 2.44, proximal interphalangeal joint) 'nodes' are osteophytes (bone over-growth at a joint) seen in osteoarthritis.
- *Gottron's papules:* purple rash on the knuckles. Look for with dilated nail-fold end-capillary loops. Seen in dermatomyositis (p549).

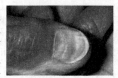

Fig 2.34 Koilonychia.

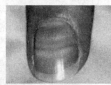

Fig 2.35 Beau's lines. Here due to chemotherapy, a new line is seen with each cycle. See p525.

Fig 2.36 Splinter haemorrhages.

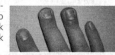

Fig 2.37 Paronychia.
Reproduced from Burge et al., Oxford Handbook of Medical Dermatology (2016), with permission from Oxford University Press.

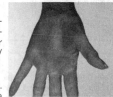

Fig 2.38 Palmar erythema.

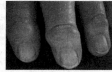

Fig 2.39 Heberden's nodes (DIP).
Reproduced from Watts et al. (eds) Oxford Textbook of Rheumatology (2013), with permission from Oxford University Press.

2 History and examination

Expose the arms and hands. Ask the patient to rest their hands on a pillow. Start by examining the dorsal surface and then turn the hands over. Always ask about pain or tender areas. Follow the 'look, move, feel' approach to avoid causing pain.

Look: skin

On both the palm and the dorsum start by inspecting the skin for:

1 **Colour** Pigmentation of creases (p75), pallor, palmar erythema (p75, fig 2.38).
2 **Consistency** Tight (sclerodactyly, fig 2.40), thick (DM, acromegaly).
3 **Characteristic lesion** Pulp infarcts, rashes, purpura, spider naevi, telangiectasia, tophi (fig 2.41), tendon xanthomata, scars (eg carpal tunnel release, joint replacement).

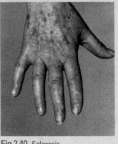

Fig 2.40 Sclerosis.

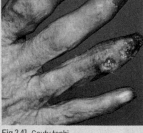

Fig 2.41 Gouty tophi.

Look: nails

See pp74–5.
• Clubbing (p74, figs 2.32, 2.33).
• Koilonychia (p75, fig 2.34).
• Leuconychia (fig 2.42).
• Pitting and onycholysis.
• Splinter haemorrhages (p75, fig 2.36).
• Nail fold infarcts.

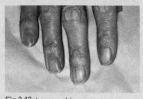

Fig 2.42 Leuconychia.

Look: muscles

Wasting and fasciculations
• Palmar surface: look particularly at the thenar (median nerve, fig 2.43) and hypothenar eminences.
• Dorsal surface: look for wasting of dorsal interossei. Generalized wasting, particularly of the interossei on the dorsum, but sparing of the thenar eminence suggests an ulnar nerve lesion.

Dupuytren's contracture (fig 2.24, p58).

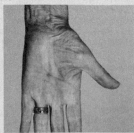

Fig 2.43 Thenar wasting.

History and examination

Look: joints

1 Look for signs of acute inflammation: swelling/erythema of joints.
2 Characteristic deformities of rheumatoid arthritis:
   • Ulnar deviation at the wrist.
   • Z deformity of the thumb.
   • Swan-neck: flexed DIP, hyperextended PIP (fig 12.2, p536).
   • Boutonnière: hyperextended DIP, flexed PIP.
3 Characteristic deformities of osteoarthritis:
   • Heberden's nodes (DIP joint, figs 2.39, 2.44).
   • Bouchard's nodes (PIP joint, fig 2.44).

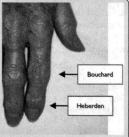

Fig 2.44 Bouchard's nodes.
Reproduced from Jolly *et al.* (eds) *Training in Medicine* (2016), with permission from Oxford University Press.

Feel

1 Using the dorsum of your hand, gently feel for warmth (and tenderness) over each joint (don't forget scaphoid: 'snuffbox' tenderness). Once pain excluded, palpate for joint effusions.
2 Palpate thenar and hypothenar muscle bulk.
3 Palpate for palmar thickening of Dupuytren's contracture (fig 2.24, p58).
4 Palpate radial and ulnar pulse to confirm blood supply to hand.
5 Sensation:
   • Median nerve: index finger, thenar eminence.
   • Ulnar nerve: little finger, hypothenar eminence.
   • Radial: first dorsal webspace.
6 *Tinel's test* (percuss over the distal skin crease of the wrist), *Phalen's test* (patient holds dorsal surfaces of both hands together for 60 seconds). Tests are positive if tingling is reported, suggesting carpal tunnel syndrome.

Move

Wrist and forearm
• Extension: prayer position.
• Flexion: reverse prayer.
• Supination and pronation.
Small muscles
• Pincer grip: finger and thumb.
• Power grip: 'Squeeze my fingers.'
• Thumb abduction: with palm facing ceiling ask patient to, 'Point your thumb to the ceiling and don't let me push down'.
• Finger abduction ('Spread your fingers') and adduction ('Grip this piece of paper between your fingers'). *Froment's sign* = flexion of the thumb during grip as ulnar nerve lesion prevents adduction (p449).
Functional assessment
• Write a sentence, undo a button, pick up a coin.

Other

• Examine the elbows: psoriatic plaque, rheumatoid nodule, surgical scar.
• Neurological examination of the upper limb (p62).
• Examination of the face for signs of connective tissue disease.

Top tips
• Cross your fingers before the patient grips them, it hurts less!
• Don't forget to palpate the radial and ulnar pulses.
• Don't forget to look at the elbows for plaques of psoriasis and rheumatoid nodules.

For symptoms of thyroid disease see **p29**, **p212**, **p214**.

If clinical examination suggests that a lump is not arising from the thyroid then examine lump like any other (**p586**; lump in the neck, **pp590–592**).

---

1 Inspect

Position patient sitting on a chair (with space behind), adequately expose neck. Inspect from front and sides:

1 Is there a goitre?
  • The normal thyroid is usually neither visible nor palpable. A midline swelling should raise your suspicion of thyroid pathology. Look for scars (eg collar incision from previous thyroid surgery).
2 What is the thyroid status?
  • *Hypothyroidism:* puffiness, pallor, dry flaky skin, xanthelasma, corneal arcus, balding, loss of the lateral third of eyebrow, slowness, lethargy, weight gain.
  • *Hyperthyroidism:* anxious, nervous, agitated, fidgety, tremor, weight loss.

NB Proptosis is better seen from above and behind so is inspected for when you move behind the patient for palpation.

---

2 Swallow test

Stand in front of the patient. Ask them to, 'Sip water... hold it in your mouth... and swallow' to see if any midline swelling moves up on swallowing. Goitres (**p592**) and thyroglossal cysts (**p590**) (and rarely lymph nodes) move up on swallowing.

---

3 Tongue protrusion test

Ask patient to 'stick out your tongue'. Does the lump move up? A thyroglossal cyst will move up on tongue protrusion.

---

4 Palpation

Stand behind the patient.
• **Proptosis (p213)** May be best seen from above and behind, so can be examined for at this stage. Ask the patient to tilt their head back slightly; this will give you a better view to assess protrusion of the eyeball anteriorly out of the orbit.
• **Thyroid gland**
  • Exclude pain prior to palpation.
  • Place middle 3 fingers of either hand along midline below chin and 'walk down' to thyroid, 2 finger breadths below the cricoid on both sides. Assess any enlargement/nodules.
  • Palpate each lobe. Determine size, *nodular* (*solitary* or *multiple*) or *smooth/diffuse*.
  • Repeating the swallow test while palpating allows you to confirm the inspection finding, but also allows an attempt to 'get below the lump'. If there is a distinct inferior border under which you can place your hand then the goitre is unlikely to have retrosternal extension.
• **Lymph nodes** Examine lymph nodes of head and neck (**p58**).
• **Trachea** Palpate for tracheal deviation from the midline.

---

5 Percussion

Percuss the sternum for the dullness of retrosternal extension of a goitre.

6 Auscultation

Listen over the goitre for a *bruit* (a continuous sound heard over the thyroid). A bruit in a smooth thyroid goitre is suggestive of Graves' disease (p212) and oc-curs due to a proliferation of the blood supply when the thyroid enlarges.

7 Hands

• **Inspect** Thyroid acropachy (clubbing) and palmar erythema in hyperthyroidism.
• **Temperature** Warm peripheries in hyperthyroidism, cool in hypothyroidism.
• **Pulse** Rate and rhythm. Tachycardia and atrial fibrillation may be seen in hyper-thyroidism, while bradycardia may be seen in hypothyroidism.
• **Fine tremor** Ask patient to, 'Hold hands out'. Place a sheet of paper over out-stretched hands to help elicit tremor.

8 Eyes

The 'normal' upper eyelid should always cover the upper eye such that the white sclera is not visible between the lid and the iris. If visible, *lid retraction* is present.

Lid-lag = the upper eyelid is higher than normal with the globe in downgaze and can be elicited with downward movement of the eye. Ask patient to, 'Follow my finger' as you move your finger from a point above the eye to below hori-zontal gaze.

Proptosis and exophthalmos are often used interchangeably. Some stick to a stricter definition: *exophthalmos = proptosis + lid retraction/lag*.

Eye movements Ask the patient to follow your finger whilst gently holding their head still, as you make an 'H' shape with your finger. Any double vision?

Lid retraction, lid-lag, exophthalmos and ophthalmoplegia are all signs of auto-immune hyperthyroidism, most commonly due to Graves' disease (p213).

9 Other

1 **Proximal myopathy** Ask patient to stand up from the chair without using their arms to assess for proximal myopathy (can occur due to both hyper- and hypothyroidism).
2 **Pretibial myxoedema** Swelling and discolouration of the lower leg above the lateral malleoli in Graves' disease.
3 **Ankle reflexes** Delayed relaxation in hypothyroidism.

Breast symptoms

Symptoms that require exclusion of breast cancer include:
►Lump or swelling in breast/upper chest/axilla.
►Breast skin changes, eg dimpling/puckering.
►Change in skin colour, erythema.
►Nipple change, eg inversion.
►Nipple rash or crusting/discharge.
►Change in size or shape of breast.

Lump

* Site (fig 2.45) and size. Change in size related to menstrual cycle?
* Associated symptoms: pain, overlying skin change, nipple change/inversion/discharge?
* Drugs (eg HRT/oestrogens)?
* Systemic symptoms: weight loss, breathlessness, back/bone pain?
* History: previous lumps? Family history of breast/ovarian cancer (p516)? Obstetric and menstrual history. Previous mammograms, clinical examinations of the breast, USS, fine-needle aspirate (FNA)/core biopsy.
* Social support.

Nipple changes

* Shape change: unilateral/bilateral, fixed, associated skin changes/discharge?
* Discharge: amount, nature, colour? Any blood? Associated symptoms: pain, skin changes, headache, visual loss, amenorrhoea/infertility.
* *Causes:* duct ectasia (green/brown/red, often multiple ducts and bilateral), intraductal papilloma/adenoma/carcinoma (bloody discharge, often single duct), lactation/galactorrhoea.
* *Management:* diagnose the cause (mammogram, ultrasound, ductogram, biopsy, serum prolactin) then treat appropriately. Cessation of smoking may reduce discharge from duct ectasia.

Breast pain

* SOCRATES (p26), bilateral/unilateral, history of trauma, related to menstrual cycle?
* Associated symptoms: mass, nipple/skin changes.
* Exclude breast cancer (rare if isolated pain).
* Rule out cardiac chest pain (p86, p764).
* If non-malignant and non-cyclical, consider:
  * Tietze's syndrome: costochondritis plus swelling of the costal cartilage.
  * Bornholm disease/Devil's grip: coxsackie B virus causing chest/abdominal pain, which may be mistaken for cardiac pain or an acute surgical abdomen. It resolves within ~2 weeks.
  * Angina.
  * Gallstones.
  * Lung disease.
  * Thoracic outlet syndrome.

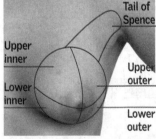

Fig 2.45 The quadrants of the breast with the axillary tail of Spence.

Reproduced from Thomas J, *et al.* (eds) *Oxford Handbook of Clinical Examination and Practical Skills* (2014), with permission from Oxford University Press.

1 Inspection

▶*Always have a chaperone present.*
* Position patient sitting at edge of bed with hands by side, exposed to waist.
* Inspect with hands on hips, then again with hands on head to accentuate asymmetrical changes.
* Inspect for: masses, contour anomalies, asymmetry, scars, ulceration, skin changes (*peau d'orange*: orange peel appearance resulting from oedema).
* Look for nipple inversion and nipple discharge.

While patient has arms raised, inspect axillae for any masses as well as inspecting under the breasts.

2 Palpation of the breast

* Position patient sitting at 45° with hand behind head (ie right hand behind head when examining right breast, fig 246).
* Ask about pain and discharge. Examine painful areas last. Ask patient to express any discharge.
* Examine each breast (asymptomatic side first). Examine each quadrant as well as axillary tail of Spence (fig 245), or use a concentric spiral method (fig 247). Use flat fingers to feel breast tissue against chest wall.
* Define lumps/lumpy areas. If you discover a lump, to examine for fixity to skin and pectoral muscles: ask patient to push against their hip to contract muscle and then try to move at right angles to the long axis of pectoralis muscle fibres.

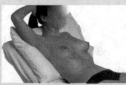

Fig 2.46 Correct patient position for breast examination.

Reproduced from Thomas J, *et al.* (eds) *Oxford Handbook of Clinical Examination and Practical Skills* (2014), with permission from Oxford University Press.

Fig 2.47 Methods for systematic breast palpation.

Reproduced from Thomas J, *et al.* (eds) *Oxford Handbook of Clinical Examination and Practical Skills* (2014), with permission from Oxford University Press.

3 Palpation of the axilla

Examine both axillae. When examining the right axilla, support the patient's right arm on your examining left arm. Similarly, examine the left axilla with your right hand, supporting the patient's left arm on your right arm.
Palpate five sets of axillary nodes:
  1 Apical: palpate against glenohumeral joint.
  2 Anterior: palpate against pectoralis major.
  3 Central: palpate against lateral chest wall.
  4 Posterior: palpate against latissimus dorsi.
  5 Medial: palpate against humerus.

4 Further examination

* Other lymphadenopathy.
* Spine for tenderness.
* Abdomen for hepatomegaly (p59).
* Respiratory examination for effusion (p49, p51).
* Neurological examination if symptoms (pp62–7).

The peripheral vascular system: examination

Arterial

▶▶The 'P's suggest acute ischaemia, which is a surgical emergency (p579, p649):

Pale   **P**ulseless   **P**ainful
Paralysed   **P**araesthetic   '**P**erishingly' cold

---

1 Inspection

- **Skin** Hair loss, pallor, shiny skin, ulceration, gangrene, cyanosis, scars.
- **Pressure points** Between toes, lift up heels to inspect for ulceration underneath.

---

2 Palpation

- **Temperature** Check thighs, legs, and feet with dorsum of hand on both legs. Is there a level above which the skin is warmer?
- **Capillary refill** Press/squeeze great toe until blanches, release, and count time for colour to return (normal <2s).
- **Peripheral pulses** Assess whether palpable bilaterally. Detect rate and rhythm (?irregularly irregular raising possibility of emboli from atrial fibrillation).
  1 *Femoral*—mid-inguinal point.
  2 *Popliteal*—flex knees slightly and press into centre of popliteal fossa (fig 2.48).
  3 *Posterior tibial*—just posterior & inferior to medial malleolus.
  4 *Dorsalis pedis*—between bases of 1st & 2nd metatarsals, lateral to extensor hallucis longus. For brachial and carotid, determine volume and character (p40).
- **Abdominal aorta** Midline above umbilicus. A pulsatile, expansile mass is an aortic aneurysm until proven otherwise (fig 2.49).

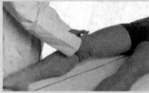

Fig 2.48 Palpation of popliteal pulse.
Reproduced from Thomas J, *et al.* (eds). *Oxford Handbook of Clinical Examination and Practical Skills* (2014), with permission from Oxford University Press.

 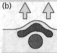

Fig 2.49 Pulses: abdominal aorta.
(a) Expansile (aneurysm?).
(b) Transmitted.
Reproduced from Thomas J, *et al.* (eds). *Oxford Handbook of Clinical Examination and Practical Skills* (2014), with permission from Oxford University Press.

---

3 Auscultation

- **Bruits** Aortic, iliac, and femoral. (Carotid and renal either now, or at the end.)

---

4 Special tests

- **Buerger's test** Lift both legs to 45° above horizontal. Allow a minute for legs to pale. Then ask patient to sit up, with lower legs off the edge of the bed. Observe for colour change: usually white to pink. Flushed red (reactive hyperaemia) may indicate more severe disease.
- **Buerger's angle** Angle above horizontal that leads to pallor (<20° = severe ischaemia).

---

5 Further examination

- Examination of peripheral vascular system outside the leg:
  - *Other pulses:* radial, brachial, carotid.
  - *Other bruits:* carotid, renal.
- Doppler probe to detect pulses and measure ankle–brachial pressure index (p648).
- Neurological examination of lower limbs (pp64–5).

1 Inspection
- **Varicosities** Inspect with patient standing. Decide whether varicosities are:
  - Long saphenous vein—medial.
  - Short saphenous vein—posterior lateral, below the knee.
  - Calf perforators—usually few varicosities but commonly show skin changes.
- **Ulcers** Around the medial malleolus are more suggestive of venous disease, whereas those at the pressure points suggest arterial pathology (p82).
- **Other skin changes**
  - *Haemosiderin deposition:* brown skin deposits due to venous hypertension.
  - Atrophy and loss of elasticity.
  - *Lipodermatosclerosis:* induration, hyperpigmentation, erythema, swelling, inverted champagne bottle appearance. Pathology is panniculitis (inflammation of subcutaneous fat) caused by a chronic innate immune response in soft tissues secondary to venous hypertension.

2 Palpation
- **Characterize** Firm and tender may suggest thrombosis, warm and tender may suggest infection.
- **Cough impulse** Ask patient to cough while you palpate for a transmitted impulse (incompetence) at the saphenofemoral junction (SFJ) and saphenopopliteal junction (SPJ).
- **Tap test** Percuss lower limit of varicosity and feel for impulse at SFJ. A transmitted percussion impulse demonstrates incompetence of superficial valves.
- **Arterial pulses** If ulceration is present, palpate to rule out arterial disease (p82).

3 Auscultation
Listen for bruits over any varicosities (occur if arteriovenous malformation).

4 Special tests
- **Doppler** Test to determine the level of incompetence. On squeezing the leg distal to the probe you should only hear one 'whoosh' if the valves are competent at the level of probe. Place probe over SFJ, squeeze calf, and listen. Repeat with probe at SPJ.
- **Brodie–Trendelenburg test** Used if Doppler is not available. Elevate leg and massage veins to empty varicosities. Apply tourniquet to upper thigh. Ask patient to stand. If not controlled, repeat, placing tourniquet below knee.
- **Perthes' test** Used to distinguish between superficial and deep venous pathology. Apply a tourniquet at mid-thigh level whilst the patient is standing (varicosities filled/partially filled). Ask the patient to walk, or alternate between tip-toes and flat feet, for 5 minutes. If the varicosities become less distended, the calf muscle is able to pump blood from superficial to the deep venous system normally. If the varicosities remain distended (or become more distended) it suggests deep venous pathology, eg thrombus. Contemporary imaging of the deep leg veins using Doppler ultrasound means this test is largely historical.

5 Further examination
- Examination of the abdomen (p58), pelvis, rectum (p59), and genitals for masses.

3 Cardiovascular medicine

Contents

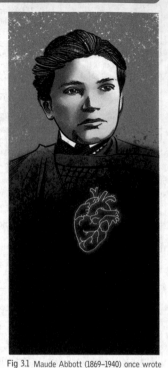

Fig 3.1 Maude Abbott (1869–1940) once wrote 'One of my daydreams, which I feel to be selfish, is that of going to school'. Overcoming both a difficult childhood and initial rejection from medical school because she was female, she later became an international authority on heart disease. Through her work as the assistant curator at the McGill Museum of Medicine, she organized systematized knowledge on congenital heart disease, laying the foundation for modern cardiac surgery. Although museum work wasn't her first choice of career, she was advised by her mentor, Sir William Osler, to look past the 'dreary and unpromising drudgery' and seize the 'splendid opportunity' to do 'wonderful things'. In 2000, Canada Post issued a forty-six-cent postage stamp entitled 'The Heart of the Matter' in her honour.

Artwork by Gillian Turner.

We thank Paul Cacciottolo, our Specialist Reader for this chapter.

Cardiovascular health

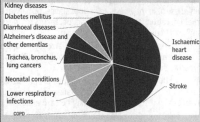

Fig 3.2 Top ten global causes of death, 2019.
■ Non-communicable disease.
■ Communicable disease.
Source: https://www.who.int/news-room/fact-sheets/detail/the-top-10-causes-of-death

Cardiovascular disease (CVD) is common in the general population, and includes ischaemic heart disease (IHD), stroke, peripheral vascular disease, and aortic aneurysms. IHD and stroke are globally the leading causes of death (fig 3.2). Risk stratification is the key to prevention. All adults age 40–75 years should undergo routine CVD assessment using a validated risk model such as QRISK3 (www.qrisk.org) or pooled cohort equation. In discussion with the patient, consider treatment if ≥10% risk of developing CVD within the next 10 years. Adults aged 20–39 years should also be assessed periodically as the prevalence of vascular risk factors such as hypertension and diabetes are increasing at a younger age. Cardiovascular disease starts silently at a young age, but those with fewer risk factors age more healthily.

Addressing modifiable risk factors[1]

• *A healthy diet* should be consumed with plenty of fruit and vegetables while minimizing trans fatty acids, saturated fats, red meat, and refined carbohydrates.

• *Regular physical activity* of moderate-intensity exercise for ≥150 minutes/week.

• *Obesity*, now a global epidemic associated with significant morbidity and mortality, should be tackled with a structured programme of caloric restriction and physical activity. Consider a glucagon-like peptide (GLP-1) agonist (eg semaglutide) or referral for bariatric surgery (p618).

• *Smoking cessation* saves lives and although sometimes it may seem futile to us, brief advice from doctors has been shown to increase the quit rate.[2] Refer to behavioural support resources. Treat hospitalized patients and continue after discharge. First-line cessation medications are nicotine replacement (gum, patches), varenicline (an oral selective nicotine receptor partial agonist; start 1 week before target stop date), and bupropion (= amfebutamone; avoid if history of seizures). Caution against vaping as the long-term effects are unknown and may include significant lung morbidity.

• ►*Hypertension* (p108) is the leading modifiable risk factor. For most at-risk patients, the goal should be <130/80mmHg.

• *Lipid-lowering therapy:* start a statin for primary prevention if >10% CVD risk in 10 years.[3]

• *Tight glycaemic control* in type 1 or 2 diabetic patients. Target HbA1c <48mmol/mol if young and not prone to hypoglycaemia.

• *Antiplatelet therapy* should not be routinely prescribed for primary prevention as the net harm may outweigh the potential benefits.

• *CKD:* prevent and treat underlying aetiology (eg diabetes, GN) where possible. Strict BP control <120/80mmHg.[4] Proteinuric patients are at much higher risk.

The randomized trial

Cardiovascular medicine has an unrivalled treasure house of randomized trials. One of the chief pleasures of cardiovascular medicine lies in integrating these with clinical reasoning in a humane way. After a cardiac event, a protocol may 'mandate' statins, aspirin, β-blockers, ACE-i (p106), and a target BP and LDL cholesterol that makes your patient feel dreadful. What to do? Inform, negotiate, and compromise. Never reject your patient because of lack of compliance with your over-exacting regimens. Keep smiling, keep communicating, and keep up to date: the latest data may show that your patient was right all along.

Chest pain ▶Cardiac-sounding chest pain may have no serious cause, but always think 'Could this be a myocardial infarction (MI), dissecting aortic aneurysm, pericarditis, or pulmonary embolism?', particularly if sudden-onset pain.

Character Constricting suggests angina, oesophageal spasm, or anxiety; a sharp pain may be from the pleura, pericardium, or chest wall. A prolonged (>30min), dull, central crushing pain or pressure suggests MI.

Radiation To shoulder, either or both arms, or neck/jaw suggests cardiac ischaemia. The pain of aortic dissection (p646) is classically instantaneous, tearing, and interscapular, but may be retrosternal. Epigastric pain may be cardiac.

Precipitants Pain associated with cold, exercise, palpitations, or emotion suggests cardiac pain or anxiety; if brought on by food, lying flat, hot drinks, or alcohol, consider oesophageal spasm/disease (but meals can also cause angina).

Relieving factors If pain is relieved within minutes by rest or glyceryl trinitrate (GTN), suspect angina (GTN relieves oesophageal spasm more slowly). If antacids help, suspect GI causes. Pericarditic pain improves on leaning forward.

Associations Dyspnoea occurs with cardiac pain, pulmonary emboli, pleurisy, or anxiety. MI may cause nausea, vomiting, or sweating. Angina is caused by coronary artery disease—and also by aortic stenosis, hypertrophic cardiomyopathy (HCM), paroxysmal supraventricular tachycardia (SVT)—and can be exacerbated by anaemia. Chest pain with tenderness suggests self-limiting Tietze's syndrome. Odd neurological symptoms and atypical chest pain—think aortic dissection.

Pleuritic pain Pain exacerbated by inspiration. Implies inflammation of the pleura from pulmonary infection, inflammation, or infarction. It causes us to 'catch our breath'. ΔΔ: musculoskeletal pain; fractured rib (pain on respiration, exacerbated by gentle pressure on the sternum); subdiaphragmatic pathology (eg gallstones).

▶▶**Chest pain & acutely unwell** (See p764.) • Admit. • Check pulse, BP in both arms (unequal in aortic dissection, p646), JVP, heart sounds; examine legs for DVT. • Give O₂ if hypoxic. • IV line. • Relieve pain (eg 2.5–5mg IV morphine). • Cardiac monitor. • 12-lead ECG. • CXR. • Arterial blood gas (ABG). **Famous traps** Aortic dissection; zoster (p400); ruptured oesophagus; cardiac tamponade (p132); opiate addiction.

Dyspnoea May be from LVF, PE, any respiratory cause, anaemia, pain, or anxiety. **Severity** ▶▶Emergency presentations: p765. Ask about shortness of breath at rest, on exertion, and on lying flat; has their exercise tolerance changed? **Associations** Specific symptoms associated with heart failure are orthopnoea (ask about number of pillows used at night), paroxysmal nocturnal dyspnoea (waking up at night gasping for breath, p46), and peripheral oedema. Pulmonary embolism is associated with acute onset of dyspnoea and pleuritic chest pain; ask about risk factors for DVT.

Palpitation(s) May be due to ectopics, sinus tachycardia, AF, SVT, VT, thyrotoxicosis, anxiety, and rarely phaeochromocytoma. See p36. **History** Characterize: do they mean their heart was beating fast, hard, or irregularly? Ask about previous episodes, precipitating/relieving factors, duration of symptoms, associated chest pain, dyspnoea, dizziness, or collapse. Did the patient check their pulse?

Syncope May reflect cardiac or CNS events. Vasovagal 'faints' are common (↓pulse, pupils dilated). The history from an observer is invaluable in diagnosis. **Prodromal symptoms** Chest pain, palpitations, or dyspnoea point to a cardiac cause, eg arrhythmia. Aura, headache, dysarthria, and limb weakness indicate CNS causes. **During the episode** Was there a pulse? Limb jerking, tongue biting, or urinary incontinence? NB: hypoxia from lack of cerebral perfusion may cause seizures. **Recovery** Was this rapid (arrhythmia) or prolonged, with drowsiness (seizure)?

Chest pain from the patient's perspective

On acute wards we are always hearing questions such as 'Is your pain sharp or dull?', followed by an equivocal answer. The doctor goes on: 'Sharp like a knife—or dull and crushing?' The doctor is getting irritated because the patient must know the answer but is not saying it. A true story paves the way to being less inquisitorial and having a more creative understanding of the nature of symptoms.

A patient came to a previous *OHCM* author saying 'Last night I dreamed I had a pain in my chest. Now I've woken up, and I'm not sure—have I got chest pain, doctor? What do you think?' How odd it is to be asked to examine a patient to exclude a symptom, not a disease. (It turned out that she did have serious chest pathology.) Odd, until one realizes that symptoms are often half-formed, and it is our role to give them a local habitation and a name. Dialogue can transform a symptom from 'airy nothingness' to a fact (fig 3.3).[1]

Patients often avoid using the word 'pain' to describe ischaemia: 'wind', 'tightening', 'pressure', 'burning', or 'a lump in the throat' (angina means to choke) may be used. They may say 'sharp' to communicate severity, and not character. So be as vague in your questioning as your patient is in their answers. 'Tell me some more about what you are feeling (long pause) ... as if someone was doing what to you?' 'Sitting on me' or 'like a hotness' might be the response (suggesting cardiac ischaemia). Do not ask 'Does it go into your left arm?' Try 'Is there anything else about it?' (pause) ... 'Does it go anywhere?' Note down your patient's exact words.

A good history, taking account of these features, is the best way to stratify patients likely to have cardiac pain. If the history is non-specific, there are no risk factors for cardiovascular diseases, and ECG and plasma troponin T (p114) are normal 6–12h after the onset of pain, discharge will probably be OK. When in doubt, get help. Features making cardiac pain unlikely:
• Stabbing, shooting pain.
• Pain lasting <30s, however intense.
• Well-localized, left sub-mammary pain ('In my heart, doctor').
• Pains of continually varying location.
• Youth.

NB: 25% of non-cardiac chest pain is *musculoskeletal:* look for pain on specific postures or activity. Aim to reproduce the pain by movement and, sometimes, palpation over the structure causing it. Focal injection of local anaesthetic helps diagnostically and is therapeutic. *Tietze's syndrome:* self-limiting costochondritis ± costosternal joint swelling. Causes: idiopathic; microtrauma; infection; psoriatic/rheumatoid arthritis. R: NSAIDs or steroid injections. Tenderness is also caused by: fibromyalgia, lymphoma, chondrosarcoma, myeloma, metastases, rib TB. Imaging: bone scintigraphy; CT.

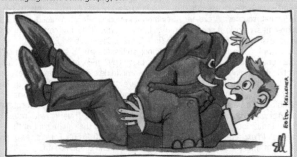

Fig 3.3 The elephant on my chest.   Image courtesy Eoin Kelleher.

1 Dialogue-transformed symptoms explain one of the junior doctor's main vexations: when patients retell symptoms to a consultant in the light of day, they bear no resemblance to what you originally heard. But do not be vexed: your dialogue may have helped the patient far more than any ward round.

3 Cardiovascular medicine

Where to place the chest leads (See fig 3.4.)

v₁ Right sternal edge, 4th intercostal space.

v₂ Left sternal edge, 4th intercostal space.

v₃ Half-way between v₂ and v₄.

v₄ 5th intercostal space, mid-clavicular line; all subsequent leads are in the same horizontal plane as v₄.

v₅ Anterior axillary line.

v₆ Mid-axillary line (v₇: posterior axillary line).

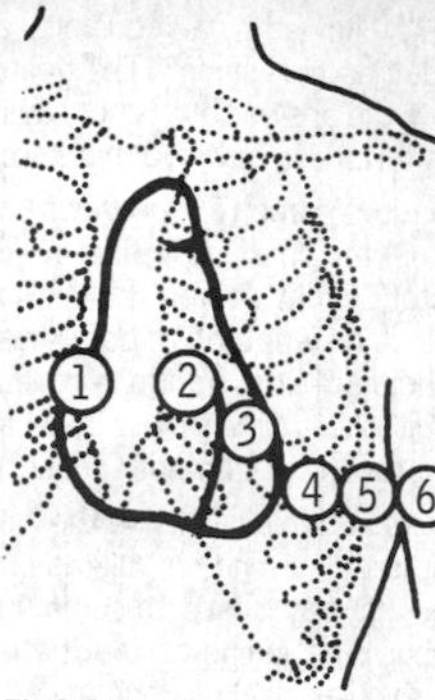

Reading an ECG

▶First confirm the patient's name and age, and the ECG date. Then (see fig 3.5).

- **Rate** At usual speed (25mm/s) each 'big square' is 0.2s and 'small square' 0.04s. To calculate the rate, divide 300 by the number of big squares between two consecutive R waves. The normal rate is 60–100bpm.

Fig 3.4 Placement of ECG leads.

- **Rhythm** If cycles are not clearly regular, use the 'card method': lay a card along the ECG, marking positions of three successive R waves. Slide the card to and fro to check that all intervals are equal. If they are not, note if:
  - there is slight but regular lengthening and then shortening (with respiration)—sinus arrhythmia, common in the young
  - there are different rates which are multiples of each other—varying block
  - it is 100% irregular—atrial fibrillation (AF) or ventricular fibrillation (VF).

Sinus rhythm is characterized by a P wave followed by a QRS complex. AF has no discernible P waves and QRS complexes are irregularly irregular. Atrial flutter (p126; fig 3.40, p127) has a 'sawtooth' baseline of atrial depolarization (~300/min) and regular QRS complexes. Ventricular rhythm has QRS complexes >0.12s with P waves following them or absent (fig 3.15, p98).

- **Axis** The overall direction of depolarization across the patient's anterior chest; this is the sum of all the ventricular electrical forces during ventricular depolarization. See BOX. Left axis deviation can result from left anterior hemiblock, inferior MI, VT from a left ventricular focus, WPW, LVH. Right axis deviation can result from RVH, PE, anterolateral MI, WPW, and left posterior hemiblock.

- **P wave** Normally precedes each QRS complex, and upright in II, III, & aVF but inverted in aVR. Absent P wave: AF, P hidden due to junctional or ventricular rhythm. P mitrale: bifid P wave, indicates left atrial hypertrophy. P pulmonale: peaked P wave, indicates right atrial hypertrophy. Pseudo-P-pulmonale seen if ↓K⁺.

- **PR interval** Measure from start of P wave to start of QRS. Normal range: 0.12–0.2s (3–5 small squares). A prolonged PR interval implies delayed AV conduction (1st-degree heart block). A short PR interval implies unusually fast AV conduction down an accessory pathway, eg WPW (see fig 3.42, p129). See heart block, p90.

- **QRS complex** See fig 3.6. Normal duration: <0.12s. QRS >0.12s suggests ventricular conduction defects, eg a bundle branch block (p92, p93), metabolic disturbance, ventricular origin or a paced rhythm. High-amplitude QRS complexes suggest ventricular hypertrophy (p92). Normal Q waves are <0.04s wide and <2mm deep; they are often seen in leads I, aVL, v₅, v₆ and reflect normal septal depolarization. Pathological Q waves (deep and wide) may occur within a few hours of an acute MI.

- **QT interval** Measure from start of QRS to end of T wave. It varies with rate. The corrected QT interval (QTc) is the QT interval divided by the square root of the R–R interval, ie QTc = QT/√RR. Normal QTc: <0.45s (M) or <0.46s (F). For causes of prolonged QT interval, see p697. Long QT can lead to VT and sudden death.

- **ST segment** Usually isoelectric. Planar elevation (>1mm) or depression (>0.5mm) usually implies infarction (p115, figs 3.12, 3.13, pp95-6) or ischaemia, respectively.

- **T wave** Normally inverted in aVR, v₁, and occasionally v₂. Normal if inverted in isolation in lead III. Abnormal if inverted in I, II, and v₄–v₆. Peaked in hyperkalaemia (fig 14.3, p667) and flattened in hypokalaemia.

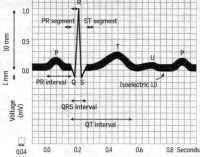

Fig 3.5 Schematic diagram of a normal ECG trace.

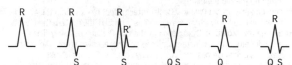

Fig 3.6 'QRS' complexes. If the first deflection from the isoelectric line is negative, it is a Q wave. Any positive deflection is an R wave. Any negative deflection after an R is an S. A second positive deflection within the same complex is R' (R prime).

Determining the ECG axis

Each 'lead' on the 12-lead ECG represents electrical activity along a particular plane (fig 3.7).

The axis lies at 90° to the direction of the lead in which the isoelectric (equally +ve and −ve) QRS complex is found. For example, if the QRS is isoelectric in lead II (+60°), the axis is either:

+60° − 90° = −30°, or

+60° + 90° = +150°.

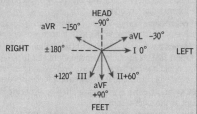

Fig 3.7 The planes represented by the limb 'leads'.

If the QRS is more positive than negative in lead I (0°) then the axis must be −30°, and vice versa.

In practice, the exact axis matters little; what you need to be able to recognize is whether the axis is normal (−30° to +90°), left-deviated (<−30°), or right deviated (>+90°). There are many ways of doing this. If the QRS in lead I (0°) is predominantly positive (the R wave is taller than the S wave is deep), the axis must be between −90° and +90°. If lead II (+60°) is mostly positive, the axis must be between −30° and +150°. So if both I and II are positive, the axis must be between −30° and +90°—the normal range. When II is negative, the axis is likely to be left-deviated (<−30°) and when I is negative, the axis is likely to be right-deviated (>+90°). One way of remembering this is:

• Lovers **L**eaving—**L**eft axis deviation—the QRS complexes in I and II point away from each other.
• Lovers **R**eturning—**R**ight axis deviation—the QRS complexes in I and III ± II point towards each other (fig 3.14, p97).

Sinus tachycardia All impulses are initiated in the sinoatrial node ('sinus rhythm') hence all QRSs are preceded by a normal P wave with a normal PR interval. Tachycardia means rate >100bpm. See p123.

Sinus bradycardia Sinus rhythm at a rate <60bpm. **Causes** Physical fitness, vasovagal syncope, sinus node dysfunction, drugs (β-blockers, digoxin, amiodarone, non-dihydropyridine CCBs), hypothyroidism, hypothermia, ↑intracranial pressure. See p118.

AF (ECG, p121) Common causes: IHD, thyrotoxicosis, hypertension, obesity, heart failure, alcohol. See p126.

Heart block (HB) (See fig 3.8.) Disrupted passage of electrical impulse through the AV node or His–Purkinje system. 1st- and 2nd-degree HB may be caused by: normal variant, athletes, sinus node dysfunction, IHD (esp. inferior MI), acute myocarditis, drugs (digoxin, β-blockers). 3rd-degree HB is always pathological.

• **1st-degree HB** Delayed AV conduction. The PR interval is prolonged and unchanging; no missed beats.
• **2nd-degree HB: Mobitz I (Wenckebach)** Intermittent block within the AV node. The PR interval progressively lengthens until a QRS is missed, the pattern then resets.
• **2nd-degree HB: Mobitz II** Dysfunction of the His–Purkinje pathway. The PR interval of the conducted beats is constant until one or more P waves is not followed by a QRS complex. This is a dangerous rhythm as it may progress to complete HB.
• **3rd-degree HB: complete heart block** No impulses are passed from atria to ventricles so P waves and QRSs appear independently of each other. As tissue distal to the AV node paces slowly, the patient becomes very bradycardic, and may develop haemodynamic compromise. Urgent treatment is required. **Causes** IHD (esp. inferior MI), idiopathic (fibrosis), congenital, infective endocarditis, cardiac surgery/trauma, digoxin toxicity, infiltration (abscesses, granulomas, tumours, parasites).

ST elevation Normal variant, widespread concave pattern in young patients due to benign early repolarization, acute MI (STEMI), Prinzmetal's angina (p696), acute pericarditis (saddle-shaped) (fig 3.45, p133), myocarditis, Takotsubo cardiomyopathy, left ventricular aneurysm.

ST depression Normal variant (upward sloping), digoxin toxicity (downward sloping), ischaemic (horizontal): angina, NSTEMI, acute posterior MI (ST depression in V_1–V_3).

T inversion In V_1–V_3: normal (black patients and children), right bundle branch block (RBBB), RV strain (eg secondary to PE). In V_2–V_5: anterior ischaemia, HCM, subarachnoid haemorrhage, lithium. In V_4–V_6 and aVL: lateral ischaemia, LVH, left bundle branch block (LBBB). In II, III and aVF: inferior ischaemia.

NB: ST- and T-wave changes are often non-specific, and must be interpreted in the light of the clinical context.

Myocardial infarction (See p114 and fig 3.27; example ECGs, figs 3.12, 3.13, pp95–6.)
• Within hours, the T wave may become peaked and ST segments may begin to rise.
• Within 24h, the T wave inverts. ST elevation rarely persists, unless a left ventricular aneurysm develops. T-wave inversion may or may not persist.
• Within a few days, pathological Q waves begin to form. Q waves usually persist, but may resolve in 10% of patients.
• The location of these changes indicates the ischaemic area location, see table 3.1.

Pulmonary embolism (See fig 3.14, p97.) ECG findings may include: sinus tachycardia (commonest), RBBB (p92), right ventricular strain pattern (R-axis deviation, dominant R wave, and T-wave inversion/ST depression in V_1 and V_2). Rarely, the 'S1Q3T3' pattern occurs: deep S waves in I, pathological Q waves in III, inverted T waves in III.

Metabolic abnormalities Digoxin effect Down-sloping ST depression and inverted T wave in V_5–V_6 ('reversed tick', see fig 3.23, p107). In digoxin toxicity, any arrhythmia may occur (ventricular ectopics and nodal bradycardia are common). **Hyperkalaemia** Tall, tented T wave, widened QRS, absent P waves, 'sine wave' appearance (see fig 14.3, p667). **Hypokalaemia** Small T waves, prominent U waves, peaked P waves. **Hypercalcaemia** Short QT interval. **Hypocalcaemia** Long QT interval, small T waves. See p697 for causes of long QT intervals.

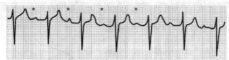

First degree AV block. P–R interval = 0.28s.

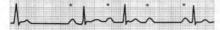

Mobitz type I (Wenckebach) AV block. With each successive QRS, the P–R interval increases until there is a non-conducted P wave.

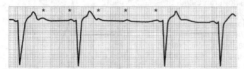

Mobitz type II AV block. Ratio of AV conduction varies from 2:1 to 3:1.

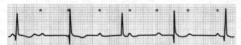

Complete AV block with narrow ventricular complex.
There is no relation between atrial and the slower ventricular activity.

Fig 3.8 Rhythm strips of heart blocks. * P wave.

Location, location, location

When considering rate and rhythm, your findings should be the same in all leads, albeit clearer in some than others. Other ECG features may vary lead by lead, both in terms of what is 'normal' and in what a change indicates. For example, ST elevation in leads II, III, and aVF suggests an inferior MI requiring immediate treatment, likely PCI to the right coronary artery, see table 3.1. ST elevation across *all* leads, however, suggests instead pericarditis which necessitates entirely different management (p132). An R wave taller than the S is deep (R dominance) is normal in V_5 and V_6 but may suggest right ventricular strain or posterior MI if seen in V_1 and V_2.

Table 3.1 ECG territories

ECG leads	Heart territory	Coronary artery
I, aVL, V_{4-6}	Lateral	Circumflex
V_{1-3}	Anteroseptal	Left anterior descending
II, III, aVF	Inferior	Right coronary artery in 80% Circumflex in 20%: 'left dominant'
V_{7-9}	Posterior	Circumflex

▶To detect posterior infarcts, which are often associated with inferior or lateral wall MI, posterior ECG leads (V_7–V_9) are applied by moving V_4–V_6 to under the left scapula. Consider if ST depression in V_{1-3} or R/S amplitude ratio in V_1 or V_2 is >1. See fig 3.29, p117.

The 'upside-down' changes seen in posterior MI are called *reciprocal changes*: changes that appear when 'looking' at ischaemic myocardium from the other side of the heart. These can arise with MIs in other locations (fig 3.12). They are particularly important in posterior MI as they may be the only changes on the 12-lead ECG.

▶See figs 3.12, 3.13, 3.29 for example ECGs. See fig 3.22 for coronary artery anatomy.

3 Cardiovascular medicine

▶ **The right-sided ECG for the right diagnosis**
(fig 3.9) If you suspect RV infarction, which complicates up to 40% of inferior MIs, place leads V_1–V_6 in a mirror-image position on the right side of the chest. Consider if patient is hypotensive, ST elevation in lead III > II, ST elevation in V_1 and ST depression in V_2 (highly specific for RV infarction), or isoelectric ST segment in V_1 with marked ST depression in V_2.

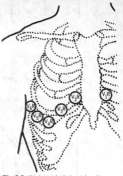

Fig 3.9 Right-sided chest leads.

QRS complexes: the long and the short

QRS complexes represent ventricular depolarization, and width represents time, so a broader QRS complex means depolarization is taking longer. Normally, a wave of depolarization reaches the ventricles via the specialist conduction pathways—the bundles of His, which ensures rapid efficient spread of charge. Hence, the QRS complex is narrow (<120ms). The septum depolarizes first, left to right, giving rise to a small Q wave in V_6. Next there is rapid simultaneous depolarization of both ventricles, from apex to outflow tracts, but voltage-wise this is dominated by the larger left ventricle, hence the S wave in V_6. Ventricular depolarization takes longer when depolarization is not initiated in this pattern. For example, if it originates in the ventricles (eg ventricular ectopics, VT) or if one or more branches of the bundles of His are blocked—bundle branch blocks—meaning depolarization is initiated in one ventricle but not the other, so it has to travel the long (in time and space) path from one ventricle to the other.

Ventricular depolarization also takes longer if all conduction is slowed. This may happen in some electrolyte imbalances, eg hyperkalaemia.

Right bundle branch block (p94, fig 3.11) QRS >0.12s, 'RSR' pattern in V_1; dominant R in V_1; inverted T waves in V_1–V_3 or V_4; wide, slurred S wave in V_6. Causes: normal variant (isolated RBBB), pulmonary embolism, cor pulmonale.

Left bundle branch block (p93, fig 3.10) QRS >0.12s, 'M' pattern in V_5, dominant S in V_1, inverted T waves in I, aVL, V_5–V_6. Causes: IHD, hypertension, cardiomyopathy, idiopathic fibrosis. ▶NB: if there is LBBB, no comment can be made on the ST segment or T wave. ▶▶New LBBB may represent a STEMI, see p782. Difficult to interpret ST-T segment changes in this context, see BOX on Sgarbossa criteria.

Bifascicular block The combination of RBBB and left bundle hemiblock, manifest as an axis deviation, eg left axis deviation in the case of left anterior hemiblock.

Trifascicular block Bifascicular block plus 1st-degree HB. ▶▶Both bifascicular and trifascicular block are important causes of syncope that may need pacing (p128).

Suspect left ventricular hypertrophy (LVH) If the R wave in V_6 is >25mm or the sum of the S wave in V_1 and the R wave in V_6 is >35mm (see fig 3.25, p111).

Suspect right ventricular hypertrophy (RVH) If dominant R wave in V_1, T-wave inversion in V_1–V_3 or V_4, deep S wave in V_6, right axis deviation.

Other causes of dominant R wave in V_1 RBBB, posterior MI, type A WPW syndrome (p129).

Causes of low-voltage QRS complex (QRS <5mm in all limb leads.) Hypothyroidism, chronic obstructive pulmonary disease (COPD), ↑haematocrit (intracardiac blood resistivity is related to haematocrit), changes in chest wall impedance (eg in renal failure & subcutaneous emphysema but not obesity), pulmonary embolism, bundle branch block, carcinoid heart disease, myocarditis, cardiac amyloid, doxorubicin cardiotoxicity, and other heart muscle diseases, pericardial effusion, pericarditis.

J wave See p831. The J point is where the S wave finishes and ST segment starts. A J wave is a notch at this point. Seen in hypothermia, SAH, and ↑Ca^{2+}.

See lifeinthefastlane.com for excellent ECG tutorials, cases, and examples.

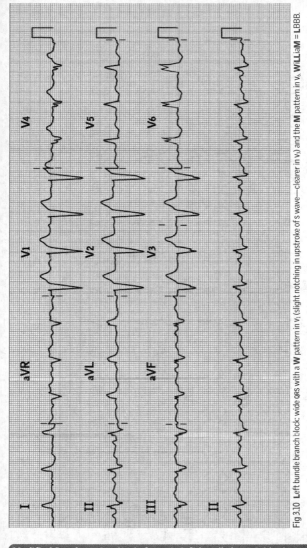

Fig 3.10 Left bundle branch block: wide QRS with a **W** pattern in V₁ (slight notching in upstroke of S wave—clearer in V₃) and the **M** pattern in V₆. WiLLiaM = LBBB.

Modified Sgarbossa's criteria for MI in left bundle branch block

- ≥1 leads with ≥1mm of concordant ST elevation.
- ≥1 leads of V₁–V₃ with ≥1mm of concordant ST depression.
- ≥1 leads anywhere with ≥1mm ST elevation and proportionally excessive discordant ST elevation, as defined by 25% or greater of the depth of the preceding S wave.
- Yes to any criteria has an 80% sensitivity and 99% specificity in diagnosis of acute MI in the context of known LBBB.[5]

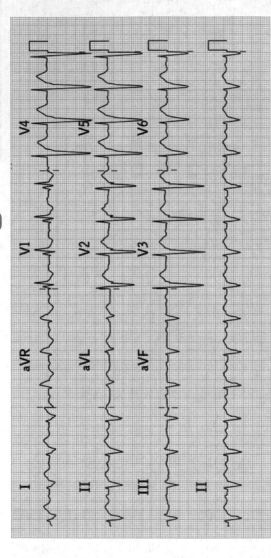

Fig 3.11 **Right bundle branch block**—broad QRS, **M** pattern in v₁ and sloped S wave (with the eye of faith, a '**W**' shape) in v₆. **MaRRoW** = RBBB.

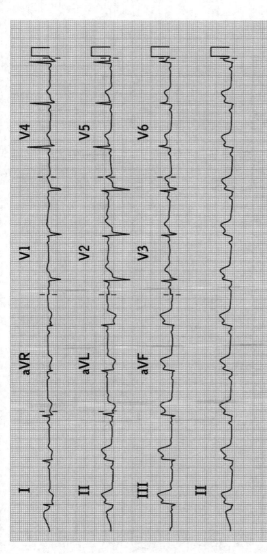

Fig 3.12 Acute inferolateral myocardial infarction: marked ST elevation in the inferior leads (II, III, aVF), but also in V₅ and V₆, indicating lateral involvement. There is a 'reciprocal change' of ST-segment depression in leads I and aVL; this is often seen with a large inferior myocardial infarction.

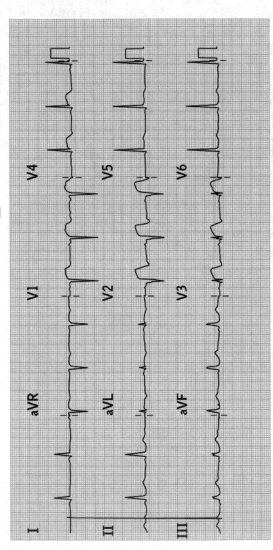

Fig 3.13 Acute anterior myocardial infarction—ST segment elevation and evolving Q-waves (the first QRS deflection is negative) in leads V₁₋₄.

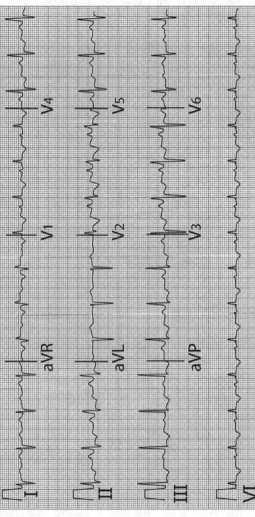

Fig 3.14 Changes seen in pulmonary hypertension (eg after a ᴾE).
- Right axis deviation (QRS more negative than positive in lead I).
- Positive QRS complexes ('dominant R-waves') in V₁ and V₂ suggesting right ventricular hypertrophy.
- ST depression and T-wave inversion in the right precordial leads (V₁₋₃) suggesting right ventricular strain.
- Peaked P waves (P pulmonale) suggesting right atrial hypertrophy.

 3 Cardiovascular medicine

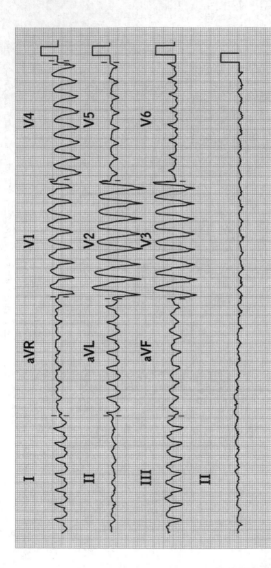

Fig 3.15 Ventricular tachycardia—regular broad complex tachycardia indicating a likely ventricular origin for the rhythm.

3 Cardiovascular medicine

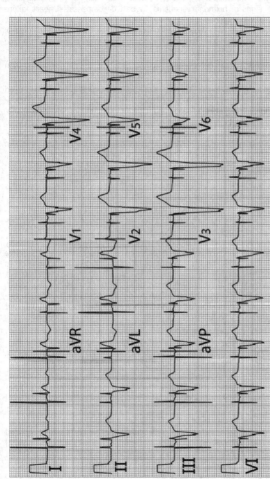

Fig 3.16 Dual-chamber pacemaker. Pacing spikes occur before each P wave and each QRS complex. QRS complexes are broad with a LBBB morphology, indicating the presence of a ventricular pacing electrode in the right ventricle. The absence of paced complexes does not always mean pacemaker failure as it may reflect satisfactory native conduction.

Reproduced from Myerson et al., Emergencies in Cardiology, 2012, with permission from Oxford University Press.

There are many heart conditions associated with structural defects, eg valve defects, congenital heart diseases, and some muscle disorders (eg hypertrophic cardiomyopathy (HCM)). Whilst clues to these can sometimes be found on history, examination, and ECG, it is imaging that gives the diagnosis.

Chest x-ray An enlarged heart (cardiothoracic ratio >0.5) suggests congestive heart failure; signs of pulmonary oedema suggest decompensated heart failure (see fig 3.46, p135); a globular heart may indicate pericardial effusion (fig 3.17); metal wires and valves will show up, evidencing previous cardiothoracic surgery; dextrocardia may explain a bizarre ECG; and rib notching may be an important clue in coarctation of the aorta (p148).

Lung ultrasound This can detect pulmonary oedema with greater sensitivity than a CXR and can be a useful adjunctive tool for the diagnosis of acute heart failure.[6]

Echocardiography This is the workhorse of cardiac imaging. Ultrasound is used to give real-time images of the moving heart. This can be transthoracic (TTE) or transoesophageal (TOE), at rest, during exercise, or after infusion of a pharmacological stressor (eg dobutamine). If the patient is too unwell to be moved, an echo machine can be brought to them and continuous TOE imaging may be used as a guide during surgery. Use of contrast can improve visualization of the endocardium in patients with poor acoustic windows and allow some estimation of myocardial perfusion. Contrast studies with Valsalva manoeuvre should be considered to exclude paradoxical embolism through a cardiac shunt from the right heart. In patients with a high clinical suspicion of a cardiac source of embolism, in whom TTE is normal, TOE is recommended. See p102.

Cardiac CT First line if stable anginal symptoms. This can provide detailed information about cardiac structure and function. CT angiography (fig 3.18) permits contrast-enhanced imaging of coronary arteries during a single breath hold with very low radiation doses. It can diagnose significant (>50%) stenosis in coronary artery disease with an accuracy of 89%. CT coronary angiography has a negative predictive value of >99%, which makes it an effective non-invasive alternative to routine transcatheter coronary angiography to rule out coronary artery disease. Medications are often given to slow the heart down and the imaging may be 'gated', meaning the scanner is programmed to take images at times corresponding to certain points on the patient's ECG. This allows characterization of the heart at different points in the cardiac cycle. See p724.

Coronary artery calcium screening With multidetector or multislice CT. Many limitations and generally only used in a select group of intermediate-risk patients.

Cardiac MR Cardiovascular MRI is the gold standard method for the three-dimensional (3D) analysis of cardiothoracic anatomy, the assessment of global and regional myocardial function, and viability imaging. MR is the first-choice imaging method to look at diseases that directly affect the myocardium (fig 3.19) and has high diagnostic accuracy for the identification of myocardial ischaemia. Patterns of late gadolinium enhancement can be helpful to diagnose cardiac amyloid, sarcoid, or myocarditis. Check pacemaker compatibility. See p724.

Myocardial perfusion scintigraphy with single photon emission computed tomography (MPS with SPECT) Offer if CT coronary angiography has shown CAD of uncertain functional significance or is non-diagnostic. Perfusion is assessed at rest and with exercise or pharmacologically induced stress. Minimally invasive and not dependent on overall exercise capacity, this test is particularly useful for assessing whether myocardium distal to a blockage is viable and so whether stenting or CABG will be of value. If hypoperfusion is 'fixed', ie present at rest and under stress, the hypoperfused area is probably scar tissue and so non-viable. If hypoperfusion is 're-versible' at rest, the myocardium may benefit from improved blood supply. See p725.

Positron emission tomography (PET). Better image quality and quantification of myocardial perfusion than MPS but very expensive. However, it is the gold standard for diagnosing cardiac sarcoidosis.

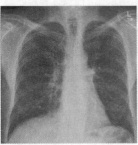
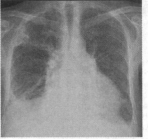

Fig 3.17 Two CXRs of the same patient, the one on the right was taken 6 months after the one on the left. On the later image, a pericardial effusion has expanded the cardiac shadow and given it a 'globular' shape.
Reproduced from Leeson, *Cardiovascular Imaging*, 2011, with permission from Oxford University Press.

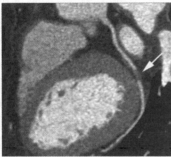
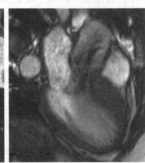

Fig 3.18 Cardiac CT demonstrating coronary artery stenosis.
Reproduced from Camm *et al.*, *ESC Textbook of Cardiovascular Medicine*, 2009, with permission from Oxford University Press.

Fig 3.19 Cardiac MRI demonstrating the asymmetrical left ventricular wall thickening typical of hypertrophic cardiomyopathy.
Reproduced from Myerson *et al.*, *Cardiovascular Magnetic Resonance*, 2013, with permission from Oxford University Press.

The story of Echo and Narcissus

Echo, in Greek mythology, was a mountain nymph, or Oread. Ovid's *Metamorphoses*, Book III, relates that Echo offended the goddess Hera by keeping her in conversation, thus preventing her from spying on her husband Zeus who was with another lover. To punish Echo, Hera deprived her of speech, except for the ability to repeat the last words of another. Echo's own hopeless love for the boy Narcissus, who fell in love with his own image, made her fade away until all that was left of her was her voice (fig 3.20).

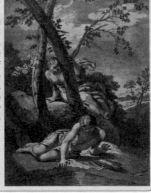

Fig 3.20 Narcissus and Echo.
Engraving by F. Bartolozzi, 1791, after B. Luti. Wellcome Collection. Public Domain Mark. Source: Wellcome Collection

This non-invasive technique uses the differing ability of various structures within the heart to reflect ultrasound waves. It not only demonstrates anatomy but also provides a continuous display of the functioning heart throughout its cycle.

Types of scan

M-mode (motion mode) A single-dimension image.

Two-dimensional (real time) A 2D, fan-shaped image of a segment of the heart is produced on the screen (fig 3.21); the moving image may be 'frozen'. Several views are possible, including parasternal long axis and short axis, apical 4-chamber, and subcostal. 2D echocardiography is good for visualizing conditions such as: congenital heart disease, LV aneurysm, mural thrombus, LA myxoma, septal defects.

3D echocardiography Now possible with matrix array probes, and is termed 4D (3D + time) if the images are moving.

Doppler and colour-flow echocardiography Different coloured jets illustrate flow and gradients across valves and septal defects (p148) (Doppler effect, p720).

Tissue Doppler imaging This employs Doppler ultrasound to measure the velocity of myocardial segments over the cardiac cycle. It is particularly useful for assessing longitudinal motion—and hence long-axis ventricular function, which is a sensitive marker of systolic and diastolic heart failure.

Contrast studies with Valsalva manoeuvre IV injection of saline after agitation between two syringes enhances the back-scatter of the ultrasound beam, thus highlighting venous blood flow. If the 'bubbles' generated are visualized in the left heart chambers, this can indicate either intracardiac or transpulmonary shunting.

Transoesophageal echocardiography (TOE) More sensitive than transthoracic echocardiography (TTE) as the transducer is nearer to the heart. Indications: diagnosing aortic dissections; assessing prosthetic valves; finding cardiac source of emboli; and IE/SBE. Contraindicated in oesophageal disease and cervical spine instability.

Stress echocardiography Used to evaluate ventricular function, ejection fraction, myocardial thickening, regional wall motion pre- and post-exercise, and to characterize valvular lesions. Dobutamine or dipyridamole may be used if the patient cannot exercise. Inexpensive and as sensitive/specific as a thallium scan (p725).

Uses of echocardiography

Quantification of global LV function Heart failure may be due to systolic or diastolic ventricular impairment (or both). Echo helps by measuring end-diastolic volume. If this is large, systolic dysfunction is the likely cause. If small, diastolic. Pure forms of diastolic dysfunction are rare. Differentiation is important because vasodilators are less useful in diastolic dysfunction as a high ventricular filling pressure is required.

Echo is also useful for detecting focal and global hypokinesia, LV aneurysm, mural thrombus, and LVH (echo is 5–10 times more sensitive than ECG in detecting this).

Estimating right heart haemodynamics Doppler studies of pulmonary artery flow and tricuspid regurgitation allow evaluation of RV function and pressures.

Valve disease The technique of choice for measuring pressure gradients and valve orifice areas in stenotic lesions. Detecting valvular regurgitation and estimating its significance is less accurate. Evaluating function of prosthetic valves is another role.

Congenital heart disease Establishing the presence of lesions, and significance.

Endocarditis Vegetations may not be seen if <2mm in size. TTE with colour Doppler is best for aortic regurgitation (AR). TOE is useful for visualizing mitral valve vegetations, leaflet perforation, or looking for an aortic root abscess.

Pericardial effusion Best diagnosed by echo. Fluid may first accumulate between the posterior pericardium and the left ventricle, then anterior to both ventricles and anterior and lateral to the right atrium. There may be paradoxical septal motion.

HCM (p130) Echo features include asymmetrical septal hypertrophy, small LV cavity, dilated left atrium, and systolic anterior motion of the mitral valve.

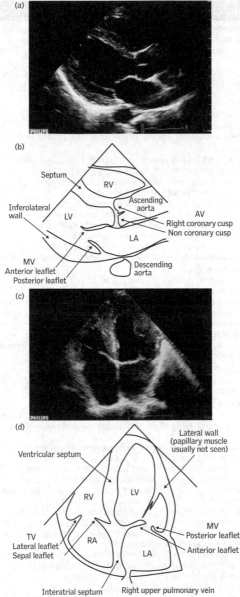

Fig 3.21 Echo images. (a) A normal heart seen with the parasternal long-axis view. (b) Diagram of what can be seen in (a). (c) A normal heart seen in apical four-chamber view. (d) Diagram of what can be seen in (c).

Reproduced from Leeson *et al.*, *Echocardiography*, 2012, with permission from Oxford University Press.

This involves the insertion of a catheter into the heart via the femoral or radial artery or venous system, and manipulating it within the heart and great vessels to:
- Inject radiopaque contrast medium to image cardiac anatomy and blood flow, see fig 3.22a.
- Perform angioplasty (ballooning and stenting), valvuloplasty (eg transcatheter aortic valve implantation (TAVI, fig 3.50, p141)), cardiac biopsies, transcatheter septal defect closure.
- Perform electrophysiology studies and radiofrequency ablations.
- Sample blood to assess oxygen saturation and measure pressures.
- Perform intravascular ultrasound or echocardiography.
- During the procedure, ECG and arterial pressures are monitored continuously.

Indications
- Coronary artery disease: diagnostic (assessment of coronary vessels and graft patency); therapeutic (angioplasty, stent insertion), see fig 3.22b.
- Valvular disease: diagnostic (pressures indicate severity); therapeutic valvuloplasty (if the patient is too ill or declines valve surgery).
- Congenital heart disease: diagnostic (assessment of severity of lesions by measuring pressures and saturations); therapeutic (balloon dilatation or septostomy).
- Other: cardiomyopathy; pericardial disease (constriction indicated by equalization of all intracardiac diastolic pressure); endomyocardial biopsy.
- Right heart catheterization: to confirm pulmonary hypertension in select cases, assess contribution of left heart disease, vasoreactive testing before therapy.

Pre-procedure checks
- Brief history/examination; NB: peripheral pulses, bruits, aneurysms.
- Investigations: FBC, U&E, LFT, clotting screen, CXR, ECG. IV access, ideally in left hand.
- Consent for procedure, including possible extra procedures, eg consent for angioplasty if you plan to do angiography as you may find a lesion that needs stenting. Explain reason for procedure and possible complications.
- Patient should be nil by mouth (NBM) from 6h before the procedure.
- Patients should take all their morning drugs (and pre-medication if needed)—but withhold oral hypoglycaemics.

Post-procedure checks
- Pulse, BP, arterial puncture site (for bruising or swelling), foot pulses.
- Investigations: FBC and clotting (if suspected blood loss), ECG.

Complications
- Haemorrhage: apply firm pressure over puncture site. If you suspect a false aneurysm, ultrasound the swelling and consider surgical repair. Haematomas are high risk for infections.
- Contrast reaction: this is usually mild with modern contrast agents.
- Loss of peripheral pulse: may be due to dissection, thrombosis, or arterial spasm. Occurs in <1% of radial catheterizations. Rare with femoral catheterization.
- Angina: may occur during or after cardiac catheterization. Usually responds to sublingual GTN; if not, give analgesia and IV nitrates. MI in <0.1% of cases.
- Arrhythmias: usually transient. Manage along standard lines.
- Pericardial effusion: suspect if unexplained continued chest pain. Arrange for urgent echo. May need drain depending on severity and haemodynamic status.
- Pericardial tamponade: rare, but should be suspected if the patient becomes hypotensive and anuric. ▶▶Urgent pericardial drain.
- Stroke: complicates 0.4% of cases. Can be ischaemic or haemorrhagic.
- Infection: post-catheter pyrexia is usually due to a contrast reaction. If it persists for >24h, take blood cultures before giving antibiotics.

Mortality <1 in 1000 patients, in most centres.

Intracardiac electrophysiology This catheter technique can determine types and origins of arrhythmias, and locate and ablate problem areas, eg aberrant pathways in WPW or arrhythmogenic foci. Arrhythmias may be induced, and the effectiveness of control by drugs assessed.

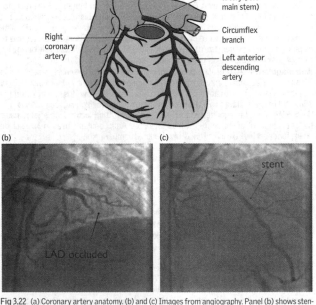

Fig 3.22 (a) Coronary artery anatomy. (b) and (c) Images from angiography. Panel (b) shows stenosis of the left anterior descending artery (LAD). In (c), the same patient has had their LAD stented, allowing contrast to flow freely through to the distal vessel. The stenting is a type of angioplasty (a procedure to widen the lumen of a blood vessel); in the context of coronary arteries, it is called PCI (percutaneous coronary intervention). PPCI (primary PCI) is PCI performed acutely for a patient with acute coronary syndrome (ACS), see p116.

Images (b) and (c) reproduced from Ramrakha *et al.*, *Oxford Handbook of Cardiology*, 2012, with permission from Oxford University Press.

Urine my heart

In 1929, fresh out of medical school, Werner Forssmann, a 25-year-old surgical trainee, performed the first cardiac catheterization on himself using a 65cm-long urethral catheter inserted via his left cubital vein. He then walked to the x-ray department, where a photograph was taken of the catheter lying in his right auricle. After rejection from a career in academic cardiology because of this style of self-experimentation, he ended up becoming a urologist. His seminal work on cardiac catheterization was later recognized when he was jointly awarded the Nobel Prize in Physiology or Medicine in 1956.

Antiplatelet drugs Aspirin irreversibly acetylates cyclo-oxygenase, preventing production of thromboxane A_2, thereby inhibiting platelet aggregation. Used in low dose (eg 75mg/24h PO) for secondary prevention following MI, TIA/stroke, and for patients with angina or peripheral vascular disease. Indicated for primary prevention in only select group as harms (bleeding risk) may outweigh benefits.[7,8] ADP receptor antagonists (eg clopidogrel, prasugrel, ticagrelor) also block platelet aggregation, but may cause less gastric irritation. They have a role if truly intolerant of aspirin; with aspirin after PCI; and in acute coronary syndrome. Ticagrelor may be preferable to clopidogrel.[9] Glycoprotein IIb/IIIa antagonists (eg tirofiban) may have a role during PCI for high-risk patients with ongoing ischaemia or large thrombus burden.

Anticoagulants See p346. Direct oral anticoagulants (DOACs, previously NOACs), eg Xa inhibitors (eg apixaban) and direct thrombin inhibitors (dabigatran), are increasingly replacing warfarin for treatment of AF and clots, see p346. Low-dose rivaroxaban (eg 2.5mg BD) may also have a role in secondary CVD prevention in high-risk polyvascular patients.[10] Warfarin (antagonizes vitamin K-dependent clotting factor synthesis) remains the anticoagulant of choice for mechanical valves. Anticoagulants used in ACS include LMWH, fondaparinux (Xa inhibitor), & bivalirudin (thrombin inhibitor).

β-blockers Block β-adrenoceptors. Blocking $β_1$-receptors is negatively inotropic and chronotropic; blocking $β_2$-receptors induces peripheral vasoconstriction and bronchoconstriction. Drugs vary in their $β_1/β_2$ selectivity (eg propranolol is non-selective, and bisoprolol relatively $β_1$ selective), but this does not seem to alter their clinical efficacy. **Uses** Angina, hypertension, anti-dysrhythmic, post-MI (↓mortality), heart failure (with caution). CI Severe asthma/COPD, heart block. SE Lethargy, erectile dysfunction, ↓joie de vivre, nightmares, headache.

ACE inhibitors (ACE-I)/angiotensin receptor antagonists (ARAs) These are used in hypertension, heart failure, and post-MI. Monitor U&E when starting (after 1–2 weeks) or raising ACE-i dose, a creatinine rise of >20% is concerning and associated with worse cardiorenal outcomes and mortality[11]—these patients should be monitored closely. If renal function deteriorates markedly, consider investigating for renal artery stenosis. Hold in AKI and hyperkalaemia. Teach patients 'sick day rules'—avoid if fever, vomiting, diarrhoea, etc. SE Include dry cough (switch to ARA) and urticaria.

Angiotensin receptor–neprilysin inhibitor (ARNI) A replacement for ACE-i/ARA in chronic symptomatic heart failure with ↓EF. May further reduce morbidity and mortality. Ensure adequate BP and GFR >30 before starting.[12]

Diuretics
- *Loop diuretics* (eg furosemide) are used in heart failure, and inhibit the Na/2Cl/K co-transporter. SE: volume depletion, ↓Na^+, ↓K^+, ↓Ca^{2+}, ototoxic.
- *Thiazides* and thiazide-like diuretics are used in hypertension (eg chlortalidone) and heart failure (eg metolazone). SE: ↓Na^+, ↓K^+, ↑Ca^{2+}, ↓Mg^{2+}, ↑urate (±gout), impotence. (NB: small doses, eg chlortalidone 25mg/24h rarely cause significant SE.)
- *Potassium-sparing diuretics:* aldosterone antagonists (eg spironolactone, eplerenone) directly block aldosterone receptors; amiloride blocks the epithelial sodium channel in the distal convoluted tubule.

Vasodilators Used in heart failure, IHD, and hypertension. Nitrates (p112) preferentially dilate veins and large arteries, ↓ filling pressure (pre-load), while hydralazine (often used with nitrates) primarily dilates the resistance vessels, thus ↓ BP (afterload). Hydralazine + nitrates are better at ↓ mortality than ACE-i for black patients.

Calcium channel antagonists These ↓ cell entry of Ca^{2+} via voltage-sensitive channels in smooth muscle, thereby promoting coronary and peripheral vasodilation and reducing myocardial oxygen consumption. All current drugs block L-type Ca^{2+} channels. However, their effects differ because of differential binding properties.
- *The dihydropyridines*, eg nifedipine, amlodipine, are mainly peripheral vasodilators (also dilate coronary arteries) and cause a reflex tachycardia, so are often used with a β-blocker. They are used mainly in hypertension and angina.
- *The non-dihydropyridines*—verapamil and diltiazem—also slow conduction at the AV and SA nodes and may be used to treat hypertension, angina, and dysrhythmias. Δ Don't give non-dihydropyridines with β-blockers (risk of severe bradycardia ± LVF).

SE Flushes, headache, ankle oedema (diuretic unresponsive), ↓LV function, gingival hypertrophy. **CI** Heart block, heart failure.

Digoxin Blocks the Na⁺/K⁺ pump. It is used to slow the pulse in fast AF (p126). As a weak +ve inotrope, it has been shown to improve symptoms, quality of life, and hospitalizations in heart failure but not mortality; its routine use is not recommended due to its narrow therapeutic window.[13] Elderly people are at ↑risk of toxicity: use lower doses. Measure plasma levels >6h post-dose (p740). **Typical dose** 500mcg stat PO, repeated after 12h, then 125mcg (if elderly) to 250mcg/d PO OD. IV dose: 0.25–0.5mg in 100ml of 0.9% NaCl over 2h. ↑Toxicity risk if: ↓K⁺, ↓Mg²⁺, or ↑Ca²⁺. **SE** Any arrhythmia, nausea, ↓appetite, yellow vision, confusion, gynaecomastia. If toxicity is suspected, do an ECG (fig 3.23), digoxin levels, and check K⁺, Mg²⁺, and Ca²⁺. If toxicity is confirmed, stop digoxin, correct electrolyte imbalances, treat arrhythmias, and consider antidote with antibody (Fab) fragments, eg IV DigiFab® (p826). **CI** HCM; WPW syndrome (p129).

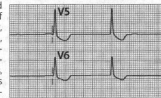

Fig 3.23 Classic 'reverse tick' associated with digoxin use: downsloping ST wave with rapid upstroke back to isoelectric line.

Sodium channel blockers Class I anti-arrhythmics. Procainamide (1a) and lidocaine (1b) can be used to terminate VT. **NB:** QT interval may be prolonged. Flecainide (1c) is useful for AF cardioversion if no CI, and for prophylaxis in patients with WPW or troublesome paroxysmal AF. **CI** Heart failure, IHD, valve disease, and heart block.

Amiodarone A class III anti-arrhythmic. Amiodarone prolongs the cardiac action potential, reducing the potential for tachyarrhythmias. Used in both supraventricular and ventricular tachycardias, including during cardiac arrest. Broad range of side effects, eg thyroid disease, liver disease, pulmonary fibrosis and peripheral neuropathy. Monitor TFTs and LFTs every 6 months.

Ivabradine Selective sinus node inhibitor, slowing pulse rate without significantly dropping blood pressure. Used in angina, heart failure, and (off licence) in autonomic tachycardia syndromes. No role in atrial tachycardia. **CI** Acute MI, bradycardia, long QT syndrome, shock. Many drug interactions, including with calcium antagonists.

Statins Statins (eg simvastatin, p682) inhibit the enzyme HMG-CoA reductase, which causes *de novo* synthesis of cholesterol in the liver. This increases LDL receptor expression by hepatocytes leading to ↓circulating LDL cholesterol. More effective if given at night, but optimum dose and target plasma cholesterol are unknown. **SE** Muscle aches, abdominal discomfort, ↑transaminases (eg ALT), ↑CK, myositis, rarely rhabdomyolysis (more common if used with fibrates). Statins are generally well tolerated. See also hyperlipidaemia, pp682–3, fig 14.12.

PCSK9 Inhibitors Reduce LDL receptor degradation. Expensive, but very effective. ↓ LDL cholesterol when combined with statin, eg alirocumab SC injection 2-weekly.

Anti-anginal drugs See p112. **Antihypertensives** See p110. **SGLT2 inhibitors** See p138. **Inotropes** See p787.

Drugs that slow conduction through the atrioventricular node

Drugs that slow conduction through the atrioventricular node (AVN) include digoxin, verapamil, and adenosine. Uses include cardioverting atrioventricular nodal re-entry tachycardia (AVNRT) and diagnosing atrial tachycardias.

Drugs that slow AVN conduction should be avoided in patients with aberrant pathways (eg WPW) as blocking the AVN can increase conduction via the alternative pathways. AVN blockers are contraindicated in patients with or at risk of VT, eg those with long QT syndrome.

Hypertension is the most important risk factor for premature death and CVD; causing ~50% of all vascular deaths (8 million per year). Usually asymptomatic, so regular screening (eg yearly) is a *vital* task—most preventable deaths are in areas without universal screening.

Defining hypertension BP has a skewed normal distribution (p735) within the population, and risk is continuously related to BP, so it is impossible to define 'hypertension' and guidelines differ in terms of thresholds.[14] There has been a general shift in clinical practice now to treat if ≥140/90mmHg, particularly if other CV risk factors present. Don't rely on a single reading—assess over a period of time. Confirm with 24h ambulatory BP monitoring (ABPM); or a week of home readings.

Whom to treat All with clinic BP ≥140/90mmHg (≥135/85mmHg on 24h ABPM) or ≥130/80mmHg if <65 years or CV risk factors present (eg diabetes, CKD, proteinuria) and see fig 3.24.[15] The HYVET study showed that there is even substantial benefit in treating the over-80s.[16] Guidelines are concordant in their recommendation to discuss with individual patients about their CV risk and the benefits of further lowering BP to <130/80mmHg.[17] Consider downstream benefits—likely ↓ dementia.

White-coat hypertension Refers to an elevated *clinic* pressure, but normal ABPM (day average <130/80mmHg). Associated with ↑risk of CVD and all-cause mortality.[18] Lifestyle modifications should be instituted and home BP readings strongly encouraged to monitor for the development of sustained hypertension.

'Malignant' or accelerated phase hypertension (p778; fig 3.25, p111) A rapid rise in BP leading to vascular damage (pathological hallmark is fibrinoid necrosis). Usually there is severe hypertension (eg systolic >200, diastolic >120mmHg) + bilateral retinal haemorrhages and exudates; papilloedema may or may not be present. Symptoms are common, eg headache ± visual disturbance. It requires urgent treatment, and may also precipitate acute kidney injury, heart failure, or encephalopathy, which are hypertensive emergencies. Untreated, 90% die in 1yr; treated, 70% survive 5yrs. It is more common in younger and in black subjects. Look hard for any underlying cause.

Primary or 'essential' hypertension Cause unknown, ~95% of cases.

Secondary hypertension ~5% of cases. Consider if severe/resistant, abrupt rise, <30yrs if no risk factors, presents with hypertensive emergency, or associated with electrolyte abnormalities (eg ↓K+, metabolic alkalosis). Causes include:
- *Kidney disease:* the most common secondary cause. 75% are from *intrinsic kidney disease:* glomerulonephritis, polyarteritis nodosa (PAN), systemic sclerosis, chronic pyelonephritis, or polycystic kidneys. 25% are due to *renovascular disease*, most frequently atheromatous (elderly ♂ cigarette smokers, eg with peripheral vascular disease) or rarely fibromuscular dysplasia (young ♀).
- *Endocrine disease:* Cushing's (p218) and Conn's syndromes (p222), bilateral adrenal hyperplasia, phaeochromocytoma (p222), acromegaly, hyperparathyroidism.
- *Others:* coarctation (p148), pregnancy (OHCS p35), liquorice, drugs: steroids, MAOI, oral contraceptive pill, cocaine, amphetamines.

Signs and symptoms Usually asymptomatic (except malignant hypertension, see earlier in topic). Headache is no more common than in the general population. Always examine the CVS fully and check for retinopathy. Are there features of an underlying cause (phaeochromocytoma, p222, etc.), signs of renal disease, radiofemoral delay, or weak femoral pulses (coarctation), renal bruits, palpable kidneys, or Cushing's syndrome? Look for end-organ damage: LVH, retinopathy and proteinuria—indicates severity and duration of hypertension and associated with a poorer prognosis.

Tests To confirm diagnosis ABPM or home BP monitoring. To help quantify overall risk Fasting glucose, cholesterol, eGFR. To look for end-organ damage ECG or echo (any LV hypertrophy? past MI?); urinalysis (protein, blood). To 'exclude' secondary causes U&E (eg ↓K+ in hyperaldosteronism); Ca2+ (↑ in hyperparathyroidism); plasma metnoradrenaline/adrenaline (p222); renin & aldosterone. **Special tests** CTA or MRA (renal artery stenosis), 24hr urinary free cortisol (p219) or overnight dexamethasone suppression test; MR aorta (coarctation).

Grading hypertensive retinopathy

I Tortuous arteries with thick shiny walls (silver or copper wiring, p558, fig 12.19).
II AV nipping (narrowing where arteries cross veins, p558, fig 12.20).
III Flame haemorrhages and cotton-wool spots.
IV Papilloedema, p558, fig 12.21.

Measuring BP with a sphygmomanometer

• Use the correct size cuff. The cuff width should be >40% of the arm circumference. The bladder should be centred over the brachial artery, and the cuff applied snugly. Support the arm in a horizontal position at mid-sternal level.
• Inflate the cuff while palpating the brachial artery, until the pulse disappears. This provides an estimate of systolic pressure.
• Inflate the cuff until 30mmHg above systolic pressure, then place stethoscope over the brachial artery. Deflate the cuff at 2mmHg/s.
• *Systolic pressure:* appearance of sustained repetitive tapping sounds (Korotkoff I).
• *Diastolic pressure:* usually the disappearance of sounds (Korotkoff V). However, in some individuals (eg pregnant women) sounds are present until the zero point. In this case, the muffling of sounds, Korotkoff IV, should be used. State which is used for a given reading. For children, see *OHCS* p267.
• For advice on using automated sphygmomanometers and a list of validated devices, see http://www.bhsoc.org/latest-guidelines/how-to-measure-blood-pressure/

Managing suspected hypertension

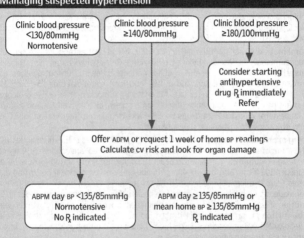

Fig 3.24 Managing suspected hypertension based on the 2019 NICE guidelines.[19]
Source: data from NICE CG127, https://www.nice.org.uk/guidance/cg127/resources/
hypertension-in-adultsdiagnosis-and-management-35109454941637.

3 Cardiovascular medicine

Look for and treat underlying causes (eg kidney disease, ↑alcohol: see fig 3.24, p109 & p112). Drug therapy reduces the risk of CVD and death. Almost any adult over 50 would benefit from antihypertensives, whatever their starting BP.[20] Essential hypertension is not 'curable' and long-term treatment is needed. Emphasize the importance of compliance and regular home BP monitoring.

Treatment goal <140/90mmHg (possibly <130/80 in selected cases, eg <40 years). Reduce BP *slowly*; rapid reduction can be fatal, especially in the context of an acute stroke. ▶▶See p778 for treatment of malignant hypertension/emergencies.

Lifestyle changes ↓Concomitant risk factors: stop smoking; low-fat diet. ↓ Alcohol and salt intake; ↑ exercise; ↓ weight if obese.

Drugs The ALLHAT trial supports the view that adequate BP reduction is more important than the specific drug used.[21] However, β-blockers were not included in the trial, and meta-analyses suggest they are less effective than other drugs at reducing major cardiovascular events, particularly stroke. Ethnicity also appears to be important, as chlortalidone is generally better at preventing events than other drugs in black patients. Many patients will require combination therapy (if >20/10mmHg above their BP target)—ideally use a single-pill strategy (caution if frail or elderly).

Monotherapy First-line agents include ACE-i, ARB, Ca²⁺-channel antagonist, and thiazide diuretics. ACE-i or ARB *may* be more effective in younger patients and have additional benefits in patients with diabetes or CKD. Conversely, thiazides (chlortalidone/indapamide) and Ca²⁺-channel antagonists are favoured in older or black patients. β-blockers are not 1st line for hypertension, but consider in patients with coexisting coronary artery disease, or stable HF.

Combination ℞ ACE-i + thiazide or ACE-i + Ca²⁺-channel antagonist are sensible dual combinations followed by ACE-i + thiazide + Ca²⁺-channel antagonist. Thiazide diuretics are particularly useful in obese patients. If BP still uncontrolled on adequate doses of three drugs, add a 4th—consider: spironolactone 25–50mg/24h or amiloride 10mg, but monitor U&E. Alternatively, β-blocker, or selective α-blocker and get help. Check compliance (urinary drug screen, or observed ℞). Add a *statin* if cholesterol raised. ▶Most drugs take 4–8wks to gain maximum effect: don't assess efficacy with just one BP measurement.

Drug examples Thiazides eg chlortalidone 25–50mg/24h PO in the morning. SE: ↓K⁺, ↓Na⁺, impotence. CI: gout. **Ca²⁺-channel antagonists** eg amlodipine 5–10mg OD. SE: fatigue, gum hyperplasia, ankle oedema; DO NOT use short-acting form. ACE-i eg lisinopril 10–40mg/24h PO (max 40mg/d). ACE-i may be 1st choice if coexisting diabetes (esp. if microalbuminuria, p310) or proteinuria. SE: cough, ↑K⁺, renal failure, angioedema. CI: bilateral renal artery stenosis; p106. ARB Candesartan (8–32mg/d); caution if valve disease or hypertrophic cardiomyopathy; monitor K⁺. SE: vertigo, urticaria, pruritus. Useful if ACE-i induces cough. **β-blockers** eg bisoprolol 2.5–5mg/24h PO. SE: bronchospasm, heart failure, cold peripheries, lethargy, impotence. CI: asthma; caution in heart failure.

Always think about secondary hypertension...

A casual conversation about lifestyle led a 40-year-old woman who had been seen for 4 years by hypertension specialists to reveal that she was addicted to *mighty imps*—liquorice sweets containing glycyrrhizinic acid which inhibits the enzyme HSD-11β. This protects the mineralocorticoid receptor from endogenous cortisol... Sure enough her BP returned to normal on stopping the *mighty imps*.

A 38-year-old pregnant normotensive woman complained of palpitations. Plasma metadrenalines were 10-fold elevated. On questioning, she complained of long-standing headaches and feeling cold all the time, 'pre-eclampsia' in her pregnancy 10 years ago followed by a cardiac arrest. Sure enough, she had a large phaeochromocytoma. This is one of the rare occasions that patients with hypertension experience symptoms—unfortunately, rather non-specific ones at that.

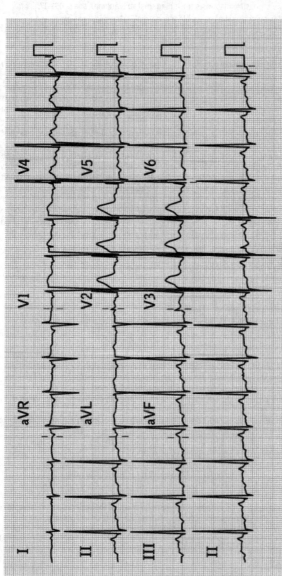

Fig 3.25 Left ventricular hypertrophy—this is from a patient with malignant hypertension—note the sum of the S wave in V₁ and R wave in v₅ is greater than 35mm (Sokolow–Lyon criteria). Other criteria include the presence of an R wave in aVL ≥11mm (Sokolow–Lyon criteria) or if the S wave in v₃ >28mm in men or >20mm in women (Cornell criteria).

▶If ACS is a possible diagnosis (including unstable angina), see pp114–17.

Angina[22] is symptomatic reversible myocardial ischaemia. Features:
1 Constricting/heavy discomfort to the chest, jaw, neck, shoulders, or arms.
2 Symptoms brought on by exertion.
3 Symptoms relieved within 5min by rest or glyceryl trinitrate (GTN).

All 3 features = *typical angina*; 2 features = *atypical angina*; 0–1 features = *non-anginal chest pain*.

Other precipitants: emotion, cold weather, and heavy meals. *Associated symptoms:* dyspnoea, nausea, sweatiness, faintness. *Features that make angina less likely:* pain that is continuous, pleuritic, or worse with swallowing; pain associated with palpitations, dizziness or tingling.

Causes Atheroma. Rarely: anaemia; coronary artery spasm; AS; tachyarrhythmias; HCM; arteritis/small vessel disease (microvascular angina/cardiac syndrome X).

Types of angina Stable angina Induced by effort, relieved by rest. Good prognosis. **Unstable angina** (Crescendo angina.) Angina of increasing frequency or severity; occurs on minimal exertion or at rest; associated with ↑↑risk of MI. **Decubitus angina** Precipitated by lying flat. **Variant (Prinzmetal) angina** (BOX 'Vasospastic angina') Caused by coronary artery spasm (rare; may coexist with fixed stenoses).

Tests ECG usually normal, but may show ST depression; flat or inverted T waves; signs of past MI. **Blood tests** FBC, U&E, TFTs, lipids, HbA1c. Consider *echo* and CXR. **Further investigations** are usually necessary to confirm an IHD diagnosis—see BOX 'Investigating patients'.

Management

Address exacerbating factors Anaemia, tachycardia (eg fast AF), thyrotoxicosis.

Secondary prevention of cardiovascular disease
• Stop smoking; exercise; dietary advice; optimize hypertension and diabetes control.
• 75mg aspirin daily if not contraindicated.
• Address hyperlipidaemia—see p682.
• Consider ACE-i, especially if hypertensive or diabetic.

PRN **symptom relief** GTN spray or sublingual tabs. Advise the patient to repeat the dose if the pain has not gone after 5min and to call an ambulance if the pain is still present 5min after the second dose. SE: headaches, ↓BP.

Anti-anginal medication (p106) First line: β-blocker and/or calcium channel blocker (▶do not combine β-blockers with non-dihydropyridine calcium antagonists). If these fail to control symptoms or are not tolerated, trial other agents.
• *β-blockers:* eg atenolol 50mg BD or bisoprolol 5–10mg OD.
• *Calcium antagonists:* amlodipine—start at 5mg OD; diltiazem—dose depends on formulation.
• *Long-acting nitrates:* eg isosorbide mononitrate—starting regimen depends on formulation. Alternatives: GTN skin patches. SE: headaches, ↓BP.
• *Ranolazine:* inhibits late Na⁺ current. Start at 375mg BD. Caution if heart failure, elderly, weight <60kg, or prolonged QT interval.
• *Ivabradine:* reduces heart rate with minimal impact on BP. Patient must be in sinus rhythm. Start with 5mg BD. Only consider if clinical HF also present.
• *Nicorandil:* a K⁺ channel activator. Start with 5–10mg BD. CI: acute pulmonary oedema, severe hypotension, hypovolaemia, LV failure.

Revascularization Considered when optimal medical therapy proves inadequate or if likely to derive survival benefit, eg left main or triple vessel disease.
• *Percutaneous coronary intervention (PCI)* (p104): a balloon is inflated inside the stenosed vessel to open the lumen. A stent is usually inserted to reduce the risk of re-stenosis. Dual antiplatelet therapy (DAPT; usually aspirin and clopidogrel) is recommended for at least 12 months after stent insertion to reduce the risk of in-stent thrombosis. Seek specialist advice regarding antiplatelets if the patient has a high bleeding risk or requires surgery.
• *CABG* (p119) compared to PCI, patients undergoing CABG are less likely to need repeat revascularization and those with multivessel disease can expect better outcomes. However, recovery is slower.

Investigating patients with possible stable angina

Investigations for ischaemic heart disease (IHD) include:
• Exercise ECG—assess for ischaemic ECG changes.
• Angiography—either using cardiac CT with contrast, or transcatheter angiography (more invasive but can be combined with stenting, p104).
• Functional imaging (p102): myocardial perfusion scintigraphy, stress echo (echo whilst undergoing exercise or receiving dobutamine), cardiac MRI.

NICE recommends the following investigations when considering stable angina.[23]

Typical angina in a patient with previously proven IHD
Treat as stable angina; if further confirmation is required, use non-invasive testing, eg exercise ECG. Offer non-invasive functional testing when there is uncertainty about whether chest pain is caused by myocardial ischaemia.

Typical and atypical angina
CT angiography, fig 3.26. If inconclusive, use functional imaging as 2nd line and transcatheter angiography as 3rd line.

Non-anginal chest pain
Does the patient have ischaemic changes on 12-lead ECG?
• Yes: investigate as per typical and atypical angina.
• No: no further investigations for IHD at this point (unless high clinical suspicion of IHD for other reasons—discuss with a specialist). Ensure alternative chest pain diagnoses are adequately explored.

Further investigations
If the patient has typical angina but few risk factors for IHD, be sure to look for possible precipitating or exacerbating factors, eg severe anaemia or cardiomyopathy.

If anginal symptoms not adequately controlled with optimal medical therapy
Offer transcatheter angiography. Additional non-invasive or invasive functional testing may be required to evaluate angiographic findings and guide R decisions.

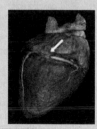

Fig 3.26 CT angiogram data has been used to construct this 3D image. The white arrow points to an obstruction of the right coronary artery.

Reprinted from *Journal of the American College of Cardiology*, 52(3), MM Henneman *et al.*, Noninvasive Evaluation With Multislice Computed Tomography in Suspected Acute Coronary Syndrome, 216–22, 2008, with permission from Elsevier.

Vasospastic angina (Prinzmetal angina)

Angina due to epicardial coronary artery spasm, which can occur even in normal coronary arteries. The pain usually occurs during rest (often at night) and resolves rapidly with short-acting nitrates (eg GTN spray). ECG during pain shows ST-segment elevation or depression.

Risks and triggers Smoking increases risk but hypertension and hypercholesterolaemia do not. Probable triggers include cocaine, amphetamine, marijuana, low magnesium, and artery instrumentation (eg during angiography).

Treatment Avoid triggers. Correct low magnesium. Stop smoking. PRN GTN. Calcium channel blockers ± long-acting nitrates. Avoid non-selective β-blockers, aspirin, and triptans. Prognosis is usually very good.

Definitions ACS includes unstable angina and myocardial infarction (MI). These share a common underlying pathology—plaque rupture, thrombosis, and inflammation. However, ACS may rarely be due to emboli, coronary spasm, or vasculitis (p554) in normal coronary arteries. *Myocardial infarction* means there is myocardial cell death, releasing troponin (see BOX 'Troponin'). *Ischaemia* means a lack of blood supply, ± cell death. *Unstable angina* refers to the presence of ischaemic symptoms suggestive of an ACS without elevation in biomarkers with or without ECG changes indicative of ischaemia. An MI may be a *STEMI*—ACS with ST-segment elevation (may only be present in V_7–V_9 if posterior STEMI) or new-onset LBBB; or an *NSTEMI*—troponin-positive ACS without ST-segment elevation—the ECG may show ST depression, T-wave inversion, non-specific changes, or be normal. The degree of irreversible myocyte death varies, and significant necrosis can occur without ST elevation.

Risk factors Non-modifiable Age, ♂ sex, family history of IHD (MI in 1st-degree relative <55yrs). **Modifiable** Smoking, hypertension, DM, hyperlipidaemia, obesity, sedentary lifestyle, cocaine use.

Incidence >100 000 admissions per annum (UK) due to MIs.

Diagnosis An increase in cardiac biomarkers (eg troponin) and either: symptoms of ischaemia, ECG changes of new ischaemia, development of pathological Q waves, new loss of myocardium, or regional wall motion abnormalities on imaging.

Symptoms Acute central chest pain, lasting >20min, often associated with nausea, sweatiness, dyspnoea, palpitations. ACS without chest pain is called 'silent'; mostly seen in elderly and diabetic patients. Can also present as a cardiac arrest (early angiography better in this setting if suggestive ECG changes). Silent MIs may present with: syncope, pulmonary oedema, epigastric pain and vomiting, post-operative hypotension or oliguria, acute confusional state, stroke, and diabetic hyperglycaemic states. MIs are also more likely to be under-diagnosed in women (↑ mortality).

Signs Distress, anxiety, pallor, sweatiness, pulse ↑ or ↓, BP ↑ or ↓, 4th heart sound. There may be signs of heart failure (↑JVP, 3rd heart sound, basal crepitations) or a pansystolic murmur (papillary muscle dysfunction/rupture, VSD). Low-grade fever may be present. Later, a pericardial friction rub or peripheral oedema may develop.

Tests ECG (See fig 3.27.) *STEMI:* classically, hyperacute (tall) T waves, ST elevation, or new LBBB occur within hours. T-wave inversion and pathological Q waves follow over hours to days (p90). *NSTEMI/unstable angina:* ST depression, T-wave inversion, non-specific changes, or the ECG may be normal. ▶In 20% of MIs, the ECG may be normal initially. Paced ECGs and ECGs with chronic bundle branch block are unhelpful for diagnosing NSTEMIs and may hinder STEMI diagnosis (see BOX 'Modified Sgarbossa's criteria', p93); in these cases, clinical assessment and troponin levels are especially important. CXR Look for cardiomegaly, pulmonary oedema, or a widened mediastinum. Don't routinely delay treatment whilst waiting for a CXR. **Blood** FBC, U&E, glucose, lipids, cardiac enzymes. **Cardiac enzymes** (See BOX 'Troponin'.) Cardiac troponin levels (cTnT and cInI) are the most sensitive and specific markers of myocardial necrosis. Different hospitals use different assays: check the required timing of troponin blood samples where you work (eg two samples 3h apart). With highly sensitive troponin assays, most patients can be diagnosed within 2–3h of presentation. Serial testing is indicated if initial −ve test and suggestive presentation. Acute MI can be excluded in most patients by 6h, but the guidelines suggest that if there is a high degree of suspicion of an ACS, a 12h sample should be obtained. Other cardiac enzymes are sensitive but less specific and not frequently used. **Echo** Regional wall abnormalities.

Differential diagnosis (p86.) Stable angina, pericarditis, myocarditis, Takotsubo cardiomyopathy (p139), aortic dissection (p647), PE, oesophageal reflux/spasm, pneumothorax, musculoskeletal pain, pancreatitis.

Management See p116, pp780–83.

Mortality 50% of deaths occur within 2h of onset of symptoms. Up to 7% die before discharge. Worse prognosis if: elderly, LV failure, and ST changes.

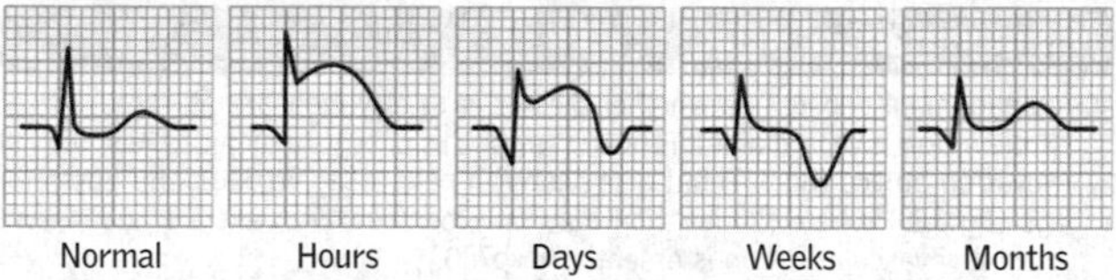

Normal   Hours   Days   Weeks   Months

Fig 3.27 Sequential ECG changes following acute MI.

Myocardial injury vs infarction

- **Myocardial injury ('troponin leak')** Elevated cTn with at least one value above the 99th percentile. Considered acute if there is a rise and/or fall of cTn values. No signs/symptoms suggestive of myocardial ischaemia.
- **Myocardial infarction (MI)** Acute myocardial injury with clinical evidence of acute myocardial ischaemia (ie ≥1 of symptoms, ECG or imaging changes).
- **Type 1 MI** Caused by acute atherothrombotic CAD and usually precipitated by atherosclerotic plaque disruption (rupture or erosion). Also includes coronary artery dissection.
- **Type 2 MI** Caused by an imbalance between myocardial oxygen supply and demand unrelated to acute atherothrombosis, eg sustained tachyarrhythmia, severe anaemia, shock, respiratory failure, coronary spasm, emboli.
- **Type 3 MI** Sudden unexpected cardiac death with symptoms/ECG suggestive of myocardial ischaemia.
- **Type 4 MI** MI associated with PCI or stent/scaffold thrombosis.
- **Type 5 MI** MI associated with cardiac surgery.[24]

Troponin

Troponins are proteins involved in cardiac and skeletal muscle contraction (fig 3.28). When myocardial cells are damaged, troponins are released and enter the bloodstream. The levels of troponin in the blood can therefore help with diagnosing myocardial damage. Troponins I and T are most specific to the heart.

Cardiac troponin is a highly sensitive biomarker of myocardial cell damage (injury), which is often, but not always, due to CAD. While it is highly specific for myocardial cell release, it is not specific for ACS as the cause. Injury to myocardial cells can arise from conditions such as myocarditis, pericarditis, infiltrative conditions, or other non-cardiac mechanisms such as following preload-induced mechanical stretch (eg heart failure), oxygen supply–demand mismatch (eg tachyarrhythmia), haemodynamic stress (eg right ventricular strain due to a massive PE), or physiological stresses in otherwise normal hearts (eg sepsis). With these conditions, the troponin levels are likely to change little hour by hour as the insults are ongoing. Troponin levels can also be raised iatrogenically, eg following CPR, DC cardioversion, ablation therapy.

A common cause of consistently elevated troponin is CKD, likely due to chronic myocardial injury or other underlying structural heart disease rather than epicardial CAD. Hence, when measuring troponin in CKD or dialysis-dependent patients, change in level is often more important than the level itself. ►Check old values and be mindful of the clinical context in which it was checked. However, although troponin has a lower sensitivity, specificity and PPV for type 1 MI in CKD, elevated levels are still associated with worse CV outcomes.[25]

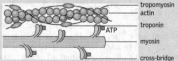

Fig 3.28 Diagram of myocardial contraction unit. The troponin complex controls when the myosin heads can bind to the actin chain, shortening the muscle fibre.

Reproduced from Barnard et al., *Cardiac Anaesthesia*, 2010, with permission from Oxford University Press.

ACS management depends on whether the ACS is 'ST elevation' or not:

1 ST elevation myocardial infarction (STEMI): this category includes ACS with ST elevation on ECG (fig 3.12) but also ACS with new LBBB (fig 3.10); and posterior MIs (fig 3.29) where ST elevation may only be seen with extra leads (V_7–V_9). Urgent revascularization is essential. ▶▶p780.

2 ACS without ST elevation: serial troponins are needed to differentiate non-ST elevation MIs (NSTEMIs) (trop rise) from unstable angina (no trop rise). ▶▶p782.

After the immediate actions described on pp780–83, treatment of ACS focuses on managing symptoms, secondary prevention of further cardiovascular disease, revascularization (if not already undertaken), and addressing complications.

Symptom control Manage chest pain with PRN GTN and opiates (IV morphine only if very severe). If this proves insufficient, consider a GTN infusion (monitor BP, omit if recent sildenafil use). If patient is deteriorating or if pain worsening, seek senior help. Manage symptomatic heart failure, p136.

Modify risk factors
• Patients should be strongly advised, and helped, to stop smoking (p85).
• Identify and treat diabetes, hypertension, hyperlipidaemia, and CKD.
• Advise a diet high in oily fish, fruit, vegetables, & fibre, and low in saturated fats.
• Encourage daily exercise. Refer to a cardiac rehab programme.
• Mental health: flag to the patient's GP if depression or anxiety are present—these are independently associated with poor cardiovascular outcomes.

Optimize cardioprotective medications
• Antiplatelets: aspirin (75mg OD) and a second antiplatelet agent (eg ticagrelor) for at least 12 months to ↓ vascular events (eg MI, stroke). Consider adding a PPI (eg lansoprazole) for gastric protection. If already taking DOAC, see BOX 'Triple therapy'.
• Anticoagulate, eg with enoxaparin 1mg/kg BD (OD if GFR <30mL/min), until discharge.
• β-blockade reduces myocardial oxygen demand. Start low and increase slowly, monitoring pulse and BP. If contraindicated, consider verapamil or diltiazem.
• ACE-i (or ARB) in all patients. Monitor renal function.
• High-dose statin, eg atorvastatin 80mg.
• Do an echo to assess LV function. Add MRA (eg spironolactone) if LV function <40%.

Revascularization
• STEMI patients and very high-risk NSTEMI patients (eg haemodynamically unstable) should receive immediate angiography ± PCI. NSTEMI patients who are high risk (eg GRACE score >140) should have angiography within 24h; intermediate risk (eg GRACE 109–140) within 3d; low-risk patients may be considered for non-invasive testing.
• Patients with multivessel disease may be considered for CABG instead of PCI (p119).

Manage complications See p118.

Discharge Address any questions the patient has. Discuss 'red flag' symptoms and where to seek medical advice should they arise. Ensure the management plan is communicated to the patient's GP. Book clinic and cardiac rehab appointments.

General advice
• **Driving**[26] Drivers with group 1 licences (car and motorcycle) can resume driving 1wk after successful angioplasty, or 4wks after ACS without successful angioplasty, if their ejection fraction is >40%. Group 2 licence holders must inform the DVLA of their ACS and stop driving; depending on the results of functional tests, they may be able to restart after 6wks.
• **Work** How soon a patient can return to work will depend on their clinical progress and the nature of their work. They should be encouraged to discuss speed of return ± changes in duties (eg to lighter work if manual labour) with their employer. Some occupations cannot be restarted post-MI: eg airline pilots & air traffic controllers. Drivers of public service or heavy goods vehicles will have to undergo functional testing (eg exercise test), as mentioned previously.

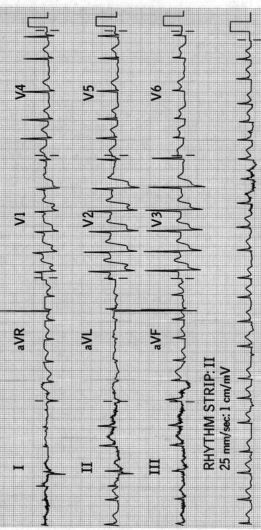

Fig 3.29 Acute posterolateral MI. The posterior infarct is evidenced by the reciprocal changes seen in V_{1-3}: dominant R waves ('upside-down' pathological Q waves) and ST depression ('upside-down' ST elevation). If extra chest leads were added (V_{7-9}), we would see the classic ST elevation pattern, see p90. The ST elevation in V_6 suggests lateral infarction. A blockage in the circumflex coronary artery could explain both the posterior and lateral changes.

RHYTHM STRIP: II
25 mm/sec: 1 cm/mV

Triple therapy

For patients post-PCI with stenting who also have an indication for long-term anticoagulation, eg pre-existing AF, decision-making needs to be individualized, taking into account both the thrombotic and bleeding risk. Seek expert cardiology advice. DOAC (rather than warfarin) + clopidogrel monotherapy may be the safest combination where necessary.[27]

Cardiac arrest (See p878, fig A3.)

Cardiogenic shock (See p786.)

Left ventricular failure (ischaemic cardiomyopathy) (See p136, p784, p786.)

Bradyarrhythmias Sinus bradycardia See p792. Patients with inferior MIs may suffer atropine-unresponsive bradycardia due to infarction of nodal tissue. **1st-degree AV block** Most commonly seen in inferior MI. Observe closely as ~40% develop higher degrees of AV block (in which case calcium channel blockers and β-blockers should be stopped). **Wenckebach phenomenon** (Mobitz type I) Does not require pacing unless poorly tolerated. **Mobitz type II block** Carries a high risk of developing sudden complete AV block; should be paced. **Complete AV block** Usually resolves within a few days. Insert pacemaker (may not be necessary after inferior MI if narrow QRS, reasonably stable and pulse ≥40–50). **Bundle branch block** Pace MI complicated by trifascicular block or non-adjacent bifascicular disease (p128).

Tachyarrhythmias NB: ↓K+, hypoxia, and acidosis all predispose to arrhythmias and should be corrected. **Sinus tachycardia** ↑ Myocardial O_2 demand, treat causes (pain, hypoxia, sepsis, etc.) and add β-blocker if not contraindicated. **SVT** See p122. **AF or flutter** If compromised, DC cardioversion. Otherwise, medical therapy as per p126. **Frequent PVCs (premature ventricular complexes) and non-sustained VT** (≥3 consecutive PVCs >100bpm and lasting <30s) are common after acute MI and are associated with increased risk of sudden death. Correct hypokalaemia and hypomagnesaemia and ensure the patient is on β-blockers, if not contraindicated **Sustained VT** (Consecutive PVCs >100bpm and lasting >30s.) Treat with synchronized DC shock (if no pulse, treat as per advanced life support algorithm, see p878, fig A3). Use anti-arrhythmics only if VT recurrent and not controlled with shocks. Consider ablation &/or ICD. **Ventricular fibrillation** 80% occurs within 12h. VF occurring after 48h usually indicates pump failure or cardiogenic shock. ℞ DC shock (see p878, fig A3), consider ICD.

Right ventricular failure (RVF)/infarction Presents with low cardiac output and ↑JVP. Fluid is key; avoid vasodilators (eg nitrates) and diuretics. Inotropes are required in some cases.

Pericarditis Central chest pain, relieved by sitting forwards. ECG: saddle-shaped ST elevation, see fig 3.45, p133. Treatment: NSAIDs. Echo to check for effusion.

Systemic embolism May arise from LV mural thrombus. After large anterior MI, consider anticoagulation with DOAC or warfarin for 3 months.

Cardiac tamponade (p786) Presents with low cardiac output, pulsus paradoxus, Kussmaul's sign,[2] muffled heart sounds. Diagnosis: echo. Treatment: pericardial aspiration (provides temporary relief, ▶▶see p757 for technique), surgery.

Mitral regurgitation May be mild (minor papillary muscle dysfunction) or severe (chordal or papillary muscle rupture secondary to ischaemia). Presentation: pulmonary oedema. Treat LVF (p784) and consider valve replacement.

LV free wall or interventricular septum rupture New holosystolic murmur in the case of VSD. Can lead to cardiogenic shock, tamponade, and sudden death. Diagnosis: echo, pericardiocentesis. Treatment: surgery. 50% mortality in first week.

Late malignant ventricular arrhythmias Occur 1–3wks post-MI and are the cardiologist's nightmare. Avoid hypokalaemia, the most easily avoidable cause. Consider 24h ECG monitoring prior to discharge if large MI.

Dressler's syndrome (p133) Recurrent pericarditis, pleural effusions, fever, anaemia, and ↑ESR 1–3wks post-MI. Treatment: consider NSAIDs; steroids if severe.

Left ventricular aneurysm This occurs late (4–6wks post-MI), and presents with LVF, angina, recurrent VT, or systemic embolism. ECG: persistent ST-segment elevation. Treatment: anticoagulate, consider excision.

---

2 JVP rises during inspiration. Adolf Kussmaul was a prominent 19th-century physician and the first to attempt gastroscopy. Inspired by a sword swallower he passed a rigid tube into the stomach; however, light technology was limited and it was not until years later that gastroscopists could visualize the stomach.

Coronary artery bypass graft (CABG)

CABG is performed in left main stem disease; multivessel disease; multiple severe stenoses; patients unsuitable for angioplasty; failed angioplasty; refractory angina.

Indications for CABG—to improve survival
• Left main stem disease.
• Triple-vessel disease involving proximal part of the left anterior descending.

Indications for CABG—to relieve symptoms
• Angina unresponsive to drugs.
• Unstable angina (sometimes).
• If angioplasty is unsuccessful.

NB: when CABG and percutaneous coronary intervention (PCI, eg angioplasty) are both clinically valid options, NICE recommends that the availability of new stent technology should push the decision towards PCI. In practice, patients with single-vessel coronary artery disease and normal LV function usually undergo PCI, and those with triple-vessel disease and abnormal LV function more often undergo CABG. Compared with PCI, CABG results in longer recovery time and length of in-patient stay. Recent RCTs indicate that early procedural mortality rates and 5-year survival rates are similar after PCI and CABG. Compared with PCI, CABG probably provides more complete long-term relief of angina in patients, and less repeated revascularization.

Procedure The heart is usually stopped and blood pumped artificially by a machine outside the body (cardiac bypass). Minimally invasive thoracotomies not requiring this are well described,[28] but randomized trials are few. The patient's own saphenous vein or internal mammary artery is used as the graft. Several grafts may be placed. >50% of vein grafts close in 10yrs (low-dose aspirin helps prevent this). Internal mammary artery grafts last longer.

Complications Bleeding, stroke, cognitive dysfunction, sternal wound infection, mediastinitis, AKI, peri-op MI, early graft occlusion, arrhythmias, vasoplegic shock, pericarditis, pericardial effusion/tamponade.

On-pump or off-pump Off-pump refers to CABG without the use of cardiopulmonary bypass. Similar short-term outcomes to on-pump surgery but higher rates of revascularization at 1 year with off-pump.[29] On-pump generally preferable unless high risk of stroke from aortic manipulation.

After CABG If angina persists or recurs (from poor graft run-off, distal disease, new atheroma, or graft occlusion) restart anti-anginal drugs, and consider angioplasty. Ensure optimal management of hypertension, diabetes, and hyperlipidaemia, and that smoking is addressed. Continue aspirin 75mg OD indefinitely; consider clopidogrel if aspirin contraindicated. Mood, sex, and intellectual problems[30] are common early. Rehabilitation helps:
• Exercise: walk→cycle→swim→jog.
• Drive at 1 month: no need to tell DVLA if non-HGV licences, p150.
• Return to work, eg at 3 months.

'We' is more important than 'I'

René Gerónimo Favaloro, an Argentinian surgeon, is known as the father of CABG surgery. Prior to this, he spent years trying to improve the health of local farming communities in his home country, educating them about preventative medicine, creating blood banks, building operating theatres, and training new doctors. In 1967, after joining the Cleveland Clinic, he performed the first successful bypass surgery. Shortly after this, he returned to Argentina where he established the Favaloro Foundation dedicated to medical research and teaching for the people of Latin America. Reminding us all of the great collective effort of past, present, and future colleagues, he once wrote humbly, 'In medicine, the advances are always the result of many efforts accumulated over the years.'

Disturbances of cardiac rhythm (arrhythmias) are:
• Common.
• Often benign (but may reflect underlying heart disease).
• Often intermittent, causing diagnostic difficulty; see BOX 'Continuous ECG monitoring'.
• Occasionally severe, causing cardiac compromise which may be fatal.
▶▶Emergency management: pp788–93.

Causes Cardiac Ischaemic heart disease (IHD); structural changes, eg left atrial dilatation secondary to mitral regurgitation; cardiomyopathy; pericarditis; myocarditis; aberrant conduction pathways. **Non-cardiac** Caffeine; smoking; alcohol; pneumonia; drugs (β_2-agonists, digoxin, tricyclics, doxorubicin); metabolic imbalance (K^+, Ca^{2+}, Mg^{2+}, hypoxia, hypercapnia, acidosis, thyroid disease); and phaeochromocytoma.

Presentation Palpitations, chest pain, presyncope/syncope, hypotension, or pulmonary oedema. Some arrhythmias may be asymptomatic, incidental findings, eg AF.

History Take a detailed history of palpitations (p36). Ask about precipitating factors, onset/offset, nature (fast or slow, regular or irregular), duration, associated symptoms (chest pain, dyspnoea, collapse). Review drug history. Ask about past medical history and family history of cardiac disease and sudden death. Syncope occurring during exercise is always concerning; the patient may have a condition predisposing them to sudden cardiac death (eg long QT syndrome).

Tests FBC, U&E, glucose, Ca^{2+}, Mg^{2+}, TSH, ECG: look for signs of IHD, AF, short PR interval (WPW syndrome), long QT interval (metabolic imbalance, drugs, congenital), U waves (hypokalaemia). 24h ECG monitoring or other continuous ECG monitoring (see BOX 'Continuous ECG monitoring'). Echo to look for structural heart disease, eg mitral stenosis, HCM. Provocation tests: exercise ECG, cardiac catheterization ± electrophysiological studies may be needed.

▶▶**Narrow complex tachycardias** See pp790–1, p126.

▶▶**Atrial fibrillation and flutter** See pp790–1, p126.

▶▶**Broad complex tachycardias** See pp788–9, p128.

▶▶**Bradycardia** See p792 (causes and management of acute bradycardia) and p90 (heart block). Intermittent, self-resolving bradycardic episodes can cause significant problems (eg recurrent syncope). Continuous ECG monitoring (BOX 'Continuous ECG monitoring') will be needed to assist the diagnosis ± specialist tests (eg tilt table testing for reflex syncope). Seek out reversible causes, eg hypothyroidism or medications such as β-blockers. In some cases, no reversible cause is found and the intermittent bradycardia is sufficiently dangerous to warrant a permanent pacemaker (p128). See BOX, 'Sinus node dysfunction'.

Management Some arrhythmias can be managed *conservatively*, eg by reducing alcohol intake. Many arrhythmias respond to *medical* management with regular tablets or a 'pill in the pocket'. *Interventional* management may include pacemakers (p128), ablation (eg of accessory pathways or arrhythmogenic foci), or implantable cardioverter defibrillators (ICDs), eg in patients with ventricular arrhythmias post-MI and in those with congenital arrhythmogenic conditions (p148).

Screening athletes The incidence of SCD among young athletes is low (1:50 000–1:100 000/yr) but it is a devastating event—likely attributable to a combination of structural heart disease, inherited arrhythmia syndrome, & CAD. Pre-participation cardiovascular screening of young competitive athletes (those who engage in >6–8 h/week of intensive sport since >6 months) is recommended by the ESC and should include a detailed personal and family history, physical examination, and a 12-lead ECG.[31] Common ECG variants found in athletes include sinus bradycardia, first-degree AV block, incomplete RBBB, isolated electrical LVH, early repolarization pattern—all of which are likely attributable to training-related changes. ECG abnormalities warranting further investigation include ventricular pre-excitation, epsilon waves, complete LBBB, pathological Q waves, ST depression, long QTC, T-wave inversion.

Continuous ECG monitoring

A simple 12-lead ECG only gives a snapshot of the heart's electrical activities. Many disorders, particularly the arrhythmias, come and go and so may be missed at the time of the ECG recording. If you feel you are missing a paroxysmal arrhythmia, there are many ways of recording the electrical activity over a longer period:

Telemetry An inpatient wears ECG leads and the signals are shown on screens being watched by staff. Thus, if a dangerous arrhythmia occurs, help is immediately available. This is very resource intensive so reserved for those at high risk of dangerous arrhythmias, eg immediately post-STEMI.

Exercise ECGs The patient exercises according to a standardized protocol (eg Bruce on a treadmill) and the BP and ECG are monitored, looking for ischaemic changes, arrhythmias, and features suggestive of arrhythmia risk, such as delta waves.

Holter monitors The patient wears an ECG monitor which records their rhythm for 24h–7d whilst they go about their normal life, and this is later analysed. These can also be used to pick up ST changes suggestive of ischaemia.

Loop recorders These record any detected arrhythmias, but can be activated by patients to correlate symptoms with recordings—useful if the arrhythmia causes loss of consciousness: the patient can press the button when they wake up. Loop recorders may be implanted just under the skin (eg Reveal* or the newer, injectable LINQ™ device), and are especially useful in patients with infrequent episodes as they can continually monitor for months or years awaiting an event (fig 3.30).

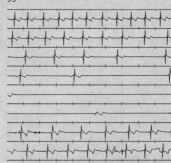

Pacemakers and ICDs These record details of cardiac electrical activity and device activity. This information can be useful for establishing an arrhythmic origin for symptoms.

Fig 3.30 This is a recording from a loop recorder, each line follows on from the one above. This tracing was recorded at the time of a syncopal episode, it shows cardiac slowing then a 15s pause: quite long enough to cause syncope! But not long enough to arrange a standard ECG, even if the patient were in hospital.

Reproduced from Camm *et al.*, *ESC Textbook of Cardiovascular Medicine*, 2009, with permission from Oxford University Press.

Sinus node dysfunction

Sinus node dysfunction, formerly known as sick sinus syndrome, is usually caused by sinus node fibrosis, typically in elderly patients. Other causes include medications (eg digoxin, donepezil), toxins, or systemic conditions. The sinus node becomes dysfunctional, in some cases slowing to the point of sinus bradycardia or sinus pauses, in others generating tachyarrhythmias such as AF and atrial tachycardia.

Symptoms Syncope, pre-syncope, light-headedness, palpitations, SOB.

Management
- Thromboembolism prophylaxis if episodes of AF are detected.
- Permanent pacemakers for patients with symptomatic bradycardia or sinus pauses.

Some patients develop a '*tachy brady syndrome*', suffering from alternating tachycardic and bradycardic rhythms. This can prove difficult to treat medically as treating one circumstance (eg tachycardia) increases the risk from the other. Pacing for bradycardic episodes in combination with rate-slowing medications for tachycardic episodes may be required if the patient is symptomatic or unstable.

Narrow complex tachycardia

Definition ECG shows rate of >100bpm and QRS complex duration of <120ms. Narrow QRS complexes occur when the ventricles are depolarized via the normal conduction pathways. The arrhythmia originates above or within the His bundle (ie a supraventricular tachycardia—SVT) (fig 3.32).

Differential diagnosis Assess rhythm and P waves (if present—atrial rate, P-wave morphology, relationship between atrial and ventricular rates, position of P wave in cardiac cycle (short vs long RP interval)).

Regular narrow complex tachycardias See fig 3.33.

Irregular narrow complex tachycardias
• Normal variant: sinus dysrhythmia (rate changes with inspiration/expiration—regularly irregular); sinus rhythm with frequent ectopic beats.
• Atrial fibrillation (AF)—no P waves present: p127, fig 3.40.
• Atrial flutter with variable block: eg P–P–P–QRS–P–P–QRS (3:1 block then 2:1 block). The atrial rhythm is regular but the ventricular rhythm (hence pulse) is irregular.
• Multifocal atrial tachycardia: like focal atrial tachycardia but there are multiple groups of atrial cells taking it in turns to initiate a cardiac cycle. P-wave morphology and P-P intervals vary. Usually associated with COPD.

Principles of management See p791.
▶▶If the patient is compromised, use DC cardioversion (p754).
• Identify and treat the underlying rhythm: eg treating sinus tachycardia secondary to volume depletion with IV fluids; treating multifocal sinus tachycardia secondary to COPD by correcting hypoxia and hypercapnia; treating focal atrial tachycardia secondary to digoxin toxicity with digoxin-specific antibody fragments; treating AV re-entry tachycardia (AVRT) secondary to WPW with flecainide, propafenone, or amiodarone; for AF and atrial flutter see p126.
• If AV nodal re-entry tachycardia (AVNRT) or AVRT are suspected, consider transiently blocking the AVN. This should break the circuit of an atrioventricular re-entry rhythm, allowing sinus rhythm to re-establish. If the underlying rhythm is actually atrial in origin (eg flutter or atrial tachycardia), AVN blockade will not treat the rhythm but the paused ventricular activity will unmask the atrial rhythm (fig 3.31), aiding diagnosis and management. AVN blockade can be achieved by:
  1 Vagal manoeuvres: carotid sinus massage, Valsalva manoeuvre (eg blowing into a syringe followed by supine repositioning with 15 seconds of passive leg raise at a 45° angle—this modified Valsalva is the most effective vagal manoeuvre).[32]
  2 IV adenosine: see p790.
• In some cases, narrow complex tachyarrhythmias cause symptomatic episodes of sufficient severity and frequency to warrant more invasive treatment, eg ablation therapy for accessory pathways.

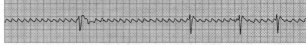

Fig 3.31 This patient was given adenosine for tachycardia thought to be due to AVRT or AVNRT. The adenosine has slowed the ventricular rate, revealing flutter waves (sawtooth appearance), disproving an AVRT/AVNRT diagnosis.   Image courtesy of Dr Ed Burns, www.lifeinthefastlane.com

Holiday heart syndrome

Binge drinking in a person *without* any clinical evidence of heart disease may result in acute cardiac rhythm and/or conduction disturbances, which is called holiday heart syndrome (note that recreational use of cannabis may have similar effects). The most common rhythm disorders are supraventricular tachyarrhythmia and AF (consider this diagnosis in patients without structural heart disease who present with new-onset AF).

The prognosis is excellent, especially in young patients without structural heart disease. As holiday heart syndrome resolves rapidly by abstinence from alcohol use, advise all patients against the excessive use of alcohol in future.

Normal conduction

Normal conduction: initiated by the sinoatrial node (SAN), electrical activity spreads around the atria. The atrioventricular node (AVN) receives this activity, pauses, then passes it on, down the bundle of His which splits into left and right bundle branches. These cause depolarization of the ventricular myocardium from bottom (apex) to top (outflow tracts).

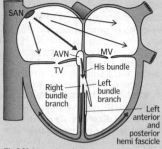

Fig 3.32 Normal conduction.

Regular rhythm tachycardia

See fig 3.33.

A. Sinus tachycardia Conduction occurs as per fig 3.32 but impulses are initiated at a high frequency. Causes include infection, pain, exercise, anxiety, volume depletion, bleed, systemic vasodilation (eg in sepsis), drugs (caffeine, nicotine, salbutamol), anaemia, fever, PE, hyperthyroidism, pregnancy, CO_2 retention, autonomic neuropathy (eg inappropriate sinus tachycardia).

B. Focal atrial tachycardia A group of atrial cells act as a pacemaker, out-pacing the SAN. P-wave morphology (shape) is different to sinus. Long RP interval.

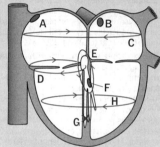

Fig 3.33 Regular tachycardias.

C. Atrial flutter Electrical activity circles the atria 300 times per minute, giving a 'sawtooth' baseline, see fig 3.40, p127. The AVN passes some of these impulses on, resulting in ventricular rates that are factors of 300 (150, 100, 75).

D. Atrioventricular re-entry tachycardia (AVRT) An accessory pathway (eg in Wolff–Parkinson–White (WPW), p129) allows electrical activity from the ventricles to pass to the resting atrial myocytes, creating a circuit: atria–AVN–ventricles– accessory pathway–atria. This conduction is called 'orthodromic' conduction and results in narrow QRS complexes as ventricular depolarization is triggered via the bundle of His. Conduction in the other direction is called 'antidromic' and results in broad QRS complexes. No or retrograde P wave and short RP interval.

E. Atrioventricular nodal re-entry tachycardia (AVNRT) Circuits form within the AVN, causing narrow complex tachycardias with no or retrograde P wave and short RP interval. This is very common.

F. Junctional tachycardia Cells in the AVN become the pacemaker, giving narrow QRS complexes as impulses reach the ventricles through the normal routes; P waves may be inverted and late.

G. SVT with aberrancy Any of the above conditions can result in broad complex tachycardias if there is bundle branch block (p92).

H. Ventricular tachycardia (VT) This can result from circuits, similar to atrial flutter, or from focuses of rapidly firing cells. The QRS is broad. When a circuit is in action and its plane rotates, the ECG shows broad complex tachycardia with regularly increasing and decreasing amplitudes; this is called *torsades de pointes*.

Definition ECG shows rate of >100 and QRS complexes >120ms. If no clear QRS complexes, it is VF or asystole (or problems with the ECG machine or stickers).

Principles of management ►► If the patient is unstable or you are uncertain of what to do, get help fast—the patient may be peri-arrest (p788).
• Identify the underlying rhythm and treat accordingly.
• If in doubt, treat as ventricular tachycardia (VT)—the commonest cause.
• Giving AVN blocking agents to treat SVT with aberrancy when the patient is in VT can cause dangerous haemodynamic instability. Treating for VT when the patient is actually in SVT has less potential for deterioration.
• If WPW is suspected, avoid drugs that slow AV conduction—see p106.

Differential diagnosis Assess rhythm (irregular rhythm suggests AF with aberrancy), QRS axis (extreme axis deviation suggests VT), whether any AV dissociation present (in keeping with VT), any known history of structural heart disease, especially CAD, or arrhythmias.
• Ventricular fibrillation—chaotic, no pattern, fig 3.34.
• VT, fig 3.15, p98; fig 3.35.
• *Torsades de pointes (polymorphic VT)*—VT with varying axis (fig 3.36), may look like VF. ↑QT interval is a predisposing factor.
• Any cause of narrow complex tachycardias (p122) when in combination with bundle branch block or metabolic causes of broad QRS.
• Antidromic AVRT (eg WPW), p123.

Differentiating VT from SVT with aberrancy This may be difficult; seek expert help. Diagnosis is based on the history (IHD increases the likelihood of a ventricular arrhythmia), a 12-lead ECG, and the response (or lack thereof) to certain medications. ECG findings in favour of VT:
• Fusion beats or capture beats (figs 3.37, 3.38).
• +ve or −ve QRS concordance in all chest leads (ie all +ve (R) or all −ve (QS)).
• QRS >160ms.
• Marked axis deviation, or 'northwest axis' (QRS positive in aVR).
• AV dissociation (Ps independent of QRSs) or 2:1 or 3:1 Mobitz II heart block.
• RSR' pattern where R is taller than R'. (R' taller than R suggests RBBB.)

Management See p789. Helpful tests include U&E, troponin, CXR.

Implantable cardioverter defibrillator (ICD) Used to prevent sudden cardiac death in patients with prior sustained VT/VF or in those at high-risk of same, eg prior MI + LVEF ≤30%, symptomatic HF (New York Heart Association (NYHA) II–III) + LVEF ≤35% (despite 3mths of optimal medical therapy), certain high-risk inherited arrhythmia syndromes. A combined ICD and biventricular pacing device (cardiac resynchronization therapy-defibrillator (CRT-D)) is recommended to reduce mortality in patients with a QRS ≥ 130ms with an LVEF ≤35% and LBBB. See ICD complications, p129. An entirely subcutaneous ICD is an alternative to the traditional transvenous ICD in patients in whom transvenous leads should be avoided (eg those at high risk of systemic infection).

Ventricular extrasystoles (ectopics) These are common and can be symptomatic—patients describe palpitations, a thumping sensation, or their heart 'missing a beat'. The pulse may feel irregular if there are frequent ectopics. On ECG, ventricular ectopics are broad QRS complexes; they may be single or occur in patterns:
• *Bigeminy:* ectopic every other beat, see fig 3.39. ECG machines may disregard the second QRS and so calculate the rate to be half the true value.
• *Trigeminy:* every third beat is an ectopic.
• *Couplet:* two ectopics together.
• *Triplet:* three ectopics together.

Occasional ventricular ectopics in otherwise healthy people are extremely common and rarely significant. Frequent ectopics (>60/h), particularly couplets and triplets, should prompt testing for underlying cardiac conditions.

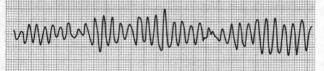

Fig 3.34 VF (p878).

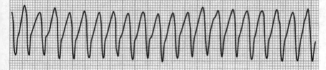

Fig 3.35 VT with a rate of 235/min.

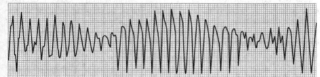

Fig 3.36 *Torsades de pointes* tachycardia.

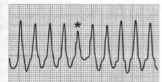

Fig 3.37 A fusion beat (*)—a 'normal beat' fuses with a VT complex creating an unusual complex.

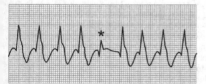

Fig 3.38 A capture beat (*)—a normal QRS amongst runs of VT. This would not be expected if the QRS breadth were down to bundle branch block or metabolic causes.

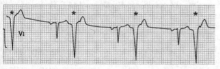

Fig 3.39 Bigeminy—a normal QRS is followed by a ventricular ectopic beat (*) then a compensatory pause, this pattern then repeats. The ectopic beats have the same morphology as each other so probably all share an origin.

3 Cardiovascular medicine

AF[33] is a chaotic, irregular atrial rhythm at 300–600bpm (fig 3.40); the AV node responds intermittently, hence an irregular ventricular rhythm. Cardiac output drops by 10–20% as the ventricles aren't primed reliably by the atria. AF is common in the elderly (≤9%). The main risk is embolic stroke. Warfarin reduces this to 1%/yr from 4%. So, *do an ECG on everyone with an irregular pulse* (opportunistic screening recommended if >65yr). If AF started more than 48h ago, intracardiac clots may have formed, necessitating anticoagulation prior to cardioversion.

Causes Hypertension; IHD (seen in 22% of MI patients); PE; mitral valve disease; heart failure; pneumonia; hyperthyroidism; caffeine; alcohol; post-op; ↓K⁺; ↓Mg²⁺.

Types Paroxysmal AF (PAF) Intermittent. **Persistent AF** Fails to self-terminate in 7d. **Long-standing persistent AF** Lasts >12mths. **Permanent AF** Decision made not to pursue rhythm control strategy. **'Lone' AF** This means no cause found.

Symptoms May be asymptomatic or cause chest pain, palpitations, dyspnoea, or faintness. **Signs** *Irregularly irregular pulse*, the apical pulse rate is greater than the radial rate, and the 1st heart sound is of variable intensity; signs of LVF (p784).
►Examine the whole patient: AF is *often* associated with non-cardiac disease.

Tests ECG Shows absent P waves, irregular QRS complexes, fig 3.40. **Blood tests** U&E, cardiac enzymes, thyroid function tests. **Echo** To look for left atrial enlargement, mitral valve disease, poor LV function, and other structural abnormalities. Ambulatory ECG may help diagnose PAF or assess AF burden.

Managing acute AF
- If the patient has adverse signs (shock, myocardial ischaemia (chest pain or ECG changes), syncope, heart failure): ►►ABCDE, get senior input ►►DC cardioversion (synchronized shock, start at 120–150J) ± amiodarone if unsuccessful (p791); do not delay treatment in order to start anticoagulation.
- If the patient is stable & AF started <48h ago: rate or rhythm control may be tried. For rhythm control, DC cardiovert or give flecainide (CI: structural heart disease, IHD) or amiodarone. Start heparin in case cardioversion is delayed (see BOX 'Anticoagulation and AF').
- If the patient is stable & AF started >48h ago or unclear time of onset: rate control (eg with bisoprolol or diltiazem). If rhythm control is chosen, the patient must be anticoagulated for >3wks first.
- Correct electrolyte imbalances (K⁺, Mg²⁺, Ca²⁺); ℞ associated illnesses (eg MI, pneumonia); and consider anticoagulation (see BOX 'Anticoagulation and AF').

Managing chronic AF The main goals are rate control and anticoagulation. Rate control is at least as good as rhythm control,[34] but rhythm control may be appropriate if • symptomatic or CCF • younger • presenting for 1st time with lone AF • AF from a corrected precipitant (eg ↑U&E). **Anticoagulation** See BOX 'Anticoagulation and AF'. **Rate control** β-blocker or rate-limiting Ca²⁺ blocker are 1st choice. Avoid Ca²⁺ blocker if LVEF <40%. If this fails, add digoxin (p107), then consider amiodarone. Digoxin as monotherapy in chronic AF is only acceptable in sedentary patients. ►Do not give β-blockers with verapamil. Aim for heart rate <110pm at rest. **Rhythm control** *Elective DC cardioversion:* do echo first to check for intracardiac thrombi. If there is ↑risk of cardioversion failure (past failure, or past recurrence) give amiodarone for 4wks before the procedure and 12 months after. *Elective pharmacological cardioversion* flecainide is 1st choice (CI if structural heart disease, eg scar tissue from MI: use IV amiodarone instead). In refractory cases, AVN ablation with pacing, pulmonary vein ablation, or the maze procedure may be considered. **Paroxysmal AF** 'Pill in the pocket' (eg flecainide or propafenone PRN) may be tried if: infrequent AF, BP >100mmHg systolic, no past LV dysfunction. Anticoagulate (see BOX 'Anticoagulation and AF'). Consider ablation if symptomatic or frequent episodes.

Atrial flutter See p127, fig 3.40. **Treatment** Similar to AF regarding rate/rhythm control and the need for anticoagulation. DC-CV is preferred to pharmacological cardioversion. IV amiodarone may be needed if rate control is proving difficult. Recurrence rates are high so ablation is often recommended for long-term management.

Anticoagulation and AF

Acute AF Use heparin until a full risk assessment for emboli (see below) is made—eg AF started <48h ago and elective cardioversion is being planned. If >48h, ensure ≥3wks of therapeutic anticoagulation before elective cardioversion + 4wks afterwards (in patients without long-term need for anticoagulation); NB: transoesophageal-guided cardioversion is an option if urgent cardioversion is required. Use a DOAC (eg apixaban) or warfarin (target INR 2–3) if high risk of emboli (past ischaemic stroke, TIA, or emboli; ≥75yrs with ↑BP, DM; coronary or peripheral arterial disease; evidence of valve disease or ↓LV function/CCF—only do echo if unsure).[35] Use *no anticoagulation* if *stable* sinus rhythm has been restored, no risk factors for emboli, and AF recurrence unlikely (ie no failed cardioversions, no structural heart disease, no previous recurrences, no sustained AF for >1yr).

Chronic AF In all cases, the need for anticoagulation should be assessed using the CHA₂DS₂-VASc score to assess embolic stroke risk (consider anticoagulation if score ♂ >0, ♀ >1), and balancing this against the risks of anticoagulation to the patient, assessed with the HAS-BLED score. Long-term anticoagulation should be with a DOAC (see p346) or warfarin. DOACs should be preferentially used except in the case of mechanical heart valves or moderate–severe mitral stenosis where warfarin is the anticoagulant of choice. Where anticoagulation is contraindicated due to high bleeding risk etc., consider a left atrial appendage occlusion device.

CHA₂DS₂-VASc—**C**ongestive cardiac failure (1 point), **H**ypertension (1), **A**ge 65–74yrs (1), **A**ge >74yrs (2), **D**iabetes (1), previous **S**troke/TIA/thromboembolism (2), **V**ascular disease (1), **S**ex **C**ategory (1 if female). A score of 2 = an annual stroke risk of 2.2%. Online calculators can be helpful (eg www.mdcalc.com).

HAS-BLED—1 point for each of: • labile INR • age >65 • use of medications that can predispose to bleeding (eg NSAIDs, antiplatelets) • alcohol abuse • uncontrolled hypertension • history of, or predisposition to, major bleeding • renal disease • liver disease • stroke history.

Pre-excited AF

In pre-excited AF, accessory pathways capable of conducting at rapid rates (eg sometimes in WPW syndrome) pass erratic electrical activity from the atria to the ventricles, unfiltered by the AVN. ECGs will show irregular, broad QRS complexes at >200bpm. High risk of VT and VF.

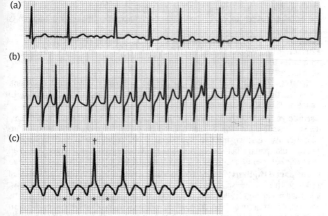

(a)

(b)

(c)

Fig 3.40 (a) AF: note the irregular spacing of QRS complexes and lack of P waves. (b) AF with a rapid ventricular response (sometimes referred to as 'fast AF'). No pattern to QRS complex spacing, and rate >100bpm. (c) Atrial flutter with 2:1 block (2 P waves (*) for every 1 QRS complex (†)). The P waves have the classic 'sawtooth' appearance. Alternate P waves are merged with the QRS complex.

In normal circumstances the SAN plays the role of pacemaker. On occasion, other areas of myocardium will set the pace (see earlier in chapter). If the heart is not pacing itself fast enough, artificial pacing may be required. Options include 'percussion pacing'—fist strikes to the precordium, used only in peri-arrest situations; transcutaneous pacing—electrical stimulation via defibrillator pads (p754); temporary transvenous pacing (p760); and a subcutaneously implanted permanent pacemaker. Leadless pacemakers are a less invasive alternative for single ventricle (RV only) pacing in patients in whom you wish to avoid transvenous pacing.

Indications for temporary cardiac pacing include

• Symptomatic bradycardia, unresponsive to atropine.
• After acute *anterior* MI, prophylactic pacing is required in:
  • complete AV block
  • symptomatic Mobitz type I AV block (Wenckebach)
  • Mobitz type II AV block
  • non-adjacent bifascicular, or trifascicular block (p92).
• After *inferior* MI, pacing may not be needed in complete AV block if reasonably stable, rate is >40–50, and QRS complexes are narrow.
• Suppression of drug-resistant tachyarrhythmias by overdrive pacing, eg SVT, VT.
• Special situations: during general anaesthesia; during cardiac surgery; during electrophysiological studies; drug overdose (eg digoxin, β-blockers, verapamil).
▶See p760 for further details and insertion technique.

Indications for a permanent pacemaker (PPM) include

• Complete AV block (Stokes–Adams attacks, asymptomatic, congenital).
• Mobitz type II AV block (p91).
• Persistent AV block after anterior MI.
• Symptomatic bradycardias (eg sinus node dysfunction, p121).
• Heart failure (cardiac resynchronization therapy).
• Drug-resistant tachyarrhythmias.

Pre-operative assessment Bloods (FBC, clotting screen, renal function), IV cannula, consent, antibiotics as per local protocol.

Post-operative management Prior to discharge, check wound for bleeding or haematoma; check lead positions and for pneumothorax on CXR; check pacemaker function. During 1st week, inspect for wound haematoma or dehiscence. The battery needs changing every 5–10 years. For driving rules see p150.

Pacemaker letter codes These enable pacemaker identification (minimum is 3 letters):

• 1st letter the chamber paced (A=atria, V=ventricles, D=dual chamber).
• 2nd letter the chamber sensed (A=atria, V=ventricles, D=dual chamber, O=none).
• 3rd letter the pacemaker response (T=triggered, I=inhibited, D=dual).
• 4th letter (R=rate modulation, P=programmable, M=multiprogrammable).
• 5th letter (P means that in tachycardia the pacemaker will pace the patient. S means that in tachycardia the pacemaker shocks the patient. D=dual ability to pace and shock. O=neither of these).

Cardiac resynchronization therapy (CRT) Improves the synchronization of cardiac contraction and reduces mortality[36] in people with symptomatic heart failure who have an ejection fraction <35% and a QRS duration >130ms.[37] It involves biventricular pacing (both septal and lateral walls of the LV) and, if required, also an atrial lead. It may be combined with a defibrillator (CRT-D).

ECG of paced rhythms (fig 3.16, p99; fig 3.41). Pacemaker input appears as a vertical 'spike' on the ECG. This spike can be very small with modern bipolar pacing systems. Ventricular pacing usually has a broad QRS morphology (similar to LBBB). Systems are usually programmed 'on demand' so will only pace when necessary. Modern systems are generally very reliable but pacing spikes with no capture afterwards suggests a problem. Programming of devices is complicated so seek help early if concerned. Many pacemakers store intracardiac electrograms which can be accessed to correlate rhythm with any symptoms.

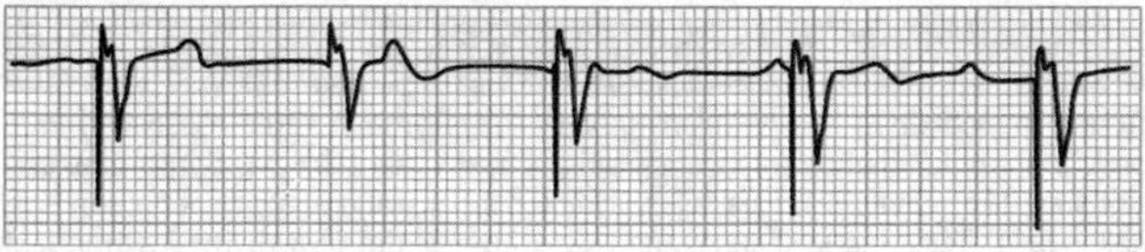

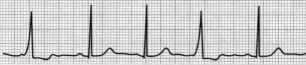

Fig 3.41 ECG of a paced rhythm.

Pacemaker/ICD complications

Peri-procedural (3–6%)
• Bleeding.
• Infection—can be life-threatening; complete removal and antibiotics needed.
• Lead dislodgement.
• Pneumothorax.
• Cardiac perforation.
• Death (rarely).

Long-term
• Infection.
• Lead failure (resulting in failure to pace/shock or inappropriate shocks).
• Tricuspid valve damage.
• Venous thrombosis.
• ↑Pacing/defibrillation thresholds.
• Device and/or lead migration or fracture.

Congenital arrhythmogenic cardiac conditions

As well as the many acquired conditions that can predispose to arrhythmias (p121), there are a number of congenital conditions. These may be clinically silent until a fatal attack and are likely to be responsible for most cases of sudden arrhythmic death syndrome (SADS). They include:

WPW syndrome (Wolff–Parkinson–White; fig 3.42.) Caused by congenital accessory conduction pathway between atria and ventricles. Resting ECG shows short PR interval, wide QRS complex (due to slurred upstroke or 'delta wave') and ST–T changes. Two types: WPW type A (+ve δ wave in V₁), WPW type B (−ve δ wave in V₁). Tachycardia can be due to an AVRT or pre-excited AF/atrial flutter (p126). Management may include ablation of the accessory pathway.

LQTS (Long QT syndromes.) These are channelopathies that result in prolonged repolarization phases, predisposing the patient to ventricular arrhythmias; classically *torsades de pointes*. ▶p788. Conditions associated with LQTS include Jervell and Lange-Nielsen syndrome (p690) and Romano–Ward syndrome (p696).

ARVC (Arrhythmogenic right ventricular cardiomyopathy.) RV myocardium is replaced with fibro-fatty material. Symptoms: palpitations and syncope during exercise. ECG changes include epsilon wave; T inversion and broad QRS in V₁–V₃.

Brugada Sodium channelopathy. Diagnosis: classic coved ST elevation in V₁–V₃ *plus* suggestive clinical history. ECG changes and arrhythmias can be precipitated by fever, medications (www.brugadadrugs.org), electrolyte imbalances, and ischaemia.

Many of these patients can be treated medically or conservatively but those at high risk may require an implantable cardiac defibrillator (ICD). Screening family members is important for picking up undiagnosed cases.

Fig 3.42 This patient has Wolff–Parkinson–White syndrome as they have delta waves (slurred QRS upstrokes) in beats 1 and 4 of this rhythm strip. The delta wave both broadens the ventricular complex and shortens the PR interval. ▶If a patient with WPW has AF, avoid AV node blockers such as diltiazem, verapamil, and digoxin—but procainamide, ibutilide, or flecainide may be used.

Acute myocarditis This is inflammation of myocardium, often associated with pericardial inflammation (myopericarditis). **Causes** See table 3.2. **Symptoms and signs** ACS-like symptoms, heart failure symptoms, palpitations, tachycardia, soft S_1, S_3 gallop (p44). **Tests** ECG: ST changes and T-wave inversion, atrial arrhythmias, transient AV block, QT prolongation. Bloods: CRP, ESR, & troponin may be raised; viral serology and tests for other likely causes. Echo: diastolic dysfunction, regional wall abnormalities. Cardiac MR if clinically stable. Endomyocardial biopsy is gold standard. ℞ Supportive. Treat the underlying cause, dysrhythmias, and heart failure (p136). Avoid NSAIDs, heavy alcohol, and exercise as these can precipitate dysrhythmias and ↑ severity. **Prognosis** 50% will recover within 4wks. 12–25% will develop DCM and severe heart failure. DCM can occur years after apparent recovery.

Dilated cardiomyopathy (DCM) Dilatation and impaired contraction of one or both ventricles. Associations: alcohol, ↑BP, chemotherapeutics, haemochromatosis, viral infection, autoimmune, pregnancy, thyrotoxicosis, genetic (50% of 'idiopathic' cases). **Prevalence** 0.2%. **Presentation** Fatigue, dyspnoea, pulmonary oedema, RVF, emboli, AF, VT. **Signs** ↑Pulse, ↓BP, ↑JVP, displaced and diffuse apex, S_3 gallop, mitral or tricuspid regurgitation (MR/TR), pleural effusion, oedema, jaundice, hepatomegaly, ascites. **Tests** *Blood:* BNP (p134), ↓Na⁺ indicates a poor prognosis. *CXR:* cardiomegaly, pulmonary oedema. *ECG:* Tachycardia, non-specific T-wave changes, poor R-wave progression. *Echo:* Globally dilated hypokinetic heart and low ejection fraction. Look for MR, TR, LV mural thrombus. ℞ Diuretics, β-blockers, ACE-i, anticoagulation, biventricular pacing, ICDs, LVADs, transplantation. **Mortality** Variable, eg 40% in 2yrs.

Hypertrophic cardiomyopathy (HCM) LV outflow tract (LVOT) obstruction from asymmetric septal hypertrophy. HCM is the leading cause of sudden cardiac death in the young. **Prevalence** 0.2%. Autosomal dominant inheritance, but 50% are sporadic. 70% have mutations in genes encoding β-myosin, α-tropomyosin, and troponin T. May present at any age. Ask about family history of sudden death. **Symptoms and signs** Sudden death may be the first manifestation of HCM in many patients (VF is amenable to implantable defibrillators), angina, dyspnoea, palpitation, syncope, CCF. Jerky pulse; *a* wave in JVP; double-apex beat; systolic thrill at lower left sternal edge; harsh ejection systolic murmur. **Tests** • *ECG:* LVH; progressive T-wave inversion; deep Q waves (inferior + lateral leads); AF; WPW (p129); ventricular ectopics; VT. • *Echo:* asymmetrical septal hypertrophy; small LV cavity with hypercontractile posterior wall; mid-systolic closure of aortic valve; systolic anterior movement of mitral valve. • *MRI:* see fig 3.19, p101. • *Cardiac catheterization* helps assess: severity of gradient; coronary artery disease or mitral regurgitation, but may provoke VT. • Electrophysiological studies may be needed (eg if WPW, p129). • Exercise test ± Holter monitor (p121) to risk stratify. ℞ β-blockers or verapamil for symptoms (the aim is reducing ventricular contractility). Amiodarone (p130) for arrhythmias (AF, VT). Anticoagulate for paroxysmal AF or systemic emboli. Septal myomectomy (surgical or chemical (with alcohol) to ↓ LV outflow tract gradient) is reserved for those with severe symptoms. Consider ICD—use http://www.doc2do.com/hcm/webHCM.html to assess risk of sudden cardiac death. **Mortality** 5.9%/yr if <14yrs; 2.5%/yr if >14yrs. *Poor prognostic factors:* age <14yrs or syncope at presentation; family history of HCM/sudden death.

Restrictive cardiomyopathy Causes Idiopathic; amyloidosis; haemochromatosis; sarcoidosis; scleroderma; Löffler's eosinophilic endocarditis; endomyocardial fibrosis. **Presentation** Is like constrictive pericarditis (p132). Features of RVF predominate: ↑JVP, with prominent *x* and *y* descents; hepatomegaly; oedema; ascites. **Diagnosis** ↑↑BNP, echo, MRI, cardiac catheterization. ℞ Treat the cause.

Cardiac myxoma (figs 3.43, 3.44) Rare benign cardiac tumour. Prevalence ≤5/10 000, ♀:♂ ≈ 2:1. Usually sporadic, but may be familial (Carney complex: cardiac and cutaneous myxomas, skin pigmentation, endocrinopathy, etc., p217). It may mimic infective endocarditis (fever, weight loss, clubbing, ↑ESR, systemic emboli), or mitral stenosis (left atrial obstruction, AF). A 'tumour plop' may be heard, and signs may vary according to posture. **Tests** Echo. ℞ Resection.

How to inflame the heart

Table 3.2 Causes of myocarditis

Idiopathic	50% of cases
Viral	Enteroviruses, adenoviruses, HHV6, EBV, CMV, influenza, hepatitis, mumps, rubeola, Coxsackie, polio, HIV, HSV
Bacterial	*Staph*, *Strep*, *Clostridia*, diphtheria, TB, meningococcus, *Mycoplasma*, brucellosis, psittacosis
Spirochaetes	Leptospirosis, syphilis, Lyme disease
Protozoa	Chagas' (p419), *Leishmania*, toxoplasmosis
Drugs	Cyclophosphamide, trastuzumab, penicillin, chloramphenicol, sulfonamides, methyldopa, spironolactone, phenytoin, carbamazepine
Toxins	Cocaine, lithium, alcohol, lead, arsenic
Immunological	SLE, sarcoid, Kawasaki, scleroderma, heart transplant rejection

Cardiac amyloidosis

Infiltration of the heart by amyloidogenic proteins including monoclonal light chains in light-chain (AL) amyloidosis presenting as heart failure, syncope, or angina. Echo shows increased thickness of the ventricular walls (± ↑echogenicity, thickened valve leaflets, interatrial septum). Diastolic dysfunction precedes ↓LVEF. CMR may be helpful. ℞ Loop diuretics, anticoagulation if AF, intracardiac thrombi, or embolic event. Chemotherapy ± autologous SCT if AL amyloidosis.

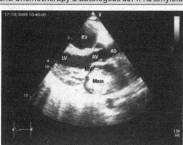

Fig 3.43 Echocardiogram of a 35yr-old patient who presented with severe exertional dyspnoea and several episodes of syncope. Look at the large mass (cardiac myxoma) in left atrium.
Reproduced with permission from Hamid Reza Taghipour.

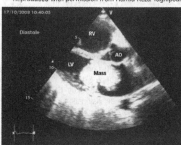

Fig 3.44 Echocardiogram of the same patient as fig 343 during diastole. Notice how the large mass of myxoma protrudes into the left ventricle during diastole, and obstructs the mitral valve almost completely.
Reproduced with permission from Hamid Reza Taghipour.

Acute pericarditis This is inflammation of the pericardium.[38] **Causes** Idiopathic (80%) or secondary to:

• Viruses: eg coxsackie, echovirus, EBV, CMV, adenovirus, mumps, varicella, HIV.
• Bacteria: eg TB—commonest cause worldwide, Lyme disease, Q fever, pneumonia, rheumatic fever, *Staphs, Streps, Mycoplasma, Legionella, Mycobacterium avium intracellulare* in HIV.
• Fungi and parasitic: v rare, usually in immunocompromised.
• Autoimmune: systemic autoimmune diseases, eg SLE, RA; vasculitides, eg Behçet's, Takayasu; IBD; sarcoidosis; amyloidosis; Dressler's (p133).
• Drugs: eg procainamide, hydralazine, penicillin, isoniazid, chemotherapy.
• Metabolic: uraemia, hypothyroidism, anorexia nervosa.
• Others: trauma, surgery, malignancy, radiotherapy, MI, chronic heart failure.

Clinical features Central chest pain worse on inspiration or lying flat ± relief by sitting forward. A pericardial friction rub (p44) may be heard. Look for evidence of a pericardial effusion or cardiac tamponade (see later in topic). Fever may occur. **Tests** ECG classically shows concave (saddle-shaped) ST-segment elevation and PR depression, but may be normal or non-specific (10%); see fig 3.45. *Blood tests:* FBC, ESR, U&E, cardiac enzymes (NB: troponin may be raised); tests relating to possible aetiologies. Cardiomegaly on CXR may indicate a pericardial effusion. *Echo* (if suspected pericardial effusion). CMR and CT may show localized inflammation. **Treatment** Aspirin or NSAIDs (ibuprofen preferred) with gastric protection for 1–2weeks if viral/idiopathic. Steroids if NSAIDs CI (eg CKD) or for autoimmune condition. Add colchicine for 3mths if not improving. Rest until symptoms resolve. Admit if any predictor of poor prognosis (see below) & aetiology search. Treat the cause.

Pericardial effusion Accumulation of fluid in the pericardial sac (normally 10–50mL).[38] **Causes** Pericarditis, myocardial rupture (haemopericardium—surgical, stab wound, post-MI); aortic dissection; pericardium filling with pus; malignancy. **Clinical features** Dyspnoea, chest pain, signs of local structures being compressed—hiccoughs (phrenic N), nausea (diaphragm), bronchial breathing at left base (Ewart's sign: compressed left lower lobe). Muffled heart sounds. Look for signs of cardiac tamponade. **Diagnosis** CXR shows an enlarged, globular heart if effusion >300mL; fig 3.17, p101. ECG shows low-voltage QRS complexes and may have alternating QRS morphologies (electrical alternans). *Echocardiography* shows an echo-free zone surrounding the heart. **Management** Treat the cause. Pericardiocentesis may be *diagnostic* (suspected bacterial pericarditis) or *therapeutic* (cardiac tamponade). See p757. Send pericardial fluid for culture, ZN stain/TB culture, and cytology.

Constrictive pericarditis The heart is encased in a rigid pericardium.[38] **Causes** Often unknown (UK); elsewhere TB, or after *any* pericarditis. **Clinical features** These are mainly of right heart failure with ↑JVP (with prominent *x* and *y* descents, p41); Kussmaul's sign (JVP rising paradoxically with inspiration); soft, diffuse apex beat; quiet heart sounds; S₃; diastolic pericardial knock; hepatosplenomegaly; ascites; and oedema. **Tests** CXR: small heart ± pericardial calcification. CT/MRI—helps distinguish from restrictive cardiomyopathy. *Echo. Cardiac catheterization.* **Management** Surgical excision. Medical ℞ to address the cause and symptoms.

Cardiac tamponade A pericardial effusion that raises intrapericardial pressure, reducing ventricular filling and thus dropping cardiac output.[38] ►►Can lead rapidly to cardiac arrest. **Signs** ↑Pulse, ↓BP, pulsus paradoxus, ↑JVP, Kussmaul's sign, muffled S₁ and S₂. **Diagnosis** *Beck's triad:* falling BP; rising JVP; muffled heart sounds. ECG: low-voltage QRS ± electrical alternans. *Echo* is diagnostic: echo-free zone (>2cm, or >1cm if acute) around the heart ± diastolic collapse of right atrium and right ventricle. **Management** Seek expert help. The pericardial effusion needs urgent drainage (p757). Send fluid for culture, ZN stain/TB culture, and cytology.

Predictors of poor prognosis in pericarditis **Major** • Fever >38°C. • Subacute onset. • Large pericardial effusion/tamponade. • Lack of response after 1wk of therapy. **Minor** • Myopericarditis. • Immunosuppression or anticoagulation. • Trauma. • Venous thrombosis. • ↑Pacing/defibrillation thresholds. • Device and/or lead migration or fracture.

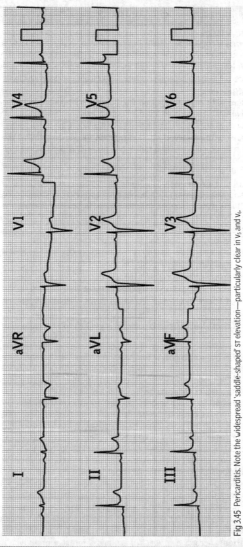

Fig 3.45 Pericarditis. Note the widespread 'saddle-shaped' ST elevation—particularly clear in V5 and V6.

Dressler's syndrome

Dressler's syndrome (named after US cardiologist William Dressler, 1890–1969) develops 2–10wks after an MI, heart surgery (or even pacemaker insertion). It is thought that myocardial injury stimulates formation of autoantibodies against heart muscle.

Symptoms Recurrent fever and chest pain ± pleural or pericardial rub (from serositis). Cardiac tamponade may occur, so avoid anticoagulants. ℞ Aspirin, NSAIDs, or steroids.

Definition A failure of the heart to meet the metabolic demands of the body. Characterized by typical symptoms (eg SOB, fatigue) ± signs (eg ↑JVP, pulmonary crackles, and SOA) caused by a structural and/or functional cardiac abnormality, resulting in a ↓cardiac output and/or ↑intracardiac pressures at rest or during stress.

Prevalence 1–3% of the general population; ~10% among elderly patients.

Key classifications[30]

Heart failure with reduced ejection fraction (HFrEF) Inability of the ventricle to contract normally, resulting in ↓cardiac output (systolic failure) with progressive chamber dilation and eccentric remodelling. EF is ≤40%. *Causes:* MI, cardiomyopathy.

Heart failure with preserved ejection fraction (HFpEF) Inability of the ventricle to relax and fill normally, causing ↑filling pressures (diastolic failure). Typically EF is ≥50%. LV concentric remodelling or hypertrophy often present. *Causes:* hypertension, CAD, CKD, obesity, infiltrative conditions, constrictive pericarditis.

Left ventricular failure (LVF) *Symptoms:* dyspnoea, poor exercise tolerance, fatigue, orthopnoea, paroxysmal nocturnal dyspnoea (PND), nocturnal cough (± pink frothy sputum), wheeze (cardiac 'asthma'), nocturia, cold peripheries, weight loss.

Right ventricular failure (RVF) *Causes:* LVF, pulmonary stenosis, lung disease (cor pulmonale, see p189). *Symptoms:* Peripheral oedema (up to thighs, sacrum, abdominal wall), ascites, nausea, anorexia, facial engorgement, epistaxis.

LVF and RVF may occur independently, or together as *congestive cardiac failure* (CCF).

Acute heart failure Often used exclusively to mean new-onset acute or decompensation of chronic heart failure (ADHF) characterized by pulmonary and/or peripheral oedema with or without signs of peripheral hypoperfusion.

Chronic heart failure Develops or progresses slowly. Venous congestion is common but arterial pressure is well maintained until very late.

Low-output heart failure Cardiac output is ↓ and fails to ↑ normally with exertion. *Causes:*
• *Excessive preload:* eg mitral regurgitation or fluid overload (eg renal failure or too rapid IV infusions, particularly in the elderly and those with established HF).
• *Pump failure:* systolic and/or diastolic HF (see above), ↓heart rate (eg β-blockers, heart block, post-MI), negatively inotropic drugs (eg most anti-arrhythmic agents).
• *Chronic excessive afterload:* eg aortic stenosis, hypertension.

Excessive preload can cause ventricular dilatation, this exacerbates pump failure. *Excessive afterload* prompts ventricular muscle thickening (ventricular hypertrophy), resulting in stiff walls and diastolic dysfunction.

High-output heart failure This is rare. Here, output is normal or increased in the face of ↑↑needs. Failure occurs when cardiac output fails to meet these needs. It will occur with a normal heart, but even earlier if there is heart disease. *Causes:* anaemia, pregnancy, hyperthyroidism, Paget's disease, arteriovenous malformation, beriberi.

Diagnosis Requires symptoms of failure (see above) and objective evidence of cardiac dysfunction at rest. For CCF, use the *Framingham* criteria.[40]

Signs As described previously plus cyanosis, ↓BP, narrow pulse pressure, pulsus alternans, displaced apex (LV dilatation), RV heave (pulmonary hypertension), signs of valve diseases. Severity can be graded using the New York classification (see BOX).

Investigations According to NICE,[41] if ECG and N-terminal pro-B-type natriuretic peptide (NT-proBNP; see BOX 'NT-proBNP') are normal, heart failure is unlikely, and an alternative diagnosis should be considered; if either is abnormal or the history/PE suggestive, then echocardiography (p102) is required.

Tests FBC; U&E; NT-proBNP; CXR (fig 3.46); ECG; echo. *ECG* may indicate cause (look for evidence of ischaemia, MI, or LVH). It is rare to get a completely normal ECG in chronic heart failure. *Echo* is the key investigation. It may indicate the cause (MI, valvular heart disease) and can confirm the presence or absence of LV dysfunction. CMR may be helpful if non-diagnostic. *Endomyocardial biopsy* is rarely needed.

New York Heart Association (NYHA) classification

I Heart disease present, but no undue dyspnoea from ordinary activity.
II Comfortable at rest; dyspnoea during ordinary activities.
III Less than ordinary activity causes dyspnoea, which is limiting.
IV Dyspnoea present at rest; all activity causes discomfort.

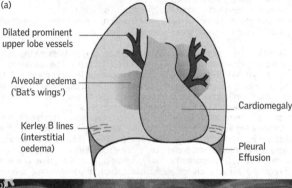

(a)

Dilated prominent upper lobe vessels

Alveolar oedema ('Bat's wings')

Kerley B lines (interstitial oedema)

Cardiomegaly

Pleural Effusion

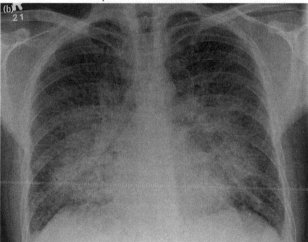

Fig 3.46 (a) The CXR in left ventricular failure. These features can be remembered as **A B C D E**. **A**lveolar oedema, classically this is perihilar 'bat's wing' shadowing. Kerley **B** lines—now known as septal lines. These are variously attributed to interstitial oedema and engorged peripheral lymphatics. **C**ardiomegaly—cardiothoracic ratio >50% on a PA film. **D**ilated prominent upper lobe veins (upper lobe diversion). Pleural **E**ffusions. Other features include peribronchial cuffing (thickened bronchial walls) and fluid in the fissures. (b) 'Bat's wing', perihilar pulmonary oedema indicating heart failure and fluid overload.

NT-proBNP—a diagnostic and prognostic marker in heart failure

An NT-proBNP level <400ng/L (47pmol/L) makes a diagnosis of heart failure less likely. Because very high levels of NT-proBNP carry a poor prognosis, refer people with suspected heart failure and an NT-proBNP level >2000ng/L (236pmol/L) urgently, to have specialist assessment and TTE within 2 weeks. Refer people with an NT-proBNP level between 400 and 2000ng/L (47–236pmol/L) to have specialist assessment and TTE within 6 weeks.

3 Cardiovascular medicine

Acute heart failure ▶▶This is a medical emergency (p784).

Chronic heart failure ▶Stop smoking. Stop drinking alcohol. Eat less salt. Optimize weight & nutrition.[41]

• Treat the cause (eg dysrhythmias; valve disease).
• Treat exacerbating factors (anaemia, thyroid disease, infection, ↑BP).
• Avoid exacerbating factors, eg NSAIDs (fluid retention) and verapamil (–ve inotrope).
• Annual 'flu vaccine, one-off pneumococcal vaccine.
• Drugs:

  1 **Diuretics** Give loop diuretics to relieve symptoms & ↓ mortality, eg furosemide 40mg/24h PO or bumetanide 1–2mg/24h PO. Increase dose as necessary. SE: K⁺↓, AKI. Monitor U&E and add K⁺-sparing diuretic (eg spironolactone) if K⁺ <3.5mmol/L, predisposition to arrhythmias, concurrent digoxin therapy, or pre-existing K⁺-losing conditions. If refractory oedema, consider adding a thiazide, eg chlortalidone 25/24h PO for sequential nephron blockade.

  2 **ACE-i** Consider in all those with left ventricular systolic dysfunction (LVSD)—start low (eg lisinopril 2.5mg/24h PO) and wind up the dose, monitor BP and U&E. Improves symptoms and prolongs life (pp106–7). If cough is a problem, an *angiotensin receptor antagonist* (ARA) may be substituted. SE: ↑K⁺.

  3 **ARNI** (eg sacubitril/valsartan) Promotes vasodilatation, natriuresis, & diuresis. *Replaces* ACE-i/ARB in chronic symptomatic heart failure NYHA II–III to further reduce morbidity and mortality. Dosing depends on prior dose of ACE-i/ARB.

  4 **β-blockers** (eg carvedilol) ↓Mortality in heart failure with systolic dysfunction. Use with caution: 'start low and go slow' once euvolemic; if in doubt seek specialist advice first; wait ≥2weeks between each dose increment. β-blocker therapy in patients hospitalized with decompensated heart failure is associated with lower post-discharge mortality risk and improved treatment rates.[42]

  5 **Mineralocorticoid receptor antagonists** Spironolactone (25mg/24h PO) ↓ mortality by 30% when added to conventional therapy.[43] Use in those still symptomatic despite optimal therapy, and in post-MI patients with LVSD. Since spironolactone is K⁺ sparing, the U&E should be monitored, particularly if the patient has known CKD.

  6 **Vasodilators** The combination of hydralazine (SE: drug-induced lupus) and isosorbide dinitrate should be used if intolerant of ACE-i and ARBs as it reduces mortality. It also reduces mortality when added to standard therapy (including ACE-i) in black patients with heart failure.[44]

  7 **SGLT2 inhibitors** Recent evidence suggests they ↓ hospitalizations and CV death regardless of diabetes status.[45] Recommended for HFrEF, eg dapagliflozin 10mg OD.

  8 **Ivabradine** May ↓ hospitalizations in patients with chronic HFrEF in sinus rhythm with a resting HR >70bpm and who are on a max tolerated dose of β-blocker.

  9 **Digoxin** ↓ Hospitalizations in symptomatic HFrEF. Mainly helpful for additional rate/symptom control in HF patients with AF. Dose example: 125mcg/24h PO Monitor U&E; maintain K⁺ at 4–5mmol/L as ↓K⁺ risks digoxin toxicity, and vice versa. Digoxin levels: p740.

HFpEF Manage contributing factors and associated conditions, eg HTN, AF. Control volume overload with diuretics. Avoid β-blockers unless other indication.

Intractable heart failure Reassess the cause. Are they taking the drugs?—at maximum dose? Switching furosemide to bumetanide (one 5mg tab ≈ 200mg furosemide) might help. Inpatient management may include:

• Minimal exertion; Na⁺ & fluid restriction (1.5L/24h PO).
• Metolazone (as above) and IV furosemide (p784).
• Opiates and IV nitrates may relieve symptoms (p784).
• Weigh daily (target 0.5–1kg reduction/24h). Do frequent U&E (beware ↓K⁺).
• Give DVT prophylaxis: heparin + TED stockings (p578).

Consider Cardiac rehabilitation, CRT (p128), LV assist device, or transplantation (see BOX 'Device therapy and transplantation').

Device therapy and transplantation

ICD See indications p128 and complications p129.

CRT See indications p128.

Short-term mechanical circulatory support devices (eg IABP, Impella, ECMO) See p784.

Long-term mechanical circulatory support devices

Left ventricular assist devices (LVAD) bridge to transplantation for selected patients with refractory HFrEF (fig 3.47). Less common indications include bridge to decision, permanent (or 'destination') therapy, or bridge to recovery. An internalized pump forces blood through tubing from the left ventricle to the aorta. Patients with continuous (rather than pulsatile) flow LVADs have no pulse (fig 3.47c) and auscultation will reveal a loud, continuous, mechanical hum. If the patient collapses and there is no hum, resuscitation should include checking the LVAD power supply!

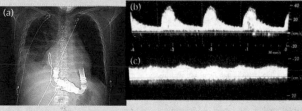

Fig 3.47 (a) CXR of a patient with a continuous flow LVAD. Blood is taken from the LV apex and pumped into the aorta. (b) Retinal flow velocity trace from a normal subject—large peaks in flow rate during systole. (c) Retinal flow velocity trace from a patient with an LVAD. The flow rate only slightly rises during systole as the flow from the LVAD is continuous.

Image in (a) reproduced from Gardener *et al.*, *Heart Failure*, 2014, with permission from Oxford University Press. (b) and (c) courtesy of Barry McDonnell.

Biventricular support (eg total artificial heart or biventricular assist device): less commonly used bridge to transplantation for selected patients with refractory biventricular HFrEF.

All patients treated with ventricular assist devices require systemic anticoagulation to reduce the risk of thrombotic complications such as device thrombosis and embolic stroke. Other complications include bleeding, infection, arrhythmias, and haemolysis.

Cardiac transplantation Consider if persistent symptoms at rest or on minimal exertion despite optimal medical therapy, recurrent admissions, recurrent symptomatic ventricular arrhythmia, refractory ischaemia not amenable to revascularization associated with severely impaired LV function. Several contraindications including infection, PVD, GFR <40mL/min, cancer, severe lung disease, and pulmonary hypertension. Lifelong immunosuppression but median survival >10 years in most centres.

Prognosis and palliative care

Prognosis Poor with ~25–50% of patients dying within 5yrs of diagnosis. If admission is needed, 5yr mortality ≈75%. Be realistic: in one study, 54% of those dying in the next 72h had been expected to live for >6mths.

Palliative care Treat/prevent comorbidities (eg 'flu vaccination). Good nutrition (↓ alcohol!). Involve GP: continuity of care and discussion of prognosis is much appreciated. Dyspnoea, pain (from liver capsule stretching), nausea, constipation, and ↓mood all need tackling. Opiates improve pain and dyspnoea. Home O_2 may help.

Mitral regurgitation (MR) Backflow through the mitral valve during systole.

Causes *Acute:* papillary muscle dysfunction/rupture (eg post-MI, trauma); ruptured chordae tendineae due to mitral valve prolapse (MVP), infective endocarditis, rheumatic fever. *Chronic:* functional (LV dilatation); annular calcification (elderly); connective tissue disorders (Ehlers–Danlos, Marfan's); cardiomyopathy (eg HCM, dilated CM); MVP; congenital (may be associated with other defects, eg ASD, AV canal); appetite suppressants (eg fenfluramine, phentermine).

Symptoms Dyspnoea; fatigue; palpitations; symptoms of causative factor (eg fever).

Signs AF; displaced, hyperdynamic apex; pansystolic murmur at apex radiating to axilla; soft S₁; split S₂; loud P₂ (pulmonary hypertension). *Severity:* the more severe, the larger the left ventricle.

Tests *ECG:* AF; P-mitrale if in sinus rhythm (may mean ↑left atrial size); LVH. *CXR:* big LA & LV; mitral valve calcification; pulmonary oedema.

Echocardiogram To assess LV function and MR severity and aetiology (transoesophageal to assess severity and suitability for repair rather than replacement). *Cardiac catheterization* to confirm diagnosis, exclude other valve disease, and assess coronary artery disease (can combine CABG with valve surgery).

Management Control rate if fast AF. Anticoagulate if: AF; history of embolism; prosthetic valve; additional mitral stenosis. Diuretics improve symptoms. Surgery if symptomatic with severe MR or if asymptomatic with severe MR and ↓LVEF; aim to repair or replace the valve before LV is irreversibly impaired. If prohibitive surgical risk and favourable anatomy, consider transcatheter mitral valve repair (MitraClip™ device).

Mitral valve prolapse Is the most common valvular abnormality (prevalence: ~5%). Occurs alone or with: ASD, patent ductus arteriosus, cardiomyopathy, Turner syndrome, Marfan's syndrome, osteogenesis imperfecta, pseudoxanthoma elasticum, WPW (p129). **Symptoms** Usually asymptomatic. May develop atypical chest pain, palpitations, and autonomic dysfunction symptoms. **Signs** Mid-systolic click and/or a late systolic murmur. **Complications** MR, cerebral emboli, arrhythmias, sudden death. **Tests** *Echo* is diagnostic. *ECG* may show inferior T-wave inversion. ℞ β-blockers may help palpitations and chest pain. Surgery if severe MR.

Mitral stenosis (MS) Causes Rheumatic fever, congenital, mucopolysaccharidoses, endocardial fibroelastosis, malignant carcinoid (p266; rare), prosthetic valve.

Presentation Normal mitral valve orifice area is ~4–6cm². Symptoms usually begin when the orifice becomes <2cm². Pulmonary hypertension causes dyspnoea, haemoptysis, chronic bronchitis-like picture; pressure from large left atrium on local structures causes hoarseness (recurrent laryngeal nerve), dysphagia (oesophagus), bronchial obstruction; also fatigue, palpitations, chest pain, systemic emboli, infective endocarditis (rare).

Signs Malar flush on cheeks (due to ↓cardiac output); low-volume pulse; AF common (due to enlarged LA); tapping, non-displaced, apex beat (palpable S₁); RV heave. On auscultation: loud S₁; opening snap (pliable valve); rumbling mid-diastolic murmur (heard best in expiration, with patient on left side). Graham Steell murmur (p44) may occur. *Severity:* the more severe the stenosis, the longer the diastolic murmur, and the closer the opening snap is to S₂.

Tests *ECG:* AF; P-mitrale; RVH; progressive RAD. *CXR:* left atrial enlargement (double shadow in right cardiac silhouette); pulmonary oedema; mitral valve calcification. *Echo* is diagnostic. Significant stenosis exists if the valve orifice is <1cm²/m² body surface area. Indications for *cardiac catheterization:* previous valvotomy; signs of other valve disease; angina; severe pulmonary hypertension; calcified mitral valve.

Management If in AF, *rate control* (p126) *is crucial*; anticoagulate with warfarin (p346). Diuretics ↓ preload and pulmonary venous congestion. If symptomatic with severe MS present, balloon valvuloplasty (if pliable, non-calcified valve), open mitral valvotomy, or valve replacement.

What becomes of the broken hearted?

From Aztec priests raising beating human hearts to the Sun God, to heart metaphors in song lyrics today, ideas of links between the heart and human psychosocial self/soul/experience-of-being have pervaded the imaginative landscapes of cultures throughout time and place.

Some of these links relate to physiological changes associated with emotion-triggered adrenaline surges—'my heart raced', for example, is a phrase we relate to both physically and emotionally. Other heart phrases result from poetic extrapolations of heart/self ideas and have no physiological explanation, eg 'he wears his heart on his sleeve'.

Evidence is building that heart/self interactions exist beyond metaphor and symptomatic 'flight-or-fight' responses. Affective disorders, certain personality types, and traumatic life experiences increase the risk of cardiac disease, even when lifestyle factors are controlled for. In 'broken heart syndrome' (stress or Takotsubo cardiomyopathy), ventricular contraction morphology changes in response to emotional or physical stress (fig 3.48). It mimics a myocardial infarction in terms of clinical history, ECG changes, and troponin rises, but the prognosis and management may be quite different so accurate diagnosis is important.

As physicians, we often focus on explainable physical aspects of disease, but the physical and psychosocial are inconveniently related and both should be assessed to determine best management. Should an IHD sufferer be offered CBT alongside their statins? Could a grieving patient's 'MI' be Takotsubo cardiomyopathy? To answer these questions we must look beyond ECGs and troponin, to the 'heart-ache' of the literary and philosophical kinds.

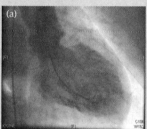 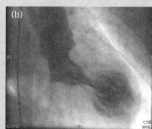

Fig 3.48 (a) Left ventriculogram of a heart in diastole. (b) The same patient's heart in systole. The apex is ballooning whilst the base contracts, causing inefficient pumping and a risk of rupture. This pattern is classic of Takotsubo cardiomyopathy.

The heartless

'How about my heart?' asked the Tin Woodman.

'Why, as for that,' answered Oz, 'I think you are wrong to want a heart. It makes most people unhappy. If you only knew it, you are in luck not to have a heart.'

'That must be a matter of opinion,' said the Tin Woodman. 'For my part, I will bear all the unhappiness without a murmur, if you will give me the heart.'

(Baum FL, *The Wonderful Wizard of Oz: Oxford World's Classics* (2008), p.191)

Aortic stenosis (AS) Causes Senile calcification is the commonest. *Others:* Congenital (bicuspid valve, Williams syndrome, p143), rheumatic heart disease.

Presentation Think of AS in any elderly person with chest pain, exertional dyspnoea, or syncope. The classic triad includes angina, syncope, and heart failure. Also: dyspnoea; dizziness; syncope; systemic emboli if infective endocarditis; sudden death. **Signs** Slow rising pulse with narrow pulse pressure (feel for diminished and delayed carotid upstroke—*parvus et tardus*); heaving, non-displaced apex beat; LV heave; aortic thrill; ejection systolic murmur (heard at the base, left sternal edge and the aortic area, radiates to the carotids). S_1 is usually normal. As stenosis worsens, A_2 is increasingly delayed, giving first a single S_2 and then reversed splitting. But this sign is rare. More common is a quiet A_2. In severe AS, A_2 may be inaudible (calcified valve). There may be an ejection click (pliable valve) or an S_4.

Tests *ECG:* LVH with strain pattern; P-mitrale; LAD; poor R-wave progression; LBBB or complete AV block (calcified ring). *CXR:* LVH; calcified aortic valve (fig 3.49); post-stenotic dilatation of ascending aorta. *Echo:* diagnostic (p102). Doppler echo can estimate the gradient across valves: severe stenosis if peak gradient ≥40mmHg (but beware the poor left ventricle not able to generate gradient—'low flow, low gradient' severe AS) and valve area <1cm². If the aortic jet velocity is >4m/s (or is increasing by >0.3m/s per year) risk of complications is increased. *Cardiac catheter:* can assess: valve gradient; LV function; coronary artery disease; risks: emboli generation. CT aortogram if bicuspid aortic valve to look for coarctation or root dilatation (BAV aortopathy).

Differential diagnosis Hypertrophic cardiomyopathy (HCM, p130); aortic sclerosis.

Management If symptomatic, prognosis is poor without surgery: 2–3yr survival if angina/syncope; 1–2yrs if cardiac failure. If moderate-to-severe and treated medically, mortality can be as high as 50% at 2yrs, therefore prompt valve replacement (p142) is usually recommended if symptomatic, ↓LVEF, or if undergoing other cardiac surgery. If the patient is not medically fit for surgery, transcatheter aortic valve implantation (TAVI; fig 3.50) may be attempted (see BOX 'TAVI').

Aortic sclerosis Senile degeneration of the valve. There is an ejection systolic murmur; but no carotid radiation, and normal pulse (character and volume) and S_2.

Aortic regurgitation (AR) Acute Infective endocarditis, ascending aortic dissection, chest trauma. **Chronic** Congenital, connective tissue disorders (Marfan's syndrome, Ehlers–Danlos), rheumatic fever, Takayasu arteritis, rheumatoid arthritis, SLE, pseudoxanthoma elasticum, appetite suppressants (eg fenfluramine, phentermine), seronegative arthritides (ankylosing spondylitis, Reiter's syndrome, psoriatic arthropathy), hypertension, osteogenesis imperfecta, syphilitic aortitis.

Symptoms Exertional dyspnoea, orthopnoea, and PND. Also: palpitations, angina, syncope, CCF. **Signs** Collapsing (waterhammer) pulse (p40); wide pulse pressure; displaced, hyperdynamic apex beat; high-pitched early diastolic murmur (heard best in expiration, with patient sat forward). **Eponyms** *Corrigan's sign:* carotid pulsation; *de Musset's sign:* head nodding with each heart beat; *Quincke's sign:* capillary pulsations in nail beds; *Duroziez's sign:* in the groin, a finger compressing the femoral artery 2cm proximal to the stethoscope gives a systolic murmur; if 2cm distal, it gives a diastolic murmur as blood flows backwards; *Traube's sign:* 'pistol shot' sound over femoral arteries; *Austin Flint murmur:* (p44) denotes *severe* AR.

Tests *ECG:* LVH. *CXR:* cardiomegaly; dilated ascending aorta; pulmonary oedema. *Echo:* is diagnostic. *Cardiac catheterization:* to assess severity of lesion; anatomy of aortic root; LV function; coronary artery disease; other valve disease.

Management The main goal of medical therapy is to reduce systolic hypertension; ACE-i are helpful. Echo every 6–12 months to monitor. Indications for surgery: severe AR with enlarged ascending aorta, increasing symptoms, enlarging LV or deteriorating LV function on echo; or infective endocarditis refractory to medical therapy. Aim to replace the valve before significant LV dysfunction occurs. Predictors of poor post-operative survival: ejection fraction <50%, NYHA class III or IV (p135), duration of CCF >12 months.

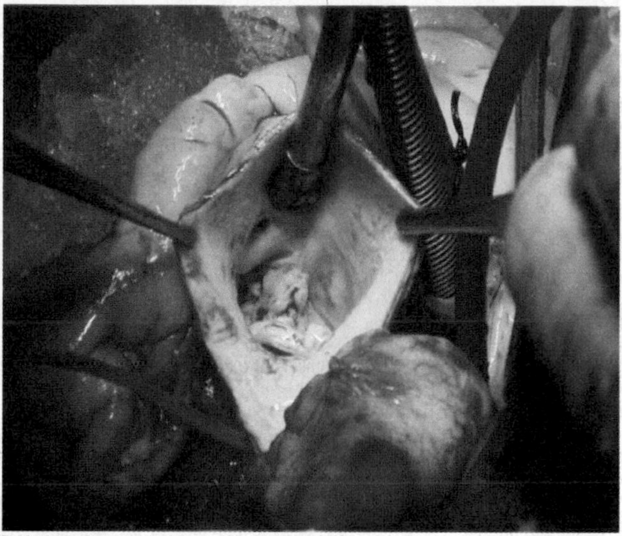

Fig 3.49 Severely calcified aortic valve.   Reproduced with permission from Hamid Reza Taghipour.

TAVI

Indications

According to ESC guidelines, mainly indicated symptomatic, severe AS patients with high surgical risk due to comorbidities, age >75 years, previous cardiac surgery, or frailty. American guidelines recommend more liberal use in intermediate-risk patients where short-term outcomes appear to be comparable. The decision should be individualized taking into account comorbidities, transfemoral access, bicuspid vs unicuspid aortic valve, severe LV outflow tract calcification, and the presence of an adverse aortic root.

Complications

Peri-procedural: bleeding, access-related complications, aortic dissection/perforation (0.12%), ventricular perforation (1%), annular rupture, TAVI malpositioning, AR, stroke (2–5%), myocardial ischaemia/injury, AKI, and arrhythmias. *Long term:* AR (12% moderate-severe), valve thrombosis (<1%), prosthetic valve endocarditis, prosthesis-patient mismatch.

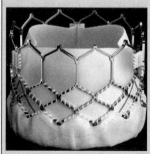

Fig 3.50 This is one of the two main types of TAVI: animal valve leaflets mounted on metal stents. This structure must be resilient against the movement of the heart walls and the powerful flow of blood; it must avoid obstructing forward flow of blood whilst providing a near-complete block to backflow; and it has surfaces of foreign material yet must avoid triggering clots or allowing microbial growth. It must also be able to fold down over a wire to allow safe passage through the arterial tree from the groin to the heart, before being opened out by an inflated balloon.

Image courtesy of Edwards Lifesciences LLC, Irvine, CA. Edwards, Edwards Lifesciences, Edwards SAPIEN, SAPIEN, SAPIEN XT and SAPIEN 3 are trademarks of Edwards Lifesciences Corporation.

Right heart valve disease

Tricuspid regurgitation Causes Functional (RV dilatation; eg due to pulmonary hypertension induced by LV failure or PE); rheumatic fever; infective endocarditis (IV drug user[3]); carcinoid syndrome; congenital (eg ASD, AV canal, Ebstein's anomaly (downward displacement of the tricuspid valve—see *OHCS* p846)); drugs (eg ergot-derived dopamine agonists, p491; fenfluramine). **Symptoms** Fatigue; hepatic pain on exertion (due to hepatic congestion); ascites; oedema and symptoms of the causative condition. **Signs** Giant *v* waves and prominent *y* descent in JVP (p41); RV heave; pansystolic murmur, heard best at lower sternal edge in inspiration; pulsatile hepatomegaly; jaundice; ascites. **Management** Drugs: diuretics for systemic congestion; drugs to treat underlying cause. Valve repair or replacement (~10% 30-day mortality). Tricuspid regurgitation resulting from myocardial dysfunction or dilatation has a mortality of up to 50% at 5yrs.

Tricuspid stenosis Causes Main cause is rheumatic fever, which almost always occurs with mitral or aortic valve disease. Also: congenital, infective endocarditis. **Symptoms** Fatigue, ascites, oedema. **Signs** Giant *a* wave and slow *y* descent in JVP (p41); opening snap, early diastolic murmur heard at the left sternal edge in inspiration. AF can also occur. **Diagnosis** Echo. **Treatment** Diuretics; surgical repair.

Pulmonary stenosis Causes Usually congenital (Turner syndrome, Noonan syndrome, Williams syndrome, Fallot's tetralogy, rubella). Acquired causes: rheumatic fever, carcinoid syndrome. **Symptoms** Dyspnoea; fatigue; oedema; ascites. **Signs** Dysmorphic facies (congenital causes); prominent *a* wave in JVP; RV heave. In mild stenosis, there is an ejection click, ejection systolic murmur (which radiates to the left shoulder); widely split S_2. In severe stenosis, the murmur becomes longer and obscures A_2. P_2 becomes softer and may be inaudible. **Tests** ECG: RAD, P-pulmonale, RVH, RBBB; echo/TOE (p102); CXR: prominent pulmonary arteries caused by post-stenotic dilatation. Cardiac catheterization is diagnostic. **Treatment** Pulmonary valvuloplasty or valvotomy.

Pulmonary regurgitation Causes Any cause of pulmonary hypertension (p188). **Signs** Decrescendo murmur in early diastole at the left sternal edge (the Graham Steell murmur if associated with mitral stenosis and pulmonary hypertension).

Cardiac surgery

Cardiac surgery has come on a long way since 1923 when Dr Henry Souttar[46,47] used his finger to open a stenosed mitral valve in a beating heart.[4] Cardiac bypass allows prolonged access to the open, static heart, during which complex and high-precision repair and replacement of valves and aortic roots can occur. Transcatheter procedures are playing an increasing role in the management of cardiovascular disease. Key open heart procedures include:

Valve replacements *Mechanical valves* may be of the ball-cage (Starr–Edwards), tilting disc (Bjork–Shiley), or double tilting disc (St. Jude) type. These valves are very durable but the risk of thromboembolism is high; patients require lifelong anticoagulation. *Xenografts* are made from porcine valves or pericardium. These valves are less durable and may require replacement at 8–10yrs but have the advantage of not necessitating anticoagulation. *Homografts* are cadaveric valves. They are particularly useful in young patients and in the replacement of infected valves. *Complications of prosthetic valves:* systemic embolism, infective endocarditis, haemolysis, structural valve failure, arrhythmias.

CABG See p119.

Cardiac transplantation Consider this when cardiac disease is *severely* curtailing quality of life, and survival is not expected beyond 6–12 months. See p137.

Surgery for congenital heart defects See p148.

Aortic root surgery Replacement/repair if dissection or aneurysmal.

---

3 Remember that it is the tricuspid valve which is the valve most vulnerable to events arriving by vein, eg pathogens from IV drug users or hormones (particularly 5HT) from carcinoid tumours.

4 Souttar's own description of this landmark case is available online: HS Souttar. The surgical treatment of mitral stenosis. *BMJ* 1925; 2(3379):603–6.

The heart in various, mostly rare, systemic diseases

This list reminds us to look at the heart *and* the whole patient, not just in exams (where those with odd syndromes congregate), but always.

Acromegaly (p232) ↑BP; LVH; hypertrophic cardiomyopathy; high-output cardiac failure; coronary artery disease.

Amyloidosis (p364) Restrictive cardiomyopathy. Bright myocardium on echo.

Ankylosing spondylitis (p546) Conduction defects; AV block; AR.

Behçet's disease (p554) Aortic regurgitation; arterial ± venous thrombi.

β thalassaemia (p338) Dilated and restrictive cardiomyopathies.

Carcinoid syndrome (p266) Tricuspid regurgitation and pulmonary stenosis.

Cushing's syndrome (p218) Hypertension.

Down's syndrome (*OHCS* p273) ASD; VSD; mitral regurgitation.

Ehlers–Danlos syndrome (*OHCS* p846) Mitral valve prolapse; aortic aneurysm and dissection; hyperelastic skin; GI bleeds. Joints are loose and hypermobile; mutations exist, eg in genes for procollagen (COL3A1); there are six types.

Friedreich's ataxia (p688) Hypertrophic cardiomyopathy, dilatation over time.

Haemochromatosis (p284) AF; cardiomyopathy.

Holt–Oram syndrome ASD or VSD with upper limb defects (eg polydactyly and triphalangeal thumb).

Human immunodeficiency virus (p394) Myocarditis; dilated cardiomyopathy; effusion; ventricular arrhythmias; SBE/IE; non-infective thrombotic (marantic) endocarditis; RVF (pulmonary hypertension); metastatic Kaposi's sarcoma.

Hypothyroidism (p214) Sinus bradycardia; low pulse pressure; pericardial effusion; coronary artery disease; low-voltage ECG.

Kawasaki disease (*OHCS* p850) Coronary arteritis similar to PAN; commoner than rheumatic fever (p146) as a cause of acquired heart disease.

Klinefelter's syndrome ♂ (*OHCS* p850) ASD. Psychopathy; learning difficulties; ↓libido; gynaecomastia; sparse facial hair and small firm testes. XXY.

Marfan's syndrome Mitral valve prolapse; AR; aortic dissection. Look for long fingers and a high-arched palate.

Myotonic dystrophy (p506) Progressive conduction system disease; arrhythmias; LV dysfunction.

Noonan syndrome (*OHCS* p854) ASD; pulmonary stenosis ± low-set ears.

Polyarteritis nodosa (PAN) (p554) Small and medium vessel vasculitis + angina; MI; arrhythmias; CCF; pericarditis and conduction defects.

Rheumatoid arthritis Conduction defects; pericarditis; LV dysfunction; aortic regurgitation; coronary arteritis. Look for arthritis signs, p542.

Sarcoidosis (p190) Infiltrating granulomas may cause complete AV block; ventricular or supraventricular tachycardia; myocarditis; CCF; restrictive cardiomyopathy. ECG may show Q waves.

Syphilis (p408) Myocarditis; ascending aortic aneurysm.

Systemic lupus erythematosus (p552) Pericarditis/effusion; myocarditis; Libman–Sacks endocarditis; mitral valve prolapse; coronary arteritis.

Systemic sclerosis (p548) Pericarditis; pericardial effusion; myocardial fibrosis; myocardial ischaemia; conduction defects; cardiomyopathy.

Thyrotoxicosis (p212) Pulse↑; AF ± emboli; wide pulse pressure; hyperdynamic apex; loud heart sounds; ejection systolic murmur; pleuropericardial rub; angina; high-output cardiac failure.

Turner syndrome ♀ Coarctation of aorta. Look for webbed neck. XO.

Williams syndrome Supravalvular aortic stenosis (↓visuospatial IQ).

▶Fever + new murmur = endocarditis until proven otherwise. Any fever lasting >1wk in those known to be at risk[5] must prompt blood cultures. *Acute* infective endocarditis (IE) tends to occur on 'normal' valves and may present with acute heart failure ± emboli; the commonest organism is *Staph. aureus*. Risk factors: skin breaches (dermatitis, IV lines, wounds); haemodialysis; immunosuppression; DM. Mortality: 5–50% (related to age and embolic events). Endocarditis on *abnormal valves* tends to run a *subacute* course. Risk factors: aortic or mitral valve disease; tricuspid valves in IV drug users; coarctation; PDA; VSD; prosthetic valves. Endocarditis on prosthetic valves may be 'early' (within 60d of surgery, usually *Staph. aureus* or *epidermidis*, poor prognosis) or 'late'.

Causes Bacteria Bacteraemia occurs all the time, eg when we chew (not just during dentistry or medical interventions—which is why routine prophylaxis for such procedures does not make sense). *Staph. aureus* is the commonest (usually subacute) followed by oral viridans group *Strep.*, non-oral *Strep.* including *Strep. bovis* (need colonoscopy ?tumour), Enterococci and *Coxiella burnetii*. Rarely: **HACEK** Gram −ve bacteria (**H**aemophilus-**A**ggregatibacter-**C**ardiobacterium-**E**ikenella-**K**ingella); diphtheroids; *Chlamydia*. **Fungi** *Candida*; *Aspergillus*; *Histoplasma*. Usually in IV drug users, immunocompromised patients or those with prosthetic valves. High mortality, need surgical management. **Other** SLE (Libman–Sacks endocarditis); malignancy.

Signs Septic signs Fever, rigors, night sweats, malaise, weight loss, anaemia, splenomegaly, and clubbing (fig 3.51). **Cardiac lesions** Any new murmur, or a change in pre-existing murmur, should raise the suspicion of endocarditis. Vegetations may cause valve destruction and severe regurgitation, or valve obstruction. An aortic root abscess causes prolongation of the PR interval, and may lead to complete AV block. LVF is a common cause of death. **Immune complex deposition** Vasculitis (p554) may affect any vessel. Microscopic haematuria is common; glomerulonephritis and acute kidney injury may occur. Roth spots (boat-shaped retinal haemorrhage with pale centre); splinter haemorrhages (fig 3.52); Osler's nodes (painful pulp infarcts in fingers or toes). **Embolic phenomena** Emboli may cause abscesses in the relevant organ, eg brain, heart, kidney, spleen, gut (or lung if right-sided IE) or skin: termed Janeway lesions (fig 3.53; painless palmar or plantar macules), which, together with Osler's nodes, are pathognomonic.

Diagnosis Use the Modified Duke criteria (see BOX 'Modified Duke criteria').[48,49] **Blood cultures** Do three sets at different times from different sites at peak of fever. 85–90% are diagnosed from the 1st two sets; 10% is culture negative. **Blood tests** Normochromic, normocytic anaemia, neutrophilia, high ESR/CRP. Rheumatoid factor positive (an immunological phenomenon). Also check U&E, Mg^{2+}, LFT. **Urinalysis** For microscopic haematuria. **CXR** Cardiomegaly, pulmonary oedema. **Regular ECGs** To look for heart block. **Echocardiogram** TTE (p102) may show vegetations, but only if >2mm. TOE (p102) is more sensitive, and better for visualizing mitral lesions and possible development of aortic root abscess. **CT** To look for emboli (spleen, brain, etc.). Cardiac CT and FDG PET/CT are emerging imaging modalities to better delineate complications, extra-cardiac sites of infection and in the setting of non-diagnostic TOE.

Treatment Liaise early with microbiologists and cardiologists.[50] Antibiotics: see BOX 'Antibiotic therapy for infective endocarditis'. Surgery if heart failure, valvular obstruction; repeated emboli; fungal IE; persistent bacteraemia; myocardial abscess; unstable infected prosthetic valve.

Prognosis 50% require surgery. 20% in-hospital mortality (*Staphs* 30%; bowel bacteria 14%; *Streps* 6%). 15% recurrence at 2yrs.

Prevention ▶ Antibiotic prophylaxis (eg oral amoxicillin 2g) is recommended for those at risk of IE undergoing invasive procedures—those with prosthetic valves (including transcatheter valves), those who have undergone valve repair in whom a prosthetic material is used, if history of previous IE, cyanotic congenital heart defects, and in patients for the first 6 months after surgical or percutaneous repair of a congenital heart disease with a prosthetic material (indefinitely in case of residual shunt or valvular regurgitation). Routine prophylaxis for low-risk individuals is not indicated.

5 Past IE or rheumatic fever; IV drug user; damaged or replaced valve; PPM or ICD; structural congenital heart disease (but not simple ASD, fully repaired VSD, or patent ductus); hypertrophic cardiomyopathy.

Modified Duke criteria for infective endocarditis

Major criteria
- Positive blood culture:
  - Typical organism in 2 separate cultures *or*
  - Persistently +ve blood cultures, eg 3 >12h apart (or majority if >3) *or*
  - Single positive blood culture for *Coxiella burnetii* or phase I IgG antibody titre >1:800.
- Endocardium involved:
  - Positive echocardiogram (vegetation, abscess, new valvular regurgitation, dehiscence of prosthetic valve) *or*
  - Abnormal activity around prosthetic valve on PET/CT or SPECT/CT *or*
  - Paravalvular lesions on cardiac CT.

Minor criteria
- Predisposition (cardiac lesion; IV drug abuse).
- Fever >38°C.
- Vascular phenomena (major arterial emboli, septic pulmonary infarcts Janeway's lesions, etc.).
- Immunological phenomena (glomerulonephritis, Osler's nodes, etc.).
- Positive blood culture that does not meet major criteria.

How to diagnose Definite infective endocarditis: 2 major *or* 1 major and 3 minor *or* all 5 minor criteria.

Antibiotic therapy for infective endocarditis

Prescribe antibiotics for infective endocarditis as follows. For more information on individual antibiotics, see tables 9.3–9.8, pp382–3.
- Blind therapy—native valve or prosthetic valve implanted >1yr ago: ampicillin, flucloxacillin, and gentamicin. Vancomycin + gentamicin if penicillin-allergic. If thought to be Gram –ve: meropenem + vancomycin.
- Blind therapy—prosthetic valve: vancomycin + gentamicin + rifampicin.
- *Staphs*—native valve: flucloxacillin for >4wks. If allergic or MRSA: vancomycin.
- *Staphs*—prosthetic valves: flucloxacillin + rifampicin + gentamicin for 6wks (review need for gentamicin after 2wks). If penicillin-allergic or MRSA: vancomycin + rifampicin + gentamicin.
- *Streps*—fully sensitive to penicillin: benzylpenicillin 1.2g/4h IV for 4–6wks.[6]
- *Streps*—less sensitive: benzylpenicillin + gentamicin; if penicillin-allergic or highly penicillin resistant: vancomycin + gentamicin.
- Enterococci: amoxicillin + gentamicin. If pen-allergic: vancomycin + gentamicin—for 4wks (6wks if prosthetic valve); review need for gentamicin after 2wks.
- HACEK organisms (*Haemophilus, Aggregatibacter, Cardiobacterium, Eikenella, Kingella*): ceftriaxone for 4wks with native valve or 6wks with prosthetic.
- Fungal: *Candida*—amphotericin. *Aspergillus*—voriconazole.

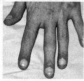

Fig 3.51 Clubbing with endocarditis.

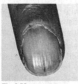

Fig 3.52 Splinter haemorrhages are normally seen under the fingernails or toenails. They are usually red-brown in colour.

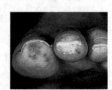

Fig 3.53 Janeway's lesions are non-tender erythematous, haemorrhagic, or pustular spots, eg on the palms or soles.

6 If *Strep bovis* is cultured, do colonoscopy, as a colon neoplasm is the likely portal of entry (table 6.4, p245).

3 Cardiovascular medicine

This systemic infection is still common in developing countries but increasingly rare in the West. Peak incidence: 5–15yrs. Tends to recur unless prevented. Pharyngeal infection with Lancefield group A β-haemolytic streptococci triggers rheumatic fever 2–4wks later, in the susceptible 2% of the population. An antibody to the carbohydrate cell wall of the streptococcus cross-reacts with valve tissue (antigenic mimicry) and may cause permanent damage to the heart valves.

Diagnosis Use the *revised Jones criteria* (may be over-rigorous). There must be evidence of recent strep infection plus 2 major criteria, or 1 major + 2 minor.

Evidence of group A β-haemolytic streptococcal infection
• Positive throat culture (usually negative by the time RF symptoms appear).
• Rapid streptococcal antigen test +ve.
• Elevated or rising streptococcal antibody titre (eg anti-streptolysin O (ASO) or DNase B titre).
• Recent scarlet fever.

Major criteria
• *Carditis:* tachycardia, murmurs (mitral or aortic regurgitation, Carey Coombs' murmur, p44), pericardial rub, CCF, cardiomegaly, conduction defects (45–70%). An apical systolic murmur may be the only sign.
• *Arthritis:* a migratory, 'flitting' polyarthritis; usually affects larger joints (75%).
• *Subcutaneous nodules:* small, mobile, painless nodules on extensor surfaces of joints and spine (2–20%).
• *Erythema marginatum:* (fig 3.54) geographical-type rash with red, raised edges and clear centre; occurs mainly on trunk, thighs, and arms in 2–10% (p560).
• *Sydenham's chorea (St Vitus' dance):* (fig 3.55) occurs late in 10%. Unilateral or bilateral involuntary semi-purposeful movements. May be preceded by emotional lability and uncharacteristic behaviour.

Minor criteria
• Fever.
• Raised ESR or CRP.
• Arthralgia (but not if arthritis is one of the major criteria).
• Prolonged PR interval (but not if carditis is major criterion).
• Previous rheumatic fever.

Management
• Bed rest until CRP normal for 2wks (may be 3 months).
• Phenoxymethylpenicillin 500mg three times daily PO for 10 days or benzylpenicillin 1.2 million units IM as single dose (if allergic to penicillin, give cephalexin or azithromycin for 10 days).
• Analgesia for carditis/arthritis: aspirin 100mg/kg/d PO in divided doses (max 4–8g/d) for 2d, then 70mg/kg/d for 6wks. Monitor salicylate level. Toxicity causes tinnitus, hyperventilation, and metabolic acidosis. Risk of Reye syndrome in children. Alternative: NSAIDs (p545). If moderate-to-severe carditis is present (cardiomegaly, CCF, or 3rd-degree heart block), add oral prednisolone to salicylate therapy. In case of heart failure, treat appropriately (p136), with severe valve disease, surgery may be required.
• Immobilize joints in severe arthritis.
• Haloperidol (0.5mg/8h PO), carbamazepine, or valproate for the chorea.

Prognosis 60% with carditis develop chronic rheumatic heart disease. This correlates with the severity of the carditis. Acute attacks last an average of 3 months. Recurrence may be precipitated by further streptococcal infections, pregnancy, or use of the oral contraceptive pill. Cardiac sequelae affect mitral (70%), aortic (40%), tricuspid (10%), and pulmonary (2%) valves. Incompetent lesions develop during the attack, stenoses years later.

Secondary prophylaxis Phenoxymethylpenicillin 250mg/12h PO. Alternatives: sulfadiazine 1g daily (0.5g if <30kg) or erythromycin 250mg twice daily (if penicillin-allergic). Duration: If carditis + persistent valvular disease, continue at least until age of 40 (sometimes lifelong). If carditis but no valvular disease, continue for 10yrs. If there is no carditis, 5yrs of prophylaxis (until age of 21) is sufficient.

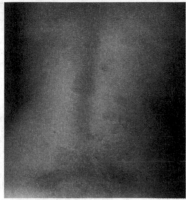

Fig 3.54 Erythema marginatum.
Image courtesy of Dr Maria Angelica Binotto.

Sydenham's chorea

The term 'chorea' comes from the ancient Greek word *choreia*, which means dance, as the quick involuntary movements of the feet or hands are comparable to dancing. The artist Pieter Bruegel is a famous contributor to the iconography of chorea and 'St. Vitus' dance'. Charcot describes fig 3.55 as 'Sufferers from St Vitus' dance going on a pilgrimage to the church of St Willibrod, Epternach, near Luxemburg'. After an outbreak of the 'dancing plague' in Strasbourg in 1418, St Vitus became the specific saint of this neurosis. The healing power of the saint's relics was thought to be especially efficacious for the sick with 'unsteady step, trembling limbs, limping knees, bent fingers and hands, paralysed hands, lameness, crookedness, and withering body'.

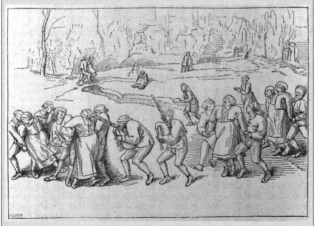

Fig 3.55 Representation of the nature of the dance of Saint Guy by P. Breughel.
Wellcome Collection. Public Domain Mark. https://wellcomecollection.org/works/uq8uykf6

Adult congenital heart disease (ACHD)

This is a growing area of cardiology as increasing numbers of children with congenital heart defects survive to adulthood, sometimes as a result of complex restructuring procedures which have their own physiological implications. ACHD patients are at increased risk of many conditions described elsewhere, for which many of the 'standard' investigations and therapies will apply: including arrhythmias (p120), heart failure (p134), and infective endocarditis (p144). Remember it is often part of a multisystem disorder.

Investigations Echocardiography (± bubble contrast) is first line. Increasingly, cardiac CT and MR are used to provide precise anatomical and functional information. Cardiac catheterization generates data on oxygen saturation and pressure in different vessels and chambers. Exercise testing assesses functional capacity.

Bicuspid aortic valve These work well at birth and go undetected. Many eventually develop aortic stenosis ± aortic regurgitation predisposing to IE/SBE ± aortic dilatation/dissection. (Do CT aortogram to look for aortopathy.) Intense exercise may accelerate complications, so do yearly echocardiograms on affected athletes.

Atrial septal defect (ASD) A hole connects the atria.
- **Ostium secundum defects** 80% cases; hole high in the septum; often asymptomatic until adulthood when a L→R shunt develops. Shunting depends on the compliance of the ventricles. LV compliance decreases with age (esp. if ↑BP), so augmenting L→R shunting; hence dyspnoea/heart failure, typically aged 40–60yrs.
- **Ostium primum defects** Associated with AV valve anomalies, eg in Down's syndrome; present in childhood.

Signs and symptoms Chest pain, palpitations, dyspnoea. Arrhythmias incl. AF; ↑JVP; wide, fixed split S₂; pulmonary systolic flow murmur. Pulmonary hypertension may cause pulmonary or tricuspid regurgitation, dyspnoea, and haemoptysis. ↑Frequency of migraine. **Simple tests** ECG: RBBB with LAD (primum defect) or RAD (secundum defect). CXR: small aortic knuckle, pulmonary plethora, atrial enlargement. **Complications** • Reversal of left-to-right shunt, ie *Eisenmenger's complex*: initial L→R shunt leads to pulmonary hypertension which increases right heart pressures until they exceed left heart pressures, hence shunt reversal. This causes cyanosis as deoxygenated blood enters systemic circulation. • Paradoxical emboli, eg causing strokes (vein→artery via ASD; rare). **Treatment** May close spontaneously. If not, primum defects are usually closed in childhood. Secundum defects should be closed if symptomatic or signs of RV overload. Transcatheter closure is more common than surgical.

Ventricular septal defect (VSD) A hole connects the ventricles. **Causes** Congenital (prevalence 2:1000 births); acquired (post-MI). **Symptoms** May present with severe heart failure in infancy, or remain asymptomatic and be detected incidentally in later life. **Signs** Classically, a harsh pansystolic murmur is heard at the left sternal edge, with a systolic thrill, ± left parasternal heave. Smaller holes, which are haemodynamically less significant, give louder murmurs. Signs of pulmonary hypertension. **Complications** AR, IE/SBE, pulmonary hypertension, Eisenmenger's complex (above), heart failure from volume overload. **Tests** ECG: normal, LAD, LVH, RVH. CXR: normal heart size ± mild pulmonary plethora (small VSD) or cardiomegaly, large pulmonary arteries and marked pulmonary plethora (large VSD). Cardiac catheter: step up in O₂ saturation in right ventricle. **Treatment** Initially medical as many close spontaneously. Indications for surgical closure: failed medical therapy, symptomatic VSD, shunt >3:1, SBE/IE. Endovascular closure may be possible.

Coarctation of the aorta Congenital narrowing of the descending aorta; usually occurs just distal to the origin of the left subclavian artery. More common in boys. **Associations** Bicuspid aortic valve; Turner syndrome. **Signs** Radiofemoral delay; weak femoral pulse; ↑BP; scapular bruit; systolic murmur (best heard over the left scapula); cold feet. **Complications** Heart failure from high afterload; IE; intracerebral haemorrhage. **Tests** CT or MRI-aortogram; CXR may show rib notching as blood diverts down intercostal arteries to reach the lower body, causing these vessels to dilate and erode local rib bone. **Treatment** Surgery, or balloon dilatation ± stenting.

Tetralogy of Fallot See p149. **Patent foramen ovale (PFO)** See p149.

Fallot's tetralogy: what the non-specialist needs to know

Tetralogy of Fallot (TOF) is the most common cyan-otic congenital heart disorder (prevalence: 3–6 per 10 000). It is also the most common cyanotic heart defect that survives to adulthood, accounting for 10% of all ACHD. It is believed to be due to abnormalities in separation of the truncus arteriosus into the aorta and pulmonary arteries early in gestation (fig 3.56).

The 'tetralogy' of features are:
1 Ventricular septal defect (VSD).
2 Pulmonary stenosis.
3 Right ventricular hypertrophy.
4 The aorta overrides the VSD, accepting right heart blood.

A few patients also have an ASD, which makes up the pentad of Fallot.

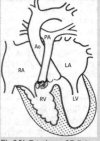

Fig 3.56 Tetralogy of Fallot.
Reproduced from Thorne et al., Adult Congenital Heart Disease, 2009, with permission from Oxford University Press.

Presentation Severity of illness depends greatly on the degree of pulmonary stenosis. Infants may be acyanotic at birth, with a pulmonary stenosis murmur as the only initial finding. Gradually (especially after closure of the ductus arteriosus) they become cyanotic due to decreasing flow of blood to the lungs and increasing right-to-left flow across the VSD. During a hypoxic spell, the child becomes restless and agitated. Toddlers may squat, which is typical of TOF, as it increases peripheral vascular resistance, thereby decreasing the degree of right-to-left shunt. Adult patients are often asymptomatic. In the unoperated adult patient, cyanosis is common, although extreme cyanosis or squatting is uncommon. In repaired patients, late symptoms include exertional dyspnoea, palpitations, clubbing, RV failure, syncope, and even sudden death.

Investigations ECG shows RV hypertrophy with a right bundle branch block. CXR may be normal, or show the hallmark of TOF, which is the classic boot-shaped heart (fig 3.57). Echocardiography can show the anatomy as well as the degree of stenosis. Cardiac CT and cardiac MRI can give valuable information for planning the surgery.

Management Surgery is usually done before 1yr of age, with closure of the VSD and correction of pulmonary stenosis.

Prognosis Without surgery, mortality rate is ~95% by age 20. After repair, 85% of patients survive to 35yrs. Common problems in adulthood include pulmonary regurgitation, causing RV dilatation and failure; RV outflow tract obstruction; AR; LV dysfunction; and arrhythmias.

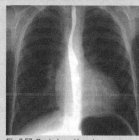

Fig 3.57 Boot-shaped heart.
Courtesy of Dr Edward Singleton.

Patent foramen ovale (PFO)

This is a congenital cardiac defect found in 25–30% of the population. After birth, left atrial pressure exceeds right atrial pressure and normally closes the PFO. However, in some cases, the valve of the foramen ovale fails to fuse with the septum. There has been a growing interest in PFOs as they are associated with cryptogenic embolic stroke in young adults, with neurological decompression sickness in divers, and with migraine with aura. Agitated saline contrast with ultrasound techniques (TTE, TOE, or transcranial Doppler) enables shunt identification. In young adults with an embolic-appearing cryptogenic ischaemic stroke and a PFO with R→L shunt detected by bubble study, percutaneous PFO closure should be considered in addition to antiplatelet therapy.

Driving and the heart

UK licences are inscribed 'You are required by law to inform Drivers Medical Branch, DVLA, Swansea SA99 1AT at once if you have any disability (physical or medical), which is, or may become likely to affect your fitness as a driver, unless you do not expect it to last more than 3 months'. It is the responsibility of drivers to inform the DVLA (the UK Driving and Vehicle Licensing Authority), and that of their doctors to advise patients that medical conditions[s1] (and drugs) may affect their ability to drive and for which conditions patients should inform the DVLA. Drivers should also inform their insurance company of any condition disclosed to the DVLA. If in doubt, ask your defence union.

The following are examples of the guidance for holders of *standard* licences; different rules apply for group 2 vehicle licence-holders (eg lorries, buses). More can be found at: https://www.gov.uk/guidance/cardiovascular-disorders-assessing-fitness-to-drive

Angina Driving must cease when symptoms occur at rest or with emotion. Driving may recommence when satisfactory symptom control is achieved. DVLA need not be notified.

Angioplasty Driving must cease for 1wk, and may recommence thereafter provided no other disqualifying condition. DVLA need not be notified.

MI If successfully treated with angioplasty, cease driving for 1wk provided urgent intervention not planned and LVEF (left ventricular ejection fraction) >40%, and no other disqualifying condition. Otherwise, driving must cease for 1 month. DVLA need not be notified.

Dysrhythmias Including sinoatrial disease, AF/flutter, atrioventricular conduction defects, and narrow or broad complex tachycardias. Driving must cease if the dysrhythmia has caused or is likely to cause incapacity. Driving may recommence 4wks after successful control provided there is no other disqualifying condition.

Pacemaker implant Stop driving for 1wk, the patient must notify the DVLA.

Implanted cardioverter defibrillator The licence is subject to annual review. Driving may occur when these criteria can be met:
• 6 months have passed since ICD implanted for secondary prevention.
• 1 month has passed since ICD implanted for primary prophylaxis.
• The device has not administered therapy (shock and/or symptomatic antitachycardia pacing) within the last 6 months (except during testing).
• No therapy (shock) in the last 2 years has been accompanied by *incapacity* (whether caused by the device or arrhythmia)—unless this was a result of device malfunction which has been corrected for at least 1 month or steps have been taken to avoid recurrence (eg ablation) which have been successful for at least 6 months.
• A period of 1 month off driving must occur following any revision of the device (generator and/or electrode) or alteration of anti-arrhythmics.
• The device is subject to regular review with interrogation.
• There is no other disqualifying condition.

Syncope Simple faint No restriction. **Unexplained syncope** With probable cardiac aetiology—4wks off driving if cause identified and treated; otherwise 6 months off. Loss of consciousness or altered awareness associated with signs of seizure requires 6 months off driving. If the patient is known to be epileptic or has had another such episode in the preceding 5yrs, they must abstain from driving for 1yr. See driving and epilepsy (BOX 'Other conditions'). Patients who have had a single episode of loss of consciousness with no cause found despite neurological and cardiac investigations, must abstain from driving for 6 months.

Hypertension Driving may continue unless treatment causes unacceptable side effects. DVLA need not be notified.

Other conditions: UK DVLA states it must be informed if a driver suffers from medical conditions including

- Epilepsy (the patient must have had at least two seizures in the last 5yrs). An epileptic patient who has suffered an epileptic attack while awake must not drive for 1yr from the date of the attack. Patients who have seizures that do not affect their consciousness (eg simple partial seizures) or seizures only during sleep may be allowed to drive. Being allowed to drive is conditional on the patient following medical advice and there not being reason to believe they are at high risk of further seizures.
- TIA or stroke. These patients should not drive for at least 1 month. There is no need to inform the DVLA unless there is residual neurological defect after 1 month, eg visual field defect. If TIAs have been recurrent and frequent, a 3-month period free of attacks may be required.
- Sudden attacks or disabling giddiness, fainting, or blackouts.
- Chronic neurological conditions including multiple sclerosis, Parkinson's (any 'freezing' or on–off effects), and motor neuron diseases.
- Severe mental disorders; including serious memory problems and severe psychiatric illness. Those with dementia should only drive if the condition is mild (do not rely on armchair judgements: on-the-road trials are better). Encourage relatives to contact DVLA if a dementing relative should not be driving. GPs may desire to breach confidentiality (the GMC approves) and inform DVLA of demented or psychotic patients (tel. 01792 783686). Many elderly drivers (~1 in 3) who die in accidents are found to have Alzheimer's.
- A pacemaker, defibrillator, or antiventricular tachycardia device fitted.
- Diabetes controlled by insulin or tablets. The main issues which may result in driving bans are impaired awareness of hypoglycaemia and impaired vision.
- Angina while driving.
- Any type of brain surgery, brain tumour. Severe head injury involving inpatient treatment at hospital.
- Continuing/permanent difficulty in the use of arms or legs which affects ability to control a vehicle.
- Dependence on or misuse of alcohol, illicit drugs, or chemical substances in the past 3yrs (do not include drink/driving offences).
- Any visual disability which affects *both* eyes (do not declare short/long sight or colour blindness).
- Vision (new drivers) should be 6/9 on Snellen's scale in the better eye and 6/12 on the Snellen scale in the other eye, wearing glasses or contact lenses if needed, and 3/60 in each eye without glasses or contact lenses.

The above-listed rules apply to standard licences only, for group 2 entitlement (eg HGV drivers) see: www.dvla.gov.uk/medical/ataglance.aspx

Flying after a stroke or MI

Patients with a recent MI may travel after 7–10 days if there are no complications. As there is the potential risk for barotrauma after CABG and other chest or thoracic surgery, these patients should wait 10–14 days. Patients with uncomplicated PCI such as angioplasty with stent placement may be fit to travel after 3 days, but individual assessment is essential. Following a stroke, patients are advised to wait 10 days following an event, although if stable may be carried within 3 days of the event. Cardiovascular contraindications to commercial airline flight include uncomplicated MI within 7 days, complicated MI (eg recurrent event, EF <40% or signs/symptoms of heart failure) within 4–6 weeks, unstable angina, decompensated CHF, uncontrolled hypertension, CABG within 10 days, stroke within 3 days, uncontrolled cardiac arrhythmia, and severe symptomatic valvular heart disease.

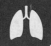

Contents

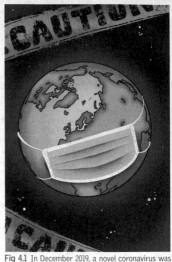

Fig 4.1 In December 2019, a novel coronavirus was identified as the cause of a cluster of pneumonia cases in Wuhan, a city in the Hubei Province of China. This outbreak spread rapidly through China and then the rest of the world, becoming the first global pandemic since Spanish 'flu. Novel coronavirus disease (COVID-19) (p172), as it was subsequently termed by the World Health Organization, is caused by severe acute respiratory syndrome (SARS) coronavirus (COV) 2 virus, primarily manifesting as an acute respiratory illness with interstitial and alveolar pneumonia, but it can affect multiple organs such as the kidney, heart, digestive tract, blood, and nervous system. To date, it has infected over 700 million people worldwide and has caused nearly 7 million deaths. In response to the pandemic, most countries around the world instituted strict lockdown measures including the closure of all non-essential businesses, schools, and shops, and restriction of all non-essential travel and movement. At-risk or vulnerable individuals were encouraged to 'cocoon' or 'shield' themselves safely at home. Though there was much sorrow and sacrifice, there was also an outpouring of generosity and solidarity. We were reminded of the words of Dr Bernard Rieux from Albert Camus' *The Plague*, 'the whole thing is not about heroism... It may seem a ridiculous idea, but the only way to fight the plague is with decency.' Pandemics aside, the art and practice of medicine should always be about decency.

Artwork by Gillian Turner.

We thank Nicola Ronan, our Specialist Reader and Gemma Smith, our Junior Reader for this chapter.

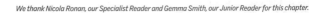

Respiratory health

The lungs provide a vital physiological function in allowing gas exchange, but are also at the vanguard of a constant battle between host, pathogens, and pollutants. Respiratory medicine exemplifies how careful epidemiology, science, and randomized controlled trials have revolutionized our understanding of common diseases, leading to preventative measures and effective treatments. However, the importance of poverty and general improvements in public health cannot be underestimated. Rates of TB in the UK declined well before the introduction of BCG vaccination and streptomycin, largely due to improvements in sanitation and less dense living conditions. Public health campaigns and taxation have helped lower smoking rates, although reductions in lung cancer will lag behind for many years. Increasing air pollution levels, diminished air quality, and climate change pose new challenges for lung function and respiratory disease.

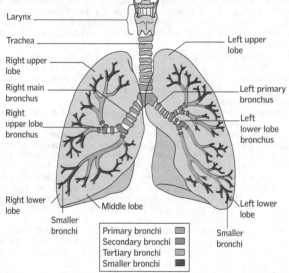

Fig 4.2 Segmental anatomy of the lungs and main bronchi. The left lung has two lobes and the right has three.

There is no substitute for careful history taking and examination in making the 'correct' diagnosis. Tests should help clarify and assess severity. When examining the chest think about the anatomy, and the location of pathology (fig 4.2).

Sputum examination Collect a good sample; if necessary ask a physiotherapist to help. Note the appearance: clear and colourless (chronic bronchitis), yellow-green or brown (pulmonary infection), red (haemoptysis), black (smoke, coal dust), or frothy white-pink (pulmonary oedema). Send the sample to the laboratory for microscopy, culture/sensitivity. If indicated, ask for ZN stain, and PCR.

Peak expiratory flow (PEF) Measured by a maximal forced expiration through a peak flow meter. It correlates well with the forced expiratory volume in 1 second (FEV_1) & is used as an estimate of airway calibre in asthma, but is effort dependent.

Pulse oximetry Allows non-invasive assessment of peripheral O_2 saturation (SpO_2). Useful for monitoring those who are acutely ill or at risk of deterioration. Target oxygen saturations are usually 94–98% in a well patient or 88–92% in those with certain pre-existing lung pathology (eg COPD with a history of type 2 respiratory failure). Oxygen saturation of <92% in a normally well person is a serious sign and arterial blood gases (ABGs) should be checked. Causes of erroneous readings: poor perfusion, movement, skin pigmentation, nail varnish, dyshaemoglobinaemias, and carbon monoxide poisoning. As with any bedside test, be sceptical, and check ABGs whenever indicated (p158).

Arterial blood gas (ABG) analysis Heparinized blood is usually taken from the radial or femoral artery (p755). The brachial artery is used less because of median nerve proximity and it is an end artery. pH, P_aO_2, P_aCO_2, HCO_3 are measured using an automated analyser. For ABG interpretation, see p159.

Lung function tests

1 **Spirometry** (See table 4.1.) Measures functional lung volumes. Forced expiratory volume in 1s (FEV_1) and forced vital capacity (FVC) are measured from a full forced expiration into a spirometer (Vitalograph®); exhalation continues until no more breath can be exhaled. FEV_1 is less effort dependent than PEF. FEV_1 gives a good estimate of the severity of airflow obstruction; and helps classify COPD severity. Bronchodilator testing may be performed if reversible airflow obstruction (eg asthma) suspected—a 12% and 200mL change in FEV_1 or FVC is defined as a response. *Obstructive defect:* (fig 4.3) asthma, bronchiectasis, COPD, cystic fibrosis. *Restrictive defect:* fibrosis, sarcoidosis, pneumoconiosis, interstitial pneumonias, connective tissue diseases, pleural effusion, obesity, kyphoscoliosis, neuromuscular problems.

2 **Lung volume measurement** *Total lung capacity* (TLC) and *residual volume* (RV) are useful in distinguishing obstructive and restrictive diseases (fig 4.4). TLC and RV are increased in obstructive airways disease and reduced in restrictive lung diseases and musculoskeletal abnormalities. Combined obstructive and restrictive defects can be seen in certain conditions such as sarcoidosis. *Flow–volume loop* (fig 4.5) measures flow at various lung volumes. Characteristic patterns are seen with intrathoracic airways obstruction (asthma, emphysema) and extrathoracic airways obstruction (tracheal stenosis).

3 **Gas exchange** The *gas transfer* coefficient (KCO) represents the carbon monoxide diffusing capacity (DLCO) corrected for alveolar volume. It is calculated by measuring carbon monoxide uptake from a single inspiration in a standard time (usually 10s) and lung volume by helium dilution. It is an indirect assessment of parenchymal lung disease, pulmonary vascular disease, and/or anaemia. Low in emphysema, interstitial lung disease, and pulmonary vascular disease; high in alveolar haemorrhage and left-to-right shunt.[1]

►Of note, obesity can affect PFTs, decreasing lung volumes and increasing DLCO.

Lung clearance index (LCI) A measure of ventilation distribution obtained from the multiple-breath washout test. The test involves following the washout of an inert tracer gas from the lungs during relaxed tidal breathing. The LCI is a sensitive marker of lung disease severity in cystic fibrosis.

Table 4.1 Spirometry results (data source NICE COPD 2010 guidelines)

	FEV₁	FVC	FEV₁/FVC ratio
Normal	>80% predicted	>80% predicted	75–80%
Restrictive	<80% predicted*	<80% predicted	>70% normal
Obstructive	<80% predicted	Normal or low	<70% predicted
*FEV₁ can also be normal in restrictive lung disease.			

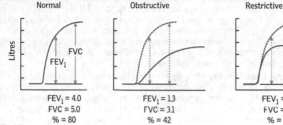
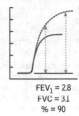

Normal

$FEV_1 = 4.0$
$FVC = 5.0$
$\% = 80$

Obstructive

$FEV_1 = 1.3$
$FVC = 3.1$
$\% = 42$

Restrictive

$FEV_1 = 2.8$
$FVC = 3.1$
$\% = 90$

Fig 4.3 Examples of spirograms.

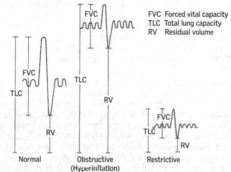

FVC Forced vital capacity
TLC Total lung capacity
RV Residual volume

Normal   Obstructive   Restrictive
                (Hyperinflation)

Fig 4.4 Lung volumes: physiological and pathological.

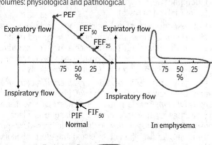

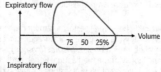

Fig 4.5 Flow–volume loops. PEF = peak expiratory flow; FEF_{50} = forced expiratory flow at 50% TLC; FEF_{25} = forced expiratory flow at 25% TLC; PIF = peak inspiratory flow; FIF_{50} = forced inspiratory flow at 50% TLC.

Radiology Chest x-ray See p706. **Ultrasound** Used in diagnosing and guiding drainage of pleural effusions (particularly loculated effusions) and empyema. **Radionuclide scans** *Ventilation/perfusion* (V/Q, p722) *scans* are occasionally used to diagnose pulmonary embolism (PE), eg in pregnancy (unmatched perfusion defects are seen). *Bone scans* are used to diagnose bone metastases. *PET scans* to assess cancer and inflammation. **Computed tomography** (CT, p714) Used for diagnosing and staging lung cancer, imaging the hila, mediastinum, and pleura, and guiding biopsies. Thin (1–1.5mm) section high-resolution CT (HRCT) is used in the diagnosis of interstitial lung disease, emphysema, and bronchiectasis. CT pulmonary angiography (CTPA) is used in the diagnosis of PE (fig 4.6). **Pulmonary angiography** Now rarely used for diagnosing pulmonary hypertension.

Fibreoptic bronchoscopy (See fig 4.7.) Performed under sedation with local anaesthetic via the nose or mouth. **Diagnostic indications** Suspected lung carcinoma, slowly resolving pneumonia, pneumonia in the immunosuppressed, interstitial lung disease. Bronchoalveolar lavage fluid may be sent to the lab for microscopy, culture, and cytology. Mucosal abnormalities may be brushed (cytology) and biopsied (histopathology). **Therapeutic indications** Aspiration of mucus plugs causing lobar collapse, removal of foreign bodies, stenting or treating tumours, eg laser. **Pre-procedure investigations** FBC, coagulation, CXR, CT, spirometry, pulse oximetry, and ABG (if indicated). **Complications** Hypoxia, bleeding, infection, pneumothorax (fig 16.44, p733). *Diagnostic sensitivity* for cancer 50–90%, depends on tumour location; gene profiling of cell sample may improve this.[z] May also be used to deliver an ultrasound probe (endobronchial ultrasound), and treatments—eg stents, or cryotherapy.

Bronchoalveolar lavage (BAL) Performed at the time of bronchoscopy by instilling and aspirating a known volume of warmed, buffered 0.9% saline into the distal airway. The scope is wedged in a segmental airway. It differs from simple *bronchial washings* as it samples cells from alveolar airspaces as opposed to just cells from the proximal airway. It can also provide a cell count and differential that can be useful to distinguish the different types of ILD. **Diagnostic indications for washings or BAL** Suspected malignancy, pneumonia in the immunosuppressed (especially HIV), bronchiectasis, suspected TB (if sputum negative), interstitial lung diseases (eg sarcoidosis, hypersensitivity pneumonitis, histiocytosis X). **Complications** Hypoxia (give supplemental O_2), transient fever, transient CXR shadow, infection (rare).

Endobronchial ultrasound (EBUS) A bronchoscopic technique that uses ultrasound to visualize structures within the airway wall, lung, and mediastinum. Most commonly used in combination with transbronchial needle aspiration (EBUS-TBNS) to sample hilar and mediastinal lymphadenopathy, endobronchial or peribronchial lesions in order to diagnose lung cancer, lymphoma, sarcoidosis, etc.

Lung biopsy May be performed in several ways. *Percutaneous needle biopsy* is performed under radiological guidance and is useful for peripheral lung and pleural lesions. *Transbronchial biopsy* performed at bronchoscopy may help in diagnosing interstitial lung diseases such as sarcoidosis or lung transplant complications. *Cryoprobe transbronchial biopsy*, a newer diagnostic procedure, provides larger biopsies that are usually crush artefact free and therefore of higher diagnostic yield. **Alternatives** If unsuccessful, consider open lung biopsy or video-assisted thoracoscopy.

Surgical procedures These are performed under general anaesthetic. *Rigid bronchoscopy* provides a wide lumen, enables larger mucosal biopsies, control of bleeding, and removal of foreign bodies. *Mediastinoscopy* and *mediastinotomy* enable examination and biopsy of the mediastinal lymph nodes/lesions. *Thoracoscopy* allows examination and biopsy of pleural lesions, drainage of pleural effusions, and talc pleurodesis and pleurectomy.

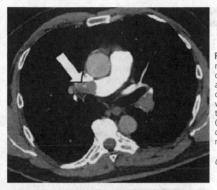

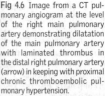

Fig 4.6 Image from a CT pulmonary angiogram at the level of the right main pulmonary artery demonstrating dilatation of the main pulmonary artery with laminated thrombus in the distal right pulmonary artery (arrow) in keeping with proximal chronic thromboembolic pulmonary hypertension.

Reproduced from Stirrup J et al. *Cardiovascular Tomography* (2019), with permission from Oxford University Press.

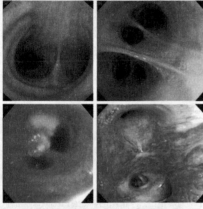

Fig 4.7 The videobronchoscopic appearance of (a) the trachea and main bronchi; (b) segmental bronchi in the right lower lobe; (c) polypoid tumour arising from a bronchial segment; and (d) submucosal disease.

Reproduced from Firth *et al.*, *Oxford Textbook of Medicine* (2020), with permission from Oxford University Press.

Echocardiography and right heart catheterization

Echocardiography This is the best screening test for significant pulmonary hypertension (p102). The tricuspid regurgitant jet velocity can be used to estimate the right ventricular systolic pressure, which in the absence of pulmonary valve stenosis, is equal to the pulmonary artery systolic pressure (PASP). In addition, the left ventricle can be assessed to determine whether there is a contribution from left ventricular systolic or diastolic dysfunction to elevated pulmonary arterial pressure. Atrial and ventricular dimensions and wall thickness can be measured, and paradoxical bowing of the intraventricular septum into the left ventricular cavity may be seen during systole as a consequence of greatly elevated right-sided pressures. **Right heart catheterization** This can confirm the diagnosis of pulmonary hypertension and provide important prognostic information. An elevated mean pulmonary arterial pressure >20mmHg at rest is the accepted definition. An elevated pulmonary capillary wedge pressure (PCWP) (>15mmHg) generally indicates left heart disease. Indicators of right heart failure, and hence poorer prognosis, include: 1 an elevated right atrial pressure (>10mmHg); 2 an elevated right ventricular end-diastolic pressure (>10mmHg); 3 a reduced mixed venous oxygen saturation (SvO$_2$ <63%); and 4 reduced cardiac output (<2.5L/min). **Vasoreactivity testing** This may be undertaken at the time of right heart catheterization, using inhaled nitric oxide or an IV infusion of epoprostenol or adenosine, to identify the subgroup of patients with pulmonary arterial hypertension who are likely to respond favourably to long-term treatment with vasodilator therapy, eg nifedipine.

Respiratory failure occurs when gas exchange is inadequate, resulting in hypoxia. It is defined as a P_aO_2 <8kPa and subdivided into two types according to P_aCO_2 level.

Type I respiratory failure Defined as hypoxia (P_aO_2 <8kPa) with a normal or low P_aCO_2. It is caused primarily by ventilation/perfusion (V/Q) mismatch, abnormal diffusion, right-to-left cardiac shunts. Examples of V/Q mismatch: PE, pneumonia, pulmonary oedema, asthma, emphysema, ARDS (p178).

Type II respiratory failure Defined as hypoxia (P_aO_2 <8kPa) with hypercapnia (P_aCO_2 >6.0kPa). This is caused by alveolar hypoventilation, with or without V/Q mismatch. Causes include:
• **Pulmonary disease** COPD, pneumonia, end-stage pulmonary fibrosis, obstructive sleep apnoea (OSA, p188), obesity hypoventilation syndrome (↑prevalence).
• **Reduced respiratory drive** Sedative drugs, CNS tumour or trauma.
• **Neuromuscular disease** Cervical cord lesion, diaphragmatic paralysis, poliomyelitis, myasthenia gravis, Guillain–Barré syndrome.
• **Thoracic wall disease** Flail chest, kyphoscoliosis.

Clinical features Features of the underlying cause together with symptoms and signs of hypoxia, with or without hypercapnia.

Hypoxia Dyspnoea; restlessness; agitation; confusion; central cyanosis. If longstanding hypoxia: polycythaemia; pulmonary hypertension; cor pulmonale.

Hypercapnia Headache; peripheral vasodilation; tachycardia; bounding pulse; tremor/flap; papilloedema; confusion; drowsiness; coma.

Investigations Aimed at determining the underlying cause:
• Blood tests: FBC, U&E, CRP, ABG. See table 4.2.
• Radiology: CXR ± CT thorax/CTPA.
• Microbiology: COVID/flu swabs, respiratory BioFire® PCR panel, sputum and blood cultures (if febrile).
• Spirometry (COPD, neuromuscular disease, Guillain–Barré syndrome).

Management Depends on the cause. Senior support essential. At an early stage, consider the appropriateness of the management setting and the ceilings of care.

Type I respiratory failure
• Treat underlying cause.
• Give oxygen (24–60%)—see BOX 'Administering oxygen'.
• Get ICU support and consider high flow nasal cannula (p159) or CPAP (continuous positive airway pressure) if requiring >40% O_2. The latter is a mask covering the nose and mouth that provides fixed positive pressure to the airways throughout the breathing cycle, to splint open the respiratory tract and improve gas exchange. The standard CPAP starting pressure is usually 5cmH$_2$O. Most useful in CHF, COPD, or OSA.

Type II respiratory failure The respiratory centre may be relatively insensitive to CO_2 and respiration could be driven by hypoxia.
• Treat underlying cause.
• Controlled oxygen therapy: target SpO$_2$ of 88–92% if COPD and history of CO_2 retention; start at 24% O_2. ▶Oxygen therapy should be given with care. Nevertheless, don't leave the hypoxia untreated.
• Recheck ABG after 20min. If P_aCO_2 is steady or lower, increase O_2 concentration to 28%. If P_aCO_2 has risen >1.5kPa and the patient is still hypoxic, consider assisted ventilation (eg NIPPV, p797, ie non-invasive positive pressure ventilation).
• If this fails, consider intubation and ventilation, if appropriate.

When to consider ABG (arterial blood gas) measurement

• Any unexpected deterioration in an ill patient. (Technique: see p755.)
• Anyone with an acute exacerbation of a chronic chest condition.
• Anyone with impaired consciousness or impaired respiratory effort.
• Signs of CO_2 retention, eg bounding pulse, drowsy, tremor (flapping), headache.
• Cyanosis, confusion, visual hallucinations (signs of ↓P_aO_2; S$_aO_2$ is an alternative).
• To validate measurements from transcutaneous pulse oximetry (p154).

ABG interpretation

Normal pH is 7.35–7.45. pH <7.35 indicates acidosis and >7.45 indicates alkalosis.

Table 4.2 Interpreting blood gas analysis

	pH	P_aCO_2	HCO_3^-
Metabolic acidosis	Low	Normal/low	Low
Respiratory acidosis	Low	High	Normal/high
Metabolic alkalosis	High	Normal/high	High
Respiratory alkalosis	High	Low	Normal/low

Steps to ABG interpretation

1 PO_2: is this normal given the FiO_2 (fraction of inspired oxygen)?
2 pH: acidosis or alkalosis?
3 Is the primary disturbance respiratory or metabolic? See table 4.2.
4 Is there any compensation (ie changes in pCO_2/HCO_3^- to try and correct an underlying imbalance)? Is this partial (pH abnormal) or complete (pH normalized)?
5 If metabolic acidosis present, calculate the anion gap: $(Na^+ + K^+) - (Cl^- + HCO_3^-)$. See p662 for causes of raised anion gap (normal 10–18mmol/L).
6 In a non-anion gap acidosis, determine the urinary anion gap: urinary $Na^+ + K^+ - Cl^-$ (should be <−40 in acidaemia; used to identify renal tubular acidosis; see p662).
7 In an anion gap acidosis, determine if there is a pre-existing metabolic disorder with the delta gap (ratio of rise in anion gap to fall in bicarbonate; see p662).

Administering oxygen

Oxygen should be prescribed. Titrate the amount guided by the patient's S_aO_2 and clinical condition. Use the lowest flow delivery system necessary to maintain SpO2 within target range. Humidification is only required for longer-term delivery of O_2 at high flow rates and tracheostomies, but may ↑ expectoration in bronchiectasis.

Nasal cannulae For mild–moderate hypoxaemia. Preferred by patients, but O_2 delivery is relatively imprecise and may cause nasal soreness. The flow rate (1–4L/min) roughly defines the concentration of O_2 (24–40%). May be used to maintain S_aO_2 when nebulizers need to be run using air, eg COPD.

Simple face mask Delivers a variable amount of O_2 depending on the rate of inflow. Less precise than venturi masks—so don't use if hypercapnia or type II respiratory failure. Risk of CO_2 accumulation (within the mask and so in inspired gas) if flow rate <5L/min. ►Be careful in those with COPD (p796).

Venturi mask For controlled oxygen therapy. Provides a precise percentage or fraction of O_2 (FiO_2) at high flow rates. Start at 24–28% in COPD. Colours of masks:
• **BLUE** = 24% at 2L/min.
• **WHITE** = 28% at 4L/min.
• **YELLOW** = 35% at 8L/min.
• **RED** = 40% at 10L/min.
• **GREEN** = 60% at 15L/min.

Non-rebreathing mask These have a reservoir bag and deliver high concentrations of O_2 (60–90%), determined by the inflow (10–15L/min) and the presence of flap valves on the side. They are commonly used in emergencies, but are imprecise and should be avoided in those requiring controlled O_2 therapy.

High-flow nasal oxygen (aka Optiflow™/AIRVO™, high-flow nasal cannula) This is humidified, warmed oxygen delivered at up to 60L per minute. The major advantages it has over standard oxygen are that it provides some positive end-expiratory pressure, which improves oxygenation by 'recruitment' of alveoli, that it can deliver an FiO_2 ~100%, and that it is well tolerated.

Promoting oxygenation Other ways to ↑ oxygenation to reach the target S_aO_2 (this should be given as a number on the drug chart):
• Treat anaemia (transfuse if essential).
• Improve cardiac output (treat heart failure).
• Chest physio to improve ventilation/perfusion mismatch.
• Consider patient positioning (eg sitting upright in pulmonary oedema etc.).

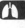

4 Chest medicine

4 Chest medicine

Asthma affects 8% of the population. It is characterized by recurrent episodes of dyspnoea, cough, and wheeze caused by reversible airways obstruction. Three factors contribute to airway narrowing: *bronchoconstriction*, triggered by a variety of stimuli; *mucosal swelling/inflammation*, caused by mast cell and basophil release of inflammatory mediators; and *increased mucus production*.

▶Occupational asthma, aspirin-sensitive asthma, and eosinophilic asthma are distinct syndromes that typically have their onset in adulthood.

Symptoms Episodic: ≥1 of wheeze, breathlessness, chest tightness, and cough occurring in episodes with periods of no (or minimal) symptoms between episodes.

Precipitants Respiratory irritants (smoke, perfume, pollution, etc.), allergens (house dust mite, pollen, fur), infection (particularly viral), drugs (NSAIDs via ↑leukotrienes, β-blockers via bronchospasm), cold air, exercise (typically after 5–15 minutes).

Diurnal variation Symptoms or peak flow may vary over the day but tend to be worse at night or in the early morning. Marked morning dipping of peak flow is common and can tip the balance into a serious attack, despite having normal peak flow (figs 4.9, 4.10, p163) at other times.

Exercise Quantify the exercise tolerance.

Disturbed sleep Quantify as nights per week (a sign of severe asthma).

Acid reflux 40–60% of those with asthma have reflux; treating it improves spirometry, but not necessarily symptoms.[3]

Other atopic disease Eczema, hay fever, allergy, or family history?

The home (especially the bedroom) Pets? Carpet? Feather pillows or duvet? Floor cushions and other 'soft furnishings'?

Job If symptoms remit at weekends or holidays, work may provide the trigger (15% of cases are work-related—more for paint sprayers, food processors, welders, and animal handlers).[4] Ask the patient to measure their peak flow at intervals at work and at home (at the same time of day) to confirm this.

Exacerbations Frequency, severity, duration, and required treatment (need for steroids, A&E visits, hospitalizations, and intubations), days per week off work or school. ▶*Adherence to treatment. Observe inhaler technique.*

Signs Tachypnoea; audible wheeze; hyperinflated chest; hyperresonant percussion note; ↓air entry; widespread, polyphonic wheeze with prolonged expiratory phase. Presence of nasal polyps, rhinitis, rash (allergic component). ▶▶Recognize signs of *a severe or life-threatening attack* on p794.

Tests The diagnosis is ultimately clinical supported by objective tests that seek to demonstrate variable airflow obstruction or the presence of airway inflammation. Compare results when asymptomatic vs symptomatic to avoid false negative results and to detect variation over time. **Initial diagnosis** Assess probability of asthma based on initial structured clinical assessment (table 4.3) and then follow the diagnostic algorithm (fig 4.8). The diagnostic indications for referral for specialist advice/investigations are shown in table 4.4. **Acute attack** See p794. PEF (or FEV₁), sputum culture, FBC, U&E, CRP, blood cultures. ABG analysis usually shows a normal or slightly ↓P_aO_2 but ↓P_aCO_2 (hyperventilation). If P_aO_2 is normal but the patient is hyperventilating, watch carefully and repeat the ABG a little later. ▶*If P_aCO_2 is normal or raised*, transfer to high-dependency unit or ITU for close monitoring ± ventilatory support, as this signifies failing respiratory effort. CXR (to exclude infection or pneumothorax). **Chronic asthma** PEF monitoring for 2–4wks (p164): a diurnal variation of >15% on ≥3d a wk for 2wks. *Spirometry:* obstructive defect (↓FEV₁/FVC, ↑RV, p164); usually ≥12% improvement in FEV₁ following β₂ agonists or steroid trial with increase in volume ≥200mL (=significant reversibility). Histamine or methacholine bronchial challenge tests. Fractional exhaled nitric oxide (FeNO) to detect eosinophilic airway inflammation or atopy. CXR: hyperinflation. **Allergy tests** Perform to confirm sensitivity to suspected allergic triggers—suggested by raised allergen-specific IgE levels, positive skin-prick tests to aeroallergens, or blood eosinophilia. Consider ABPA and check *Aspergillus* serology if eosinophilia, a positive skin test to *Aspergillus*, mucus plugging, or central bronchiectasis on CXR.

Differential diagnosis Pulmonary oedema ('cardiac asthma'); COPD (may coexist); large airway obstruction (eg foreign body, tumour—consider if focal, monophonic wheeze); SVC obstruction (wheeze/dyspnoea not episodic); pneumothorax; PE; bronchiectasis; obliterative bronchiolitis (suspect in elderly); post-viral tussive syndrome; Churg–Strauss syndrome (asthma may precede the vasculitic phase by 8–10 years); hyperventilation and panic attack.

▶**Coexistent conditions** Allergic rhinitis (in most; postnasal drip—'integrated airway hypothesis'), sinus disease (as per allergic rhinitis, inflammation in the upper airways can drive inflammation in the lower airways, exacerbating asthma), obesity (may worsen perception of symptom severity), gastro-oesophageal reflux disease (GORD). All can worsen asthma symptoms.

▶**Be aware** Difficult asthma may be associated with psychological morbidity.[1]

Treatment Chronic asthma (p164). Emergency treatment (p794).

Natural history Most childhood asthmatics (see *OHCS* p212) either grow out of asthma in adolescence or suffer much less as adults. 'New-onset' asthma in adulthood sometimes has its origin in undiagnosed childhood asthma. The risk of progressive clinical deterioration in adults is small, and asthma in the absence of other comorbidities does not appear to decrease life expectancy. Patients with severe asthma and one or more adverse psychosocial factors are at risk of death.

Mortality 1320 asthma deaths in the UK in 2017, 20% increase in last 5 years.

Table 4.3 Initial structured clinical assessment of the probability of asthma

	Features	Testing strategy
High probability	• Episodic symptoms ('attacks') • Wheeze • Variable airflow obstruction • History of atopy • No features suggestive of alternative diagnosis	1 Commence monitored treatment (6 weeks of inhaled corticosteroids) 2 Assess status with symptom questionnaire and/or lung function tests 3 Confirm diagnosis with response to treatment 4 If response is poor, check inhaler technique and arrange further tests
Intermediate probability	• Some but not all typical features of asthma • Does not respond well to a monitored initiation of treatment	1 Spirometry with reversibility tests and/or a monitored initiation of treatment 2 Assess the response by repeating lung function tests. 3 If normal spirometry results, do challenge tests and/or measurement of FeNO to identify eosinophilic inflammation
Low probability	• No typical features (eg no lung function abnormalities, onset >50 years) • Symptoms suggest alternative diagnosis	1 Investigate for alternative diagnosis 2 Undertake/refer for further asthma tests

Source: data from BTS/SIGN Guideline for the management of asthma 2019: https://www.brit-thoracic.org.uk/quality-improvement/guidelines/asthma/

1 During the 1930s to 1950s, asthma was known as one of the 'holy seven' psychosomatic illnesses. Its cause was considered to be psychological, with treatment often based on psychoanalysis and other talking cures. As these psychoanalysts interpreted the asthmatic wheeze as the suppressed cry of the child for its mother, they considered the treatment of depression to be especially important for individuals with asthma.

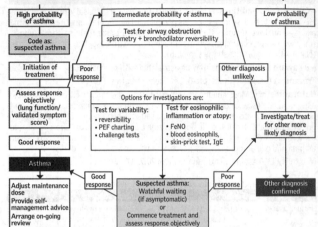

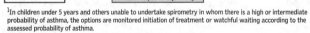

[1] In children under 5 years and others unable to undertake spirometry in whom there is a high or intermediate probability of asthma, the options are monitored initiation of treatment or watchful waiting according to the assessed probability of asthma.

Fig 4.8 BTS/SIGN Guideline for the diagnosis of asthma (2019).

Reproduced from BTS/SIGN Guideline for the management of asthma. SIGN 158 revised 2019.

Table 4.4 Diagnostic indications for specialist referral and 'red flag' features (BTS/SIGN 2019)

Diagnostic indications for referral for specialist advice/investigations
Referral for tests not available in primary care
• Diagnosis unclear
• Suspected occupational asthma (symptoms that improve when patient is not at work, adult-onset asthma, and workers in high-risk occupations)
• Poor response to asthma treatment
• Severe/life-threatening asthma attack
'Red flags' and indicators of other diagnoses
• Prominent systemic features (myalgia, fever, weight loss)
• Unexpected clinical findings (eg crackles, clubbing, cyanosis, cardiac disease, monophonic wheeze or stridor)
• Persistent invariable breathlessness
• Chronic sputum production
• Unexplained restrictive spirometry
• CXR shadowing
• Marked blood eosinophilia

Source: data from BTS/SIGN Guideline for the management of asthma 2019: https://www.brit-thoracic.org.uk/quality-improvement/guidelines/asthma/

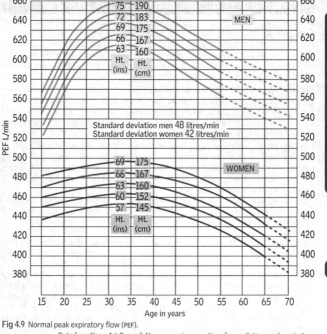

Fig 4.9 Normal peak expiratory flow (PEF).

Data from Nunn AJ, Gregg I. New regression equations for predicting peak expiratory flow in adults. *BMJ* 1989;298:1068–70.

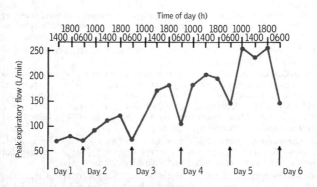

Recovery from severe attack of asthma
Predicted PEF was 320 L/min
Arrows point to early morning 'dips'

Fig 4.10 Example of serial peak flow chart.

4 Chest medicine

Lifestyle Help to quit smoking (p85). Avoid precipitants. Weight loss if overweight. Check inhaler technique. Teach use of a peak flow meter to monitor PEF twice a day. Offer self-management education which should include a written personalized asthma action plan with specific advice about what to do in an emergency and how to alter their medication in the light of symptoms or PEF. Breathing exercise programmes have been shown to improve quality of life (QOL) & reduce symptoms.

Global Initiative for Asthma guidelines (GINA³) Start at the step most appropriate to severity; moving up if needed, or down if control is good for >3 months. Before initiating a new therapy, check adherence with existing therapies, check inhaler technique, and eliminate trigger factors. Treat modifiable risk factors and comorbidities. For drug examples see table 4.5.

▶Treatment with short-acting $β_2$-agonists (SABA) alone without inhaled corticosteroids (ICS) is no longer recommended as this appears to ↑exacerbations. All adults with asthma should now receive ICS. This can be either symptom-driven (in mild asthma, GINA steps 1 to 2) or daily (GINA steps 2 to 5), to reduce the risk of serious exacerbations and to control symptoms.

• **Step 1: intermittent asthma (symptoms < twice/month)** Use a combination inhaler of low-dose ICS and long-acting $β_2$-agonist (LABA) (eg budesonide-formoterol) as needed for symptoms relief. Alternatively, use low-dose ICS whenever a SABA is needed.

• **Step 2: mild persistent (symptoms ≥ twice a month but < than daily)** Daily low-dose ICS + as-needed SABA or as-needed low-dose ICS-LABA. Leukotriene receptor antagonists (LTRA) are an alternative if avoiding ICS, but less efficacious.

• **Step 3: moderate persistent (symptoms most days, or waking with asthma once a week or more)** Low-dose ICS-LABA maintenance and reliever therapy (preferred) or daily low-dose ICS-LABA maintenance plus as-needed SABA. Consider addition of long-acting muscarinic antagonist (LAMA) (eg tiotropium) if LABA contraindicated/not tolerated. Less effective alternatives include medium dose of inhaled ICS + as-needed SABA or low-dose ICS with LTRA.

• **Step 4: severe persistent (symptoms most days, or waking with asthma once a week or more, or low lung function)** Medium-dose ICS-LABA as maintenance and reliever therapy. Alternative options include high-dose ICS, add-on tiotropium, or add-on LTRA.

• **Step 5** High-dose ICS-LABA. Refer for phenotypic assessment ± add-on therapy, eg tiotropium, anti-IgE, anti-IL-5/5R, anti-IL-4R. Some patients may benefit from low-dose oral corticosteroids but long-term SE are common and serious.

▶At each step, every patient should also have a reliever inhaler, either low-dose ICS-formoterol (preferred) or SABA.

Drugs Corticosteroids Best inhaled to minimize systemic effects, eg beclometasone via spacer (or powder), but may be given PO or IV. They act over days to ↓ bronchial mucosal inflammation. Rinse mouth after inhaled steroids to prevent oral candidiasis. Oral steroids are used acutely (high-dose, short courses, eg prednisolone 40mg/24h PO for 7d) and longer term in lower dose (eg 5–10mg/24h) if control is not optimal on inhalers. Warn about SE: p373.

$β_2$-adrenoceptor agonists Relax bronchial smooth muscle (↑cAMP), acting within minutes. Salbutamol is best given by inhalation (aerosol, powder, nebulizer), but may also be given PO or IV. SE: tachyarrhythmias, ↓K⁺, tremor, anxiety.

Anticholinergics (Eg tiotropium (Spiriva®Respimat®), 2 puffs (2.5 mcg) once daily.) May ↓muscle spasm synergistically with $β_2$-agonists. An add-on option at step 4 or 5 by mist inhaler for patients with a history of exacerbations despite ICS ± LABA. SE: dry mouth, URTI.

Leukotriene receptor antagonists (Eg oral montelukast, zafirlukast.) Block the effects of cysteinyl leukotrienes in the airways by antagonizing the CystLT₁ receptor.

Cromoglicate (Mast cell stabilizer.) Very limited role in long-term treatment of asthma. Weak anti-inflammatory effect, less effective than low-dose ICS. Require meticulous inhaler maintenance. SE: cough upon inhalation, pharyngeal discomfort.

Anti-IgE monoclonal antibody Omalizumab[6] may be of use in highly selected patients with persistent allergic asthma who have a serum IgE level of 30–700IU/mL and documented sensitivity to a perennial allergen. Given as a subcutaneous injection every 2–4wks depending on dose. Specialists prescribe only.

Anti-IL-5 therapy Anti-IL-5 monoclonal antibodies (eg mepolizumab, reslizumab) or anti-IL-5 receptor alpha antibody (eg benralizumab). Reduce exacerbations in severe eosinophilic asthma.

Anti-IL-4 receptor alpha-subunit antibody (eg dupilumab), similarly reduces exacerbations in moderate-to-severe, eosinophilic asthma.

Table 4.5 Adult doses of common inhaled drugs used in bronchoconstriction

	Inhaled aerosol	Inhaled powder	Nebulized (supervised)
Salbutamol (SABA)			
Dose example:	100–200mcg/6h	200–400mcg/6h	2.5–5mg/6h
Formoterol (LABA)			
Single dose		12mcg	
Recommended regimen		12mcg/12h	
Steroids			
Budesonide			
Doses available/puff		100–800mcg/12h	250mcg
Recommended regimen		200–400mcg/24h	0.25–1mg/12h
Budesonide–formoterol combination			
		100/6, 200/6, 400/12 mcg	
Recommended regimen	For maintenance therapy, initially 1–2 puffs/12h. For maintenance and reliever therapy, 2 puffs daily in 1–2 divided doses + 1 puff as required for relief of symptoms, increased if necessary up to 6 puffs as required		
Fluticasone			
Doses available/puff	50, 100, 250, & 500mcg	As for aerosol	250mcg/mL
Recommended regimen	100–250mcg/12h	100–250mcg/12h max 1mg/12h	0.5–2mg/12h
Tiotropium bromide (COPD)			
Dose/puff	2.5mcg	9mcg	—
Recommended regimen	25mcg daily	18mcg daily	—

Systemic absorption (via the throat) is less if inhalation is through a large-volume device, eg Volumatic® or AeroChamber Plus® devices. The latter is more compact. Static charge on some devices reduces dose delivery, so wash in water before dose; leave to dry (don't rub). It's pointless to squirt many puffs into a device: it is best to repeat single doses, and be sure to inhale *as soon as the drug is in the spacer*. SE: local (oral) candidiasis (p373); ↑rate of cataract if lifetime dose ≥2g beclometasone.[7]

▶Prescribe beclometasone by brand name, because, dose for dose, Qvar® is twice as potent as the other available CFC-free brand (Clenil Modulite®).
Any dose ≥250mcg ≈significant steroid absorption: carry a steroid card; this recommendation is being widened, and lower doses (beclometasone) are now said to merit a steroid card (manufacturer's information).

Definitions COPD is a common, preventable, and treatable disease that is characterized by persistent respiratory symptoms and airflow limitation (FEV₁ <80% predicted; FEV₁/FVC <0.7; see p155) that is due to airway and/or alveolar abnormalities usually caused by significant exposure to noxious particles or gases. COPD subtypes include chronic bronchitis and emphysema though there is significant overlap. *Chronic bronchitis* is defined *clinically* as cough, sputum production on most days for 3 months of 2 successive years. Symptoms improve if they stop smoking. There is no excess mortality if lung function is normal. *Emphysema* is defined *histologically* as enlarged air spaces distal to terminal bronchioles, with destruction of alveolar walls but often visualized on CT. *Asthma-COPD overlap* is characterized by persistent airflow limitation with several features usually associated with asthma and several features usually associated with COPD.

Prevalence 251 million cases globally; 4th leading cause of death.[8]

Risk factors Tobacco smoking (most commonly), indoor and outdoor air pollution, occupational exposures (eg chemicals and fumes), genetic factors (α₁-antitrypsin deficiency), ageing, female sex, low socioeconomic status, asthma, severe childhood respiratory infections.

Assessment of COPD Assess symptoms, degree of airflow limitation using spirometry, risk of exacerbations, and comorbidities.

Symptoms Chronic cough; sputum; dyspnoea; wheeze. Recurrent LRTIs. **Signs** Tachypnoea; use of accessory muscles of respiration; hyperinflation; ↓cricosternal distance (<3cm); ↓expansion; resonant or hyperresonant percussion note; quiet breath sounds (eg over bullae); wheeze; cyanosis; cor pulmonale.

Complications Acute exacerbations ± infection; polycythaemia; respiratory failure; cor pulmonale (oedema; ↑JVP); pneumothorax (ruptured bullae); lung carcinoma.

Concomitant chronic diseases CVD, metabolic syndrome, osteoporosis, depression, anxiety.

Tests FBC ↑PCV. α₁-antitrypsin <20% highly suggestive of homozygous deficiency CXR Hyperinflation; flat hemidiaphragms; large central pulmonary arteries; ↓peripheral vascular markings; bullae. **CT** Bronchial wall thickening; scarring; air space enlargement. **ECG** Right atrial and ventricular hypertrophy (cor pulmonale). **ABG** Recommended in severe COPD. ↓P_aO_2 ± hypercapnia. **Spirometry** (p154, p155) Obstructive + air trapping (FEV₁ <80% of predicted, FEV₁:FVC ratio <70% post-bronchodilator, ↑TLC, ↑RV, ↓DLCO in emphysema—see p154). Learn how to do spirometry from an experienced person: ensure *maximal* expiration of the full breath (it takes >4s; it's *not* a quick puff out). **6-minute walk test** Evaluate disability, rehab assessment. **Assess complications/comorbidities** TTE if signs of RHF, low threshold to evaluate for coronary artery disease, screen for lung cancer, osteoporosis, depression, GORD, etc.

Treatment Multidisciplinary. *Chronic stable:* see BOX and fig 4.11; be aware of ↑SE risk (including pneumonia) with ICS.[2] ►►*Emergency R̶:* p794. ►*Smoking cessation advice* (p85). *Encourage exercise:* consider physio or OT referral. BMI is often low; *diet advice ± supplements*[9] may help (p584). *Mucolytics* (BNF 3.7) may help chronic productive cough (NICE).[10] Disabilities may cause serious, treatable *depression;* screen for this (p15). *Oedema:* diuretics. ►*Flu and pneumococcal vaccinations:* p169 and p392. Assess inhaler technique and medication compliance regularly. *Azithromycin* ↓ exacerbations. Consider in sputum-producing non-smokers, optimized on other therapies, if ≥4 exacerbations/year, prolonged exacerbation, or exacerbation requiring hospitalization. Check QTc before prescribing. *Theophylline* is an older, oral bronchodilator; less commonly used now due to risk of toxicity.

Long-term O₂ therapy (LTOT) An MRC trial showed that if P_aO_2 was maintained ≥8.0kPa for 15h a day, 3yr survival improved from 30% to 50%. UK NICE guidelines suggest LTOT should be given for: 1 Clinically stable non-smokers with P_aO_2 <7.3kPa—despite maximal R̶. These values should be stable on two occasions >3wks apart. 2 If P_aO_2 7.3–8.0 *and* pulmonary hypertension (eg RVH; loud s₂), or polycythaemia, or peripheral oedema, or nocturnal hypoxia. 3 O₂ can also be prescribed for terminally ill patients.

Severity assessment in COPD

Severity assessment has implications for therapy and prognosis. The Global Initiative for COPD (GOLD) categorizes COPD into four stages based on post-bronchodilator FEV1% predicted. Later versions ('ABCD') also include symptom burden and risk of exacerbation. But, neither predict outcome. The BODE index (Body mass index, air-flow Obstruction, Dyspnoea and Exercise capacity) does have some predictive value for outcomes, and number and severity of exacerbations—4-year survival for those scoring 7–10 is only 20% and likely to have even poorer survival if offered mechanical ventilation. Similarly, being house-, bed-, or chair-bound carries a very poor prognosis and it would be difficult to justify mechanical ventilation in this group.

NICE COPD guidelines

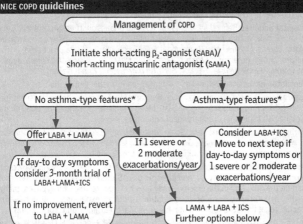

Fig 4.11 Chronic obstructive pulmonary disease in over 16s: non-pharmacological management and use of inhaled therapies. * Asthmatic features/features suggesting steroid responsiveness: previous diagnosis of asthma/atopy, ↑blood eosinophil count, substantial variation in FEV1 (>400mL) or diurnal variation in PEF (>20%).

© National Institute for Health and Care Excellence 2019. NNG115 *Chronic obstructive pulmonary disease in over 16s: diagnosis and management.* Available from https://www.nice.org.uk/guidance/ng115. NICE guidance is prepared for the National Health Service in England. All NICE guidance is subject to regular review and may be updated or withdrawn.

More advanced COPD

► Pulmonary rehabilitation improves symptoms, QOL, and reduces hospitalizations.
• Consider LTOT if P_aO_2 <7.3kPa (see 'Long-term O_2 therapy', earlier in topic).
• Surgery may be appropriate in selected patients, eg recurrent pneumothoraces; isolated bullous disease. Lung volume reduction/endobronchial valve/transplant.
• NIV may be appropriate if hypercapnic on LTOT.
• NB: may need an oxygen assessment pre-flight as air travel is risky if very hypoxic.
• Consider palliative care input.

Indications for specialist referral

• Uncertain diagnosis, or suspected severe COPD, or a rapid decline in FEV1.
• Onset of cor pulmonale.
• Bullous lung disease (to assess for surgery).
• Assessment for oral corticosteroids, nebulizer therapy, or LTOT.
• <10 pack-years smoking (= the number of packs/day × years of smoking) or COPD in patient <40yrs (eg is the cause α_1-antitrypsin deficiency? p286).
• Symptoms disproportionate to lung function tests.
• Frequent infections (to exclude bronchiectasis) or haemoptysis.

2 Cochrane meta-analyses (2007) of trials (including TORCH) favour steroids + LABA (long-acting β-agonist) vs either alone. LABA alone may ↑ exacerbation rates, but no excess hospitalizations or mortality; steroid inhalers alone are associated with ↑mortality (by 33%) compared with steroids + LABA.[11]

4 Chest medicine

An acute lower respiratory tract infection associated with fever, symptoms and signs in the chest, and abnormalities on the chest x-ray—fig 16.2, p707. Incidence: 5–11/1000, ↑ if very young or old (30% are under 65yrs). Mortality: ~10% in hospital.[12]

Classification and causes

Community-acquired pneumonia (CAP) May be primary or secondary to underlying disease. Typical organisms: *Streptococcus pneumoniae* (commonest), *Haemophilus influenzae*, *Moraxella catarrhalis*. Atypicals: *Mycoplasma pneumoniae*, *Staphylococcus aureus*, *Legionella* species, and *Chlamydia*. Gram-negative bacilli, *Coxiella burnetii* and anaerobes are rarer (?aspiration). Viruses account for up to 24%. 'Flu may be complicated by community-acquired MRSA pneumonia.[13]

Hospital-acquired Defined as >48h after hospital admission. If early onset (<5d) and no other risk factors for multidrug-resistant (MDR) organisms: *Strep. pneumoniae*, *Staph. aureus*, *H. influenzae*, Gram-negative enterobacteria. If late onset (≥5d) or risk factors for MDR organisms: *Staph. aureus* (often MRSA), Gram-negative enterobacteria (eg *Pseudomonas*, *Klebsiella*, *E. coli*, *Serratia marcescens*, *Enterobacter*).

Ventilator-associated Defined as >48h after endotracheal intubation.

Aspiration Those with stroke, myasthenia, bulbar palsies, ↓consciousness (eg postictal or intoxicated), oesophageal disease (achalasia, reflux), or poor dental hygiene risk aspirating oropharyngeal anaerobes.

Immunocompromised patient *Strep. pneumoniae*, *H. influenzae*, *Staph. aureus*, *M. catarrhalis*, *M. pneumoniae*, Gram −ve bacilli, and *Pneumocystis jirovecii* (formerly named *P. carinii*, p397). Other fungi, viruses (CMV, HSV), and mycobacteria.

Clinical features Symptoms Fever, rigors, malaise, anorexia, dyspnoea, cough, purulent sputum, haemoptysis, and pleuritic pain. Signs Pyrexia, cyanosis, confusion (can be the only sign in the elderly—may also be hypothermic), tachypnoea, tachycardia, hypotension, signs of consolidation (reduced expansion, dull percussion, ↑tactile vocal fremitus/vocal resonance, bronchial breathing), and a pleural rub.

Tests *Assess oxygenation:* oxygen saturation, p154 (ABGs if S_aO_2 <92% or severe pneumonia) and BP. *Blood tests:* FBC, U&E, LFT, CRP. *CXR* (fig 16.2, p707): lobar or multilobar infiltrates, cavitation, or pleural effusion. *Sputum* for microscopy and culture. Nasal MRSA screen can help predict presence/absence of MRSA pneumonia. *Urine:* check for *Legionella/Pneumococcal* urinary antigens. Atypical organism/viral serology (PCR sputum/BAL, complement fixation tests acutely, paired serology). *COVID/influenza* swabs ± respiratory *BioFire® PCR* panel. *Pleural fluid* may be aspirated for culture. Consider *bronchoscopy/BAL* if patient is immunocompromised or on ITU.

Severity 'CURB-65' is a simple, validated severity scoring system.[14,15] 1 point for each of:
• **C**onfusion (abbreviated mental test ≤8).
• **U**rea >7mmol/L.
• **R**espiratory rate ≥30/min.
• **B**P <90mmHg systolic and/or 60mmHg diastolic.
• **A**ge ≥65.
0–1, PO antibiotic/home treatment; 2, hospital therapy; ≥3, severe pneumonia indicates mortality 15–40%—consider ITU assessment. It may 'underscore' the young—use clinical judgement. Other features increasing the risk of death are: comorbidity; bilateral/multilobar; P_aO_2 <8kPa.

Management ▸▸p796. *Antibiotics*—refer to your local hospital antibiotic policy. When none exists, consult table 4.6. If pneumonia not severe and not vomiting (CURB-65 1–2) give PO antibiotic; severe (CURB-65 >2) give IV. *Oxygen:* keep P_aO_2 >8.0 and/or saturation ≥94%. *IV fluids* (anorexia, volume depletion, shock) and VTE prophylaxis. *Analgesia* if pleurisy. Consider ITU if shock, hypercapnia, or remains hypoxic. Consider adjunctive *steroids* in significant hypoxia (eg requiring NIV), refractory septic shock, COVID-19, or COPD. *Follow-up:* at 6 weeks (± CXR).

Complications (See p175.) Pleural effusion, empyema, lung abscess, respiratory failure, septicaemia, brain abscess, pericarditis, myocarditis, cholestatic jaundice.

Table 4.6 Empirical treatment of pneumonia (check local policy)

Clinical setting	Organisms	Antibiotic (further dosage details: pp382–3)[16]
Community-acquired		
Mild not previously R̶ CURB 0–1	*Streptococcus pneumoniae* *Haemophilus influenzae*	Oral amoxicillin 500mg–1g/8h or clarithromycin 500mg/12h or doxycycline 200mg loading then 100mg/day (initially 5-day course)
Moderate CURB 2	*Streptococcus pneumoniae* *Haemophilus influenzae* *Mycoplasma pneumoniae*	Oral amoxicillin 500mg–1g/8h + clarithromycin 500mg/12h or doxycycline 200mg loading then 100mg/12h. If IV required: amoxicillin 500mg/8h + clarithromycin 500mg/12h (5–7-day course)
Severe CURB >3	As above	Co-amoxiclav 1.2g/8h IV or cephalosporin IV (eg ceftriaxone 2g/24h IV) AND clarithromycin 500mg/12h IV (5–7 days)
		Add flucloxacillin ± rifampicin if *Staph* suspected; vancomycin (or teicoplanin) if MRSA suspected. Treat for 10d (14–21d if *Staph*, *Legionella*, or Gram −ve enteric bacteria suspected)
	Panton–Valentine leucocidin-producing *Staph. aureus* (PVL-SA)	Seek urgent help. Consider adding IV linezolid, clindamycin, and rifampicin
Atypical	*Legionella pneumophilia*	Fluoroquinolone combined with clarithromycin, or rifampicin, if severe. See p170
	Chlamydophila species	Tetracycline
	Pneumocystis jirovecii	High-dose co-trimoxazole (p397)
Hospital-acquired		
	Staph. aureus (often MRSA) Gram-negative bacilli *Pseudomonas* Anaerobes	Co-amoxiclav PO/IV if non-severe symptoms or signs and not at higher risk of resistance. If severe or higher risk of resistance, antipseudomonal penicillin IV (eg piperacillin-tazobactam 4.5g/8h) or 3rd-generation cephalosporin IV (eg ceftriaxone 2g/24h IV) or levofloxacin 750mg IV/PO/ 24h (p383). Add vancomycin if risk of MRSA
Aspiration		
	Streptococcus pneumoniae Anaerobes Gram-negative bacilli	Co-amoxiclav IV OR cephalosporin IV (eg ceftriaxone 2g/24h IV) + metronidazole IV
Neutropenic patients		
	Gram-positive cocci Gram-negative bacilli	Aminoglycoside IV + antipseudomonal penicillin IV or 3rd-generation cephalosporin IV
	Fungi (p174)	Consider antifungals after 48h

4 Chest medicine

Pneumococcal vaccine

At-risk groups
- All adults ≥65yrs old.
- Chronic heart, liver, kidney, or lung conditions.
- Diabetes mellitus not controlled by diet.
- Immunosuppression, eg ↓spleen function, AIDS, or on chemotherapy or prednisolone >20mg/d, cochlear implant, occupation risk (eg welders), CSF fluid leaks. Vaccinate every 5yrs.

CI Pregnancy, lactation, ↑T°, previous anaphylaxis to vaccine or one of its components.

4 Chest medicine

Pneumococcal pneumonia The commonest bacterial pneumonia. Affects all ages, but is commoner in the elderly, alcoholics, post-splenectomy, immunosuppressed, and patients with chronic heart failure or pre-existing lung disease. **Clinical features** Fever, pleurisy, herpes labialis. CXR shows lobar consolidation. If mod/severe check for urinary antigen. **Treatment** Ceftriaxone (preferred), fluoroquinolone eg levofloxacin or vancomycin. ↑ resistance to β-lactams—check with Microbiology if in doubt.

Staphylococcal pneumonia May complicate influenza infection or occur in the young, elderly, intravenous drug users, or patients with underlying disease, eg leukaemia, lymphoma, cystic fibrosis (CF). It causes a bilateral cavitating bronchopneumonia. **Treatment** MSSA: flucloxacillin; MRSA: vancomycin or linezolid.

***Klebsiella* pneumonia** Rare. Community-acquired in elderly, diabetics, and alcoholics, otherwise often HAP. Causes a cavitating pneumonia, particularly of the upper lobes, often drug resistant. **Treatment** Ceftriaxone or meropenem (if resistant).

Pseudomonas A common pathogen in bronchiectasis and CF. It also causes hospital-acquired infections, particularly on ITU or after surgery. **Treatment** Antipseudomonal penicillin eg piperacillin-tazobactam, ceftazidime, meropenem, or ciprofloxacin + aminoglycoside. Consider dual therapy until susceptibility is known.

Mycoplasma pneumoniae Occurs in epidemics about every 4yrs. It presents insidiously with 'flu-like symptoms (headache, myalgia, arthralgia) followed by a dry cough. CXR: reticular-nodular shadowing or patchy consolidation often of one lower lobe, and worse than signs suggest. **Diagnosis** PCR sputum or serology. Cold agglutinins may cause an autoimmune haemolytic anaemia. **Complications** Skin rash (erythema multiforme, fig 12.23, p561), Stevens–Johnson syndrome, meningoencephalitis, or myelitis; Guillain–Barré syndrome, GN. **Treatment** Clarithromycin (500mg/12h) or doxycycline (200mg loading then 100mg OD) or a fluroquinolone (eg levofloxacin or moxifloxacin).

Legionella pneumophila Colonizes water tanks kept at <60°C (eg hotel air-conditioning and hot water systems) causing outbreaks. Immunocompromise, smoking and comorbidities are risk factors. 'Flu-like symptoms (fever, malaise, myalgia) precede a dry cough and dyspnoea. Extrapulmonary features include anorexia, D&V, hepatitis, AKI, confusion, and coma. CXR shows bi-basal consolidation. **Blood tests** may show lymphopenia, hyponatraemia, and deranged LFTs. Urinalysis may show haematuria. **Diagnosis** Urine antigen/culture, PCR sputum/BAL. **Treatment** fluoroquinolone (eg levofloxacin) for 2–3wks or azithromycin (p383). 10% mortality.

Chlamydophila pneumoniae The commonest chlamydial infection. Person-to-person spread, biphasic illness: pharyngitis, hoarseness, otitis, followed by pneumonia. **Diagnosis** *Chlamydophila* complement fixation test, PCR invasive samples.[17] **Treatment** Doxycycline or azithromycin.

Chlamydophila psittaci Causes psittacosis (also known as ornithosis), acquired from infected birds (typically parrots). Symptoms include headache, fever, dry cough, lethargy, arthralgia, anorexia, and D&V. Extrapulmonary features are legion but rare, eg meningoencephalitis, infective endocarditis, hepatitis, nephritis, rash, splenomegaly. CXR shows patchy consolidation. **Diagnosis** *Chlamydophila* serology. **Treatment** Doxycycline or azithromycin.

Viral pneumonia Influenza commonest (p392 and BOX), but 'swine flu' (H1N1) is now considered seasonal and covered by the annual 'flu vaccine. Others: measles, CMV, varicella zoster.

***Pneumocystis* pneumonia** Causes life-threatening pneumonia in the immunosuppressed (eg HIV, high-dose steroids). The organism responsible was previously called *Pneumocystis carinii*, and now *P. jirovecii*.[18] It presents with a dry cough, exertional dyspnoea, ↓P_aO_2, fever, bilateral crepitations. CXR may be normal or show bilateral perihilar interstitial shadowing. **Diagnosis** Visualization of the organism in induced sputum, bronchoalveolar lavage, or in a lung biopsy specimen. Sputum PCR. **Drugs** High-dose co-trimoxazole (p397), or pentamidine by slow IVI for 2–3 weeks (p397). Steroids are beneficial if severe hypoxaemia. Prophylaxis is indicated if the CD4 count is <200 × 10⁶/L or after the 1st attack.[19]

Avian (pandemic) influenza

Avian influenza A viruses rarely infect humans and most follow direct or close contact with infected poultry. The issue remains a public health priority because of the ability of the virus to mutate. Symptoms range from conjunctivitis to influenza-like illness (low pathogenic forms) to severe respiratory illness and multi-organ failure (highly pathogenic forms). H7N9 and H5N1 have been responsible for most human illnesses worldwide. Highly pathogenic avian H5N1 influenza viruses are endemic among bird and poultry populations in Eurasia. ▶Suspect avian flu if fever (>38°C), chest signs or consolidation on CXR, or life-threatening infection, and contact with poultry or others with similar symptoms.[20] NB: D&V, abdominal pain, pleuritic pain, and bleeding from the nose and gums are reported to be an early feature in some patients.[21]

Diagnosis Viral culture ± reverse transcription PCR with H5- & N1-specific primers of respiratory specimens.[22] **Management** ▶Get help. Contain the outbreak, p393, in the UK, via your consultant in communicable disease control.[23] Ventilatory support + O_2 and antivirals may be needed. Most viruses are susceptible to oseltamivir, peramivir, and zanamivir. Nebulizers and high-air flow O_2 masks are implicated in nosocomial spread.[21,24] Antigenic diversity and uncertainty of the next pandemic virus subtype render vaccine preparedness difficult.

Precautions for close contacts of infected patients

Hand hygiene, avoid shared utensils and face-to-face contact, wear high-efficiency masks and eye protection. Start empirical antiviral treatment (oseltamivir within 48h of exposure and zanamivir within 36h). Monitor for fever, cough, shortness of breath, diarrhoea, or other systemic symptoms developing.

Coronaviruses COVID-19, SARS, and MERS

Coronavirus disease 2019 (COVID-19) See p172.

Severe acute respiratory syndrome (SARS[25]) Caused by SARS-COV virus—a coronavirus. Major features are persistent fever (>38°C), chills, rigors, myalgia, dry cough, headache, diarrhoea, and dyspnoea—with an abnormal CXR and ↓WCC. Respiratory failure is a complicating feature: ~20% progress to acute respiratory distress syndrome requiring invasive ventilation.[26] Mortality is 1–50%, depending on age, but no cases since 2004. Close contacts, or travel to an area with known cases should raise suspicion. The mechanism of transmission of SARS-COV is human–human. *Management:* seek expert help. Largely supportive with good infection control measures.

Middle East respiratory syndrome (MERS) A viral respiratory disease caused by novel coronavirus (MERS CoV) and first identified in 2012 in Saudi Arabia. Symptoms include fever, cough, shortness of breath, and gastrointestinal upset. Incubation period 14 days. Human-to-human transmission has been reported in most cases, but camels play a pivotal host role in animal-to-human transmission. Large outbreaks linked to healthcare facilities have been reported in the Middle East and South Korea. The WHO has reported mortality up to 36%.[23]

Coronavirus disease 2019 (COVID-19) was caused by a novel coronavirus, designated SARS-COV-2 virus. The first outbreak of COVID-19 acute respiratory illness occurred in China, and quickly spread globally to become a pandemic that affected >700 million people. Several variants of SARS-COV-2 have since emerged, eg Omicron, that continue to generate some concern because of their potential for increased transmissibility, more breakthrough infections in vaccinated individuals, and reinfection risk in those previously infected with other variants. Fortunately, these variants have been associated with less severe illness.

Natural history Varies from mild or asymptomatic infection to critical, life-threatening illness with ARDS. Male sex, hypertension, CVD, DM, chronic lung disease, pregnancy, and immunosuppression are all associated with more severe illness.[27] Severe disease affects ~15–20% of unvaccinated individuals. The incubation period for COVID-19 may extend to 14 days, with a median time of 4–5 days from exposure to symptom onset.[28]

Mode of transmission Direct person-to-person transmission via respiratory droplet secretion (eg coughing, sneezing, talking) is the main means of transmission. Transmission most likely occurs during the early stage of infection (even prior to symptom onset) and in enclosed, poorly ventilated spaces.

Clinical features **Symptoms** Most symptomatic infections are mild. Major features are cough, breathlessness, fever, myalgia, headache, and anosmia/ageusia. **Signs** Pyrexia, hypoxia. The degree of hypoxia can be out of keeping with clinical signs and symptoms.

Complications Respiratory failure, secondary bacterial infections (20%), arrythmias, heart failure, VTE (10–40%), encephalopathy, Guillain–Barré syndrome (GBS), AKI. The frequency and pathophysiology of 'long COVID' (persistent post-viral/critical illness symptoms such as fatigue, cough, anxiety, poor memory & concentration) is unclear.

Tests Diagnosis is via nasopharyngeal and oropharyngeal swabs (reverse transcription (RT)-PCR) with serology more useful to confirm past infection. Antigen testing (lateral flow tests) is faster and may be an acceptable alternative in some settings but it is less sensitive than RT-PCR. *Blood tests:* ↓lymphocytes, ↑CRP, ↑fibrinogen, ↑D-dimer, ↑LFTs. **CXR/CT thorax** Consolidation and ground-glass opacities, with bilateral, peripheral, and lower lung zone distributions (fig 4.12).

Management High-flow nasal cannula (HFNC) oxygen or NIV. Dexamethasone (6mg) for all hypoxic patients as it ↓ mortality ± tocilizumab or baricitinib if high O_2 requirements.[29] There is some evidence that remdesivir may reduce time to recovery and risk of mechanical ventilation in patients with risk factors for severe illness but no mortality benefit. ▶VTE prophylaxis. Prone positioning may be helpful. In severe cases, mechanical ventilation ± ECMO. Infection control measures.

Prevention Physical distancing, and isolation have some role. The effectiveness of routine non-FFP3 mask wearing in public is less clear. In clinical areas FFP3 masks/respirators appear effective in reducing transmission and general infection control measured in should be strictly adhered to. Isolation for COVID +ve patients and staff also helps reduce nosocomial infection.

Vaccines & immunity Following infection, individuals will have a protective immune response for at least 6–8 months. ▶▶Vaccination is highly effective against severe illness and essential for all. Several are now available including 2 mRNA vaccines (Pfizer & Moderna; SE: rarely myocarditis) and 2 adenoviral vector vaccines (AstraZeneca & Johnson & Johnson; SE: vaccine-induced ITP (VITT—see p343) and possibly GBS). Due to the possibility of waning immunity over time and the risk of immune escape by new variants, a booster dose is recommended 2–3 months after completion of the primary series to further reduce the risk of symptomatic or severe infection. Additional doses may be needed in immunocompromised individuals, eg those receiving chemotherapy and those who are dialysis dependent to maximize immune response.

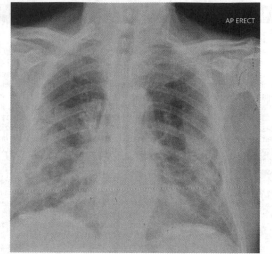

AP ERECT

Fig 4.12 CXR: bilateral patchy and/or confluent, bandlike ground-glass consolidation in a peripheral and mid to lower lung zone distribution consistent with pneumonitis. Note also the presence of chronic pleural plaques.

The Valley of the Shadow of Death

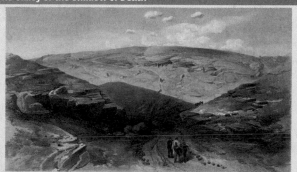

Fig 4.13 Crimean War: ambulancemen carrying the wounded in the Valley of the Shadow of Death. Coloured lithograph by J. Needham, 1855, after W. Simpson.

Wellcome Collection. Public Domain Mark. https://wellcomecollection.org/works/ynmygsd2

Most of the time we are unaware of our place in this world. It takes a pandemic or war (fig 4.13) to remind us that we have a responsibility or role that extends far beyond the reaches of a job description. As doctors, we may sometimes feel like gatekeepers in this endless cycle of life and death but more often than we would care for, we are helpless bystanders with just a closer view than most. To bear witness to so much tragedy and grief takes a very personal toll, not least in the midst of a pandemic, but within this pain, there remains a great privilege that we can offer support and comfort during these dark hours. Let us find solace in the words of the poet Seamus Heaney that 'Hope is not optimism, which expects things to turn out well, but something rooted in the conviction that there is good worth working for.'

Aspergillus This group of fungi affects the lung in five ways:

1 **Asthma** Type I hypersensitivity reaction to fungal spores (p160).

2 **Allergic bronchopulmonary aspergillosis (ABPA)** Results from type I and III hypersensitivity reactions to *Aspergillus fumigatus*. Affects 1–5% of asthmatics, 2–25% of CF patients.[30] Initially bronchoconstriction, then permanent damage occurs causing bronchiectasis (fig 4.14). *Symptoms:* wheeze, cough, sputum (plugs of mucus containing fungal hyphae, see p404), dyspnoea, and 'recurrent pneumonia'. *Diagnosis:* in a predisposed patient, *Aspergillus*-specific I_gE RAST (radioallergosorbent test), positive *Aspergillus* skin test, and serum ↑I_gE. Other criteria: positive serum precipitins, typical radiological findings (eg transient segmental collapse or consolidation, central proximal bronchiectasis), and eosinophilia. *Treatment:* mainstay is oral corticosteroids with a tapering course. Antifungal therapy, eg voriconazole added for steroid weaning. Bronchodilators for asthma.

3 **Aspergilloma (mycetoma)** A fungus ball within a pre-existing cavity (often caused by TB or sarcoidosis). It is usually asymptomatic but may cause cough, haemoptysis (may be torrential), lethargy ± weight loss. *Investigations:* CXR/CT (round opacity within a cavity, usually apical); sputum culture; strongly positive serum precipitins; *Aspergillus* skin test (30% +ve). *Treatment* antifungal therapy if symptomatic or growing in size and consider surgical resection if this fails. Use antifungal therapy adjunctively postresection and in those with progressive radiological findings/symptoms who are unable to undergo surgery. If massive haemoptysis, may need to consider embolization.

4 **Invasive aspergillosis** *Risk factors:*[31] immunocompromise, eg HIV, leukaemia, burns, ANCA vasculitis (p700), and SLE, or after broad-spectrum antibiotic therapy. However, also increasingly recognized in immunocompetent, critically ill patients. *Investigations:* serum biomarkers including galactomannan (an *Aspergillus* antigen) and β-D-glucan (non-specific; a cell wall component of many fungi), sputum for fungal staining and culture; CXR/CT (consolidation, abscess); bronchoscopy with BAL, transbronchial, CT-guided or VATS biopsy. *Treatment:* voriconazole is superior to IV amphotericin.[32] Consider adding echinocandin for first 1–2 weeks if severe or progressive disease. *Prognosis:* 30% mortality.

5 **Hypersensitivity pneumonitis (extrinsic allergic alveolitis)** See p193.

Other fungal infections *Candida* and *Cryptococcus* may cause pneumonia in the immunosuppressed (p404).

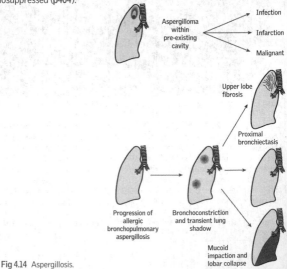

Fig 4.14 Aspergillosis.

Respiratory failure (See p158.) Type I respiratory failure (P_aO_2 <8kPa) is relatively common. Treatment is with high-flow (60%) oxygen. *Transfer the patient to ITU if hypoxia does not improve with O_2 therapy or P_aCO_2 rises to >6kPa.* Be careful with O_2 in COPD patients; check ABGs frequently, and consider elective ventilation if rising P_aCO_2 or worsening acidosis. Aim to keep SaO_2 at 94–98%, P_aO_2 ≥8kPa.

Hypotension and septic shock May be due to a combination of volume depletion and vasodilation due to sepsis. If systolic BP is <90mmHg, give an IV fluid challenge of 500mL crystalloid over 15min. If systolic BP remains <90mmHg despite adequate fluid resuscitation (ie 30mL/kg over 3h period), this may indicate septic shock—request urgent ITU assessment for vasopressor support.

Atrial fibrillation (See p126.) Common in the elderly. It usually resolves with treatment of the pneumonia but the patients may still require long-term anticoagulation depending on CHA_2DS_2-VASc score and other risk factors. β-blocker or digoxin may be required to slow the ventricular response rate in the short term.

(Parapneumonic) pleural effusion Inflammation of the pleura by adjacent pneumonia may cause fluid exudation into the pleural space. If this accumulates faster than it is reabsorbed, a pleural effusion develops. If small, it may be of no consequence. If larger and patient symptomatic, or infected (empyema), drainage is required (p176, p750).

Empyema Pus in the pleural space. It should be suspected if a patient with a resolving pneumonia develops a recurrent fever. Clinical features: CXR indicates a pleural effusion. The aspirated pleural fluid is typically yellow and turbid with a pH <7.2, ↓glucose, and ↑LDH. The empyema should be drained using a chest drain, inserted under radiological guidance. Adhesions and loculation can make this difficult.

Lung abscess A cavitating area of localized, suppurative infection within the lung.
Causes •Most commonly, aspiration (eg alcoholism, oesophageal obstruction, bulbar palsy). •Inadequately treated pneumonia. •Bronchial obstruction (tumour, foreign body). •Pulmonary infarction. •Septic emboli (septicaemia, right heart endocarditis, IV drug use). •Subphrenic or hepatic abscess.
Clinical features Swinging fever; cough; purulent, foul-smelling sputum; pleuritic chest pain; haemoptysis; malaise; weight loss. Look for: finger clubbing; anaemia; crepitations. Empyema develops in 20–30%
Tests *Blood:* FBC (anaemia, neutrophilia), ESR, CRP, blood cultures. Sputum microscopy, culture, and cytology. *CXR:* walled cavity, often with a fluid level. Consider CT scan to exclude obstruction, and bronchoscopy to obtain diagnostic specimens.
Treatment Antibiotics as indicated by sensitivities; empiric regimens should target both strict anaerobes and facultatively anaerobic species (ie streptococci); continue until healed (4–6wks). Postural drainage. Repeated aspiration, antibiotic instillation, or surgical excision may be required.

Septicaemia May occur as a result of bacterial spread from the lung parenchyma into the bloodstream. This may cause metastatic secondary infection, eg infective endocarditis, meningitis. Treat with IV antibiotic according to sensitivities.

Pericarditis and myocarditis May also complicate pneumonia.

Jaundice This is usually cholestatic, and may be due to sepsis or secondary to antibiotic therapy (particularly flucloxacillin and co-amoxiclav).

Definitions A pleural effusion is fluid in the pleural space. Effusions can be divided by their protein concentration into *transudates* (<25g/L) and *exudates* (>35g/L), see table 4.7. Blood in the pleural space is a *haemothorax*, pus in the pleural space is an *empyema*, and chyle (lymph with fat) is a *chylothorax*. Both blood and air in the pleural space is called a *haemopneumothorax*.

Causes *Transudates* may be due to ↑venous pressure (cardiac failure, constrictive pericarditis, fluid overload), or hypoproteinaemia (cirrhosis, nephrotic syndrome, malabsorption). Also occur in hypothyroidism and Meigs' syndrome (right pleural effusion and ovarian fibroma). *Exudates* are mostly due to increased leakiness of pleural capillaries secondary to infection, inflammation, or malignancy. Causes: pneumonia; TB; pulmonary infarction; rheumatoid arthritis; SLE; bronchogenic carcinoma; malignant metastases; lymphoma; mesothelioma; lymphangitic carcinomatosis.

Symptoms Asymptomatic—or dyspnoea, pleuritic chest pain.

Signs *Decreased expansion; stony dull percussion note; diminished breath sounds* occur on the affected side. Tactile vocal fremitus and vocal resonance are ↓ (inconstant and unreliable). Above the effusion, where lung is compressed, there may be *bronchial breathing*. With large effusions there may be *tracheal deviation* away from the effusion. Look for aspiration marks and signs of associated disease: malignancy (cachexia, clubbing, lymphadenopathy, radiation marks, mastectomy scar); stigmata of chronic liver disease; cardiac failure; hypothyroidism; rheumatoid arthritis; butterfly rash of SLE.

Tests CXR Small effusions blunt the costophrenic angles, larger ones are seen as water-dense shadows with concave upper borders (fig 4.15). A completely flat horizontal upper border implies that there is also a pneumothorax.

Ultrasound Useful in identifying the presence of pleural fluid and in guiding diagnostic or therapeutic aspiration. Detects pleural fluid septations with greater sensitivity than CT scanning.[33]

Diagnostic aspiration BTS recommend that all aspirates should be ultrasound-guided to improve success rate, reduce complications (including pneumothorax), and reduce the risk of organ puncture. Infiltrate down to the pleura with 5–10mL of 1% lidocaine. Attach a 21G needle to a syringe and insert it just above the upper border of an appropriate rib (avoids neurovascular bundle). Draw off 10–30mL of pleural fluid and send it to the lab for *clinical chemistry* (protein, glucose, pH, LDH, amylase), *bacteriology* (microscopy & culture, auramine stain, TB culture), *cytology* (malignant effusions can be diagnosed based on pleural fluid cytology results in 60% of cases), and, if indicated, *immunology* (rheumatoid factor, ANA, complement). Send adenosine deaminase if a TB effusion is suspected. Light's criteria should be used to distinguish between a pleural fluid exudate and transudate. In order to apply Light's criteria, the total protein and LDH values should be measured in both blood and pleural fluid. See table 4.7.

CT thorax With pleural phase contrast enhancement should be considered in all patients with an undiagnosed exudative pleural effusion. Useful in distinguishing malignant from benign pleural thickening.

Pleural biopsy If pleural fluid analysis is inconclusive, consider parietal pleural biopsy. Thoracoscopic or CT-guided pleural biopsy increases diagnostic yield (by enabling direct visualization of the pleural cavity and biopsy of suspicious areas).

Management is of the underlying cause.
- *Drainage:* if the effusion is symptomatic or if empyema is present (pH <7.2), drain it, repeatedly if necessary. Fluid is best removed slowly (0.5–1.5L/24h). It may be aspirated in the same way as a diagnostic tap, or using an intercostal drain (p750).
- *Pleurodesis* with talc may be helpful for recurrent effusions. Thoracoscopic mechanical pleurodesis is most effective for malignant effusions. Empyemas (p175) are best drained using a chest drain, inserted under ultrasound or CT guidance.
- *Intra-pleural alteplase and dornase alfa* may help with empyema.
- *Surgery:* persistent collections and increasing pleural thickness requires surgery.[34]

Table 4.7 Pleural fluid analysis

Gross appearance	Cause
Clear, straw-coloured	Transudate, exudate
Turbid, yellow	Empyema, parapneumonic effusion
Haemorrhagic	Trauma, malignancy, pulmonary infarction
Cytology	
Neutrophils ++	Parapneumonic effusion, PE
Lymphocytes ++	Malignancy, TB, RA, SLE, sarcoidosis
Mesothelial cells ++	Pulmonary infarction
Abnormal mesothelial cells	Mesothelioma
Multinucleated giant cells	RA
Lupus erythematosus cells	SLE
Malignant cells	Malignancy
Clinical chemistry	
*Protein<25g/L	Transudate
>35g/L	Exudate
25–35g/L	Use Light's criteria: if pleural fluid protein/serum protein >0.5 or pleural LDH/serum LDH >0.6, effusion is an exudate
Glucose <3.3mmol/L	Empyema, malignancy, TB, RA, SLE
pH <7.2	Empyema, malignancy, TB, RA, SLE
*↑LDH (pleural:serum >0.6)	Empyema, malignancy, TB, RA, SLE
↑Amylase	Pancreatitis, carcinoma, bacterial pneumonia, oesophageal rupture
Immunology	
Rheumatoid factor	RA
Antinuclear antibody	SLE
↓Complement levels	RA, SLE, malignancy, infection

* Light's criteria for defining an exudate: effusion protein/serum protein >0.5; effusion LDH/serum LDH >0.6; effusion LDH >⅔ upper reference range for serum LDH. 98% sensitive and 83% specific.

4 Chest medicine

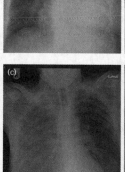
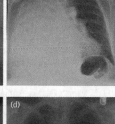
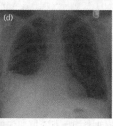

Fig 4.15 CXR appearances of a free-flowing left pleural effusion imaged erect (a); a massive right pleural effusion with mediastinal shift (b); and a pleural effusion radiographed supine (c) and erect (d) in the same patient.

Reproduced from Firth J *et al.*, *Oxford Textbook of Medicine* 2020, with permission from Oxford University Press.

ARDS is a type of respiratory failure characterized by the acute onset of bilateral alveolar infiltrates and hypoxaemia. Lung injury causes increased capillary permeability resulting in excess fluid in both the interstitium and alveoli. This leads to impaired gas exchange, decreased compliance, increased pulmonary arterial pressure, and non-cardiogenic pulmonary oedema, often accompanied by multiorgan failure. The myriad of causes are listed below and on p179, the most common of which are pneumonia, sepsis, and aspiration.

Causes Pulmonary Pneumonia; gastric aspiration; inhalation injury; vasculitis (p554); contusion. **Other** Shock; sepsis; haemorrhage; multiple transfusions; DIC (p350); pancreatitis; acute liver failure; trauma; head injury; malaria; fat embolism; burns; obstetric events (eclampsia; amniotic fluid embolus); drugs/toxins (aspirin, heroin, paraquat).

Clinical features Cyanosis; tachypnoea; tachycardia; peripheral vasodilation; bilateral fine inspiratory crackles. **Investigations** FBC, U&E, LFT, amylase, clotting, CRP, blood cultures, troponin, BNP, D-dimer, lactate, ABG. COVID/influenza swab. Sputum culture, respiratory BioFire® PCR ± BAL. CXR shows bilateral diffuse alveolar opacities with dependent atelectasis. There are usually widespread patchy and/or coalescent airspace opacities, particularly in the dependent lung zones on CT. TTE may be helpful if uncertainty whether cardiogenic vs non-cardiogenic pulmonary oedema. Occasionally, pulmonary artery catheter was used in the past to measure pulmonary capillary wedge pressure (PCWP) but this is associated with ↑ complications/mortality so is no longer routinely indicated.[35]

Differential diagnoses Cardiogenic pulmonary oedema, bilateral pneumonia, diffuse alveolar haemorrhage, vasculitis, cryptogenic organizing pneumonia.

Diagnostic criteria Are as follows: 1 Respiratory symptoms must have begun within 1 week of a known clinical insult. 2 CXR or CT: bilateral infiltrates (fig 4.16). 3 Respiratory failure not fully explained by cardiac failure or fluid overload. 4 A moderate to severe impairment of oxygenation must be present, as defined by the ratio of arterial oxygen tension to fraction of inspired oxygen (P_aO_2/FiO$_2$). The P_aO_2: FiO$_2$ is typically ≤300mmHg (or <40kPa) for ARDS and is classified as severe if ≤100mmHg (<14kPa).[36]

Management Admit to ITU; give supportive therapy; treat the underlying cause.
- **Respiratory support** In early ARDS, high-flow oxygen can be provided through a face mask or high-flow nasal cannulae (HFNC). Continuous positive airway pressure (CPAP) with 40–60% oxygen may be adequate to maintain oxygenation. But most patients need mechanical ventilation. The large tidal volumes (10–15mL/kg) produced by conventional ventilation plus reduced lung compliance in ARDS may lead to high peak airway pressures leading to barotrauma ± pneumothorax. Lung protective ventilation with a tidal-volume of 6–8mL/kg IBW, pressure-limited approach, with either low or moderate high positive end-expiratory pressure (PEEP), improves outcome.[37] Consider proning (>16h per day—improves oxygenation in the majority), neuromuscular blockade or ECMO (for patients with severe but potentially reversible acute respiratory failure—p784).
- **Circulatory support** Invasive haemodynamic monitoring with an arterial line and central venous catheter. A conservative fluid management approach improves outcome. Maintain cardiac output and O$_2$ delivery with inotropes, vasodilators, and blood transfusion. Consider using nitric oxide, a pulmonary vasodilator that improves oxygenation due to better V/Q matching and helps ameliorate pulmonary hypertension.
- **Sepsis** Identify organism(s) and treat. If septic, but no organisms cultured, use empirical broad-spectrum antibiotics (p169). Nosocomial pneumonia develops in 60% of severe ARDS patients.
- **Other** Nutritional support: enteral is best: p584 & p585, with high-fat, antioxidant formulations. Steroids may have a mortality benefit in moderate–severe refractory ARDS to standard therapies.[38] DVT and GI bleeding prophylaxis. Glucose control.

Prognosis Mortality has declined over time but remains at least 25–40%. However, prognosis varies with age of patient, cause, and number of organs involved.[39,40]

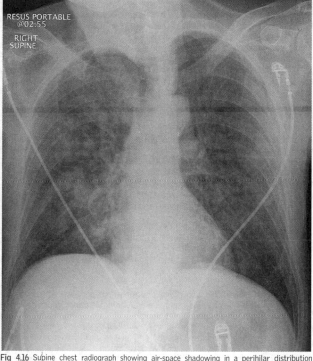

Fig 4.16 Supine chest radiograph showing air-space shadowing in a perihilar distribution spreading into the peripheries. This appearance can also be seen with infection and cardiogenic pulmonary oedema, but clues from the history, the heart size, and lack of pleural effusions can suggest ARDS over the latter. Remember though that this is a supine projection—the patient is lying flat with the x-ray beam anteroposterior—causing the cardiac shadow to be artificially enlarged and pleural effusions to level out on the posterior chest wall so they will not obscure the costophrenic angles unless very large.

Image courtesy of Nottingham University Hospitals NHS Trust Radiology Department.

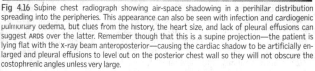

Risk factors for ARDS	
• Sepsis	• Massive transfusion
• Hypovolaemic shock	• Burns (p828)
• Trauma	• Smoke inhalation
• Pneumonia	• Near drowning
• Diabetic ketoacidosis	• Acute pancreatitis
• Gastric aspiration	• DIC (p350)
• Pregnancy	• Head injury
• Eclampsia	• ↑ICP
• Amniotic fluid embolus	• Fat embolus
• Drugs/toxins	• Heart/lung bypass
• Paraquat, heroin, aspirin	• Tumour lysis syndrome (p525)
• Pulmonary contusion	• Malaria

Bronchiectasis

Pathology Chronic inflammation of the bronchi and bronchioles leading to permanent dilatation and thinning of these airways. The induction of bronchiectasis requires an infectious insult plus impairment of drainage, airway obstruction, and/or a defect in host defence. Exacerbations are caused by acute bacterial infections, typically *H. influenzae; Strep. pneumoniae; Staph. aureus; Pseudomonas aeruginosa.*

Causes Congenital Cystic fibrosis (CF); Young's syndrome; primary ciliary dyskinesia; Kartagener's syndrome (OHCS p850). **Post-infection** Measles; pertussis; bronchiolitis; pneumonia; TB; HIV. **Other** Bronchial obstruction (tumour, foreign body); allergic bronchopulmonary aspergillosis (ABPA, p174); hypogammaglobulinaemia; rheumatoid arthritis; ulcerative colitis; idiopathic.

Clinical features Symptoms Persistent cough; copious purulent sputum; intermittent haemoptysis. **Signs** Finger clubbing; coarse inspiratory crepitations; wheeze (asthma, COPD, ABPA). **Complications** Pneumonia, pleural effusion; pneumothorax; haemoptysis; cerebral abscess; amyloidosis.

Tests *Sputum* culture. CXR: cystic shadows, thickened bronchial walls (tramline and ring shadows); see **fig 4.17.** HRCT *chest* (p156) is required to diagnose and to assess extent and distribution of disease. Typical findings include airway dilatation, lack of airway tapering, bronchial thickening, and cysts. *Spirometry* often shows an obstructive pattern; reversibility should be assessed. *Bronchoscopy* to exclude obstruction and obtain samples for culture. **Other tests** CT angiogram to investigate site of bleeding/embolizable target if significant haemoptysis. Serum immunoglobulins; CF sweat test or CFTR genotyping; test for primary ciliary dyskinesia, eg saccharin, nasal brushings, nasal NO; *Aspergillus* precipitins or skin-prick test RAST and total IGE.

Management • *Treat the underlying disease where possible,* eg certain immunodeficiencies, CF, recurrent aspiration. • *Airway clearance techniques and mucolytics:* chest physiotherapy and devices such as a flutter valve may aid sputum expectoration and mucus drainage. • *Antibiotics* should be prescribed according to bacterial sensitivities but azithromycin is frequently used prophylactically. *Pseudomonas* will require either oral ciprofloxacin or suitable IV antibiotics. If ≥3 exacerbations a year consider long-term antibiotics (may be nebulized). • *Bronchodilators* (eg nebulized salbutamol) may be useful in patients with asthma, COPD, CF, ABPA (p174). • *Corticosteroids* (eg prednisolone) and itraconazole for ABPA. • *Surgery* may be indicated in localized disease or to control severe haemoptysis. Bronchial artery embolization may be needed for patients with brisk haemoptysis. • *Other:* immunizations, PPI if GORD present, pulmonary rehabilitation for patients with moderate-to-severe airflow limitation on PFTs.

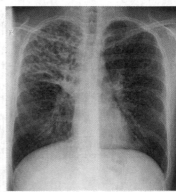

Fig 4.17 Posteroanterior (PA) chest radiograph showing marked abnormal dilatation of the airways throughout the right upper lobe, subtle similar changes throughout the rest of the lung (particularly periphery of the left upper zone). The fine background reticular pattern in the lungs suggests that there may also be some interstitial lung disease present.

Image courtesy of Nottingham University Hospitals NHS Trust Radiology Department.

One of the commonest life-threatening autosomal recessive conditions (1:2000 live births) affecting Caucasians. 1:25 people carry a copy of the faulty gene. All UK babies are screened at birth. Caused by mutations in the CF transmembrane conductance regulator (CFTR) gene on chromosome 7 (>1500 mutations have been identified). This is a Cl⁻ channel, and the defect leads to a combination of defective chloride secretion and increased sodium absorption across airway epithelium. The changes in the composition of airway surface liquid predispose the lung to chronic pulmonary infections and bronchiectasis. Deranged transport of Cl⁻ and/or other CFTR-affected ions, such as sodium and bicarbonate, leads to thick, viscous secretions in other organs as well including the pancreas, liver, intestine, and reproductive tract and to increased salt content in sweat gland secretions See *OHCS* ('Paediatrics', p178) for more detail.

Clinical features Neonate Failure to thrive; meconium ileus; rectal prolapse. **Children and young adults** *Respiratory:* cough; wheeze; recurrent infections; bronchiectasis; pneumothorax; haemoptysis; respiratory failure; cor pulmonale. *Gastrointestinal:* pancreatic insufficiency (diabetes mellitus, steatorrhoea); distal intestinal obstruction syndrome (meconium ileus equivalent); gallstones; cirrhosis. *Other:* male infertility; osteoporosis; arthritis; vasculitis (p554); nasal polyps; sinusitis; and hypertrophic pulmonary osteoarthropathy (HPOA). *Signs:* cyanosis; finger clubbing; bilateral coarse crackles.

Diagnosis Sweat test Sweat chloride ≥60mmol/L **Genetics** CFTR genotyping (CFTR modulation now possible). *Faecal elastase* is a simple and useful screening test for exocrine pancreatic dysfunction.

Tests Blood FBC, U&E, LFT; clotting; vitamin A, D, E, K levels; annual glucose tolerance test (p200). **Bacteriology** Cough swab, sputum culture. **Radiology** CXR; hyperinflation; bronchiectasis. **Abdominal ultrasound** Fatty liver; cirrhosis; chronic pancreatitis. **Spirometry** Obstructive defect. *Aspergillus serology/skin test* (20% develop ABPA, p174). **Biochemistry** Faecal fat analysis.

Management Management should be multidisciplinary, eg physician, GP, physiotherapist, specialist nurse, and dietician, with attention to psychosocial as well as physical wellbeing. **CFTR modulators** If suitable variant present. **Chest** Physiotherapy (postural drainage, airway clearance techniques). Antibiotics are given for acute infective exacerbations and prophylactically. Chronic *Pseudomonas* infection is an important predictor of survival and should be treated with nebulized antibiotics. Mucolytics may be useful (eg DNase, ie dornase alfa, 2.5mg daily nebulized, or nebulized hypertonic saline). Bronchodilators. Annual CXR surveillance is recommended. **Gastrointestinal** Malabsorption, GORD, distal obstruction syndrome. Pancreatic enzyme replacement; fat-soluble vitamin supplements (A, D, E, K); ursodeoxycholic acid for impaired liver function; cirrhosis may require liver transplantation. **Other** Treatment of CF-related diabetes (screen annually with OGTT from 12yrs); screening/treatment of osteoporosis (DEXA bone scanning); arthritis, sinusitis, and vasculitis; fertility and genetic counselling. **Advanced lung disease** Oxygen, diuretics (cor pulmonale); non-invasive ventilation; lung transplant (post-transplant survival 10yrs). **Prognosis** Median survival is now ~47yrs in the UK.

Mutation-specific therapies for cystic fibrosis

CFTR correctors (eg elexacaftor, lumacaftor, tezacaftor) correct the processing and trafficking defect of the F508del-CFTR protein to enable it to reach the cell surface where the CFTR potentiator, ivacaftor, can further enhance the ion channel function of the CFTR protein. Ivacaftor increases the open probability of CFTR channels and has been shown to improve clinical outcomes (lung function, weight, lung disease stability) in CF patients >6 years old.[41] Corrector and potentiator combination therapy (eg elexacaftor–tezacaftor–ivacaftor) for patients with F508del, have been shown to improve lung function and reduce pulmonary exacerbations.[42]

Gene therapy (transfer of CFTR gene using liposome or adenovirus vectors): phase IIb studies show modest but significant improvement in FEV1 in those receiving gene therapy.[43] Further work into vectors for gene transfer is ongoing.

4 Chest medicine

Carcinoma of the bronchus Third most common cancer in the UK, accounting for 13% of all new cancer cases and 21% of cancer deaths (35 300 cases/yr in UK).[44,45] Incidence is increasing in women. **Risk factors** Cigarette smoking (causes 90% of lung ca). Others: passive smoking, asbestos, chromium, arsenic, iron oxides, prior radiation for, eg Hodgkin's lymphoma, breast cancer, pulmonary fibrosis, and HIV.

Histology Clinically the most important division is between small cell (SCLC) and non-small cell (NSCLC). NSCLC Squamous (35%); adenocarcinoma (27%); large cell (10%); adenocarcinoma *in situ* (rare, <1%). **Small cell (20%)** Arise from endocrine cells (Kulchitsky cells), often secreting polypeptide hormones resulting in paraneoplastic syndromes (eg production of ACTH, Cushing's syndrome). Most (70%) SCLC are disseminated at presentation.

Symptoms Cough (80%); haemoptysis (70%); dyspnoea (60%); chest pain (40%); recurrent or slowly resolving pneumonia; lethargy, anorexia; weight loss.

Signs Cachexia; anaemia; clubbing; HPOA (hypertrophic pulmonary osteoarthropathy, causing wrist pain); supraclavicular or axillary nodes. *Chest signs:* none, or consolidation; collapse; pleural effusion. *Metastases:* bone tenderness; hepatomegaly; confusion; seizures; focal CNS signs; cerebellar syndrome; proximal myopathy; peripheral neuropathy.

Complications *Local:* recurrent laryngeal nerve palsy; phrenic nerve palsy; SVC obstruction; Horner's syndrome (Pancoast's tumour); rib erosion; pericarditis; AF. *Metastatic:* brain; bone (bone pain, anaemia, ↑Ca²⁺); liver; adrenals (Addison's). *Non-metastatic neurological:* confusion; fits; cerebellar syndrome; proximal myopathy; neuropathy; polymyositis; Lambert–Eaton syndrome (p508). See table 4.8.

Tests CXR: peripheral nodule (fig 4.18); hilar enlargement; consolidation; lung collapse; pleural effusion; bony secondaries. *Cytology:* sputum and pleural fluid (send at least 20mL). *Fine needle aspiration* or *biopsy* (peripheral lesions/lymph nodes). CT TAP to stage the tumour (p184) and guide bronchoscopy. *Bronchoscopy:* to give histology and assess operability, ± endobronchial ultrasound for assessment and biopsy. ¹⁸F-deoxyglucose PET or PET/CT scan to help in staging. *Radionuclide bone scan:* and CT brain if suspected metastases. *Lung function tests:* help assess suitability for lobectomy.

Management See p184 for treatment and prognosis.

Other lung tumours Bronchial adenoma Rare, slow-growing. 90% are carcinoid tumours; 10% cylindromas. ℞: surgery. Hamartoma Rare, benign; CT: lobulated mass ± flecks of calcification; ?excise to exclude malignancy.

Malignant mesothelioma A tumour of mesothelial cells that usually occurs in the pleura, and rarely in the peritoneum or other organs. It is associated with occupational exposure to asbestos but the relationship is complex.[46] 90% report previous exposure to asbestos, but only 20% of patients have pulmonary asbestosis. The latent period between exposure and development of the tumour may be up to 45yrs. Compensation is often available.

Clinical features Chest pain, dyspnoea, weight loss, finger clubbing, recurrent pleural effusions. Signs of metastases: lymphadenopathy, hepatomegaly, bone pain/tenderness, abdominal pain/obstruction (peritoneal malignant mesothelioma).

Tests CXR/CT: pleural thickening/effusion. Bloody pleural fluid.

Diagnosis Made on histology, usually following a thoracoscopy. Often the diagnosis is only made postmortem.

Management Surgery (pleurectomy/decortication or radical extrapleural pneumonectomy), radiotherapy, and systemic chemotherapy each may be beneficial as single modalities in selected situations, but the prognosis for prolonged survival is poor as disease is usually locally extensive on presentation. Pemetrexed + cisplatin chemotherapy can improve survival.[47] Pleurodesis and indwelling intra-pleural drain may help symptomatically for malignant effusions.

Prognosis Poor (especially without pemetrexed, eg <2yrs). >2500 deaths/yr in UK.

Differential diagnosis of nodule in the lung on a CXR

- Malignancy (1° or 2°).
- Abscesses (p175).
- Granuloma.
- Carcinoid tumour.
- Pulmonary hamartoma.
- Arterio-venous malformation.
- Encysted effusion (fluid, blood, pus).
- Cyst.
- Foreign body.
- Skin tumour (eg seborrhoeic wart).

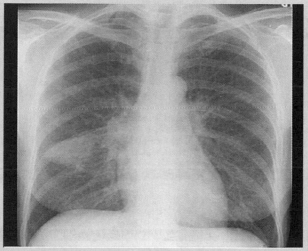

Fig 4.18 A wedge-shaped density in the right middle lobe. Also note a coin lesion at the right costophrenic angle. Right hilar lymphadenopathy.

Courtesy of Janet E. Jeddry, Yale Medical School.

Table 4.8 Non-metastatic extrapulmonary manifestations of bronchial cancer

System	Manifestations
Endocrine	Ectopic secretion, ACTH (Cushing's), ADH (hyponatraemia), PTH (hypercalcaemia), HCG (gynaecomastia)
Neurological	Cerebellar degeneration, myopathy, polyneuropathy, myasthenic syndrome
Vascular	Thrombophlebitis migrans (p560), anaemia, DIC
Cutaneous	Dermatomyositis, herpes zoster, acanthosis nigricans
Skeletal	Clubbing, HPOA

Screening for lung cancer

Although there is no national screening programme for lung cancer in the UK, Lung Health Checks are offered in some areas of England for those registered with a GP, who have ever smoked and who are between 55–75 years. They are screened for lung cancer with a low-dose CT which has a radiation dose exposure less than a third of a standard-dose diagnostic chest CT examination. Several trials have demonstrated that screening in this way is associated with a 24% reduction in lung cancer deaths along with a reduction in all-cause mortality. The risks include false-positive imaging requiring follow-up, incidental findings, radiation exposure, anxiety associated with screening and follow-up, and over-diagnosis. Ultimately, prevention through the promotion of smoking cessation is likely to have far greater impact on lung cancer mortality than is screening. [48,49]

4 Chest medicine

Assessing the extent of tumour spread (staging) is vital to determining the best course of treatment and also prognosis (figs 4.19, 4.20). All patients who may be suitable for surgery with curative intent should be offered PET-CT before treatment.[50] Some patients may undergo endobronchial ultrasound-guided transbronchial needle aspirations for mediastinal masses. TNM staging classification for non-small cell lung cancer is shown in table 4.9. You do not need to memorize this!

Table 4.9 TNM staging for non-small cell lung cancer

Primary tumour (T)	
TX	Malignant cells in bronchial secretions, no other evidence of tumour
T0	None evident
TIS	Carcinoma *in situ*
T1	≤3cm, surrounded by lung or visceral pleura, not in main bronchus
T2	>3cm and ≤5cm + any one of: involving main bronchus but not carina, invading visceral pleura, atelectasis, or obstructive pneumonitis
T3	>5cm and ≤7cm or associated with separate tumour nodules in same lobe or directly invading chest wall, phrenic nerve, parietal pericardium
T4	>7cm or associated with separate tumour nodules in different ipsilateral lobe or directly invading diaphragm, mediastinum, heart, great vessels, trachea, RLN, oesophagus, vertebral body, and carina
Regional nodes (N)	
N0	None involved
N1	Ipsilateral peribronchial and/or ipsilateral hilum
N2	Ipsilateral mediastinum or subcarinal
N3	Contralateral mediastinum or hilum, scalene, or supraclavicular
Distant metastasis (M)	
M0	None
M1	(a) Nodule in other lung, pleural or pericardial lesions, or malignant effusion (b) Single extrathoracic metastasis (c) Multiple extrathoracic metastases in ≥1 organs
Stages	
The overall stage of the tumour (stage I through IV) is determined by the combination of T, N, and M descriptors	

Adapted from: Goldstraw P, Chansky K, Crowley J, *et al.* The IASLC Lung Cancer Staging Project: Proposals for Revision of the TNM Stage Groupings in the Forthcoming (Eighth) Edition of the TNM Classification for Lung Cancer. *J Thorac Oncol* 2016; 11:39.

Treatment *NSCLC* Lobectomy (open or thoracoscopic) is the treatment of choice if medically fit and aim is curative intent or parenchymal-sparing operation for patients with borderline fitness and smaller tumours (T1a–b, N0, M0). *Radical radiotherapy* for patient with stage I, II, III NSCLC. *Chemotherapy ± radiotherapy* for more advanced disease. Specific targeted therapies are widely used for patients with advanced disease with specific molecular features, see BOX 'Novel targeted therapies'. For those without a targetable driver alteration and <50% PD-L1 expression, platinum-based chemotherapy combined with pembrolizumab is often used. *SCLC* Consider surgery with limited stage disease. *Chemotherapy ± radiotherapy* if well enough. *Palliation: radiotherapy* is used for bronchial obstruction, SVC obstruction, haemoptysis, bone pain, and cerebral metastases. *SVC stent* + radiotherapy and dexamethasone for SVC obstruction. *Endobronchial therapy:* tracheal stenting, cryotherapy, laser, brachytherapy (radioactive source is placed close to the tumour). *Pleural drainage/pleurodesis* for symptomatic pleural effusions. *Drugs:* analgesia; steroids; anti-emetics; cough linctus; bronchodilators; antidepressants.

Prognosis *Non-small cell:* 65% 5yr survival without spread; 9% with spread. *Small cell:* 30% 5yr survival without spread; 3% with spread.

Prevention Stop smoking (p85). Prevent occupational exposure to carcinogens.

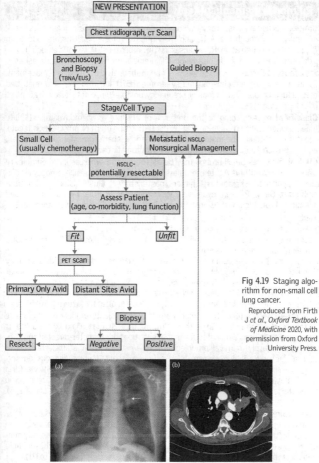

Fig 4.19 Staging algorithm for non-small cell lung cancer.

Reproduced from Firth J *et al., Oxford Textbook of Medicine* 2020, with permission from Oxford University Press.

Fig 4.20 (a) Chest radiograph showing an ill-defined parenchymal mass (arrow) in the left upper lobe; (b): CT scan of the chest of the same patient as in (a), confirming a large central mass (arrow) encasing the left upper lobe bronchus.

Reproduced from Firth J *et al., Oxford Textbook of Medicine* 2020, with permission from Oxford University Press.

Novel targeted therapies for lung cancer

Activating mutations in EGFR define a subset of patients with adenocarcinoma and more frequently affect patients who are never-smokers, women, and/or of Asian ethnicity. These patients are generally highly responsive to EGFR tyrosine kinase inhibitors (eg erlotinib, gefitinib). Another subset of patients with NSCLC may have the ROS1 or EML4-ALK fusion oncogene. Classically, these are more frequent in non-smokers or former smokers and occur at a younger age. These patients may respond to ALK inhibitors (eg alectinib, crizotinib). Immune checkpoint inhibitors targeting either programmed cell death protein 1 (PD-1) or programmed cell death ligand 1 (PD-L1) have become routinely part of the management of NSCLC where there is high PD-L1 expression (≥50%).

Pulmonary embolism (PE)

Causes PEs usually arise from a venous thrombosis in the pelvis or legs. Clots break off and pass through the veins and the right side of the heart before lodging in the pulmonary circulation. Rare causes: RV thrombus (post-MI); septic emboli (right-sided endocarditis); fat, air, or amniotic fluid embolism; neoplastic cells; parasites.

Risk factors Recent surgery, especially abdominal/pelvic or hip/knee replacement, thrombophilia, eg antiphospholipid syndrome (p371), leg fracture, prolonged bed rest/reduced mobility, malignancy, pregnancy/postpartum, combined contraceptive pill, HRT, previous PE.

Classification According to the presence or absence of haemodynamic stability (haemodynamically unstable or stable), the temporal pattern of presentation (acute, subacute, or chronic), the anatomical location (saddle, lobar, segmental, subsegmental), and the presence or absence of symptoms (symptomatic or asymptomatic).

Clinical features Small emboli may be asymptomatic, whereas large emboli are often fatal. **Symptoms** Acute breathlessness, pleuritic chest pain, haemoptysis; dizziness; syncope. Ask about risk factors, past history or family history of thromboembolism. **Signs** Pyrexia; cyanosis; tachypnoea; tachycardia; hypotension; raised JVP; pleural rub; pleural effusion. Look for signs of a cause, eg deep vein thrombosis.

Tests
• Depends on pretest probability assessment—see fig 4.21.[51]
• FBC, U&E, baseline clotting, D-dimers (BOX). ABG may show $\downarrow P_aO_2$ and $\downarrow P_aCO_2$. Troponin may help risk stratification.
• Imaging: CTPA or, less commonly, V/Q scan are the definitive diagnostic tests. CXR may be normal, or show oligaemia of affected segment, dilated pulmonary artery, linear atelectasis, small pleural effusion, wedge-shaped opacities, or cavitation (rare).
• ECG may be normal, or show tachycardia, right bundle branch block, right ventricular strain (inverted T in V_1 to V_4). The classical **SI QIII TIII** pattern (p90) is rare.

Treatment ▶▶See p802. If haemodynamically unstable, thrombolyse for massive PE (alteplase 10mg IV over 1min, then 90mg IVI over 2h; max 1.5mg/kg if <65kg). If thrombolysis is contraindicated for massive PE, consider catheter-directed thrombectomy or (rarely) surgical embolectomy. Haemodynamically stable: start LMWH or oral factor Xa inhibitors (apixaban or rivaroxaban)—choice depends on setting, bleeding risk, & associated comorbidities. After bridging with LMWH, warfarin (p346) may be needed in certain cases, eg GFR <15mL/min. For warfarin, stop heparin when INR is 2–3, due to initial prothrombotic effect of warfarin (target INR of 2–3). Consider placement of a *vena caval filter* if CI to anticoagulation.

Unprovoked PE In patients with no known provoking risk factors, consider investigation for possible underlying malignancy. Undertake full history, examination (including breast), CXR, FBC, calcium, LFTs, U&E, PT, APTT, urinalysis. Otherwise only age-appropriate malignancy unless suggestive symptoms. Consider antiphospholipid and thrombophilia testing if family history positive or recurrent episode (p371).

Prevention Give LMWH to all inpatients. Stop HRT and the oestrogen-based contraceptive pill pre-op (may need alternative form of contraception for peri-op period).

Pneumothorax

Causes Often spontaneous (especially in young, thin men) due to rupture of a subpleural bulla. Other causes: asthma; COPD; TB; pneumonia; lung abscess; carcinoma; cystic fibrosis; lung fibrosis; sarcoidosis; connective tissue disorders (Marfan's syn., Ehlers–Danlos), trauma; iatrogenic (subclavian central line insertion, pleural aspiration/biopsy, transbronchial biopsy, liver biopsy, +ve pressure ventilation).

Clinical features Symptoms May be asymptomatic (fit, young, and small pneumothorax) or there may be sudden onset of dyspnoea and/or pleuritic chest pain. Patients with asthma or COPD may present with a sudden deterioration. Mechanically ventilated patients may present with hypoxia or an increase in ventilation pressures. **Signs** Reduced expansion, hyperresonance to percussion, and diminished breath sounds on the affected side. With a *tension pneumothorax*, the trachea will be deviated away from the affected side, p733, p799. **Management** See p799.

Investigating suspected PE

Diagnosis of PE is improved by adopting a stepwise approach, combining an objective probability score, with subsequent investigations, as follows.

Assess the clinical probability of a PE If clinical suspicion of PE is low, consider using the pulmonary embolism rule-out criteria (PERC) to help determine whether any further investigations are necessary. These criteria are age ≥50 years, HR ≥100, O_2 sats <95%, unilateral leg swelling, haemoptysis, recent surgery or trauma. If none of the following criteria are present, no further workup is required as there is <2% chance of a PE. If any of these criteria are positive or a PE is clinically suspected, use the modified Wells criteria to guide further testing (table 4.10).

Table 4.10 Modified two-level PE Wells score

Feature	Score
Clinical signs and symptoms of DVT (leg pain and pain on deep palpation of veins)	3
Heart rate >100 beats per minute	1.5
Recently bed-ridden (>3 days) or major surgery (<4 weeks)	1.5
Previous DVT or PE	1.5
Haemoptysis	1
Cancer receiving active treatment, treated in last 6/12, palliative	1
An alternative diagnosis is less likely than PE	3
Score <4 = PE unlikely; score >4 = PE likely	

Wells PS, Anderson DR, Rodger M, *et al.* 'Derivation of a Simple Clinical Model to Categorize Patients Probability of Pulmonary Embolism: Increasing the Models Utility with the SimpliRED D-dimer'. *Thromb Haemost* 2000; 83: 416–20.

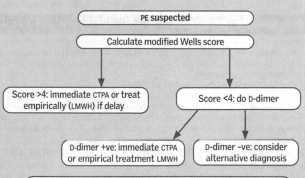

PE suspected

Calculate modified Wells score

Score >4: immediate CTPA or treat empirically (LMWH) if delay

Score <4: do D-dimer

D-dimer +ve: immediate CTPA or empirical treatment LMWH

D-dimer -ve: consider alternative diagnosis

Length of treatment
- Provoked: 3 months and then reassess risk to benefit profile (depends on whether risk factor persists)
- Unprovoked: treatment is usually continued for >3 months (people with no identifiable risk factor)
- Malignancy: continue treatment with LMWH for 6 months or until cure of cancer
- Pregnancy: LMWH is continued until delivery/end of pregnancy

Fig 4.21 Investigation and management of PE.

Prognosis There is an up to 30% risk of death if untreated. Prognostic models such as the Pulmonary Embolism Severity Index and/or biochemical markers that indicate right ventricle strain (BNP, troponin) can predict early death and/or recurrence.

4 Chest medicine

Obstructive sleep apnoea syndrome

Obstructive sleep apnoea (OSA) is characterized by intermittent closure/collapse of the pharyngeal airway causing apnoeic episodes during sleep. These are terminated by partial arousal. These recurrent episodes lead to chronic intermittent hypoxia, sleep fragmentation, and inflammatory activation.

Risk factors Age, male sex, obesity, craniofacial/upper airway abnormalities, obesity hypoventilation syndrome, pregnancy, stroke, CHF, hypothyroidism.

Clinical features Loud snoring, gasping, choking, snorting, or apnoeic episodes during sleep, daytime somnolence + ↓cognitive performance, poor sleep quality, morning headache, decreased libido, nocturia. Check Epworth Sleepiness Scale—a score >9 indicates abnormal sleepiness and should prompt further testing.

Complications Pulmonary hypertension/right heart failure (RHF); type II respiratory failure (p158); hypertension; arrhythmias; stroke; IHD; metabolic syndrome & type II DM; depression, attention and memory deficits, motor vehicle accidents.

Investigations Offer home respiratory polygraphy to people with suspected OSA. If unavailable/impractical, arrange in-hospital polysomnography (which monitors oxygen saturation, airflow at the nose and mouth, ECG, EMG chest, and abdominal wall movement during sleep) which is diagnostic. The occurrence of ≥5 episodes of apnoea/hypopnoea during 1h of sleep indicates sleep apnoea (>30 = severe).

Management
- Weight reduction, exercise, changing sleep position.
- Avoidance of tobacco and alcohol.
- Mandibular advancement device.
- CPAP during sleep is effective and recommended by NICE for those with moderate to severe disease.[52]
- Surgery to relieve pharyngeal or nasal obstruction, eg tonsillectomy or polypectomy.

Pulmonary hypertension

Pulmonary hypertension (PH) is a disease characterized by elevated pulmonary artery pressure (mean pulmonary artery pressure (PAP) ≥20mmHg at rest. It can complicate many cardiovascular and respiratory diseases, and is classified into 5 groups based on aetiology:[53]
- Group 1—pulmonary arterial hypertension (PAH).
- Group 2—PH due to left heart disease (eg congenital heart disease, LVSD).
- Group 3—PH due to chronic lung disease and/or hypoxaemia (eg COPD, ILD).
- Group 4—PH due to pulmonary artery obstructions (eg chronic VTE).
- Group 5—PH due to unclear multifactorial mechanisms (eg haemolytic anaemia).

Clinical features Symptoms include progressive exertional dyspnoea, fatigue, and syncope. Signs: raised JVP with prominent 'a' wave; loud P_2 ± features of RHF (p189).

Investigations Echo will give estimation of PAP (+ evaluate LV/RV function/valves) but right heart catheterization is the gold standard for diagnosis (mild = 20–40mmHg, moderate = 41–55mmHg, severe ≥55mmHg)—may not be needed though if clear evidence of left heart disease, chronic lung disease and/or hypoxia, or VTE. To evaluate further, consider PFTs (DLCO <60% in pulmonary venous disease), HRCT, 6-minute walk test, V/Q scan or CTPA, HIV, LFTs, CTD screen. If PAH diagnosed, the patient should undergo vasoreactivity testing with short-acting vasodilator, eg inhaled NO.

Management
- *Treat underlying cause*—eg pulmonary thromboendarterectomy for chronic thromboembolic pulmonary hypertension.
- *Specific PAH therapy*— prostanoids (eg epoprostenol), phosphodiesterase type 5 inhibitors (eg sildenafil), endothelin antagonists (eg bosentan), and riociguat.
- Refer/consider if appropriate candidate for lung transplantation.
- *Treat heart failure* with diuretics such as furosemide. Monitor U&E and give amiloride or K^+ supplements if necessary. Alternative: spironolactone.

Prognosis Depends on the cause but generally poor. 50% die within 5yrs.

Cor pulmonale

Cor pulmonale refers to PH-induced altered structure (eg RVH or dilatation) and/ or impaired RV function that is associated with chronic lung disease and/or hypoxaemia (see BOX). These RV changes result from chronic hypoxic pulmonary vasoconstriction and subsequent PH, leading to increased RV work and stress.

Clinical features Symptoms include dyspnoea, fatigue, and syncope. Signs: cyanosis; tachycardia; raised JVP with prominent a and v waves; RV heave; loud P₂, pansystolic murmur (tricuspid regurgitation); early diastolic Graham Steell murmur (pulmonary regurgitation); hepatomegaly and oedema.

Investigations *FBC:* Hb and haematocrit ↑ (secondary polycythaemia). *ABG:* hypoxia, with or without hypercapnia. *CXR:* enlarged right atrium and ventricle, prominent pulmonary arteries (**fig 4.22**). *ECG:* P pulmonale; right axis deviation; right ventricular hypertrophy/strain.

Management
• *General supportive care*—LTOT if hypoxaemic, optimize volume status with fluid/ salt restriction & diuretics, manage arrhythmias.
• *Treat underlying cause*—eg ASD closure for significant left-to-right shunt.
• *Pulmonary vasodilatory therapy* in group 1 PAH.
• *Refractory HF*—options include mechanical circulatory support, heart or combined heart–lung transplantation, or palliative care.

Causes of cor pulmonale

Lung disease
• COPD
• Bronchiectasis
• Pulmonary fibrosis
• Severe chronic asthma
• Lung resection.

Pulmonary vascular disease
• Pulmonary emboli
• Pulmonary vasculitis
• Primary pulmonary hypertension
• ARDS (p178)
• Sickle cell disease.

Thoracic cage abnormality
• Kyphoscoliosis
• Thoracoplasty.

Neuromuscular disease
• Myasthenia gravis
• Poliomyelitis
• Motor neuron disease.

Hypoventilation
• Sleep apnoea
• Obesity hypoventilation syndrome
• Central alveolar hypoventilation.

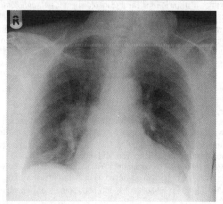

Fig 4.22 PA chest radiograph showing enlarged pulmonary arteries from pulmonary artery hypertension. When caused by interstitial lung disease and leading to right heart failure, this would be termed cor pulmonale. No signs of interstitial lung disease are identifiable in this image.
Image courtesy of Derby Hospitals NHS Foundation Trust Radiology Department.

4 Chest medicine

A multisystem granulomatous disorder of unknown cause. Prevalence highest in Northern Europe, eg UK: 10–20/10⁵ population. Usually affects adults aged 20–40yrs, more common in women. Black people are affected more frequently and more severely than Caucasians, particularly by extrathoracic disease. Associated with HLA-DRB1 and DQB1 alleles. For other causes of granuloma see **table 4.11**.

Clinical features In 20–40%, the disease is discovered incidentally, after a routine CXR, and is thus asymptomatic. *Acute sarcoidosis* often presents with fever, erythema nodosum (fig 12.22, p561),[3] polyarthralgia, and bilateral hilar lymphadenopathy (BHL), also called Löfgren syndrome, which usually resolves spontaneously.

Pulmonary disease 90% have abnormal CXRs with BHL (fig 4.23) ± pulmonary infiltrates or fibrosis; see later in topic for staging. *Symptoms:* dry cough, progressive dyspnoea, ↓exercise tolerance, and chest pain. In 10–20%, symptoms progress, with concurrent deterioration in lung function.

Non-pulmonary signs These are legion: lymphadenopathy; hepatomegaly; splenomegaly; uveitis; conjunctivitis; keratoconjunctivitis sicca; glaucoma; terminal phalangeal bone cysts; enlargement of lacrimal & parotid glands (fig 8.53, p353); Bell's palsy; neuropathy; meningitis; brainstem and spinal syndromes; space-occupying lesion; erythema nodosum (fig 12.22, p561); lupus pernio; subcutaneous nodules; cardiomyopathy; arrhythmias; hypercalcaemia; hypercalciuria; renal stones; pituitary dysfunction.

Tests Blood ↑ESR, lymphopenia, ↑LFT, ↑serum ACE in ∼60% (non-specific[4]), ↑Ca²⁺, ↑Igs. **24h urine** ↑Ca²⁺. **CXR** is abnormal in 90%: *stage 0:* normal. *Stage 1:* BHL. *Stage 2:* BHL + peripheral pulmonary infiltrates. *Stage 3:* peripheral pulmonary infiltrates alone. *Stage 4:* progressive upper lobe pulmonary fibrosis; bulla formation (honeycombing); pleural involvement. **ECG** May show arrhythmias or bundle branch block. **Lung function tests** May be normal or show ↓lung volumes, impaired gas transfer, & a restrictive ventilatory defect. **Tissue biopsy** (Lung, liver, lymph nodes, skin nodules, or lacrimal glands.) Is diagnostic and shows non-caseating granulomata. **Bronchoalveolar lavage (BAL)** Shows ↑lymphocytes in active disease; ↑neutrophils with pulmonary fibrosis. **Transbronchial biopsy** May be diagnostic. **Ultrasound** May show nephrocalcinosis or hepatosplenomegaly. **Hand x-rays** Show 'punched out' lesions in terminal phalanges. **CT/MRI** May be useful in assessing severity of pulmonary disease or diagnosing neurosarcoidosis. ECG, and cardiac MRI or PET-CT if suspicion for cardiac involvement. *Ophthalmology assessment* (slit lamp examination, fluorescein angiography) is indicated in ocular disease.

Management ▶Patients with *BHL* alone don't need treatment as most recover spontaneously.[54,55] *Acute sarcoidosis:* steroids if significant respiratory disease/compromise or end-organ damage, NSAIDs for joint disease or Löfgren syndrome.

Indications for corticosteroids
• Parenchymal lung disease (symptomatic, static, or progressive).
• Uveitis.
• Hypercalcaemia.
• Neurological or cardiac involvement.

Prednisolone (40mg/24h) PO for 4–6wks, then ↓dose over 1yr according to clinical status. A few patients relapse and may need a further course or long-term therapy.

Other therapy In severe illness, IV methylprednisolone or immunosuppressants (methotrexate, azathioprine, leflunomide, and mycophenolate) may be needed. Anti-TNFα therapy (eg infliximab or adalimumab) may be tried in refractory cases. Lung transplantation may be needed in advanced pulmonary fibrosis with or without PH.

Prognosis Variable rates (30–80%) of spontaneous remission depending on stage.

3 A detailed history and exam (including for synovitis) + CXR, ASO (antistreptolysin-O) titres and a tuberculin skin test are usually enough to diagnose erythema nodosum.

4 ACE is also ↑ in: hyperthyroidism, Gaucher's, silicosis, TB, hypersensitivity pneumonitis, asbestosis, pneumocystosis.[56] ↑ACE levels in CSF help diagnose CNS sarcoidosis (when serum ACE may be normal).[57] ACE is *lower* in: Caucasians; and anorexia.[58]

Table 4.11 Differential diagnosis of granulomatous diseases

Infections	Bacteria	TB, leprosy, syphilis, cat scratch fever
	Fungi	*Cryptococcus neoformans* *Coccidioides immitis*
	Protozoa	*Schistosomiasis*
Autoimmune	Primary biliary cholangitis Granulomatous orchitis	
Vasculitis (p554)	Giant cell arteritis Polyarteritis nodosa Takayasu's arteritis Granulomatosis with polyangiitis	
Organic dust disease	Silicosis, berylliosis	
Idiopathic	Crohn's disease De Quervain's thyroiditis Sarcoidosis	
Extrinsic allergic alveolitis		

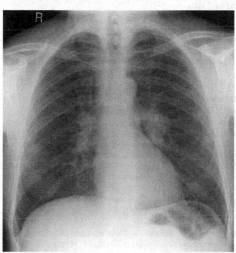

Fig 4.23 PA chest radiograph showing bilateral hilar lymphadenopathy. The important differentials for this appearance are: sarcoidosis, TB, lymphoma, pneumoconioses, and metastatic disease. This patient has sarcoidosis but there are no other stigmata (such as the presence of infiltrates, fibrosis, and honeycombing) on this image.

Image courtesy of Norfolk and Norwich University Hospitals NHS Trust Radiology Department.

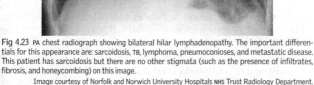

Causes of bilateral hilar lymphadenopathy (BHL)
- Sarcoidosis.
- Infection, eg TB, mycoplasma.
- Malignancy, eg lymphoma, carcinoma, mediastinal tumours.
- Organic dust disease, eg silicosis, berylliosis.
- Hypersensitivity pneumonitis.
- Histiocytosis X (Langerhans cell histiocytosis).

Interstitial lung disease (ILD)

This is the generic term used to describe a number of heterogeneous conditions that cause diffuse parenchymal lung disease.[55] They are characterized by chronic inflammation and/or progressive interstitial fibrosis (table 4.12), and share a number of clinical and pathological features. See table 4.12 and fig 4.24.

Pathological features Fibrosis and remodelling of the interstitium; chronic inflammation; hyperplasia of type II epithelial cells or type II pneumocytes.

Classification The ILDs can be grouped into the following categories:

Exposure related
- Occupational/environmental, eg asbestosis, berylliosis, silicosis, cotton worker's lung (byssinosis).
- Drugs, eg nitrofurantoin, bleomycin, amiodarone, sulfasalazine, busulfan.
- Hypersensitivity reactions, eg hypersensitivity pneumonitis.
- Infections, eg TB, fungi, viral.

Those associated with a connective tissue disorder (CTD-ILD)
- Scleroderma, rheumatoid arthritis.
- SLE, mixed connective tissue disease, Sjögren's syndrome.
- Polymyositis, dermatomyositis.

Granulomatous disease
- Sarcoidosis.

Idiopathic interstitial pneumonia (IIP)
- Idiopathic pulmonary fibrosis (IPF, p194), non-specific interstitial pneumonitis (NSIP), acute interstitial pneumonia, and smoking-related ILD including desquamative interstitial pneumonia & respiratory bronchiolitis-associated ILD.

Other forms
- Pulmonary Langerhans cell histiocytosis, lymphangioleiomyomatosis.

Clinical features Clubbing; progressive dyspnoea on exertion; non-productive paroxysmal cough; abnormal breath sounds ± crackles.

Tests ▶NB: careful history—ask about potential exposures (eg inorganic or organic dusts, drugs, radiation), features of CTD (eg joint pain, dry eyes/mouth, myalgia, Raynaud's), hobbies, home and work environment. Check autoantibodies for specific CTD if clinical suspicion (ANA, RF/CCP, JO-1, CK, SA-A, SA-B, SCL-70, PM1). Add CK and myositis blot as indicated. Abnormal CXR (reticular, nodular, or mixed pattern of interstitial markings) or high-resolution CT (to assess pattern of ILD ± guide potential BAL/biopsy); restrictive pulmonary spirometry with ↓DLCO (p154).

Management
- Specific treatment depending on the underlying condition, eg immunosuppression for CTD-ILD or sarcoidosis.
- Antifibrotic for IPF or for progressive fibrosing ILD, eg pirfenidone, nintedanib.
- Supportive care: supplemental oxygen if indicated, pulmonary rehabilitation.
- Assess and treat comorbidities and complications, eg GORD and PH.
- Manage acute exacerbations with, eg antibiotics, steroids as indicated.
- Progressive disease: refer for lung transplant; if not a candidate, discuss future ventilation decisions, and consider palliative care involvement if appropriate.

Table 4.12 Causes of fibrotic shadowing on a CXR

Upper zone	Lower zone
TB	Idiopathic interstitial pneumonias, eg IPF
Sarcoidosis	CTD, eg RA
Hypersensitivity pneumonitis	Aspiration
Ankylosing spondylitis	Asbestosis
Radiotherapy	Medications, eg amiodarone, methotrexate
Silicosis, berylliosis	Infection
Pneumoconiosis (coal workers)	

Hypersensitivity pneumonitis (HP) represents an immunological reaction occurring within the lung parenchyma caused by hypersensitivity to an inhaled agent, such as microbial, avian, and animal antigens and, less commonly, organic compounds. In the acute phase, the alveoli are infiltrated with acute inflammatory cells. Early diagnosis and prompt allergen removal can halt and reverse disease progression, so prognosis can be good. With chronic exposure, granuloma formation and obliterative bronchiolitis occur.

Causes
- Bird-fancier's and pigeon-fancier's lung (proteins in bird droppings).
- Farmer's and mushroom worker's lung (*Micropolyspora faeni, Thermoactinomyces vulgaris*).
- Malt worker's lung (*Aspergillus clavatus*).
- Bagassosis or sugar worker's lung (*Thermoactinomyces sacchari*).

Classification Acute, subacute, and chronic. Non-fibrotic (purely inflammatory) vs fibrotic (mixed inflammatory plus fibrotic or purely fibrotic) phenotypes based on the predominant presence or absence of fibrosis on imaging or histopathologic examination.

Clinical features Acute (less frequent; associated with non-fibrotic HP) Fever, rigors, myalgia, dry cough, dyspnoea, fine bibasal crackles. **Chronic (fibrotic HP)** Finger clubbing (50%), increasing dyspnoea, ↓weight, exertional dyspnoea, type I respiratory failure, cor pulmonale.

Tests [59] **Acute** *Blood*: FBC (neutrophilia); ↑ESR; ABGs; serum antibodies (may indicate exposure/previous sensitization rather than disease). *CXR:* upper-zone mottling/consolidation; hilar lymphadenopathy (rare). *Lung function tests:* restrictive defect; reduced gas transfer during acute attacks. **Chronic** Blood tests: serum antibodies. *CXR:* upper-zone fibrosis; honeycomb lung. *CT chest:* mid-to-upper zone predominance of centrilobular ground-glass or nodular opacities ± fibrotic changes. *Lung function tests:* restrictive defect. Bronchoalveolar lavage (BAL) fluid shows ↑lymphocytes and ↑mast cells.

Management Acute Remove allergen, PO prednisolone (0.5mg/kg/24h (up to 30mg) PO), reducing course. **Chronic** Allergen avoidance, or wear a facemask or +ve pressure helmet. Trial of steroids. Azathioprine/MMF sometimes effective in steroid-resistant cases. Lung transplant for advanced fibrotic disease. Compensation (UK Industrial Injuries Act) may be payable.

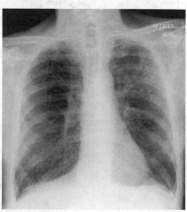

Fig 4.24 AP chest radiograph showing air-space shadowing in the left upper zone. Although this appearance often represents infection, it is non-specific. Differential diagnosis for this distribution of shadowing include lymphoma, alveolar cell carcinoma (both to be considered if not resolving in appearance on follow-up imaging), and haemorrhage.

Image courtesy of Nottingham University Hospitals NHS Trust Radiology Department.

Idiopathic pulmonary fibrosis (IPF)

IPF (also known as usual interstitial pneumonia (UIP)) is the most common type of idiopathic interstitial pneumonia (IIP). Risk factors include genetic predisposition, smoking, environmental pollutants, and possibly chronic microaspiration. Repetitive alveolar epithelial injury triggers the early development of fibrosis. It is the commonest cause of interstitial lung disease. The age of onset is typically 60+ years (♂ > ♀).

Symptoms Dry cough; exertional dyspnoea; malaise; ↓weight; arthralgia.

Signs Cyanosis; finger clubbing; fine end-inspiratory crepitations.

Complications Respiratory failure; PH; ↑risk of lung cancer; comorbid emphysema and obstructive sleep apnoea.

Tests Blood ABG (↓P_aO_2; if severe, ↑P_aCO_2); ↑CRP; ↑immunoglobulins; ANA or rheumatoid factor may be +ve if associated with CTD. **Imaging** (fig 4.25) *CXR:* increase in reticular markings. *HRCT:* characteristic features include an apicobasal gradient of peripheral (subpleural), reticular opacities associated with architectural distortion, including honeycomb changes and traction bronchiectasis or bronchiolectasis. **Spirometry** Restrictive (p154); ↓transfer factor. **BAL** Limited role in diagnosis and usually only indicated to rule out alternative diagnosis, eg sarcoidosis. May indicate activity of alveolitis: ↑lymphocytes (good response/prognosis) or ↑neutrophils and ↑eosinophils (poor response/prognosis). **Lung biopsy** All patients must have MDT discussion. Biopsy may be required for diagnosis depending on MDT consensus if clinical and imaging features are inconclusive. The histology observed on biopsy in UIP is a heterogeneous appearance with alternating areas of normal lung, fibrosis, fibroblast foci, and honeycomb change.

Management Supportive care: oxygen, pulmonary rehabilitation, influenza and pneumococcal vaccination, treat GORD. Give antifibrotic therapies—pirfenidone or nintedanib—which have been shown to slow disease progression.[60,61] All patients should be considered for current clinical trials or early referral for lung transplantation (for those with progressive disease and minimal comorbidities).[55] It is strongly recommended that high-dose steroids are not used except where the diagnosis of IPF is in doubt or as a short course to treat acute exacerbations along with broad-spectrum antibiotics.

Prognosis Median survival ranges from 2–5 years.

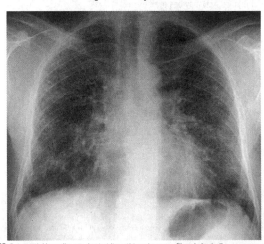

Fig 4.25 Interstitial lung disease due to idiopathic pulmonary fibrosis (a similar appearance to the interstitial oedema of moderate left heart failure, but without a big heart).

Courtesy of Prof P Scally.

Coal worker's pneumoconiosis (CWP) A common dust disease in countries that have or have had underground coal mines. It results from inhalation and deposition of coal dust particles (1–3μm in diameter) over 15–20yrs. These are ingested by macrophages which die, releasing their enzymes and causing fibrosis.

Clinical features Asymptomatic, but coexisting chronic bronchitis is common. CXR: many round opacities (1–10mm), especially in upper zone.

Management Avoid exposure to coal dust; smoking cessation; vaccination; treat coexisting chronic bronchitis; claim compensation (in the UK, via the Industrial Injuries Act).

Progressive massive fibrosis (PMF) Due to progression of CWP, which causes progressive dyspnoea, fibrosis, and, eventually, cor pulmonale. CXR: usually bilateral, upper-mid zone fibrotic masses (1–10cm), develop from periphery towards hilum.

Management Avoid exposure to coal dust; claim compensation (as for CWP).

Caplan's syndrome The association between rheumatoid arthritis, pneumoconiosis, and pulmonary rheumatoid nodules.

Silicosis (See fig 4.26.) Caused by inhalation of silica particles, which are very fibrogenic. A number of jobs may be associated with exposure, eg metal mining, stone quarrying, sandblasting, and pottery/ceramic manufacture.

Clinical features Progressive dyspnoea, ↑incidence of TB, CXR shows diffuse miliary or nodular pattern in upper and mid-zones and eggshell calcification of hilar nodes. Spirometry: restrictive ventilatory defect.

Management Avoid exposure to silica; claim compensation (as for CWP).

Asbestosis Caused by inhalation of asbestos fibres. Asbestos was commonly used in the building trade for fire proofing, pipe lagging, electrical wire insulation, and roofing felt. Most patients are asymptomatic for 20–30 years after the initial exposure. Degree of asbestos exposure is related to degree of pulmonary fibrosis.

Clinical features Similar to other fibrotic lung diseases with progressive dyspnoea, clubbing, and fine end-inspiratory crackles. Also causes pleural plaques, ↑risk of bronchogenic carcinoma and mesothelioma.

Management Symptomatic. Patients are often eligible for compensation through the UK Industrial Injuries Act.

Mesothelioma See p182.

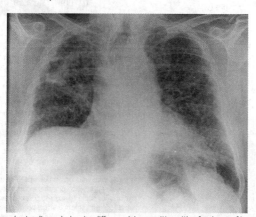

Fig 4.26 PA chest radiograph showing diffuse nodular opacities with a focal area of irregular soft tissue shadowing in the right upper zone, consistent with silicosis and developing progressive massive fibrosis (PMF).

Image courtesy of Derby Hospitals NHS Foundation Trust Radiology Department.

4 Chest medicine

5   Endocrinology

Contents

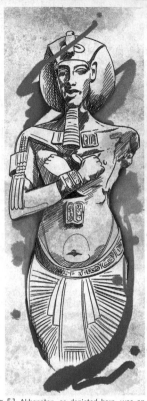

Fig 5.1 Akhenaten, as depicted here, was an important Egyptian pharaoh of the 18th dynasty, reigning from 1365 to 1348 BC. Akhenaten made radical changes in Egypt including establishing a new capital and forming a new religion associated with a pacifist philosophy and a deep respect for nature. He also encouraged a new concept of art in which sculptures or reliefs portraying the pharaoh were no longer highly idealized. Akhenaten was then often portrayed as a person with a prominent jaw, sunken chest, bulky abdomen, and gynecoid fat distribution. Several authors have suggested that Akhenaten suffered from acromegaly, with or without hypogonadism, isolated hypogonadism, or rickets. His sometimes androgynous portrayal, with wide hips, an elongated head, almond eyes, square jaw, gynaecomastia, and no male genitalia have also led some to suggest possible diagnoses of Klinefelter's syndrome or even gender dysphoria.

Artwork by Gillian Turner.

We thank Helen Turner, Rustam Rea, and Michael Matheou, our Specialist Readers and Oliver Mowforth, our Junior Reader for this chapter. We also thank Michael Matheou for contributing to this chapter.

The essence of endocrinology

For scientists

- Define a syndrome, and match it to a gland malfunction.
- Measure the gland's output in the peripheral blood. Define clinical syndromes associated with too much or too little secretion (*hyper-* and *hypo-*syndromes, respectively; *eu-* means normal, neither ↑ nor ↓, as in *euthyroid*). Note factors that may make measurement variable, eg diurnal release of cortisol.
- If suspecting hormone deficiency, test by stimulating the gland that produces it (eg short ACTH stimulation test or *Synacthen®* test in Addison's). If the gland is not functioning normally, there will be a blunted response to stimulation.
- If suspecting hormone excess, test by inhibiting the gland that produces it (eg dexamethasone suppression test in Cushing's). If there is a hormone-secreting tumour then this will fail to suppress via normal feedback mechanisms.
- Find a way to image the gland. NB: non-functioning tumours or 'incidentalomas' may be found in health, see p218. Imaging alone does not make the diagnosis.
- Aim to halt disease progression; diet and exercise can stop progression of impaired fasting glucose to frank diabetes.[1,2] For other glands, halting progression will depend on understanding autoimmunity, and the interaction of genes and environment. In thyroid autoimmunity (an archetypal autoimmune disease), it is possible to track interactions between genes and environment (eg smoking and stress) via expression of immunologically active molecules (HLA class I and II, adhesion molecules, cytokines, CD40, and complement regulatory proteins).[3]

Endocrinologists love this reductionist approach, but have been less successful at understanding *emergent phenomena*—those properties and performances of ours that cannot be predicted from full knowledge of our perturbed parts. We understand the diurnal nature of cortisol secretion, for example, but the science of relating this to dreams, the consolidation of memory, and the psychopathology of families and other groups (such as the endocrinology ward round you may be about to join) is in its infancy. But as doctors we are steeped in the hormonal lives of patients (as they are in ours)—and we may as well start by recognizing this now.

For those doing exams

'What's wrong with *him*?' your examiner asks, boldly. While you apologize to the patient for this rudeness by asking, 'Is it alright if we speak about you as if you weren't here?', think to yourself that if you were a betting person you would wager that the diagnosis will be endocrinological. In no other discipline are gestalt impressions so characteristic. To get good at recognizing these conditions, spend time in endocrinology outpatients and looking at collections of clinical photographs. Also, specific cutaneous signs are important, as follows.

Thyrotoxicosis: hair loss; pretibial myxoedema (confusing term, p212); onycholysis (nail separation from the nailbed); bulging eyes (exophthalmos/proptosis).

Hypothyroidism: hair loss; eyebrow loss; cold, pale skin; characteristic face. You might, perhaps should, fail your exam if you blurt out 'Toad-like face'.

Cushing's syndrome: central obesity and wasted limbs (= 'lemon on sticks' see fig 5.2); proximal myopathy; moon face; buffalo hump; supraclavicular fat pads; striae.

Addison's disease: hyperpigmentation (face, neck, palmar creases), postural hypotension.

Acromegaly: acral (distal) + soft tissue overgrowth; big jaws (macrognathia), hands, and feet; the skin is thick; facial features are coarse.

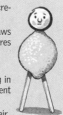

Hyperandrogenism (♀): hirsutism; temporal balding; acne.

Hypopituitarism: pale or yellow-tinged thinned skin, resulting in fine wrinkling around the eyes and mouth, making the patient look older.

Hypoparathyroidism: dry, scaly, puffy skin; brittle nails; coarse hair.

Pseudohypoparathyroidism: short stature, short neck, and short 4th and 5th metacarpals.

Fig 5.2 'Lemon on sticks.'

Hormones are chemical messengers which act directly on nearby cells (paracrine effect), on the cell of origin (autocrine effect), at a distant site (endocrine effect), or as neurotransmitters (brain and gastrointestinal tract). Thirst, thermal regulation, appetite, sleep cycles, menstrual cycle, and stress/mood are all controlled by the hypothalamus. Releasing factors produced by the hypothalamus reach the pituitary via the portal system (pituitary stalk), see **fig 5.3**. The releasing factors stimulate or inhibit the production of hormones from the anterior pituitary, **fig 5.4**. Vasopressin and oxytocin are produced in the hypothalamus and stored and released from the posterior pituitary.

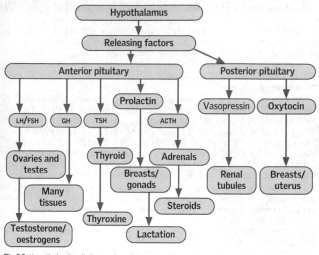

Fig 5.3 Hypothalamic–pituitary axis.

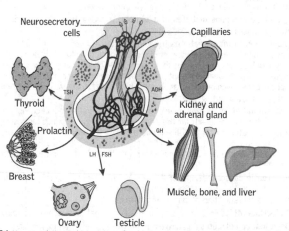

Fig 5.4 Neuroregulation and integration of endocrine axes makes us who we are—and who we are and what we do feeds back into our hormonal milieu. Multifactorial disruptions within the growth hormone (GH), luteinizing hormone (LH)–testosterone, adrenocorticotropin (ACTH)–cortisol, and insulin axes play a major role in healthy maturation and ageing.

DM results from lack, or reduced effectiveness, of endogenous insulin. Hyperglycaemia is one aspect of a far-reaching metabolic derangement, which causes serious microvascular (retinopathy, nephropathy, neuropathy) or macrovascular problems: stroke, MI, renovascular disease, limb ischaemia. *So think of DM as a vascular disease:*[1] adopt a holistic approach and consider other cardiovascular risk factors too.

Categories of diabetes

1 Type 1 DM Usually adolescent onset but may occur at *any* age. *Cause:* insulin deficiency from autoimmune destruction of insulin-secreting pancreatic β cells. Patients must have insulin, and are prone to ketoacidosis and weight loss. Associated with other autoimmune diseases (>90% HLA DR3 ± DR4). Concordance is only ~30% in identical twins, indicating environmental influence. >90% of people with type 1 DM at diagnosis will have positive islet cell antibodies (ICA) or other islet autoantibodies (antibodies to glutamic acid decarboxylase 65 (GAD65), the tyrosine phosphatases, insulinoma-associated protein 2 (IA-2) and IA-2 beta; and zinc transporter (ZnT8)).

2 Type 2 DM (Formerly non-insulin-dependent DM.) This is at 'epidemic' levels in many places, mainly due to changes in lifestyle, but also because of better diagnosis and improved longevity.[4] Higher prevalence in Asians, men, and the elderly (up to 18%). Most are over 40yrs, but teenagers are now getting type 2 DM (*OHCS* p246). *Cause:* ↓insulin secretion ± ↑insulin resistance. It is associated with obesity, lack of exercise, calorie and alcohol excess. ≥80% concordance in identical twins, indicating stronger genetic influence than in type 1 DM. Typically progresses from a preliminary phase of impaired glucose tolerance (IGT) or impaired fasting glucose (IFG). (▶This is a unique window for lifestyle intervention.)

3 Latent autoimmune diabetes of adulthood (LADA) A form of type 1 DM, with slower progression to insulin dependence in later life.

4 Monogenic forms of diabetes Including maturity-onset diabetes of the young (MODY), and other genetic forms of diabetes, eg mitochondrial diabetes, genetic lipodystrophies. MODY is thought to account for 1–2% of people with diabetes, inherited in an autosomal dominant pattern; MODY is most commonly caused by mutations in genes encoding the transcription factors HNF1A, HNF4A, and HNF1B, and the glycolytic enzyme glucokinase (GCK).

5 Gestational diabetes May develop when there is failure to balance insulin secretion with the composite of prepregnancy and pregnancy-induced insulin resistance (created by the anti-insulin hormones secreted by the placenta). It is an increasingly prevalent condition (affecting between 2% and 38% of pregnant women worldwide) and is associated with multiple adverse maternal and fetal outcomes.[5]

6 Pancreatic causes Diseases of the exocrine pancreas, eg pancreatitis; surgery (where >90% pancreas is removed); trauma; pancreatic destruction (haemochromatosis, cystic fibrosis); pancreatic cancer.

7 Endocrinopathies Eg Cushing's syndrome, acromegaly, phaeochromocytoma.

8 Drug-induced diabetes Eg steroids, anti-HIV drugs, newer antipsychotics.

Categories of increased risk for diabetes (prediabetes)

- Impaired fasting glucose: fasting plasma glucose (5.6–6.9mmol/L).
- Impaired glucose tolerance: 2-hour post glucose load on the 75g oral glucose tolerance test 7.8–11.0mmol/L.
- Non-diabetic hyperglycaemia: impaired fasting glucose, or HbA1c 6.0–6.4% (42–46mmol/mol).

Incidence of DM if IFG and HbA1c at high end of normal (42–46mmol/mol) is ~25%.[6]

---

1 Chicken or egg? Most type 2 diabetes-associated genes have a function in the vasculature, and stress in β-cells can result from vascular defects in the pancreas, so maybe vascular events trigger DM.[7]

Diagnosis of diabetes mellitus (DM): NICE guidelines

Persistent hyperglycaemia is defined as:
* HbA1c of 48mmol/mol (6.5%) or more.
* Fasting plasma glucose level of 7.0mmol/L or more.
* Random plasma glucose of 11.1mmol/L or more in the presence of symptoms or signs of diabetes.

If the person is symptomatic (eg polyuria, polydipsia, unexplained weight loss), a single abnormal HbA1c or fasting plasma glucose level can be used, although repeat testing is sensible to confirm the diagnosis.

If the person is asymptomatic, do not diagnose diabetes on the basis of a single abnormal HbA1c or plasma glucose result. Arrange repeat testing, preferably with the same test, to confirm the diagnosis. If the repeat test result is normal, arrange to monitor the person for the development of diabetes, the frequency depending on clinical judgement.

Differentiating type 1 and 2 DM

Occasionally it may be difficult to differentiate whether a patient has type 1 or 2 DM, although they can present differently (table 5.1). Features of type 1 include weight loss; lean body habitus; acute presentation; persistent hyperglycaemia despite diet and medications; presence of autoantibodies: islet cell antibodies (ICA) and anti-glutamic acid decarboxylase (GAD) antibodies; ketoacidosis.

Table 5.1 Differences between type 1 and type 2 diabetes

	Type 1 DM	Type 2 DM
Epidemiology	Often starts before puberty	Older patients (usually)
Islet autoantibodies	>90% positive, eg GAD, IA2, ZnT8, islet cell	Negative
Cause	Autoimmune β-cell destruction	Insulin resistance/β-cell dysfunction
Presentation	Usually acute with polydipsia, polyuria, ↓weight, ketosis	Asymptomatic/complications, eg MI

►Not all new-onset DM in older people is type 2: if ketotic ± a poor response to oral hypoglycaemics (and patient is slim or has a family or personal history of autoimmunity), think of latent autoimmune diabetes in adults (LADA) and measure islet cell antibodies. There is also the entity of ketosis-prone diabetes which is a heterogeneous syndrome characterized by patients who present with DKA or un-provoked ketosis but who do not have the typical phenotype of autoimmune type 1 DM. They are usually obese, islet autoantibody negative, and have features of both impaired insulin secretion and action.

Non-diabetic hyperglycaemia and diabetes prevention

High-risk individuals, including those with impaired fasting glucose, impaired glucose tolerance, obesity, family history of type 2 DM, or certain vulnerable ethnic groups (Asian, Hispanic, black), should be targeted for preventative interventions. Lifestyle modifications including healthy diet, regular exercise, weight loss, and smoking cessation decrease the risk of future diabetes. For selected patients (eg <60 years and/or BMI >35), metformin may be useful for diabetes prevention. Overweight or obese individuals with prediabetes may benefit from semaglutide which helps delay or prevent the onset of overt diabetes. In the UK, the Healthier You programme identifies people with non-diabetic hyperglycaemia who are at risk of developing type 2 DM and refers them onto a 9-month, evidence-based lifestyle change programme (either face-to-face or digital). It has been shown to reduce the risk of developing type 2 DM by >33%.

5 Endocrinology

General ▶*Focus on education and lifestyle advice* (eg exercise to ↑ insulin sensitivity), healthy eating: p238—For patients with type 2 DM advise high fibre, low-glycaemic-index sources of carbohydrate, and controlling intake of saturated and trans-fatty acids. Consider referral for bariatric surgery if BMI >35kg/m² in patients with type 2 DM despite lifestyle interventions. Be prepared to negotiate HbA1c target and review every 3–6 months. Assess *global* vascular risk; start a high-intensity statin (p107), eg atorvastatin as tolerated, control BP (p205). Give foot care (p206). (Pre-)pregnancy care should be in a multidisciplinary clinic (*OHCS* p26). Advise informing DVLA and not to drive if hypoglycaemic spells (p150; loss of hypoglycaemia awareness may lead to loss of licence; permanent if HGV). More detailed guidance available at https://www.gov.uk/guidance/diabetes-mellitus-assessing-fitness-to-drive

Type 1 DM Insulin (see BOX 'Using insulin').

Type 2 DM See fig 5.5.

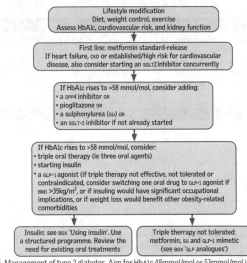

Lifestyle modification
Diet, weight control, exercise
Assess HbA1c, cardiovascular risk, and kidney function

First line: metformin standard-release
If heart failure, CKD or established/high risk for cardiovascular disease, also consider starting an SGLT2 inhibitor concurrently

If HbA1c rises to >58 mmol/mol, consider adding:
• a DPP4 inhibitor OR
• pioglitazone OR
• a sulphonylurea (SU) OR
• an SGLT-2 inhibitor if not already started

If HbA1c rises to >58 mmol/mol, consider:
• triple oral therapy (ie three oral agents)
• starting insulin
• a GLP-1 agonist (if triple therapy not effective, not tolerated or contraindicated, consider switching one oral drug to GLP-1 agonist if BMI >35kg/m², or if insuling would have significant occupational implications, or if weight loss would benefit other obesity-related comorbidities)

Insulin: see BOX 'Using insulin'. Use a structured programme. Review the need for existing oral treatments

Triple therapy not tolerated: metformin, SU and GLP-1 mimetic (see BOX 'GLP analogues')

Fig 5.5 Management of type 2 diabetes. Aim for HbA1c 48mmol/mol or 53mmol/mol if ≥2 agents.
Data from Algorithm for blood glucose lowering therapy in adults with type 2 diabetes,
https://www.nice.org.uk/guidance/ng28

Oral hypoglycaemic agents

Metformin A biguanide. ↑ insulin sensitivity and weight neutral. SE: nausea; diarrhoea (try modified-release version); abdominal pain; not hypoglycaemia. Avoid if eGFR <30mL/min (due to risk of lactic acidosis).

DPP4 inhibitors/gliptins (Eg sitagliptin.) Weight neutral. Block the action of DPP4, an enzyme which destroys the hormone incretin.

Glitazone ↑ insulin sensitivity. SE: bone fractures, bladder cancer, weight gain, fluid retention, ↑LFT (monitor LFTs periodically based on clinical judgement). CI: past or present CCF; osteoporosis; monitor weight, and stop if ↑ or oedema.

Sulfonylurea ↑ insulin secretion; eg gliclazide 40mg/d. SE: hypoglycaemia (monitor glucose); it ↑ weight.

SGLT2i Selective sodium–glucose co-transporter-2 inhibitor. Blocks the reabsorption of glucose in the kidneys and promotes weight loss and excretion of excess glucose in the urine (eg empagliflozin, shown to reduce mortality from cardiovascular disease and CKD progression in patients with type 2 DM, when compared to placebo).

Glucagon-like peptide (GLP) analogues (semaglutide, dulaglutide, liraglutide)

Incretin mimetics. Incretins are gut peptides that work by augmenting insulin release and reducing appetite and food intake. Given by subcutaneous injection. Used for type 2 diabetes as monotherapy, if metformin inappropriate, or in combination with other agents. May also be used to treat obesity in combination with lifestyle measures, eg BMI >35 plus 1 obesity-related comorbidity, or 30–35 if needs specialist referral for weight management. Generally leads to 5–15% weight loss.

Using insulin

Vital to educate to self-adjust doses in the light of exercise, finger-prick glucose, calorie intake, and carbohydrate counting. • Phone support (trained nurse 7/24). • Can modify diet wisely and avoid binge drinking (danger of delayed hypoglycaemia). • Partner can abort hypoglycaemia: sugary drinks; GlucoGel® PO if coma (no risk of aspiration). • Dose titration to target—eg by 2–4 UNIT steps.
▶▶It is vital to write UNITS in full when prescribing insulin to avoid misinterpretation of U for zero!

Subcutaneous insulins Short-, medium-, or long-acting.
1 Rapid-acting insulin (eg Humalog®; Novorapid®)—prandial insulins to be injected 15min before meals.
2 Isophane insulin (variable peak at 4-12h): favoured by NICE (it's cheap!).
3 Pre-mixed insulins (eg NovoMix® 30 = 30% short-acting and 70% long-acting).
4 Long-acting recombinant human insulin analogues (*insulin glargine*) are used at bedtime in type 1 or 2 DM. There is no awkward peak, so good if nocturnal hypoglycaemia is an issue. *Insulin detemir* is similar and has a role in intensive insulin regimens for overweight type 2 DM.

Common insulin regimens ▶*Plan the regimen to suit the lifestyle, not vice versa.* Disposable pens: dial dose; insert needle 90° to skin. Vary injection site (outer thigh/abdomen); change needle with each injection.
• 'BD biphasic regimen': twice-daily premixed insulins by pen (eg NovoMix 30®)—useful in type 2 DM.
• 'QDS regimen': before meals rapid-acting insulin + bedtime long-acting analogue: useful in type 1 DM for achieving a flexible lifestyle (eg for adjusting doses with size of meals, or exercise).
• Once-daily before-bed long-acting insulin: a good initial insulin regimen when intensifying treatment in type 2 DM, eg initial starting dose of 10 units or 0.2 units/kg—and uptitrate as needed.

Dose adjustment for normal eating (DAFNE) multidisciplinary teams promoting autonomy can save lives. DAFNE found that training in flexible, intensive insulin dosing improved glycaemic control as well as wellbeing. It is resource intensive.

Subcutaneous insulin dosing during intercurrent illnesses (eg influenza) (Advice leaflets with sick day rules for patients with type 1 and 2 diabetes available at https://trenddiabetes.online/trend-uk-releases-updated-sick-day-rules-leaflets/)
▶▶Advise patients to avoid stopping insulin during acute illness.
• Illness often increases insulin requirements despite reduced food intake.
• Maintain calorie intake, eg using milk.
• Check blood glucose ≥4 times a day and look for ketonuria. Increase insulin doses if glucose rising. Advise to get help from a specialist diabetes nurse or GP if concerned (esp. if glucose levels are rising or ketonuria). One option is 2-hourly ultra fast-acting insulin (eg 6–8U) preceded by a fingerprick glucose check.
• Admit if vomiting, dehydrated, ketotic (▶▶p816), a child, or pregnant.
• Stop SGLT2 inhibitors in type 2 DM during acute illness or pre-surgery to avoid risk of euglycaemic ketoacidosis. Check ketone levels in such cases.
• Metformin should be stopped in acute illness if diarrhoea and vomiting or AKI present (due to greater risk of lactic acidosis).

Insulin pumps (continuous subcutaneous insulin) Consider only in type 1 DM when attempts to reach HbA1c with multiple daily injections have resulted in disabling hypoglycaemia or person has been unable to achieve target HbA1c despite careful management.

5 Endocrinology

Prospective studies show that good control of hyperglycaemia is key to preventing microvascular complications in type 1 and 2 DM.[8] ▶*Find out what problems are being experienced* (eg glycaemic control, morale, erectile dysfunction—p224).

Assess vascular risk BP control (see BOX 'Controlling blood pressure in diabetes') is crucial for preventing macrovascular disease and ↓mortality. Refer to *smoking cessation* services. Check *plasma lipids*.

Look for complications • Check injection sites for infection or lipohypertrophy (fatty change): advise on rotating sites of injection if present.

• **Vascular disease** Chief cause of death. MI is 4-fold commoner in DM and is more likely to be 'silent'. Stroke is twice as common. Women are at high risk—DM removes the vascular advantage conferred by the female sex. Address other risk factors—diet, smoking, hypertension (p85). Suggest a statin (eg offer atorvastatin 20mg daily for primary prevention in T2D if QRISK >10%, or in type 1 DM if they have had diabetes >10yrs, age >40yrs, established nephropathy or other CVD risk factors), even if no overt IHD, vascular disease, or microalbuminuria. Aspirin 75mg reduces vascular events (in context of secondary prevention). Safe to use in diabetic retinopathy.[9] Aspirin is not indicated for primary prevention; only used for secondary prevention. Offer atorvastatin 20mg daily for primary prevention in T2D if QRISK >10%, or in T1D if they have had diabetes >10 years, or if age >40 years, or if established nephropathy or other CVD risk factors.

• **Nephropathy** (p310) Microalbuminuria is when urine dipstick is −ve for protein but the urine albumin:creatinine ratio (uACR) is ≥3mg/mmol (units vary, check lab) reflecting early kidney disease and ↑vascular risk. If uACR >3, inhibiting the renin–angiotensin system with an ACE-i or ARA (titrate the max dose as tolerated), even if BP is normal, protects the kidneys. Titrate ACE-i to maximum tolerated dose. Consider referral to renal team if progressive ↓ in eGFR by >15mL/min in a year, ↓ eGFR of ≥25% + change in eGFR category within 12mths, when eGFR <30, or if marked albuminuria, eg uACR >70mg/mmol. SGLT2 inhibitors reduce diabetic kidney disease progression.

• **Diabetic retinopathy** Blindness is *preventable*. ▶*Annual retinal screening mandatory for all patients.* Most referrals to ophthalmologists now come from the retinopathy screening service. Refer to an ophthalmologist if any evidence of diabetic retinopathy or if any uncertainty at or near the macula (the only place capable of 6/6 vision). ▶Pre-symptomatic screening enables laser photocoagulation to be used, aimed to stop production of angiogenic factors from the ischaemic retina. Indications: maculopathy or proliferative retinopathy. See figs 5.6–5.9. ℞ Support treatment by aiming for HbA1c 6.5%, BP <130/80mmHg, and possibly consider fibrate therapy.

  • **Background retinopathy** Microaneurysms (dots), haemorrhages (blots), and hard exudates (lipid deposits). Refer if near the macula, eg for intravitreal triamcinolone.
  • **Pre-proliferative retinopathy** IRMAs, venous beading, venous reduplication, and multiple blot haemorrhages are features of pre-proliferative retinopathy. Refer to a specialist.
  • **Proliferative retinopathy** New vessels form. Needs urgent referral.
  • **Maculopathy** (Hard to see in early stages.) Suspect if ↓acuity. Prompt laser, intravitreal steroids, or anti-angiogenic agents may be needed in macular oedema.[2]

• **Cataracts** May be juvenile 'snowflake' form, or 'senile'—which occur earlier in diabetic subjects. Osmotic changes in the lens induced in acute hyperglycaemia reverse with normoglycaemia (so wait before buying glasses).
• **Rubeosis iridis** New vessels on iris: occurs late and may lead to glaucoma.
• **Metabolic complications** See p816.
• **Diabetic feet** See p206.
• **Neuropathy** See p206.

Controlling blood pressure in diabetes

Type 1 DM Treat BP if >135/85mmHg, unless albuminuria or two or more features of metabolic syndrome, in which case it should be 130/80mmHg (NICE 2015). Use an ACE-i 1st line or ARA if intolerant. If hypertensive and underlying renal involvement, see local guidance, p300.

Type 2 DM Target BP <135/85mmHg or <130/80mmHg kidney, eye, or cerebrovascular damage. 1st-line drug treatment should be an ACE-i. African-Caribbean patients with T2D are also offered ACE-i/ARBs first line but with the caveat that they may be less effective, and may need to progress to Step 2 treatment (ie addition of diuretic or CCB) if initial treatment less effective. ARBs are generally preferred to ACE-i in people of African-Caribbean origin as ACE inhibitors have a higher risk of angioedema in this population. ACE-i contraindicated in pregnancy. Consider switching to alternate agents pre-pregnancy, eg labetalol, CCBs. Do not combine an ACE-i with an angiotensin receptor antagonist.

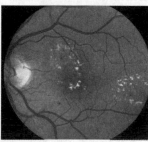

Fig 5.6 Background retinopathy, with micro-aneurysms and hard exudates.
Courtesy of Prof J Trobe.

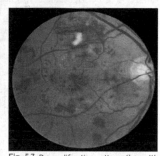

Fig 5.7 Pre-proliferative retinopathy, with haemorrhages and a cotton-wool spot.
Reproduced from Warrell et al., *Oxford Textbook of Medicine*, 2010, with permission from Oxford University Press.

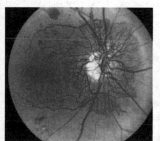

Fig 5.8 Proliferative retinopathy, with new vessel formation and haemorrhages.
Courtesy of Prof J Trobe.

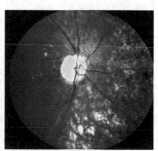

Fig 5.9 Scars from previous laser photo-coagulation.
Courtesy of Prof J Trobe.

►Refer *early* to foot services (podiatry, imaging, vascular surgery). Multidisciplinary input essential.

Amputations are common (135/week)—and preventable: *good care saves legs.* Examine feet regularly. Distinguish between ischaemia (critical toes ± absent foot pulses and worse outcome) and peripheral neuropathy (injury or infection over pressure points, eg the metatarsal heads). In practice, many have both.

Neuropathy ↓Sensation in 'stocking' distribution: test sensation with a 10g monofilament fibre (sensory loss is patchy so examine all areas), absent ankle jerks, neuropathic deformity (Charcot joint, fig 5.11): pes cavus, claw toes, loss of transverse arch, rocker-bottom sole. Caused by loss of pain sensation, leading to ↑mechanical stress and repeated joint injury. Swelling, instability, and deformity. ►Early recognition is vital (cellulitis or osteomyelitis are often misdiagnosed).

Ischaemia If the foot pulses cannot be felt, do Doppler pressure measurements. Any evidence of neuropathy or vascular disease raises risk of foot ulceration. *Educate* (daily foot inspection—eg with a mirror for the sole; comfortable shoes). *Regular podiatry* to remove callus, as haemorrhage and tissue necrosis may occur below, leading to ulceration. *Treat fungal infections* (p404). *Surgery* (including endovascular angioplasty balloons, stents, and subintimal recanalization) has a role.

Foot ulceration Typically painless, punched-out ulcer (fig 5.10) in an area of thick callus ± superadded infection. Causes cellulitis, abscess ± osteomyelitis.

Assess degree of
1 Neuropathy (clinically).
2 Ischaemia (clinically + Doppler ± angiography).
3 Bony deformity, eg Charcot joint (clinically + x-ray). See fig 5.11.
4 Infection (swabs, blood culture, x-ray, and MRI for osteomyelitis, probe ulcer to reveal depth).

Management Multidisciplinary approach required, involving podiatrist, diabetologists, diabetes specialist nurses, vascular surgeons, orthopaedic surgeons, microbiologists. Management principles are: 1 optimizing diabetes control, 2 ongoing podiatry for wound care, regular debridement of callus and dead tissue, 3 off-loading the wound—consider therapeutic shoes, 4 treat any superadded infection—refer to local infection guidance, 5 consider whether revascularization procedures required, eg angioplasty, vascular bypass grafting. Diabetic foot infections: include a drug predictably active against MRSA. Empiric drug regimes should cover both *Staph* and *Strep* but, if severe limb and/or life-threatening infection, will need broader cover against Gram +ve cocci, coliforms and other aerobic Gram –ve rods and anaerobes (eg vancomyin + piperacillin-tazobactam). Oral augmentin may be reasonable if superficial infection (eg ulcer with superficial inflammation). Risk of osteomyelitis increased if ulcer area >2cm², positive probe to bone, ESR >70 or abnormal x-ray. Consider admission if failing oral antibiotic therapy, scoring for sepsis markers, evidence for urgent surgery, eg abscess, deep or spreading infection, wet gangrene.

►**Absolute indications for surgery** Abscess or deep infection; osteomyelitis; spreading anaerobic infection; gangrene/rest pain; suppurative arthritis.

Diabetic neuropathies **Symmetric sensory polyneuropathy** ('Glove & stocking' numbness, tingling, and pain, eg worse at night.) *R*: first-line pharmacotherapy options for *painful* diabetic neuropathy include duloxetine, amitriptyline, pregabalin, and gabapentin, eg amitriptyline 10mg nocte—titrating in steps of 10–25mg up to 75mg; eg duloxetine commence at 30mg daily and uptitrate to 60–120mg daily. May take 2–3mths to gauge response to treatment. If inadequate effect, consider switching or adding in a second-line agent. Consider referral to pain specialist. Avoid use of opioids to treat painful diabetic neuropathy because of lack of evidence for long-term efficacy and concern about addiction. **Autonomic neuropathy** (p501) Postural BP drop; ↓cerebrovascular autoregulation; loss of respiratory sinus arrhythmia (vagal neuropathy); gastroparesis; urine retention; erectile dysfunction; gustatory sweating; diarrhoea (may respond to codeine phosphate). Gastroparesis (see p264). Postural hypotension may respond to fludrocortisone (SE: oedema, ↑BP)/midodrine (α-agonist; SE: ↑BP).

Preventing loss of limbs: primary or secondary prevention?

Traditionally prevention involves foot care advice in diabetic clinics (eg 'Don't go bare-foot'), promoting euglycaemia and normotension. But despite this, the sight of a diabetic patient minus one limb is not rare, and must prompt us to redouble our commitment to primary prevention, ie stopping those at risk from ever getting diabetes. The sequelae of diabetic neuropathy can lead to gangrene, amputation, and the impact on quality of life can be profound. As one patient post amputation said, 'I begin again to walk, on crutches. What nuisance, what fatigue, what sadness, when I think about all my ancient travels, and how active I was just 5 months ago! Where are the runnings across mountains, the walks, the deserts, the rivers, and the seas? And now, the life of a legless cripple. For I begin to understand that crutches, wooden and articulated legs, are a pack of jokes … Goodbye to family, goodbye to future! My life is gone, I'm no more than an immobile trunk' (Arthur Rimbaud. Letter to his sister Isabelle, 10 July 1891).

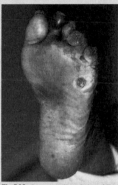

Fig 5.10 Gangrene (toes 2, 4, and 5).
Reproduced from Warrell *et al.*,
Oxford Textbook of Medicine, 2010,
with permission from Oxford
University Press.

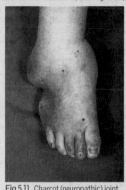

Fig 5.11 Charcot (neuropathic) joint.
Reproduced from Warrell *et al.*,
Oxford Textbook of Medicine, 2010,
with permission from Oxford
University Press.

Special situations in diabetes

Pregnancy (*OHCS* p26) 4% are complicated by DM: either pre-existing (<0.5%), or new-onset gestational diabetes (GDM) (>3.5%).
- All forms carry an increased risk to mother and fetus: miscarriage, pre-term labour, pre-eclampsia, congenital malformations, macrosomia, and a worsening of diabetic complications, eg retinopathy, nephropathy.
- Risk of GDM ↑ if: aged over 25; family history; +ve; ↑weight; non-Caucasian; HIV+ve; previous gestational DM.
- Pre-conception: offer general advice and discuss risks. Control/reduce weight, aim for HbA1c 6.5%, offer folic acid 5mg/d until 12 weeks.
- Screen for GDM with OGTT if risk factors at booking (16–18 weeks if previous GDM).
- Oral hypoglycaemics other than metformin should be discontinued. Metformin may be used as an adjunct or alternative to insulin in type 2 DM or GDM.

6wks postpartum with GDM, do a fasting glucose. Even if −ve, 50% go on to develop DM.

Surgery Optimal blood sugar control pre-, peri-, and post-operatively is important to minimize risk of infection and balance catabolic response to surgery. Type 1 diabetics should ideally be first on the list and blood glucose levels should have been stabilized 1–2 days pre major surgery. Consult local policy for how to manage insulin-treated/non-insulin-treated patients on morning of surgery (eg setting up glucose/insulin infusion).

▶▶**Hypoglycaemia** Commonest endocrine emergency—see p818. Prompt diagnosis and treatment essential—brain damage & death can occur if severe or prolonged.

Definition Blood glucose level <3.9mmol/L = hypoglycaemia in non-diabetic individuals. However, some guidelines use <3.3mmol/L. Severe hypoglycaemia indicates severe cognitive impairment requiring external assistance for recovery. See BOX.

Symptoms Autonomic Sweating, anxiety, hunger, tremor, palpitations, dizziness. **Neuroglycopenic** Confusion, drowsiness, visual trouble, seizures, coma. Rarely focal symptoms, eg transient hemiplegia. Mutism, personality change, restlessness, and incoherence may lead to misdiagnosis of alcohol intoxication or even psychosis.

Fasting hypoglycaemia Causes The chief cause is insulin or sulfonylurea treatment in a diabetic, eg ↑activity, missed meal, accidental or non-accidental overdose (check for circulating oral hypoglycaemics). In diabetic patients, you can assess awareness of hypoglycaemia with scoring systems like the GOLD score. In *non-diabetics* you must EXPLAIN mechanism: •**Ex**ogenous drugs, eg insulin, oral hypoglycaemics (p202)? Access through diabetic in the family? Body-builders may misuse insulin to help stamina. Also: alcohol, eg a binge with no food; aspirin poisoning; ACE-i; β-blockers; pentamidine; quinine sulfate; aminoglutethamide; insulin-like growth factor.[10] •**Pit**uitary insufficiency. •**L**iver failure, plus some rare inherited enzyme defects. •**A**ddison's disease. •**I**slet cell tumours (insulinoma) and immune hypoglycaemia (eg anti-insulin receptor antibodies in Hodgkin's disease). •**N**on-pancreatic neoplasms due to overproduction of IGF-2, eg fibrosarcomas and haemangiopericytomas.

When to investigate
- Whipple answered this (*Whipple's triad*): symptoms or signs of hypoglycaemia (due to overproduction of IGF-2) + ↓plasma glucose + resolution of symptoms or signs post glucose rise.
- Document blood glucose levels during attack and lab glucose if in hospital (monitors often not reliable at low readings).
- Take a drug history and exclude liver failure and adrenal insufficiency. Consider assay for presence of sulfonylureas.
- 72h fasting may be needed (monitor closely). Bloods: glucose, insulin, c-peptide, and plasma ketones if symptomatic. If endogenous hyperinsulinism suspected, do insulin, c-peptide, proinsulin, β-hydroxybutyrate. Consider measuring IGF-2 and insulin antibodies.

Interpreting results
- Hypoglycaemic hyperinsulinaemia (HH). *Causes:* insulinoma, sulfonylureas, insulin injection (no detectable c-peptide—only released with endogenous insulin); non-insulinoma pancreatogenous hypoglycaemia syndrome, mutation in the insulin-receptor gene. Congenital HH follows mutations in genes involved in insulin secretion (ABCC8, KCNJ11, GLUD1, CGK, HADH, SLC16A1, HNF4A, ABCC8, & KCNJ11).[11]
- Insulin low or undetectable, no excess ketones. *Causes:* non-pancreatic neoplasm; anti-insulin receptor antibodies.
- ↓Insulin, ↑ketones. *Causes:* alcohol, pituitary insufficiency, Addison's disease.

Post-prandial hypoglycaemia May occur after gastric/bariatric surgery ('dumping', p618), and in type 2 DM. **Investigation** Mixed meal test.

Treatment ▶▶See p818. If episodes are often, advise many small high-starch meals. If post-prandial ↓glucose, give slowly absorbed carbohydrate (high fibre). Consider acarbose—sometimes used in post-prandial hypoglycaemia. In diabetics, rationalize hypoglycaemic agents (p203).

The definition of hypoglycaemia is context dependent

The brain stops working if plasma glucose levels get too low, so we are nervous of levels ≤3mmol/L. But some are asymptomatic at this level. So what is definitely abnormal? The answer may be 4mmol/L, allowing for inaccuracies in fingerprick blood glucose levels (NB: whole blood glucose is 10–15% < plasma glucose.) Think: 'In this ill patient when can I be sure that a low glucose is not contributing to their illness?' If <4mmol/L, you may be wise to treat (p818)—just in case. Consider, is the patient on hypoglycaemics, have they binged on alcohol 24h pre-test? Skipped meals? Is there an underlying illness, eg insulinoma? Unlikely, but possible. Keep an open mind; let the GP know. Counsel patient and relative about warning signs of hypoglycaemia. Be more inclined to investigate if the effects of even mild hypoglycaemia might be disastrous (eg in pilots) or if there are unexplained symptoms.

Insulinoma

This often benign (90–95%) pancreatic islet cell tumour is sporadic or seen with MEN-1 (p217). It presents as fasting hypoglycaemia, with Whipple's triad:
1 Symptoms associated with fasting or exercise.
2 Recorded hypoglycaemia with symptoms.
3 Symptoms relieved with glucose.

Screening test Hypoglycaemia + ↑plasma insulin with ↑c-peptide/proinsulin and negative sulfonylurea screen.

Imaging CT/MRI ± endoscopic pancreatic US ± intra-arterial calcium stimulation test with hepatic venous sampling (IACS) (see BOX; all fallible, so don't waste too much time before proceeding to intra-operative visualization ± intra-operative ultrasound). ^{18}F-L-3,4-dihydroxyphenylalanine PET-CT can help guide laparoscopic surgery. Somatostatin receptor scintigraphy (gallium DOTATATE scans) have been shown to be useful in detecting insulinomas when conventional imaging studies do not identify them.

Treatment Excision. Medical treatment to control symptoms for insulinoma, eg diazoxide, octreotide in those pending surgery.

Pursuing a voyage to the islets of Langerhans to the bitter end

A 50-year-old had episodic early-morning sweats and tremors and was found to have hyperinsulinaemic hypoglycaemia (a rare condition known as nesidioblastosis). Selective IACS showed a 2-fold increase in insulin secretion after infusion of the splenic and superior mesenteric arteries, so setting the stage for 'hunt the insulinoma'.

But cross-sectional imaging and endoscopic ultrasound were normal. At laparotomy, no lesion was found despite mobilization of the pancreas, or during intra-operative ultrasound. 'Time to sew up and go home?' 'No!' said the surgeon, 'I'm going to do a distal pancreatectomy'. Histology showed no discrete insulinoma, but diffuse islet cell hyperplasia (nesidioblastosis). How much pancreas to resect? Too little and nothing is gained: too much spells pancreatic endocrine disaster. Luckily the surgeon guessed right, and the patient was cured by the procedure.[12]

Physiology

Thyroid-stimulating hormone (TSH = thyrotropin), a glycogenin, is produced from the anterior pituitary (fig 5.12). The thyroid produces mainly T_4, which is 5-fold less active than T_3. 85% of T_3 is formed from peripheral conversion of T_4. Most T_3 and T_4 in plasma is protein bound, eg to thyroxine-binding globulin (TBG). The unbound portion is the active part. T_3 and T_4 ↑ cell metabolism, via nuclear receptors, and are thus vital for growth and mental development. They also ↑ catecholamine effects. Thyroid hormone abnormalities are usually due to problems in the thyroid gland itself, and rarely caused by the hypothalamus or the anterior pituitary.

TRH from the hypothalamus acts on the pituitary gland

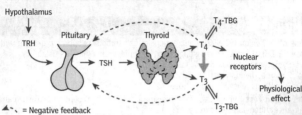

◄▾◂ = Negative feedback
Fig 5.12 Pathways involved in thyroid function.

Basic tests

See table 5.3. Free T_4 and T_3 are more useful than total T_4 and T_3 as the latter are affected by TBG. Total T_4 and T_3 are ↑ when TBG is ↑ and *vice versa*. TBG is ↑ in pregnancy, oestrogen therapy (HRT, oral contraceptives), and hepatitis. TBG is ↓ in nephrotic syndrome and malnutrition (both from protein loss), drugs (androgens, corticosteroids, phenytoin), chronic liver disease, and acromegaly. TSH is very useful:

- **Hyperthyroidism suspected** Ask for T_3, T_4, and TSH. All will have ↓TSH (except the rare TSH-secreting pituitary adenoma). Most have ↑T_4, but ~1% have only raised T_3.
- **Hypothyroidism suspected or monitoring replacement ℞** Ask for only T_4 and TSH. T_3 does not add any extra information. TSH varies through the day: trough at 2PM; 30% higher during darkness, so during monitoring, try to do at the same time.

Sick euthyroidism In any systemic illness, TFTs may become deranged. The typical pattern is for 'everything to be low'. The test should be repeated after recovery.

Assay interference is caused by antibodies in the serum, interfering with the test.

Other tests

Thyroid autoantibodies Antithyroid peroxidase (TPO; formerly called microsomal) antibodies or antithyroglobulin antibodies may be increased in autoimmune thyroid disease: Hashimoto's or Graves' disease. If +ve in Graves', there is an increased risk of developing hypothyroidism at a later stage.
- **TSH receptor antibody** Useful to diagnose Graves' disease.
- **Serum thyroglobulin** Useful in monitoring the treatment of carcinoma (p592), and in detection of factitious (self-medicated) hyperthyroidism, where it is low.
- **Isotope scan** (^{123}Iodine, ^{99}technetium pertechnetate, etc.; see fig 13.21, p593.) Useful for determining the cause of hyperthyroidism and to detect retrosternal goitre, ectopic thyroid tissue, or thyroid metastases (+ whole body CT). If there are suspicious nodules, the question is: does the area have increased (hot), decreased (cold), or the same (neutral) uptake of isotope as the remaining thyroid (fig 5.13)? Few neutral and almost no hot nodules are malignant. 20% of 'cold' nodules are malignant. Surgery is most likely to be needed if: • rapid growth • compression signs • dominant nodule on scintigraphy • nodule ≥3cm • hypo-echogenicity. See also p722.
- **Ultrasound** This distinguishes cystic (usually, but not always, benign) from solid (possibly malignant) nodules. If a solitary (or dominant) large nodule, in a multinodular goitre, do a fine-needle aspiration to look for thyroid cancer; see fig 13.22, p593.

Screen the following for abnormalities in thyroid function

- Patients with atrial fibrillation.
- Patients with hyperlipidaemia (4–14% have hypothyroidism).
- Diabetes mellitus—on annual review.
- Women with type 1 DM during 1st trimester and post delivery (3-fold rise in incidence of postpartum thyroid dysfunction).
- Patients on amiodarone or lithium (6-monthly).
- Patients with Down's or Turner's syndrome, or Addison's disease (yearly).
- Pregnant women/women planning a pregnancy if >30 years, have a history of goitre, family history of thyroid disease, or other autoimmune disease.
- As part of a dementia screen.

Table 5.3 Interpreting TFTs

Hormone profile	Diagnosis
↑TSH, ↓T₄	Hypothyroidism
↑TSH, normal T₄	Treated hypothyroidism or subclinical hypothyroidism (p215)
↑TSH, ↑T₄	Poor compliance with levothyroxine; TSH-secreting tumour or thyroid hormone resistance
↑TSH, ↑T₄, and ↓T₃	Slow conversion of T₄ to T₃ (deiodinase deficiency; euthyroid hyperthyroxinaemia*) or thyroid hormone antibody artefact
↓TSH, ↑T₄ or ↑T₃	Hyperthyroidism
↓TSH, normal T₄ and T₃	Subclinical hyperthyroidism
↓TSH, ↓T₄	Central hypothyroidism (hypothalamic or pituitary disorder)
↓TSH, ↓T₄, and ↓T₃	Sick euthyroidism or pituitary disease
Normal TSH, abnormal T₄	Consider changes in thyroid-binding globulin, assay interference, amiodarone, or pituitary TSH tumour

* In 'consumptive hypothyroidism' deiodinase activity is ↑↑; suspect if thyroxine doses have to be ↑↑.

5 Endocrinology

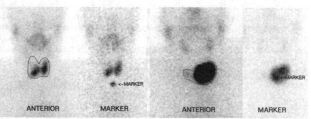

Fig 5.13 The images are from an isotope scan, with and without markers placed over the sternal notch. We can see on the left that the nodule is metabolically inactive ('cold'). The hot nodule (right pair) is a very avid nodule causing background thyroid suppression.

Image courtesy of Dr Y.T. Huang.

5 Endocrinology

The clinical effect of excess thyroid hormone, usually from gland hyperfunction.

Symptoms Diarrhoea; ↓weight; ↑appetite (if ↑↑, paradoxical weight *gain* in 10%); overactive; sweats; heat intolerance; palpitations; tremor; irritability; labile emotions; oligomenorrhoea ± infertility. Rarely psychosis; chorea; panic; itch; alopecia; urticaria.

Signs Pulse fast/irregular (AF or SVT; VT rare); warm moist skin; fine tremor; palmar erythema; thin hair; lid lag; lid retraction (exposure of sclera above iris; causing 'stare') (fig 5.14; eyelid lags behind eye's descent as patient watches your finger descend slowly). There may be goitre (fig 5.15); thyroid nodules; or bruit depending on the cause. **Signs of Graves' disease** 1 *Eye disease* (see BOX 'Thyroid eye disease'): exophthalmos, ophthalmoplegia. 2 *Pretibial myxoedema*: oedematous swellings above lateral malleoli; the term *myxoedema* is confusing here. 3 *Thyroid acropachy*: extreme manifestation, with clubbing, painful finger and toe swelling, and periosteal reaction in limb bones.

Tests ↓TSH (suppressed), ↑↑T₄, and ↑↑T₃. There may be mild normocytic anaemia, mild neutropenia (in Graves'), ↑ESR, ↑Ca²⁺, ↑LFT. **Also** Check thyroid autoantibodies (TSH receptor antibody). If antibody negative, and cause of hyperthyroidism unclear—consider thyroid uptake scan. If ophthalmopathy, test visual fields, acuity, and eye movements (see BOX 'Thyroid eye disease').

Causes Graves' disease Prevalence: 0.5% (⅔ of cases of hyperthyroidism). ♀:♂≈9:1. Typical age: 40–60yrs (younger if maternal family history). Cause: circulating IgG autoantibodies binding to and activating G-protein-coupled thyrotropin receptors, which cause smooth thyroid enlargement and ↑hormone production (esp. T₃), and react with orbital autoantigens. Triggers: stress; infection; childbirth. Patients are often hyperthyroid but may be, or become, hypo- or euthyroid. It is associated with other autoimmune diseases: vitiligo, type 1 DM, Addison's (table 5.4). **Toxic multinodular goitre** Seen in the elderly and in iodine-deficient areas. There are nodules that secrete thyroid hormones. Surgery is indicated for compressive symptoms from the enlarged thyroid (dysphagia or dyspnoea). **Toxic adenoma** There is a solitary nodule producing T₃ and T₄. On isotope scan, the nodule is 'hot' (p210), and the rest of the gland is suppressed. **Ectopic thyroid tissue** Metastatic follicular thyroid cancer, or struma ovarii: ovarian teratoma with thyroid tissue. **Exogenous** Iodine excess, eg food contamination, contrast media (►►thyroid storm, p820, if already hyperthyroid). Levothyroxine excess causes ↑↑T₄, ↓T₃, ↓thyroglobulin. **Others** 1 *Subacute de Quervain's thyroiditis:* self-limiting post-viral with painful goitre, ↑↑T° ± ↑ESR. Low isotope uptake on scan. ℞ NSAIDs. 2 *Drugs:* amiodarone (p214), lithium (hypothyroidism more common), immunotherapy. 3 *Postpartum.* 4 *TB* (rare). 5 Hydatidiform mole (consider if hyperemesis).

Treatment Varies depending on cause.

1 **Drugs** β-blockers (eg propranolol 40mg/6h) for rapid control of symptoms. *Anti-thyroid medication:* two strategies (equally effective):[13] **A** *Titration*, eg carbimazole 20–40mg/24h PO; check TFTs every 6wks and adjust dose; once TFTs in range, monitor 3-monthly. **B** *Block-replace:* give carbimazole + levothyroxine simultaneously (less risk of iatrogenic hypothyroidism). In Graves', maintain on either regimen for 12–18 months then withdraw. ~50% will relapse, requiring radioiodine or surgery. Carbimazole SE: agranulocytosis (↓↓neutrophils, can lead to dangerous sepsis; rare (0.03%)); warn to stop and get an urgent FBC if signs of infection, eg T°↑, sore throat/mouth ulcers.

2 **Radioiodine (¹³¹I)** Most become hypothyroid post-treatment. There is no evidence for ↑cancer, birth defects, or infertility in women. CI: pregnancy, lactation. Caution in active hyperthyroidism as risk of thyroid storm, and avoid if active thyroid eye disease (p821).

3 **Thyroidectomy (usually total)** Carries a risk of damage to recurrent laryngeal nerve (hoarse voice) and hypoparathyroidism (transient/permanent). Patients will become hypothyroid, so thyroid replacement needed.

4 **In pregnancy and infancy** Get expert help. See *OHCS* p28 & *OHCS* p251.

Complications Heart failure (thyrotoxic cardiomyopathy, ↑ in elderly), angina, AF (seen in 10–25%: control hyperthyroidism and warfarinize if no contraindication), osteoporosis, ophthalmopathy, gynaecomastia. ►►Thyroid storm (p821).

Thyroid eye disease

Seen in 25–50% of people with Graves' disease. The main known risk factor is smoking. The eye disease may not correlate with thyroid disease and the patient can be euthyroid, hypothyroid, or hyperthyroid at presentation. Eye disease may be the first presenting sign of Graves' disease, and can also be worsened by treatment, typically with radioiodine (usually a transient effect). Retro-orbital inflammation and lymphocyte infiltration results in swelling of the orbit.

Symptoms Eye discomfort, grittiness, ↑tear production, photophobia, diplopia, ↓acuity, afferent pupillary defect (p68) may mean optic nerve compression: ►*seek expert advice at once as decompression may be needed*. Nerve damage does not necessarily go hand-in-hand with protrusion. Indeed, if the eye cannot protrude for anatomical reasons, optic nerve compression is more likely—a paradox!

Signs Exophthalmos—appearance of protruding eye; proptosis—eyes protrude beyond the orbit (look from above in the same plane as the forehead); conjunctival oedema; corneal ulceration; papilloedema; loss of colour vision. Ophthalmoplegia (especially of upward gaze) occurs due to muscle swelling and fibrosis.

Tests Diagnosis is clinical. CT/MRI of the orbits may reveal enlarged eye muscles.

Management Get specialist help. Treat hyper- or hypothyroidism. Advise to stop smoking (worse prognosis). Most have mild disease that can be treated symptomatically (artificial tears, sunglasses, avoid dust, elevate bed when sleeping to ↓ periorbital oedema). Diplopia may be managed with a Fresnel prism stuck to one lens of a spectacle (aids easy changing as the exophthalmos changes). Oral selenium supplementation at 200mcg daily may be beneficial in mild disease. In more severe disease, try high-dose steroids (IV methylprednisolone) and mycophenolate mofetil. Surgical decompression is used for severe sight-threatening disease, or for cosmetic reasons once the activity of eye disease has reduced (via an inferior orbital approach, using space in the ethmoidal, sphenoidal, and maxillary sinuses). Eyelid surgery may improve cosmesis and function. Orbital radiotherapy can be used to treat ophthalmoplegia but has little effect on proptosis. *2nd line:* rituximab, tocilizumab.

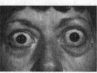

Fig 5.14 Thyroid eye disease: lid retraction causing a 'staring' appearance.

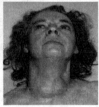

Fig 5.15 Goitre.

Causes of goitre

Diffuse
- Physiological
- Graves' disease
- Hashimoto's thyroiditis
- Subacute (de Quervain's) thyroiditis (painful).

Nodular
- Multinodular goitre
- Adenoma
- Carcinoma.

Table 5.4 Manifestations of Graves' disease—and pathophysiology

Pituitary	Suppressed TSH	↓Expression of thyrotropin β subunit
Heart	↑Rate; ↑contractility	↑Serum atrial natriuretic peptide
Liver	↑Peripheral T₃; LDL↓ (p682)	↑Type 1 5'-deiodinase; LDL receptors
Bone	↑Bone turnover; osteoporosis	↑Osteocalcin; ↑ALP; ↑urinary N-telopeptide
Genital ♂	↓Libido; erectile dysfunction	↑Sex hormone globulin; ↓testosterone
Genital ♀	Irregular menses	Oestrogen antagonism
Metabolic	↑Thermogenesis; ↑O₂ use	↑Fatty acid oxidation; ↑Na-K ATPase
White fat	↓Fat mass	↑Adrenergic-mediated lipolysis
CNS	Stiff person syndrome (rare)*	Antibodies to glutamic acid decarboxylase
Muscle	Proximal myopathy	↑Sarcoplasmic reticulum Ca²⁺-activated ATPase
Thyroid	↑Secretion of T₃ and T₄	↑Type 2 5'-deiodinase activity in thyroid

* Emotional or tactile stimuli cause spasms; seen in any autoimmune state (eg type 1 DM); ℞: baclofen± IV Ig.

The clinical effect of lack of thyroid hormone. It is common (4/1000/yr). If treated, prognosis is excellent; untreated it is disastrous (eg heart disease, dementia). ▶*As it is insidious, both you and your patient may not realize anything is wrong*, so be alert to subtle, non-specific symptoms, esp. in women ≥40yrs old (♀:♂ ≈ 6:1).

Symptoms Tiredness; sleepy, lethargic; ↓mood; cold-disliking; ↑weight; constipation; menorrhagia; hoarse voice; ↓memory/cognition; dementia; myalgia; cramps; weakness.

Signs BRADYCARDIC: **R**eflexes relax slowly; **A**taxia (cerebellar); **D**ry thin hair/skin; **Y**awning/drowsy/coma (p820); **C**old hands ± ↓T°; **A**scites ± non-pitting oedema (lids; hands; feet) ± pericardial or pleural effusion; **R**ound puffy face/double chin/obese; **D**efeated demeanour; **I**mmobile ± ileus; **C**CF. Also: neuropathy; myopathy; goitre (fig 5.16).

Diagnosis (p210) ▶Have a low threshold for doing TFTs! ↑TSH (eg ≥4mu/L);[2] ↓T₄ (in rare secondary hypothyroidism: ↓T₄ and ↓TSH or ↔ due to lack from the pituitary, p226). Cholesterol and triglyceride ↑; macrocytosis (less often normochromic anaemia too).

Causes of primary autoimmune hypothyroidism
• **Primary atrophic hypothyroidism** ♀:♂ ≈ 6:1. Common. Diffuse lymphocytic infiltration of the thyroid, leading to atrophy, hence no goitre.
• **Hashimoto's thyroiditis** Goitre due to lymphocytic and plasma cell infiltration. Commoner in women aged 60–70yrs. May be hypothyroid or euthyroid; rarely initial period of hyperthyroidism ('Hashitoxicosis'). Autoantibody titres are very high.

Other causes of primary hypothyroidism
▶Worldwide the chief cause is *iodine deficiency*.
• *Post-thyroidectomy or radioiodine treatment*.
• *Drug-induced:* antithyroid drugs, amiodarone, lithium, iodine, immunotherapy.
• *Subacute thyroiditis:* temporary hypothyroidism after hyperthyroid phase.
Secondary hypothyroidism Not enough TSH (due to hypopituitarism); very rare.

Hypothyroidism's associations Autoimmune is seen with other autoimmune diseases (type 1 DM, Addison's, and PA, p330). Turner's and Down's syndromes, cystic fibrosis, primary biliary cholangitis, ovarian hyperstimulation (*OHCS* p146); POEMS syndrome—polyneuropathy, organomegaly, endocrinopathy, M-protein band (plasmacytoma) + skin pigmentation/tethering. **Genetic** Dyshormonogenesis: genetic (often autosomal recessive) defect in hormone synthesis, eg Pendred's syndrome (with deafness): there is ↑uptake on isotope scan, which is displaced by potassium perchlorate.

Pregnancy problems Poorly treated hypothyroidism may be associated with pre-eclampsia, preterm delivery, low birth weight, postpartum haemorrhage, cognitive impairment in the child. Often needs increased dose of levothyroxine in pregnancy.

Treatment
• **Healthy and young** Start levothyroxine (T₄) at 1.6mcg/kg PO; review at 12wks. Aim for TSH in the lower half of the reference range. Consider measuring TSH every 3 months and titrating levothyroxine as needed—until TSH is on target—thereafter monitor TSH once a year. Enzyme inducers (p681) ↑ metabolism of levothyroxine.
• **Elderly or ischaemic heart disease** Start with 25mcg/24h; ↑dose by 25mcg/4wks according to TSH (▶cautiously, as levothyroxine may precipitate angina or MI).
• **If diagnosis is in question and T₄ already given** Stop T₄; recheck TSH in 6 weeks.

Amiodarone An iodine-rich drug structurally like T₄; 2% of users will get significant thyroid problems from it. Hypothyroidism can be caused by toxicity from iodine excess (T₄ release is inhibited). Thyrotoxicosis may be caused by a destructive thyroiditis or due to ↑ thyroid hormone synthesis from the excess iodine content of amiodarone. Radioiodine uptake scans or gland vascularity on thyroid ultrasound may help distinguish the causes and strategy of treatment. Seek expert help. Patients are often treated with a combination of antithyroid medications and steroids whilst the cause is identified. Thyroidectomy may be needed if resistant to medical therapy.

▶▶**Myxoedema coma** The ultimate hypothyroid state before death. See p820.

2 ▶*Treat the patient not the blood level!* No exact cut-off in TSH can be given partly because risk of death from heart disease mirrors TSH even when in the normal range in women. Risk ≈ 1.4 if TSH 1.5–2.4 vs 1.7 if TSH 2.5–3.5. If TSH >3.65 and possibly symptomatic, a low dose of levothyroxine may be tried. Monitor symptoms, TSH, and T₄ carefully. Overexposure to thyroxine may cause osteoporosis ± AF.

Why are symptoms of thyroid disease so various, and so subtle?

Almost all our cell nuclei have receptors showing a high affinity for T_3: that known as TRα-1 is abundant in muscle and fat; TRα-2 is abundant in brain; and TRβ-1 is abundant in brain, liver, and kidney. These receptors, via their influence on various enzymes, affect the following processes:
• The metabolism of substrates, vitamins, and minerals.
• Modulation of all other hormones and their target-tissue responses.
• Stimulation of O_2 consumption and generation of metabolic heat.
• Regulation of protein synthesis, and carbohydrate and lipid metabolism.
• Stimulation of demand for co-enzymes and related vitamins.

Subclinical thyroid disease

Subclinical hypothyroidism Defined by a raised TSH with normal T_4 and T_3. It is common: ~10% of those >55yrs have ↑TSH. Risk of progression to frank hypothyroidism is ~2%, and increases as ↑TSH; risk doubles if thyroid peroxidase antibodies are present, and is also increased in men.

Management:
• Confirm that raised TSH is persistent (recheck in 2–4 months).
• Recheck the history: if any non-specific features (eg depression), discuss benefits of treating (p214) with the patient—maybe they will function better.
• Have a low threshold for carefully supervised treatment as your patient may not be so asymptomatic after all, and cardiac deaths *may* be prevented. Treat if: 1 TSH ≥10mu/L. 2 +ve thyroid autoantibodies. 3 Past (treated) Graves'. 4 Other organ-specific autoimmunity (type 1 DM, myasthenia, pernicious anaemia, vitiligo), as they are more likely to progress to clinical hypothyroidism. *If TSH 4–10, and vague symptoms*, treat for 6 months—only continue if symptoms improve (or the patient is trying to conceive). If the patient does not fall into any of these categories, monitor TSH yearly.
• Risks from well-monitored treatment of subclinical hypothyroidism are small (but there is an ↑risk of atrial fibrillation and osteoporosis if overtreated).

Subclinical hyperthyroidism Occurs when ↓TSH, with normal T_4 and T_3. There is an increased risk of AF, heart failure, and osteoporosis.

Management:
• Confirm that suppressed TSH is persistent (recheck in 2–4 months).
• Check for a non-thyroidal cause: illness, pregnancy, pituitary or hypothalamic insufficiency (suspect if T_4 or T_3 are at the lower end of the reference range), use of TSH-suppressing medication, eg thyroxine, steroids.
• If TSH <0.1, treat on an individual basis, eg if aged >65 years, concurrent cardiovascular disease or osteoporosis, symptoms of hyperthyroidism, or a toxic nodule.
• Options are carbimazole or propylthiouracil—or radioiodine therapy.
• If no symptoms, recheck 6-monthly.

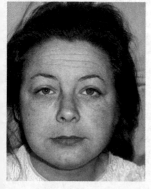

Fig 5.16 Facial appearance in hypothyroidism. Look for: pallor; coarse, brittle, diminished hair (scalp, axillary, and pubic); dull or blank expression lacking sparkle; coarse features; puffy lids. These signs are subtle: ►have a low threshold for measuring TSH.

Reproduced from Cox and Roper, *Clinical Skills*, 2005, with permission from Oxford University Press.

5 Endocrinology

Parathyroid hormone (PTH) is normally secreted in response to low ionized Ca^{2+} levels, by four parathyroid glands situated posterior to the thyroid (p593). The glands are controlled by −ve feedback via Ca^{2+} levels. PTH acts by: • ↑osteoclast activity releasing Ca^{2+} and PO_4^{3-} from bones • ↑Ca^{2+} and ↓PO_4^{3-} reabsorption in the kidney • active 1,25 dihydroxy-vitamin D_3 production is ↑. Overall effect is ↑Ca^{2+} and ↓PO_4^{3-}.

Primary hyperparathyroidism Causes ~80% solitary adenoma, ~20% hyperplasia of all glands, <0.5% parathyroid cancer. **Presentation** Often 'asymptomatic' (►*not in retrospect!*), with ↑Ca^{2+} on routine tests. Signs relate to: 1 ↑Ca^{2+} (p668): weak, tired, depressed, thirsty, dehydrated-but-polyuric; also renal stones, abdominal pain, pancreatitis, and ulcers (duodenal:gastric ≈ 7:1). 2 Bone resorption effects of PTH can cause pain, fractures, and osteopenia/osteoporosis. 3 ↑BP: ►so check Ca^{2+} in *everyone* with hypertension. *Association:* MEN-1 (see BOX 'Multiple endocrine neoplasia'). **Tests** ↑Ca^{2+} & ↑PTH or inappropriately normal with normal vit D (other causes of this: thiazides, lithium, familial hypocalciuric hypercalcaemia, tertiary hyperparathyroidism). Also ↓PO_4^{3-} (unless in renal failure), ↑ALP from bone activity, 24h urinary ↑Ca^{2+}. *Imaging: osteitis fibrosa cystica* (due to severe resorption; rare) may show up as subperiosteal erosions, cysts, or brown tumours of phalanges ± acro-osteolysis (fig 5.17) ± 'pepper-pot' skull. *DEXA* (p675; for osteoporosis, p674). ℞ If mild: ↑fluid intake to prevent stones; avoid thiazides + high Ca^{2+} intake. *Indications for parathyroidectomy:* symptomatic hypercalcaemia, serum Ca^{2+} >2.85, osteoporosis, renal calculi, ↓renal function, age ≤50yrs, hypercalciuria. *Complications:* hypoparathyroidism, recurrent laryngeal nerve damage (∴ hoarse), symptomatic Ca^{2+}↓ (hungry bones syndrome). Pre-op US and MIBI scan may localize an adenoma; intra-op PTH sampling may be used to confirm removal. *Recurrence:* ~8% over 10yrs.[14] Cinacalcet (a 'calcimimetic') ↑sensitivity of parathyroid cells to Ca^{2+} (∴ ↓PTH secretion); mainly indicated for management of symptomatic hyperparathyroidism in those not fit for surgical intervention; monitor Ca^{2+} within 1 week of dose changes; SE: gastrointestinal, myalgia.

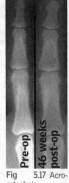

Fig 5.17 Acro-osteolysis.
© Dr I Maddison
myweb.lsbu.ac.uk

Pre-op
46 weeks post-op

Secondary hyperparathyroidism ↓Ca^{2+}, ↑PTH (appropriately). **Causes** ↓Vit D intake, chronic renal failure. ℞ Correct causes. Phosphate binders; vit D; cinacalcet if PTH ≥85pmol/L and parathyroidectomy tricky.

Tertiary hyperparathyroidism ↑Ca^{2+}, ↑↑PTH (inappropriately). Occurs after prolonged secondary hyperparathyroidism, causing glands to act autonomously having undergone hyperplastic or adenomatous change. This causes ↑Ca^{2+} from ↑↑secretion of PTH unlimited by feedback control. Seen in chronic renal failure.

Malignant hyperparathyroidism Parathyroid-related protein (PTHrP) is produced by some squamous cell lung cancers & breast and renal cell carcinomas. This mimics PTH resulting in ↑Ca^{2+} (PTH is ↓, as PTHrP is not detected in the assay).

Hypoparathyroidism

Primary hypoparathyroidism PTH secretion is ↓ due to gland failure. **Tests** ↓Ca^{2+}, usually with ↓ or inappropriately normal PTH; ↑PO_4^{3-}or ↔, ↔ALP. **Signs** Those of hypocalcaemia, p670, ± autoimmune comorbidities (see BOX 'Autoimmune polyendocrine syndromes'). **Causes** Autoimmune; congenital (Di George syn., OHCS p846). ℞ Activated vitamin D (calcitriol/alfacalcidol) combined with Ca^{2+} supplements. Aim for a low–normal Ca^{2+}. Daily recombinant synthetic PTH injections are available—emerging treatment option.

Secondary hypoparathyroidism Radiation, surgery (thyroidectomy, parathyroidectomy), hypomagnesaemia (magnesium is required for PTH secretion).

Pseudohypoparathyroidism Failure of target cell response to PTH. **Signs** Short metacarpals (esp. 4th and 5th, fig 5.18), round face, short stature, calcified basal ganglia (fig 5.19), ↓IQ. **Tests** ↓Ca^{2+}, ↑PTH, ↔ or ↑ALP. ℞ As for 1° hypoparathyroidism.

Multiple endocrine neoplasia (MEN types 1, 2a, and 2b)

In MEN syndromes there are functioning hormone-producing tumours in multiple organs (they are inherited as autosomal dominants).[15] They comprise: MEN-1 and -2.
• Neurofibromatosis (p510). • Von Hippel–Lindau and Peutz–Jeghers syndromes (p698 & p694). • Carney complex (spotty skin pigmentation, schwannomas, myxoma of skin, mucosa, or heart, especially atrial myxoma), and endocrine tumours: eg pituitary adenoma, adrenal hyperplasia, and testicular tumour.

MEN-1
• Parathyroid hyperplasia/adenoma (~95%; most ↑Ca^{2+}).
• Pancreas endocrine tumours (70%)—gastrinoma (p267) or insulinoma (p209) or, rarely, somatostatinoma (DM + steatorrhoea + gallstones/cholangitis), VIPoma (p255), or glucagonomas (±glucagon syndrome: migrating rash; glossitis; cheilitis, fig 8.21, p327; anaemia; ↓weight; ↑plasma glucagon; ↑glucose).
• Pituitary prolactinoma (~50%) or GH secreting tumour (acromegaly,[18] p232); also, adrenal and carcinoid tumours are associated.

The MEN-1 gene is a tumour suppressor gene. Menin, its protein, alters transcription activation. Many are sporadic, presenting in the 3rd–5th decades.

MEN-2a
• Thyroid: medullary thyroid carcinoma (seen in ~100%, p592).
• Adrenal: phaeochromocytoma (~50%, usually benign and bilateral).
• Parathyroid hyperplasia (~80%, but less than 20% have ↑Ca^{2+}).

MEN-2b Has similar features to MEN-2a plus mucosal neuromas and Marfanoid appearance, but no hyperparathyroidism. Mucosal neuromas consist of 'bumps' on: lips, cheeks, tongue, glottis, eyelids, and visible corneal nerves.

The gene involved in MEN-2a and b is the ret proto-oncogene, a receptor tyrosine kinase. Tests for ret mutations are revolutionizing MEN-2 treatment by enabling a prophylactic thyroidectomy to be done before neoplasia occurs, usually before 3yrs of age. NB: ret mutations rarely contribute to sporadic parathyroid tumours.

Autoimmune polyendocrine syndromes

Autoimmune disorders cluster into two defined syndromes:
Type 1 Autosomal recessive, rare.
Cause Mutations of AIRE (Auto ImmuneREgulator) gene on chromosome 21.
Features • Addison's disease. • Chronic mucocutaneous candidiasis. • Hypoparathyroidism.
Also associated with hypogonadism, pernicious anaemia, autoimmune primary hypothyroidism, chronic active hepatitis, vitiligo, alopecia.
Type 2 HLA D3 and D4 linked, common.
Cause Polygenic.
Features • Addison's disease. • Type 1 diabetes mellitus (in 20%).
• Autoimmune thyroid disease—hypothyroidism or Graves' disease.
Also associated with primary hypogonadism, vitiligo, alopecia, pernicious anaemia, chronic atrophic gastritis, coeliac disease, dermatitis herpetiformis.

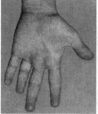

Fig 5.18 Pseudohypoparathyroidism: short 4th and 5th metacarpals.

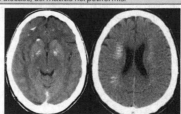

Fig 5.19 Cerebral calcification in pseudohypoparathyroidism: periventricular (left) and basal ganglia (right).
Courtesy of Professor Peter Scally.

5 Endocrinology

Physiology The adrenal cortex produces steroids: 1 *Glucocorticoids* (eg cortisol), which affect carbohydrate, lipid, and protein metabolism. 2 *Mineralocorticoids*, which control sodium and potassium balance (eg aldosterone, p660). 3 *Androgens*, sex hormones which have weak effect until peripheral conversion to testosterone and dihydrotestosterone. Corticotropin-releasing factor (CRF) from the hypothalamus stimulates ACTH secretion from the pituitary, which in turn stimulates cortisol and androgen production by the adrenal cortex. Cortisol is excreted as urinary free cortisol and various 17-oxogenic steroids.

Cushing's syndrome This is the clinical state produced by chronic glucocorticoid excess + loss of the normal feedback mechanisms of the hypothalamic–pituitary–adrenal axis and loss of circadian rhythm of cortisol secretion (normally highest on waking). The chief cause is oral steroids. Endogenous causes are rare: 80% are due to ↑ACTH; of these a pituitary adenoma (Cushing's disease) is the commonest cause.

1 **ACTH-dependent causes (↑ACTH)**
   - **Cushing's disease** Bilateral adrenal hyperplasia from an ACTH-secreting pituitary adenoma (usually a microadenoma, p228). ♀:♂ >1:1. Peak age: 30–50yrs. A low-dose dexamethasone test (see BOX 'Investigating suspected Cushing's disease') leads to no change in plasma cortisol, but 8mg may be enough to more than halve morning cortisol (as occurs in normals).
   - **Ectopic ACTH production** Especially small cell lung cancer and carcinoid tumours, p266. Specific features: pigmentation (due to ↑↑ACTH), hypokalaemic metabolic alkalosis (↑↑cortisol leads to mineralocorticoid activity), weight loss, hyperglycaemia. Classical features of Cushing's are often absent. Dexamethasone even in high doses (8mg) fails to suppress cortisol production.
   - **Rarely, ectopic CRF production** Some thyroid (medullary) and prostate cancers.
2 **ACTH-independent causes (↓ACTH due to −ve feedback)**
   - **Iatrogenic** Pharmacological doses of steroids (common).
   - **Adrenal adenoma/cancer** (May cause abdo pain ± virilization in ♀, p224.) Because the tumour is autonomous, dexamethasone in any dose won't suppress cortisol.
   - **Adrenal nodular hyperplasia** (As for adrenal adenoma, no dexamethasone suppression.)
   - **Rarely** *Carney complex*, p217. *McCune–Albright syndrome*, see OHCS p854.

Symptoms ↑Weight; mood change (depression, lethargy, irritability, psychosis); proximal weakness; gonadal dysfunction (irregular menses; hirsutism; erectile dysfunction); acne; recurrent Achilles tendon rupture; occasionally virilization if ♀.

Signs Central obesity; plethoric, moon face; buffalo hump; supraclavicular fat distribution; skin & muscle atrophy; bruises; purple abdominal striae (fig 5.20); osteoporosis; ↑BP; ↑glucose; infection-prone; poor healing. Signs of the cause (eg abdo mass).

Tests Random plasma cortisols may mislead, as illness, time of day, and stress (eg venepuncture) influence results. Also, don't rely on imaging to localize the cause: non-functioning 'incidentalomas' occur in ~5% on adrenal CT and ~10% on pituitary MRI. MRI detects only ~70% of pituitary tumours causing Cushing's (many are too small).

Treatment Depends on the cause.
- **Iatrogenic** Stop medications if possible.
- **Cushing's disease** Selective removal of pituitary adenoma (trans-sphenoidally). Bilateral adrenalectomy if source unlocatable, or recurrence post-op (complication: *Nelson's syndrome*: ↑skin pigmentation due to ↑↑ACTH from an enlarging pituitary tumour, as adrenalectomy removes −ve feedback; responds to pituitary radiation).
- **Adrenal adenoma or carcinoma** Adrenalectomy: 'cures' adenomas but rarely cures cancer. Radiotherapy & adrenolytic drugs (mitotane) follow if carcinoma.
- **Ectopic ACTH** Surgery if tumour is located and hasn't spread. Metyrapone, ketoconazole, and fluconazole ↓cortisol secretion pre-op or if awaiting effects of radiation. Intubation + mifepristone (competes with cortisol at receptors) + etomidate (blocks cortisol synthesis) may be needed, eg in severe ACTH-associated psychosis.

Prognosis Untreated Cushing's has ↑vascular mortality.[17] Treated, prognosis is good (but myopathy, obesity, menstrual irregularity, ↑BP, osteoporosis, subtle mood changes and DM often remain—so follow up carefully, and manage individually).

Investigating suspected Cushing's syndrome

First, confirm the diagnosis (a raised plasma cortisol), then localize the source on the basis of laboratory testing. Use imaging studies to confirm the likely source.

1st-line tests *Overnight dexamethasone suppression test:* a good outpatient test. Dexamethasone 1mg PO at midnight; do serum cortisol at 9AM. Normally, cortisol suppresses to <50nmol/L; no suppression in Cushing's syndrome. False −ve rate: <2%; false +ves: 2% normal, 13% obese, and 23% of inpatients. *NB:* false +ves (*pseudo-Cushing's*) are seen in depression, obesity, alcohol excess, and inducers of liver enzymes (↑rate of dexamethasone metabolism, eg phenytoin, phenobarbital, rifampicin, p681). *24h urinary free cortisol:* (normal: <280nmol/24h) is an alternative.

2nd-line tests If 1st-line tests abnormal: *48h dexamethasone suppression test:* give dexamethasone 0.5mg/6h PO for 2d. Measure cortisol at 0 and 48h (last test at 6h after last dose). Again, in Cushing's syndrome, there is a failure to suppress cortisol. *48h high-dose dexamethasone suppression test:* (2mg/6h) may distinguish pituitary (suppression) from other causes (no/part suppression). *Midnight cortisol:* admit (unless salivary cortisol used). Often inaccurate due to measurement issues. Normal circadian rhythm (cortisol *lowest* at midnight, *highest* early morning) is lost in Cushing's syndrome. Midnight blood, via a cannula during sleep, shows cortisol ↑ in Cushing's. Late night salivary cortisol can also be used as a 2nd-line test.

Localization tests (Where is the lesion?) If the 1st- and 2nd-line tests are +ve— *plasma ACTH. If ACTH is undetectable,* an adrenal tumour is likely → CT/MRI adrenal glands. If no mass, proceed to *adrenal vein sampling. If ACTH is detectable,* distinguish a pituitary cause from ectopic ACTH production by high-dose suppression test or *corticotropin-releasing hormone (CRH) test:* 100mcg ovine or human CRH IV. Measure cortisol at 120min. Cortisol rises with pituitary disease but not with ectopic ACTH production.

If tests indicate that cortisol responds to manipulation, Cushing's disease is likely. Image the pituitary (MRI) and consider *bilateral inferior petrosal sinus blood sampling.*

If tests indicate that cortisol does not respond to manipulation, hunt for the source of ectopic ACTH—eg IV contrast CT of chest, abdomen, and pelvis ± MRI of neck, thorax, and abdomen, eg for small ACTH-secreting carcinoid tumours.

5 Endocrinology

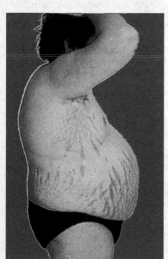

Fig 5.20 Hypercortisolism weakens skin; even normal stretching (or the pressure of obesity, as here) can make its elastin break—on healing we see these depressed purple scars (striae). Cortisone or rapid growth contributes to striae in other contexts: pregnancy, adolescence, weight lifting, sudden-onset obesity, or from strong steroid creams. Striae mature into silvery crescents looking like the underside of willow leaves. Unsightly immature striae may be improved by YAG lasers.

5 Endocrinology

Primary adrenocortical insufficiency (Addison's disease) is rare (~0.8/100 000), but can be fatal. Destruction of the adrenal cortex leads to glucocorticoid (cortisol) and mineralocorticoid (aldosterone) deficiency (fig 5.21). Signs are capricious: it is *'the unforgiving master of non-specificity and disguise'*.[18] You may diagnose a viral infection or anorexia nervosa in error (K+ is ↓ in the latter but ↑ in Addison's).

Physiology See fig 5.21.

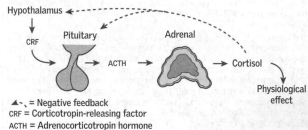

▲-◟ = Negative feedback
CRF = Corticotropin-releasing factor
ACTH = Adrenocorticotropin hormone

Fig 5.21 Pathways involved in adrenal function.

Causes 80% are due to autoimmunity in the UK. **Other causes** TB (commonest cause worldwide), adrenal metastases (eg from lung, breast, renal cancer), lymphoma, opportunistic infections in HIV (eg CMV, *Mycobacterium avium*, p396); adrenal haemorrhage (▶▶Waterhouse–Friderichsen syndrome, p698; antiphospholipid syndrome; SLE), congenital (late-onset congenital adrenal hyperplasia).

Secondary adrenal insufficiency The commonest cause is iatrogenic, due to long-term steroid therapy leading to suppression of the pituitary–adrenal axis. This only becomes apparent on withdrawal of the steroids. Other causes are rare and include hypothalamic–pituitary disease leading to ↓ACTH production. Mineralocorticoid production remains intact, and there is no hyperpigmentation as ↓ACTH.

Symptoms Often diagnosed late: lean, tanned, tired, tearful ± weakness, anorexia, dizzy, faints, flu-like myalgias/arthralgias. *Mood:* depression, psychosis. *GI:* nausea/vomiting, abdominal pain, diarrhoea/constipation. *Think of Addison's in all with unexplained abdominal pain or vomiting.* Pigmented palmar creases & buccal mucosa (↑ACTH; cross-reacts with melanin receptors). Postural hypotension. Vitiligo. ▶▶*Signs of critical deterioration* (p819): shock (↓BP, tachycardia), T°↑, coma.

Tests ↓Na+ & ↑K+ (due to ↓mineralocorticoid), ↓glucose (due to ↓cortisol). Also: uraemia, ↑Ca²⁺, eosinophilia, anaemia. Δ *Short ACTH stimulation test (Synacthen® test):* do plasma cortisol before and ½h after tetracosactide (Synacthen®) 250mcg IM/IV. Addison's is excluded if 30min cortisol >~550nmol/L (but exact threshold varies depending on laboratory assay). Steroid drugs may interfere with assays: ask lab. NB: in pregnancy and contraceptive pill, cortisol levels may be reassuring but falsely ↑, due to ↑cortisol-binding globulin. **Also** •*ACTH:* in Addison's, 9AM ACTH is ↑ (>300ng/L: inappropriately high). It is low in secondary causes. • *21-Hydroxylase adrenal autoantibodies:* +ve in autoimmune disease in >80%. • *Plasma renin & aldosterone:* to assess mineralocorticoid status. **Adrenal CT/MRI** consider adrenal imaging if autoantibodies are negative—eg to look for TB or metastatic disease.

Treatment ▶▶See p819 for Addisonian crisis (shocked). Replace steroids: ~15–25mg hydrocortisone daily, in 2–3 doses, eg 10mg on waking, 5mg at lunchtime, and 5mg in late afternoon. Avoid giving late (may cause insomnia). Mineralocorticoids to correct postural hypotension, ↓Na+, ↑K+: fludrocortisone PO from 50–200mcg daily. Adjust both on clinical grounds. If there is a poor response, suspect an associated autoimmune disease (check thyroid, do coeliac serology: p262).

Steroid use Advise wearing a bracelet declaring steroid use. Add 5–10mg hydro-cortisone to daily intake before strenuous activity/exercise. Double steroids in fe-brile illness, injury, or stress. Give out syringes and in-date IM hydrocortisone, and show how to inject 100mg IM if vomiting prevents oral intake (seek medical help; admit for IV fluids if dehydrated).

Follow-up Yearly (BP, U&E); watch for autoimmune diseases (pernicious anaemia).[3]

Prognosis (treated) Adrenal crises and infections do cause excess deaths: mean age at death for men is ~65yrs (11yrs <estimated life expectancy; women lose ~3yrs).

⚠️ **Exogenous steroid use**

Replacement steroids are vital in those taking long-term steroids when acutely unwell. Adrenal insufficiency may develop with deadly hypovolaemic shock, if additional steroid is not given. ▶▶See p819.

Steroid use Warn against abruptly stopping steroids. Emphasize that prescribing doctors/dentists/surgeons *must* know of steroid use: give *steroid card* (https://www.endocrinology.org/adrenal-crisis).

Excerpt from the notes of Miss E.L.R., 92 days before her death from undiagnosed Addison's disease. From the Coroner's Court …

'Typical day—wakes up at 11.30, still feels tired, then will have some breakfast and usually fall asleep on the couch. The most energy req. activity in last 1 month is—cooking herself a pasta meal. Then, totally exhausted will sleep more in pm, then eat some dinner. Goes to bed at 11pm—latest. Not able to concentrate... Used to weigh 45kg. Now weighs 42kg.'[19]

Placed on a page about Addison's disease, we might think there are sufficient clues to raise the suspicion of Addison's (even though her electrolytes were not particularly awry, and her pigmentation was barely perceptible). But change the context to our last busy clinic. We are a little distracted. The memory of Addison's is fading. Who among us will hear the alarm bell ring?

3 Autoimmune polyglandular syndromes types 1–4: 1 Monogenic syndrome (AIRE gene on chromosome 21); signs: candidiasis, hypoparathyroidism + Addison's. 2 (Schmidt syndrome.) Adrenal insufficiency + auto-immune thyroid disease ± DM ± pleuritis/pericarditis. 3 Autoimmune thyroid disease + other autoimmune conditions but *not* Addison's. 4 Autoimmune combinations not included in 1–3.

Primary hyperaldosteronism Excess production of aldosterone, independent of the renin–angiotensin system, causing ↑sodium and water retention, and ↓renin release. Consider if: hypertension, hypokalaemia, or alkalosis in someone not on diuretics. Commonest cause of secondary hypertension.

Symptoms Often asymptomatic or signs of hypokalaemia (p666): weakness (even quadriparesis), cramps, paraesthesiae, polyuria, polydipsia. ↑BP but not always.

Causes ~1/3 due to a solitary aldosterone-producing adenoma (some are linked to mutations in K^+ channels)[4]—*Conn's syndrome*. ~2/3 due to bilateral adrenocortical hyperplasia. Rare causes: adrenal carcinoma; or glucocorticoid-remediable aldosteronism (GRA)—the ACTH regulatory element of the 11β-hydroxylase gene fuses to the aldosterone synthase gene, ↑aldosterone production, & bringing it under the control of ACTH.

Tests Initial screening test with U&E, renin:aldosterone ratio. If positive, consider confirmatory saline infusion test, imaging of adrenals and adrenal vein sampling. Do not rely on a low K^+, as >20% are normokalaemic. For GRA (suspect if there is a family history of early hypertension), genetic testing is available. **Treatment** •*Conn's*: laparoscopic adrenalectomy is treatment of choice. Medical therapy with mineralocorticoid receptor antagonists (spironolactone) is an option for bilateral hyperplasia, or those with Conn's who are unfit for surgery or express preference for medical mgmt. Other drugs include amiloride. •*GRA:* dexamethasone 1mg/24h PO for 4wks, normalizes biochemistry but not always BP. If BP is still ↑, use spironolactone as an alternative. •*Adrenal carcinoma:* surgery ± post-operative adrenolytic therapy with mitotane—prognosis is poor.

Secondary hyperaldosteronism Due to a high renin from ↓renal perfusion, eg in renal artery stenosis, accelerated hypertension, diuretics, CCF, or hepatic failure.

Bartter's syndrome This is a major cause of congenital (autosomal recessive) salt wasting—via a sodium and chloride leak in the loop of Henle via mutations in channels and transporters. Presents in childhood with failure to thrive, polyuria, and polydipsia. BP is *normal*. Sodium loss leads to volume depletion, causing ↑renin and aldosterone production, leading to hypokalaemia and metabolic alkalosis, ↑urinary K^+ and Cl^-. **Treatment** K^+ replacement, NSAIDs (to inhibit prostaglandins), and ACE-i.

Phaeochromocytoma

Rare catecholamine-producing tumours. They arise from sympathetic paraganglia cells (= phaeochrome bodies), which are collections of chromaffin cells. They are usually found within the adrenal medulla. Extra-adrenal tumours (paragangliomas) are rarer, and often found by the aortic bifurcation (the organs of Zuckerkandl). Traditionally, phaeochromocytomas were roughly thought to follow the 10% rule: 10% malignant, 10% are extra-adrenal, 10% bilateral. Historically, it was also thought that 10% were familial—but it is now thought that ~30% are due to genetic mutations. Thus, family history is crucial and referral for genetic screening (particularly <50 years old). A dangerous but treatable cause of hypertension (in <0.1%).

Associations ~70% are sporadic; 30% are part of hereditary cancer syndromes (p209), eg MEN-2A and 2B, neurofibromatosis, von Hippel–Lindau syndrome, and associated with mutations in succinate dehydrogenase (SDH).

Classic triad Episodic headache, sweating, and tachycardia (± ↑, ↓, or ↔BP, see BOX 'Features of phaeochromocytoma').

Tests • *Biochemical:* plasma free metanephrines is first line. 24h urine for metanephrines/metadrenaline is an alternative if unavailable. • *Localization:* abdominal CT/MRI, or meta-iodobenzylguanidine (MIBG; chromaffin-seeking isotope) scan (can find extra-adrenal tumours, p722). **Treatment Surgery** α-blockade pre-op: phenoxybenzamine or doxazosin (α-blockers) is used before β-blocker to avoid crisis from unopposed α-adrenergic stimulation, β-block too if heart disease or tachycardic. *Consult the anaesthetist.* Post-op Do 24h urine metanephrine 2wks post-op, monitor BP (risk of ↓↓BP). ▶▶**Emergency** R p820. If malignant, chemotherapy or therapeutic radiolabelled MIBG may be used. **Follow-up** Lifelong: malignant recurrence may present late, genetic screening.

Hypertension: a common context for hyperaldosteronism tests

Think of Conn's in these contexts:
• Hypertension associated with hypokalaemia.
• Refractory hypertension, eg despite ≥3 antihypertensive drugs.
• Hypertension occurring before 40yrs of age (especially in women).

The approach to investigation remains controversial, but the simplest is to look for a suppressed renin and ↑aldosterone (may be normal if there is severe hypokalaemia). This is followed by a confirmatory saline infusion test, prior to proceeding with imaging. A CT or MRI of the adrenals is then performed to localize the cause. This should be done after hyperaldosteronism is proven, due to the high number of adrenal incidentalomas. If imaging shows a unilateral adenoma, *adrenal vein sampling* may be done (venous blood is sampled from both adrenals). If one side reveals increased aldosterone:cortisol ratio compared with the other (>3-fold difference), an adenoma is likely, and surgical excision is indicated. If no nodules or bilateral nodules are seen, think about adrenal hyperplasia or GRA.

▶NB: renal artery stenosis is a more common cause of refractory ↑BP and ↓K⁺ (p311).

Features of phaeochromocytoma (often episodic and often vague)

Try to diagnose before death: suspect if BP hard to control, accelerating, or episodic.
• **Heart** ↑Pulse; palpitations/VT; dyspnoea; faints; angina; MI/LVF; cardiomyopathy.[5]
• **CNS** Headache; visual disorder; dizziness; tremor; numbness; fits; encephalopathy; Horner's syndrome (paraganglioma); subarachnoid/CNS haemorrhage.
• **Psychological** Anxiety; panic; hyperactivity; confusion; episodic psychosis.
• **Gut** D&V; abdominal pain over tumour site; mass; mesenteric vasoconstriction.
• **Others** Sweats/flushes; heat intolerance; pallor; ↑T°; backache; haemoptysis.

Symptoms may be precipitated by straining, exercise, stress, abdominal pressure, surgery, or by agents such as β-blockers, IV contrast agents, metoclopramide, or the tricyclics. The site of the tumour may determine precipitants, eg if pelvic, precipitants include sexual intercourse, parturition, defecation, and micturition. Adrenergic crises may last minutes to days. Suddenly patients feel 'as if about to die'—and then get better, or go on to develop a stroke or cardiogenic shock. On examination, there may be no signs, or hypertension ± signs of heart failure/cardiomyopathy (± paradoxical shock, similar to Takotsubo's[6]), episodic thyroid swelling, glycosuria during attacks, or terminal haematuria from a bladder phaeochromocytoma.

---

4 Tumours from the zona **g**lomerulosa, zona **f**asciculata, or zona **r**eticularis associate with syndromes of ↑ **miner**alocorticoids, **g**lucocorticoids, or **a**ndrogens respectively, usually; remember '**GFR** ≈ **miner GA**'.
5 *Takotsubo cardiomyopathy* (= stress- or catecholamine-induced cardiomyopathy/broken heart syndrome) may cause sudden chest pain mimicking MI, with ↑ST segments, and its signature apical ballooning on echo (also ↓ejection fraction) occurring during catecholamine surges. It is a cause of MI in the presence of normal arteries. The stress may be medical (SAH, p474) or psychological.

Hirsutism Common (10% of women) and usually benign. It implies male pattern hair growth in women. Causes are familial, idiopathic, or are due to ↑androgen secretion by the *ovary* (eg polycystic ovarian syndrome, ovarian cancer, *OHCS* p174), the *adrenal gland* (eg non-classic congenital adrenal hyperplasia, *OHCS* p115, Cushing's syndrome, adrenal cancer), or *drugs* (eg steroids). **Polycystic ovarian syndrome (PCOS)** causes secondary oligo- or amenorrhoea, infertility, obesity, acne, and hirsutism (*OHCS* p116). Ultrasound: bilateral polycystic ovaries. Blood tests: ↑testosterone (if ≥5nmol/L, look for an androgen-producing adrenal or ovarian tumour), ↓sex-hormone binding globulin, ↑LH:FSH ratio (not consistent), TSH, lipids. Address any feelings of lack of conformity to society's perceived norms of feminine beauty. **Management** Healthy eating, optimize weight, shaving; laser photoepilation; wax; creams, eg eflornithine, or electrolysis (expensive/time-consuming, but effective).
- Oestrogens: combined contraceptive pill (*OHCS* p152)—third-generation are first line. Yasmin® and co-cyprindiol contain progestins with lower androgenicity (desogestrel and cyproterone) but may have higher rate of VTE so use second line. Stop co-cyprindiol 3–4 months after hirsutism has completely resolved because of increased VTE risk. If COCs are contraindicated or have not worked (after 6/12), refer the woman to secondary care for specialist treatment.
- Metformin (helps with insulin resistance) and spironolactone are sometimes tried.
- Clomifene is used for infertility (a fertility expert should prescribe).

Virilism Onset of amenorrhoea, clitoromegaly, deep voice, temporal hair recession + hirsutism. Look for an androgen-secreting adrenal or ovarian tumour.

Gynaecomastia (Ie abnormal amount of breast tissue in men; may occur in normal puberty.) Oestrogen/androgen ratio↑ (vs galactorrhoea in which prolactin is ↑). **Causes** Hypogonadism (see BOX 'Male hypogonadism'), liver cirrhosis (↑oestrogens), hyperthyroidism, tumours (oestrogen-producing, eg testicular, adrenal; human chorionic gonadotropin-producing, eg testicular, bronchial); drugs: oestrogens, spironolactone, digoxin, testosterone, marijuana; if stopping is impossible, consider testosterone if hypogonadism ± anti-oestrogen (tamoxifen).

Erectile dysfunction Erections result from neuronal release of nitric oxide (NO) which, via cGMP and Ca²⁺, hyperpolarizes and thus relaxes vascular and trabecular smooth muscle cells, allowing engorgement. Common after 50yrs, and often multifactorial. A psychological facet is common (esp. if erectile dysfunction occurs only in some situations, if onset coincides with stress, and if early morning erections still occur: these also persist in early organic disease). **Organic causes** The big three: smoking, alcohol, and diabetes (reduce NO + autonomic neuropathy). Also *endocrine:* hypogonadism, hyperthyroidism, ↑prolactin; *neurological:* cord lesions, MS, autonomic neuropathy; *pelvic surgery:* eg bladder-neck, prostate; *radiotherapy;* *atheroma*; *renal* or *hepatic failure*; *prostatic hyperplasia*; *penile anomalies:* eg postpriapism, or Peyronie's (p694); *drugs:* digoxin, β-blockers, diuretics, antipsychotics, antidepressants, oestrogens, finasteride, narcotics. **Workup** After a full sexual and psychological history do: U&E, LFT, fasting glucose, HbA1c, TFT, LH, FSH, lipids, 9AM fasting testosterone ± prolactin. Other specialized tests such as Doppler rarely required. **R** • Treat causes. • Counselling. • Oral phosphodiesterase (PDE5) inhibitors ↑cGMP. Erection isn't automatic (depends on erotic stimuli). Sildenafil 25–100mg ½–1h pre-sex (food and alcohol upset absorption). SE Headache (16%); flushing (10%); dyspepsia (7%); stuffy nose (4%); transient blue-green tingeing of vision (inhibition of retinal PDE6). CI See BOX 'Contraindications and cautions to PD5 inhibitors'. Tadalafil (long *t½*) 10–20mg ½–36h pre-sex. Don't use > once daily. Vardenafil (5–20mg). • Vacuum aids (ideal for penile rehabilitation after radical prostatectomy), intracavernosal injections, transurethral pellets, and prostheses (inflatable or malleable; partners may receive unnatural sensations). • Corpus cavernosum tissue engineering (eg on acellular collagen scaffolds) is in its infancy.

Contraindications and cautions to PD5 inhibitors

►►Contraindications
- Concurrent use of nitrates.
- BP high or systolic <90mmHg/arrhythmia.
- Degenerative retinal disorders, eg retinitis pigmentosa.
- Unstable angina/stroke <6 months ago.
- Myocardial infarction <90 days ago.

Cautions ► Angina (especially if during intercourse).
- Bleeding; peptic ulcer (sildenafil).
- Marked hepatic or renal impairment.
- Peyronie's disease or cavernosal fibrosis.
- Risk of priapism (sickle cell anaemia, myeloma, leukaemia).
- Concurrent complex antihypertensive regimens.
- Dyspnoea on minimal effort (sexual activity may be unsupportable).

Use in coronary artery disease has been a question, but is probably OK.[20]

Interactions Nitrates (contraindication); cytochrome P450 (CYP3A) inducers: macrolides, protease inhibitors, theophyllines, azole antifungals, rifampicin, phenytoin, carbamazepine, phenobarbital, grapefruit juice (↑bioavailability). Caution if α-blocker use; avoid vardenafil with type 1A (eg quinidine; procainamide) and type 3 anti-arrhythmics (sotalol; amiodarone)—as well as nitrates as above-mentioned.

Male hypogonadism

Hypogonadism is failure of testes to produce testosterone, sperm, or both. Features: small testes, ↓libido, erectile dysfunction, loss of pubic hair, ↓muscle bulk, ↑fat, gynaecomastia, osteoporosis, ↓mood. If prepubertal: ↓virilization; incomplete puberty; eunuchoid body; reduced secondary sex characteristics. Causes include:

Primary hypogonadism Due to testicular failure, eg from: • Local trauma, torsion, chemotherapy/irradiation. • Post-orchitis, eg mumps, HIV, brucellosis, leprosy. • Renal failure, liver cirrhosis, or alcohol excess (toxic to Leydig cells). • Chromosomal abnormalities, eg Klinefelter's syndrome (47XXY)—delayed sexual development, small testes, and gynaecomastia. Anorchia is rare.

Secondary hypogonadism ↓Gonadotropins (LH & FSH), eg from: • Hypopituitarism. • Prolactinoma. • Kallman's syndrome—isolated gonadotropin-releasing hormone deficiency, often with anosmia and colour blindness. • Systemic illness (eg COPD; HIV; DM). • Laurence–Moon–Biedl and Prader–Willi syndromes (OHCS p852 & p856). • Age.

℞ (p226) If total testosterone ≤8nmol/L, on 2 mornings (or <15 if ↑LH too) and ↓muscle bulk, testosterone may help, eg 1% dermal gel (Testogel®). Heart, bladder, and sexual function may perk up in age-related hypogonadism. Beware medicalizing ageing!

CI Severe CKD; polycythaemia; prostate, breast, or liver ca. Monitor PSA and Hct.

5 Endocrinology

Hypopituitarism entails ↓secretion of anterior pituitary hormones and/or posterior pituitary hormones (figs 5.3, p199, 5.22). They are affected in this order: growth hormone (GH), gonadotropins: follicle-stimulating hormone (FSH) and luteinizing hormone (LH), thyroid-stimulating hormone (TSH), and adrenocorticotrophic hormone (ACTH), prolactin (PRL). Panhypopituitarism is deficiency of all anterior hormones, usually caused by irradiation, surgery, or pituitary tumour.

Causes are at three levels. 1 **Hypothalamus** Kallman's syndrome (p225), tumour, inflammation, infection (meningitis, TB), ischaemia. 2 **Pituitary stalk** Trauma, surgery, tumour (craniopharyngioma, p228), meningioma, carotid artery aneurysm, inflammation. 3 **Pituitary** Tumour, irradiation, inflammation, autoimmunity,[6] infiltration (haemochromatosis, amyloid, metastases), ischaemia (pituitary apoplexy, p228; DIC[7]; Sheehan's syndrome[8]).

Features Due to:

1 **Hormone lack** •*GH:* central obesity, atherosclerosis, dry wrinkly skin, ↓strength, ↓balance, ↓wellbeing, ↓exercise ability, ↓cardiac output, osteoporosis, ↓glucose. •*Gonadotropin (FSH; LH):* ♀: oligomenorrhoea or amenorrhoea, ↓fertility, ↓libido, osteoporosis, breast atrophy, dyspareunia. ♂: erectile dysfunction, ↓libido, ↓muscle bulk, hypogonadism (↓hair, all over; small testes; ↓ejaculate volume; ↓spermatogenesis). •*Thyroid:* as for hypothyroidism (p214). •*Corticotropin:* as for adrenal insufficiency (p220). NB: no ↑skin pigmentation as ↓ACTH. •*Prolactin:* rare: absent lactation.

2 **Causes** Eg pituitary tumour (p228), causing mass effect, or hormone secretion with ↓secretion of other hormones—eg prolactinoma, acromegaly, rarely Cushing's.

Tests (The triple stimulation test is now rarely done.)
• **Basal tests** LH and FSH (↓ or ↔), testosterone or oestradiol (↓); TSH (↓ or ↔), T₄ (↓); prolactin (may be ↑, from loss of hypothalamic dopamine that normally inhibits its release), insulin-like growth factor-1 (IGF-1; ↓—used as a measure of GH axis, p232), cortisol (↓). Also do U&E (↓Na⁺from dilution), ↓Hb (normochromic, normocytic).
• **Dynamic tests** 1 Short Synacthen® test: (p220) to assess the adrenal axis.
2 Insulin tolerance test (ITT): done in specialist centres to assess the adrenal and GH axes. CI: epilepsy, heart disease, adrenal failure. Consult lab first. It involves IV insulin to induce hypoglycaemia, causing stress to ↑ cortisol and GH secretion. It is done in the morning (water only taken from 22:00h the night before). Have 50% glucose and hydrocortisone to hand and IV access. Glucose must fall below 2.2mmol/L and the patient should become symptomatic when cortisol and GH are taken. Normal: GH >20mu/L & peak cortisol >550nmol/L (exact threshold varies locally).
3 Arginine + growth hormone-releasing hormone test.
4 Glucagon stimulation test is alternative when ITT is contraindicated.
• **Investigate cause** MRI scan to look for a hypothalamic or pituitary lesion.

Treatment Refer to an endocrinologist for assessment of pituitary function and to oversee hormone replacement and treatment of underlying cause.
• *Hydrocortisone* for 2° adrenal failure (p220) ►before other hormones are given. Risk of precipitation of adrenal crisis if thyroxine given before hydrocortisone.
• Thyroxine if hypothyroid (p214, but TSH is useless for monitoring).
• Hypogonadism (for symptoms and to prevent osteoporosis). ♂: options include topical testosterone gels (eg Testogel®), or testosterone undecanoate 1000mg IM every 12 weeks. ♀: (premenopausal): *Hormone replacement therapy:* transdermal oestradiol patches, or oral HRT (this needs a progestogenic component in women with intact uterus) ± testosterone or dehydroepiandrosterone (DHEA, in hypoandrogenic women; a small amount may improve wellbeing and sexual function, and help bone mineral density and lean body mass).
• *Gonadotropin* therapy is needed to induce fertility in both men and women.
• Growth hormone (GH). Somatotrophin mimics human GH. It addresses problems of ↑fat mass, ↓bone mass, ↓lean body mass (muscle bulk), ↓exercise capacity, and problems with heat intolerance.

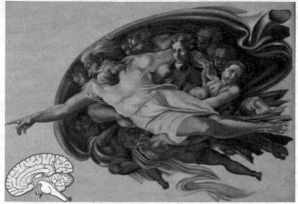

Fig 5.22 Neuroendocrinology: emotions ⇄ thoughts ⇄ actions. As Michelangelo foretold (in his *Creation of Adam*) 'all gods and demons that have ever existed are within us as possibilities, desires, and ways of escape'. Within the dark red vault of our skull we see human and god-like forms reaching out, as thoughts escape into actions—with legs extending into our brainstem (b) and a fist is pushing from our hypothalamus into the pituitary stalk (p). Above the pituitary we have thoughts, ideas, impulses, and neurotransmitters. Below we have hormones. Between is the realm of neuroendocrinology—the neurosecretory cells which turn emotions into the releasing factors for the pituitary hormones (**fig 54, p199**).

Image courtesy of Gary Bevans; quote from Frank Lynn Meshberger.
Michelangelo, Renaissance Man of the Brain, Too?

6 Autoimmune hypophysitis (= inflamed pituitary) mimics pituitary adenoma. It may be triggered by pregnancy or immunotherapy blocking CTLA-4 and PD-1. No pituitary autoantigen is yet used diagnostically.
7 Snake bite is a common cause in India (eg when associated with acute kidney injury).
8 Sheehan's syndrome is pituitary necrosis after postpartum haemorrhage.

Pituitary tumours (almost always benign adenomas) account for 10% of intracranial tumours (figs 5.23, 5.24). They may be divided by size: a microadenoma is a tumour <1cm across, and a macroadenoma is >1cm. There are three histological types (table 5.5):

1 *Chromophobe* 70%. Many are non-secretory,[9] some cause hypopituitarism. Half produce prolactin (PRL); a few produce ACTH or GH. Local pressure effect in 30%.
2 *Acidophil* 15%. Secrete GH or PRL. Local pressure effect in 10%.
3 *Basophil* 15%. Secrete ACTH. Local pressure effect rare.

Symptoms are caused by pressure, hormones (eg galactorrhoea), or hypopituitarism (p226). FSH-secreting tumours can cause macro-orchidism in men, but are rare.

Features of local pressure Headache, visual field defects (bitemporal hemianopia, due to compression of the optic chiasm), palsy of cranial nerves III, IV, VI (pressure or invasion of the cavernous sinus; fig 5.25). Also, diabetes insipidus (DI; p234; more likely from hypothalamic disease or post-pituitary surgery); disturbance of hypothalamic centres of T°, sleep, and appetite; erosion through floor of sella leading to CSF rhinorrhoea.

Tests MRI defines intra- and supra-sellar extension; accurate assessment of visual fields; screening tests: PRL, IGF-1 (p232), ACTH, 9AM cortisol, TFTs, LH/FSH, testosterone in ♂, short Synacthen® test. OGTT if acromegaly suspected (p232). If Cushing's suspected, see p219. Urine/serum osmolality ± water deprivation test if DI is suspected (p234).

Treatment Start hormone replacement as needed (p226). Ensure steroids are given before levothyroxine, as thyroxine may precipitate an adrenal crisis. For Cushing's disease see p219, prolactinoma p230, acromegaly p232.

• **Surgery** (fig 5.26) Most pituitary surgery is trans-sphenoidal, but if there is supra-sellar extension, a trans-frontal approach may be used. For prolactinoma, 1st-line treatment is medical with a dopamine agonist, p230. *Pre-op:* ensure hydrocortisone 100mg IV/IM. Subsequent cortisol replacement and reassessment varies with local protocols: get advice. *Post-op:* retest pituitary function (p226) to assess replacement needs. Repeating dynamic tests for adrenal function ≥6 weeks post-op.

• **Radiotherapy** (Eg stereotactic.) Good for residual or recurrent adenomas (good rates of tumour control and normalization of excess hormone secretion).[11]

Post-op Recurrence may occur late after surgery, so long-term follow-up is required. Fertility should be discussed: this may be reduced post-op due to ↓gonadotropins.

Pituitary apoplexy Infarction of the pituitary gland due to either haemorrhage or ischaemia. Suspect if acute-onset headache, meningism, ↓GCS, ophthalmoplegia/ visual field defect, especially if there is a known tumour (may present like subarachnoid haemorrhage). Apoplexy is a medical emergency—as prompt administration of steroids may be life-saving. ℞ Urgent steroids (hydrocortisone 100mg IV); involve a pituitary multidisciplinary team; if marked neuro-ophthalmic signs, early surgery (within 8 days) is usually indicated.

Craniopharyngioma Not strictly a pituitary tumour: it originates from Rathke's pouch so is situated between the pituitary and 3rd ventricle floor. They are rare, but are the commonest childhood intracranial tumour. Over 50% present in childhood with growth failure; adults may present with amenorrhoea, ↓libido, hypothalamic symptoms (eg DI, hyperphagia, sleep disturbance) or tumour mass effect. **Tests** CT/ MRI (calcification in 50%, may also be seen on skull x-ray). **Treatment** Surgery ± post-op radiation; test pituitary function post-op.

Table 5.5 Frequency of hormones secreted by pituitary adenomas based on immunohistochemistry

Hormone	%	Hormone	%
PRL only (→prolactinoma)	35%	ACTH (→Cushing's disease)	7%
GH only (→acromegaly)	20%	LH/FSH/TSH	≥1%*
PRL and GH	7%	No obvious hormone	30%

* Sensitive methods of TSH measurement have improved recognition of TSH-secreting tumours. These are now more frequently found at microadenoma stage, medially located, and *without* associated hormone hypersecretion. In these tumours, somatostatin analogues (p232) are very helpful. See also Socin *et al.*, *Eur J Endocrinol.* 2003;148:433–42.

9 If <1cm, usually 'incidentaloma'; most non-functioning macroadenomas are revealed by mass effect and/ or hypopituitarism. Here, recurrence after surgery is common, so follow carefully with MRIs.

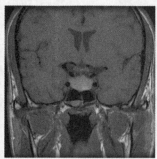 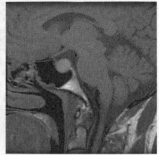

Fig 5.23 Coronal T1-weighted MRI of the brain (no gadolinium contrast) showing a lesion in the pituitary fossa, most likely a haemorrhagic pituitary adenoma. Differential diagnosis includes a Rathke's cleft cyst.

Courtesy of Norwich Radiology Dept.

Fig 5.24 Sagittal T1-weighted MRI of the brain (no gadolinium contrast) showing a lesion in the pituitary fossa (see fig 5.23).

Courtesy of Norwich Radiology Dept.

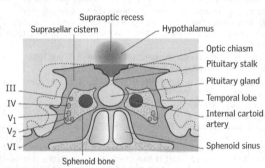
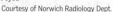

Fig 5.25 The pituitary gland's relationships to cranial nerves III, IV, V, and VI.

Supraoptic recess

Suprasellar cistern — Hypothalamus

Optic chiasm

Pituitary stalk

Pituitary gland

III
IV — Temporal lobe
V₁
V₂ — Internal cartoid artery
VI

Sphenoid sinus

Sphenoid bone

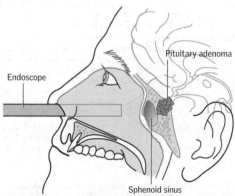

Endoscope

Pituitary adenoma

Sphenoid sinus

Fig 5.26 Endoscopic surgery is now possible for pituitary surgery.

5 Endocrinology

This is the commonest hormonal disturbance of the pituitary. It presents earlier in women (menstrual disturbance) but later in men (eg with erectile dysfunction and/or mass effects). Prolactin stimulates lactation.[10,11] Raised levels lead to hypogonadism, infertility, and osteoporosis, by inhibiting secretion of gonadotropin-releasing hormone (hence ↓LH/FSH and ↓testosterone or oestrogen).

Causes of raised plasma prolactin PRL is secreted from the anterior pituitary and release is inhibited by dopamine produced in the hypothalamus. Hyperprolactinaemia may result from: 1 Excess production from the pituitary, eg prolactinoma. 2 Disinhibition, by compression of the pituitary stalk, reducing local dopamine levels. 3 Use of a dopamine antagonist. A PRL of 1000–5000mU/L may result from any, but >5000 is likely to be due to a prolactinoma, with macroadenomas (>10mm) having the highest levels, eg 10 000–100 000.
- **Physiological** Pregnancy; breastfeeding; stress. Acute rises occur post-orgasm.[10]
- **Drugs (most common cause)** Metoclopramide; haloperidol; methyldopa; oestrogens; ecstasy/MDMA;[11] antipsychotics (a reason for 'non-compliance': sustained hyperprolactinaemia may cause ↓libido, anorgasmia, and erectile dysfunction).
- **Diseases** *Prolactinoma:* micro- or macroadenoma. *Stalk damage:* pituitary adenomas, surgery, trauma. *Hypothalamic disease:* craniopharyngioma, other tumours. *Other:* hypothyroidism (due to ↑TRH), chronic renal failure (↓excretion).

Symptoms ♀ Amenorrhoea or oligomenorrhoea; infertility; galactorrhoea (fig 5.27). Also: ↓libido, ↑weight, dry vagina. ♂ Erectile dysfunction, ↓facial hair, galactorrhoea. May present late with osteoporosis or local pressure effects from the tumour (p228).

Tests Basal PRL: non-stressful venepuncture between 09.00 and 16.00h. Do a pregnancy test, TFT, U&E. MRI pituitary if other causes are ruled out.

Management Refer to a specialist endocrinology clinic. Dopamine agonists (bromocriptine or cabergoline) are 1st line.

Microprolactinomas A tumour <10mm on MRI (~25% of us have asymptomatic microprolactinomas). Cabergoline, a dopamine agonist, ↓PRL secretion, restores menstrual cycles and ↓tumour size. The initial dose is 0.25mg twice a week or 0.5mg once a week. SE: nausea, depression, postural hypotension (minimize by giving at night), or rarely, impulse-control disorders. If pregnancy is planned, use barrier contraception until 2 periods have occurred. If subsequent pregnancy occurs, stop cabergoline after the 1st missed period. An alternative dopamine agonist is bromocriptine: less effective but better safety data in pregnancy. NB: ergot alkaloids (bromocriptine and cabergoline) can cause fibrosis (eg echocardiograms are needed). Trans-sphenoidal surgery may be considered if intolerant of dopamine agonists. It has a high success rate, but there are risks of permanent hormone deficiency and prolactinoma recurrence, and so it is usually reserved as a 2nd-line treatment.

Macroprolactinomas A tumour >10mm diameter on MRI. As they are near the optic chiasm, there may be ↓acuity, diplopia, ophthalmoplegia, visual-field loss, and optic atrophy. Treat initially with a dopamine agonist (cabergoline if fertility is the goal). Surgery is rarely needed, but consider if visual symptoms or pressure effects which fail to respond to medical treatment. Cabergoline, and in some cases radiation therapy, may be required post-op as complete surgical resection is uncommon. If pregnant, monitor closely ideally in a combined endocrine/antenatal clinic as there is ↑risk of expansion.

Follow-up Monitor PRL. If headache or visual loss, check fields (? do MRI). Medication can be decreased after 2yrs, but recurrence of hyperprolactinaemia and expansion of the tumour may occur, and so these patients should be monitored carefully.

---

10 The prolactin increase (♂ and ♀) after coitus is ~400% greater than after masturbation; post-orgasmic prolactin is part of a feedback loop decreasing arousal by inhibiting central dopaminergic processes. The size of post-orgasmic prolactin increase is a neurohormonal index of sexual satisfaction.
11 MDMA also ↑oxytocin; prolactin + oxytocin are thought to mediate post-orgasmic wellbeing.

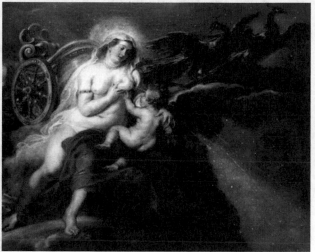

Fig 5.27 Galactorrhoea can be prolific enough to create medium-sized galaxies (bottom right). In the *Birth of the Milky Way* Hera is depicted by Rubens in her chariot, being drawn through the night sky by ominous black peacocks. Between journeys, she enjoyed discussing difficult endocrinological topics with her husband Zeus (who was also her brother), such as whether women or men find sexual intercourse more enjoyable. Hera inclined to the latter—and it is on this flimsy evidence, and her gorgeous galactorrhoea, that we diagnose her hyperprolactinaemia (which is known to decrease desire, lubrication, orgasm, and satisfaction). In the end, this issue was settled, in favour of Zeus's view, by Tiresias, who had unique insight into this intriguing question: every time this soothsayer saw two snakes entwined, (s)he changed sex, so coming to know a thing or two about sex and sexual pleasure. This is a primordial example of an 'N-of-1' trial, where the subject is their own control. Generalizability can be a problem with this methodology.

Image is in the public domain.

This is due to ↑secretion of GH (growth hormone) from a pituitary tumour (99%) or very rarely hyperplasia, eg via ectopic GH-releasing hormone from a carcinoid tumour. ♀:♂≈1:1. Incidence: UK 3/million/yr. ~5% are associated with MEN-1 (p217). GH stimulates bone and soft tissue growth through ↑secretion of insulin-like growth factor-1 (IGF-1).

Symptoms Acroparaesthesia (akron = extremities); amenorrhoea; ↓libido; headache; ↑sweating; snoring; arthralgia; backache; fig 5.28: 'My rings don't fit, nor my old shoes, and now I've got a wonky bite (malocclusion) and curly hair. I put on lots of weight, all muscle and looked good for a while; now I look so haggard'.

Signs (See BOX 'Signs of acromegaly'.) Often predate diagnosis by >4yrs. If acromegaly occurs before bony epiphyses fuse (rare), gigantism occurs.

Complications (May present with CCF or ketoacidosis.)
• Impaired glucose tolerance (~40%), DM (~15%).
• Vascular: ↑BP, left ventricular hypertrophy (±dilatation/CCF), cardiomyopathy, arrhythmias. There is ↑risk of ischaemic heart disease and stroke (?due to ↑BP ± insulin resistance and GH-induced increase in fibrinogen and decrease in protein S).
• Neoplasia: ↑colon cancer risk; colonoscopy may be needed.[16]

Acromegaly in pregnancy (Subfertility is common.) Pregnancy may be normal; signs and chemistry may remit. Monitor glucose.

Tests ↑IGF-1: preferred screening test. GH Don't rely on random GH as secretion is pulsatile and during peaks acromegalic and normal levels overlap. GH also ↑ in: stress, sleep, puberty, and pregnancy. Normally GH secretion is inhibited by high glucose, and GH hardly detectable. In acromegaly GH release fails to suppress.
• If ↑IGF-1 (p226), an oral glucose tolerance test (OGTT) is needed. If the lowest GH value during OGTT is above 1mcg/L (3mIU/L), acromegaly is confirmed. With general use of very sensitive assays, it has been said that this cut-off be decreased to 0.3mcg/L (0.9mIU/L).[22] **Method** Collect samples for GH glucose at: 0, 30, 60, 90, 120, 150min. Possible false +ves: puberty, pregnancy, hepatic and renal disease, anorexia nervosa, and DM.
• MRI scan of pituitary fossa. • Look for hypopituitarism (p226).
• Visual fields and acuity. • ECG, echo. Old photos if possible. Check HbA1c.

Treatment Aim to correct (or prevent) tumour compression by excising the lesion; aim for a GH level of <1mcg/L and normal IGF-1. A 3-part strategy: 1 Trans-sphenoidal surgery is often 1st line. 2 If surgery fails to correct GH/IGF-1 hypersecretion, try somatostatin analogues (SSAs) and/or radiotherapy, SSAs being generally preferred. Example: octreotide (Sandostatin LAR®, given monthly IM), or lanreotide (Somatuline LA®). SE: pain at the injection site; gastrointestinal: abdominal cramps, flatulence, loose stools, ↑gallstones; impaired glucose tolerance. 3 The GH antagonist pegvisomant (recombinant GH analogue) is used if resistant or intolerant to SSA. It suppresses IGF-1 to normal in 90%, but GH levels may rise; rarely tumour size increases, so monitor closely. **Radiotherapy** If unsuited to surgery or as adjuvant; may take years to work. **Follow-up** Yearly GH, IGF-1 ± OGTT, cardiovascular risk reduction, intermittent colonoscopy, photos (fig 5.29). **Prognosis** May return to normal (any excess mortality is mostly vascular). 16% get diabetes with SSAs vs ~13% after surgery.

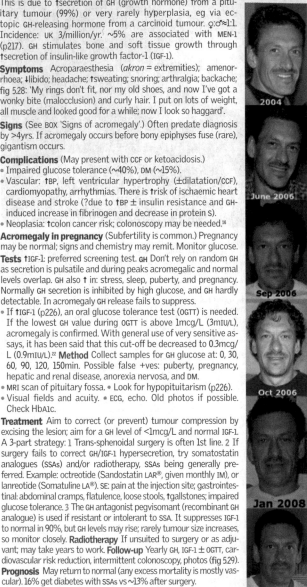

Fig 5.28 Acromegaly. Courtesy of Omar Rio.
My life with acromegaly. (http://odelrio.blogspot.com)

2004
June 2006
Sep 2006
Oct 2006
Jan 2008
Aug 2008
2 weeks Post Op

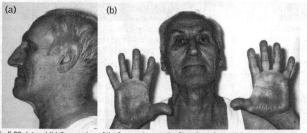

Fig 5.29 (a) and (b) Coarsening of the face and ↑growth of hands and mandible (prognathism).

Signs of acromegaly

- ↑Growth of hands (fig 5.29b; may be spade-like), jaw (fig 5.29a), and feet (sole may encroach on the dorsum).
- Coarsening face; wide nose.
- Big supraorbital ridges.
- Macroglossia (big tongue).
- Widely spaced teeth.
- Puffy lips, eyelids, and skin (oily and large-pored); also skin tags.
- Scalp folds (*cutis verticis gyrata*; due to expanding but tethered skin).
- Skin darkening (fig 5.29).
- Acanthosis nigricans (fig 12.29, p561).
- Laryngeal dyspnoea (fixed cords).
- Obstructive sleep apnoea.
- Goitre (↑thyroid vascularity).
- Proximal weakness + arthropathy.
- Carpal tunnel signs in 50%, p497.
- Signs from any pituitary mass: hypopituitarism ± local mass effect (p226; ↓vision; hemianopia); fits.

Physiology This is the passage of large volumes (>3L/day) of dilute urine due to impaired water resorption by the kidney, because of reduced ADH secretion from the posterior pituitary (cranial DI) or impaired response of the kidney to ADH (nephrogenic DI).

Symptoms Polyuria; polydipsia; dehydration; symptoms of hypernatraemia (p664). *Polydipsia* can be uncontrollable and all-consuming, with patients drinking anything and everything to hand: in such cases, if beer is on tap, disaster will ensue!

Causes of cranial DI • *Idiopathic* (≤50%). • *Congenital:* defects in ADH gene, **DIDMOAD**.[12] • *Tumour* (may present with DI + hypopituitarism): metastases, craniopharyngioma, pituitary tumour. • *Trauma:* temporary if distal to pituitary stalk as proximal nerve endings grow out to find capillaries in scar tissue and begin direct secretion again. • Hypophysectomy. • Autoimmune hypophysitis (p226). • *Infiltration:* histiocytosis, sarcoidosis.[13] • *Vascular:* haemorrhage.[14] • *Infection:* meningoencephalitis.

Causes of nephrogenic DI •Inherited. •*Metabolic:* low potassium, high calcium. •*Drugs:* lithium, demeclocycline. •Chronic renal disease. •Post-obstructive uropathy.

Tests U&E, Ca^{2+}, glucose (exclude DM), serum and urine osmolalities. Serum osmolality estimate ≈ 2 × (Na^+ + K^+) + urea + glucose (all in mmol/L). Normal plasma osmolality is 285–295mOsmol/kg, and urine can be concentrated to more than twice this concentration. Significant DI is excluded if urine to plasma (U:P) osmolality ratio is more than 2:1, provided plasma osmolality is no greater than 295mOsmol/kg. In DI, despite raised plasma osmolality, urine is dilute with a U:P ratio <2. In primary polydipsia there may be dilutional hyponatraemia—and as hyponatraemia may itself cause mania, be cautious of saying 'It's water intoxication from psychogenic polydipsia'.

Diagnosis Water deprivation test See BOX 'The 8-hour water deprivation test'. NB: it is often difficult to differentiate primary polydipsia from partial DI. ΔΔ DM; diuretics or lithium use; *primary polydipsia* causes symptoms of polydipsia and polyuria with dilute urine. Its cause is poorly understood;[15] it may be associated with schizophrenia or mania (± Li^+ therapy), or, rarely, hypothalamic disease (neurosarcoid; tumour; encephalitis; brain injury; HIV encephalopathy). As part of this syndrome, the kidneys may lose their ability to fully concentrate urine, due to a wash-out of the normal concentrating gradient in the renal medulla. In the absence of a water deprivation test, if available, plasma copeptin (a surrogate marker of vasopressin secretion) can be used to diagnose nephrogenic DI (>21.4pmol/L).

Treatment Cranial DI MRI (head); test anterior pituitary function (p226). Give desmopressin, a synthetic analogue of ADH. It is available in multiple formulations including IV, intranasal, sublingual, and oral preparations.

Nephrogenic Treat the cause. If it persists, try bendroflumethiazide 5mg PO/24h. NSAIDs lower urine volume and plasma Na^+ by inhibiting prostaglandin synthase: prostaglandins locally inhibit the action of ADH.

▶▶Emergency management
• Seek urgent Endocrinology or Nephrology advice.
• Do urgent plasma U&E, and serum and urine osmolalities. Monitor urine output carefully and check U&E twice a day initially.
• IVI to keep up with urine output. If severe hypernatraemia, do not lower Na^+ rapidly as this may cause cerebral oedema and brain injury. If Na^+ is ≥170, use 0.9% saline initially—this contains 150mmol/L of sodium. Aim to reduce Na^+ at a rate of less than 10mmol/L per day. Use of 0.45% saline can be dangerous.
• Desmopressin 2mcg IM (lasts 12–24h) may be used as a therapeutic trial if polyuric.

---

12 **DIDMOAD** is a rare autosomal recessive disorder: **D**iabetes **I**nsipidus, **D**iabetes **M**ellitus, **O**ptic **A**trophy and **D**eafness (also known as Wolfram's syndrome).
13 Suspect neurosarcoidosis if ↑CSF protein (seen in 34%), facial nerve palsy (25%), CSF pleocytosis (23%), diabetes insipidus (21%), hemiparesis (17%), psychosis (17%), papilloedema (15%), ataxia (13%), seizures (12%), optic atrophy (12%), hearing loss (12%), or nystagmus (9%).
14 Sheehan's syndrome is pituitary infarction from shock, eg postpartum haemorrhage. It is rare.
15 Most of us could drink 20L/d and not be hyponatraemic; some get hyponatraemic drinking 5L/d; they may have **P**sychosis, **I**ntermittent hyponatraemia, and **P**olydipsia (PIP syndrome), ?from ↑intravascular volume leading to ↑atrial natriuretic peptide, p135, hence natriuresis and hyponatraemia.

The 8-hour water deprivation test

Tests the ability of kidneys to concentrate urine for diagnosis of DI (dilute urine in spite of dehydration), and then to localize the cause (table 5.6). Do not do the test before establishing that urine volume is >3L/d (output less than this with normal plasma Na+ and osmolality excludes significant disturbance of water balance).
- Stop test if *urine* osmolality >~600mOsmol/kg in stage 1 (DI is excluded).
- Free fluids until 07.30. Light breakfast at 06.30, no tea, no coffee, no smoking.

Stage 1 Fluid deprivation (0–8h): for diagnosis of DI. Start at 08.00.
- Empty bladder, then no drinks and only dry food.
- Weigh hourly. If >3% weight lost during test, order urgent serum osmolality. If >300mOsmol/kg, proceed to stage 2. If <300, continue test.
- Collect urine every 2h; measure its volume and osmolality.
- Venous sample for osmolality every 4h.
- Stop test after 8h (16.00) if urine osmolality >600mOsmol/kg (ie normal).

Stage 2 Differentiate cranial from nephrogenic DI.
- Proceed if urine still dilute—ie urine osmolality <600mOsmol/kg.
- Give desmopressin 2mcg IM. Water can be drunk now.
- Measure urine osmolality hourly for the next 4h.

Table 5.6 Interpreting the water deprivation test

Diagnosis	Urine osmolality
Normal	Urine osmolality >600mOsmol/kg in stage 1 U:P ratio >2 (normal concentrating ability)
Primary polydipsia	Urine concentrates, but less than normal, eg >400–600mOsmol/kg
Cranial DI	Urine osmolality increases to >600mOsmol/kg *after* desmopressin (if equivocal an extended water deprivation test may be tried (no drinking from 18:00 the night before))
Nephrogenic DI	No increase in urine osmolality after desmopressin

Syndrome of inappropriate ADH secretion (SIADH)

In SIADH, ADH continues to be secreted in spite of low plasma osmolality or large plasma volume. Diagnosis requires concentrated urine (Na+ >20mmol/L and osmolality >100mOsmol/kg) In the presence of hyponatraemia and low plasma osmolality, having excluded adrenal insufficiency and hypothyroidism. Causes are numerous. See p665.

6 Gastroenterology

Contents

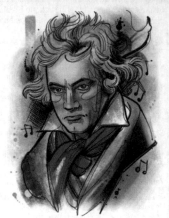

Fig 6.1 Suffering in silence: Ludwig van Beethoven's gastrointestinal symptoms began in his late teens, soon after the death of his mother from tuberculosis and the lapse of his father into alcoholism. Like the stark rhythmic motifs that increasingly characterized his compositions, a pattern of recurrent abdominal cramping and alternating bouts of severe diarrhoea and constipation emerged as an underlying constant in his life. The affliction rose to a stifling crescendo with prostration, anorexia, a host of rheumatic problems, and even jaundice and ascites proving debilitating modulations. His renowned deafness began with high-frequency loss and tinnitus at the age of 28, becoming relentlessly progressive. Multiple theories to explain his hearing loss have been proposed. Beethoven's own supposition that his deafness had its root in the abdomen may well have been correct, despite his physicians' uniform dismissal. Bilateral sensorineural hearing loss in the context of immunopathy is well described. Inflammatory bowel disease, with its weaving counterpoint of extra-intestinal manifestations and the oft-associated primary sclerosing cholangitis provides an all-encompassing source. A source not only of his symptoms but quite possibly the suffering as a wellspring of his genius, bubbling with emotion and gushing with harmonious floods of the most profound and inspiring sounds yet conceived.

Reproduced from Baldwin A. *Oxford Handbook of Clinical Specialties* (2020), with permission from Oxford University Press.

We thank Simon Campbell, our Specialist Reader for this chapter.

Lumen

We learn about gastroenterological diseases as if they were separate entities, in-dependent species collected by naturalists, each kept in its own dark matchbox—collectors' items collecting dust in a desiccated world on a library shelf. But this is not how illness works. Otto had diabetes, but refused to see a doctor until it was far advanced, and an amputation was needed. He needed looking after by his wife Aurelia. But she had her children Warren and Sylvia to look after too. And when Otto was no longer the bread-winner, she forced herself to work as a teacher, an accountant, and at any other job she could get. Otto's illness manifested in Aurelia's duodenum—as an ulcer. The gut often bears the brunt of other people's worries. Inside every piece of a gut is a lumen[1]—the world is in the gut, and the gut is in the world. But the light does not always shine. So when the lumen filled with Aurelia's blood, we can expect the illness to impact the whole family. Her daughter knows where blood comes from ('straight from the heart … pink fizz'). After Otto died, Sylvia needed long-term psychiatric care, and Aurelia moved to be near her daughter. The bleeding duodenal ulcer got worse when Sylvia needed electroconvulsive therapy. The therapy worked and now, briefly, Sylvia, before her own premature death, is able to look after Aurelia, as she prepares for a gastrectomy.

The story of each illness told separately misses something; but even taken in its social context, this story is missing something vital: the poetry, in most of our patients lived rather than written—tragic, comic, human, and usually obscure—but in the case of this family not so obscure. Welling up, as unstoppable as the bleeding from her mother's ulcer came the poetry of Sylvia Plath.

1 *Lumen* is Latin for light (hence its medical meaning of a tubular cavity open to the world at both ends), as well as being the SI unit of light flux falling on an object—ie the power to illuminate. All doctors have this power, whether by insightfully interpreting patients' lives and illnesses to them, or by acts of kindness—even something so simple as bringing a cup of tea.

Nutritional science is plagued by its own media success. Even the lowest quality research enjoys an editorial queue jump to the headlines. The result is a diet both rich and varied in contradictory advice served directly to an increasingly confused and frustrated public. A study on the latest diet, ground-breaking 'superfood', or newly purported harm/benefit of something we eat is sure to whet journalistic appetite. Guidelines on healthy eating must also be updated when diet-outcome associations are revised. Observational research at the heart of nutritional epidemiology is particularly prone to bias from measurement error (typically we cannot remember what we ate yesterday, never mind details on exact portion sizes), confounding, reverse causation, and biomarkers that poorly represent intake. Eggs went from shunned one day to encouraged the next. Red meat and a daily glass of red wine rapidly followed the opposite trajectory. In the ensuing confusion, we risk rejecting simple and undisputed tenets of healthy eating based on large, high-quality prospective epidemiological studies. In particular, balancing intake across food groups and eating less (for the majority of the population) should be encouraged.

The urgent problems at both ends of the dietary spectrum
• 2 in 3 UK adults and 1 in 3 children are overweight or obese.
• The prevalence of obesity has doubled in the last two decades.
• More than 3 million people in the UK are malnourished/at risk of malnutrition.
• The cost to health services of obesity and malnutrition exceeds that of smoking.

Important components of a healthy diet
Balancing energy in and out Energy intake should equal expenditure for those of normal weight (BMI 18.5–25; table 6.1). UK guidelines recommend 2500 kcal/d for men and 2000 for women. Physical activity should be encouraged for all; 1 in 2 adults are inactive, making caloric balance more difficult.

Carbohydrate Aim for around ⅓ of energy consumed to derive from starchy carbohydrate (pasta, rice, potatoes, bread); low-carbohydrate diets with meat replacement are associated with higher mortality.[1]

Protein Good sources include lean meat, fish, eggs, beans, and nuts. Processed and red meat consumption has been associated with increased mortality compared with white meats. Aim for 2 servings of fish per week, including oily fish rich in omega-3 fatty acids (probable reductions in vascular risk).

Fibre 30g per day is recommended, and there is a dose–response relationship with higher consumption associated with greater reduction in vascular disease, type 2 diabetes, colorectal cancer, and breast cancer risk.[2]

Fat The type of fat consumed is more important than the quantity; avoid trans fats completely (not yet banned in the UK and present in some spreads, fried and baked goods) and limit saturated fat (replace with mono- and polyunsaturates).

Eat enough fruit and vegetables Aiming for 5 portions of a variety per day.

Eat some dairy produce/alternatives Lower fat & sugar options where possible.

Limit alcohol ≤14u/wk for both men and women, spread over 3 or more days. There is no 'safe' level (apparent protective effects largely artefactual).

Caffeine There is insufficient evidence to either promote or discourage tea/coffee consumption, despite possible mortality benefits in cohort studies. Beware the 'tea and toast' diet, a common form of malnutrition in the elderly.

Supplements There is scant evidence for most nutritional supplements in those able to follow a balanced diet. Women attempting to conceive should take 400mcg/day folic acid from (pre-)conception until 13wks. Vitamin D supplements (10mcg/day) should be considered by all in the UK during autumn and winter.

▶This diet is not appropriate for all • <5yrs old. • At risk of malabsorption or dietary deficiency (eg IBD, p260). • Special diet (coeliac disease, p262). **Emphasis may be different in** Dyslipidaemia (p682); DM (p200); obesity; constipation (p256); liver failure (p270); chronic pancreatitis (p262); renal failure (less protein) (p296); ↑BP (p110).

Screening for malnutrition

Impact of malnutrition The notion that malnutrition is a problem restricted to the developing world is a myth. It affects ⅓ of UK hospital inpatients and 10% of those aged >65yrs in the community. Malnutrition increases mortality, prolongs hospital stay, and increases healthcare use.

Malnutrition Universal Screening Tool The MUST is a validated screening tool to identify adults at risk of malnutrition. Patients should be screened at hospital admission or at their first outpatient appointment. BMI, % unplanned weight loss, and the presence of acute disease are used to calculate a simple risk score. A score of ≥2 should prompt referral to a dietitian.

Losing weight—why and how?

Health consequences of obesity The risks have been appreciated since the time of Hippocrates. Obesity is a disease associated with a significant increase in mortality, vascular disease, type 2 diabetes, hypertension, cancer, hepatobiliary disease, sleep apnoea, osteoarthritis, depression, and social stigma.

Losing weight Motivational and behaviour-modification therapy, in combination with dietary adherence (regardless of the type of diet). Exercise is less successful for weight loss but is a powerful predictor of loss maintenance.

Drugs or surgery for obesity? The most desirable treatment for obesity is still primary prevention, but pharmacotherapy does work. *Orlistat* lowers fat absorption (hence SE of oily faecal incontinence)—see *OHCS* p830. *Surgery:* carries potential for significant weight loss in appropriately selected patients but also significant morbidity (see p618). *Endoscopic management:* may replicate some of the anatomical and physiological effects of weight loss surgery but with less morbidity.

Calculating body mass index

Table 6.1 BMI = (weight in kg)/(height in m)^2

BMI	State	Some implications within the categories
<18.5	Underweight	Consider pathology (incl. eating disorder)
18.5–24.9	Healthy range	
25–29.9	Overweight	Weight loss should be considered
30–39.9	Obesity	>32 is unsuitable for day-case general surgery
≥40	Extreme/morbid obesity	≥40 is an indication for bariatric surgery

Caveats: BMI is reliable and easy to measure, but does not take into account the distribution of body fat, overestimates body fat mass in those who are very muscular, and is harder to interpret for children and adolescents. This classification underestimates risk in Asian populations; guidelines define overweight as BMI 23–25 and obesity as BMI >25. Waist circumference is especially useful to measure in those with a BMI 25–35; >94cm in men and >80cm in women reflects omental fat and correlates better with risk than does BMI.

Vitamin deficiency syndromes are making a worrying return in Western countries, even in obese individuals. ►Always consider their co-occurrence (table 6.2).

Scurvy This is due to lack of vitamin C. Is the patient poor, pregnant, or on an odd diet? **Signs** 1 Listlessness, anorexia, cachexia (p35). 2 Gingivitis, loose teeth, halitosis. 3 Bleeding from gums, nose, hair follicles (fig 6.2), or into joints, bladder, gut. 4 Muscle pain/weakness. 5 Oedema. **Diagnosis** No test is completely satisfactory. WBCs: ↓ascorbic acid. ℞ Dietary education;[2] ascorbic acid ≥250mg/24h PO.

Beriberi There is heart failure with oedema (wet beriberi) or peripheral neuropathy (dry beriberi) due to lack of vitamin B_1 (thiamine, present in yeast, whole grains, *brown* rice, legumes). For treatment and diagnostic tests, see Wernicke's encephalopathy (p700).

Pellagra = Lack of nicotinic acid (meat, yeast, grains, seeds, nixtamalized maize). Classical triad: **D**iarrhoea, **D**ementia, photosensitive **D**ermatitis (Casal's necklace, fig 6.3) ± neuropathy, depression, insomnia, tremor, rigidity, ataxia, fits. It may occur in carcinoid syndrome and anti-TB drugs (isoniazid). It is endemic in China and Africa (non-treated corn). ℞ Education, nicotinamide 100mg/4h.

Xerophthalmia This vitamin A (liver, egg yolk, butter) deficiency syndrome is a major cause of blindness in the Tropics. Conjunctivae become dry and develop oval/triangular spots (Bitôt's spots). Corneas become cloudy and soft. Night blindness. Give vitamin A (OHCS p374). ►Get special help if pregnant: vitamin A embryopathy must be avoided. Re-educate and monitor diet.

Table 6.2 Deficiency syndromes and the sites of nutrient absorption

Vitamin/nutrient	Site of absorption	Deficiency syndrome
A[F]	Small intestine	Xerophthalmia
B_1 (thiamine)	Small intestine	Beriberi; Wernicke's encephalopathy (p700)
B_2 (riboflavin)	Proximal small intestine	Angular stomatitis; cheilitis (p242)
B_3 (niacin)	Jejunum	Pellagra
B_6 (pyridoxine)	Small intestine	Polyneuropathy
B_{12}	Terminal ileum	Macrocytic anaemia (p328); neuropathy; glossitis (p242)
C	Proximal ileum	Scurvy
D[F]	Jejunum as free vitamin	Rickets (p676); osteomalacia (p676)
E[F]	Small intestine	Haemolysis; neurological deficit
K[F]	Small intestine	Bleeding disorders (p342)
Folic acid	Jejunum	Macrocytic anaemia (p328), glossitis (p242)
Mineral		
Calcium	Duodenum + jejunum	p668
Copper	Stomach + jejunum	Menkes' kinky hair syndrome
Fluoride	Stomach	Dental caries
Iodide	Small intestine	Goitre; hypothyroidism
Iron	Duodenum + jejunum	Microcytic anaemia (p326)
Magnesium	Small intestine	p671
Phosphate	Small intestine	Osteoporosis; anorexia; weakness
Selenium	Small intestine	Cardiomyopathy (p671); myopathy
Zinc	Jejunum	Acrodermatitis enteropathica; poor wound healing (p671)

[F] = fat-soluble vitamin, thus deficiency is likely if there is fat malabsorption.

2 That oranges and lemons prevent 'the scurvy' was noted by the naval surgeon James Lind in 1753. In what may rank as the first ever clinical trial, he randomly divided 12 sailors with scurvy into 6 groups, given the same basic diet but each group received a unique dietary intervention. The 2 sailors receiving oranges and lemons both made a good recovery.

'The sweet smell is a great sorrow on the land. Men who can graft the trees and make the seed fertile and big can find no way to let the hungry people eat their produce… The works of the roots of the vines, of the trees, must be destroyed to keep up the price …

There is a crime here that goes beyond denunciation. There is a sorrow here that weeping cannot symbolize. There is a failure here that topples all our success. The fertile earth, the straight tree rows, the sturdy trunks, and the ripe fruit. And children dying of pellagra must die because a profit cannot be taken from an orange. And coroners must fill in the certificates—died of malnutrition—because the food must rot, must be forced to rot.

The people come with nets to fish for potatoes in the river, and the guards hold them back; they come in rattling cars to get the dumped oranges, but the kerosene is sprayed. And they stand still and watch the potatoes float by, listen to the screaming pigs being killed in a ditch and covered with quicklime, watch the mountains of oranges slop down to a putrefying ooze; and in the eyes of the people there is a failure; and in the eyes of the hungry there is a growing wrath. In the souls of the people the grapes of wrath are filling and growing heavy, growing heavy for the vintage.' J Steinbeck, *The Grapes of Wrath*.

How do John Steinbeck's grapes grow in our 21st-century soil? Too well; a double harvest, it turns out, as not only is much of the world starving, amid plenty (for those who can pay) but also there is a new 'sorrow in our land that weeping cannot symbolize': pathological 'voluntary' *self-starvation*, again amid plenty, in pursuit of the body-beautiful according to images laid down by media gods. If gastroenterologists had one wish it might not be the ending of all their diseases, but that humankind stand in a right relationship with Steinbeck's fertile earth, his straight trees, his sturdy trunks, and his ripe fruit.

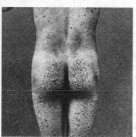

Fig 6.2 Petechiae and perifollicular haemorrhage due to scurvy.

Scurvy; male figure. Wellcome Collection. Attribution 4.0 International (CC BY 4.0).

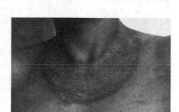

Fig 6.3 Dermatitis caused by chronic pellagra.

Courtesy of the CDC (https://phil.cdc.gov/Details. aspx?pid=3757).

The mouth

The diagnosis will often come out of your patient's mouth, so open it! So many GI investigations are indirect... now is your chance for direct observation.

Leucoplakia (fig 6.4) An oral mucosal white plaque that will not rub off and is not attributable to any other known disease. It is a premalignant lesion, with squamous cell carcinoma transformation rates ranging from <1% to 36% (tongue lesions are riskier). Oral hairy leucoplakia is a shaggy white patch on the side of the tongue seen in HIV, caused by EBV, and is not premalignant. ►When in doubt, refer all intra-oral white lesions (see BOX).

Aphthous ulcers (fig 6.5) 20% of us get these shallow, painful ulcers on the tongue or oral mucosa that heal without scarring. **Causes of severe ulcers** Crohn's and coeliac disease; Behçet's (p554); erythema multiforme; lichen planus; infections (herpes simplex, syphilis, Vincent's angina, p698). *R̃ Minor ulcers:* avoid oral trauma (eg hard toothbrushes) and acidic foods or drinks. *Tetracycline* or antimicrobial mouthwashes (eg chlorhexidine) with topical steroids (eg triamcinolone gel) and topical analgesia. *Severe ulcers:* consider systemic corticosteroids or thalidomide (absolutely contraindicated in pregnancy). ►Biopsy ulcers not healing after 3 weeks to exclude malignancy; refer if uncertain.

Candidiasis (thrush) (fig 6.6) Causes white patches or erythema of the buccal mucosa. Patches may be hard to remove and bleed if scraped. **Risk factors** Extremes of age; DM; antibiotics; immunosuppression (long-term corticosteroids, including inhalers; cytotoxics; malignancy; HIV). *R̃ Nystatin* suspension 400 000u (4mL swill and swallow/6h). *Oral fluconazole* for non-responders or oropharyngeal thrush.

Cheilitis (angular stomatitis) Fissuring of the mouth's corners is caused by denture problems, candidiasis, or deficiency of iron or riboflavin (vitamin B₂) (fig 8.21, p327.)

Gingivitis Gum inflammation ± hypertrophy occurs with poor oral hygiene, drugs (phenytoin, ciclosporin, nifedipine), pregnancy, vitamin C deficiency (scurvy, p240), acute myeloid leukaemia (p354), or Vincent's angina (p698).

Microstomia (fig 6.7) The mouth is too small, eg from thickening and tightening of the perioral skin after burns or in epidermolysis bullosa (destructive skin and mucous membrane blisters ± ankyloglossia) or systemic sclerosis (p548).

Oral pigmentation Perioral brown spots characterize Peutz–Jeghers' (p694). Pigmentation anywhere in the mouth suggests Addison's disease (p220) or drugs (eg antimalarials). Consider malignant melanoma. **Telangiectasia** Systemic sclerosis; Osler–Weber–Rendu syndrome (p694). **Fordyce glands** (Creamy yellow spots at the border of the oral mucosa and the lip vermilion.) Sebaceous cysts, common and benign. *Aspergillus niger* colonization may cause a black tongue.

Teeth (fig 6.8) A blue line at the gum–tooth margin suggests lead poisoning. Prenatal or childhood tetracycline exposure causes a yellow–brown discolouration.

Tongue This may be furred or dry (xerostomia) in dehydration, drug therapy,[3] after radiotherapy, in Crohn's disease, Sjögren's (p548), and Mikulicz's syndrome (p692). **Glossitis** Means a smooth, red, sore tongue, eg caused by iron, folate, or B₁₂ deficiency (fig 8.29, p331). If local loss of papillae leads to ulcer-like lesions that change in colour and size, use the term *geographic tongue* (harmless migratory glossitis). **Macroglossia** The tongue is too big. Causes: myxoedema; acromegaly; amyloid (p364). A *ranula* is a bluish salivary retention cyst to one side of the frenulum, named after the bulging vocal pouch of frogs' throats (genus *Rana*). **Tongue cancer** The most common site for oral cavity SCC. Appears as a raised ulcer with firm edges. Risk factors: smoking, alcohol.[4] Spread: anterior ⅓ of tongue drains to submental nodes; middle ⅓ to submandibular nodes; posterior ⅓ to deep cervical nodes. *Treatment:* radiotherapy or surgery. Surgery is recommended if good functional reconstruction can be achieved. 5yr survival (early disease): 70%. ►When in doubt, refer.

---

3 Drugs causing xerostomia: ACE-i; antidepressants; antihistamines; antipsychotics; antimuscarinics/anti-cholinergics; bromocriptine; diuretics; loperamide; nifedipine; opiates; prazosin; prochlorperazine, etc.
4 Betel nut (*Areca catechu*) chewing, common in South Asia, may be an independent risk factor.

White intra-oral lesions

- Idiopathic keratosis.
- Leucoplakia.
- Lichen planus.
- Poor dental hygiene.
- Candidiasis.
- Squamous papilloma.
- Carcinoma.
- Hairy oral leucoplakia.
- Lupus erythematosus.
- Smoking.
- Aphthous stomatitis.
- Secondary syphilis.

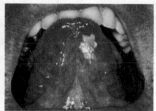

Fig 6.4 Leucoplakia on the underside of the tongue. It is important to refer leucoplakia because it is premalignant.

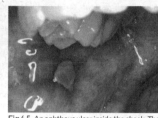

Fig 6.5 An aphthous ulcer inside the cheek. The name is tautological: *aphtha* in Greek means ulceration.

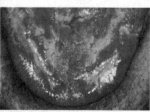

Fig 6.6 White fur on an erythematous tongue caused by oral candidiasis. Oropharyngeal candidiasis in an apparently fit patient may suggest underlying HIV infection.

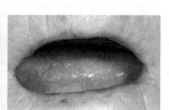

Fig 6.7 Microstomia (small, narrow mouth), eg from hardening of the skin in scleroderma which narrows the mouth. It is cosmetically and functionally disabling.

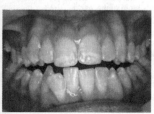

Fig 6.8 White bands on the teeth can be caused by excessive fluoride intake.

▶Consent is needed for all these procedures; see p566.

Upper GI endoscopy Indications See table 6.3. **Pre-procedure** Stop PPIs 2wks pre-op if possible (∴ pathology-masking). Nil by mouth for 6h before. Don't drive for 24h if sedation is used. **Procedure** Sedation optional, eg midazolam 1–5mg slowly IV (to remain conscious; if deeper sedation is needed, propofol via an anaesthetist (narrow therapeutic range)); nasal prong O_2 (eg 2L/min; monitor respirations & oximetry). The pharynx may be sprayed with local anaesthetic before the endoscope is passed. Continuous suction must be available to prevent aspiration. **Complications** Sore throat; amnesia from sedation; perforation (<0.1%); bleeding (if on aspirin, clopidogrel, warfarin, or DOACs, these need stopping only if therapeutic procedure). **Duodenal biopsy** The gold standard test for coeliac disease (p262); also useful in unusual causes of malabsorption, eg giardiasis, lymphoma, Whipple's disease.

Sigmoidoscopy Views the rectum + distal colon (to ∼splenic flexure). Flexible sigmoidoscopy has largely displaced rigid sigmoidoscopy for diagnosis of distal colonic pathology, but ∼25% of cancers are still out of reach. It can also be used for the rapid assessment of severe ulcerative colitis, and can be used therapeutically, eg for polypectomy or decompression of sigmoid volvulus (p603). **Preparation** Phosphate enema PR 1–2 hours prior. **Procedure** Learn from an expert; do PR exam first. Do biopsies—macroscopic appearances may be normal, eg amyloidosis, microscopic colitis.

Colonoscopy Indications See table 6.4. **Preparation** Stop iron 1wk prior; low-fibre diet on preceding day; split-dose laxative bowel preparation (± simethicone to reduce bubbles). **Procedure** Do PR first. Sedation (see earlier in topic) and analgesia are given before colonoscope is passed and guided around the colon. **Complications** Abdominal discomfort; incomplete examination; haemorrhage after polypectomy (1 in 150); perforation (<0.1%). See figs 6.9–6.13. Post-procedure: no alcohol, and no operating machinery/driving for 24h, no flying for 1wk post-polypectomy.

Video capsule endoscopy (VCE) 1st line for evaluating obscure GI bleeding (p326) and to detect small bowel pathology. This is a rapidly evolving area; while it is the gold standard for small bowel visualization, there are now colonic and upper GI capsule alternatives to traditional endoscopy. Use small bowel imaging (eg contrast) or patency capsule test ahead of VCE if patient has abdominal pain or symptoms suggesting small bowel obstruction. **Preparation** Clear fluids only the evening before then nil by mouth from morning until 4h after capsule

Fig 6.14 PillCam®.

swallowed. **Procedure** Capsule is swallowed (fig 6.14)—this transmits video wirelessly to capture device worn by patient. Normal activity can take place for the day. **Complications** Capsule retention in 1% (endoscopic or surgical removal is needed)—avoid MRI for 2 wks after unless AXR confirms capsule has cleared; obstruction, incomplete exam (eg slow transit, achalasia). **Problems** No therapeutic options; poor localization of lesions; may miss more subtle lesions.

Liver biopsy Route *Percutaneous* if INR in range else *transjugular* with FFP. **Indications 1** Diagnosis—chronic ↑LFT of unknown aetiology; suspected hepatic lesions/cancer, pyrexia of unknown origin, suspected cirrhosis. **2** Staging fibrosis—gold standard for severity (this indication being replaced by ultrasound-based elastography). **Pre-op** Nil by mouth for 8h. Are INR <1.5 and platelets >50 × 10⁹/L? Give analgesia. **Procedure** Sedation may be given. The liver borders are percussed and where there is dullness in the mid-axillary line in expiration, lidocaine 2% is infiltrated down to the liver capsule. Consider US/CT guidance. Breathing is rehearsed and a needle biopsy is taken with the breath held in expiration. Afterwards lie on the right side for 2h, then in bed for 4h; check pulse and BP every 15min for 1h, every 30min for 2h, then hourly until discharge 4h post-biopsy. **Complications** Local pain; pneumothorax; bleeding (<0.5%); death (<0.1%).

Table 6.3 Indications for upper GI endoscopy

Diagnostic indications	Therapeutic indications
Haematemesis/melaena	Treatment of bleeding lesions
Dysphagia	Variceal banding and sclerotherapy
Dyspepsia (≳55yrs old + alarm symptoms or treatment refractory, p248)	Argon plasma coagulation for suspected vascular abnormality
Duodenal biopsy (?coeliac)	Stent insertion, laser therapy
Persistent vomiting and weight loss	Stricture dilatation, polyp resection
Iron-deficiency anaemia	Treatment of achalasia
Barrett's oesophagus surveillance	

Table 6.4 Indications for colonoscopy

Diagnostic indications	Therapeutic indications
Rectal bleeding—when settled, if acute	Haemostasis (eg by clipping vessel)
Iron-def. anaemia (♂/non-menstruating ♀)	Bleeding angiodysplasia lesion (argon beamer photocoagulation)
Persistent diarrhoea of unexplained cause	Colonic stent deployment (cancer)
Positive faecal immunochemical test (FIT)	Volvulus decompression (flexi sig)
Assessment or suspicion of IBD	Pseudo-obstruction
Colon cancer surveillance	Polypectomy

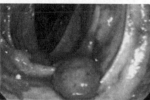

Fig 6.9 A big polyp seen on colonoscopy. An advantage of colonoscopy over barium enema is the ability to biopsy or intervene at the same time—in this case, polypectomy.

Image courtesy of Dr Anthony Mee.

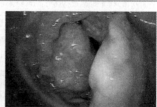

Fig 6.10 Colonoscopic image of an adenocarcinoma—p608. Compared with a colonic polyp (fig 6.9), the carcinoma is irregular in shape and colour, larger, and more aggressive.

Image courtesy of Dr J Simmons.

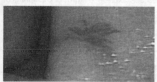

Fig 6.11 Angiodysplasia lesion seen at colonoscopy. Bleeding may be brisk. ℞: endoscopic obliteration. It is associated with aortic stenosis (Heyde's syndrome).[3]

Image courtesy of Dr Anthony Mee.

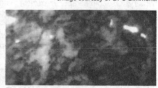

Fig 6.12 Colonic mucosa in active UC (p258); it is red, inflamed, and friable (bleeds on touching). Signs of severity: mucopurulent exudate, mucosal ulceration ± spontaneous bleeding. If quiescent, there may only be a distorted or absent mucosal vascular pattern.

Image courtesy of Dr J Simmons.

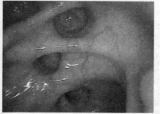

Fig 6.13 Colonoscopic image showing diverticulosis (p620). Navigating safely through the colon, avoiding the false lumina of the diverticula, can be a challenge. Don't go there if diverticula are inflamed (diverticulitis): perforation is a big risk. *Other CI to colonoscopy:* MI in last month; ischaemic colitis (*Oxford Handbook of Gastroenterology and Hepatology*, Second Edition (Bloom *et al.*), p165).

Image courtesy of Dr J Simmons.

Dysphagia

Dysphagia is a sensation of difficult swallowing or food sticking after swallowing and should prompt urgent investigation to exclude malignancy.

Causes Oropharyngeal or oesophageal? Structural or motility related? (See BOX.)

Five questions to ask to help determine the cause

1 Is the problem initiating a swallow, or a feeling of food sticking seconds later?
   Initiating: oropharyngeal, associated coughing/choking. *Sticking:* oesophageal.
2 Was there difficulty swallowing solids *and* liquids from the start?
   Yes: neuromuscular (motility) disorder of the oesophagus.
   No: solids *then* liquids: structural—suspect a stricture (benign or malignant).
3 Is the dysphagia progressive or intermittent?
   Progressive: structural, slowly (peptic) or rapidly (malignant) stricture.
   Intermittent: suspect oesophageal spasm.
4 Is swallowing painful (odynophagia)?
   Yes: suspect oesophagitis (severe reflux, alcohol, viral infection, *Candida* in im-munocompromised or poor steroid inhaler technique, medications) or spasm.
5 Does the neck bulge or gurgle? *Yes:* suspect a pharyngeal pouch (see *OHCS* p420).

Signs Is the patient cachectic or anaemic? Examine the mouth; feel for supraclavicular nodes (left supraclavicular node = Virchow's node—suggests intra-abdominal malignancy); look for signs of systemic disease, eg systemic sclerosis (p548), CNS disease.

Tests FBC (anaemia); U&E (dehydration). Upper GI endoscopy ± biopsy (fig 6.15). If suspicion of pharyngeal pouch consider contrast swallow (± ENT opinion). Video fluor-oscopy may help identify neurogenic causes. Oesophageal manometry for dysmotility.

Specific conditions **Oesophagitis** See p252. **Distal oesophageal spasm** Causes intermittent dysphagia ± chest pain. Contrast swallow/manometry: abnormal con-tractions.[5] **Achalasia** Coordinated peristalsis is lost and the lower oesophageal sphincter fails to relax (due to degeneration of the myenteric plexus), causing dys-phagia, regurgitation, and ↓weight. Characteristic findings on manometry or contrast swallow showing dilated tapering oesophagus. *Treatment:* endoscopic balloon dilata-tion, or Heller's cardiomyotomy—then proton pump inhibitors (PPIs, p248). Botulinum toxin injection if a non-invasive procedure is needed (repeat every few months). Calcium channel blockers and nitrates may also relax the sphincter. **Benign oesopha-geal stricture** Caused by gastro-oesophageal reflux disease (GORD, p250), corrosives, surgery, or radiotherapy. *Treatment:* endoscopic balloon dilatation. **Oesophageal cancer** (p610.) Associations: ♂, GORD, tobacco, alcohol, Barrett's oesophagus (p251), tylosis (palmar hyperkeratosis), Plummer–Vinson syndrome (post-cricoid dysphagia, upper oesophageal web + iron-deficiency). **CNS causes** Ask for help from a speech and language therapist. **Globus sensation** 'I've got a lump in my throat'; functional oesophageal disorder. Rule out a structural or motility cause and reassure.

Nausea and vomiting

Consider pregnancy where appropriate! Other causes, p52.

What's in the vomit? Reports of 'coffee grounds' *may* indicate upper GI bleeding but represent one of the most over-called signs in clinical medicine—always verify yourself and look for other evidence of GI bleeding (melaena, anaemia, ↑urea); rec-ognizable food ≈ gastric stasis; feculent ≈ small bowel obstruction.

Timing Morning ≈ pregnancy or ↑ICP; 1h post food ≈ gastric stasis/gastroparesis (DM); vomiting that relieves pain ≈ peptic ulcer; preceded by loud gurgling ≈ GI obstruction.

Tests Bloods FBC, U&E, LFT, Ca^{2+}, glucose, amylase. ABG A metabolic (hypochloraemic) alkalosis from loss of gastric contents (pH >7.45, ↑HCO_3^-) indicates severe vomiting. **Plain** AXR If suspected bowel obstruction (p712). **Upper** GI endoscopy (See p244). If suspicion of bleed or persistent vomiting. Consider head CT in case ↑ICP.

Treatment Identify and *treat underlying causes.* Symptomatic relief: table 6.5. Be pre-emptive, eg pre-op for post-op symptoms. Try oral route first. 30% need a 2nd-line anti-emetic, so be prepared to prescribe more than one. Give IV fluids with K^+ replacement if severely dehydrated or nil by mouth, and monitor electrolytes and fluid balance.

Causes of dysphagia

Oropharyngeal

Structural:
- Pharyngeal pouch
- Cervical web
- Cricopharyngeal bar
- Oropharyngeal tumour.

Neuromuscular:
- Cortical (pseudobulbar palsy (p503)):
  - Stroke (p466)
  - Multiple sclerosis (p492)
  - Motor neuron disease (p502)
  - Wilson's or Parkinson's disease
- Bulbar palsy (p503):
  - Syringobulbia (p512)
  - Motor neuron disease (p502)
- Peripheral:
  - Myasthenia gravis (p508)
  - Poliomyelitis (p432)
  - Guillain–Barré syndrome (p500).

Oesophageal

Structural:
- Benign stricture:
  - Oesophageal web or ring
  - Peptic stricture
  - Oesophagitis
- Malignant stricture (fig 6.15):
  - Oesophageal/gastric tumour
- Extrinsic pressure:
  - Lung cancer
  - Mediastinal lymph nodes
  - Aortic aneurysm
  - Left atrial enlargement
  - Retrosternal goitre.

Neuromuscular:
- Achalasia (see p246)
- Distal oesophageal spasm
- Systemic sclerosis (p548)
- Chagas' disease (p419).

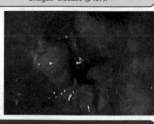

Fig 6.15 A malignant lower oesophageal stricture seen at endoscopy. Note the asymmetry and heaped edges. Benign strictures have a smoother appearance and tend to be circumferential.

Reproduced from Bloom *et al.*, *Oxford Handbook of Gastroenterology and Hepatology*, 2012, with permission from Oxford University Press.

Remembering your anti-emetics

One way of recalling anti-emetics involves using (simplified) pharmacology.

Table 6.5 Pharmacology of common anti-emetics

Receptor	Antagonist	Dose	Notes
H_1	Cyclizine	50mg/8h PO/IV/IM	GI causes
	Cinnarizine	30mg/8h PO	Vestibular disorders
D_2	Metoclopramide	10mg/8h PO/IV/IM	GI causes; also prokinetic
	Domperidone	60mg/12h PR; 20mg/6h PO	Also prokinetic
	Prochlorperazine	12.5mg IM; 5mg/8h PO	Vestibular/GI causes
	Haloperidol	1.5mg/12h PO	Chemical causes, eg opioids
$5HT_3$	Ondansetron	4–8mg/8h IV slowly	Doses can be higher for, eg emetogenic chemotherapy
Others	Hyoscine hydrobromide	200–600mcg SC/IM	Antimuscarinic ∴ also antispasmodic and antisecretory (don't prescribe with a prokinetic)
	Dexamethasone	6–10mg/d PO/SC	Unknown mode of action; an adjuvant
	Midazolam	2–4mg/d SC (syringe driver)	Unknown action; anti-emetic effect outlasts sedative effect[4]

► All antidopaminergics can cause dystonias and oculogyric crisis, especially in younger patients.

5 Non-propulsive contractions manifest as tertiary contractions or 'corkscrew oesophagus' (fig 16.35, p727) and suggest a motility disorder and may lead to ↓acid clearance. Symptoms and radiology may not match. Nutcracker oesophagus denotes distal peristaltic contractions >180mmHg. It may cause pain, relieved by nitrates or sublingual nifedipine.

War The stomach is a battle ground between the forces of attack (acid, pepsin, *Helicobacter pylori*, bile salts) and defence (mucin secretion, cellular mucus, bicarbonate secretion, mucosal blood flow, cell turnover). Gastric antisecretory agents, eg H$_2$ receptor antagonists (H2RAs), and proton pump inhibitors (PPIs) may only work if you have optimized cytoprotection (antacids and sucralfate work this way). Success may depend on you being not just a brilliant general, but also a tactician, politician, and diplomat. Plan your strategy carefully[5] (fig 6.16). As in any war, neglecting psychological factors can prove disastrous. The aim is not outright victory but *maintaining the balance of power* so all may prosper.

Symptoms Epigastric discomfort often related to hunger, specific foods, or time of day, fullness after meals, heartburn (retrosternal pain); tender epigastrium. Beware **ALARM** symptoms: **A**naemia (iron deficiency); **L**oss of weight; **A**norexia; **R**ecent onset/progressive symptoms; **M**elaena/haematemesis; **S**wallowing difficulty.

H. pylori (See table 6.6.) If ≤55yrs old 'Test and treat' for *H. pylori*;[6] if +ve give appropriate PPI and 2-antibiotic combination, eg lansoprazole 30mg/12h PO, clarithromycin 250mg/12h PO, and amoxicillin 1g/12h PO for 1wk. If –ve give acid suppression alone. ►Refer for urgent endoscopy (p244) *all* with dysphagia, as well as those ≥55yrs with *alarm symptoms* or with treatment-refractory dyspepsia.

Peptic ulcer disease Duodenal (DU, fig 6.17) are 4-fold more common than gastric ulcers (GU occur mainly in the elderly, on the lesser curve—ulcers elsewhere are more often malignant). Although there are some distinct features, these usually cannot be distinguished by the history alone. **Major risk factors** *H. pylori* (80–90%); drugs (NSAIDs; steroids; SSRI). **Minor** ↑Gastric acid secretion (eg gastrinoma, p267); ↑gastric emptying (DU) ↓emptying (GU); blood group O; smoking; stress, eg neurosurgery or burns (Cushing's or Curling's ulcers). **Symptoms** Asymptomatic or epigastric pain immediately (GU) or a few hours (DU) after meals (relieved by antacids) ± ↓weight. Nocturnal pain is more common with DU. **Signs** Epigastric tenderness. **Diagnosis** Upper GI endoscopy with biopsy, and to exclude malignancy (fig 6.16). Test for **H. pylori**. Repeat endoscopy after 6–8 weeks to confirm healing and exclude malignancy. Measure gastrin concentrations when off PPIs if Zollinger–Ellison syndrome (p267) is suspected. ΔΔ Non-ulcer dyspepsia; duodenal Crohn's; TB; lymphoma; pancreatic cancer (p612). **Follow-up** None; if good response to R (eg PPI).

Gastritis Risk factors Alcohol, NSAIDs, *H. pylori*, reflux/hiatus hernia, atrophic gastritis, granulomas (Crohn's; sarcoidosis), CMV, Zollinger–Ellison syndrome & Ménétrier's disease (p267 & p692). **Symptoms** Epigastric pain, vomiting. **Tests** Upper GI endoscopy only if suspicious features (fig 6.16).

Treatment Lifestyle ↓Alcohol and tobacco.

H. pylori eradication Triple therapy is 80–85% effective at eradication.[7]

Drugs to reduce acid PPIs are effective, eg lansoprazole 30mg/24h PO for 4 (DU) or 8 (GU) wks. H$_2$ blockers have a place (ranitidine 300mg each night PO for 8wks).

Drug-induced ulcers Stop drug if possible. PPIs may be best for treating and preventing GI ulcers and bleeding in patients on NSAID or antiplatelet drugs. Misoprostol is an alternative with different SE. If symptoms persist, re-endoscope, retest for *H. pylori*, and reconsider differential diagnoses (eg gallstones). **Surgery** See p614.

Complications ►►Bleeding (p252), ►►perforation (p598), malignancy, ↓gastric outflow.

Functional (non-ulcer) dyspepsia Common. *H. pylori* eradication (only after a +ve result) *may* help. Some evidence favours PPIs (only short-term courses) and psychotherapy. Low-dose amitriptyline (10–20mg each night PO) may help. Antacids, antispasmodics, H$_2$ blockers, misoprostol, prokinetic agents, bismuth, or sucralfate all have less evidence.

---

6 *H. pylori* is the commonest bacterial pathogen found worldwide (>50% of the world population over 40yrs has it). It's a class I carcinogen causing gastritis, duodenal/gastric ulcers, & gastric cancer/lymphoma (MALT, p360), also associated with coronary artery disease, B$_{12}$ and iron deficiency.

7 1 week of therapy sufficient; 2 weeks increases eradication rates by ~5% but also increases SE. For resistant infections switch to a 2nd-line antibiotic combination (see BNF).

Table 6.6 Tests (other than serology) should be performed after >2wks off PPI

		Sensitivity	Specificity
Invasive tests	CLO test	95%	95%
	Histology	95%	95%
	Culture	90%	100%
Non-invasive	¹³C breath test*	95%	95%
	Stool antigen	95%	94%
	Serology	92%	83%

* The ¹³C breath test is the most accurate non-invasive *Helicobacter* test.

Differential diagnosis of dyspepsia

- Functional dyspepsia (70%).
- Duodenal/gastric ulcer (15%).
- Duodenitis.
- Oesophagitis/GORD (15%).
- Gastric malignancy.
- Gastritis (p248).

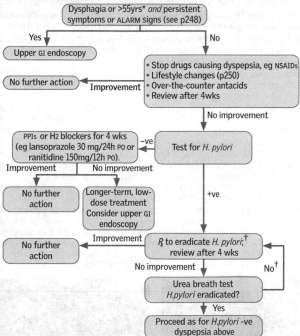

Fig 6.16 See NICE dyspepsia guidelines.⁵ * Nothing magical happens on the 55th birthday—this is simply an inflection point in population risk data. US and Canadian guidelines have increased the age to 60. We should not be overly rigid in applying these rules to the patient in front of us—though those who hold the purse strings may at time seek to reduce costs by strict enforcement of such guidelines.
† Don't treat +ve cases of *H. pylori* more than twice. If still +ve refer for specialist opinion.

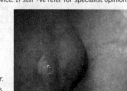

Fig 6.17 Endoscopic image of a duodenal ulcer.
© Dr Jon Simmons.

GORD is common, and caused by reflux of stomach contents (acid ± bile)[8] causing troublesome symptoms and/or complications. If reflux is prolonged, it may cause oesophagitis (fig 6.18), benign oesophageal stricture, or Barrett's oesophagus (fig 6.19 and BOX; it is pre-malignant). **Causes** Lower oesophageal sphincter hypotension, hiatus hernia (see BOX), oesophageal dysmotility (eg systemic sclerosis), obesity, gastric acid hypersecretion, delayed gastric emptying, smoking, alcohol, pregnancy, drugs that reduce lower oesophageal sphincter pressure or affect motility (tricyclics, anticholinergics, nitrates, Ca^{2+} channel blockers), *Helicobacter pylori*?[9]

Symptoms Oesophageal Heartburn (burning, retrosternal discomfort after meals, lying, stooping, or straining, relieved by antacids); belching; acid brash (acid or bile regurgitation); waterbrash (↑↑salivation: 'My mouth fills with saliva'); odynophagia (painful swallowing, eg from oesophagitis or ulceration). **Extra-oesophageal** Nocturnal asthma, chronic cough, laryngitis (hoarseness, throat clearing), sinusitis.

Complications Oesophagitis, ulcers, benign stricture, iron-deficiency. **Metaplasia →dysplasia→neoplasia** GORD may lead to Barrett's oesophagus (fig 6.19 and BOX).

ΔΔ Oesophagitis from corrosives, NSAIDs, herpes, *Candida*; duodenal or gastric ulcers or cancers; non-ulcer dyspepsia; oesophageal spasm; cardiac disease; functional heartburn/reflux hypersensitivity.

Tests Endoscopy if dysphagia, or if ≥55yrs old with *alarm symptoms* (p248) or with treatment-refractory dyspepsia. 24h oesophageal pH monitoring ± manometry help diagnose GORD when endoscopy is normal.

Treatment Lifestyle Weight loss; smoking cessation; small, regular meals; reduce hot drinks, alcohol, citrus fruits, tomatoes, onions, fizzy drinks, spicy foods, caffeine, chocolate; avoid eating <3h before bed. Raise the bed head.

Drugs Antacids, eg magnesium trisilicate mixture (10mL/8h), or alginates, eg Gaviscon® (10–20mL/8h PO) relieve symptoms. Add a PPI, eg lansoprazole 30mg/24h PO. For refractory symptoms, add an H_2 blocker and/or try twice-daily PPI. Avoid drugs affecting oesophageal motility (as *causes* above) or that damage mucosa (NSAIDs, K^+ salts, bisphosphonates, tetracyclines). Monitor for ↓Mg on long-term PPI treatment, and use the shortest course possible (discontinue if asymptomatic).

Surgery (eg laparoscopic Nissen fundoplication, or novel options including laparoscopic insertion of a LINX® magnetic sphincter prothesis or endoscopic radiofrequency-induced hypertrophy.) These all aim to ↑ lower oesophageal sphincter tone. Consider in PPI-refractory GORD (if confirmed by pH monitoring/manometry, surgery is superior to medical management[6]). Atypical symptoms (cough, laryngitis) are less likely to improve with surgery than typical symptoms.

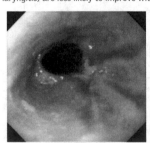

Fig 6.18 Upper GI endoscopy showing longitudinal mucosal breaks in severe oesophagitis.
© Dr A Mee.

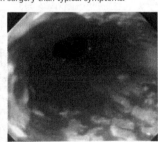

Fig 6.19 Barrett's oesophagus.
© Dr A Mee.

8 The reflux of duodenal fluid, pancreatic secretions and bile may be as important as acid; it may respond to similar lifestyle measures, sucralfate (2g/12h PO), domperidone, or metoclopramide.
9 *H. pylori* association with GORD controversial, but eradication may help symptoms especially if antral-predominant gastritis is present.

Barrett's oesophagus

Barrett's oesophagus is metaplasia of the normal stratified squamous epithelium of the distal oesophagus to a columnar epithelium, as a result of chronic GORD. Prevalence estimates vary widely; ≈8% in patients with symptomatic GORD, ≈6% in *asymptomatic* individuals. Population-based screening is not recommended, but is advised in those with chronic GORD symptoms and *multiple* risk factors (>50 years old, hiatus hernia, obesity, ♂, white race, smoking, family history of Barrett's or oesophageal adenocarcinoma). **Diagnosis** Biopsy of endoscopically visible columnarization, or the newly-developed Cytosponge® (encapsulated sponge which is swallowed and retrieved). The length should be recorded (using the Prague criteria). **Management** ►Focus on detecting and preventing the most significant associated morbidity: oesophageal adenocarcinoma. The relative risk of progression is 30× that of the general population, but the absolute risk is low (0.1–0.4% per patient per year). Risk factors for malignant transformation include ↑age, ♂, long segment involved, and evidence of dysplasia. Daily PPI for all patients. Endoscopic surveillance for dysplasia is recommended but supportive evidence is lacking. For patients without intestinal metaplasia (IM) or dysplasia and with a short (<3cm) segment, encourage discharge.[7] For those with IM, survey every 3–5 years, and >3cm segments every 2–3 years. Low-grade dysplasia warrants repeat endoscopy in 6 months and mucosal radiofrequency ablation (RFA), if confirmed. RFA or *endoscopic resection* for high-grade dysplasia or intramural carcinoma.

Hiatus hernia

Sliding hiatus hernia (95%) The gastro-oesophageal junction slides up into the chest—see fig 6.20. Acid reflux often happens as the lower oesophageal sphincter becomes less competent in many cases.

Paraoesophageal hernia (rolling hiatus hernia) (5%) The gastric fundus herniates up into the chest alongside the oesophagus—see figs 6.20, 6.21. In the majority of types where the gastro-oesophageal junction remains intact, GORD is less common. *Clinical features:* common: 30% of patients >50yrs, especially obese women. Although most small hernias are asymptomatic, patients with large hernias may develop GORD. *Imaging:* upper GI endoscopy visualizes the mucosa (?oesophagitis) but cannot reliably exclude a hiatus hernia. *Treatment:* lose weight. Treat GORD. Surgery indications: intractable symptoms despite aggressive medical therapy, complications (see p252). Although paraoesophageal hernias may strangulate the risk of this drops dramatically after 65yrs. Prophylactic repair is only undertaken in those considered at high risk, due to operative mortality (≈1–2%).

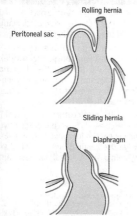

Fig 6.20 Hiatus hernia—sliding and rolling.

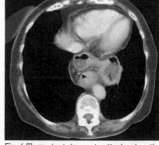

Fig 6.21 CT chest (IV contrast) showing the rolling components of a hiatus hernia anterior to the oesophagus. Between the oesophagus and the vertebral column on the left-hand side is the aorta.

© Dr S Golding.

Upper gastrointestinal bleeding

Haematemesis is vomiting of blood. It may be bright red or look like coffee grounds. *Melaena* (Greek *melas* = black) means black stool, often like tar, and has a characteristic smell of altered blood. Both indicate upper GI bleeding.

Take a brief history and examine to assess severity.

Ask about Past GI bleeds; dyspepsia/known ulcers; known liver disease or oesophageal varices; dysphagia; prolonged vomiting/retching (can cause an oesophageal mucosal 'Mallory-Weiss' tear); weight loss. Check drugs (NSAIDs, aspirin,

Common causes	Rare causes
• Peptic ulcers	• Angiodysplasia
• Severe gastritis/ oesophagitis/duodenitis	• Dieulafoy lesion[10]
• Oesophageal varices	• Gastric antral vascular ectasia[11]
• Portal hypertensive gastropathy	• Aorto-enteric fistula[12]
• Mallory-Weiss tear	• Haemobilia
• Malignancy	• Bleeding disorders
• No obvious cause.	• Osler-Weber-Rendu syndrome.

steroids, thrombolytics, anticoagulants) and alcohol use. Is there serious comorbidity (bad prognosis), eg cardiovascular disease, respiratory disease, hepatic or renal impairment, or malignancy? *Look for* signs of chronic liver disease (p272) and do a PR to check for melaena. Is the patient shocked? Also:
• Peripherally cool/clammy; capillary refill time >2s; urine output <0.5mL/kg/h.
• ↓GCS (tricky to assess in decompensated liver disease) or encephalopathy (p272).
• Tachycardic (pulse >100bpm).
• Systolic BP <100mmHg; postural drop >20mmHg.
• Calculate the *Rockall score* (tables 6.7, 6.8).

Acute management (p804). Skill in resuscitation determines survival, so get good at this! Endoscopy comes only after initial resuscitation.

Further management ►Anatomy is important in assessing risk of rebleeding. Posterior DU are highest risk as they are nearest to the gastroduodenal artery.
• Re-examine after 4h and consider the need for FFP if >4 units transfused.
• Hourly pulse, BP, CVP, urine output (4hrly if haemodynamically stable may be OK).
• A restrictive transfusion strategy has better outcomes,[8] transfuse only if Hb <80g/L; ensure a current valid group & save sample.
• Check FBC, U&E, LFT, and clotting daily.
• Keep nil by mouth if at high rebleed risk (see BOX 'Management of peptic ulcer bleeds' and 'Risk scoring for upper GI bleeds')—ask the endoscopist.

Gastro-oesophageal varices

Submucosal venous dilatation 2° to ↑portal pressures (►may not have documented liver disease—suspect varices if alcohol history); bleeding can be brisk, particularly if underlying coagulopathy 2° to loss of hepatic synthesis of clotting factors.

Causes of portal hypertension **Pre-hepatic** Thrombosis (portal or splenic vein). **Intra-hepatic** Cirrhosis (80% in UK); schistosomiasis (commonest worldwide); sarcoid; myeloproliferative diseases; congenital hepatic fibrosis. **Post-hepatic** Budd–Chiari syndrome (p686); right heart failure; constrictive pericarditis; veno-occlusive disease. **Risk factors for variceal bleeds** ↑Portal pressure, variceal size, endoscopic features of the variceal wall and advanced liver disease.

Management Endoscopic banding (oesophageal) or sclerotherapy (gastric). **Prophylaxis** *1°:* ~30% of cirrhotics with varices bleed vs ~15% with non-selective β-blockade (propranolol 20–40mg/12h PO) or repeat endoscopic banding. *2°:* after a 1st variceal bleed, 60% rebleed within 1yr. Use banding and non-selective β-blockade; transjugular intrahepatic portosystemic shunt (TIPS) for resistant varices.

---

10 A Dieulafoy lesion is the rupture of an unusually big arteriole, eg in the fundus of the stomach.
11 Also known as 'watermelon stomach', red bands of ectatic submucosal vessels radiate from the pylorus.
12 A patient with an aortic graft repair and upper GI bleeding is considered to have an aorto-enteric fistula until proven otherwise: CT abdomen is usually required as well as endoscopy.

Risk-scoring for upper GI bleeds

Glasgow Blatchford score (GBS) Used pre-endoscopy, so can be calculated when the patient first presents. The score ranges from 0–23, with higher scores predicting an increased risk of requiring endoscopic intervention. If GBS ≈ 0, the likelihood ratio for needing urgent endoscopy is 0.02, therefore admission can be avoided—ie Hb ≥130g/L (or ≥120g/L if ♀); systolic BP ≥110mmHg; pulse <100/min; urea <6.5mmol/L; no melaena or syncope + no past/present liver disease or heart failure.

Rockall score Initial Rockall score is based on pre-endoscopy criteria; these are added to post-endoscopy criteria for final score which predicts risk of rebleeding and death (table 6.8).

Table 6.7 Rockall score calculation

	0pts	1pt	2pts	3pts
Pre-endoscopy				
Age	<60yrs	60–79yrs	≥80yrs	
Shock: systolic BP & pulse rate	systolic BP >100mmHg Pulse <100/min	BP >100mmHg Pulse >100/min	BP <100mmHg	
Comorbidity	Nil major	Heart failure; ischaemic heart disease	Renal failure Liver failure	Metastases
Post-endoscopy				
Diagnosis	Mallory–Weiss tear; no lesion; no sign of recent bleeding	All other diagnoses	Upper GI malignancy	
Signs of recent haemorrhage on endoscopy	None, or dark red spot		Blood in upper GI tract; adherent clot; visible vessel	

Table 6.8 GI bleed mortality by Rockall score

Score	Mortality with initial scoring	Mortality after endoscopy
0	0.2%	0%
1	2.4%	0%
2	5.6%	0.2%
3	11.0%	2.9%
4	24.6%	5.3%
5	39.6%	10.8%
6	48.9%	17.3%
7	50.0%	27.0%
8+	–	41.1%

Management of peptic ulcer bleeds based on endoscopic findings

High-risk *Active bleeding, adherent clot, or non-bleeding visible vessel:* achieve endoscopic haemostasis (2 of: clips, cautery, adrenaline). Admit to monitored bed; start PPI (eg omeprazole 40mg/12h IV/PO; meta-analyses show 72h IV omeprazole 80mg bolus then 8mg/h *not* superior). If haemodynamically stable start oral intake of clear liquids 6h after endoscopy. Treat if positive for *H. pylori* (p248).

Low-risk *Flat, pigmented spot or clean base:* no need for endoscopic haemostasis. Consider early discharge if patient otherwise low risk. Give oral PPI (p248). Regular diet 6h after endoscopy if stable. Treat if positive for *H. pylori* (p248).

Diarrhoea is characterized by increased stool frequency and volume and decreased consistency relative to the usual habit of the individual.

History As ever, a careful history will help narrow myriad causes to just a few.

Acute or chronic? If acute (<2wks) suspect gastroenteritis—any risk factors: travel (p425)? Diet change? Contact with D&V? Any fever/pain? Pregnant (20× risk of listeriosis)? HIV; achlorhydria (eg PA, p330), or on acid suppressants, eg PPI? Chronic diarrhoea alternating with constipation suggests IBS (p264). ↓Weight, nocturnal diarrhoea, or anaemia mandate close follow-up (coeliac/UC/Crohn's?). Chronic is ≥4wks (fig 6.22).

Inflammatory? Small volume, high frequency, urgency, pre-defecation lower abdominal cramping, tenesmus. May be nocturnal, bloody, and associated with fever and shock. (See fig 6.22 for causes.) Non-inflammatory diarrhoea is watery and large volume, upper abdominal cramping.

Bloody? *Campylobacter*, *Shigella/Salmonella* (p427), *E. coli*, amoebiasis (p428), UC, Crohn's, colorectal cancer (p608), colonic polyps, pseudomembranous colitis, ischaemic colitis (p617). *Fresh PR bleeding*: p621.

Mucus Occurs in IBS (p264), colorectal cancer, and polyps.

Frank pus Suggests IBD, diverticulitis, or a fistula/abscess.

Explosive Eg cholera; *Giardia*; *Yersinia* (p427); *Rotavirus*.

Steatorrhoea (See fig 6.22.)

Drugs? (Many potentially to blame, see *BNF*.) Eg antibiotics,[13] cytotoxics, laxative abuse, propranolol, digoxin, PPIs, NSAIDs. The latter two are particularly associated with microscopic colitis.[14]

Look for Dehydration—dry mucous membranes, ↓skin turgor; capillary refill >2s; shock. Any fever, ↓weight, clubbing, anaemia, oral ulcers (p242), rashes or abdominal mass or scars? Any goitre/hyperthyroid signs? Do rectal exam for masses (eg rectal cancer) or impacted faeces:

- **Blood** *FBC:* ↓MCV/Fe deficiency, eg coeliac or colon ca; ↑MCV if alcohol abuse or ↓B12 absorption, eg in coeliac or Crohn's; eosinophilia if parasites. ↑ESR/CRP: infection, Crohn's/UC, cancer. *U&E:* ↓K+ ≈ severe D&V. ↓TSH: thyrotoxicosis. *Coeliac serology:* p262.
- **Stool** *MC&S:* bacterial pathogens, ova cysts, parasites, *C. diff* toxin (CDT, see BOX '*Clostridium difficile*'), viral PCR. *Faecal calprotectin:* highly sensitive for inflammatory causes (p258, p260). *Faecal elastase:* if suspect chronic pancreatitis (malabsorption, steatorrhoea).
- **Lower GI endoscopy** (Malignancy? Colitis?) ▶If acutely unwell, limited flexible sigmoidoscopy with biopsies. Full colonoscopy (including terminal ileum) can assess for more proximal disease If normal, consider small bowel radiology or video capsule.

Management Treat cause. Food handlers: no work until stool samples are –ve. If a hospital outbreak, wards may need closing. *Oral rehydration* is better than IV, but ▶if sustained diarrhoea or vomiting, IV fluids with appropriate electrolyte replacement may be needed. Codeine phosphate 30mg/8h PO or loperamide 2mg PO after each loose stool (max 16mg/day) ↓stool frequency (▶avoid in colitis; both may precipitate toxic megacolon). Avoid antibiotics unless infective diarrhoea is causing systemic upset, but consider metronidazole if *C. diff* is suspected (see BOX). *Antibiotic-associated diarrhoea*[13] may respond to probiotics (eg lactobacilli).

13 Erythromycin is prokinetic, others cause overgrowth of bowel organisms, or alter bile acids.
14 Think of this in any chronic watery diarrhoea; diagnosis by biopsy. Associated with a range of drugs including NSAIDs and PPIs. Stop the offending drug where possible. Treat with budesonide.

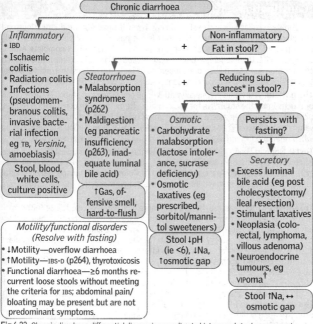

Fig 6.22 Chronic diarrhoea differential diagnosis according to history and stool assessment.
* Non-absorbed carbohydrate; lab tested with stool electrolytes, pH, and osmotic gap in watery diarrhoea.
† Vasoactive intestinal polypeptide-secreting tumour; suspect if ↓K⁺ and acidosis; ↑Ca²⁺; ↓Mg²⁻

Clostridium difficile: the cause of pseudomembranous colitis

First isolated from stools of healthy neonates, *C. difficile* was named owing to difficulties in culture. Today, '*difficile*' might better refer to challenges of containment.

Signs ↑T°; colic; diarrhoea with systemic upset—↑↑CRP, ↑WCC, ↓albumin, and colitis (with yellow adherent plaques on inflamed non-ulcerated mucosa—the pseudomembrane) progressing to toxic megacolon and multi-organ failure.

Asymptomatic carriage 2–5% of all adults. Only problematic with gut ecology disrupted by, eg antibiotics, leading to rapid proliferation and toxin expression.

Predictors of fulminant *C. diff* colitis >70yrs; past *C. diff* infection; use of antiperistaltic drugs; severe leucocytosis; haemodynamic instability.

Detection Urgent testing of suspicious stool (characteristic smell—ask the nurses). Two-stage process with rapid screening test for *C. diff* protein (or PCR) followed by specific ELISA for toxins. AXR for toxic megacolon.

℞ Stop causative antibiotic if possible. Mild disease: metronidazole 400mg/8h PO for 10–14d (vancomycin 125mg/6h PO is better in severe disease). Intensive regimens of vancomycin 500mg/6h with IV and PR vancomycin may be needed for non-responders. ►Urgent colectomy may be needed if toxic megacolon, ↑LDH, or if deteriorating.

Recurrent disease Common (≈20%). After a first recurrence, the risk of another rises to ≈50%. Fidaxomicin (200mg/12h PO), a minimally absorbed oral antibiotic, is associated with lower relapse rates and is recommended. Faecal transplantation (introduction of a suspension prepared from the faeces of a screened donor via endoscopy or via NG/NJ tube) is a highly effective, if aesthetically unappealing, treatment.

Preventing spread Meticulous cleaning and appropriate bed management policies, use of disposable gloves and aprons, hand-washing (not just gel—kill the spores).

Constipation

Constipation reflects pelvic dysfunction or ↑transit time. Accepted definitions and reported rates vary, but a place to start is the passage of ≤2 bowel motions/wk, often passed with difficulty, straining, or pain, and a sense of incomplete evacuation. ♀:♂≈2:1. Doctors' chief concerns are to find pointers to major pathology, eg constipation + rectal bleeding ≈ cancer; constipation + distension + active bowel sounds ≈ stricture/GI obstruction; constipation + menorrhagia ≈ hypothyroidism.

The patient Ask about frequency, nature, and consistency of stools. Is there blood or mucus in/on the stools? Is there diarrhoea alternating with constipation (eg IBS, p264)? Has there been recent change in bowel habit? Is she digitating the rectum or vagina to pass stool?[15] Ask about diet and drugs. ►PR examination is essential even when referring (refer if signs of colorectal ca, eg ↓weight, pain, or anaemia).

Tests None in young, mildly affected patients. Threshold for investigation diminishes with age; triggers include:[9] ↓weight, abdominal mass, +PR blood, iron deficiency anaemia. **Blood** FBC, ESR, U&E, Ca^{2+}, TFT. **Colonoscopy** If suspected colorectal malignancy. Transit studies; anorectal physiology; biopsy for Hirschsprung's are occasionally needed.

Treatment Often reassurance, drinking more, and diet/exercise advice (p239) is all that is needed. Treat causes (BOX 'Causes of constipation'). A high-fibre diet is often advised, but may cause bloating without helping constipation. ►Only use drugs if these measures fail, and try to use them for short periods only. Often, a stimulant such as senna ± a bulking agent is more effective and cheaper than agents such as lactulose. **Bulking agents** ↑Faecal mass, so stimulating peristalsis. They must be taken with plenty of fluid and may take a few days to act. CI: difficulty in swallowing; GI obstruction; colonic atony; faecal impaction. Bran powder 3.5g 2–3 times/d with food (may hinder absorption of dietary trace elements if taken with every meal). Ispaghula husk, eg 1 Fybogel® sachet after a meal, mixed in water and swallowed promptly (or else it becomes an unpleasant sludge). Methylcellulose, eg Celevac® 3–6 tablets/12h with ≥300mL water. Sterculia, eg Normacol® granules, 10mL sprinkled on food daily. **Stimulant laxatives** Increase intestinal motility, so do not use in intestinal obstruction or acute colitis. Avoid prolonged use as it *may* cause colonic atony. Abdominal cramps are an important SE. Pure stimulant laxatives are bisacodyl tablets (5–10mg at night) or suppositories (10mg in the mornings) and senna (2–4 tablets at night). Docusate sodium and dantron[16] have stimulant and softening actions. Glycerol suppositories act as a rectal stimulant. Sodium picosulfate (5–10mg at night) is a potent stimulant. Phosphate enemas are useful for rapid bowel evacuation prior to procedures. **Stool softeners** Particularly useful when managing painful anal conditions, eg fissure. Arachis oil enemas lubricate and soften impacted faeces. Liquid paraffin should not be used for a prolonged period (SE: anal seepage, lipoid pneumonia, malabsorption of fat-soluble vitamins). **Osmotic laxatives** Retain fluid in the bowel. Lactulose, a semisynthetic disaccharide, produces osmotic diarrhoea of low faecal pH that discourages growth of ammonia-producing organisms. It is useful in hepatic encephalopathy (initial dose: 30–50mL/12h). SE: bloating, so its role in treating constipation is limited. Macrogol (eg Movicol®) is a better tolerated example. Magnesium salts (eg magnesium hydroxide; magnesium sulfate) are useful when rapid bowel evacuation is required. Sodium salts (eg Microlette® and Micralax® enemas) should be avoided as they may cause sodium and water retention.

If these don't help Prucalopride is a selective 5HT$_4$ agonist with prokinetic properties; lubiprostone is a chloride-channel activator that increases intestinal fluid secretion; linaclotide is a guanylate cyclase-c agonist that also increases fluid secretion and decreases visceral pain. Naloxegol (an opioid blocker bound to macrogol) has recently been authorized for laxative-resistant opioid-induced constipation. A multidisciplinary approach with behaviour therapy, habit training ± sphincter biofeedback may help.

15 *Rectocele:* front wall of the rectum bulges into the back wall of the vagina.
16 Dantron causes colon & liver tumours in animals, so reserve use for the very elderly or terminally ill.

Causes of constipation

General
- Poor diet ± lack of exercise.
- Poor fluid intake/dehydration.
- Irritable bowel syndrome.
- Old age.
- Post-operative pain.
- Hospital environment (↓privacy; having to use a bed pan).

Anorectal disease (Esp. if painful.)
- ▶▶ Anal or colorectal cancer.
- Fissures (p622), strictures, herpes.
- Rectal prolapse.
- Proctalgia fugax (p622).
- Mucosal ulceration/neoplasia.
- Pelvic muscle dysfunction/levator ani syndrome.

Intestinal obstruction
- ▶▶ Colorectal carcinoma (p608).
- Strictures (eg Crohn's disease).
- Pelvic mass (eg fetus, fibroids).
- Diverticulosis (rectal bleeding is a commoner presentation).
- Pseudo-obstruction (p603).

Metabolic/endocrine
- Hypercalcaemia (p668).
- Hypothyroidism (rarely presents with constipation).
- Hypokalaemia (p666).
- Porphyria.
- Lead poisoning.

Drugs (Pre-empt by diet advice.)
- Opiates (eg morphine, codeine).
- Anticholinergics (eg tricyclics).
- Iron.
- Some antacids, eg with aluminium.
- Diuretics, eg furosemide.
- Calcium channel blockers.

Neuromuscular (Slow transit from decreased propulsive activity.)
- Spinal or pelvic nerve injury (eg trauma, surgery).
- Aganglionosis (Chagas' disease, Hirschsprung's disease).
- Systemic sclerosis.
- Diabetic neuropathy.

Other causes
- Chronic laxative abuse (rare—diarrhoea is commoner).
- Idiopathic slow transit.
- Idiopathic megarectum/colon.
- Functional constipation.

6 Gastroenterology

6 Gastroenterology

UC is a relapsing and remitting inflammatory disorder of the colonic mucosa. It may affect just the rectum (proctitis, as in ~30%) or extend to involve part of the colon (left-sided colitis, in ~40%) or the entire colon (pancolitis, in ~30%). It 'never' spreads proximal to the ileocaecal valve (except for backwash ileitis). **Cause** Inappropriate immune response against (?abnormal) colonic flora in genetically susceptible individuals. **Pathology** Hyperaemic/haemorrhagic colonic mucosa ± pseudopolyps formed by inflammation. Punctate ulcers may extend deep into the lamina propria—inflammation is normally not transmural. Continuous inflammation limited to the mucosa differentiates it from Crohn's disease. **Prevalence** 200–1000/100 000. **Incidence** 10–20/100 000/yr; typically presents ~15–40yrs. **Associations** UC is 3-fold as common in non-smokers (opposite is true for Crohn's disease)—symptoms may relapse on stopping smoking.

Symptoms Episodic or chronic diarrhoea (± blood & mucus); crampy abdominal discomfort; bowel frequency relates to severity (table 6.9); urgency/tenesmus ≈ proctitis. Systemic symptoms in attacks: fever, malaise, anorexia, ↓weight.

Signs May be none. In acute, severe UC there may be fever, tachycardia, and a tender, distended abdomen. **Extra-intestinal signs** Clubbing; aphthous oral ulcers; erythema nodosum (fig 6.23, p261); pyoderma gangrenosum; conjunctivitis; episcleritis; iritis; large joint arthritis; sacroiliitis; ankylosing spondylitis; PSC (p278); nutritional deficits.

Complications Acute Toxic dilatation of colon (mucosal islands, colonic diameter >6cm) with risk of perforation; venous thromboembolism: give prophylaxis to all inpatients regardless of rectal bleeding (p34); ↓K⁺ **Chronic** Colonic cancer: risk related to disease extent and activity ≈5–10% if uncontrolled pancolitis for 20yrs. Neoplasms may occur in flat, normal-looking mucosa. To spot precursor areas of dysplasia, surveillance colonoscopy, eg 1–5yrs (depending on risk), with multiple random biopsies or biopsies guided by differential uptake by abnormal mucosa of dye sprayed endoscopically.

Tests Blood FBC, ESR, CRP, U&E, LFT, blood culture. Consider performing pretreatment tests early (see BOX). **Stool MC&S/CDT** (See p254.) To exclude *Campylobacter*, *C. difficile*, *Salmonella*, *Shigella*, *E. coli*, amoebae. **Faecal calprotectin** A simple, non-invasive test for GI inflammation with high sensitivity. **AXR** No faecal shadows; mucosal thickening/islands (fig 16.9, p713); colonic dilatation (see 'Complications'). **Lower GI endoscopy** Limited flexible sigmoidoscopy if acute to assess and biopsy; full colonoscopy once controlled to define disease extent (see p245, fig 6.12).

Table 6.9 Assessing severity in UC (Truelove & Witts criteria modified to include CRP)

Variable	Mild UC	Moderate UC	Severe UC
Motions/day	≤4	5	≥6
Rectal bleeding	Small	Moderate	Large
T°C	Apyrexial	37.1–37.8°C	>37.8°C
Resting pulse	<70 beats/min	70–90 beats/min	>90 beats/min
Haemoglobin	>110g/L	105–110g/L	<105g/L
ESR (do CRP too)	<30		>30 (or CRP >45mg/L)

Data from Truelove et al., 'Cortisone in ulcerative colitis', BMJ; 2(4947): 1041–8.

Treatment Goals are to induce, then maintain disease remission. Management is based on the severity and anatomical extent of disease.

Inducing remission
Mild to moderate UC: • For distal disease (proctitis and proctosigmoiditis) topical 5-ASA,[17] eg mesalazine is the mainstay; suppositories or enemas, eg Pentasa® 1g daily. If remission is not achieved after a month, consider adding PO 5-ASA treatment (eg Pentasa® 2g daily) and/or a topical steroid (eg hydrocortisone as Colifoam®, or prednisolone 20mg retention enemas as Predsol®). • For extensive disease combine PR + PO 5-ASA. If no remission after 1 month stop the topical treatment and add a course of oral *prednisolone* 40mg/d for 1wk, then taper by 5mg/week over following 7wks, then maintain on 5-ASA.

17 5-aminosalicylic acid (5-ASA or mesalazine) must be stabilized in oral preparations to survive gastric pH. Alternatively, olsalazine is a dimer of 5-ASA or balsalazide is a prodrug, both of which are cleaved in the colon. Rare hypersensitivity reactions: worsening colitis, pancreatitis, pericarditis, nephritis.

Severe UC: admit for: IV hydration/electrolyte replacement; IV steroids, eg hydrocortisone 100mg/6h or methylprednisolone 40mg/12h; rectal steroids, eg hydrocortisone 100mg in 100mL 0.9% saline/12h PR; thromboembolism prophylaxis (p346); ensure multiple stool MC&S/CDT to exclude infection.

- Monitor T°, pulse, and BP—and record stool frequency/character on a stool chart.
- Twice-daily exam: document distension, bowel sounds, and tenderness.
- Daily FBC, ESR, CRP, U&E ± AXR. Consider blood transfusion (eg if Hb <80g/L).
- If on day 3–5 CRP >45 or >6 stools/d, ▶▶action is needed.[18] *Rescue therapy* with ciclosporin or infliximab, can avoid colectomy, but involve surgeons early in shared care.
- If improving, transfer to prednisolone PO (40mg/24h). Schedule maintenance infliximab if used for rescue, or azathioprine if ciclosporin rescue.
- If failure to improve then refer for urgent colectomy by d7–10—the challenge is not to delay surgery so long as to accumulate significant steroid exposure and debilitation that will delay post-surgical recovery.

Maintaining remission

Mild to moderate: PO (and/or PR if distal) 5-ASA is first line maintenance therapy, decreasing relapse rates from 80% to 20% at 1 year. Once-daily dosing is as effective as split dose and may improve adherence. ▶Nephrotoxicity risk; monitor U&E at the start, then after 2–3 months, then annually.

Moderate to severe: consider maintenance treatment escalation with immunomodulation in patients who flare on steroid tapering or require ≥2 courses of steroids/year, eg azathioprine (2–2.5mg/kg/d PO). 30% of patients will develop SE requiring treatment cessation including abdominal pain, nausea, pancreatitis, leucopenia, abnormal LFTs. Monitor FBC, U&E, LFT weekly for 4wks, then every 4wks for 3 months, then at least 3-monthly. Biologics were once reserved for those intolerant of immunosuppressive therapy, but with the availability of agents with less risk of toxicity and high efficacy they are being increasingly used both to induce and maintain remission (see BOX 'Therapies in Crohn's disease', p261). *Monoclonal antibodies to TNFα* (infliximab, adalimumab, golimumab), to gut-selective integrins (vedolizumab), to interleukin 12/23 (ustekinumab) play an important role. Small molecule drugs including Janus kinase (JAK) inhibitors (tofacitinib, filgotinib, upadacitinib) offer effective oral options.

Surgery This is needed at some stage in ~20%, eg *subtotal colectomy + terminal ileostomy* for failure of medical therapy or fulminant colitis with toxic dilatation/perforation. Subsequently *completion proctectomy* (permanent stoma) vs *ileo–anal pouch*. Pouches mean stoma reversal and the possibility of long-term continence but pouch opening frequency may still be around 6×/day and recurrent pouchitis can be troublesome (give antibiotics, eg metronidazole + ciprofloxacin for 2wks).

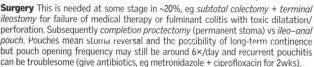

Immunomodulator and biologics pretreatment screening

All newly diagnosed IBD patients should be screened for infection risk, both as preparation for immunosuppressive treatment and because of the overall increased risk.

- TB screening—ask about prior infection and exposures. CXR and interferon-gamma release assay (IGRA) (p390) in those considered for biologic therapy.
- Vaccination history—consider updating vaccinations in all patients prior to treatment, at least 4 weeks before starting. Pneumococcal and annual flu vaccine. VZV vaccination if immunosuppression planned.
- Serology—screen for HCV, HBV, HIV. Varicella IgG testing in patients without a clear history of chickenpox, shingles, or vaccination.
- Azathioprine precautions—test for ↓TPMT activity[19] (↓ dose if low activity; avoid if no activity), ensure cervical screening is up to date and provide skin cancer risk advice.

18 Day 3 stool frequency >8×/day *or* frequency 3–8×/day & CRP >45 = 85% chance of colectomy *this admission.*

19 Inherited ↓thiopurine methyltransferase in <1% is associated with an increased risk of potentially life-threatening bone marrow suppression.

A chronic inflammatory disease characterized by transmural granulomatous inflammation affecting any part of the gut from mouth to anus (esp. terminal ileum in ~70%). Unlike with UC, there may be unaffected bowel between areas of active disease (skip lesions). **Cause** As with UC an inappropriate immune response against the (?abnormal) gut flora in a genetically susceptible individual.[20] **Prevalence** 200–1000/100 000. **Incidence** 10–20/100 000/yr; typically presents ~15–40yrs. **Associations** Smoking ↑risk ×3–4; NSAIDs may exacerbate disease.

Symptoms Diarrhoea, abdominal pain, weight loss/failure to thrive. Systemic symptoms: fatigue, fever, malaise, anorexia.

Signs Bowel ulceration (fig 6.24); abdominal tenderness/mass; perianal abscess/fistulae/skin tags; anal strictures; aphthous ulcers (p242). **Beyond the gut** (fig 6.23) Clubbing, skin, joint, & eye problems.

Complications Small bowel obstruction; toxic dilatation (colonic diameter >6cm, toxic dilatation is rarer than in UC); abscess formation (abdominal, pelvic, or perianal); fistulae (present in ~10%), eg entero-enteric, colovesical (bladder), colovaginal, perianal, enterocutaneous; perforation; colon cancer; PSC (p278); malnutrition.

Tests Blood FBC, ESR, CRP, U&E, LFT, INR, ferritin, TIBC, B₁₂, folate. Biologics pretreatment tests (see BOX 'Immunomodulator and biologics pretreatment screening' p259) **Stool** MC&S and CDT (p254) to exclude, eg *C. difficile*, *Campylobacter*, *E. coli*; faecal calprotectin is a simple, non-invasive test for GI inflammation with high sensitivity. **Colonoscopy + biopsy** Even if mucosa looks normal. **Small bowel** To detect isolated proximal disease by, eg *capsule endoscopy* (p244, use dummy patency capsule 1st that disintegrates if it gets stuck); MRI increasingly used to assess pelvic disease and fistulae, small bowel disease activity and strictures; US in skilled hands can provide small bowel imaging.

Treatment Find out how your patient deals with what may be a brutal disease (no intimacy... no sex... no hope... 'I live with this alone and will die alone'). With a collaborative approach, courage, attention to detail, and psychological support, this can change. Help quit smoking. ►*Optimize nutrition.* Assess severity: ↑T°, ↑pulse, ↑ESR, ↑WCC, ↑CRP, + ↓albumin may merit admission for IV steroids.

Inducing remission

Mild to moderate: symptomatic but systemically well. Prednisolone 40mg/d PO for 1wk, then taper by 5mg every wk for next 7wks. Budesonide (an enteric-coated steroid with extensive 1st-pass metabolism) has fewer side effects so is useful if there are contraindications, but is less effective. Exclusive enteral nutrition (EEN) is an alternative dietary approach based upon a liquid diet with polymeric (whole protein) or semi-elemental (peptide)-based feeds (more palatable than the elemental diet), is effective in children but used less in adults.

Severe: consider admission for IV hydration/electrolyte replacement; IV steroids and similar initial care to severe UC (p259). If improving switch to oral prednisolone (40mg/d). A 'top-down' approach with the early introduction of biologics may be considered in patients with an aggressive disease course or poor prognostic factors (see BOX 'Therapies in Crohn's disease'). Consider abdominal sepsis complicating Crohn's disease especially if abdominal pain (ultrasound, CT, & MRI are often required to assess this). Seek surgical advice; laparoscopic resection should be considered for those with relapsing localized ileocaecal disease.

Maintaining remission

Steroids are not effective in maintaining remission, regardless of how it is induced, and expose patients to toxicity risk. Monotherapy with azathioprine is effective (see BOX 'Therapies in Crohn's disease'). Methotrexate (at least 15mg weekly, subcutaneous dosing preferred) is an alternative. Combination therapy with infliximab should be considered in more severe cases, but there are long-term safety issues (eg increased lymphoma risk). Biologics may be considered in those refractory to immunomodulators (see BOX 'Therapies in Crohn's disease').

20 Much of the genetic risk is shared with UC—small differences in genetics combined with environmental modifiers may explain the very different phenotypes.

Therapies in Crohn's disease

Azathioprine (AZA) (2–2.5mg/kg/d PO) used if refractory to steroids, relapsing on steroid taper, or requiring ≥2 steroid courses/yr. Takes 6–10wks to work. 30% will develop SE requiring treatment cessation including abdominal pain, nausea, pancreatitis, leucopenia, abnormal LFTs. Monitor FBC, U&E, LFT weekly for 4wks, then every 4wks for 3 months, then at least 3-monthly. Alternative immunomodulators include 6-mercaptopurine and methotrexate (CI: ♀ of reproductive age).

5-ASA Unlike in UC, has no role in the management of Crohn's.

Biologics Anti-TNFα: TNFα plays an important role in pathogenesis of Crohn's disease, therefore monoclonal antibodies to TNFα, eg infliximab and adalimumab, can ↓ disease activity. They counter neutrophil accumulation and granuloma formation and cause cytotoxicity to CD4+ T cells, thus clearing cells driving the immune response. CI: sepsis, active/latent TB, ↑LFT >3-fold above top end of normal. SE: rash. Avoid in people with known underlying malignancy. **Anti-integrin:** monoclonal antibodies targeting adhesion molecules involved in gut lymphocyte trafficking, eg vedolizumab, reduce disease activity and have a more gut-specific mechanism of activity. **Anti-IL12/23:** another key pathogenic cytokine target with favourable safety profile, eg ustekinumab.

Nutrition Enteral is preferred (with tube feeding if malnourished and poor intake); consider TPN only if no enteral options. **Elemental diets:** (eg E028®.) Contain amino acids and can induce remission.

Surgery 50–80% need ≥1 operation in their life. It never cures. Indications: drug failure (most common); GI obstruction from stricture; perforation; fistulae; abscess. Surgical aims are: 1 Resection of affected areas—but beware short bowel syndrome (p580). 2 To control perianal or fistulizing disease. 3 Defunction (rest) distal disease, eg with a temporary ileostomy. Pouch surgery is avoided in Crohn's (∵ ↑ risk of recurrence).

Perianal disease Occurs in about 50%. MRI and examination under anaesthetic (EUA) are an important part of assessment. Treatment includes oral antibiotics, immunosuppressant therapy ± anti-TNFα, and local surgery ± seton insertion.

Poor prognosis Age <40yrs at diagnosis; steroids needed at 1st presentation; perianal disease; isolated terminal ileitis; smoking.

Diagnosing IBD-unclassified (IBD-U)

After full investigation, IBD may not obviously be Crohn's or UC in 5–15% of patients. IBD-U refers to isolated colonic IBD where the diagnosis remains unknown (small bowel involvement = Crohn's). This situation is rare in adults but commoner in children. Over time the phenotype tends to become clearer (generally UC > Crohn's). Colectomy ± pouch formation may be needed, though pouch failure rate is higher than in UC.

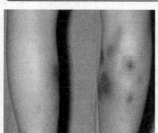

Fig 6.23 Beyond the gut... 'I hate how this stupid illness is crippling me...' As well as erythema nodosum on the shins (above; also caused by sarcoid, drugs, streptococci, and TB), Crohn's can associate with sero −ve arthritis of large or small joints, spondyloarthropathy, ankylosing spondylitis, sacroiliitis, pyoderma gangrenosum, conjunctivitis, episcleritis, and iritis.

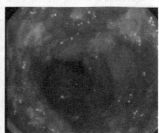

Fig 6.24 Deep fissured ulcers seen at colonoscopy. The end result? 'My family does not or will not even talk to me about the disease... I don't know when urgency to race for the bathroom will happen so I don't go out and have been living a hermit life...'

© Dr A Mee.

Impaired absorption of nutrients, including electrolytes and water, but the term is also used to incorporate maldigestion, the necessary precursor. **Causes** See BOX.

Symptoms Diarrhoea; ↓weight; lethargy; steatorrhoea; bloating. **Deficiency signs** Anaemia (↓Fe, B₁₂, folate); bleeding disorders (↓vit K); oedema (↓protein); metabolic bone disease (↓vit D); neurological features, eg neuropathy.

Tests FBC (↓ or ↑MCV); ↓Ca²⁺; ↓Fe; ↓B₁₂ + folate; ↑INR; lipid profile; coeliac tests (see 'Coeliac disease'). **Stool** Sudan stain for fat globules; stool microscopy (infestation); elastase. **Breath hydrogen analysis** For bacterial overgrowth.[21] Take samples of end-expired air; take more samples at ½h intervals; early ↑exhaled hydrogen = overgrowth. **Endoscopy + small bowel biopsy.**

Infectious malabsorption *Giardia, Cryptosporidium, Isospora belli, Cyclospora cayetanensis*, microsporidia. **Tropical sprue** Villous atrophy + malabsorption occurring in the Far and Middle East and Caribbean—the cause is unknown. Tetracycline 250mg/6h PO + folic acid 5mg/d PO for 3–6mths may help.

Coeliac disease

▶Suspect this if diarrhoea + weight loss or anaemia (esp. if iron or B₁₂ ↓). T-cell responses to gluten (alcohol-soluble proteins in wheat, barley, rye ± oats) in the small bowel causes villous atrophy and malabsorption. **Associations** HLA DQ2 in 95%; the rest are DQ8; autoimmune disease; dermatitis herpetiformis (*OHCS* p438).

Prevalence 1 in 100–300 (commoner if Irish). Any age (peaks in childhood and 50–60yrs). ♀:♂ >1:1. Relative risk in 1st-degree relatives is 6×.

Presentation Steatorrhoea; diarrhoea; abdominal pain; bloating; nausea + vomiting; aphthous ulcers; angular stomatitis (p327, fig 8.21); ↓weight; fatigue; weakness; osteomalacia; failure to thrive (children). ~30% less severe: may mimic IBS.

Diagnosis ↓Hb; ↑RCDW (p325); ↓B₁₂; ↓ferritin. Antibodies: anti-transglutaminase is single preferred test (but is an IgA antibody—check IgA levels to exclude subclass deficiency). Where serology positive or high index of suspicion proceed to duodenal biopsy while on a gluten-containing diet: expect subtotal villous atrophy, ↑intra-epithelial WBCs + crypt hyperplasia. Where doubt persists, HLA DQ2 and DQ8 genotyping may help.

Treatment *Lifelong gluten-free diet*—patients become experts. Rice, maize, soya, potatoes, and sugar are OK. Limited consumption of oats (≤50g/d) may be tolerated in patients with mild disease. Gluten-free biscuits, flour, bread, and pasta are prescribable. Monitor response by symptoms and repeat serology.[10]

Complications Anaemia; osteopenia/osteoporosis; hyposplenism (offer 'flu and pneumococcal vaccinations); GI T-cell lymphoma (rare; suspect if refractory symptoms or ↓weight); ↑malignancy (lymphoma, gastric, oesophageal, colorectal); neuropathies.

Chronic pancreatitis

Epigastric pain 'bores' through to the back, eg relieved by sitting forward or hot water bottles on epigastrium/back (look for skin mottling of *erythema ab igne*); bloating; steatorrhoea; ↓weight; diabetes mellitus. Symptoms relapse and worsen.

Causes Alcohol; smoking; autoimmune; rarely: familial; cystic fibrosis; haemochromatosis; pancreatic duct obstruction (stones/tumour); congenital (*pancreas divisum*).

Tests *Ultrasound* ± CT: pancreatic calcifications confirm the diagnosis, MRCP; AXR: speckled calcification; faecal elastase.

Treatment *Drugs* Give analgesia (coeliac-plexus block may give relief); lipase, eg Creon®; fat-soluble vitamins. Insulin needs may be high or variable (beware hypoglycaemia). *Diet* No alcohol; low fat may help. Medium-chain triglycerides (MCT oil) may be tried (no lipase needed for absorption, but diarrhoea may be worsened). *Surgery* For unremitting pain; narcotic abuse (beware of this); ↓weight: eg pancreatectomy or pancreaticojejunostomy (a duct drainage procedure).

Complications Pseudocyst; diabetes; biliary obstruction; local arterial aneurysm; splenic vein thrombosis; gastric varices; pancreatic carcinoma.

Causes of gastrointestinal malabsorption

Malabsorption results from a failure of any of the phases of digestion and absorption; luminal digestion, mucosal absorption, and postabsorptive transport into the circulation. Disorders with diffuse mucosal involvement cause global malabsorption of almost all nutrients (eg coeliac disease), while certain disorders result in malabsorption that is selective to particular nutrients (eg pernicious anaemia).

Luminal phase
• *Pancreatic insufficiency:* chronic pancreatitis; pancreatic cancer; cystic fibrosis.
• *↓Bile:* primary biliary cholangitis; ileal resection; biliary obstruction; colestyramine.

Mucosal phase
• *Small bowel mucosa:* coeliac disease; Crohn's disease; Whipple's disease (see BOX); radiation enteritis; tropical sprue; small bowel resection; brush border enzyme deficiencies (eg lactase insufficiency); drugs (metformin, neomycin, alcohol); amyloid (p364).
• *Bacterial overgrowth:*[21] spontaneous (esp. in elderly); in jejunal diverticula; post-op blind loops. DM & PPI use are also risk factors. Try metronidazole 400mg/8h PO. Don't confuse with afferent loop syndrome (p614).
• *Infection:* giardiasis; diphyllobothriasis (B_{12} malabsorption); strongyloidiasis.

Postabsorptive phase
• *Lymphatic system obstruction:* congenital (eg intestinal lymphangiectasia, Milroy disease (p692)), acquired (eg lymphoma, Whipple's disease (see BOX)).

Whipple's disease

A rare disease[11] featuring GI malabsorption which usually occurs in middle-aged white males, most commonly in Europe. It is fatal if untreated and is caused by *Tropheryma whippelii*, which, combined with defective cell-mediated immunity, produces a systemic disease.

Features Often starts insidiously with arthralgia (chronic, migratory, seronegative arthropathy affecting mainly peripheral joints). GI symptoms commonly include colicky abdominal pain, weight loss, steatorrhoea/diarrhoea, which leads to malabsorption. Systemic symptoms such as chronic cough, fever, sweats, lymphadenopathy, and skin hyperpigmentation also occur. Cardiac involvement may lead to endocarditis, which is typically blood culture negative. CNS features include a reversible dementia, ophthalmoplegia, and facial myoclonus (if all together, they are highly suggestive)—also hypothalamic syndrome (hyperphagia, polydipsia, insomnia). NB: CNS involvement may occur without GI involvement.

Tests Diagnosis requires a high level of clinical suspicion. Jejunal biopsy shows stunted villi. There is deposition of macrophages in the lamina propria-containing granules which stain positive for periodic acid–Schiff (PAS). Similar cells may be found in affected samples, eg CSF, cardiac valve tissue, lymph nodes, synovial fluid. The bacteria may be seen within macrophages on electron microscopy. PCR of bacterial RNA can be performed on serum or tissue. MRI may demonstrate CNS involvement.

℞ Should include antibiotics which cross the blood–brain barrier. Current recommendations: IV ceftriaxone (or penicillin + streptomycin) for 2wks then oral co-trimoxazole for 1 year. Shorter courses risk relapse. A rapid improvement in symptoms usually occurs.

---

21 Bacterial overgrowth proximal to the colon causes diarrhoea, abdominal pain, and vitamin malabsorption. Causes: old age, autonomic neuropathy (eg diabetic), ileocaecal valve resection, PPI usage, amyloidosis.

Gastrointestinal motility disorders

Gut motility is essential to sustain life. As a result, there are multiple overlapping mechanisms to ensure that the carefully synchronized wave of smooth muscle contraction and relaxation continues to propel food and facilitate absorption of nutrients in a variety of circumstances (even in the case of vagotomy or sympathectomy). Disorders of this coordinated peristaltic activity can occur in association with abnormalities in a range of organ systems.

Gastroparesis Delayed gastric emptying in the absence of obstruction, resulting in post-prandial bloating, nausea/vomiting, abdominal pain, and early satiety. **Causes** ⅓ cases are due to diabetes (p200), ⅓ idiopathic, and ⅓ related to a range of conditions: post-surgical; post-viral (norovirus, rotavirus); medication-induced (opioids); neurological and systemic disorders (systemic sclerosis, SLE, amyloidosis, hypothyroidism). **Signs** Look for signs of any underlying condition. There may be epigastric distension/tenderness and a succussion splash. **Diagnosis** Gastric scintigraphy with a ^{99}technetium-labelled meal **Treatment** Alter diet (↓fat, ↓fibre), prokinetics (eg metoclopramide), anti-emetics, PEG decompression if refractory.

Intestinal pseudo-obstruction This resembles mechanical GI obstruction (p602) but in the absence of an obstructing lesion. *Acute* colonic pseudo-obstruction is called Ogilvie's syndrome (p694) and usually involves the caecum and right hemicolon. *Chronic* intestinal pseudo-obstruction is rare, presents with recurrent or chronic abdominal pain/distension and weight loss from malabsorption, and has similar pathogenic mechanisms to gastroparesis. Impaired motility is confirmed with scintigraphy. Nutritional support and electrolyte replacement are important.

Irritable bowel syndrome (IBS)

IBS is the most commonly diagnosed gastrointestinal condition. It is a chronic functional disorder of the GI tract characterized by recurrent abdominal pain associated with altered bowel habits. The pathophysiology is uncertain but likely involves altered intestinal motility, visceral hypersensitivity, intestinal inflammation, or microbial dysbiosis. Several diagnostic criteria exist.

Prevalence 10–20%, but depends on the criteria used; age at onset: ≤40yrs; ♀:♂ ≥2:1.

Diagnosis The diagnosis is defined by symptom-based criteria but symptoms are not specific for IBS, therefore these must use the frequency and duration to distinguish from transient gut symptoms. Rome IV criteria[12] (see BOX 'Defining gastrointestinal dysfunction', fig 6.25): recurrent abdominal pain ≥ 1 day/week on average in the last 3 months, associated with ≥2 of: • relieved or worsened by defecation • altered stool frequency • altered stool form. Other features: urgency; incomplete evacuation; abdominal bloating/distension; mucus PR; worsening of symptoms after food. Symptoms are chronic (onset ≥6 months prior to diagnosis), and often exacerbated by stress, menstruation, or gastroenteritis (post-infectious IBS). **Subtypes** IBS-C predominant constipation; IBS-D predominant diarrhoea; IBS-M mixed; unclassified. **Signs** Examination is usually normal, but mild abdominal tenderness is common. Insufflation of air during lower GI endoscopy (*not* usually needed) may reproduce the pain. **Associated conditions** The presence of other functional bowel disorders, eg functional dyspepsia (p248), and other commonly associated conditions, eg migraine (p454), chronic fatigue syndrome (p556), fibromyalgia (p556), depression, dyspareunia, adds further support to the diagnosis.

When to investigate Diagnostic tests are rarely required when the criteria are met and alarm features are absent; FBC, CRP or faecal calprotectin (p260), and coeliac serology (p262) in IBS-D & IBS-M are sufficient. Colonoscopy in the presence of alarm features: age of onset >50yrs; history <6 months; unexplained ↓weight or anaemia; nocturnal diarrhoea; family history of IBD or colorectal cancer, abnormal CRP, ESR. **Refer if** 1 Diagnostic uncertainty (you or the patient!). 2 Changing symptoms in 'known IBS'. 3 Refractory to management (here, NICE favours cognitive therapy, OHCS p754).

Initial treatment Like the diagnosis, treatment is based on the type and severity of symptoms. All patients should be given a positive diagnosis, an explanation of the condition, and reassurance about its benign natural history. In patients with mild intermittent symptoms, lifestyle/dietary measures are sufficient. Since it is non-fatal, safety of treatment is a priority.

Lifestyle advice Exercise (inverse association with colonic transit time), stress reduction, and sleep hygiene.

Dietary modification Take a careful dietary history; 9/10 patients report that certain foods trigger symptoms. Much of the evidence is weak, but some specific dietary interventions may be recommended under dietician supervision: 1 Low FODMAP (fermentable carbohydrates; poorly absorbed and gas producing) diet, but stop if no improvement after 1 month of strict adherence. 2 Fibre supplementation; potential benefits are restricted to soluble fibre (psyllium/ispaghula), avoid increasing wheat bran intake. 3 Dietary exclusions; spicy foods and excess fat if these are triggers, gluten-free diet not recommended. 4 Probiotics; 1-month trials can be considered, but may not provide substantial benefit.

Pharmacotherapy

- *IBS-C:* if there is no response to soluble fibre, try osmotic laxatives (polyethelene glycol preferred to lactulose which can aggravate bloating). If this fails, try prosecretory agents linaclotide, prucalopride, or plecanatide.
- *IBS-D:* try loperamide 2mg 45 minutes before meals.
- *Colic/bloating:* oral antispasmodics: mebeverine 135mg/8h or hyoscine butyl-bromide 10mg/8h (over the counter).
- *Psychological symptoms/visceral hypersensitivity:* emphasize the positive! You have excluded sinister pathology and over time, symptoms tend to improve. Consider cognitive behavioural therapy (OHCS p754), hypnosis, and tricyclics, eg amitriptyline 10–20mg at night (SE: drowsiness, dry mouth); explain that this is at a low dose for visceral pain (ie you are not prescribing the higher licensed dose for depression), and that it improves IBS-D by slowing GI transit.

Defining gastrointestinal dysfunction—all roads lead to Rome

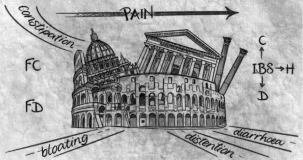

Fig 6.25 There is nothing romantic about functional bowel disorders, other than the association of the definitions of these conditions with the eternal city. The fourth iteration of the Rome criteria classifies these into 5 distinct groups (IBS, functional constipation (FC) and diarrhoea (FDR), functional bloating/distension, and unspecified) but they exist on a continuum; a predominance of pain or diarrhoea versus constipation can help to point us in the right direction. Following patients' journeys through multiple evolving symptoms and negative investigations that lead to apparent dead ends can be complex, and arriving at a clear clinical diagnosis is therapeutically invaluable.

Artwork by Gillian Turner.

A diverse group of epithelial neoplasms with neuroendocrine differentiation that can form almost anywhere. Well-differentiated tumours arise predominantly in the GI tract, are of enterochromaffin cell (neural crest) origin, and are capable of producing 5HT. These have been known as carcinoid tumours (appendix (45%), ileum (30%), rectum (20%)[22]) and islet cell tumours (pancreas). They also occur elsewhere in the GI tract, ovary, testis, and bronchi. 80% of tumours >2cm across will metastasize.

Symptoms and signs Initially few. GI tumours can cause appendicitis, intussusception, or obstruction. Hepatic metastases may cause RUQ pain. Tumours may secrete bradykinin, tachykinin, substance P, VIP, gastrin, insulin, glucagon, ACTH (∴ Cushing's syndrome), parathyroid, and thyroid hormones. 10% are part of MEN-1 syndrome (p217); 10% occur with other neuroendocrine tumours.

Carcinoid syndrome Occurs in ~5% and implies metastatic hepatic involvement (>90%, ↓inactivation of bioactive substances secreted into the portal circulation).

Symptoms and signs Bronchoconstriction; paroxysmal flushing especially in upper body (± migrating weals); diarrhoea; CCF (tricuspid incompetence and pulmonary stenosis from 5HT-induced fibrosis). ►**Carcinoid crisis** See BOX.

Tests ↑24h urine 5-hydroxyindoleacetic acid (5-HIAA, a 5HT metabolite; levels change with drugs and diet: discuss with lab). CXR + chest/pelvis MRI/CT help locate and stage primary tumours. Plasma chromogranin A (reflects tumour mass); PET/CT (p722) with novel tracers; [111]Indium octreotide scintigraphy (Octreoscan™) also have a role. Echocardiography and BNP (p135) can be used to investigate carcinoid heart disease.

Treatment Carcinoid syndrome Octreotide (somatostatin analogue) blocks release of tumour mediators and counters peripheral effects. Long-acting alternative: lanreotide. Loperamide for diarrhoea. **Tumour therapy** Resection is the only cure for carcinoid tumours so it is vital to find the primary site. At surgery, tumours are an intense yellow. Procedures depend on site, eg rectal carcinoid tumours <1cm can be resected endoscopically. Debulking (eg enucleating), embolization, or radiofrequency ablation of hepatic metastases can ↓ symptoms. Give octreotide cover to avoid precipitating a massive carcinoid crisis.

Median survival 5–8yrs (~3yrs if metastases are present, but may be up to 20yrs; so beware of giving up too easily, even in metastatic disease).

> ►►**Carcinoid crisis**
>
> When a tumour outgrows its blood supply or is handled too much during surgery, mediators flood out. There is life-threatening vasodilation, hypotension, tachycardia, bronchoconstriction, and hyperglycaemia. It is treated with high-dose octreotide, supportive measures, and careful management of fluid balance.

22 Some are never clinically detected: 1 in 300 autopsies have a small bowel carcinoid tumour.

Zollinger-Ellison syndrome

This is the association of peptic ulcers with a gastrin-secreting adenoma (gastrinoma), a neuroendocrine tumour arising in the pancreas, stomach, or duodenum. Gastrin excites excessive gastric acid production, which may produce multiple ulcers in the duodenum and stomach. **Incidence** ~0.1% of patients with peptic ulcer disease. Suspect in those with multiple peptic ulcers, ulcers distal to the duodenum, or a family history of peptic ulcers (or of islet cell, pituitary, or parathyroid adenomas). Most cases are sporadic; 20% are associated with multiple endocrine neoplasia, type 1 (MEN1, p217). 60% are malignant; metastases are found in local lymph nodes and the liver. **Symptoms** Include abdominal pain and dyspepsia, from the ulcers, and chronic diarrhoea due to inactivation of pancreatic enzymes (also causes steatorrhoea) and damage to intestinal mucosa. **Tests** (fig 6.26) ↑Fasting serum gastrin level (>1000pg/mL). Measure three fasting levels on different days and off PPI therapy. Hypochlorhydria (reduced acid production, eg in chronic atrophic gastritis) should be excluded as this also causes a raised gastrin level: gastric pH should be <2. The secretin stimulation test is useful in suspected cases with only mildly raised gastrin levels (100–1000pg/mL). The adenoma is often small and difficult to image; a combination of somatostatin receptor scintigraphy, endoscopic ultrasound, and CT is used to localize and stage the adenoma. OGD evaluates gastric/duodenal ulceration. **R** High-dose proton pump inhibitors, eg omeprazole: start with 60mg/d and adjust according to response. Measuring intragastric pH helps determine the best dose (aim to keep pH at 2–7). All gastrinomas have malignant potential and require resection (with lymph node clearance generally recommended if >2cm in size). Surgery may be avoided in MEN1, as adenomas are often multiple, and metastatic disease is rare. If well-differentiated (G1 and G2) somatostatin analogues may be 1st line and chemotherapy with streptozotocin (if available) + doxorubicin/fluorouracil is 2nd line. In G3, etoposide + cisplatin is possible.[13] Selective embolization may be done for hepatic metastases. **Prognosis** 5yr survival: 80% if single resectable lesion, ~20% with hepatic metastases. Screen all patients for MEN1.

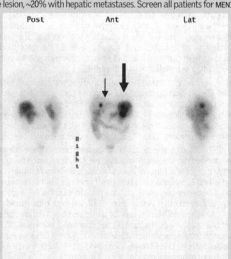

WHOLEBODY IN-111 OCTREOTIDE SCAN

Fig 6.26 Octreoscan™ in patient with metastatic MEN1 gastrinoma. Solitary hepatic metastatic deposit (thin arrow), gastric neuroendocrine tumour (thick arrow).

Reproduced from Wass *et al.*, *Oxford Textbook of Endocrinology and Diabetes*, 2011, with permission from Oxford University Press.

Jaundice refers to yellowing of skin, sclerae, and mucosae from ↑plasma bilirubin (visible at ≥60μmol/L; fig 6.27). Jaundice is classified by the site of the problem (pre-hepatic, hepatocellular, or cholestatic/obstructive) or by the type of circulating bilirubin (conjugated or unconjugated; fig 6.28).

Unconjugated hyperbilirubinaemia
Overproduction Haemolysis (p334, eg malaria/DIC, etc.); ineffective erythropoiesis.

Impaired hepatic uptake Drugs (paracetamol, rifampicin), ischaemic hepatitis.

Impaired conjugation *Gilbert's syndrome:* ↓UGT activity (see BOX) due to a defect in the gene promoter. A common (9% prevalence) benign condition that may go unnoticed for many years. Usually presents in adolescence with intermittent jaundice occurring during illness, exercise or fasting. Mild ↑bilirubin; normal FBC and reticulocytes (ie no haemolysis). *Crigler–Najjar syndrome:* two rare syndromes of inherited unconjugated hyperbilirubinaemia presenting in the 1st days of life with jaundice ± CNS signs. Gene mutations causing ↓UGT activity result in absent (type 1) or impaired (type 2) ability to excrete bilirubin. T1: phototherapy and plasmapheresis; liver transplant before irreversible kernicterus (*OHCS* p294) develops. T2: usually no R̲ needed.

Conjugated hyperbilirubinaemia Dark urine, pale stools. When severe, it can be associated with an intractable pruritus (best treated by relief of the obstruction).

Hepatocellular dysfunction There is hepatocyte damage, usually with some cholestasis. *Causes:* viruses: hepatitis (p274), CMV (p401), EBV (p401); drugs (table 6.10; alcohol; cirrhosis (see BOX 'Causes of jaundice'); liver metastases/abscess; haemochromatosis; autoimmune hepatitis (AIH); septicaemia; leptospirosis; syphilis; α₁-antitrypsin deficiency (p286); Budd–Chiari (p686); Wilson's disease (p281); failure to excrete conjugated bilirubin (Dubin–Johnson & Rotor syndromes, p688, p696); right heart failure; toxins, eg carbon tetrachloride; fungi (fig 6.29).

Impaired hepatic excretion (cholestasis) Primary biliary cholangitis; primary sclerosing cholangitis; drugs (table 6.10); common bile duct gallstones; pancreatic cancer; compression of the bile duct, eg lymph nodes at the porta hepatis; cholangiocarcinoma; choledochal cyst; Caroli's disease;[23] Mirrizi's syndrome (obstructive jaundice from common bile duct compression by a gallstone impacted in the cystic duct, often associated with cholangitis).

The patient Ask About blood transfusions, IV drug use, body piercing, tattoos, sexual activity, travel abroad, jaundiced contacts, family history, alcohol use, and *all* medications (eg old drug charts; GP records). **Examine** For signs of chronic liver disease (p272), hepatic encephalopathy (p271), lymphadenopathy, hepatomegaly, splenomegaly, ascites, and a palpable gallbladder (if seen with painless jaundice the cause is not gallstones—Courvoisier's law).[24] Pale stools + dark urine ≈ cholestatic jaundice.

Tests See p272 for screening tests in suspected liver disease. **Urine** Bilirubin is absent in pre-hepatic causes; in obstructive jaundice, urobilinogen is absent. **Haematology** FBC, clotting, film, reticulocyte count, Coombs test and haptoglobins for haemolysis (p332), malaria parasites (eg if unconjugated bilirubin/fever); Paul Bunnell (EBV). **Chemistry** U&E, LFT, γ-GT, total protein, albumin.[25] Paracetamol levels. **Microbiology** Blood and other cultures; hepatitis serology. **Ultrasound** Are the bile ducts dilated? Are there gallstones, hepatic metastases, or a pancreatic mass? ERCP (See p726.) If bile ducts are dilated and LFT not improving. MRCP (See p726.) or endoscopic ultrasound (EUS) if conventional ultrasound shows gallstones but no definite common bile duct stones. **Liver biopsy** (See p244.) If bile ducts are normal. Consider abdominal *CT/MRI* if abdominal malignancy is suspected.

What to do? ▸▸ *Treat the cause promptly.* Ensure adequate hydration; broad-spectrum antibiotics if obstruction. Monitor for ascites, encephalopathy; call a hepatologist.

---

23 Multiple segmental cystic or saccular dilatations of intrahepatic bile ducts with congenital hepatic fibrosis. It may present in 20yr-olds, with portal hypertension ± recurrent cholangitis/cholelithiasis.
24 Pancreatic or gallbladder cancer is more likely, as stones lead to a fibrotic, unexpandable gallbladder.
25 Albumin & INR are the best indicators of hepatic synthetic function. ↑Transaminases (ALT, AST) indicate hepatocyte damage. ↑ALP suggests obstructive jaundice, but also occurs in hepatocellular jaundice, malignant infiltration, pregnancy (placental isoenzyme), Paget's disease, and childhood (bone isoenzyme).

Fig 6.27 It's easy to miss mild jaundice, especially under fluorescent light, so take your patient to the window, and as you both gaze at the sky, use the opportunity to broaden the horizons of your enquiries... where have you been... where are you going... who are you with... what are you taking...? In the gaps, your patient may tell you the diagnosis—alcohol or drug abuse, sexual infections/hepatitis, or worries about the side effects of their TB or HIV medication or a spreading cancer 'from this lump here which I haven't told anyone about yet'. Reproduced from Roper, *Clinical Skills*, 2014, with permission from Oxford University Press.

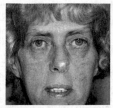

The pathway of bilirubin metabolism

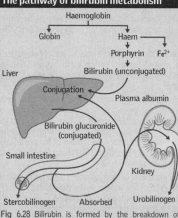

Unconjugated bilirubin is water-insoluble. In the liver, bilirubin is conjugated with glucuronic acid by hepatocytes mediated by a family of enzymes called uridine-diphosphoglucuronate glucuronosyltransferase (UGT), making it water-soluble. Conjugated bilirubin is secreted in bile and passes into the gut. Some is taken up again by the liver (via the enterohepatic circulation) and the rest is converted to urobilinogen by gut bacteria. Urobilinogen is either reabsorbed and excreted by the kidneys, giving urine its colour, or converted to stercobilin, which colours faeces brown.

Fig 6.28 Bilirubin is formed by the breakdown of haemoglobin in a 3-step process: hepatic uptake, conjugation, and excretion.

Causes of jaundice in a previously stable patient with cirrhosis

- Sepsis (esp. UTI, pneumonia, or peritonitis).
- Malignancy: eg hepatocellular carcinoma.
- Alcohol; drugs (table 6.10).
- GI bleeding.

Signs of decompensation Jaundice; ascites; UGI bleed; encephalopathy.

Table 6.10 Examples of drug-induced jaundice

Haemolysis	• Antimalarials (eg dapsone)	
Hepatitis	• Paracetamol overdose (p824)	• Sodium valproate
	• Isoniazid, rifampicin, pyrazinamide	• Halothane
	• Monoamine oxidase inhibitors	• Statins
Cholestasis	• Flucloxacillin (may be weeks after Rx)	• Sulfonylureas
	• Fusidic acid, co-amoxiclav, nitrofurantoin	• Prochlorperazine
	• Steroids (anabolic; the Pill)	• Chlorpromazine

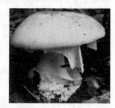

Fig 6.29 *Amanita phalloides* (Latin for 'phallic toadstool'; also known as the 'death cap') is a lethal cause of jaundice. It is the most toxic mushroom known. After ingestion (its benign appearance is confusing), amatoxins induce hepatic necrosis leaving few options other than transplantation.

© Ian Herriott. NB: don't use this image for identification!

6 Gastroenterology

Definitions Liver failure may be recognized by the development of coagulopathy (INR >1.5) and encephalopathy. This may occur suddenly in the previously healthy liver = *acute liver failure* (hyperacute = onset ≤7d; acute = 8–21d; subacute = 4–26wks.) More often it occurs on a background of cirrhosis = *chronic liver failure*. *Fulminant hepatic failure* is a clinical syndrome resulting from massive necrosis of liver cells leading to severe impairment of liver function.

Causes **Infections** Viral hepatitis (esp. B, C, CMV), yellow fever, leptospirosis. **Drugs** Paracetamol overdose, halothane, isoniazid. **Toxins** *Amanita phalloides* mushroom (fig 6.29, p269), carbon tetrachloride. **Vascular** Budd–Chiari syn. (p686), veno-occlusive disease. **Others** Alcohol, fatty liver disease, primary biliary cholangitis, primary sclerosing cholangitis, haemochromatosis, autoimmune hepatitis, α₁-antitrypsin deficiency, Wilson's disease, fatty liver of pregnancy (OHCS p29), malignancy.

Signs Jaundice, hepatic encephalopathy (see BOX 'Hepatic encephalopathy'), *fetor hepaticus* (smells like pear drops), asterixis/flap (p48), constructional apraxia (cannot copy a 5-pointed star?). Signs of chronic liver disease (p272) suggest acute-on-chronic hepatic failure.

Tests **Blood** FBC (?infection,[26] ?GI bleed), U&E,[27] LFT, clotting (↑PT/INR), glucose, paracetamol level, hepatitis, CMV and EBV serology, ferritin, α₁-antitrypsin, caeruloplasmin, autoantibodies (p550). **Microbiology** Blood culture; urine culture; ascitic tap for MC&S of ascites—neutrophils >250/mm³ indicates spontaneous bacterial peritonitis (p272). **Radiology** CXR; abdominal ultrasound; Doppler flow studies of the portal vein (and hepatic vein in suspected Budd–Chiari syndrome, p686). **Neurophysiology** EEG, evoked potentials (and neuroimaging) have a limited role.

Management ►► Beware sepsis, hypoglycaemia, GI bleeds/varices, & encephalopathy:
- Nurse with a 20° head-up tilt in ITU. Protect the airway with intubation and insert an NG tube to avoid aspiration and remove any blood from stomach.
- Insert urinary and central venous catheters to help assess fluid status.
- Monitor T°, respirations, pulse, BP, pupils, urine output hourly. Daily weights.
- Check FBC, U&E, LFT, and INR daily.
- 10% glucose IV, 1L/12h to avoid hypoglycaemia. Do blood glucose every 1–4h.
- Treat the cause, if known (eg GI bleeds, sepsis, paracetamol poisoning, p824).
- If malnourished, get dietary help: good nutrition can decrease mortality. Give thiamine and folate supplements (p700).
- Treat seizures with phenytoin (p810).[14]
- Haemofiltration or haemodialysis, if renal failure develops (BOX 'What is hepatorenal syndrome?').
- Try to avoid sedatives and other drugs with hepatic metabolism (BOX 'Prescribing in liver failure' and BNF).
- Consider PPI as prophylaxis against stress ulceration, eg omeprazole 40mg/d IV/PO.
- Liaise early with nearest transplant centre regarding appropriateness.

Treat complications

Cerebral oedema On ITU: 20% mannitol IV; hyperventilate.

Ascites Restrict fluid, low-salt diet, weigh daily, diuretics (p272).

Bleeding Vitamin K 10mg/d IV for 3d, platelets, FFP + blood as needed ± endoscopy.

Blind ℞ of infection Ceftriaxone 1–2g/24h IV, *not* gentamicin (↑risk of renal failure).

↓Blood glucose If ≤2mmol/L or symptomatic, ℞ 50mL of 50% glucose IV; check often.

Encephalopathy Avoid sedatives; 20° head-up tilt in ITU; correct electrolytes; lactulose 30–50mL/8h (aim for 2–4 soft stools/d) is catabolized by bacterial flora to short-chain fatty acids which ↓ colonic pH and trap NH₃ in the colon as NH₄⁺; Rifaximin 550mg/12h is a non-absorbable oral antibiotic that ↓ numbers of nitrogen-forming gut bacteria.

Worse prognosis if Grade III–IV encephalopathy, age >40yrs, albumin <30g/L, ↑INR, drug-induced liver failure, late-onset hepatic failure worse than fulminant failure.

Prescribing in liver failure

Avoid drugs that constipate (↑risk of encephalopathy), oral hypoglycaemics, and saline-containing IVIS. *Warfarin* effects are enhanced. **Hepatotoxic drugs include** Paracetamol, methotrexate, isoniazid, azathioprine, phenothiazines, oestrogen, 6-mercaptopurine, salicylates, tetracycline, mitomycin.

Hepatic encephalopathy: letting loose some false neurotransmitters

As the liver fails, nitrogenous waste (as ammonia) builds up in the circulation and passes to the brain, where astrocytes clear it (by processes involving the conversion of glutamate to glutamine). This excess glutamine causes an osmotic imbalance and a shift of fluid into these cells—hence cerebral oedema. Grading:

I   Altered mood/behaviour; sleep disturbance (eg reversed sleep pattern); dyspraxia ('Please copy this 5-pointed star'); poor arithmetic. No liver flap.
II Increasing drowsiness, confusion, slurred speech ± liver flap, inappropriate behaviour/personality change (ask the family—don't be too tactful).
III Incoherent; restless; liver flap; stupor.
IV Coma.

►What else could be clouding consciousness? Hypoglycaemia; sepsis; trauma; postictal.

What is hepatorenal syndrome (HRS)?

Cirrhosis + ascites + renal failure ≈ HRS—*if other causes of renal impairment have been excluded.* Abnormal haemodynamics causes splanchnic and systemic vasodilation, but renal *vasoconstriction*. Bacterial translocation, cytokines, and mesenteric angiogenesis cause splanchnic vasodilation, and altered renal autoregulation is involved in the renal vasoconstriction.

Types of HRS *HRS 1* is a rapidly progressive deterioration in circulatory and renal function (median survival <2wks), often triggered by other deteriorating pathologies. Terlipressin resists hypovolaemia. Haemodialysis may be needed. *HRS 2* is a more steady deterioration (survival ~6 months). Transjugular intrahepatic portosystemic stent shunting may be required (TIPS, p252).

Other factors in cirrhosis may contribute to poor renal function (p272).

Transplants Liver transplant may be required. After >8–12wks of pre-transplant dialysis, some may be considered for combined liver–kidney transplantation.

King's College Hospital criteria in acute liver failure

Paracetamol-induced liver failure	Non-paracetamol liver failure
• Arterial pH <7.3 24h after ingestion.	• PT >100s.
Or all of the following:	*Or 3 out of 5 of the following:*
• Prothrombin time (PT) >100s.	1 Drug-induced liver failure.
• Creatinine >300µmol/L.	2 Age <10 or >40yrs old.
• Grade III or IV encephalopathy.	3 >1wk from 1st jaundice to encephalopathy.
	4 PT >50s.
	5 Bilirubin ≥300µmol/L.

Fulfilling these criteria predicts poor outcome in acute liver failure and should prompt consideration for transplantation (p273).

Based on O'Grady J *et al.* 'Early indicators of prognosis in fulminant hepatic failure.'
Gastroenterology, 97(2):439–45, 1989.

26 Neutrophilic leucocytosis need not mean a secondary infection: alcoholic hepatitis may be the cause.
27 Urea is synthesized in the liver, so is a poor test of renal function in liver failure; use creatinine instead.

Cirrhosis (Greek *kirrhos* = yellow) implies irreversible liver damage. Histologically, there is loss of normal hepatic architecture with bridging fibrosis and nodular regeneration.

Causes Most often fatty liver disease (chronic alcohol use and non-alcoholic), HBV, or HCV infection. Others: see BOX 'Causes of cirrhosis'.

Signs Leuconychia: white nails with lunulae undemarcated, from hypoalbuminaemia; Terry's nails—white proximally but distal ⅓ reddened by telangiectasias; clubbing; palmar erythema; hyperdynamic circulation; Dupuytren's contracture; spider naevi (fig 6.30); xanthelasma; gynaecomastia; atrophic testes; loss of body hair; parotid enlargement (alcohol); hepatomegaly, or small liver in late disease; ascites; splenomegaly.

Complications **Hepatic failure** Coagulopathy (failure of hepatic synthesis of clotting factors); encephalopathy (p271); hypoalbuminaemia (oedema); sepsis (pneumonia; septicaemia); spontaneous bacterial peritonitis (SBP); hypoglycaemia. **Portal hypertension** Ascites (fig 6.31); splenomegaly; portosystemic shunt including oesophageal varices (± life-threatening upper GI bleed) and *caput medusae* (enlarged superficial periumbilical veins). HCC ↑ risk.

Tests **Blood** LFT: ↔ or ↑bilirubin, ↑AST, ↑ALT, ↑ALP, ↑γGT. Later, with loss of synthetic function, look for ↓albumin ± ↑PT/INR. ↓WCC & ↓platelets indicate hypersplenism. *Find the cause:* ferritin, iron/total iron-binding capacity (p326); hepatitis serology (p274); immunoglobulins (p286); autoantibodies (ANA, AMA, SMA, p550); α-fetoprotein (p282); caeruloplasmin in patients <40yrs old (p281); α₁-antitrypsin (p286). **Liver ultrasound + duplex** May show a small liver or hepatomegaly, splenomegaly, focal liver lesion(s), hepatic vein thrombus, reversed flow in the portal vein, or ascites. MRI ↑Caudate lobe size, smaller islands of regenerating nodules, and the presence of the right posterior hepatic notch are more frequent in alcoholic cirrhosis than in virus-induced cirrhosis. **Ascitic tap** Should be performed and fluid sent for urgent MC&S—neutrophils >250/mm³ indicates spontaneous bacterial peritonitis (see later in topic for treatment). **Liver biopsy** (See p244.) Confirms the clinical diagnosis.

Management **General** Good nutrition is vital. Alcohol abstinence (p276). Avoid NSAIDs, sedatives, and opiates. Colestyramine helps pruritus (4g/12h PO, 1h after other drugs). Consider ultrasound ± α-fetoprotein every 6 months to screen for HCC (p282) in those whose this information will change management. **Specific** For hepatitis-induced cirrhosis see p274. High-dose ursodeoxycholic acid in PBC (p278) may improve LFT and improve transplant-free survival. Penicillamine for Wilson's disease (p281). **Ascites** Fluid restriction (<1.5L/d), low-salt diet (40–100mmol/d). Give *spironolactone* 100mg/24h PO; ↑ dose as tolerated (max 400mg/24h)—it counters deranged renin–angiotensin–aldosterone (RAA) axis. Chart daily weight and aim for weight loss of ≤½kg/d. If response is poor, add furosemide ≤120mg/24h PO; do U&E (watch Na⁺) often. Therapeutic paracentesis with concomitant albumin infusion (6–8g/L fluid removed) may be required. **Spontaneous bacterial peritonitis (SBP)** ►Must be considered in any patient with ascites who deteriorates suddenly (may be asymptomatic). Common organisms are *E. coli*, *Klebsiella*, and streptococci. ℞: eg piperacillin with tazobactam 4.5g/8h for 5d or until sensitivities known. Give prophylaxis for high-risk patients (↓albumin, ↑PT/INR, low ascitic albumin) or those who have had a previous episode: eg ciprofloxacin 500mg PO daily. **Encephalopathy** Recurrent episodes may be reduced in frequency with prophylactic lactulose and rifaximin (p270). **Renal failure** ↓Hepatic clearance of immune complexes leads to trapping in kidneys (∴ IgA nephropathy ± hepatic glomerulosclerosis). See also p271 for hepatorenal syndrome.

Prognosis Overall 5yr survival is ~50%. Poor prognostic indicators: encephalopathy; serum Na⁺ <110mmol/L; serum albumin <25g/L; ↑INR.

Liver transplantation The only definitive treatment for cirrhosis (p273). **Acute indications** Acute liver failure meeting King's College criteria (see BOX 'King's College Hospital criteria in acute liver failure', p271) **Chronic indications** Advanced cirrhosis of any cause; hepatocellular cancer (1 nodule <5cm or ≤5 nodules <3cm).

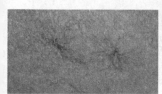

Fig 6.30 Spider naevi: a central arteriole, from which numerous vessels radiate (like the legs of a spider). These fill from the centre unlike telangiectasias that fill from the edge. They occur most commonly in skin drained by the superior vena cava. ≤5 are normal (especially in ♀). Causes include liver disease, OCP, and pregnancy (ie changes in oestrogen metabolism).

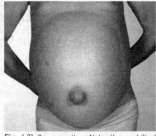

Fig 6.31 Gross ascites. Note the umbilical hernia (p605), gynaecomastia, and veins visible on the anterior abdominal wall.

Causes of cirrhosis

- Chronic alcohol use.
- Chronic HBV or HCV infection.[28]
- Non-alcoholic steatohepatitis (NASH).
- Genetic disorders: haemochromatosis (p284); α₁-antitrypsin deficiency (p286); Wilson's disease (p281).
- Hepatic vein events (Budd–Chiari, p686).
- Autoimmunity: primary biliary cholangitis (p278); primary sclerosing cholangitis (p278); autoimmune hepatitis (p280).
- Drugs: eg amiodarone, methyldopa, methotrexate.

Is cirrhosis becoming decompensated? ►►Prepare to make an arrest...

Cirrhosis may lie in wait for years before committing one of its three great crimes against the person: jaundice, ascites, or encephalopathy. There are almost always accomplices who, if arrested *now*, may stop a killing from unfolding. These usual suspects are: ►dehydration ►constipation ►covert alcohol use ►infection (eg spontaneous peritonitis, see earlier in topic) ►opiate over-use—or ►an occult GI bleed. If all have alibis, think of portal vein thrombosis, and call in the Chief Inspector.

Liver transplantation

The first liver transplant was in Denver, USA, in 1963. Now 800–1000 are performed each year in the UK (for indications see p271). The limiting step for the procedure is often the waiting list for a donor organ, which may be *cadaveric* (heart-beating or non-heart-beating) or from *live donors* (right lobe). *Contraindications* include extrahepatic malignancy; severe cardiorespiratory disease, systemic sepsis; expected non-compliance with drug therapy; ongoing alcohol consumption (in those with alcohol-related liver disease). Refer earlier rather than later, eg when ascites is refractory or after a 1st episode of bacterial peritonitis. Prioritization in the UK is based upon the UKELD (UK end-stage liver disease) score, calculated from serum Na⁺, creatinine, bilirubin, and INR.[29]

Post-op 12–48h on ITU, with enteral feeding starting as soon as possible and close monitoring of LFT. Immunosuppression examples: tacrolimus ± mycophenolate mofetil (or azathioprine) + prednisolone. Hyperacute rejection is a result of ABO incompatibility. Acute rejection (T-cell mediated, at 5–10d): the patient feels unwell with pyrexia and tender hepatomegaly—often managed by altering the immunosuppressives. Other complications: sepsis (esp. Gram −ve and CMV), hepatic artery thrombosis, chronic rejection (at 6–9 months), disease recurrence, and, rarely, graft-versus-host disease. Average patient survival at 1yr is ~80% (5yr survival 60–90%; depends on the pre-op disease).

28 Clues as to which patients with chronic HCV will get cirrhosis: platelet count ≤140 × 10⁹/L, globulin/albumin ratio ≥1, and AST/ALT ratio ≥1—100% +ve predictive value but lower sensitivity (~30%).
29 Online calculators available, eg at www.odt.nhs.uk.

6 Gastroenterology

Hepatitis A RNA virus. **Spread** Faecal–oral or shellfish. Endemic in Africa and S America, so a problem for travellers. Most infections are in childhood. **Incubation** 2–6wks.

Symptoms Fever, malaise, anorexia, nausea, arthralgia—then: jaundice (rare in children), hepatosplenomegaly, and adenopathy. **Tests** AST and ALT rise 22–40d after exposure (ALT may be >1000IU/L), returning to normal over 5–20wks. IGM rises from day 25 and means recent infection. IgG is detectable for life. ℞ Supportive. Avoid alcohol. Rarely, interferon alfa for fulminant hepatitis. **Active immunization** With inactivated viral protein. 1 IM dose gives immunity for 1yr (20yrs if further booster is given at 6–12 months). **Prognosis** Usually self-limiting. Fulminant hepatitis is rare. Chronicity doesn't occur.

Hepatitis B virus (HBV, a DNA virus.) **Spread** Blood products, IV drug abusers (IVDU), sexual, direct contact. **Deaths** 1 million/yr. **Risk groups** IV drug users and their sexual partners/carers; health workers; haemophiliacs; men who have sex with men; haemodialysis (and chronic renal failure); sexually promiscuous; foster carers; close family members of a carrier or case; staff or residents of institutions/prisons; babies of HBsAg +ve mothers; adopted child from endemic area. **Endemic in** Far East, Africa, Mediterranean. **Incubation** 1–6 months. **Signs** Resemble hepatitis A but arthralgia and urticaria are commoner. **Tests** HBsAg (surface antigen) is present 1–6 months after exposure. HBeAg (e antigen) is present for 1½–3 months after acute illness and implies high infectivity. HBsAg persisting for >6 months defines carrier status and occurs in 5–10% of infections; biopsy may be indicated unless ALT ↔ and HBV DNA <2000IU/mL. Antibodies to HBcAg (anti-HBc) imply past infection; antibodies to HBsAg (anti-HBs) alone imply vaccination. HBV PCR allows monitoring of response to therapy. See fig 6.32 and table 6.11. **Vaccination** See p283. Passive immunization (specific anti-HBV immunoglobulin) may be given to non-immune contacts after high-risk exposure.

Complications Fulminant hepatic failure, cirrhosis, HCC, cholangiocarcinoma, cryoglobulinaemia, membranous nephropathy, polyarteritis nodosa (p554). ℞ Avoid alcohol. Immunize sexual contacts. Refer all with chronic liver inflammation (eg ALT ≳30IU/L), cirrhosis, or HBV DNA >2000IU/mL for antivirals (oral nucleos(t)ide analogues, eg tenofovir, entecavir are preferred 1st line based on their better side effect profile and predictable efficacy than 48wks subcutaneous pegylated (PEG) interferon alfa-2a but are required long-term). The aim is to clear HBsAg and ►prevent cirrhosis and HCC (risk is ↑↑ if HBsAg and HBeAg +ve).

Hepatitis C virus (HCV) RNA flavivirus. **Spread** Blood: transfusion, IV drug abuse, sexual contact. UK prevalence: ~80 000 (and falling, see BOX). Early infection is often mild/asymptomatic. ~85% develop silent chronic infection; ~25% get cirrhosis in 20yrs—of these, ≤4% develop HCC/yr. **Risk factors for progression** Male, older, higher viral load, use of alcohol, HIV, HBV. **Tests** LFT (AST:ALT <1:1 until cirrhosis develops, p272), anti-HCV antibodies confirm exposure; HCV-PCR confirms ongoing infection/chronicity; liver biopsy or non-invasive elastography if HCV-PCR +ve to assess liver damage and need for treatment. Determine HCV genotype (1–6). ℞ BOX 'The virologists' triumph'; quit alcohol. **Other complications** Glomerulonephritis; cryoglobulinaemia; thyroiditis; autoimmune hepatitis; PAN; polymyositis; porphyria cutanea tarda.

Hepatitis D virus (HDV) Incomplete RNA virus (needs HBV for its assembly). HBV vaccination prevents HDV infection. 5% of HBV carriers have HDV co-infection. It may cause acute liver failure/cirrhosis. **Tests** Anti-HDV antibody (only ask for it if HBsAg +ve). ℞ As interferon alfa has limited success, liver transplantation may be needed.

Hepatitis E virus (HEV) RNA virus. Similar to HAV; common in Indochina (commoner in older men and also commoner than hepatitis A in UK); mortality is high in pregnancy. It is associated with pigs. Epidemics occur (eg Africa). Vaccine is available in China (not Europe). Δ Serology. ℞ Nil specific.

Other infective causes of hepatitis EBV; CMV; leptospirosis; malaria; Q fever; syphilis; yellow fever.

Table 6.11 Serological markers of HBV infection

	Incubation	Acute	Carrier	Recovery	Vaccinated
LFT		↑↑↑	↑	Normal	Normal
HBsAg	+	+	+		
HBeAg	+	+	+/−		
Anti-HBs				+	+
Anti-HBe			+/−		
Anti-HBc IgM		+	+/−		
Anti-HBc IgG		+	+	+	

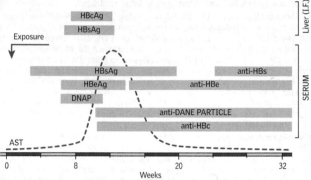

Fig 6.32 Viral events in hepatitis B in relation to AST peak. IF=immunofluorescence; Ag=antigen; HBs=hep. B surface; HBc=hep. B core; HBe=hep. B e antigen; DNAP=DNA polymerase.

The virologists' triumph: curing HCV

Since the original isolation of HCV in the late 1980s, riding the wave of the AIDS scare, less than three decades have elapsed. In this time, the comparatively simple genome of HCV has proven far easier than HIV to combat and the treatment of HCV has undergone nothing less than a revolution to the point where many common genotypes are considered curable.

All patients with sustained detectable HCV should be considered for treatment. Options are evolving rapidly, but centre on the use of inhibitors of non-structural viral proteins (eg ledipasvir + sofosbuvir) which are much better tolerated than the previous mainstay of treatment, pegylated interferon. Interferon-free regimens therefore eliminate major barriers to compliance including treatment duration and SE, as well as achieving superior results: contemporary antiviral regimens can now realistically achieve the complete absence of PCR-detectable virus in the blood 6 months post-treatment in almost 100% of genotype 1 patients, including patients with established cirrhosis. Ribavirin, a nucleoside analogue, can also increasingly be avoided in genotype 1, though it remains a useful treatment for the harder-to-treat genotypes 2 and 3. Here, reported rates of sustained undetectable viral levels now routinely exceed 90%. The costs of treatment are high, but cost-effectiveness analysis is favourable given the cure rates and the significant public health burden of HCV. Genotypes 4, 5, or 6 are prevalent in lower-income countries and have received less attention but limited data where resources do exist suggest similarly good response rates.

Meanwhile, the threat of HIV remains. HCV prevalence is ~7% for sexually transmitted HIV and >90% for IV transmission. Untreated HIV may accelerate progress of HCV-induced liver fibrosis. All HIV/HCV co-infected patients should be assessed for combination antiviral therapy. Given the potential for toxicities and viral resistance mutation, such therapies should be planned and delivered through expert services.

Alcohol use is the leading risk factor for death and disability among the global population aged 15–50 years. **Screening** Several screening tools for hazardous use have been validated (eg AUDIT) but for simplicity, a single-item question has much to recommend it, such as 'How many times in the past year have you had five (four for ♀) or more drinks in a day?' (+ve if >0; 82% sensitive, 79% specific). This can be followed up with the CAGE questions for dependence: ever felt you ought to **c**ut down? Have people **A**nnoyed you by criticizing your drinking? Ever felt **G**uilty about your drinking? Ever had an **E**ye-opener in the morning? 'Yes' to ≥2 may predict dependency (sensitivity 43–94%; specificity 70–97%). Those who refuse, or give unconvincing answers may have more to tell in their blood: look for ↑γGT, ↑ALT, ↑MCV, AST:ALT >2, ↓urea, ↓Mg²⁺, ↓platelets.

Withdrawal Starts within 10h of last drink. Consider it in any new (≤3d) ward patient with acute confusion. **Signs** ↑Pulse; ↓BP; tremor; confusion; seizures; hallucinosis (usually visual, but sometimes tactile/auditory); *delirium tremens*—occurs in 5%, begins >48h after the last drink, hallucinations, disorientation, ↑BP, ↑HR. **Management** There is almost no role for hospital inpatient 'detox' as a sole indication for admission however attractive the idea of a 'quick fix' may be—community-based services are much better placed to support cessation. Admit only if complicating or coexisting medical problems require inpatient treatment. Check BP + HR/4h. For the 1st 3d give generous chlordiazepoxide, eg 10–50mg/6h PO with additional doses PRN, then plan weaning regimen over 5–7d. Thiamine and glucose should be given to prevent Wernicke's encephalopathy (p700).

Chronic complications ▶Don't forget the risk of trauma while intoxicated.
The liver Normal in 50%; ↑ or ↑↑γGT³⁰—but may be ↑↑ in *any* type of liver inflammation, eg fatty liver, AIH (p280), HBV. **Fatty liver (steatosis)** Present in 90% of heavy drinkers, occurs acutely but is rapidly reversible with abstinence. Inflammation (steatohepatitis) may occur if drinking continues, and the risk of progression to cirrhosis is increased. **Alcoholic hepatitis** See BOX. 80% progress to cirrhosis (hepatic failure in 10%). **Cirrhosis** (See p272.) 5yr survival is 48% if drinking continues (if not, 77%). Biopsy: Mallory bodies ± neutrophils (can be indistinguishable from NASH, p281).
Gut Obesity; D&V; gastric erosions; peptic ulcers; varices (p252); pancreatitis (acute or chronic); cancer (many types); oesophageal rupture (∴ vomiting against a closed glottis; suspect if shock and surgical emphysema in the neck: Boerhaave's syndrome).
Nervous system ↓Memory/cognition; ▶high-potency vitamins IM or IV may reverse it (p700); cortical/cerebellar atrophy; retrobulbar neuropathy; seizure; falls; wide-based gait; neuropathy; confabulation/Korsakoff's (p690) ± Wernicke's encephalopathy (p700). Symmetrical polyneuropathy; alcoholic myopathy.
Blood ↑MCV anaemia from: marrow depression, GI bleeding, alcoholism-associated folate deficiency, haemolysis; sideroblastic anaemia. See p326.
Cardiovascular Arrhythmias; ↑BP; cardiomyopathy; sudden death in binge drinkers.
Reproduction Testicular atrophy; ↓testosterone/progesterone; ↑oestrogen; fetal alcohol syndrome—↓IQ, short palpebral fissure, absent philtrum, and small eyes.

Alcohol dependence Problematic pattern of alcohol use leading to clinically significant impairment or distress. Other addictions may coexist. Lifetime prevalence: ♂ ≈ 10% (♀ ≈ 4%). ▶Denial is a leading feature, so be sure to question relatives. **Management** Group therapy or self-help (eg Alcoholics Anonymous) may be useful—especially if self-initiated and determined. Encourage the will to change.
Relapse 50% will relapse soon after starting treatment. Acamprosate (p445) may help intense anxiety, insomnia, and craving. CI: pregnancy, severe liver failure, creatinine >120μmol/L. SE: D&V, ↑ or ↓libido; dose example: 666mg/8h PO if >60kg and <65yrs old. It should be started as soon as acute withdrawal is complete and continued for ~1yr. Disulfiram can be used to treat chronic alcohol dependence. It causes acetaldehyde build-up (like metronidazole) with extremely unpleasant effects to *any* alcohol ingestion—eg flushing, throbbing headache, palpitations. Care must be taken to avoid alcohol (eg toiletries, food, medicines) since severe reactions can occur. ▶Confer with experts if drugs are to be used.

30 γGT is ↑ in 52% of alcoholics; it is also ↑ in 50% of those with non-alcoholic fatty livers. Its best use is not in diagnosing alcoholism but in seeing if a raised ALP is likely to be from liver, not bone.

Addressing the behaviour of harmful drinking

The Green Fairy was an incongruous nickname given to the bearer of social degradation in 19th-century France. Parisians would spill onto the boulevards at 5pm ('*l'heure verte*') to the nearest café for their absinthe. Rather than the havoc it wreaked, absinthe became symbolic of rebellious artistic enlightenment and bohemian lifestyle. But Degas portrayed a grimly realistic view of the behaviour induced by alcohol. *Dans un café* (fig 6.33) depicts a desolate scene. A couple, lethargic, dishevelled, and trapped in vacant isolation despite their proximity, sit before a murky yellow-green glass of absinthe. Why would this well-dressed woman return to her cage of numbed misery and loneliness every evening? How might we help our patients similarly bound by entrenched behaviour from their Green Fairy?

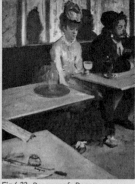

Fig 6.33 *Dans un cafe*, Degas.
Peter Barritt/Alamy Stock Photo.

Referral to specialist alcohol services is the only intervention of proven efficacy in those who are alcohol dependent. But the 'brief intervention', a structured, motivational conversation about alcohol consumption, is effective in those drinking at hazardous levels. Start by asking permission to talk about alcohol consumption and normalize the discussion 'lots of people are concerned about their drinking patterns ... '. Ascertain their level of motivation to change, and explain the health benefits or risks (depending on their responses). Follow this with open-ended questions asking what they think of these benefits/risks and their alcohol use. Emphasize that they have the responsibility for changing this and establish goals (cutting down or abstinence) and strategies to achieve these (eg not having alcohol at home, or avoiding friends who drink too much).

Managing alcoholic hepatitis

The patient Usually an acute onset of symptomatic hepatitis in those with long-standing heavy drinking, possibly with a recent ↑ intake. Malaise; anorexia; fever; D&V; tender hepatomegaly; jaundice; ascites. **Blood** ↑WCC; ↓platelets (toxic effect or ∴ hypersplenism); ↓albumin (malnutrition or ↓synthesis); ↑INR; ↑AST (*moderately* raised, usually <300IU/L). ►Jaundice, encephalopathy, or coagulopathy ≈ *severe* hepatitis. ►Rule out other causes of acute hepatitis; infectious screen; transabdominal ultrasound, ± ascitic tap and treat for SBP (p272).

- Most need hospitalizing; fluid resuscitation (albumin ideally), urinary catheter and CVP monitoring may be needed.
- Determine severity; the Maddrey discriminant function (DF) = (4.6 × PT − control PT) + (bilirubin(μmol/L)/17.1) reflects mortality.
- Stop alcohol consumption (many have stopped due to symptoms), treat withdrawal.
- Vitamins: vit K: 10mg/d IV for 3d. Thiamine 100mg/d PO (high-dose B vitamins can also be given IV as Pabrinex®—1 pair of ampoules in 50mL 0.9% saline IVI over ½h).
- Optimize nutrition (35–40kcal/kg/d non-protein energy). Use ideal body weight for calculations, eg if malnourished. Don't use low-protein diets.
- Daily weight; LFT; U&E; INR. If creatinine ↑, get help with this—HRS (p271).
- Steroids may confer benefit in those with severe disease. If DF >31 then consider prednisolone 40mg/d for 5d tapered over 3wks. ►CI: sepsis; variceal bleeding. The largest study to date (STOPAH) showed only a non-significant trend towards benefit.
- Pentoxifylline 400mg TDS (lower dose in renal dysfunction) is an alternative in those with steroid CI, but data are also inconsistent.

Prognosis Mild episodes hardly affect mortality; if severe, mortality ≈50% at 30d. 1yr after admission for alcoholic hepatitis, 40% are dead... a sobering thought.

Primary biliary cholangitis (PBC)

Interlobular bile ducts are damaged by chronic autoimmune granulomatous[31] inflammation causing cholestasis which may lead to fibrosis, cirrhosis, and portal hypertension.

Cause Unknown environmental triggers (?pollutants, xenobiotics, non-pathogenic bacteria) + genetic predisposition (eg IL12A locus) leading to loss of immune tolerance to self-mitochondrial proteins.

Antimitochondrial antibodies (AMA) These are the hallmark of PBC.

Prevalence ≤4/100 000. ♀:♂ ≈ 9:1.

Risk ↑ if: +ve family history (seen in 1–6%); many UTIs; smoking; past pregnancy; other autoimmune diseases; ↑ use of nail polish/hair dye.

Typical age at presentation ~50yrs.

The patient Often asymptomatic and diagnosed after incidental finding ↑ALP. Lethargy, sleepiness, and pruritus may precede jaundice by years. **Signs** Jaundice; skin pigmentation; xanthelasma (fig 14.12, p683); xanthomata; hepatosplenomegaly. **Complications** Those of cirrhosis (p272); osteoporosis is common. Malabsorption of fat-soluble vitamins (A, D, E, K) due to cholestasis and ↓bilirubin in the gut lumen results in osteomalacia and coagulopathy; HCC (p282).

Tests Blood ↑ALP, ↑γGT, and mildly ↑AST & ALT; late disease: ↑bilirubin, ↓albumin, ↑prothrombin time. 98% are AMA M2 subtype +ve, eg in a titre of 1:40 (see earlier in topic). Other autoantibodies (p550) may occur in low titres. Immunoglobulins are ↑ (esp. IgM). TSH & cholesterol ↑ or ↔. **Ultrasound** Excludes extrahepatic cholestasis. **Biopsy** Not usually needed (unless drug-induced cholestasis or hepatic sarcoidosis need excluding); look for granulomas around bile ducts ± cirrhosis.[31]

Treatment Symptomatic Pruritus: try colestyramine 4–8g/24h PO; naltrexone and rifampicin may also help. Diarrhoea: codeine phosphate, eg 30mg/8h PO. Osteoporosis prevention: p674. **Specific** *Fat-soluble vitamin prophylaxis:* vitamin A, D, and K. High-dose *ursodeoxycholic acid* (UDCA) with meals and at bedtime—the only recommended medication aimed at the condition itself; it may improve survival and delay transplantation. SE: ↑weight. Obeticholic acid can be added if the response is deemed inadequate. **Monitoring** Regular LFT; ultrasound ± AFP twice-yearly if cirrhotic. **Liver transplantation** (See p273.) For end-stage disease or intractable pruritus. Histological recurrence in the graft: ~17% after 5yrs; although graft failure can occur as a result of recurrence, it is rare and unpredictable.

Prognosis Highly variable. The Mayo survival model is a validated predictor of survival that combines age, bilirubin, albumin, PT time, oedema, and need for diuretics.

Primary sclerosing cholangitis (PSC)

Progressive cholestasis with bile duct inflammation and strictures (figs 6.34, 6.35).

Symptoms/signs Pruritus ± fatigue; if advanced: ascending cholangitis, cirrhosis, and hepatic failure. **Associations** • ♂ sex. • HLA-A1; B8; DR3. • AIH (p280); >80% of Northern European patients also have IBD, usually UC; this combination is associated with ↑↑risk of colorectal malignancy.

Cancers Bile duct, gallbladder, liver, and colon cancers are more common, so do yearly colonoscopy + ultrasound; consider cholecystectomy for gallbladder polyps.[32]

Tests ↑ALP, then ↑bilirubin; hypergammaglobulinaemia and/or ↑IgM; AMA −ve, but ANA, SMA, and ANCA may be +ve; see BOX and p550. ERCP (fig 6.34) or MRCP (fig 6.35) reveal duct anatomy and damage. *Liver biopsy* shows a fibrous, obliterative cholangitis.

Treatment *Liver transplant* is the mainstay for end-stage disease; recurrence occurs in up to 30%; 5yr graft survival is >60%. Prognosis is worse for those with IBD, as 5–10% develop colorectal cancer post-transplant. Endoscopic therapy to dilate/stent strictures. *Ursodeoxycholic acid* may improve LFT but has not shown evidence of survival benefit. High doses, eg 25–30mg/kg/d, may be harmful. Colestyramine 4–8g/24h PO for pruritus (naltrexone and rifampicin may also help). Antibiotics for bacterial cholangitis.

Testing for autoantibodies—the anguish of partial understanding

The diagnostic approach to several inflammatory conditions includes the measurement of autoantibodies. Consequently, and all too often, attempts to acquire (and test) medical knowledge may promote these antibody panels to a position as the final arbiter of disease diagnosis which, with their varying sensitivities and specificities, they are quite unfit to assume. Indeed, often just such a workup shows strange overlap conditions between apparently different diseases: strange until we realize that these markers are just surrogates for processes that we lack a complete aetiological explanation for and in which the antibodies themselves may just be bystanders. Process that we lack the tools to visualize, as cells of the immune system continue their onslaught against their perceived enemies, driven by reasons that none present seem willing to reveal to our crude probing with blood tests, x-rays, and biopsies. While the body knows no diseases, only pain and death, our minds attempt to impose a unitary disease on unsuspecting and sometimes innocent cells.

For example, clinically we observe that autoimmune hepatitis (AIH) frequently overlaps with PSC and IBD. A battery of antibody tests may sometimes help understand the dominant process, but equally may mystify matters still further if we attempt to apply our inadequate classifiers ('*But why is the ANCA not positive?*' cries the student, enraged at the failure of the miserable patient's B lymphocytes to do the honourable thing). As ever, management should be individualized dependent on liver and bowel histology, serum immunoglobulin levels, the degree of biochemical cholestasis, cholangiography, and, yes, autoantibodies.

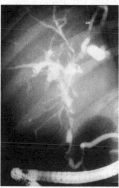

Fig 6.34 ERCP showing many strictures in the biliary tree with a characteristic 'beaded' appearance.

© Dr Anthony Mee.

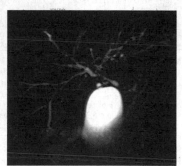

Fig 6.35 MRCP showing features of PSC. The intrahepatic ducts show multifocal strictures. Strictures can be hard to differentiate from cholangiocarcinoma (coexistence of UC may promote this development). Stenting may be needed.

© Norwich Radiology Department.

6 Gastroenterology

---

31 Other causes of liver granulomas: TB, sarcoid, infections with HIV (eg toxoplasmosis, CMV, mycobacteria), PAN, SLE, granulomatosis with polyangiitis, lymphoma, syphilis, isoniazid, quinidine, carbamazepine, allopurinol. Signs: PUO; ↑LFT.
32 Usually gallbladder polyps are an incidental finding on ultrasound, and they can often be left if <1cm diameter, but in PSC they are much more likely to become malignant.

An inflammatory liver disease of unknown cause[33] characterized by abnormal T-cell function and autoantibodies directed against hepatocyte surface antigens. Classification is by autoantibodies (table 6.12). AIH predominantly affects young or middle-aged women (bimodal, ie 10–30yrs—or >40yrs old). Up to 40% present with acute hepatitis and signs of autoimmune disease, eg fever, malaise, urticarial rash, polyarthritis, pleurisy, pulmonary infiltration, or glomerulonephritis. The remainder present with gradual jaundice or are asymptomatic and diagnosed incidentally with signs of chronic liver disease. Amenorrhoea is common and disease tends to attenuate during pregnancy.

Complications Those associated with cirrhosis (p272) and drug therapy.

Tests Serum bilirubin, AST, ALT, and ALP all usually ↑, hypergammaglobulinaemia (esp. IgG), +ve autoantibodies (table 6.12). Anaemia, ↓WCC, and ↓platelets indicate hypersplenism. **Liver biopsy** (See p244.) Mononuclear infiltrate of portal and periportal areas and piecemeal necrosis ± fibrosis; cirrhosis ≈ worse prognosis. MRCP (See p726.) Helps exclude PSC if ALP ↑ disproportionately.

Diagnosis Depends on excluding other diseases (no lab test is pathognomonic). Diagnostic criteria based on IgG levels, autoantibodies, and histology in the absence of viral disease are helpful. Sometimes diagnosis is a challenge—there is overlap with other chronic liver disease: eg PBC (p278), PSC (p278), and chronic viral hepatitis.

Table 6.12 Classifying autoimmune hepatitis: types I–II

I	Seen in 80%. Typical patient: ♀ <40yrs. ♀:♂ ≈ 4:1 Antinuclear antibody (ANA) is +ve in ≈70% with titres >1:160. Antismooth muscle antibodies (ASMA) +ve in up to 90% but are poorly specific. ↑IgG in 97%. Good response to immunosuppression in 80%. 25% have cirrhosis at presentation.
II	Commoner in Europe than USA. ♀:♂ ≈ 10:1. More often seen in children, and more commonly progresses to cirrhosis and less treatable. Typically anti-liver/kidney microsomal type 1 (LKM1) antibodies +ve. ASMA and ANA typically −ve.

Management Immunosuppressant therapy Prednisolone 30mg/d PO for 1 month; ↓ by 5mg a month to a maintenance dose of 5–10mg/d PO. Corticosteroids can sometimes be stopped after 2yrs but relapse occurs in 50–86%. Azathioprine (50–100mg/d PO) may be used as a steroid-sparing agent to maintain remission. Remission is achievable in 80% of patients within 3yrs. 10- and 20yr survival rates are >80%. SE are a big problem (p373)—partly ameliorated by a switch to budesonide, eg in non-cirrhotic AIH. **Liver transplantation** (See p273.) Indicated for decompensated cirrhosis or if there is failure to respond to medical therapy, but recurrence may occur. It is effective (actuarial 10yr survival is 75%).

Prognosis Appears not to matter whether symptomatic or asymptomatic at presentation (10yr survival ~80% for both). The presence of cirrhosis at presentation reduces 10yr survival from 94% to 62%. Overlap syndromes: AIH-PBC (primary biliary cholangitis) overlap is worse than AIH-AIC (autoimmune cholangitis).

Associations of autoimmune hepatitis

- Pernicious anaemia.
- Ulcerative colitis.
- Glomerulonephritis.
- Autoimmune thyroiditis.
- Autoimmune haemolysis.
- Diabetes mellitus.
- PSC (p278).
- HLA A1, B8, and DR3 haplotype.

---

33 Hepatotropic viruses (eg measles, herpes viruses) and some drugs appear to trigger AIH in genetically predisposed individuals exposed to a hepatotoxic *milieu intérieur*. Viral interferon can inactivate cytochrome P450 enzymes (∴ ↓ metabolism of ex- or endogenous hepatotoxins). Resulting modifications to proteins may generate autoantigens driving CD4 T-helper cell activation.

The most common liver disorder in Western countries (prevalence ≈30%) and now the leading cause of chronic liver disease worldwide, NAFLD[15] can be thought of as the hepatic manifestation of the metabolic syndrome. It will soon overtake HCV as the most common indication for liver transplantation (p273). It represents ↑fat in hepatocytes (steatosis) visualized, eg on ultrasound *that cannot be attributed to other causes* (most commonly alcohol so consider NAFLD if drink ♂ <18u/wk, ♀ <9u).

The patient Most patients are asymptomatic, but some report persistent fatigue, right upper quadrant pain or malaise, and hepatomegaly is common on exam. If inflammation is also present (↑LFT, typically ↑ALT) = non-alcoholic steatohepatitis (NASH). Rule out other causes of liver disease (p280) and check for associated metabolic disorders (obesity, dyslipidaemia, diabetes, hypertension). Progression to cirrhosis may occur—biopsy or elastography may be needed (p244).

Risk factors for progression ↑age; obesity; DM; NASH.

Treatment Control risk factors including obesity; weight loss is the mainstay of management (bariatric surgery helps). Address cardiovascular risk (commonest cause of death, see p85). Avoid alcohol consumption. No drug is of proven benefit or licences in the UK, though vitamin E may improve histology in fibrosis (eg 800IU/d—higher doses associated with excess mortality). Pioglitazone improves fibrosis and inflammation in patients with concurrent DM. Daily aspirin appears to reduce risk of progression to NASH in observational studies. **Follow-up** Monitor for complications (NASH, cirrhosis, DM). If cirrhotic, screen for HCC with ultrasound ± AFP twice-yearly.

Wilson's disease/hepatolenticular degeneration

Wilson's disease is a rare (3/100 000) inherited disorder of copper excretion with excess deposition in liver and CNS (eg basal ganglia). It is treatable, so screen all with cirrhosis.
Genetics An autosomal recessive disorder of a copper transporting ATPase, ATP7B.
Physiology Total body copper content is ~125mg. Intake ≈ 3mg/day (absorbed in proximal small intestine). In the liver, copper is incorporated into caeruloplasmin. In Wilson's disease, copper incorporation into caeruloplasmin in hepatocytes and excretion into bile are impaired. Copper accumulates in liver, and later in other organs.

Signs Children present with *liver disease* (hepatitis, cirrhosis, fulminant liver failure); young adults often start with *CNS signs*: tremor; dysarthria; dysphagia; dyskinesias; dystonias; Parkinsonism; ataxia/clumsiness. **Mood** Depression/mania; labile emotions; ↑↓libido; personality change. ►Ignoring these may cause years of needless misery: often the doctor who is good at combining the analytical and integrative aspects will be the first to make the diagnosis. **Cognition** ↓Memory; slow to solve problems; ↓IQ; delusions; mutism. **Kayser–Fleischer (KF) rings** Copper in iris; they are not invariable. **Also** Haemolysis; blue lunulae (nails); arthritis; hypermobile joints; grey skin.

Tests ►Equivocal copper studies need expert interpretation.
1 *Urine:* 24h copper excretion is *high*, eg >100mcg/24h (normal <40mcg).
2 *↑LFT:* non-specific (but ALT >1500 is *not* part of the picture).
3 *Serum copper:* typically <11μmol/L.
4 *↓Serum caeruloplasmin:* <200mg/L (<140mg/L is pathognomonic)—beware incidental low values in protein-deficiency states (eg nephrotic syndrome, malabsorption).
5 *Molecular genetic testing* can confirm the diagnosis.
6 *Slit lamp exam:* KF rings: in iris/Descemet's membrane (see fig 4.53 OHCS p368).
7 *Liver biopsy:* ↑hepatic copper (copper >250mcg/g dry weight); hepatitis; cirrhosis.
8 *MRI:* degeneration in basal ganglia, frontotemporal, cerebellar, and brainstem.

Management **Diet** Avoid foods with high copper content (eg liver, chocolate, nuts, mushrooms, legumes, and shellfish). Check water sources (eg wells, pipes) for copper. **Drugs** Lifelong penicillamine (500mg/6–8h PO for 1yr, maintenance 0.75–1g/d). SE: nausea, rash, ↓WCC, ↓Hb, ↓platelets, haematuria, nephrosis, lupus. Monitor FBC and urinary copper and protein excretion. **Liver transplantation** (See p273.) If severe liver disease. **Screen siblings** Asymptomatic homozygotes need treating.

Prognosis Pre-cirrhotic liver disease is reversible; CNS damage less so. There are no clear clinical prognostic indicators. Fatal events: liver failure, bleeding, infection.

The most common (90%) liver tumours are metastases (fig 6.36), eg from breast, bronchus, or the gastrointestinal tract (table 6.14). Primary hepatic tumours are much less common and may be benign or malignant (table 6.13).

Symptoms Fever, malaise, anorexia, ↓weight, RUQ pain (∵ liver capsule stretch). Jaundice is late, except with cholangiocarcinoma. Benign tumours are often asymptomatic. Tumours may rupture causing intraperitoneal haemorrhage.

Signs Hepatomegaly (smooth, or hard and irregular, eg metastases, cirrhosis, HCC). Look for signs of chronic liver disease (p272) and evidence of decompensation (jaundice, ascites). Feel for an abdominal mass. Listen for a bruit over the liver (HCC).

Tests Blood FBC, clotting, LFT, hepatitis serology, α-fetoprotein (↑ in 50–80% of HCC, though levels do not correlate with size, stage, or prognosis). **Imaging** US or CT to identify lesions and guide biopsy. MRI is better at distinguishing benign from malignant lesions. Do ERCP (p726) and biopsy if cholangiocarcinoma is suspected. **Liver biopsy** (See p244.) May achieve a histological diagnosis; ►careful multidisciplinary discussion is required if potentially resectable, as bleeding or seeding along the biopsy tract can occur. If the lesion could be a metastasis, find the primary, eg by CXR, mammography, colonoscopy, CT, MRI, or marrow biopsy.

Liver metastases Signify advanced disease. Treatment and prognosis vary with the type and extent of primary tumour. Chemotherapy may be effective (eg lymphomas, germ cell tumours). Small, solitary metastases may be amenable to resection (eg colorectal cancer). In most, treatment is palliative. **Prognosis** Often <6 months.

Hepatocellular carcinoma (HCC) Primary hepatocyte neoplasia accounts for 90% of primary liver cancers; it is common in China & Africa (40% of cancers vs 2% in UK). **The patient** Fatigue, ↓appetite, ↓weight, jaundice, ascites, haemobilia.[34] ♂:♀≈3. **Causes** HBV is the leading cause worldwide (esp. if high viral load; p274). HCV;[35] AIH (p280); cirrhosis (alcohol, haemochromatosis, PBC); non-alcoholic fatty liver; aflatoxin; *Clonorchis sinensis*; anabolic steroids. Δ3-phase CT (delayed wash-out of contrast in a suspect mass); MRI; biopsy. **Treatment** Laparoscopic resection of solitary tumours <3cm across ↑ 3yr survival from 13% to 59%; but ~50% have recurrence by 3yrs.[36] Liver transplant gives a 5yr survival rate of 70%.[37] Percutaneous ablation, tumour embolization (TACE[38]) are options. The anti-VEGF drug sorafenib is given for advanced disease or earlier stage tumours unsuitable for local therapy. **Prevention** ►HBV vaccination (BOX 'Vaccinating to prevent hepatitis' and table 6.15). ►Don't reuse needles. ►Screen blood. ►↓Aflatoxin exposure (sun-dry maize). Encourage coffee consumption (↓risk HCC in cirrhosis).[16] **6-monthly US screen** Consider if at ↑risk: eg all with cirrhosis; or chronic HBV in Africans or older Asians.

Cholangiocarcinoma (Biliary tree cancer.) ~10% of liver primaries. **Causes** Flukes (*Clonorchis*, p431); PSC (screening by CA19–9 may be helpful, p278); biliary cysts; Caroli's disease, p268; HBV; HCV; DM; N-nitroso toxins. **The patient** Fever, abdominal pain (± ascites), malaise, ↑bilirubin; ↑↑ALP. **Pathology** Usually slow-growing. Most are distal extrahepatic or perihilar. **Management** 70% inoperable at presentation. Of those that are, 76% recur. *Surgery:* eg major hepatectomy + extrahepatic bile duct excision + caudate lobe resection + adjuvant chemotherapy. 5yr survival ~30%. Post-op complications include liver failure, bile leak, and GI bleeding. *Stenting* of obstructed extrahepatic biliary tree, percutaneously or via ERCP (p726), improves quality of life.

Benign tumours Haemangiomas The most common benign liver tumours. ♀:♂≈4:1. Often an incidental finding on US (hyperechoic) or CT and don't require treatment. Avoid biopsy! May be part of von Hippel–Lindau syndrome; surgery if diagnosis is uncertain (may be confused with HCC) or they are enlarging on 6-monthly US. Adenomas Causes: anabolic steroids, oral contraceptive pill; pregnancy. Only treat if symptomatic, or >5cm.

---

34 Haemobilia is late in HCC. Think of bleeding into the biliary tree whenever Quincke's triad occurs: RUQ pain, upper GI haemorrhage, and jaundice. It may be life-threatening.

35 5yr cumulative risk if cirrhosis is present is 30% in Japan and 17% in USA.

36 Operative mortality: 1.6%. Recurrence is more likely if histology showed neoplastic emboli in small vessels. Get early warning of recurrence by arranging imaging, eg AFP >5.45mcg/L (esp. if trend is rising). Fibrolamellar HCC, which occurs in children and young adults, has a better prognosis.

37 Milan criteria for liver transplantation in HCC: 1 nodule <5cm or 2–3 nodules <3cm.

38 TACE=transarterial chemoembolization, eg with drug-eluting beads; it causes fever and abdo pain in 50%.

Table 6.13 Primary liver tumours

Malignant (prognosis—regardless of type—is poor)	Benign
HCC	Cysts*
Cholangiocarcinoma	Haemangioma
Angiosarcoma	Adenoma
Hepatoblastoma	Focal nodular hyperplasia†
Fibrosarcoma & hepatic gastrointestinal stromal tumour (GIST‡, formerly leiomyosarcoma)	Fibroma
	Benign GIST (=leiomyoma)

* Simple cysts (no communication with the biliary tree) are present in 1%, but rarely cause symptoms. ♀:♂≈9:1 if large or symptomatic.

† 2nd most common benign solid lesion; hyperplastic hepatocytes around a stellate scar, possibly a response to an anomalous vessel. Solitary lesion, 90% found in ♀.

‡ GISTs are mesenchymal tumours that are more likely to be found in the gut as a spherical mass arising from the muscularis propria, eg with GI bleeding. If unresectable, imatinib ↑ 2yr survival from 26% to 76%.

Table 6.14 Origins of secondary liver tumours

Common in men	Common in women	Less common (either sex)
Stomach	Breast	Pancreas
Lung	Colon	Leukaemia
Colon	Stomach	Lymphoma
	Uterus	Carcinoid tumours

Vaccinating to prevent hepatitis B (and associated complications)

Use hepatitis B vaccine 1mL into deltoid; repeat at 1 & 6 months (child: 0.5mL ≈ 3 into the anterolateral thigh). **Indications** Everyone (WHO advice, even in areas of 'low' endemicity—in 2014 this meant that 82% of the world's children received protection against HBV). This contrasts with the approach in, eg the UK and USA of targeting at-risk groups (p274). The immunocompromised and others may need further doses. Serology helps time boosters and finds non-responders (correlates with older age, smoking, and ♂ sex). ►*Know your own antibody level!*

Table 6.15 Post-immunization anti-HBs titres and actions

Anti-HBs (IU/L)	Actions and comments (advice differs in some areas)
>1000	Good level of immunity; retest in ~4yrs
100–1000	Good level of immunity; if level approaches 100, retest in 1yr
<100	Inadequate; give booster and retest
<10	Non-responder; give another set of 3 vaccinations. Retest; if <10 get consent to check hepatitis B status: HBsAg +ve means chronic infection; anti-HB core +ve represents past infection and immunity. If a non-responder is deemed susceptible to HBV, and has recently come in contact with risky bodily fluids, offer 2 doses of anti-hep B immunoglobulin

NB: protection begins some weeks after dose 1, so it won't work if exposure is recent; here, specific anti-hepatitis B immunoglobulin is best if not already immunized.

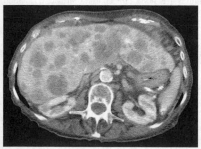

Fig 6.36 Axial CT of the liver after IV contrast showing multiple round lesions of varying size, highly suggestive of hepatic metastases.
Courtesy of Norwich Radiology Dept.

6 Gastroenterology

6 Gastroenterology

An autosomal recessive disorder of iron metabolism in which ↑intestinal iron absorption leads to iron deposition in joints, liver, heart, pancreas, pituitary, adrenals, and skin. Middle-aged men are more frequently and severely affected than women, in whom the disease tends to present ~10yrs later (menstrual blood loss is protective).

Genetics

HH is one of the commonest inherited conditions in those of Northern European (especially Celtic) ancestry (carrier rate of ~1 in 10 and a frequency of homozygosity of ~1 in 200–400). The gene responsible for most HH is HFE: the 2 commonest mutations are termed C282Y and H63D. C282Y accounts for 60–90% of HH, and H63D accounts for 1–3%, with compound heterozygotes accounting for 4–7%. Penetrance is variable—a significant fraction of C282Y homozygotes will not develop signs of iron overload during follow-up, complicating screening decisions.

The patient

Early on Nil—or tiredness; arthralgia (2nd + 3rd MCP joints + knee pseudogout); ↓libido. **Later** Slate-grey skin pigmentation; signs of chronic liver disease (p276); hepatomegaly; cirrhosis (esp. if drinks alcohol); dilated cardiomyopathy. **Endocrinopathies** DM ('bronze diabetes' from iron deposition in pancreas); hypogonadism (p226) from ↓pituitary dysfunction.

Tests

Blood ↑LFT, ↑ferritin (♂ > 200/♀ > 150ng/mL; but inflammation will also ↑ferritin); ↑transferrin saturation[39] should all trigger suspicion. Confirm by HFE genotyping. **Images** Chondrocalcinosis (fig 6.37). Liver & cardiac MRI: Fe overload. **Liver biopsy** Perl's stain quantifies iron loading[40] and assesses disease severity.

Management

Venesect ~0.5–2 units/1–2wks, until ferritin ≤50mcg/L (may take 2yrs). Iron will continue to accumulate, so maintenance venesection is needed for life (1U every 2–3 months to maintain haematocrit <0.5, ferritin <100mcg/L, and transferrin saturation <40%). No randomized evidence, but survival benefit has been shown in observational studies. Consider desferrioxamine, an iron chelator (p338), if intolerant of this.

Monitor LFT and glucose/diabetes (p200). HbA1c levels may be falsely low as venesection ↓ the time available for Hb glycosylation. If cirrhotic, screen for HCC with ultrasound ± AFP twice-yearly.

Over-the-counter drugs Ensure vitamin preparations contain no iron.

Diet A well-balanced diet should be encouraged—there is no need to avoid iron-rich foods. Avoid alcohol. Avoid uncooked seafood (may contain bacteria that thrive on increased plasma iron concentrations, eg *Listeria monocytogenes*, *Vibrio vulnificus*).

Screening Serum ferritin, transferrin saturation, and HFE genotype. ►Screen 1st-degree relatives by genetic testing even if they are asymptomatic and have normal LFT ideally prior to age where significant iron deposition likely to have occurred (eg 18–30yrs). Since C282Y homozygotes may never develop iron overload, population screening should not be performed.

Prognosis

Venesection returns life expectancy to normal if non-diabetic and non-cirrhotic (and liver histology *can* improve). Arthropathy may improve or worsen. Gonadal failure may reverse in younger men. ►If cirrhosis, 22–30% get hepatocellular cancer, especially if: age >50yrs (risk ↑ ×13), HBsAg +ve (risk ↑ ×5), or alcohol abuse (risk ↑ ×2).

---

39 Transferrin saturation >45% is a sensitive threshold for further screening but will lead to some false +ves.
40 Although generally not required, biopsy quantifies hepatic iron loading and fibrosis. This helps determine the severity of liver disease, particularly in those with other underlying causes of chronic liver disease.

A bit about iron metabolism

60% of body iron is in haemoglobin, and erythropoiesis requires ~5–30mg iron/day—provided by macrophages (recycling of haeme iron after phagocytosis of old RBCs). Intestinal iron absorption (1–2mg/day) compensates for daily iron losses.

Red meats, liver, seafoods, enriched breakfast cereals and pulses, and some spices (eg paprika) are iron-rich. Most dietary iron is in Fe^{3+}, which is reduced by low gastric pH and ascorbic acid (vitamin c) to better-absorbed Fe^{2+}. Absorption occurs mainly in the duodenum and jejunum, though very small amounts are absorbed in the stomach and ileum. Iron requirements are greater for women (menstrual loss), when growing, in pregnancy, and in chronic infection.

Hepcidin, a peptide synthesized in hepatocytes, secreted in plasma, is a negative regulator of gut iron absorption and haeme iron recycling by macrophages. Hepcidin synthesis is stimulated by iron and repressed by iron deficiency and by ↑ marrow erythropoiesis (eg in anaemia, bleeding, haemolysis, dyserythropoiesis, or erythropoietin injections). Defects in the normal triggering of hepcidin by iron excess is a rare cause of haemochromatosis unrelated to HFE mutations, whereas a defect in hepcidin repression is responsible for an iron refractory iron deficiency anaemia. More commonly excessive dosing with oral iron will lead to upregulation of hepcidin and reduce iron absorption—once daily or even alternate day oral iron replacement is now the preferred strategy for patients requiring iron supplementation.[17]

In HH, the total body iron is up to 10-fold that of a normal person, with loading found particularly in the liver and pancreas (≈100). Hepatic disease classically starts with fibrosis, progressing to cirrhosis as a late feature.

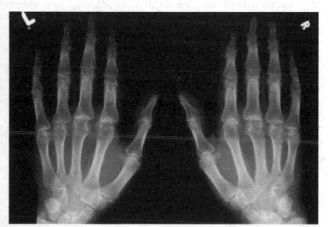

Fig 6.37 Haemochromatosis causes stressed joints to deteriorate faster than resting joints: the 2nd and 3rd MCP joints have osteophytes and narrowed joint spaces compared to the normal hand (right image) in this man who only used his dominant hand for his production line job.
Reproduced from Watts *et al.*, *Oxford Desk Reference: Rheumatology*, 2009, with permission from Oxford University Press.

6 Gastroenterology

A1AT deficiency is an inherited disorder affecting lung (emphysema) and liver (cirrhosis and HCC). A1AT is a glycoprotein and one of a family of **ser**ine **p**rotease **in**hibitors made in the liver that control inflammatory cascades. Deficiency is called a **serpin**opathy. It makes up 90% of serum α_1-globulin on electrophoresis (p679). A1AT deficiency is the chief genetic cause of liver disease in children. In adults, its lack is more likely to cause emphysema, and all those with persistent air-flow obstruction should be tested. Lung A1AT protects against tissue damage from neutrophil elastase—a process that is also induced by cigarette smoking (p166).

Prevalence
~1:4000 (higher in Caucasians).

Genetics
Autosomal co-dominant. Genetic variants of A1AT are typed by electrophoretic mobility as *medium* (M), *slow* (S), or *very slow* (Z). S and Z types are due to single amino acid substitutions and result in ↓production of α_1-antitrypsin (S = 60%, Z = 15%). The normal genotype is PiMM, the high-risk homozygote is PiZZ; heterozygotes are PiMZ and PiSZ (at low risk of developing liver disease).

The patient
Symptomatic patients usually have the PiZZ genotype: dyspnoea from emphysema; cirrhosis; cholestatic jaundice. Cholestasis often remits in adolescence.

Tests
Serum A1AT levels ↓, usually (eg <11μmol/L or <75% of lower limit of normal, which is ~0.9g/L; labs vary). Note the 'usually'. Because A1AT is part of the acute-phase response, inflammation may make a low level. Unless you do genotyping, you will inevitably mislabel some cirrhosis as cryptogenic.

Lung function testing Shows reductions in FEV_1 with obstructive pattern (p154). There may be some bronchodilator reversibility.

Liver biopsy (See p244.) Periodic acid Schiff (PAS) +ve; diastase-resistant globules.

Phenotyping By isoelectric focusing requires expertise to distinguish SZ and ZZ phenotypes. Phenotyping can miss null phenotypes.

Prenatal diagnosis Possible by DNA analysis of chorionic villus samples obtained at 11–13wks' gestation.

Management
Smoking cessation, avoid passive exposure. Prompt treatment/preventative vaccination for lung infections. Giving IV A1AT pooled from human plasma is expensive but COPD exacerbations *may* be prevented (no good randomized trials).

Liver transplantation Needed in decompensated cirrhosis.

Lung transplantation Improves survival and has a comparable survival to transplantation in non-A1AT-deficient COPD.

Inhaled A1AT Has been tried in lung disease.

Prognosis
Some patients have life-threatening symptoms in childhood, whereas others remain asymptomatic and healthy into old age. Worse prognosis if male, a smoker, or obese. Emphysema is the cause of death in most, liver disease in ~5%. In adults, cirrhosis ± HCC affect 25% of A1AT-deficient adults >50yrs.

Approaches to abnormal liver function tests (LFTs)

Abnormal LFTs can be found in ~17% of the asymptomatic general population. Also, remember that normal LFTs do not exclude liver disease.

Tests of hepatocellular injury or cholestasis

Aminotransferases (AST, ALT): released in the bloodstream after hepatocellular injury. ALT is more specific for hepatocellular injury (but also expressed in kidney and muscle). AST is also expressed in the heart, skeletal muscle, and RBCs.

Alkaline phosphatase: may originate from liver, bone (so raised in growing children) or placenta; isoenzyme testing (where available) may differentiate source.

Gamma-glutamyl transferase (GGT; γGT): present in liver, pancreas, renal tubules, and intestine—but not bone, so it helps tell if a raised ALP is from bone (GGT↔) or liver (GGT↑). NB: it is not specific to alcohol damage to the liver.

Tests of hepatic function

Serum albumin, serum bilirubin, PT (INR).

Hepatocellular predominant liver injury

↑AST & ↑ALT. Evaluate promptly, consider medications, collateral history from family ('Could he be consuming ↑alcohol?'); ultrasound for fatty liver, metastases, viral serology (hepatitis A, B, C, E, EBV, CMV).

Alcoholic liver disease: AST/ALT ratio is typically 2:1 or more. When the history is not reliable, normal ALP, ↑GGT, and macrocytosis suggest this condition.

Acute viral hepatitis: ↑ALT; bilirubin may be ↔. NB: AST may be ↑↑, p274, p277.

Chronic viral hepatitis: ↑ALT; HBV & HCV are a leading cause worldwide.

Autoimmune hepatitis (AIH): occurs mainly in young and middle-aged females.

Fatty infiltration of the liver: (see p281.) Probably the chief cause of mildly raised LFTs in the general population and may be recognized on ultrasound.

Ischaemic hepatitis: can be seen in conditions when effective circulatory volume is low (eg MI, hypotension, haemorrhage). ↑↑↑ALT, as well as LDH.

Drug-induced hepatitis: as no specific serology identifies most culprits, a good history is vital. Paracetamol overdose causes most acute liver failure in the UK.

Cholestasis predominant liver injury

ALP and GGT are ↑; AST and ALT mildly ↑.

Management

For each specific diagnosis, manage accordingly. If asymptomatic and other tests are −ve, try lifestyle modification. Help reduce weight and alcohol use (p276 & *OHCS* p826); control DM & dyslipidaemia; stop hepatotoxic drugs.

Follow-up

Repeat tests after 1–2 months; if still ↑, do US (± abdominal CT). If diagnosis still unclear, get help: is biopsy needed? Consider (if you haven't already) A1AT levels, serum caeruloplasmin (Wilson's disease), coeliac serology, ANA, and ASMA (AIH, p280).

6 Gastroenterology

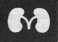

7 Kidney medicine

Contents

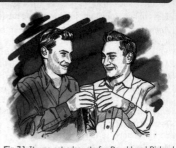

Fig 7.1 It was not adequate for Ronald and Richard Herrick to tell the world that they were identical twins. Instead, 17 formal genetic tests were undertaken, as well as an examination of their fingerprints, coordinated at a local police station, witnessed by journalists. When a reciprocal skin graft, in the absence of any immunosuppressive armoury, remained well healed it was declared that 'the probability of identity was excellent'. During this time, Richard was dying of kidney failure. He was erratic, uncooperative, and disorientated. The psychiatric evaluation concluded uraemic encephalopathy: 'Offhand, I feel the patient will recover from his psychosis with... removal of toxic agents.' He was hypertensive and fluid overloaded with primitive dialysis leading to uncontrolled electrolyte shifts and arrhythmias. But would Ronald's kidney fit inside Richard? A test run was required to ensure anatomy and logistics did not compromise the planned surgery. On 20 December 1954, Dr Joseph Murray abandoned his preparation of Christmas eggnog for 75 guests and travelled to a post-mortem room where a cadaver had finally become available for practice. Three days later the first successful human kidney transplant was performed. Although advances in dialysis, surgery, and immunosuppression over the intervening 70 years have transformed the lives of those with kidney transplants, the bravery of living donors remains. Richard knew this: 'Get out of here and go home', he wrote on the eve of the surgery. 'I am here and I am going to stay', was Ronald's reply. Ronald not only gifted a kidney to Richard, but also days he should not have had, a wife he had not yet met, and two children who glomerulonephritis had decreed should not have been born.

Artwork by Gillian Turner.

We thank Andrew Mooney, our Specialist Reader for this chapter.

Kidney disease presents as:

1 Asymptomatic disease

- **Non-visible haematuria** (NVH, microscopic haematuria) Detected on urine dip-stick. Confirm with repeat testing. Most is not due to kidney disease. Urological investigation is first line for all aged >40 years. See p290.
- **Asymptomatic proteinuria** Normal kidney protein excretion is <150mg/24h (non-pregnant). Quantification by 24h urine collection is unreliable and not used in clin-ical practice. Spot urinary albumin to creatinine ratio (uACR) >2.5(♂) or 3.5(♀)mg/mmol, or urinary protein to creatinine ratio (uPCR) >15mg/mmol may signify glom-erular (common) or tubular (rare) pathology.
- **Abnormal kidney function (GFR)** The glomerular filtration rate (GFR) is a measure of how much blood the kidneys are cleaning per minute. Direct measurement is invasive and time-consuming. Estimates derived from equations based on serum creatinine are widely used to give an eGFR (see p661). Errors in eGFR are caused by non-steady-state conditions (eg AKI), and conditions which alter serum creatinine (diet, muscle mass). eGFR is less accurate at higher levels of GFR (>60mL/min/1.73m^2), which require other evidence of kidney disease.
- **High blood pressure** Kidney disease should be excluded if hypertension occurs with any of haematuria, proteinuria, ↓eGFR.
- **Electrolyte abnormalities** Disorders of sodium, potassium, and acid–base balance (p297, pp662–7) may be due to underlying kidney disease.

2 Kidney tract symptoms

- **Urinary symptoms** *Dysuria* is a sensation of discomfort with micturition and may be accompanied by *urgency*, *frequency*, and *nocturia*. Urinary tract infec-tion (UTI) is the primary differential. Consider prostatic aetiology if there is dif-ficulty initiating voiding, poor stream, and dribbling. *Oliguria* (<400mL/24h or <0.5mL/kg/h) and *anuria* should trigger assessment and investigation for *acute kidney injury* (AKI) (see p294–5). *Polyuria* is the voiding of abnormally high volumes of urine, usually from high fluid intake but consider also DM, diabetes insipidus (p234), hypercalcaemia (p668), renal medullary disorders (impaired concentration of urine).
- **Loin pain** For pain confined to the loin consider pyelonephritis, kidney cyst path-ology, and kidney infarct. Ureteric colic is severe and radiates anteriorly from the loin to the groin. It can be caused by caliculi, clot, or a sloughed papilla.
- **Visible haematuria** (VH, macroscopic) Urological investigation is required to ex-clude renal tract malignancy. Nephrological causes include polycystic kidney dis-ease and glomerular disease: IgA (p307), anti-glomerular basement membrane (anti-GBM) disease (p307), Alport syndrome (p316).
- **Nephrotic syndrome** Proteinuria >3g/24h (= uPCR >300mg/mmol) with hypoalbuminaemia (<30g/L) and oedema. Kidney biopsy is usual in adults (p306).
- **Symptomatic chronic kidney disease (CKD)** Dyspnoea, anorexia, weight loss, pruritus, bone pain, sexual dysfunction, cognitive decline (pp298–301).

3 A systemic disorder with kidney involvement

- **DM** (See p310.)
- **Metabolic** Sickle cell disease (p311), tuberous sclerosis (p316), Fabry disease (p316), cystinosis (p317).
- **Immune-mediated** ANCA-associated vasculitis (p310, p554), SLE (p310), Henoch–Schönlein purpura (p307), systemic sclerosis (p311), sarcoid (p314), Sjögren's syn-drome (p314, p548).
- **Infection** Sepsis is a common cause of AKI. Systemic infections leading to CKD in-clude TB (p388), malaria, chronic hepatitis (p274), HIV (pp394–9).
- **Malignancy** Obstruction, hypercalcaemia, direct toxicity, eg myeloma (p310).
- **Pregnancy** Pre-eclampsia.
- **Medication** NSAIDs, aminoglycosides, chemotherapy. ACE-i, ARB are used to preserve kidney function by reducing intraglomerular pressure. They may exacerbate AKI if kidney perfusion is reduced, eg sepsis, volume depletion, but remember to re-start ACE-i/ARB following acute illness.

Perform dipstick urinalysis whenever you suspect kidney disease. This is a quick way of checking whether the urine contains anything that it should not, eg protein, blood, glucose. Abnormalities can indicate intrinsic kidney disease or kidney tract abnormalities and usually require further investigation.

▶A dipstick test of a catheter sample is difficult to interpret.

▶Look for a urine dip result (before the catheter was inserted). A positive result may need specialist advice from nephrology/urology. A negative result *may* help to reassure you about the absence of intrinsic kidney disease.

Proteinuria

Requires quantification. 24h collection of urine is not used due to inaccuracy. Urinary albumin:creatinine ratio (uACR) or protein:creatinine ratio (uPCR) is performed on a random spot urine sample. Normal uACR is <2.5(♂) or <3.5(♀) and is more sensitive than uPCR <15. Approximate equivalent levels of proteinuria are given in table 7.1.

Table 7.1 Conversion factors

Protein excretion g/24h	UACR mg/mmol	UPCR mg/mmol
0.15(physiological)	2.5♂ or 3.5 ♀	15
0.5	30	50
1	70	100
3 (nephrotic range)	250	300

Raised uACR/uPCR The higher the proteinuria, the greater the chance of glomerular disease, eg glomerulonephritis, DM, amyloidosis. Proteinuria is associated with ↑risk of cardiovascular disease and death. **False positive** Postural (repeat using an early morning sample), post-exercise, fever, heart failure. ↑ in pregnancy: uPCR <30mg/mmol and uACR <8mmg/mmol are considered normal for pregnancy.

Microalbuminuria Ultra-sensitive dipsticks are available to measure microalbuminuria (albumin excretion 30–300mg/24h). Suggests early glomerular disease, eg DM.

Haematuria

Blood in the urine may arise from anywhere in the renal tract. Transient causes should be excluded, eg UTI, menstruation. Classified as:
• Visible (macroscopic, frank).
• Invisible (microscopic): detected on dipstick testing or microscopy.

Causes Malignancy (kidney, ureter, bladder), calculi, IgA nephropathy, Alport syndrome (p316), other glomerulonephritides (p306), polycystic kidney disease (p316), schistosomiasis. Do not attribute haematuria to anticoagulation without investigation.

False positive Myoglobin triggers dipstick reaction but microscopy will be negative for red blood cells.

Management Refer for urological assessment: imaging, and cystoscopy, to exclude renal tract malignancy/calculi if aged 45 or over. Consider intrinsic kidney disease and referral to nephrology for invisible haematuria with:
• eGFR <60mL/min/1.73m².
• Coexistent proteinuria (uACR >30mg/mmol or uPCR >50mg/mmol).
• Hypertension >140/90mmHg.
• Family history of kidney disease.
No cause is found in 19–68% of invisible haematuria. If there is no proteinuria, monitor BP, eGFR, and repeat uACR/uPCR annually. Proteinuria and/or deteriorating eGFR warrant referral to nephrology.

Others

Glucose DM, pregnancy, sepsis, proximal renal tubular pathology (p312). **Ketones** Starvation, ketoacidosis. **Leucocytes** UTI (p292), vaginal discharge. **Nitrites** UTI (enteric Gram−ve organism). **Bilirubin** Haemolysis. **Urobilinogen** Liver disease, haemolysis. **Specific gravity** Normal range: 1.005–1.030, surrogate for urine osmolality, affected by proteinuria. **pH** Normal range: 4.5–9, usually acidic with meat-containing diet (acid–base balance, p662; renal tubular acidosis, pp312–13).

Urine microscopy

Urine microscopy is operator dependent and many consider it to be a dying art.

Cells

Red blood cells:
- >2 red cells/mm³ is abnormal.
- Can come from anywhere in the urinary tract. Isomorphic red cells are similar to circulating red cells and suggest bleeding from an extrarenal source. Dysmorphic red cells are abnormal in size/shape. Although they may indicate bleeding from the glomerulus (especially in exam questions), assessment is subjective and dysmorphism also occurs due to changes in pH, osmolality, protein, and due to tubular passage.

White blood cells (fig 7.2a):
- >10 white cells/mm³ or 3 or more white cells/high power film are abnormal.
- Causes include UTI, glomerulonephritis, tubulointerstitial nephritis, papillary necrosis, diabetes, kidney transplant rejection, malignancy, calculi, STI.

Squamous epithelial cells:
- Often seen, not pathological.

Casts
- Casts are cylindrical bodies formed in the lumen of distal tubules. They are formed of Tamm–Horsfall protein combined with cells.
- Hyaline casts (fig 7.2b)—seen in normal urine, fever, exercise.
- Red cell casts (fig 7.2c)—signify an inflammatory process causing bleeding in the glomerulus, eg glomerulonephritis (p307).
- White cell casts (fig 7.2d)—pyelonephritis, interstitial nephritis (p314), glomerulonephritis (p307).
- Granular casts (fig 7.2e)—formed from degenerated tubular cells, non-specific in kidney disease.

Crystals
Crystals are common in old or cold urine and may not signify pathology. They are important in renal stone disease.
- Uric acid (fig 7.2f, and p672)—stones, tumour lysis syndrome.
- Calcium oxalate (fig 7.2g)—stones (p630), oxalate nephropathy (p315), high oxalate diet, ethylene glycol poisoning.
- Cystine (fig 7.2h)—cystinuria (p317).

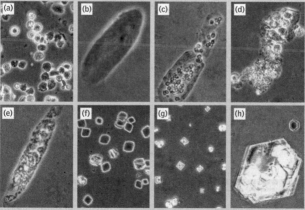

Fig 7.2 (a) White cells; (b) hyaline cast; (c) red cell cast; (d) white cell cast; (e) granular cast; (f) uric acid crystals; (g) calcium oxalate crystals; (h) cystine crystal.
Images (a) to (h) reproduced from Turner *et al.*, *Oxford Textbook of Clinical Nephrology*, 2005, with permission from Oxford University Press.

Definitions Bacteriuria Bacteria in the urine. May be asymptomatic or symptomatic. Bacteriuria is not a disease. **UTI**[1] A combination of bacteriuria and clinical features including: *Lower UTI* infection of bladder (cystitis), prostate (prostatitis); *Upper UTI* infection of kidney/renal pelvis (pyelonephritis). The aim of treatment is symptom relief and/or prevention of complications. **Abacterial cystitis/urethral syndrome** Diagnosis of exclusion in patients with dysuria and frequency, without demonstrable infection. **Urethritis** See pp408–9.

Incidence Annual incidence of UTI in ♀ is 10–20%. 10% of ♂ and 20% of ♀ >65 years have asymptomatic bacteriuria (>65 years MSU is not diagnostic in isolation and clinical assessment is mandatory). Pyelonephritis = 3 per 1000 patient-years.

Classification
• *Uncomplicated:* normal renal tract structure and function.
• *Complicated:* structural/functional abnormality of genitourinary tract, eg obstruction, catheter, stones, neurogenic bladder, kidney transplant.

Risk factors
• ↑**Bacterial inoculation** Sexual activity, urinary/faecal incontinence, constipation.
• ↑**Binding of uropathogenic bacteria** Spermicide use, ↓oestrogen, menopause.
• ↓**Urine flow** Dehydration, obstructed urinary tract (p632).
• ↑**Bacterial growth** DM, immunosuppression, obstruction, stones, catheter, renal tract malformation.

Symptoms
• **Key symptoms** Dysuria, new nocturia, cloudy urine.
• **Other symptoms** Urgency, frequency, suprapubic tenderness, haematuria.
• **Prostatitis** Pain: perineum, rectum, scrotum, penis, bladder, lower back. Fever, malaise, nausea, urinary symptoms, swollen or tender prostate on PR (p637).
• **Acute pyelonephritis** Fever, rigor, vomiting, loin pain/tenderness, costovertebral pain, associated cystitis symptoms, myalgia, septic shock.

Signs Suprapubic/loin tenderness, fever. Check for a distended bladder/enlarged prostate. If *vaginal discharge*, 80% do not have UTI, consider PID (p409).

Tests
• **Dipstick** Not needed if two or three key symptoms. Use in ♀ <65yrs if one key or other symptoms. Nitrites make UTI more likely. If only leucocytes then other diagnoses equally likely. Less useful in ♂. Do not use >65yrs. No diagnostic value in catheterized sample.
• **MSU culture** Conventional cut off >10^4–10^5 colony-forming units (cfu)/mL but if symptomatic best diagnostic criterion may be >10^2–10^3cfu/mL. Send in ♀ <65yrs if nitrite-positive dipstick and risk of resistance or leucocyte only positive, ♀ >65yrs, ♂, pregnancy. If catheterized and new urinary symptoms (not cloudy urine), change catheter first.
• **Blood tests** If systemic symptoms: FBC, U&E, CRP, and blood culture (positive in only 10–25% of pyelonephritis). Treat sepsis. Consider fasting glucose.
• **Imaging** Consider USS and referral to urology for assessment (cystoscopy, urodynamics, CT) in pyelonephritis, failure to respond to treatment, recurrent unexplained UTI, unusual organism, prostatitis, persistent haematuria.

Organisms Usually anaerobes and Gram-negative bacteria from bowel and vaginal flora. *E. coli* is the main organism (70–95% in community but ↓ in hospital). *Staphylococcus saprophyticus* (a skin commensal) in 5–10%. Other Enterobacteriaceae such as *Proteus mirabilis* and *Klebsiella pneumonia*. For sterile pyuria see **table 7.2**.

Table 7.2 Causes of sterile pyuria (↑numbers of white cells but sterile with standard culture)

Infection related	Non-infection related	
►TB	Calculi	Polycystic kidney
Recently treated UTI	Renal tract tumour	Recent catheter
Inadequately treated UTI	Papillary necrosis	Pregnancy
Fastidious culture requirement	Tubulointerstitial nephritis	SLE
Appendicitis, prostatitis, chlamydia	Chemical cystitis	Drugs, eg steroids

Managing UTI

►Do not use antibiotics for the treatment of asymptomatic bacteriuria in non-pregnant ♀, ♂, and adults with catheters.

►Treatment should be based on culture/sensitivity results, according to local guidance. The below is merely a guide.

Non-pregnant women
* Self-care advice for all: ↑fluid intake, analgesia (↓evidence for cranberry/alkali).
* May not need immediate antibiotic depending on severity and risk of complications. Back-up antibiotic if worsening symptoms or no improvement within 48h.
* First-line: 3-day course of nitrofurantoin MR (eGFR >45) 100mg BD or trimethoprim 200mg BD. Alternative: pivmecillinam 400mg stat, then 200mg TDS for 3 days or fosfomycin 3g single dose.

Pregnancy
* Treat UTI and asymptomatic bacteriuria due to risk of pyelonephritis and preterm delivery. 7-day course of antibiotics recommended.
* First-line: nitrofurantoin 100mg BD if pre-pregnancy eGFR >45 and remote from term (neonatal haemolysis). Alternatives: amoxicillin (if sensitive), cefalexin.

Men
* Treat with a 7-day course of trimethoprim 200mg BD or nitrofurantoin 100mg BD (if eGFR >45 and no clinical suspicion of prostatitis).
* If prostatitis then needs 14-day course with review for ongoing treatment. Options: ciprofloxacin, ofloxacin, trimethoprim, co-trimoxazole.

Pyelonephritis
* Treat in hospital if suspicion or risk (immunosuppression, DM) of sepsis, unable to tolerate oral medication/fluid, recurrence, abnormal renal tract, pregnancy.
* Antibiotic options: cephalexin, co-amoxiclav, trimethoprim (not in 1st trimester), ciprofloxacin (avoid in pregnancy).

Catheter associated
* Remove/change catheter if in place for >7 days.
* Cloudy urine is not a useful sign. Exclude alternative focus of infection/cause of delirium in the absence of new urinary symptoms.

Urinary tract tuberculosis

* Sterile pyuria, dysuria, frequency, suprapubic pain but negative standard culture. Ask about malaise, fever, night sweats, weight loss, back/flank pain, visible haematuria.
* Can also cause an interstitial nephritis (p314) and amyloidosis (p311). Glomerulonephritis is rare.
* Diagnose by microscopy with acid-fast techniques (↓sensitivity) and mycobacterial culture of an early morning MSU and/or urinary tract tissue.
* Treat according to local guidance, typically rifampicin and isoniazid for 6 months, with pyrazinamide and ethambutol for 2 months (p390).

The 'piss prophets'

Beware the fallacies, deceit and juggling of the piss-pot science used by all those who pretend knowledge of diseases by the urine.　　　　Thomas Brian, 1655.

Medieval texts[1] give the following maxims regarding urinary change and disease:
* White or straw-coloured urine = weak and cold liver and stomach.
* Foamy urine = eructation (belching).
* Light-coloured, turbid urine = mucus.
* Lead circle on thin urine = pathological melancholy.
* Bubbles on the surface = disease of the head.
* Watery urine = love sickness.
* Swampy, black, stinking urine = fatal.
* Lead-coloured urine = a disintegrating uterus.
* Reddish, cloudy urine with bubbles = asthma or an irregular heartbeat.

1 *Uroscopy in Early Modern Europe* by Michael Stolberg, Routledge, 2016, pp53–6.

Definition

Acute kidney injury (AKI) is a syndrome of decreased kidney function, measured by serum creatinine or urine output, occurring over hours–days. It includes different aetiologies and may be multifactorial.

AKI definitions have been amalgamated into a single definition and staging system. Kidney Diseases: Improving Global Outcomes (KDIGO) guidelines[2] define AKI as:
• Rise in creatinine >26.5μmol/L within 48h *or*
• Rise in creatinine >1.5 × baseline (pre-AKI) within 7 days *or*
• Urine output <0.5mL/kg/h for >6 consecutive hours.

The severity of AKI is then staged according to peak creatinine or period/severity of oliguria (table 7.3). A clinical approach to AKI is shown in fig 7.3.[3]

Table 7.3 KDIGO staging system for AKI

Stage	Serum creatinine	Urine output
1	>26.5μmol/L (0.3mg/dL) or 1.5–1.9 × baseline	<0.5mL/kg/h for 6–12h
2	2.0–2.9 × baseline	<0.5mL/kg/h for >12h
3	>353.6μmol/L (4.0mg/dL) or >3.0 × baseline or new renal replacement therapy	<0.3mL/kg/h for >24h or anuria for >12h

Limitations Serum creatinine does not rise above the upper reference limit until up to 50% of kidney function is lost. It is also affected by non-glomerular factors: muscle mass, protein intake, tubular secretion, pregnancy. But other AKI biomarkers (eg KIM-1, NGAL) have failed to demonstrate superiority over serum creatinine to date.

Epidemiology

AKI affects up to 18% of hospital patients and ~1 in 3 patients in intensive care. Risk factors for AKI include pre-existing CKD, age, and comorbidity (DM, cardiovascular disease, malignancy, chronic liver disease, complex surgery).

Causes

Commonest causes:
1 Sepsis.
2 Cardiogenic shock.
3 Hypovolaemia: haemorrhage, D&V, diuresis, 3rd space, eg pancreatitis.
4 Nephrotoxic medication.
5 Renal tract obstruction.
6 Hepatorenal syndrome.

Aetiology can be divided according to site (table 7.4) as:
• Pre-renal: ↓perfusion to the kidney.
• Renal: intrinsic kidney disease.
• Post-renal: obstruction to urine (bilateral if two working kidneys, unilateral if single functioning kidney).

Table 7.4 Aetiology of AKI

Where?	Pathology	Example
Pre-renal	↓Vascular volume	Haemorrhage, D&V, burns, pancreatitis
	↓Cardiac output	Cardiogenic shock, MI
	Systemic vasodilation	Sepsis, drugs
	Renal vasoconstriction	NSAIDs, ACE-i, ARB, hepatorenal syndrome
Renal	Glomerular (pp306–7)	Glomerulonephritis, ATN (prolonged kidney hypoperfusion causing intrinsic kidney damage)
	Interstitial (p314)	Drug reaction, infection, infiltration (eg sarcoid)
	Vessels	Vasculitis, HUS, TTP, DIC
Post-renal	Within renal tract	Stone, renal tract malignancy, stricture, clot
	Extrinsic compression	Pelvic malignancy, prostatic hypertrophy, retroperitoneal fibrosis

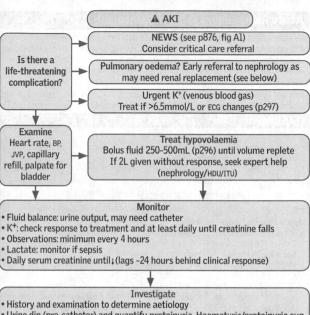

Monitor
* Fluid balance: urine output, may need catheter
* K⁺: check response to treatment and at least daily until creatinine falls
* Observations: minimum every 4 hours
* Lactate: monitor if sepsis
* Daily serum creatinine until↓ (lags ~24 hours behind clinical response)

Investigate
* History and examination to determine aetiology
* Urine dip (pre-catheter) and quantify proteinuria. Haematuria/proteinuria suggest intrinsic kidney disease
* USS within 24 hours if aetiology unclear and AKI not improving. Small kidneys (<9cm): consider CKD. Asymmetry: consider renovascular disease
* ↓Platelet count: blood film/LDH/haptoglobin to exclude haemolysis (HUS/TTP)
* Investigate for intrinsic kidney disease if indicated: Igs, paraprotein/serum light chains, autoantibodies (ANA, ANCA, anti-GBM, dsDNA), complement.

Support
* Optimize haemodynamic status. Treat sepsis (p772)
* Stop nephrotoxic medication: NSAIDs, aminoglycosides
* Stop drugs that may make things worse: (K-sparing) diuretics, metformin, antihypertensives, ACE-i/ARB (withhold temporarily, remember long-term benefit)
* Check drug dosages are appropriate for kidney impairment
* Consider gastroprotection (H2 antagonist, PPI) and nutrition

Fig 7.3 The clinical approach to AKI.[3]

Referring to a nephrologist

Request that advice/review is necessary due to:
* AKI not responding to treatment.
* AKI with complications: ↑K⁺, acidosis, fluid overload, hypertension.
* Stage 3 AKI (table 7.3).
* AKI with difficult fluid balance (eg hypoalbuminaemia, heart failure, pregnancy).
* AKI due to possible intrinsic kidney disease (table 7.4).
* AKI with hypertension.

Know Baseline creatinine and trend (not eGFR which is only for steady state), K⁺, bicarbonate/lactate, Hb, platelet count (+ film), urine dip (before catheter), observations (NEWS) since admission, fluid input/output, examination (hypo/hypervolaemia), USS result, comorbidity (eg DM), drugs given (what? when? nephrotoxic?).

Acute kidney injury (AKI): management

Management of AKI requires diagnosis and treatment of the underlying aetiology:
- Pre-renal: correct volume depletion and/or ↑kidney perfusion via circulatory/cardiac support, treat underlying sepsis, stop drugs causing hypotension.
- Renal: refer for diagnosis (biopsy) and treatment of intrinsic kidney disease.
- Post-renal: catheter, nephrostomy, urological intervention.

Common to all aetiologies of AKI are management of fluid balance, acidosis, hyperkalaemia, and the timely recognition of those who require renal replacement (p297).

Fluid balance

Volume status
- Hypovolaemia: ↑pulse, ↓BP, postural BP drop, ↓urine volume, non-visible JVP, ↓tissue turgor, ↓capillary refill, daily weight loss.
- Overload: ↑BP, ↑JVP, ↑RR, ↓O₂ saturation, lung crepitations, oedema, gallop rhythm.
- ►Hypotension may be relative if old age, vascular stiffness, chronic hypertension.
- ►JVP does not reflect intravascular volume if right-sided heart disease/failure.
- ►BP, skin turgor, capillary refill changes may be late—do not wait for them.

Hypovolaemia, fluid resuscitation
- If hypovolaemic, kidney perfusion requires volume replacement.[4]
- Care in cardiac disease (↓kidney perfusion despite adequate circulating volume) and sepsis/third-spacing (↑extravascular volume).
- *Dynamic assessment is essential:* examine before and after fluid is given to ensure an adequate response and to reduce the risk of fluid overload.
  1 Give 500mL crystalloid over 15min.
  2 Reassess fluid state. Get expert help if unsure or if patient remains shocked.
  3 Further boluses of 250–500mL crystalloid with clinical review after each.
  4 Stop when euvolaemic or seek expert help if 2L given without response.

Which crystalloid? Any crystalloid can be used (follow local guidelines). 0.9% ('normal') saline is non-buffered, contains ↑chloride, and may cause hyperchloraemic acidosis. 'Balanced' crystalloids include Hartmann's, Ringer's lactate, and Plasma-Lyte®. They are closer in composition to extracellular fluid and are often used preferentially.

What about colloid? Blood components should be used in resuscitation due to haemorrhage. Human albumin solutions may be given only under specialist advice in hepatorenal syndrome. Colloids do not improve mortality in the critically ill.

Hypervolaemia, fluid overload
Occurs due to aggressive fluid resuscitation, oliguria, and in sepsis due to ↑capillary permeability. Monitor weight daily in patients receiving IV fluids. Treat with:
- Oxygen supplementation if required.
- Fluid restriction including oral and IV volumes. Give antibiotics in minimal fluid and consider concentrated nutritional support preparations.
- Diuretics in symptomatic fluid overload.
- ►Do not use diuretics to treat oliguria without fluid overload.
- Renal replacement therapy (p302). Oligo/anuric AKI with fluid overload needs urgent referral to nephrology/critical care.

Acidosis

- Mild = pH 7.30–7.36 (~bicarbonate >20mmol/L).
- Moderate = pH 7.20–7.29 (~bicarbonate 10–19mmol/L).
- Severe = pH <7.2 (~bicarbonate <10mmol/L): refer to nephrology/critical care.

Treatment is of the underlying disorder to stop acid production. If treatment is delayed, acidosis will persist and renal replacement may be needed (p302).

Bicarbonate in *acute* acidosis is controversial. Adequate ventilation is needed to prevent respiratory acidosis. A sodium load may also precipitate fluid overload in vulnerable patients.

Chronic acidosis is treated in CKD with bicarbonate <22mmol/L due to evidence of benefit in CKD progression.

Hyperkalaemia

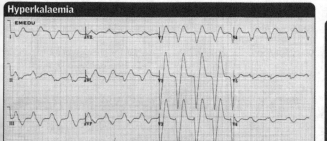

Fig 7.4 ECG changes with severe hyperkalaemia; note broad QRS complexes.

ECG changes In order: tall 'tented' T waves; increased PR interval; small or absent P wave; widened QRS complex (fig 7.4); 'sine wave' pattern; asystole. There is considerable inter-individual susceptibility. ►The ECG may be normal

►*Don't wait for a lab result: use point-of-care (blood gas) testing if available.*

►►Treat[5] if K+ >6.5mmol/L or ECG changes (look at an ECG for all K+ >6.0mmol/L):

1 **Protect the heart** 10mL of 10% calcium chloride[2] (or 30mL of 10% calcium gluconate) IV over 5–10min, repeated if necessary and if ECG changes persist. This is cardioprotective (for 30–60min) but does not treat K+ concentration.

2 **Shift K+** 10u soluble insulin in 25g glucose (e.g 125mL of 20% glucose) IV. Insulin stimulates intracellular uptake of K+, lowering serum K+ by 0.65–1.0mmol/L (varies with kidney function and DM) over 30–60min and works for up to 2h. Salbutamol can be used in addition but high doses are required: 10–20mg via nebulizer (SE: tremor, palpitations, headache).

3 **Remove K+** Sodium zirconium cyclosilicate is a non-absorbed binder that exchanges H+ and Na+ for K+ and ammonium in the gut. Data come from stable out-patients but 10g TDS is approved for use in the acute setting. Onset is within 1h, lowering serum K+ by 1.1mmol/L within 48h. Calcium resonium and patiromer have slower onsets of action (>4h) so utility is limited in acute treatment. Renal replacement may be indicated. Safe inter-hospital transfer requires K+ <6.5mmol/L—discuss with nephrology and critical care.

4 **Monitor** K+ and glucose. Hypoglycaemia occurs in 11–75%, most commonly at 2–3.5h after insulin (up to 6h in CKD). Consider 10% glucose IV at 50mL/h if pretreatment blood glucose <7.0mmol/L.

5 **Prevent recurrence** Withhold drugs which ↑K+: ACE-i, ARB, spironolactone, amiloride, eplerenone, trimethoprim, digoxin (remember to re-start when safe).

IV sodium bicarbonate is not routinely used in the treatment of ↑K+ as risks outweigh (unproven) benefit. Follow local guidelines in hyperkalaemic cardiac arrest.

Renal replacement therapy (RRT) in AKI

RRT options in AKI include haemodialysis and haemofiltration (p302). Peritoneal dialysis is rare for AKI in adults and in high-income countries but can be used. No clear benefit has been demonstrated for any RRT modality though haemofiltration is preferred if haemodynamic instability, acute brain injury, or cerebral oedema.

Possible indications for RRT

• Symptomatic fluid overload unresponsive to medical treatment.
• Severe/prolonged acidosis.
• Recurrent/persistent hyperkalaemia despite medical treatment.
• Uraemia, eg pericarditis, encephalopathy (more likely if underlying CKD).

The decision to start RRT is individualized. The aim is to prevent complications: do not wait for them to occur. Fluid overload is a predictor of worse outcomes.

Possible complications of RRT Risks of dialysis catheter insertion and maintenance, procedural hypotension, bleeding, altered nutrition, and drug clearance.

2 Calcium chloride contains 3× calcium than the same volume of gluconate. Concern exists about the bioavailability of calcium gluconate. Both salts carry a risk of tissue necrosis with extravasation.

Chronic kidney disease (CKD)

Definition Abnormal kidney structure or function, present for >3 months, with implications for health.[6]

Classification Based on GFR category (table 7.5), the presence of albuminuria as a marker of kidney damage (table 7.6), and the cause of kidney disease (table 7.7). (Problems with eGFR formulae used to stage kidney disease, p661.)

Table 7.5 Classification of CKD by GFR (mL/min/1.73m²)

Category	GFR	Notes
G1	>90	Only CKD *if other evidence of kidney damage*: protein/haematuria,
G2	60–89	pathology on biopsy/imaging, tubule disorder, transplant
G3A	45–59	Mild–moderate ↓GFR
G3B	30–44	Moderate–severe ↓GFR
G4	15–29	Severe ↓GFR
G5	<15	Kidney failure

Table 7.6 Classification of CKD by albuminuria

Category	Albumin excretion (mg/24h)	Albumin:creatinine ratio (ACR) (mg/mmol)
A1	<30	<3
A2	30–300	3–30
A3	>300	>30

Table 7.7 Classification of CKD based on underlying disease

Kidney pathology	Examples	
	Primary kidney disease	**Systemic disease**
Glomerular	Minimal change, membranous	Diabetes, amyloid
Tubulointerstitial	UTI, pyelonephritis, stones	Drugs, toxins, sarcoid
Blood flow/vessels	Kidney limited vasculitis	Heart failure, TTP
Congenital/genetic	Renal dysplasia	Alport syndrome, Fabry disease
Transplant	Recurrence of primary kidney disease	Calcineurin inhibitor toxicity

Epidemiology 10% of adults and up to 45 000 premature deaths per year in UK. Commonest aetiologies: diabetes, glomerulonephritis, ↑BP/renovascular disease. ↓GFR and albuminuria are independently associated with an ↑risk of:
• All-cause mortality.
• Cardiovascular mortality.
• Progressive kidney disease and kidney failure.
• AKI.

Patients with CKD are more likely to die of CVD than to need RRT. The risk of adverse outcomes in CKD can be represented as a 'heat map' according to GFR and albuminuria categories (fig 7.5).

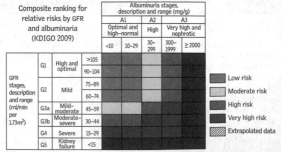

Fig 7.5 Composite risk of adverse outcome by GFR and albuminuria.
Reprinted from *Kidney International*, 80, AS Levey *et al.*, Chronic kidney disease: definition, classification, and prognosis, 17–28, 2011, with permission from Elsevier

The patient with CKD: a clinical approach

History
- *Does the patient really have CKD?* Does the eGFR reflect the true GFR (p661)? Consider non-steady state, eg AKI, drugs (eg trimethoprim alters creatinine concentration but not GFR), pregnancy (eGFR formulae underestimate), malnutrition. Evidence of chronicity >3 months—is there a previous creatinine on record?
- *Possible cause* Ask about ↑BP, DM, IHD, UTI, lower urinary tract symptoms, systemic symptoms, renal colic. Check drug history and when medications started. Family history including kidney disease and subarachnoid haemorrhage. Systems review: look out for more than immediately obvious, consider rare causes, ask about eyes, skin, joints, symptoms suggestive of systemic disorder ('When did you last feel well?'), and malignancy.
- *Current state* Patients may or may not have symptoms of CKD. Symptoms are more common once eGFR <15: fluid overload (SOB, oedema), anorexia, nausea, vomiting, restless legs, fatigue, pruritus, bone pain, amenorrhoea, impotence.

Examination
- *Periphery* Oedema, signs of peripheral vascular disease or neuropathy, vasculitic rash, gouty tophi, joint disease. Arteriovenous fistula (thrill, bruit, recent needling?). Signs of immunosuppression: bruising from steroids, skin changes/malignancy. Uraemic flap/encephalopathy are late signs.
- *Face* Anaemia, xanthelasma, yellow tinge (uraemia), jaundice (hepatorenal), gum hypertrophy (ciclosporin), Cushingoid (steroids), periorbital oedema (nephrotic syndrome), taut skin/telangiectasia (scleroderma), facial lipodystrophy (glomerulonephritis).
- *Neck* JVP for fluid state, tunnelled line (small scar over internal jugular vein and a larger scar in 'breast pocket' area), parathyroidectomy scar, lymphadenopathy.
- *Cardiovascular* BP, sternotomy, cardiomegaly, stigmata of endocarditis. If right-sided heart failure/tricuspid regurgitation, JVP may not reflect fluid state.
- *Respiratory* Pulmonary oedema or effusion.
- *Abdomen* PD catheter or scars from previous catheter (small scars just below umbilicus and to side of midline), signs of transplant (scar, palpable graft), ballotable polycystic kidneys ± palpable liver.

Investigation
- *Blood* Serum creatinine and U&E (compare with previous), Hb (normochromic, normocytic anaemia), glucose (DM), ↓Ca²⁺, ↑PO₄³⁻, ↑PTH (renal osteodystrophy). Directed investigation for intrinsic kidney disease: ANA, dsDNA, ANCA, antiphospholipid antibodies, serum light chains and paraprotein, complement, cryoglobulin, anti-GBM, hepatitis serology, anti-PLA2R. (ESR is not sensitive, ↑ in CKD and proteinuric states.)
- *Urine* Dipstick (may not detect albumin), uACR/uPCR, MC&S (p290).
- *Imaging* USS for anatomy, size, symmetry, corticomedullary differentiation (non-specific), and to exclude obstruction. CKD kidneys may be small (<9cm) except in infiltrative disorders (amyloid, myeloma), APKD, and DM. If asymmetrical consider renovascular disease. Isotope scans are more sensitive for scarring.
- *Histology* Consider kidney biopsy (p306) in nephrotic syndrome, systemic disease with kidney involvement, progressive disease, AKI without recovery, CKD without obvious cause. DM may not need biopsy unless atypical, ie haematuria, systemic symptoms, no other microvascular disease (retinopathy/neuropathy).

Monitoring kidney function in CKD
Consider patient view/preference. GFR and albuminuria should be monitored at least annually, according to risk. If high risk, monitor every 6 months (fig 7.5, orange); if very high risk, monitor at least every 3–4 months (fig 7.5, red). A change in eGFR stage with ↓eGFR ≥25% is significant. Rapid progression is ↓eGFR >15mL/min/1.73m²/yr.

Risk factors for disease progression ↑BP, DM, proteinuria, metabolic disturbance, volume depletion, infection, NSAIDs, smoking, obstruction. ↑Risk of superimposed AKI: treat illness promptly, monitor fluid balance and kidney function.

CKD encompasses a range of disease from mild disease without progression to advanced, symptomatic disease requiring renal replacement.

Management of CKD[6,7] requires:
1 Information and education for people with CKD.
2 Treatment to slow kidney disease progression.
3 Treatment of complications of CKD.
4 Management of cardiovascular risk in CKD.
5 Preparation for renal replacement therapy (dialysis/transplantation) (p302).

Referral to nephrology
• 5-year risk of renal replacement >5% using four-variable Kidney Failure Risk Equation: https://kidneyfailurerisk.co.uk
• Moderate proteinuria UACR >70mg/mmol unless due to DM and already treated.
• Proteinuria UACR >30mg/mmol with haematuria.
• Kidney disease progression:
  • ↓eGFR by ≥25% + ↓eGFR category within 12 months (table 7.5).
  • Sustained ↓eGFR >15mL/min/1.73m² within 12 months.
• Hypertension despite four agents, or suspected renal artery stenosis.
• Known or suspected rare or genetic cause of CKD.

Treatment to slow kidney disease progression
BP UACR <70: systolic <140mmHg (range 120–139mmHg) and diastolic <90mmHg.
DM or UACR ≥70: systolic <130mmHg (range 120–129) and diastolic <80mmHg.

Renin–angiotensin inhibition Offer treatment with a renin–angiotensin system antagonist (ACE-i, ARB) for:
• DM and UACR >3mg/mmol.
• Hypertension and UACR >30mg/mmol.
• Any CKD with UACR >70mg/mmol.

Do not combine agents due to risk of hyperkalaemia and hypotension. Check K^+ and kidney function prior to, and 1–2 weeks after starting treatment, or a change in dose. Stop if K^+ >6mmol/L, ↓eGFR >25%, or ↑creatinine >30%: exclude other possible causes of ↓eGFR and use lowest tolerated dose.

SGLT2 inhibitors eGFR >25 + UACR >25 + type 2 DM (caution DKA) or CKD not due to DM (insufficient data in polycystic kidney disease and after a kidney transplant). This is a fast-moving field: check up-to-date eGFR, UACR, and disease criteria for use.

Glycaemic control in DM Target HbA1c of ~53mmol/mol (7.0%) unless risk of hypoglycaemia, comorbidity, or limited life expectancy.

Lifestyle Exercise, healthy weight, and smoking cessation. Salt intake should be reduced to <2g of sodium/day (≤5g sodium chloride/day).

Treatment of complications of CKD
Anaemia Investigate (especially if anaemic with eGFR >60) and treat other deficiencies: iron (hypochromic red cells >6%, reticulocyte Hb content >29pg, transferrin saturation <20%, ferritin <100mcg/L), B₁₂, and folate. Do not miss chronic blood loss. IV iron therapy may be needed. Treat with an erythropoietic stimulating agent (ESA, 'Epo') to maintain Hb 100–120g/L. Pure red cell aplasia with ESA treatment is due to anti-erythropoietin antibodies and usually causes Hb <60g/L. It is very rare: exclude more likely causes of anaemia first. Avoid blood transfusions whenever possible, especially if kidney transplantation is predicted. Care with ESA in sickle cell disease as may increase sickle cell %.

Acidosis Consider sodium bicarbonate supplements for patients with eGFR <30 and low serum bicarbonate (<22mmol/L). Caution in hypertension and fluid overload.

Oedema Restrict fluid and sodium intake if clinically indicated. Loop diuretics can be used. A high dose may be required in advanced CKD. A loop and thiazide diuretic combination can be potent: distal tubule sodium excretion (and inhibition by a thiazide) is increased when treated with a loop diuretic (fig 7.13, p312). Monitor clinical fluid state and kidney function.

CKD **bone-mineral disorders** CKD causes ↑ in serum phosphate and reduced hydroxylation of vitamin D. Measure calcium, phosphate, ALP, PTH, and 25-OH vit D if eGFR <30 (though optimal concentrations are unknown).

- Avoid overt hyperphosphataemia (target phosphate in advanced CKD is higher than the upper reference limit), whilst avoiding hypercalcaemia. Treatment is with dietary restriction ± phosphate binders, eg calcium acetate (avoid in hypercalcaemia), sevelamer, sucroferric oxyhydroxide, lanthanum.
- Give vitamin D supplements (colecalciferol, ergocalciferol) if deficient. If ↑PTH persists or is increasing, treat with an activated vit D analogue, eg 1α-calcidol/ calcitriol.
- Calcimimetics, eg cinacalcet. Used to treat refractory ↑PTH, and ↑PTH in combination with ↑Ca.
- Bisphosphonates can be given if clinically indicated and eGFR ≥30.

Restless legs/cramps Exclude iron deficiency as a possible exacerbating factor. Sleep hygiene. Treatment for severe cases with gabapentin/pregabalin/dopamine agonists is off licence: beware of SE (falls, cognitive impairment).

Diet Expert dietary advice should be available regarding phosphate restriction and K⁺ if hyperkalaemic, whilst avoiding malnutrition.

Management of cardiovascular risk in CKD

CKD confers ↑risk of CVD due to ↑BP, vascular stiffness, inflammation, oxidative stress, and abnormal endothelial function. CV risk is often higher than the risk of kidney failure.

- Consider antiplatelets (low-dose aspirin) if risk for atherosclerotic events, unless bleeding risk outweighs benefit (mortality benefit unclear in CKD).
- Atorvastatin 20mg (higher dose if GFR >30) for primary and secondary prevention of CVD (no consistent benefit demonstrated for patients on dialysis).
- SGLT2 inhibitors if eGFR >25 + indicated for CVD or heart failure.
- CKD should not affect treatment for heart failure but ↑ monitoring of GFR and K⁺.
- GFR <60 may affect troponin and BNP concentrations. Interpret results cautiously.

Preparation for renal replacement therapy (RRT)

Planning for RRT should begin in progressive CKD when clinical judgement predicts that RRT will be required within 12 months. Shared-decision making, psychological preparation, work-up for transplantation, modality choice, and access take time.

All suitable patients should be informed about the advantages of a pre-emptive living kidney transplant and efforts made to find a donor (p304). All suitable patients without a donor should be listed for deceased donor transplantation 6 months before the anticipated start of RRT.

Prescribing in CKD

▶Never prescribe in kidney disease without checking how administration should be altered due to ↓GFR. This will be determined largely by the extent to which a drug is excreted by the kidney. This is significant for aminoglycosides, penicillins, cephalosporins, heparin, lithium, opiates, and digoxin.

▶Loading doses should not be changed.

If precision is required for dosing (eg chemotherapy) then GFR should not be estimated from creatinine and a standard reference measure should be used: inulin, 51Cr-EDTA, 125I-iothalamate, iohexol.

If the patient is receiving renal replacement (haemofiltration, peritoneal, or haemodialysis), dose modification depends on the extent to which a drug is cleared from the circulation by dialysis/filtration.

The best prescribing guide to consult is the *Renal Drug Database/Handbook* (www.renaldrugdatabase.com), an invaluable resource detailing dose modification in kidney failure and in renal replacement for almost any drug you could wish to use. All hospitals should have access: speak to your pharmacist.

Long-term dialysis is started when the complications of dialysis are less than symptoms and complications of advanced CKD. Indications for RRT may include:
• Inability to control volume status, including BP and pulmonary oedema.
• Acid–base or electrolyte abnormalities resistant to medical treatment.
• Serositis, eg pericarditis.
• Pruritus with anticipated benefit from dialysis.
• Nausea/vomiting or a deterioration in nutritional status.
• Cognitive impairment due to advanced CKD.

►RRT is a misnomer for dialysis: kidney function is not replaced, rather there is provision of just enough clearance to ameliorate the symptoms of kidney failure.

GFR at commencement of dialysis is usually ~5–10. When transplantation is awaited or not possible, there are two main options: haemodialysis and peritoneal dialysis.

Haemodialysis (HD) (fig 7.6) Blood is passed over a semi-permeable membrane against dialysis fluid flowing in the opposite direction. Diffusion of solutes occurs down the concentration gradient. A hydrostatic gradient is used to clear excess fluid as required (ultrafiltration). Access is preferentially via an arterio-venous fistula which provides ↑blood

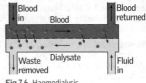

Fig 7.6 Haemodialysis.

flow and access longevity. It should be created in advance of RRT start to avoid the infection risk associated with central venous catheters. HD is usually needed 3 times/week. More frequent HD increases the 'dose' and improves outcomes. Home HD should be offered to all suitable patients. **Problems** Quality of life, access (arteriovenous fistula: thrombosis, stenosis, steal syndrome; tunnelled venous line: infection, blockage, recirculation of blood), dialysis disequilibrium (between cerebral and blood solutes leading to cerebral oedema ∴ start HD gradually), hypotension.

Peritoneal dialysis (PD) Uses the peritoneum as a semi-permeable membrane. A catheter is inserted into the peritoneal cavity and fluid (dialysate) infused. Solutes diffuse between blood and dialysate. Ultrafiltration occurs due to osmotic agents (glucose, glucose polymers) in the dialysate. It is a continuous process with intermittent drainage and refilling of the peritoneal cavity, performed at home. **Problems** Catheter site infection, PD peritonitis, hernia, ↓membrane function over time.

Haemofiltration (fig 7.7) Water is cleared by positive pressure, dragging solutes by convection. The ultrafiltrate (waste) is replaced with an appropriate volume of ('clean') fluid either before (pre-dilution) or after (post-dilution) the membrane. ↓Haemodynamic instability so used in critical care. Only used (= chronic RRT in combination with HD (= haemodiafiltration, HDF). May offer haemodynamic stability and ↑middle molecule clearance, eg β₂-microglobulin. Requires sufficient water quality.

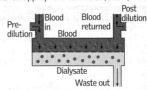

Fig 7.7 Haemofiltration.

Complications of RRT
• **Cardiovascular disease** ↑BP, vascular stiffness, inflammation, oxidative stress, endothelial dysfunction, mortality is ×20 compared to general population.
• **Protein-calorie malnutrition** Increases morbidity and mortality.
• **Renal osteodystrophy** ↑Bone turnover, osteitis fibrosa, vascular calcification.
• **Infection** Access infection, granulocyte and T-cell dysfunction may ↑ mortality.
• **Amyloid** β₂-microglobulin deposition: carpal tunnel syndrome, arthralgia.

Conservative management This is for those who opt not to receive RRT due to lack of benefit on quality or quantity of life. Dialysis does not prolong life for everyone, especially if frail with significant comorbidity. Focus is on preserving residual kidney function, symptom control, and advanced planning for end of life care.

When a patient on dialysis presents...

1 Do they *need dialysis* now? Examine for fluid overload and check K⁺. If on PD are they well enough to perform it themselves? Refer urgently to nephrology.

2 When will they need dialysis? When are they due to dialyse next? Weigh them. All patients on dialysis have a *target weight* at which they are considered euvolaemic. How much are they above it? Do they have any useful urine output that may help excrete volume/K⁺? Refer to nephrology in a timely manner.

3 What is your diagnosis? History and examination as for any other patient. *Do not measure BP on fistula arm.* Remember ↑risk for CVD but troponin concentrations have ↓specificity for cardiac injury in advanced CKD and dialysis.

4 Treat. Remember to *dose adjust for kidney function.* This includes antibiotics, opiates, insulin, and low-molecular-weight heparin (see www.renaldrugdatabase.com, p301). Care with fluid replacement in sepsis: be guided by clinical examination and target weight. If unsure get expert help. If volume depleted give a 250mL bolus of crystalloid over 15min with close observation. Avoid maintenance fluids in those who normally have a fluid restriction. *Do not use a dialysis line or fistula for IV access.* If a cannula is necessary, preferentially use the back of the hand, save other vessels for future access.

5 Surgery needs senior anaesthetic and nephrology input. Aim for pre-op K⁺ <5.5mmol/L (<5.0mmol/L if major surgery with risk of tissue breakdown/haemolysis). *Check K+ urgently* via point-of-care testing (venous blood gas) in recovery. In elective surgery, plan for dialysis provision pre- and post-operation.

Warning: there is no normal

'Ten years is a long time. For those ten years, or just over 3,650 times, I attached myself to a peritoneal dialysis machine and underwent nine hours and fifty minutes of nightly therapy. I subsequently learned to do a lot of crosswords and read a ridiculous amount of books. In ten years I had just three incidents: an inguinal hernia due to thinking that I could move a sofa (I could not), a parathyroidectomy (my knees were much happier afterwards), and one unfortunate bout of peritonitis (once was enough). Statistically speaking, I am an anomaly: the 'average' life span of a peritoneal dialysis patient is four years.

Admittedly, I did not initially cope well with needing to be on dialysis. After having lived successfully with a transplant, a return to dialysis felt like failure. I did not want the hassle of treatment. I did not want piles of boxes cluttering up our home. Mostly, I did not want a PD catheter jutting out of my belly. But what I originally believed to be unacceptable, gradually became tolerable. This took time. It took care and support. It took experiencing relative health, and seeing that dialysis life, although different to existing with a transplant, could be lived well.'

Natasha Boone, author and illustrator

The man in a red canoe who saved a million lives

Mostly we commute to work each day driven by motives we would rather not look at too deeply. But one kidney physician used a red canoe to commute each day from his houseboat to the hospital. He could have been a very rich man but instead Belding Scribner gave his invention away, and continued his modest existence.

He invented the Scribner shunt—a U of Teflon™ connecting an artery to a vein, allowing haemodialysis to be repeated as often as needed. Before Scribner, glass tubes were inserted painfully into vessels, which would be damaged, limiting haemodialysis to only a few cycles. Clyde Shields was his first patient in 1960, and said that his first treatment 'took so much of the waste I'd stored up out of me that it was just like turning on the light from darkness'. Scribner transformed a fatal condition to one with 90% survival.

On 19 June 2003, his canoe was found empty. And like those ancient Indian burial canoes found at Wiskam which have been polished to an unimaginable lustre by the action of the shifting sands around the Island of the Dead, so we polish and cherish the image of this man who gave everything and took nothing.

Transplantation (figs 7.8, 7.9) should be considered for every patient with, or progressing towards, stage G5 kidney disease (p298). It is the treatment of choice for kidney failure provided risks do not exceed benefits.

Contraindications
- Absolute: cancer with metastases.
- Temporary: active infection, HIV with viral replication, unstable CVD.
- Relative: heart failure, CVD, other comorbidities/frailty.

Types of graft
- **Living donor** Better graft function and survival, especially if HLA matched.
- **Deceased donor** (p13)
  1 Donor after brain death (DBD, heart-beating donor).
  2 Expanded criteria donor (ECD) from an older donor or one with CVA, BP, or CKD. Impacts long-term outcome but better anticipated survival/quality of life than dialysis.
  3 Donor after cardiac death (DCD, non-heart-beating donor) with ↑risk of delayed graft function.

Immunosuppression
A combination of drugs are used. Aim is to use the minimal effective dose with the lowest drug-related toxicity. Protocol depends upon the immunological risk of the recipient and type of donated kidney.

Monoclonal antibodies eg basiliximab, daclizumab (selectively block activated T cells via CD-25), alemtuzumab (T- and B-cell depletion). Used at the time of transplantation ('induction'). ↓Acute rejection and graft loss. SE: ↑infection risk if non-selective.

Calcineurin inhibitors eg tacrolimus, ciclosporin. Inhibit T-cell activation and proliferation. ↑Inter-individual variation and narrow therapeutic window so monitoring of drug concentrations is required. Clearance via cytochrome P450 isoenzymes so beware of drug interactions including macrolide antibiotics and antifungal drugs. SE: nephrotoxicity, ↑BP, ↑cholesterol, new-onset diabetes after transplantation (NODAT).

Anti-metabolites eg mycophenolic acid (MPA), azathioprine. Inhibit T- and B-cell proliferation. MPA is now used preferentially to ↓ acute rejection and ↑ graft survival (not in pregnancy, MPA is teratogenic). SE: anaemia, leucopenia, GI toxicity.

Mammalian target of rapamycin (mTOR) inhibitor eg sirolimus. May replace anti-metabolite/CNI. Theoretical ↓cancer risk but data conflicting. SE: ↓wound healing.

Glucocorticoids ↓Transcription of inflammatory cytokines. Significant SE (BP, hyperlipidaemia, DM, impaired wound healing, osteoporosis, cataracts, skin fragility) have led to protocols with early withdrawal of steroids and the use of steroid-free immunosuppression regimens.

Complications
Surgical Bleeding, thrombosis, infection, urinary leak, lymphocele, hernia.

Delayed graft function Up to 40% of grafts, more common in DCD.

Rejection Presents with ↓kidney function. Diagnosed on transplant biopsy. Can be acute or chronic. *Acute rejection* can be antibody- (rare unless known pre-sensitized recipient, check for donor specific antibodies) or T-cell-mediated (most common). Treat with (short-term) ↑immunosuppression. *Chronic rejection* is better termed 'chronic allograft nephropathy' and is a major cause of transplant loss. Slow immune-mediated damage to the microcirculation leads to inflammation, remodelling, and irreversible tissue injury. CNI-mediated nephrotoxicity, recurrent disease, and infection may also contribute. Umbrella terminology and a lack of controlled studies mean optimum treatments are not known.

Infection ↑Risk of all infections. Typically hospital acquired/donor derived in month 1, opportunistic in months 1–6 (prophylactic treatment for CMV and *Pneumocystis jirovecii* given), usual spectrum of infection after 6–12 months. Late viral infection should be considered: eg CMV, HSV.

Malignancy Up to 25× ↑risk of cancer with immunosuppression, particularly skin, post-transplant lymphoproliferative disorder (PTLD), and gynaecological.

CVD 3–5× ↑risk of premature CVD compared to population (but ~80% less than dialysis). BP, NODAT, rejection, and kidney history (uraemic cardiomyopathy) contribute.

Prognosis

Acute rejection <15%, 1-year graft survival >90%. Longer-term graft loss ~4%/year. Factors contributing to graft loss:

• Donor factors: age, comorbidity, living/deceased, DBD/DCD.
• Rejection.
• Infection.
• BP/CVD.
• Recurrent kidney disease in graft.

Most common outcome is death with a functioning transplant (ie transplant 'outlives' the patient).

When a patient with a kidney transplant presents...

1 Inform the local kidney transplant unit: they will be happy to advise, review, transfer, and follow-up all kidney transplant recipients.
2 What is the eGFR/creatinine? How does this compare with previous results? If you do not have any previous results, ask the transplant unit.
3 Examine for and treat any reversible cause of AKI. Fluid state assessment (p296) is important—if you are unsure, get expert help. Correction of volume depletion and treatment of sepsis should be prompt.
4 Consider viral/opportunistic infections and atypical presentations due to immunosuppression, eg CMV, *Pneumocystis jirovecii*.
5 *Do not stop immunosuppressive medication.* Change in immunosuppression is led by the transplant unit. If the patient is unable to tolerate oral medication then immunosuppression should be given NG or converted to an IV dose (conversion depends on drug: check with your pharmacist).
6 Check for medication interactions: eg macrolide antibiotics (erythromycin, clarithromycin) can cause calcineurin inhibitor toxicity.
7 Dose all drugs according to kidney function: penicillins, cephalosporins, aminoglycosides, insulin, opiates, and low-molecular-weight heparin.
8 Check with the transplant unit before you give low-molecular-weight heparin for VTE prophylaxis: they may need to do a transplant biopsy.

Thank you for life

Dear Donor Family,

I always knew I wanted to write to you. Before I received my transplant, I had been unwell for many years, and was undergoing dialysis every day. I knew a transplant wouldn't cure me, but I hoped it would give me back so many things I'd lost through being sick. I want you to know that I do the best I can every day to look after myself and my new kidney. I know how lucky I am to have it and taking care of it helps me to honour the huge gift your loved one has given me. I've thought of him, and of you, every single day since I had my transplant. I never imagined that people I know so little about would become such an important part of my life, but you have. I want you to know that although I am cautious over my health, I am determined to not be so fearful I miss out on living. Anything less would be a waste. Because of you, I'm healthier than I ever thought I would be. For the first time in a really long time, I'm excited about what's in my future. Thank you for helping me find that hope. With love and gratitude, Holly.

Reproduced with kind permission from Holly Loughton.

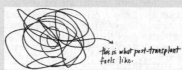

Fig 7.8 'Alive' by Natasha Boone.
www.natashaboone.com

Fig 7.9 Post-transplant scribble by Natasha Boone.
www.natashaboone.com

this is what post-transplant feels like.

The term glomerulonephritis (GN) encompasses a number of conditions which:
• are caused by pathology in the glomerulus.
• present with proteinuria, haematuria, or both.
• are diagnosed on a kidney biopsy.
• cause CKD.
• can progress to kidney failure (except minimal change disease).
The names of the diseases come from either histological appearance (eg membranous glomerulonephritis); or the associated systemic condition (eg lupus nephritis).

Nephrotic or nephritic? The glomerulonephritides classically present on a spectrum ranging from nephrosis (proteinuria due to podocyte pathology, p308), to nephritis (haematuria due to inflammatory damage, p307). This is illustrated in fig 7.10. However, proteinuria can occur in any GN that causes scarring. Proteinuria can therefore complicate the longer-term clinical picture of any GN, including those that are classically 'nephritic'.

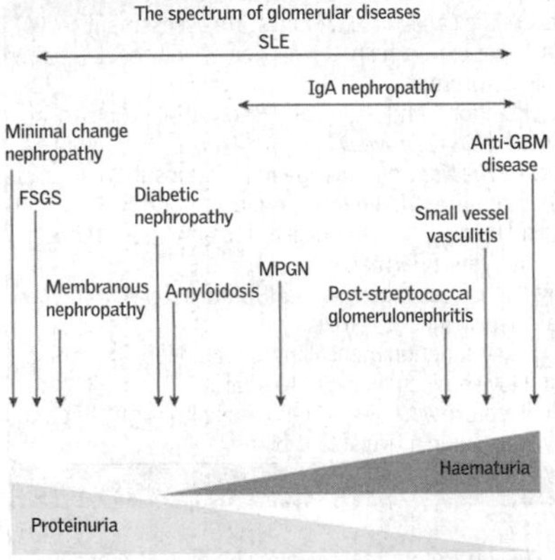

Fig 7.10 Spectrum of glomerular disease from proteinuria (nephrosis) to haematuria (nephritis).
Figure adapted from Turner et al., *Oxford Textbook of Clinical Nephrology*, 2015, with permission from Oxford University Press.

Investigation Assess damage and potential cause.
Blood FBC, U&E, LFT, CRP, immunoglobulins, serum light chains, C3, C4. Autoantibodies (p550): ANA, ANCA, anti-dsDNA, anti-GBM, anti-PLA2R. Blood culture, ASOT, hepatitis and HIV serology.
Urine UACR/UPCR (p290), RBC casts (p291), MC&S.
Imaging Ultrasound (size and anatomy for biopsy), CXR (pulmonary haemorrhage).
Kidney biopsy Required for diagnosis in most (adult) cases.

Kidney biopsy

►Follow local protocol for kidney biopsy.
Pre-procedure BP (<160/95), FBC (Hb >9, plt >100), clotting (PT and APTT <1.2), G&S. Written informed consent including complications: mild back/loin pain, visible haematuria (~5%, usually clears), bleeding, need for transfusion (~1%), angiographic intervention (~ ≤0.5%). Stop anticoagulants (aspirin 1 week, warfarin to PT <1.2, low-molecular-weight heparin 24h).
Post-procedure Bed rest for a minimum of 4h. Monitor HR, BP, symptoms, and urine. Do not discharge home until macroscopic haematuria has settled. Aspirin or warfarin can be restarted the next day if procedure uncomplicated.
Result Proportion of glomeruli involved (focal vs diffuse), how much of each glomerulus is involved (segmental vs global), hypercellularity, sclerosis. Also examines tubulointerstitium (atrophy, fibrosis, inflammation) and any vessels. Immunohistology for deposits (Ig, light chains, complement). Electron microscopy for ultrastructure: precise location of deposits, podocyte appearance.

Management General management as for CKD (pp298–301) including BP control, and renin–angiotensin & SGLT2 inhibition. Specific treatment including immunosuppression depends on histological diagnosis, disease severity, disease progression, and comorbidity.

Nephritic glomerulonephritis (GN)

Nephritic glomerulonephritides[a] include:

IGA nephropathy

Commonest primary GN in high-income countries. Historically: Berger's disease. *Presentation:* asymptomatic non-visible haematuria, or episodic visible haematuria which may be 'synpharyngitic': within 12–72h of infection. ↑BP. Proteinuria usually <1g. Indolent: 20–50% progress to kidney failure over 30yrs. Worse prognosis in ♂, ↑BP, ↑creatinine, proteinuria. *Diagnosis:* IgA deposition in mesangium. *Treatment* ACE-i/ARB and SGLT2 inhibitor (p300). Limited evidence for immunosuppression. Immune suppression may be considered if persistent significant proteinuria despite ACE-i/ARB, or progressive CKD, but beware SE.

Henoch–Schönlein purpura (HSP)

Small vessel vasculitis and systemic variant of IgA nephropathy with IgA deposition in skin/joints/gut in addition to kidney. *Presentation:* purpuric rash on extensor surfaces (typically legs), flitting polyarthritis, abdominal pain, and nephritis. *Diagnosis:* clinical. Confirmed with positive IF for IgA and C3 in skin. Kidney biopsy is identical to IgA nephropathy. *Treatment:* supportive. Steroids may be used for gut involvement. Kidney disease managed as IgA nephropathy.

Post-streptococcal GN

Occurs after a throat (~2 weeks) or skin (~3–6 weeks) infection. Streptococcal antigen deposits in the glomerulus lead to immune complex formation and inflammation. *Presentation:* varies from haematuria to acute nephritis, ie haematuria, oedema, ↑BP, and oliguria. *Diagnosis:* evidence of streptococcal infection: ↑ASOT, ↑anti-DNAse B. ↓C3. Subepithelial humps on electron microscopy. *Treatment:* supportive, antibiotics to prevent spread of nephritogenic bacteria.

Anti-glomerular basement membrane (anti-GBM) disease

Rare. Antibodies to type IV collagen in glomerular and alveolar basement membranes. Historically: Goodpasture's disease. *Presentation:* kidney disease (oliguria/anuria, haematuria, AKI) and lung disease (alveolar haemorrhage in 40–60% ∴ SOB, haemoptysis). Oligoanuria, dialysis dependence, ↑crescents on biopsy predict poor prognosis. *Diagnosis:* anti-GBM in circulation/kidney (fig 7.11). *Treatment:* plasma exchange (remove circulating antibody), corticosteroids, and cyclophosphamide (stop antibody production).

Rapidly progressive GN

Aggressive GN, rapidly progressing to kidney failure over days/weeks. Causes include small vessel/ANCA vasculitis (p310), lupus nephritis (p310), anti-GBM disease. Other GN may 'transform' to become rapidly progressive including IgA, membranous. *Diagnosis:* breaks in the GBM allow an influx of inflammatory cells so that crescents are seen on kidney biopsy (crescentic GN) (fig 7.12). *Treatment:* corticosteroids and cyclophosphamide. Rituximab increasingly used. Other treatments depend on aetiology, eg plasma exchange for anti-GBM, mycophenolate for lupus nephritis (p310).

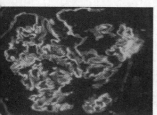

Fig 7.11 Immunofluorescence for IgG, showing linear staining characteristic of anti-GBM disease.

Reproduced from Barratt *et al.*, *Oxford Desk Reference: Nephrology*, 2008, with permission from Oxford University Press.

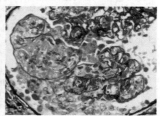

Fig 7.12 Crescentic GN: a proliferation of epithelial cells and macrophages with rupture of Bowman's capsule.

Reproduced from Turner *et al.*, *Oxford Textbook of Nephrology*, 2016, with permission from Oxford University Press.

Nephrotic syndrome

▶If there is oedema, dipstick the urine to avoid missing kidney disease.

Definition The nephrotic syndrome is a triad of:
- Proteinuria >3g/24h (uPCR >300mg/mmol, uACR >250mg/mmol, p290).
- Hypoalbuminaemia (usually <30g/L, can be <10g/L).
- Oedema.

Aetiology
- **Primary kidney disease** Minimal change disease, membranous nephropathy (may be associated with underlying inflammation/malignancy), focal segmental glomerulosclerosis (FSGS), membranoproliferative GN.
- **Secondary kidney disease** DM, lupus nephritis, myeloma, amyloid, pre-eclampsia.

Pathophysiology The filtration barrier of the kidney is formed of podocytes, the glomerular basement membrane (GBM), and endothelial cells. Proteinuria is due to:
- Podocyte pathology: abnormal function in minimal change disease, immune-mediated damage in membranous nephropathy, podocyte injury/death in FSGS.
- GBM/endothelial cell pathology: membranoproliferative GN, inherited abnormalities in membrane proteins causing disease (Alport's, p316) or treatment resistance.

Presentation Generalized, pitting oedema, which can be rapid and severe. Check dependent areas (ankles if mobile, sacral pad/elbows if bed-bound) and areas of low tissue resistance, eg periorbitally. **History** Ask about systemic symptoms, eg joint, skin. Consider malignancy and chronic infection. **ΔΔ** CCF (↑JVP, pulmonary oedema), liver disease (↓albumin).

Management
1 Reduce oedema
Fluid and salt restriction. Diuresis with loop diuretics, eg furosemide. Give IV if oral absorption affected. Use daily weights to guide. Aim for 0.5–2kg weight loss per day depending on severity/size to try and avoid intravascular volume depletion and secondary AKI. Thiazide diuretics can be added if resistant. Albumin infusion ↑ proteinuria—data that it benefits outcomes are limited and of low quality.

2 Treat underlying cause
Adults need a kidney biopsy (p306) if cause unclear. It may not be indicated if DM + microvascular complications, positive PLA2-R (p309). Diuresis may be required first if orthopnoea or subcutaneous oedema at biopsy site. Histology may direct disease-specific treatment, eg immunosuppression in minimal change disease/lupus nephritis. In children, minimal change disease is the commonest aetiology and steroids induce remission in the majority. Biopsy is avoided in children unless steroid resistant, or if atypical features: age <1yr, family history, extrarenal disease, kidney failure, haematuria.

3 Reduce proteinuria
ACE-i/ARB reduce proteinuria (may not be needed in minimal change if treatment response is rapid). SGLT2 in proteinuric CKD: eGFR >25 + uACR >25 at the time of press but criteria are likely to expand, so seek contemporary guidance.

4 Complications
- *Thromboembolism*: hypercoagulable due to ↑clotting factors, ↓anti-thrombin III, and platelet abnormalities. ↑Risk of VTE including DVT/PE (~10% adult patients) and renal vein thrombosis (loin pain, haematuria, ↑LDH, AKI if bilateral). If low bleeding risk, consider prophylaxis when albumin <25g/L.
- *Infection*: urine losses of immunoglobulins and immune mediators lead to ↑risk of urinary, respiratory, and CNS infection. Infection also seen in areas of fluid accumulation: cellulitis, peritonitis, empyema. Ensure pneumococcal vaccination given. ↑Risk of varicella with steroid treatment: post-exposure prophylaxis in non-immune, do not give live vaccine if immunosuppressed.
- *Hyperlipidaemia*: ↑cholesterol (often >10mmol/L), ↑LDL, ↑triglycerides, ↓HDL. Attributed to ↑hepatic synthesis in response to ↓oncotic pressure and defective lipid breakdown. Proportional to proteinuria. The benefits of statins in CKD are extrapolated to nephrotic syndrome where there is ↓evidence.

Nephrotic glomerulonephritis

Nephrotic glomerulonephritides[a] include:

Minimal change disease

~25% of adult nephrotic syndrome. Idiopathic (most). Rarely in association with drugs (NSAIDs, lithium) or paraneoplastic (haematological malignancy, usually Hodgkin's lymphoma). Does not cause kidney failure (if CKD consider missed FSGS).

Diagnosis: light microscopy is normal (hence the name). Electron microscopy shows effacement of podocyte foot processes (non-specific finding in proteinuria).

Treatment: prednisolone 1mg/kg 75% of adults will respond within 16 weeks, >50% relapse. Relapses may need longer-term immunosuppression. Tacrolimus is an alternative for both *de novo* and relapsed disease.

Focal segmental glomerulosclerosis (FSGS)

Commonest glomerulonephritis on kidney biopsy. Primary (idiopathic) or secondary (HIV, heroin, lithium, lymphoma, any cause of ↓kidney mass/nephrons, scarring due to another glomerulonephritis). Risk of progressive CKD and kidney failure: ↑proteinuria worsens prognosis. Primary disease recurs in 30–50% of transplants.

Diagnosis: glomeruli have scarring of certain segments (ie focal sclerosis). May miss early disease if <10 glomeruli in biopsy sample.

Treatment: ACE-i/ARB and blood pressure control in all. SGLT2 inhibitor (p306). Corticosteroids in primary disease: remission in ~25%, partial remission in up to 50%. Calcineurin inhibitors used second line or if SE of steroids are significant. Plasma exchange and rituximab have been used for recurrence in transplants.

Membranous nephropathy

~25% of adult nephrotic syndrome. Primary (anti-phospholipase A2 receptor (PLA2-R) antibody in 70–80%, thrombospondin type 1 domain-containing 7A antibodies in 3–5%), or secondary to:

• Malignancy: lung, breast, GI, prostate, haematological.
• Infection: hepatitis B/C, *Streptococcus*, malaria, schistosomiasis.
• Immunological disease: SLE, rheumatoid arthritis, sarcoidosis, Sjögren's.
• Drugs: gold, penicillamine.

Indolent disease with spontaneous complete remission in ~20%, partial in 20%.

Diagnosis: PLA2-R antibody concentrations are prognostic. Biopsy: diffusely thickened GBM, subepithelial deposits (IgG4 dominant in idiopathic, other IgGs in secondary disease), 'spikes' on silver stain where GBM grows between deposits.

Treatment: ACE-i/ARB, blood pressure control, and lipid management. SGLT2 inhibitor (p306). Consider VTE prophylaxis if albumin <25g/L. Observation for spontaneous remission. Immunosuppression for high-risk primary disease, eg nephrosis/ progressive CKD despite ACE-i/ARB inhibition. Options include: rituximab, alternating steroids/cytotoxics for 6 months ('Ponticelli regimen'), steroids plus calcineurin inhibitors. PLA2-R antibody concentrations may correlate with disease activity. Treat underlying cause if secondary disease.

Membranoproliferative glomerulonephritis

~10% of adult nephrotic syndrome (higher in low- and middle-income countries due to infection). Divided into:

• *Immune-complex associated:* increased or abnormal immune complexes deposit in the kidney and activate complement. An underlying cause can be found in most adult cases, eg infection, cryoglobulinaemia, monoclonal gammopathy, autoimmunity
• *C3 glomerulopathy:* due to a genetic or acquired defect in the alternative complement pathway, eg C3 nephritic factor. Progressive kidney disease is common.

Diagnosis: proliferative glomerulonephritis with electron-dense deposits. Immunoglobulin deposition distinguishes immune-complex-associated disease from C3 glomerulopathy.

Treatment: ACE-i/ARB and blood pressure control in all. SGLT2 inhibitor (p306). Expert evaluation of complement pathways may offer utility in tailoring treatment according to aetiology. Underlying cause in immune-complex disease. Targeted C3 therapies awaited.

Diabetic nephropathy

DM nephropathy[9] is the commonest cause of end-stage kidney failure: ~30–40% of patients requiring renal replacement. Predicted prevalence ↑ by 25–40% over next 20 years. Hyperglycaemia leads to ↑growth factors, renin–angiotensin–aldosterone activation, production of advanced glycosylation end-products, and oxidative stress. Causes ↑glomerular capillary pressure, podocyte damage, and endothelial dysfunction. Microalbuminuria is first clinical sign. Later scarring (glomerulosclerosis), nodule formation (Kimmelstiel–Wilson lesions), and fibrosis with progressive loss of kidney function. Coexisting ↑BP and poor DM control accelerate disease. **Diagnosis** Microalbuminuria = uACR 3–30mg/mmol ('moderately increased') (p290, p298). Regression at this level of disease is possible. Not detected on standard dipstick ∴ must send uACR. Screen annually.

Treatment

- Intensive DM control prevents microalbuminuria and reduces risk of progression to macroalbuminuria = uACR >30mg/mmol ('severely increased'). HbA1c of 53mmol/mol (7%) reduces development of microvascular complications (less impact on CVD and kidney outcomes). Consider risk of hypoglycaemia.
- BP <130/80mmHg. Use ACE-i/ARB for CV and nephroprotection above BP control. Can prevent progression from normoalbuminuria to microalbuminuria to macroalbuminuria in hypertensive DM. (Less clear benefit in normotensive DM but recommended if uACR >30mg/mmol.) No head-to-head studies of ACE-i/ARB in DM but equivalence outside DM. If cough with ACE-i, switch to ARB. No benefit to dual therapy and ↑risk of ↑K⁺. No benefit for direct renin inhibitors above ACE-i/ARB.
- SGLT2 inhibitors improve glycaemic control and kidney outcomes (3×DS: death, dialysis, doubling of creatinine) in type 2 DM. Risk of (euglycaemic) DKA in type 1 DM.
- Finerenone slows disease progression when added to ACE-i/ARB in type 2 DM with CKD stages 3–4. Used in addition to SGLT2 inhibitors. CI: hyperkalaemia.
- Statins reduce CV risk. Unclear benefit on dialysis but continue if tolerated.

Lupus nephritis

Systemic autoimmune disease with antibodies against nuclear components, eg double-stranded (ds)DNA. Deposition of antibody complexes causes inflammation and tissue damage. **Presentation** Rash, photosensitivity, ulcers, arthritis, serositis, CNS disease, cytopenia, and kidney disease. Nephropathy is common (50% in first year, 75% overall). Can present as nephritis (p306) or nephrosis (p308). **Diagnosis** Clinical. Antibody profile: ANA is sensitive but not specific. Anti-dsDNA has a specificity of 75–100% and titres correlate with disease activity. Consider biopsy if uACR >30, uPCR >50. **Treatment** Depends on histological class. Classes I and II show mild changes with little risk of kidney disease progression: ACE-i/ARB for nephroprotection and hydroxychloroquine for extrarenal disease. Classes III–V require immunosuppression: mycophenolate, glucocorticoids, cyclophosphamide, rituximab, belimumab. Ofatumumab may offer more B-cell depletion than rituximab.

ANCA-associated vasculitis (AAV)

Occurs with or without specificity for proteinase 3 (PR3) and myeloperoxidase (MPO). **Presentation** Usually >60yrs, 20% of kidney biopsies >80yrs. Lethargy, fever, myalgia, anorexia, SOB, haemoptysis. Ask: 'When did you last feel well?' **Diagnosis** Clinical + ANCA + biopsy: rapidly progressive GN (p307) without immune deposits ('pauci-immune'), alveolar haemorrhage. **Treatment** High-dose glucocorticoids plus cyclophosphamide/rituximab. Benefit of plasma exchange is not clear: no reduction in death or end-stage kidney disease in a randomized trial (PEXIVAS). Avacopan (C5a receptor inhibitor) has shown non-inferiority to oral steroids.

Myeloma (p366)

Kidney disease in up to 40%: tubular obstruction due to light chain casts ('myeloma kidney'), deposition of Ig/light chains in glomerulus (proteinuria), hypercalcaemia, renal tract infection due to immunoparesis. **Treatment** Hydration, bisphosphonates for hypercalcaemia (eGFR ≥30), anti-myeloma chemotherapy. Light chain removal (plasma exchange, large pore haemodialysis) unproven over standard chemotherapy.

Amyloid

Pathological folding of proteins leads to extracellular accumulation and organ dysfunction including kidney disease. Classified according to protein: light chains in myeloma = AL amyloid; serum amyloid A in chronic inflammation = AA amyloid; also rare familial types. **Diagnosis** Congo red staining on biopsy, SAP scan. **Treatment** Underlying condition. New therapies target amyloid production, aggregation, and breakdown.

Haemolytic uraemic syndrome (HUS)

Presents with a microangiopathic haemolytic anaemia (Hb <100g/L, ↑LDH, ↓haptoglobin, fragments on blood film), ↓platelets, and AKI due to thrombosis of the glomerular capillaries (microangiopathy). In children, primarily associated with haemorrhagic colitis due to Shiga toxin-producing *E. coli* (STEC) eg 0157:H7. Atypical HUS (aHUS) is caused by dysregulation/uncontrolled activation of complement = ~5% of HUS. Can be precipitated by pregnancy. **Diagnosis** Triad of haemolytic anaemia, ↓platelets, and AKI with haematuria/proteinuria. ?Evidence of STEC. Look for abnormalities in the complement pathway: C3, C4, factors H and I, complement mutation screen. **Treatment** STEC-HUS: supportive. aHUS: eculizumab/ravulizumab (anti-C5) in England via the national aHUS centre, individual patient requests in rest of UK.

Thrombotic thrombocytopenic purpura (TTP)

Clinical overlap with HUS. Pentad: microangiopathic haemolytic anaemia, ↓platelets, AKI, neurological symptoms (headache, palsies, seizure, confusion, coma), and fever. Due to a congenital deficiency of, or acquired antibodies to, ADAMTS13 protease which normally cleaves multimers of von Willebrand factor (VWF). Large VWF multimers cause platelet aggregation and fibrin deposition in small vessels, leading to multisystem thrombotic microangiopathy. **Diagnosis** Clinical. ADAMTS13 activity. **Treatment** ►*TTP is a haematological emergency: get expert help.* Plasma infusion/exchange removes antibodies/replaces ADAMTS13 and may be life-saving. Corticosteroids. Consider rituximab for non-responders/relapse.

Atherosclerotic renovascular disease

Part of systemic atheromatous vascular disease that includes cardio-, cerebro-, and peripheral vascular disease (ask about claudication, check foot pulses), ↑BP, and ↑lipids. Leads to renin–angiotensin upregulation which causes treatment-resistant ↑BP and/or a deterioration in kidney function with ACE-i/ARB. Acute decompensated heart failure (no LV impairment on echo) with flash pulmonary oedema in up to 10%. **Diagnosis** >1.5cm asymmetry in kidney size (but ↓sensitivity and ↓specificity). CT or MR angiography. Doppler studies are not consistently accurate for diagnosis. **Treatment** Modification of CV risk factors: statin, aspirin, antihypertensive treatment. Historically, ACE-i/ARB were considered contraindicated due to concern about renin–dependent kidney perfusion and deterioration in function. However, ↓mortality seen with ACE-i/ARB so ↓eGFR by <25% 'sacrificed' for longer-term kidney and cardiac outcomes. Large RCTs of medical treatment vs revascularization have failed to show an advantage to revascularization ∴ only considered in flash pulmonary oedema, rapid/oligo-anuric kidney failure.

Scleroderma kidney crisis

Occurs in ~5% of systemic sclerosis. ↑Risk with: diffuse disease, anti-RNA polymerase III antibodies, and <2yrs from diagnosis. ↓Incidence with widespread use of ACE-i/ARB. **Diagnosis** Accelerated hypertension and AKI (↓eGFR by >30%). Biopsy: collapsed glomeruli, onion-skin thickening of arterioles. **Treatment** ACE-i/ARB. Vasodilators for digital ischaemia. May recover kidney function after many months so listing for transplantation is delayed for up to 2 years.

Sickle cell nephropathy

HbSS is associated with hyperfiltration (lower than expected creatinine) and albuminuria. Although up to 75% of patients will have some degree of CKD, progression to kidney failure is usually associated with another trigger, eg papillary necrosis, infection. **Diagnosis** Clinical. Biopsy only if looking for another diagnosis, eg AKI without clinical cause, nephrotic syndrome. **Treatment** ACE-i/ARB. Inconsistent data re hydroxycarbamide and ↓hyperfiltration. ↑Mortality on dialysis: aim to transplant. Care with erythropoietin-stimulating agents due to ↑ % sickle cells.

Tubular disorders and the action of diuretics can be classified by the segment of the nephron affected (fig 7.13 and table 7.8).

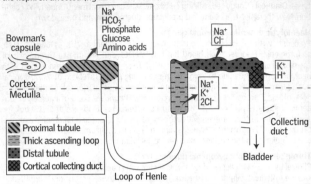

Fig 7.13 The nephron divided into segments (proximal tubule, thick ascending loop of Henle, distal tubule, collecting duct) with key solute movement (red).

Table 7.8 Summary table of tubular disorders and diuretic action (RTA = renal tubular acidosis)

Nephron segment	Solute movement	Tubular pathology	Diuretic
Proximal tubule	Reabsorption: Na⁺, HCO₃⁻, phosphate, sugars, amino acids	Fanconi syndrome Proximal (type 2) RTA	SGLT2 inhibitor, mannitol, carbonic anhydrase inhibitor
Thick ascending loop	Reabsorption: Na⁺, K⁺, Cl⁻	Bartter syndromes	Loop
Distal tubule	Reabsorption: Na⁺, Cl⁻	Gitelman syndrome	Thiazide
Cortical collecting duct	Excretion: K⁺, H⁺	Distal (type 1) RTA Type 4 RTA	K⁺-sparing
Collecting duct	Excretion: water	Diabetes insipidus (p234)	V2 antagonists ('vaptan') (p316)

Proximal tubule

Physiology
Reabsorbs Na⁺ (~70%), bicarbonate, phosphate, amino acids, sugars, uric acid.

Pathology
Fanconi syndrome: impairment of proximal tubular function. Glycosuria without DM, phosphaturia, uricosuria, aminoaciduria, and tubular-proteinuria. Can be genetic or acquired, eg cystinosis, Wilson disease. Phosphate loss from bone, demineralization, and growth impairment. *Treatment:* underlying cause. Correct volumetric and phosphate/electrolytic deficiencies. *Proximal (type 2) renal tubular acidosis (RTA):* failure of bicarbonate reabsorption. Distal reabsorption intact so bicarbonate usually ≥12mmol/L. Accompanied by Fanconi syndrome unless rare familial cause. *Aetiology:* light chain disease, drugs (eg tenofovir), heavy metals. *Diagnosis:* IV bicarbonate increases bicarbonate loss in urine with rapid rise in urine pH to ~7.5. *Treatment:* bicarbonate and potassium replacement.

Diuretics
SGLT2 inhibitors: ↓glucose reabsorption and Na⁺ co-transport. ↑Na⁺ delivery to macula densa leads to afferent arteriolar vasoconstriction and ↓glomerular pressure. *Mannitol:* Freely filtered and ↓reabsorbed, holding water by osmosis. ↓ICP and intra-ocular pressure. Risk of pulmonary oedema if oligo/anuric. *Carbonic anhydrase inhibitor, eg acetazolamide:* Metabolic acidosis due to ↑bicarbonate excretion. Used in altitude sickness, glaucoma. Risk of nephrocalcinosis.

Thick ascending loop of Henle

Physiology
Reabsorbs Na^+ (~10–30%) and other electrolytes. Key transport via electro-neutral $Na^+/K^+/2Cl^-$ co-transporter.

Pathology
Bartter syndromes: genetic mutations lead to impaired salt reabsorption. Phenotype includes low-normal BP, ↓K^+, metabolic alkalosis, ↓Cl. Also hypercalciuria, ↓Ca^{2+}, and secondary hyperparathyroidism. Fluid wasting causes activation of the renin–angiotensin–aldosterone axis: ↑renin, ↑aldosterone. Divided into subtypes depending on transport molecule defect. Type 1 mimics a loop diuretic. Elevated prostaglandin concentrations may be a feature. Treatment is with electrolyte replacement and use of NSAIDs (after volume repletion).

Diuretics
Loop diuretics (eg furosemide, bumetanide): block the $Na^+/K^+/2Cl^-$ co-transporter increasing the solute load of the filtrate and reducing water resorption. Increase excretion of water, Na^+, Cl^-, phosphate, Mg^{2+}, Ca^{2+}, K^+, and H^+. Readily absorbed from the GI tract (unless it is oedematous when IV may be needed), peak concentration within 30–120min. Widely used in oedematous states: heart failure, ascites, nephrotic syndrome. Also used to treat hypercalcaemia. Side effects include hypokalaemic metabolic alkalosis, hypovolaemia, and ototoxicity.

Distal tubule

Physiology
Reabsorbs Na^+ (~5–10%) and other electrolytes. Key transport via NaCl co-transporter.

Pathology
Gitelman syndrome: loss of function of the NaCl co-transporter. Milder than Bartter syndrome: usually presents in adolescence/adulthood with incidental finding of electrolyte abnormalities. Mimics thiazide diuretic administration. Treat with electrolyte supplementation.

Diuretics
Thiazide (eg bendroflumethiazide) and thiazide-like diuretics (eg indapamide, chlortalidone, metolazone): inhibit the NaCl transporter ∴ decrease NaCl reabsorption and increase water loss. Used to treat ↑BP. Side effects: hyponatraemia, hypokalaemia, and hypomagnesaemia. Calcium excretion is reduced (in contrast to loop diuretics) ∴ can be used to treat recurrent kidney stones in patients with hypercalciuria. Excretion of uric acid is reduced so care in gout. Glucose intolerance can occur (hypokalaemia and changes to renin–aldosterone are hypothesized mechanisms) so care in DM. ↑LDL cholesterol is not significant with chronic use at low dose, especially in the context of beneficial BP reduction.

Cortical collecting duct

Physiology
Acid–base and K^+ homeostasis. Aldosterone acts to retain Na^+ and excrete K^+.

Pathology
Distal (type 1) renal tubular acidosis (RTA): failure of acid (H^+) excretion. Primary genetic disease or secondary to autoimmune disease (eg Sjögren's syndrome, SLE), toxins (eg lithium). Can cause, or be caused by, nephrocalcinosis (eg medullary sponge kidney, sarcoid). Leads to bone demineralization, kidney stones. Hypokalaemia can be severe. Diagnosis: urine fails to acidify (pH >5.3) despite metabolic acidosis. Treat with bicarbonate replacement and management of underlying disease. *Type 4 RTA:* hyperkalaemia and acidosis due to (real or relative) hypoaldosteronism, eg adrenal insufficiency, DM, ACE-i/ARB, K^+-sparing diuretics.

Diuretics
K^+-sparing amiloride, aldosterone antagonists, eg spironolactone, eplerenone: used in hyperaldosteronism, hypertension, heart failure, cirrhosis, K^+-wasting states. Decreased Na^+ resorption, increased K^+ resorption. Can cause ↑K^+, acidosis. Oestrogenic effects with spironolactone.

The tubules and the interstitium make up ~80% of the kidney. Damage to one is usually associated with damage to the other = tubulointerstitial disease.

Acute tubulointerstitial nephritis (ATIN)
Presents with AKI. Eosinophilia in ~30%. An 'allergic triad' of fever, rash, and arthralgia occurs in ~10%. Should be considered in all cases of AKI for which there is no obvious pre-renal or post-renal precipitant (p294). Biopsy shows an inflammatory cell infiltrate in the interstitium ± tubule ('tubulitis'). Prognosis improves with early recognition although residual CKD in up to 40%.

▶Take a full drug history including over-the-counter and herbal preparations.

Aetiology
- Drugs: antibiotics, NSAIDs, PPIs, diuretics, ranitidine, anticonvulsants, warfarin.
- Infection: *Streptococcus*, *Pneumococcus*, *Staphylococcus*, *Campylobacter*, *E. coli*, *Mycoplasma*, CMV, EBV, HSV, hepatitis A–C.
- Autoimmune disease: SLE, sarcoid, Sjögren's syndrome, ANCA.
- Tubulointerstitial nephritis and uveitis syndrome (TINU): interstitial and uveal inflammation do not need to occur simultaneously. Presumed immune mediated and responds to steroids. Rarely drug/infection induced.

Treatment Stop causative agent/treat underlying cause. Steroids (↓RCT evidence).

Chronic tubulointerstitial nephritis (CTIN)
Insidious onset and slowly progressive kidney impairment. Biopsy shows interstitial fibrosis and tubular atrophy. Most commonly due to drugs (>70%) or infection. Possible causes include:
- Drugs: NSAIDs (p315), lithium, calcineurin inhibitors, aminosalicylates (eg mesalazine, sulfasalazine), chemotherapy (eg cisplatin).
- Infection: TB, pyelonephritis, leptospirosis, HIV.
- Immune disease: sarcoid, Sjögren's syndrome.
- Specific nephrotoxins: lead, cadmium, mercury, aristolochic acid (p315).
- Haematological disorders: myeloma.
- Genetic interstitial disease.

Treatment Stop causative agent or treat underlying cause. Reduce risk of progression as per CKD management: ACE-i/ARB, BP control, glucose, lipids (pp300–1).

Nephrotoxins

Many agents may be toxic to the kidneys either by direct damage to the tubules, or by causing an interstitial nephritis. Examples (not an exhaustive list and idiosyncratic reactions are possible):

Analgesics NSAIDs (p315).

Antimicrobials Aminoglycosides (p315), sulfamethoxazole (in co-trimoxazole), penicillins, rifampicin, amphotericin, aciclovir.

Anticonvulsants Lamotrigine, valproate, phenytoin.

Other drugs PPIs, cimetidine, furosemide, thiazides, ACE-i/ARB, lithium, iron, calcineurin inhibitors, cisplatin.

Anaesthetic agents Methoxyflurane, enflurane.

Radiocontrast material (See p315.)

Proteins Igs in myeloma, light chain disease, Hb in haemolysis, myoglobin in rhabdomyolysis (p315).

Crystals Urate (p315), oxalate (p315).

Bacteria Streptococci, *Legionella*, *Brucella*, *Mycoplasma*, *Chlamydia*, TB, *Salmonella*, *Campylobacter*, *Leptospira*, syphilis.

Viruses EBV, CMV, HIV, polyomavirus, adenovirus, measles.

Parasites *Toxoplasma*, *Leishmania*.

Other Ethylene glycol, radiation (p315), aristolochic acid (p315).

Analgesic nephropathy

Caused by NSAIDs, aspirin. ↓Prevalence since phenacetin withdrawn. Risk determined by frequency and duration of use. **Presentation** History of chronic pain. Often silent until advanced CKD. **Diagnosis** Urinalysis: normal or sterile pyuria, proteinuria. USS: small and irregular kidneys. Historically classic 'cup and spill' appearance on IVU. Non-contrast CT: ↓kidney mass, papillary calcification. Biopsy: CTIN, papillary necrosis. **Treatment** Discontinue analgesia whenever possible. Manage CKD (pp300–1). USS/CT urogram if sudden flank pain to exclude obstruction from sloughed papilla.

Aminoglycosides (gentamicin > tobramycin > amikacin > streptomycin)

Toxic to renal tubules. AKI due to tubular necrosis. Risk factors: ↑dose, prolonged use, CKD, volume depletion, other nephrotoxins. **Presentation** Typically non-oliguric AKI 1–2 weeks after therapy. Recovery can be delayed/incomplete. **Treatment** Prevention. Single daily dose may be less nephrotoxic. ►Check levels (p740).

Radiocontrast-associated AKI

Presentation AKI 2–7 days after IV contrast. Risk factors: CKD, DM, ↑dose of contrast, volume depletion, other nephrotoxins. Cause/association debated: comparable rates of AKI after procedures without contrast. Do not delay a necessary test. **Treatment** None. Pre-hydration with IV crystalloid has ↓evidence, and care with any fluid load in advanced CKD. Consider discontinuation of nephrotoxic medication for 24h pre- and post-procedure if possible. Use lowest dose of low/iso-osmolar contrast.

Rhabdomyolysis

Skeletal muscle breakdown with release of intracellular contents. Myoglobin is filtered causing obstruction and inflammation. ↑Cytokines and ↓nitric oxide cause vasoconstriction. **Presentation** History: trauma, surgery, limb ischaemia/embolism, immobility, hyperthermia, seizure. Muscle pain, swelling, AKI. Red-brown urine. **Diagnosis** Serum myoglobin: short half-life, may be missed. Plasma CK ×5. False +ve blood on dipstick (ie *no* RBC on microscopy). ↑K⁺, ↑↑PO₄³⁻, ↓Ca²⁺. **Treatment** Supportive. Treat hyperkalaemia (p297). May need dialysis/filtration (p302). Avoid Ca²⁺ supplementation due to myocyte entry and ↑cell destruction. IV fluid to maintain volume and urine output until myoglobinuria ceased. Alkalinization of urine hypothesized to ↓crystallization but no RCT evidence and may exacerbate ↓Ca²⁺.

Urate nephropathy

Presentation Uric acid crystals precipitate within the tubulointerstitium causing inflammation. Seen in tumour lysis syndrome: ↑tumour burden and sensitivity to chemotherapy, ↑phosphate. ↑Serum uric acid is associated with CKD progression but association/causation unclear. **Treatment** Tumour lysis: aggressive hydration, allopurinol/rasburicase to ↓synthesis of uric acid. CKD: no evidence for chronic treatment to ↓uric acid (allopurinol, febuxostat).

Oxalate nephropathy

Deposition of calcium oxalate crystals (fig 7.2g, p291) in tubules causing tubular injury/interstitial nephritis/fibrosis. **Presentation** Enteric hyperoxaluria (fat malabsorption due to Crohn's, UC, bariatric surgery): calcium bound by free fatty acids is unavailable for oxalate binding so ↑oxalate is absorbed. High dietary oxalate, eg high-dose vit C. **Treatment** Underlying cause. Hydration. Citrate may ↓crystallization (↓data).

Radiation nephritis

Kidney impairment due to ionizing radiation. Exclude obstruction due to strictures. **Presentation** Months–years after total body irradiation, local field radiotherapy, or targeted radionucleotide therapy. Presents with ↑BP, proteinuria/haematuria, progression to kidney failure. Prognosis linked to ↑BP. **Treatment** Use lowest therapeutic dose. As CKD (pp300–1), with strict BP control.

Aristolochic acid nephropathy

Progressive CKD due to herbal preparations containing aristolochic acid. **Presentation** Disproportionate anaemia, proteinuria, and kidney dysfunction. Biopsy: fibrosis and tubular atrophy. Risk of urothelial malignancy ×5, occurs in up to 40%. *Balkan endemic nephropathy:* cluster of CKD/kidney failure in Balkan areas where aristolochic acid is detected in wheat. **Treatment** Avoid exposure. Treat as CKD (pp300–1). Screen for malignancy. Consider therapeutic trial of steroids (limited data).

7 Kidney medicine

Autosomal dominant polycystic kidney disease (ADPKD)

1 in 400–1000 (~7 million worldwide). *De novo* mutation in ~10%. 2/3 will require renal replacement. 85% have mutations in PKD1 (chromosome 16) and often reach ESRF by 50s. Mutation in PKD2 (chromosome 4) has a slower course, often reaching ESRF by 70s. **Presentation** May be clinically silent unless cysts become symptomatic due to size/haemorrhage (fig 7.14). Loin pain, visible haematuria, cyst infection, calculi, ↑BP, progressive kidney failure. *Extrarenal:* liver cysts, intracranial aneurysm→SAH (p474), mitral valve prolapse, ovarian cyst, diverticular disease. **Diagnosis** USS. Kidney cysts are common and ↑prevalence with age so diagnostic criteria are age specific: 15–39yrs ≥3 cysts, 40–59yrs >2 cysts in each kidney give a positive predictive value of 100% for PKD1 and PKD2. Sensitivity is >93% for PKD1 but only 69% for diagnosis of PKD2 <30 years. Liver (90% by age 50) and pancreatic cysts (~10%) support the diagnosis. Genetic testing available but ~1500 different mutations are described so use limited to diagnostic uncertainty, potential donors, and pre-implantation diagnosis. CT for renal colic as cysts obscure view on USS. Screening for intracranial aneurysms (MRI) recommended for age <65yrs if personal/family history of aneurysm/SAH. **Treatment** Water intake 3–4L/day (if eGFR >30) may suppress cyst growth. Tolvaptan is recommended to slow progression of cysts in CKD stages G2 and G3 if evidence of progressive disease. ↑BP should be treated to target <130/80mmHg using ACE-i/ARB. Calcium channel blockers are avoided unless resistant hypertension due to theoretical concern that ↓Ca²⁺ accelerates cyst proliferation (no outcome data). Treat infection. Haematuria usually managed conservatively. Persistent/severe pain may need cyst decompression. Plan for RRT including pre-emptive transplantation.

Autosomal recessive polycystic kidney disease

1 in 20 000, chromosome 6. Presents ante/perinatally with kidney cysts ('salt and pepper' appearance on USS), congenital hepatic fibrosis→portal hypertension. Poor prognosis if neonatal respiratory distress. No specific therapy. Tolvaptan under investigation. See OHCS p228.

Kidney phakomatoses

Tuberous sclerosis complex 1 in 6000, autosomal dominant. Two genes: TSC1 (chromosome 9) and TSC2 (chromosome 16). Variable phenotype. Multisystem disorder with hamartoma formation in skin, brain (→epilepsy), eye, heart, and lung (see OHCS p842). In kidney: angiomyolipomata with risk of aneurysm and haemorrhage, cystic disease in 50%, replacement of kidney tissue leads to kidney failure, renal cell carcinoma (rare). mTOR inhibitors (eg sirolimus, everolimus) block pathological cell signalling and reduce tumour volume.

Von Hippel–Lindau syndrome 1 in 36 000, autosomal dominant (p698). Mutation in VHL gene (chromosome 3) leads to uncontrolled activation of growth factors. Phenotype is a familial, multisystem cancer syndrome including kidney cysts and clear cell carcinoma at mean age 40s, ~70% risk by age 60 (VHL tumour-suppressor gene is inactivated in most sporadic renal cell cancers). Manage by screening for tumours.

Alport syndrome

1 in 5000. ~80–85% x-linked. Mutations in COL4A3, COL4A4, or COL4A5 gene, which encode the α–chain of type IV collagen. Haematuria, proteinuria, and progressive kidney disease. Average age of kidney failure in ♂ 30–40yrs. ♀ are no longer considered 'carriers' as kidney failure in ~30% by 60yrs. High-tone sensorineural hearing loss. Anterior lenticonus: bulging of lens on slit-lamp examination (see OHCS p842). Type IV collagen is the antigen in anti-GBM disease (p307) so there is a risk of anti-GBM disease following transplantation as graft type IV collagen is recognized as 'foreign'. Managed with ACE-i/ARB, BP control, lipid management and transplantation. Newer therapies (bardoxolone, anti-microRNA, stem-cell therapy) are under investigation.

Fabry disease

1 in 40 000–120 000. x-linked. Lysosomal storage disorder due to a deficiency of the enzyme α-galactosidase-A. Proteinuria and progressive kidney disease in most ♂ and some ♀ 'carriers'. Lipid deposits in urine and on kidney biopsy ('zebra body'). Treatment with IV enzyme replacement can stabilize early kidney disease.

Cystinuria

1 in 17 000. Autosomal recessive defect prevents reabsorption of cystine and di-basic amino acids in proximal tubule. Leads to cystinuria and cystine stone forma-tion. May present with kidney failure requiring renal replacement. Treatment: diet, ↑fluid intake, and urine alkalinization to pH 6.5–7.0. α-mercaptopropionyl glycine makes cystine more soluble and reduces crystal and stone formation and is better tolerated than D-penicillamine.

Cystinosis

1 in 100 000–200 000. Autosomal recessive lysosomal storage disorder with accu-mulation of cystine. Proximal tubule dysfunction in nephropathic forms. Fanconi syndrome (p312), and progressive kidney impairment. Also visual impairment, my-opathy, hypothyroidism. Oral cysteamine ↓intralysosomal cystine and delays kidney failure, but may be poorly tolerated due to GI symptoms and foul smell and taste.

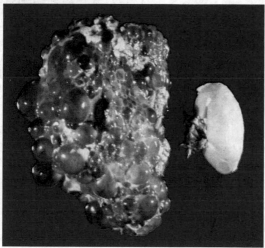

Fig 7.14 A polycystic kidney (left) compared with a normal-sized kidney (right). The progressive increase in size can lead to abdominal discomfort. There may be haemorrhage into a cyst causing haematuria, or infection.

Courtesy of the PKD Foundation.

8 Haematology

Contents

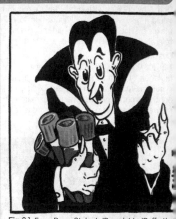

Fig 8.1 From Bram Stoker's 'Dracula' to 'Buffy the Vampire Slayer' and the 'Twilight' series, we have been fascinated by the undying allure of vampires. Many times, perched by the unsuspecting patient's antecubital fossa in the middle of the night, armed with a cannula and a variable degree of competency, we may have often felt like one ourselves. One theory regarding the origin of the vampire legend is that the hysteria arose because of outbreaks of infectious diseases that were associated with abnormal bleeding. For example, it is thought that the epidemic of supposed vampirism in the Serbian village of Medvegia in 1731 was in fact due to anthrax whereby affected individuals developed disseminated intravascular coagulation (DIC), causing them to bleed from their nose and mouth.

Image courtesy of Eoin Kelleher

We thank Drew Provan and Siobhan Glavey, our Specialist Readers for this chapter.

A sense of humourism

Whilst our understanding of blood has changed emphatically with the advent of medical research, its importance in health and disease is a common theme throughout human history and culture. Hippocrates (460–370BC) first described the four bodily fluids, or humours (Latin *umor* = body fluid): blood, phlegm, and yellow and black bile. This is not bile and phlegm as we know it; rather, it was postulated by Fahraeus (1921, the Swedish physician who pioneered the ESR, p368) that humourism arose from watching blood coagulate *in vitro*: distilling into layers of bilious yellow serum floating on a scurf of white cells, with the dark red-black clot of erythrocytes lurking in the depths of the sample.

These four humours were later elaborated by Roman physician, surgeon, and philosopher Claudius Galen (c.129–c.201AD) who attributed physical and behavioural traits to each humour: sanguine people are warm hearted and confident, the phlegmatic practical and rational, those with a choleric nature are fiery and passionate, while the melancholic (melas = black, khole = bile) are depressed yet creative.[1] It was thought that an imbalance of any of these elements was the source of disease, a belief which led to the wide-scale recommendation of the removal of the excess bodily fluid: expectoration, purging, and most popularly, bloodletting. William Harvey, Sydenham, and Dupuytren are among the famous names who celebrated this cure, with Harvey stating that 'daily experience satisfies us that bloodletting has a most salutary effect in many diseases, and is indeed the foremost among all the general remedial means'. Many tools were developed to aid this procedure, notably a collecting bowl with a convenient notch for the antecubital fossa or neck: the predecessor of the modern kidney dish.

Such was the conviction of the healing brought about by bloodletting that 'haematomania' reigned despite a suspicious degree of mortality. Indeed, it may have even killed inaugural US president George Washington in 1799: on developing laryngitis he was enthusiastically bled four times by his personal physician, and died 24 hours after symptom onset.

Eventually, the credibility of this practice waned, and by 1860 it had virtually disappeared. However, venesection still plays an important role in the management of haemochromatosis (p284) and polycythaemia rubra vera (p362).

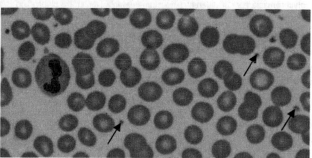

Fig 8.2 A normal blood film, with a neutrophil, red cells, and platelets (arrows).
© Prof. K Lewandowski & Dr H Jastrow.

1. Compare these personalities with those of the 2015 anthropomorphic Pixar film *Inside Out*.

8 Haematology

▶Many haematological (and other) diagnoses are made by careful examination of the peripheral blood film. It is also necessary for interpretation of the FBC indices.

Features Include:

Acanthocytes (fig 8.3) Spicules on RBCs (∴ unstable RBC membrane lipid structure); causes: splenectomy, alcoholic liver disease, abetalipoproteinaemia, spherocytosis.

Anisocytosis Variation in RBC size, eg megaloblastic anaemia, thalassaemia, IDA.

Basophilic RBC stippling (fig 8.4) Denatured RNA found in RBCs, indicating accelerated erythropoiesis or defective Hb synthesis. Seen in lead poisoning, megaloblastic anaemia, myelodysplasia, liver disease, haemoglobinopathy, eg thalassaemia.

Blasts Nucleated precursor cells. They should not normally appear in peripheral blood but do in myelofibrosis, leukaemia, and malignant marrow infiltration.

Burr cells (echinocytes) RBC projections (less marked than in acanthocytes); fig 8.5.

Cabot rings Seen in: pernicious anaemia; lead poisoning; bad infections (fig 8.6).[1]

Dimorphic picture Two populations of red cells. Seen after treatment of Fe, B₁₂, or folate deficiency, in mixed deficiency (↓Fe with ↓B₁₂ or folate), post-transfusion, or with primary sideroblastic anaemia, where a clone of abnormal erythroblasts produce abnormal red cells, alongside normal red cell production.

Howell–Jolly bodies DNA nuclear remnants in RBCs, which are normally removed by the spleen (fig 8.7). Seen post-splenectomy and in hyposplenism (eg sickle cell disease, coeliac disease, congenital, UC/Crohn's, myeloproliferative disease, amyloid). Also in dyserythropoietic states: myelodysplasia, megaloblastic anaemia.

Hypochromia (p326) Less dense staining of RBC due to ↓Hb synthesis, seen in IDA, thalassaemia, and sideroblastic anaemia (iron stores unusable, p362).

Left shift Immature neutrophils released from the marrow, eg in infection (fig 8.8).

Leukoerythroblastic film Immature cells (myelocytes, promyelocytes, metamyelocytes, normoblasts) ± teardrop RBCs from haemolysis or marrow infiltration/infection (malignancy; TB; brucella; visceral leishmaniasis; parvovirus B19).

Leukaemoid reaction A marked leucocytosis (WCC >50 × 10⁹/L). Seen in severe illness, eg with infection or burns, and also in leukaemia.

Pappenheimer bodies Granules of siderocytes containing iron. Seen in lead poisoning, carcinomatosis, and post-splenectomy.

Poikilocytosis Variation in RBC shape, eg in IDA, myelofibrosis, thalassaemia.

Polychromasia RBCs of different ages stain unevenly (young are bluer). This is a response to bleeding, haematinic replacement (ferrous sulfate, B₁₂, folate), haemolysis, or marrow infiltration. Reticulocyte count is raised.

Reticulocytes (Normal range: 0.8–2%; or <85 × 10⁹/L). (fig 8.10) Young, larger RBCs (contain RNA) signifying active erythropoiesis. Increased in haemolysis, haemorrhage, and if B₁₂, iron, or folate is given to marrow that lack these.

Right shift Hypermature white cells: hypersegmented polymorphs (>5 lobes to nucleus) seen in megaloblastic anaemia, uraemia, and liver disease. See p329, fig 8.26.

Rouleaux formation (fig 8.11) Red cells stack on each other (causing a raised ESR; p368). Seen with chronic inflammation, paraproteinaemia, and myeloma.

Schistocytes Fragmented RBCs sliced by fibrin bands, in intravascular haemolysis (p335, fig 8.34). Look for microangiopathic anaemia, eg DIC (p350), haemolytic uraemic syndrome, thrombotic thrombocytopenic purpura (TTP: p311), or pre-eclampsia.

Spherocytes Spherical cells found in hereditary spherocytosis and autoimmune haemolytic anaemia. See p334.

Target cells (Also known as Mexican hat cells, fig 8.7 and fig 8.44, p339.) These are RBCs with central staining, a ring of pallor, and an outer rim of staining seen in liver disease, hyposplenism, thalassaemia—and, in small numbers, in IDA.

Teardrop RBCs Seen in extramedullary haematopoiesis; see leukoerythroblastic film.

---

2 Cabot 'figure-of-eight' rings may be microtubules from mitotic spindles. It is easy to confuse them with malaria parasites, p412 (especially if stippling gives a 'chromatin dot' artefact, as here). Richard Clarke Cabot (1868–1939) liked diagnostic challenges: he founded the notoriously hard but beautifully presented clinicopathological conference of the Massachusetts General Hospital which made the *New England Journal of Medicine* so famous. He also wisely recommended that: 'before you tell the truth to the patient, be sure you know the truth, and that the patient wants to hear it'.

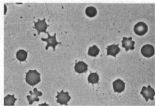

Fig 8.3 Acanthocytosis.
© Dr N Medeiros.

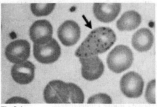

Fig 8.4 Basophilic stippling.
From the *New England Journal of Medicine*, Bain, B, 'Diagnosis from the blood smear', 353(5), 498. Copyright © 2005 Massachusetts Medical Society. Reprinted with permission from Massachusetts Medical Society.

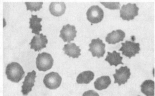

Fig 8.5 Burr cells: the cause may be kidney or liver failure, or an EDTA storage artefact.
© Prof. Christine Lawrence.

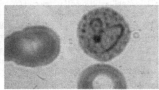

Fig 8.6 A Cabot ring.[2]
© Crookston Collection.

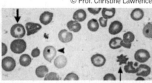

Fig 8.7 Film in hyposplenism: target cell (short arrow), acanthocyte (long arrow), and a Howell–Jolly body (arrow head).
From the *New England Journal of Medicine*, Bain, B, 'Diagnosis from the blood smear', 353(5), 498. Copyright © 2005 Massachusetts Medical Society. Reprinted with permission from Massachusetts Medical Society.

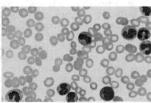

Fig 8.8 Left shift: presence of immature neutrophils in the blood. See p324.
© Prof. Krzysztof Lewandowski.

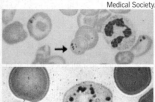

Fig 8.9 Pappenheimer bodies.
Top image © Prof. Christine Lawrence, bottom image © Crookston Collection.

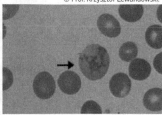

Fig 8.10 Reticulocytes. RNA in RBCs; supravital staining (azure B; cresyl blue) is needed.
© Dr N Medeiros.

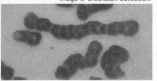

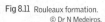

Fig 8.11 Rouleaux formation.
© Dr N Medeiros.

Neutrophils (figs 8.12, 8.13) 2–7.5 × 10⁹/L (40–75% of white blood cells: but absolute values are more meaningful than percentages).

Increased in (ie *neutrophilia*)
• Bacterial infections.
• Inflammation, eg myocardial infarction, polyarteritis nodosa.
• Myeloproliferative disorders.
• Drugs (steroids).
• Disseminated malignancy.
• Stress, eg trauma, surgery, burns, haemorrhage, seizure.

Decreased in (ie *neutropenia*—see p350–1)
• Viral infections.
• Drugs: post-chemotherapy, cytotoxic agents, carbimazole, sulfonamides.
• Severe sepsis.
• Neutrophil antibodies (SLE, haemolytic anaemia)—↑destruction.
• Hypersplenism (p369), eg Felty's syndrome (p688).
• Bone marrow failure—↓production (p348).

Other neutrophil responses to infection These include: • Vacuoles in the cytoplasm (the most specific sign of bacterial infection). • Döhle bodies: inconspicuous grey-blue areas of cytoplasm (residual ribosomes). Up to 17% of neutrophils from females show a drumstick-shaped Barr body (arrow, fig 8.13d). It is the inactivated x chromosome.

Lymphocytes (fig 8.14) 1.5–4.5 × 10⁹/L (20–45%).

Increased in (ie *lymphocytosis*)
• Acute viral infections.
• Chronic infections, eg TB, brucellosis, hepatitis, syphilis.
• Leukaemias and lymphomas, especially chronic lymphocytic leukaemia (CLL).

Large numbers of abnormal ('atypical') lymphocytes are characteristically seen with EBV infection: these are T cells reacting against EBV-infected B cells. They have a large amount of clearish cytoplasm with a blue rim that flows around neighbouring RBCs. Other causes of 'atypical' lymphocytes: see p401.

Decreased in (ie *lymphopenia*)
• Steroid therapy; SLE; uraemia; Legionnaire's disease; HIV infection; marrow infiltration; post chemotherapy or radiotherapy.

T-lymphocyte subset reference values: CD4 count: 537–1571/mm³ (low in HIV infection). CD8 count: 235–753/mm³; CD4/CD8 ratio: 1.2–3.8.

Eosinophils (fig 8.15) 0.04–0.4 × 10⁹/L (1–6%).

Increased in (ie *eosinophilia*)
• Drug reactions, eg with erythema multiforme, p560.
• Allergies: asthma, atopy.
• Parasitic infections (especially invasive helminths).
• Skin disease: especially pemphigus, eczema, psoriasis, dermatitis herpetiformis.

Also seen in malignancy (eg lymphomas), PAN, adrenal insufficiency, irradiation, Löffler syndrome (p692), eosinophilic granulomatosis with polyangiitis (Churg–Strauss) (p686), and during the convalescent phase of any infection.

The hypereosinophilic syndrome (HES) occurs where eosinophilia >1.5 × 10⁹/L is sustained for >6 weeks leading to end-organ damage (endomyocardial fibrosis and restrictive cardiomyopathy, skin lesions, thromboembolic disease, lung disease, neuropathy, and hepatosplenomegaly). The cause is often unknown, though if FIP1L1-PDFRA genotype, diagnose myeloproliferative HES or eosinophilic leukaemia. ℞ PO steroids ± mepolizumab (anti-interleukin-5 monoclonal antibody). Imatinib is 1st choice for myeloproliferative HES.

Monocytes (fig 8.16) 0.2–0.8 × 10⁹/L (2–10%). **Increased in** (ie *monocytosis*) the aftermath of chemo- or radiotherapy, chronic infections (eg malaria, TB, brucellosis, protozoa), malignant disease (including M4 and M5 acute myeloid leukaemia (p354), and Hodgkin's disease), myelodysplasia.

Basophils (fig 8.17) 0–0.1 × 10⁹/L (0–1%). **Increased in** (ie *basophilia*) myeloproliferative disease, viral infections, IgE-mediated hypersensitivity reactions (eg urticaria, hypothyroidism), and inflammatory disorders (eg UC, rheumatoid arthritis).

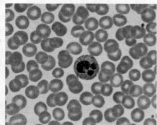

Fig 8.12 Neutrophil. These ingest and kill bacteria, fungi, and damaged cells.
Courtesy of Prof. Krzysztof Lewandowski.

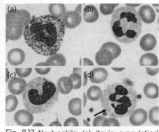

Fig 8.13 Neutrophils: (a) 'toxic granulation' seen in infection or pregnancy; (b) normal appearances; (c) 'left shift': immature forms are released with few lobes to their nuclei, seen in infection; (d) Barr body (arrow, see text).
Courtesy of Prof. Tangün and Dr Köroğlu.

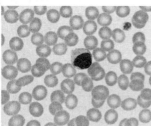

Fig 8.14 Lymphocyte: divided into T & B types, which have important roles in cell-mediated immunity and antibody production.
Courtesy of Prof. Krzysztof Lewandowski.

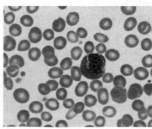

Fig 8.15 Eosinophil: these mediate allergic reactions and defend against parasites.
Courtesy of Prof. Krzysztof Lewandowski.

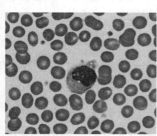

Fig 8.16 Monocyte: precursors of tissue macrophages.
Courtesy of Prof. Krzysztof Lewandowski.

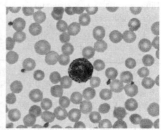

Fig 8.17 Basophil. The cytoplasm is filled with dark-staining granules, containing histamine, myeloperoxidase, and other enzymes. On binding IgE, histamine is released from the basophil.
Courtesy of Prof. Krzysztof Lewandowski.

Anaemia is defined as a low haemoglobin (Hb) concentration, and may be due either to a low red cell mass or increased plasma volume (dilutional as in pregnancy). A low Hb is <135g/L for men and <120g/L for women. Low red cell mass may reflect reduced production or increased loss of RBCs and has many causes. These will often be distinguishable by history, examination, and inspection of the blood film (fig 8.2, p319).

Symptoms Often a combination of underlying cause and anaemia *per se*: fatigue, dyspnoea, light-headedness, palpitation, headache, tinnitus, anorexia—and angina if there is pre-existing coronary artery disease. Are there symptoms suggestive of malignancy (eg weight loss, fever/night sweats) or chronic conditions (eg RA, CKD)?

Signs May be absent even in severe anaemia. There may be pallor (eg of the conjunctivae, see fig 8.18, although this is not a reliable sign). In severe anaemia (Hb <80g/L), there may be signs of a hyperdynamic circulation, eg tachycardia, flow murmurs (ejection-systolic loudest over apex), and cardiac enlargement; or retinal haemorrhages (rarely). Later, heart failure may occur: here, rapid blood transfusion can be fatal.

Types of anaemia The first step in diagnosis is to look at the mean cell volume (MCV). *Normal* MCV is 76–96 femtolitres (×10^{-15} L) (fig 8.19).

Low MCV (microcytic anaemia) check iron studies (Fe, TIBC, ferritin)
1 Iron-deficiency anaemia (IDA), the most common cause: see p326.
2 Thalassaemia (suspect if the MCV is 'too low' for the Hb level and the red cell count is raised, though definitive diagnosis needs DNA analysis): see p338.
3 Sideroblastic anaemias (very rare, heterogeneous group): p326.

NB: there is iron accumulation in the last two conditions, and so tests will show increased serum iron and ferritin with a low total iron-binding capacity (TIBC).

Normal MCV (normocytic anaemia) Further tests (eg smear, retics, LDH, creatinine).
1 Acute blood loss.   5 Hypothyroidism (or ↑MCV).
2 Anaemia of chronic disease (or ↓MCV).   6 Haemolysis (or ↑MCV).
3 Bone marrow failure.   7 Pregnancy.
4 Chronic kidney disease.

NB: if ↓WCC or ↓platelets in normocytic anaemia, suspect marrow failure: see p348.

High MCV (macrocytic anaemia) Further tests (eg B$_{12}$, folate, LFTs).
1 B$_{12}$ or folate deficiency.   5 Myelodysplastic syndromes.
2 Alcohol excess—or liver disease.   6 Marrow infiltration.
3 Reticulocytosis (p320, eg with haemolysis). 7 Hypothyroidism.
4 Cytotoxics, eg hydroxycarbamide.   8 Antifolate drugs (eg phenytoin).

Haemolytic anaemias These do not fit into the above-mentioned classification as the anaemia may be normocytic or, if there are many young (hence larger) RBCs and reticulocytes, macrocytic (p328). Suspect if there is a reticulocytosis (>2% of RBCs; or reticulocyte count >100 × 10^9/L), mild macrocytosis, ↓haptoglobin, ↑bilirubin, ↑LDH, ↑urobilinogen, or positive direct antiglobulin test (DAT). These patients will often be mildly jaundiced.

Does the patient need a blood transfusion? Probably not if Hb >70g/L. Chronic anaemia in particular can be well tolerated (though it is crucial to ascertain the cause), and in IDA, iron supplements will raise the Hb more safely and cost-effectively. In *acute* anaemia (eg haemorrhage with active peptic ulcer), transfusion for those with Hb <70g/L may be indicated. Other factors to consider include comorbidities and whether the patient is symptomatic. A higher transfusion threshold of <80g/L is appropriate in a patient with pre-existing IHD.

In severe anaemia with heart failure, transfusion is vital to restore Hb to a safe level, eg 80g/L, but this must be done with great care. Give it *slowly* with 40mg furosemide IV/PO with alternate units (dose depends on previous exposure to diuretics; do not mix with blood). Check for signs of worsening overload: rising JVP and basal crackles: in this eventuality, stop and treat.

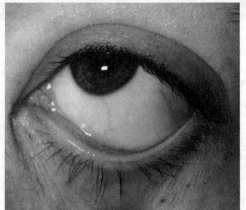

Fig 8.18 'Conjunctival pallor', *the* classic sign of anaemia, is a confusing term as the conjunctiva is translucent, transmitting the colour of structures under it. The 'pallor' refers to the vasculature on the inner surface of the lid which is lacking Hb. It is this colour [   ] but it should be: [   ]

Red cell distribution width (RCDW or RDW)

In health or in unifactorial anaemia, all the red cells in a sample are about the same size, and the graph of their volume distribution forms a narrow peak. In mixed anaemias, however, this peak broadens, reflecting an abnormally large RDW—this may be the first clue to dual pathology. In coeliac disease, for example, poor absorption of iron (↓MCV) and folate (↑MCV) may occur simultaneously, resulting in a combination of microcytes and macrocytes in the circulation. The visual analogue of this is anisocytosis (p320) on a blood film. The laboratory measure is an ↑RDW, where RDW = the standard deviation of MCV divided by the mean MCV, multiplied by 100. Reference interval: 11.5–14.6%. If the MCV is high and the RDW is *normal*, the cause is likely to be alcohol, liver disease, or a marrow problem (chemotherapy or aplastic anaemia).

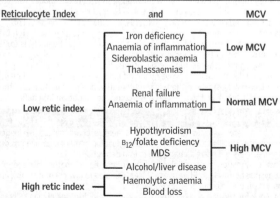

Fig 8.19 Evaluation of anaemia: consider both a combined morphological (MCV) and kinetic (reticulocyte index/count) approach. Anaemia can be due to one or more of these mechanisms: ↓red cell production (low retic count), ↑red cell destruction (high retic count), or red cell loss (high retic count).

This is common—according to the WHO, one-third of all women of reproductive age are anaemic, the majority of these are IDA.[2]

Causes •Blood loss (▶assume to be the cause until proven otherwise, eg menor-rhagia or GI bleeding (upper p252; lower p621)).
• Poor diet or poverty may cause IDA in babies or children (but rarely in adults).
• Malabsorption (eg coeliac disease) is a cause of refractory IDA.
• In the tropics, hookworm (GI blood loss) is the most common cause.

Signs Chronic IDA (signs very rare): koilonychia (fig 8.20 and p75), atrophic glossitis, an-gular cheilosis (fig 8.21), and, rarely, post-cricoid webs (Plummer–Vinson syndrome).

Tests Blood film: microcytic, hypochromic anaemia with anisocytosis and poikilo-cytosis (figs 8.22, 8.23). ↓MCV, ↓MCH, and ↓MCHC. Confirmed by ↓ferritin (also ↓serum iron with ↑TIBC, but these are less reliable, see table 8.1). ▶NB: ferritin is an acute phase protein, ↑ with inflammation, eg infection, malignancy, and therefore may be 'falsely normal' in iron-deficient patients with comorbidities. Transferrin saturation (TSAT) is the ratio of serum iron to TIBC. TSAT <20% indicates iron deficiency. Check coeliac serology in all (p262): if negative then refer all males and post-menopausal females for gastroscopy *and* colonoscopy. Consider stool microscopy for ova if relevant travel history. Faecal occult blood is not recommended as sensitivity is poor. ▶IDA with no obvious source of bleeding mandates careful GI workup.

Treatment Treat the cause. Oral iron, eg ferrous sulfate 200mg/8h PO. SE: nausea, abdominal discomfort, diarrhoea or constipation, black stools. Hb should rise by 1g/L/week, with a modest reticulocytosis (young RBC, p320). Continue for at least 3 months after Hb normalizes to replenish stores. Oral iron should be effective for most patients but consider IV iron if likely to be poorly tolerated (eg older patients, IBD), if rapid correction/resolution of symptoms required, or where oral iron is likely to be ineffective (eg functional iron deficiency in CKD, malabsorption or inflamma-tory states).

Check compliance if IDA fails to respond to therapy. Is the reason for the problem GI disturbance? Modifying the dose of elemental iron with a different preparation or alternate-day dosing may help. Alternatively, there may be continued blood loss, malabsorption, anaemia of chronic disease, or misdiagnosis.

Anaemia of chronic disease (ACD)

The commonest anaemia in hospital patients (and the 2nd commonest, after IDA, worldwide). It arises from three problems (in which the polypeptide, hepcidin, plays a key role): 1 Poor use of iron in erythropoiesis. 2 Cytokine-induced shortening of RBC survival. 3 ↓Production of and response to erythropoietin.

Causes Many, eg chronic infection, vasculitis, rheumatoid, malignancy, CKD.

Tests Ferritin normal or ↑ in mild normocytic or microcytic anaemia (see table 8.1). Often ↑ ESR/CRP. Check blood film, B₁₂, folate, TSH, and tests for haemolysis (p332).

Treatment Treating the underlying disease may help, as may an erythropoietin-stimulating agent (ESA—SE: 'flu-like symptoms, hypertension, mild ↑ platelets and thromboembolism). It may improve quality of life in non-haematological malignan-cies (or low-risk MDS) where there is symptomatic anaemia due to chemotherapy (seek expert advice). IV iron can safely overcome the functional iron deficiency.

Sideroblastic anaemia

Refers to a heterogeneous group of rare anaemias characterized by ineffective erythropoiesis, leading to ↑iron absorption, iron loading in marrow ± haemosiderosis (endocrine, liver, and heart damage due to iron deposition).

Causes Congenital (rare, x-linked) or acquired, eg idiopathic as one of the myelodysplastic/myeloproliferative diseases, can also follow chemotherapy, anti-TB drugs, irradiation, alcohol or lead excess.

Tests Look for ↑ferritin, a hypochromic blood film, and disease-defining sideroblasts in the marrow (figs 8.24, 8.25; table 8.1).

Treatment Remove the cause. Pyridoxine ± repeated transfusions for severe anaemia.

Table 8.1 Interpreting plasma iron studies

	Iron	TIBC	Ferritin
Iron deficiency	↓	↑	↓
Anaemia of chronic disease[3]	↓	↓	↑
Chronic haemolysis	↑	↓	↑
Haemochromatosis	↑	↓ (or ↔)	↑
Pregnancy	↑	↑	↔
Sideroblastic anaemia	↑	↔	↑

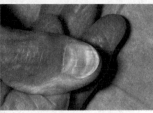

Fig 8.20 Koilonychia: spoon-shaped nails.

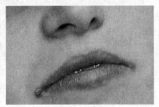

Fig 8.21 Angular cheilosis (also known as stomatitis): ulceration at the side of the mouth. Also a feature of vitamin B₁₂ and B₂ (riboflavin) deficiency, and glucagonoma (p217).
Courtesy of Dr Joseph Thompson: AskAnOrthodontist.com.

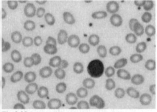

Fig 8.22 Microcytic hypochromic cells.
Courtesy of Prof. Krzysztof Lewandowski.

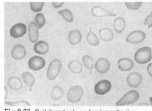

Fig 8.23 Poikilocytosis and anisocytosis.
Courtesy of Prof. Christine Lawrence.

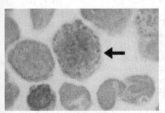

Fig 8.24 Ring sideroblasts in the marrow, with a perinuclear ring of iron granules, found in sideroblastic anaemia.
Courtesy of Prof. Christine Lawrence.

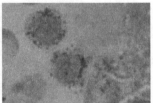

Fig 8.25 Two ringed sideroblasts showing how the distribution of perinuclear mitochondrial ferritin can vary. The problem in congenital sideroblastic anaemia is disordered mitochondrial haem synthesis.
Courtesy of Prof. Tangün and Dr Köroğlu.

3 There is also an acute variant of ACD known as 'acute event-related anaemia' which may occur after major surgery, trauma, or in the setting of severe sepsis (a condition known as 'anaemia of critical illness'). It shares many features of ACD including low serum iron, high ferritin, and blunted response to EPO. Several mechanisms may be involved including inflammation inducing a functional iron deficiency, shorted red cell survival and chronic blood loss from ongoing procedures, repeated phlebotomy etc. Dx of exclusion.

Macrocytosis (increased RBC size; MCV >96fL) is common, and may not always be accompanied by anaemia (eg in alcohol excess). Due to abnormal RBC production in the bone marrow, altered RBC membrane composition, or reticulocytosis (reticulocytes are immature RBCs larger than mature RBC).

Causes of macrocytosis (MCV >96fL)

►The three most common are alcohol, B₁₂/folate deficiency, and reticulocytosis.
* **Megaloblastic** (fig 8.26) A megaloblast is a cell in which nuclear maturation is delayed compared with the cytoplasm (note only seen on bone marrow biopsy, not in the peripheral smear). This occurs with B₁₂ (p330) and folate deficiency: both are required for DNA synthesis. (Haematopoietic precursor cells are among the most rapidly dividing cells in the body and hence sensitive to abnormal DNA synthesis.) Certain medications may also cause this including cytotoxic drugs, hydroxycarbamide, antiretroviral or anti-epileptic drugs.
* **Non-megaloblastic** Alcohol excess, reticulocytosis (eg in haemolysis, bone marrow, or following EPO treatment).
* **Other haematological disease** Myelodysplasia (fig 8.27).

Tests Ask about alcohol, diet, and medications. Severe macrocytosis MCV >110fL is usually associated with megaloblastic anaemias. B₁₂ and folate deficiency result in similar blood film and bone marrow biopsy appearances. ►If the B₁₂ or folate level is borderline/normal and high suspicion for deficiency, test methylmalonic acid (MMA) and homocysteine levels (intermediates in B₁₂ and folate metabolism). If both are elevated, this indicates B₁₂ deficiency. If homocysteine is elevated and MMA normal, this suggests folate deficiency.

Blood film Hypersegmented neutrophils (fig 8.28) in B₁₂ and folate deficiency. Target cells if liver disease; see fig 8.7, p321 and fig 8.44, p339.

Other tests Reticulocyte count, LFT (include γGT), TFT, serum B₁₂, and serum folate (or red cell folate—a more reliable indicator of folate status, as serum folate only reflects *recent* intake; not routinely used as costly). Test copper if recent gastric bypass or history of excessive zinc intake.

Bone marrow biopsy is indicated if the cause is not revealed by the above tests, in the setting of other cytopenias, or the presence of immature white cells on peripheral smear. It is likely to show one of the following four states:

1 Megaloblastic marrow.
2 Normoblastic marrow (eg in liver disease, alcohol abuse, hypothyroidism).
3 Abnormal erythropoiesis (eg sideroblastic anaemia, p326).
4 Increased erythropoiesis (eg haemolysis).

Folate Found in green vegetables, nuts, yeast, and liver; it is synthesized by gut bacteria. Body stores can last for 4 months. Maternal folate deficiency causes fetal neural tube defects. It is absorbed by duodenum/proximal jejunum.

Causes of deficiency

* Poor/restricted diet, eg poverty, alcoholics, elderly.
* Increased demand, eg pregnancy or ↑cell turnover (seen in haemolysis, malignancy, inflammatory disease, and dialysis).
* Malabsorption, eg coeliac disease, tropical sprue.
* Alcohol.
* Drugs: anti-epileptics (phenytoin, valproate), methotrexate, trimethoprim.

Treatment Assess for an underlying cause, eg poor diet, malabsorption. Treat with folic acid 5mg/day PO for 4 months, ►never without B₁₂ unless the patient is known to have a normal B₁₂ level, as in low B₁₂ states it may precipitate, or worsen, subacute combined degeneration of the cord (p330). In pregnancy, prophylactic doses of folate (400mcg/day) are given from ≥1 month preconception until at least 12wks; this helps prevent spina bifida, as well as anaemia.

NB: in unwell patients (eg CCF) with megaloblastic anaemia, it may be necessary to treat before serum B₁₂ and folate results are known. Do tests then treat with large doses of hydroxocobalamin, eg 1mg/48h IM—see *BNF*, with folic acid 5mg/24h PO.

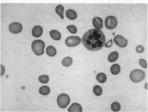
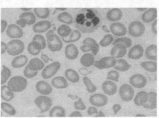

Fig 8.26 Megaloblastic anaemia: peripheral blood film showing many macrocytes and one hypersegmented neutrophil (normally there should be ≤5 segments).

From the *New England Journal of Medicine*, Bain, B, 'Diagnosis from the blood smear', 353(5), 498. Copyright © 2005 Massachusetts Medical Society. Reprinted with permission from Massachusetts Medical Society.

Fig 8.27 Oval macrocytes seen here in myelodysplastic syndromes. Note aniso- and poikilocytosis with small fragmented cells (schistocytes). NB: B_{12} and folate deficiencies also cause oval macrocytes, but macrocytes caused by alcohol and liver disease are usually round.

Courtesy of Prof. Tangün and Dr Köroğlu.

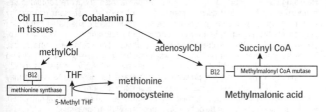

DNA (thymine) Synthesis   for the TCA cycle

Fig 8.28 Physiology of B_{12}.

Marvellous Marmite®

In 1928, a British haematologist called Lucy Wills travelled to India to investigate macrocytic anaemia in pregnancy, prevalent in female textile workers in Bombay. Since the anaemia was most frequent in poorer populations with diets deficient in protein, fruit, and vegetables, Wills extrapolated that a nutritional deficiency may be the root cause. She studied the effects of changes in diet on the macrocytic anaemia of albino rats produced by a deficient diet and *Bartonella* infection. The anaemia was prevented by yeast added to a B vitamin-deplete diet. Yeast or yeast extract (Marmite®) was then found to correct the macrocytic anaemia in the pregnant Bombay patients. It was the folic acid contained in the extract, a discovery initially dubbed the 'Wills factor', that corrected the anaemia and thus changed the face of preventive prenatal care for women. Wills also undertook a placebo trial of routine iron supplementation in pregnant women in London during the World War II, unhampered by bombing interruptions and restrictions.

Folinic acid

Folinic acid, also known as leucovorin, is a naturally occurring form of reduced folate. It is typically used as a folic acid antagonist in the case of methotrexate overdose or to potentiate cytotoxicity of fluorouracil (FU) in chemotherapy regimens for colon cancer. It is rapidly converted to the metabolically active form of folate required in cells (tetrahydrofolate) without the need for dihydrofolate reductase, which is inhibited by methotrexate.

Vitamin B₁₂ deficiency is common, occurring in up to 15% of older people. B₁₂ helps synthesize thymidine, and hence DNA, so in deficiency RBC production is slow. Untreated, it can lead to megaloblastic anaemia (p328) and irreversible CNS complications. ▶Body stores of B₁₂ are sufficient for 4yrs.

Causes of deficiency • Dietary (eg vegans: B₁₂ is found in meat, fish, and dairy products, but not in plants). • Malabsorption: during digestion, intrinsic factor (IF) in the stomach binds B₁₂, enabling it to be absorbed in the terminal ileum. Malabsorption can therefore arise in the *stomach* due to lack of IF (pernicious anaemia, post gastrectomy) or the *terminal ileum* (ileal resection, Crohn's disease, bacterial overgrowth, tropical sprue, tapeworms). • Medications (eg PPI, H₂ antagonists, metformin). • Congenital metabolic errors.

Features General Symptoms of anaemia (p324), other cytopenias, 'lemon tinge' to skin due to combination of pallor (anaemia) and mild jaundice (due to haemolysis), glossitis (beefy-red sore tongue; fig 8.29), angular cheilosis (p326).

Neuropsychiatric Irritability, depression, psychosis, dementia.

Neurological Paraesthesiae, peripheral neuropathy. Also *subacute combined degeneration of the spinal cord*, a combination of peripheral sensory neuropathy with both upper *and* lower motor neuron signs due to ↓B₁₂. The patient may display the classical triad of: • extensor plantars (UMN) • absent knee jerks (LMN) • absent ankle jerks (LMN). The onset is insidious (*subacute*) and signs are symmetrical. There is a *combination* of posterior (dorsal) column loss, causing the sensory and LMN signs, and corticospinal tract loss, causing the motor and UMN signs (p442). The spinothalamic tracts are preserved so pain and temperature sensation may remain intact even in severe cases. Joint-position and vibration sense are often affected first leading to ataxia, followed by stiffness and weakness if untreated. ▶The neurological signs of B₁₂ deficiency can occur without anaemia.

Pernicious anaemia (PA) This is an autoimmune condition caused by autoantibodies against IF leading to atrophic gastritis. Dietary B₁₂ therefore remains unbound and consequently cannot be absorbed by the terminal ileum.

Incidence 1:1000; ♀:♂≈1.6:1; usually >40yrs; higher incidence if blood group A.

Associations Other autoimmune diseases (p550): thyroid disease (~25%), vitiligo, Addison's disease, hypoparathyroidism. Carcinoma of stomach is ~3-fold more common in pernicious anaemia, so have a low threshold for upper GI endoscopy.

Tests • ↓Hb. • ↓MCV. • WCC and ↓platelets if severe. • ↓Serum B₁₂[4] • Reticulocytes may be ↓ as production impaired. • Hypersegmented neutrophils (p328). • Megaloblasts in the marrow. • Specific tests for PA: 1 Parietal cell antibodies: found in 90% with PA, but also in 3–10% without. 2 IF antibodies: specific for PA, but lower sensitivity.

Treatment Treat the cause if possible and treat urgently if symptomatic, neuropsychiatric symptoms or pregnant. If pernicious or other macrocytic anaemia, give hydroxocobalamin 1 mg IM 3 times a week for 2 weeks, then 1 mg every 2–3 months. If neurological involvement, give 1 mg IM once daily on alternate days until no further improvement, then 1 mg every 2 months. Can treat orally with cyanocobalamin (50mcg daily for 4 weeks then recheck) if malabsorption due to diet etc.

Practical hints • Beware of diagnosing PA if <40yrs old: look for GI malabsorption.
• Watch for hypokalaemia due to uptake into new haematopoietic cells.
• Transfusion is best avoided, but PA with high-output CCF may require transfusion, after doing tests for FBC, folate, B₁₂, and marrow sampling.
• As haematopoiesis accelerates on treatment, additional iron may be needed.
• Hb rises ~10g/L per week; WCC and platelet count should normalize in 1wk.

Prognosis Supplementation usually improves peripheral neuropathy within the first 3–6 months, but has little effect on cord signs. Patients do best if treated as soon as possible after the onset of symptoms: don't delay!

---

4 Serum B₁₂ levels are normal in many patients with subclinical B₁₂ deficiency. Measuring homocysteine or methylmalonic acid (↑ if B₁₂ low) may be helpful, but these are non-standard tests (pp328, 329).

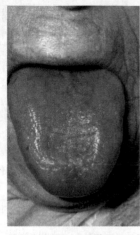

Fig 8.29 The big, beefy tongue of B12 deficiency glossitis. Other causes of glossitis: iron (or Zn) deficiency, pellagra, contact dermatitis/specific food intolerances, Crohn's disease, drugs (minocycline, clarithromycin, some ACE-i), TB of the tongue. Glossitis may be the presenting feature of coeliac disease or alcoholism.

Fanconi anaemia

Autosomal recessive disorder caused by mutations in key DNA repair genes (>21 identified), leading to defective stem cell repair & chromosomal fragility and thus aplastic anaemia, ↑risk of AML and breast ca (BRCA2), skin pigmentation, absent radii, short stature, microcephaly, syndactyly, deafness, ↓IQ, hypopituitarism, and cryptorchidism. ℞ Stem-cell transplant. Guido Fanconi, 1892–1979 (Swiss paediatrician).

Paroxysmal nocturnal haemoglobinuria: the darkest hour

In paroxysmal nocturnal haemoglobinuria (PNH, also known as Marchiafava–Micheli syndrome), surface proteins are missing in all blood cells due to a somatic mutation in the X-linked PIG-A gene. Cells lack the glycosyl-phosphatidylinositol (GPI) anchor that binds the surface proteins to cell membranes. This causes uncontrolled amplification of the complement system and leads to destruction of the RBC membrane and release of haemoglobin into the circulation (fig 8.30). NB: the phenomenon of haemoglobinuria[5] is not all that reliable. A much better test even than a marrow biopsy (right-hand panel, showing a clone of PNH cells) is flow cytometric analysis of GPI-anchored proteins on peripheral blood cells. This can determine the size of the PNH clone and type of GPI deficiency (complete or partial). ℞ Most benefit from supportive measures—but allogeneic stem cell transplantation is the only cure. Eculizumab is a monoclonal antibody that targets the C5 protein of the complement system. Blockade prevents activation of the complement distal pathway, reducing haemolysis, stabilizing haemoglobin, and reducing transfusion requirements.

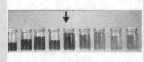
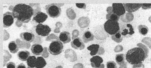

Fig 8.30 Urine and blood in PNH. In this 24h urine sample, the darkest hour is before dawn. Haemolysis occurs throughout the day and night, but the urine concentrated overnight produces the dramatic change in colour.

Courtesy of the Crookston Collection.

5 In haemoglobinuria, urine dipstick will be positive for blood but microscopy of urine does not show RBCs (thus differentiating it from haematuria, but not myoglobinuria—where CK ± AST will be high).

8 Haematology

Haemolysis is the premature breakdown of RBCs, before their normal lifespan of ~120d. It usually happens in the reticuloendothelial system, ie macrophages of liver, spleen, and bone marrow (*extravascular*), or less commonly in the circulation. In sickle cell anaemia, lifespan may be only 5d. Haemolysis may be asymptomatic, but if the bone marrow does not compensate sufficiently, a haemolytic anaemia results.

An approach is first to confirm haemolysis and then find the cause—try to answer these four questions:

1 **Is there evidence of increased red cell breakdown?**
   • Anaemia with normal or ↑MCV.
   • ↑Bilirubin: unconjugated, from haem breakdown (pre-hepatic jaundice).
   • ↑Urinary urobilinogen (no urinary conjugated bilirubin).
   • ↑Serum LDH, as it is released from red cells.

2 **Is there increased red cell production?**
   • ↑Reticulocytes, causing ↑MCV (reticulocytes are large immature RBCs) and polychromasia—ensure not related to recent bleeding or EPO treatment etc.

3 **Is the haemolysis mainly extra- or intravascular?**
   Extravascular haemolysis may lead to splenic hypertrophy and splenomegaly. Features of intravascular haemolysis are:
   • ↑Free plasma haemoglobin: released from RBCs.
   • Methaemalbuminaemia: some free Hb is broken down in the circulation to produce haem and globin; haem combines with albumin to make methaemalbumin.
   • ↓Plasma haptoglobin: mops up free plasma Hb, then removed by the liver.
   • Haemoglobinuria: causes red-brown urine, in absence of red blood cells.
   • Haemosiderinuria: occurs when haptoglobin-binding capacity is exceeded, and free Hb is filtered in glomeruli, with absorption of free Hb via the renal tubules and storage in the tubular cells as haemosiderin. This is detected in the urine in sloughed tubular cells by Prussian blue staining ~1 week after onset (implying a chronic intravascular haemolysis). Free haemoglobin or haeme in the circulation can cause an AKI, trigger DIC, and increase risk of clotting.

4 **Why is there haemolysis?** Causes are on p334. ▶ Life-threatening ones that require urgent identification include acute transfusion reaction, DIC, or thrombotic thrombocytopenic purpura (TTP). The direct antiglobulin (Coombs) test (DAT, fig 8.31) identifies red cells coated with antibody or complement, the presence of which indicates an immune cause.

History Family history, race, jaundice, dark urine, drugs, previous anaemia, travel.

Examination Jaundice, hepatosplenomegaly, gallstones (pigmented, due to ↑bilirubin from haemolysis), leg ulcers (due to poor blood flow).

Tests FBC, reticulocytes, bilirubin, LDH, haptoglobin, urinary urobilinogen. Thick and thin films for malaria screen if history of travel. The blood film may show polychromasia and macrocytosis due to reticulocytes, or point to the diagnosis:
• Hypochromic microcytic anaemia (thalassaemia).
• Sickle cells (sickle cell anaemia).
• Schistocytes (fig 8.33, p335; TTP, haemolytic uraemic syndrome (HUS), or other cause of microangiopathic haemolytic anaemia).
• Abnormal cells in haematological malignancy.
• Spherocytes (hereditary spherocytosis or autoimmune haemolytic anaemia).
• Elliptocytes (fig 8.39, p335; hereditary elliptocytosis).
• Heinz bodies, 'bite' cells (fig 8.35, p335; glucose-6-phosphate dehydrogenase deficiency).

Further tests (if the cause is still not obvious)
• Osmotic fragility testing will confirm the presence of membrane abnormalities which have been identified on the film, eg in hereditary spherocytosis.
• Hb electrophoresis will detect haemoglobinopathies.
• Enzyme assays are reserved for when other causes have been excluded.
• Paroxysmal nocturnal haemoglobinuria (PNH) test by flow cytometry of peripheral blood (p334).

Direct Coombs test/Direct antiglobulin test

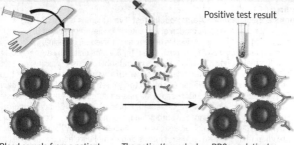

Positive test result

Blood sample from a patient with immune mediated haemolytic anaemia: antibodies are shown attached to antigens on the RBC surface.

The patient's washed RBCs are incubated with antihuman antibodies (Coombs reagent).

RBCs agglutinate: antihuman antibodies form links between RBCs by binding to the human antibodies on the RBCs.

Indirect Coombs test/Indirect antiglobulin test

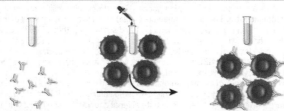

Recipient's serum is obtained, containing antibodies (Ig's).

Donor's blood sample is added to the tube with serum.

Recipient's Ig's that target the donor's red blood cells form antibody-antigen complexes.

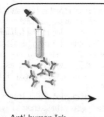

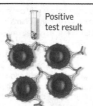

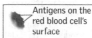

Positive test result

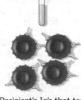

	Antigens on the red blood cell's surface
Y	Human anti-RBC antibody
Y	Antihuman antibody (Coombs reagent)

Anti-human Ig's (Coombs antibodies) are added to the solution.

Agglutination of red blood cells occurs, because human Ig's are attached to red blood cells.

Fig 8.31 The *direct* Coombs test detects antibodies on RBCs. The *indirect* Coombs test is used in prenatal testing and before blood transfusion. It detects antibodies against RBCs that are free in serum—serum is incubated with RBCs of known antigenicity. If agglutination occurs, the indirect Coombs test is positive.

With kind permission of Aria Rad.

8 Haematology

Acquired

1 **Immune-mediated/direct antiglobulin test +ve** (Coombs test, p333.)
  - *Drug-induced:* causing formation of RBC autoantibodies from binding to RBC membranes (eg penicillin) or production of immune complexes (eg quinine).
  - *Autoimmune haemolytic anaemia (AIHA; fig 8.32):* mediated by autoantibodies causing mainly extravascular haemolysis and spherocytosis. Classify according to optimal binding temperature to RBCs: *warm AIHA:* IgG-mediated, bind at body T° 37°C. *R:* steroids/rituximab (± splenectomy if refractory to medical therapy). Crossmatching is difficult because of pan-agglutinating Abs. ►Use closest match possible. *Cold AIHA:* IgM-mediated, bind at ↓T° (<4°C), activating cell-surface complement. Causes a chronic anaemia made worse by cold, often with Raynaud's or acrocyanosis. *R:* keep warm. Chlorambucil may help. *Causes:* most are idiopathic; 2° causes of warm AIHA include lymphoproliferative disease (CLL, lymphoma), drugs (eg methyldopa), autoimmune disease (eg SLE). Cold AIHA may follow infection (mycoplasma; EBV).
  - *Paroxysmal cold haemoglobinuria:* seen with viruses/syphilis. It is caused by Donath–Landsteiner antibodies sticking to RBCs in the cold, causing self-limiting complement-mediated haemolysis on rewarming.
  - *Isoimmune:* acute transfusion reaction (p345); haemolysis of the newborn.
2 **Direct antiglobulin/Coombs −ve AIHA** (2% of all AIHA.) Autoimmune hepatitis; hepatitis B & C; post flu and other vaccinations (piperacillin, rituximab).
3 **Microangiopathic haemolytic anaemia (MAHA)** Mechanical damage to RBCs in circulation, causing intravascular haemolysis and schistocytes (figs 8.33, 8.31). Causes include haemolytic uraemic syndrome (HUS), TTP (p311), DIC, pre-eclampsia, and eclampsia. Prosthetic heart valves can also cause mechanical damage.
4 **Infection** Malaria (p412): RBC lysis and 'blackwater fever' (haemoglobinuria). ►All infections can exacerbate haemolysis.
5 **Paroxysmal nocturnal haemoglobinuria** Very rare acquired stem cell disorder, with chronic haemolysis (esp. at night→haemoglobinuria, fig 8.30, p331), marrow failure + thrombophilia (can cause both arterial and venous clots). *Tests:* urinary haemosiderin +ve; if suspect in Coombs −ve intravascular haemolysis, seek confirmation by flow cytometry (absence of CD55 & CD59). *R:* anticoagulation; monoclonal anticomplement antibodies (eg eculizumab); stem cell transplantation.

Hereditary

1 **Enzyme defects**
  - *Glucose-6-phosphate dehydrogenase (G6PD) deficiency (X-LINKED):* the chief RBC enzyme defect, affects 100 million (mainly ♂) in Mediterranean, Africa, Middle/Far East. Most are asymptomatic, but may get oxidative crises due to ↓glutathione production, precipitated by drugs (eg primaquine, sulfonamides, aspirin), exposure to *Vicia faba* (broad beans/favism), or illness. In attacks, there is rapid anaemia and jaundice. Film: bite- and blister-cells (figs 8.35, 8.33). *Tests:* enzyme assay (>8wks after crisis as young RBCs may have enough enzyme so results normal). *R:* avoid precipitants (eg henna, fig 8.37); transfuse if severe.
  - *Pyruvate kinase deficiency (AUTOSOMAL RECESSIVE):* ↓ATP production causes ↓RBC survival. Homozygotes have neonatal jaundice; later, haemolysis with splenomegaly ± jaundice. *Tests:* enzyme assay. *R:* often not needed; splenectomy may help.
2 **Membrane defects** All are Coombs −ve and need folate; splenectomy may help.
  - *Hereditary spherocytosis (AUTOSOMAL DOMINANT):* prevalence: 1:3000. Less deformable spherical RBCs, so trapped in spleen→extravascular haemolysis. *Signs:* splenomegaly, jaundice. *Tests:* mild if Hb >110g/L and reticulocytes <6%; film: fig 8.38. ↑ Bilirubin (→gallstones). Confirm with eosin-5-maleimide binding test by flow cytometry. *R:* folic acid, splenectomy (limits haemolysis).
  - *Hereditary elliptocytosis (AUTOSOMAL DOMINANT):* film: fig 8.39. Mostly asymptomatic (somewhat protects from malaria). 10% display a more severe phenotype (± death *in utero*).
  - *Hereditary ovalocytosis and stomatocytosis* are rarer. Refer to a haematologist.
3 **Haemoglobinopathy** • *Sickle cell disease* (p336). • *Thalassaemia* (p338).

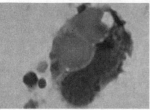

Fig 8.32 Autoimmune haemolytic anaemia: antibody-coated red cells undergoing phagocytosis by monocytes.

© Prof. C Lawrence.

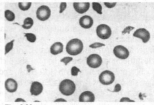

Fig 8.33 Microangiopathic anaemia, eg from DIC: numerous cell fragments (schistocytes) are present.

From the *New England Journal of Medicine*, Bain, B, 'Diagnosis from the blood smear', 353(5), 498. Copyright © 2005 Massachusetts Medical Society. Reprinted with permission from Massachusetts Medical Society.

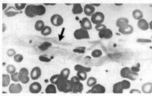

Fig 8.34 Fibrin strands, deposited in HUS and TTP (p311), slicing up RBCs (microangiopathy).

From the *New England Journal of Medicine*, Bain, B, 'Diagnosis from the blood smear', 353(5), 498. Copyright © 2005 Massachusetts Medical Society. Reprinted with permission from Massachusetts Medical Society.

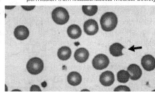

Fig 8.35 A bite-cell in G6PD, after removal of a Heinz body by the spleen; these are formed from denatured Hb during oxidative crises.

From the *New England Journal of Medicine*, Bain, B, 'Diagnosis from the blood smear', 353(5), 498. Copyright © 2005 Massachusetts Medical Society. Reprinted with permission from Massachusetts Medical Society.

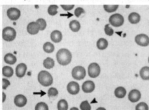

Fig 8.36 Blister-cells (arrows) in G6PD, following removal of Heinz bodies. Also contracted red cells (arrowheads).

From the *New England Journal of Medicine*, Bain, B, 'Diagnosis from the blood smear', 353(5), 498. Copyright © 2005 Massachusetts Medical Society. Reprinted with permission from Massachusetts Medical Society.

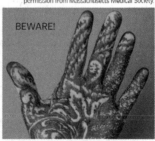

Fig 8.37 Avoid henna use in G6PD deficiency!
© Catherine Cartwright-Jones (artist) and Roy Jones (photographer).

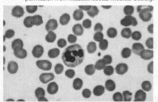

Fig 8.38 Hereditary spherocytosis. Osmotic fragility tests: RBCs show ↑fragility in hypotonic solutions.

From the *New England Journal of Medicine*, Bain, B, 'Diagnosis from the blood smear', 353(5), 498. Copyright © 2005 Massachusetts Medical Society. Reprinted with permission from Massachusetts Medical Society.

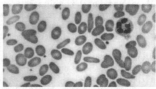

Fig 8.39 Hereditary elliptocytosis.

From the *New England Journal of Medicine*, Bain, B, 'Diagnosis from the blood smear', 353(5), 498. Copyright © 2005 Massachusetts Medical Society. Reprinted with permission from Massachusetts Medical Society.

Sickle cell anaemia is an autosomal recessive disorder in which production of abnormal haemoglobin results in haemolysis and vaso-occlusive crises. It is most commonly seen in people of African and African-Caribbean ethnicity, and arises from an amino acid substitution in the gene coding for the β chain (Glu→Val at position 6) leading to production of HbS rather than HbA (HbA$_2$ and HbF are still produced). Homozygotes (ss) have sickle cell *anaemia* (HbSS), and heterozygotes (HbAS) have sickle cell *trait*, which causes no disability (and protects from *falciparum* malaria). Heterozygotes may still, however, experience symptomatic sickling in hypoxia, eg in unpressurized aircraft or anaesthesia (so all those of African descent need a pre-op sickle cell test).

Pathogenesis HbS polymerizes when deoxygenated, causing RBCs to deform, producing sickle cells, which are fragile and haemolyse, and also block small vessels.

Prevalence 1 out of every 2000 live births in the UK. Approximately 8% of black people carry the sickle cell gene.

Tests Haemolysis is variable. Hb ≈ 60–90g/L, ↑reticulocytes 10–20%, ↑bilirubin. *Film:* sickle cells and target cells (fig 8.40). *Sickle solubility test:* +ve, but does not distinguish between HbSS and HbAS. *Hb electrophoresis:* confirms the diagnosis and distinguishes ss, as states, and other Hb variants. ►Aim for diagnosis *at birth* (cord blood) to aid prompt pneumococcal prophylaxis (vaccine, p169 ± penicillin v).

Signs/symptoms Chronic haemolysis is usually well tolerated (except in crises; see BOX 'Managing sickle cell crises').

Vaso-occlusive 'painful' crisis Common, due to microvascular occlusion. Often affects the marrow, causing severe pain, triggered by cold, volume depletion, infection, or hypoxia. Hands and feet are affected if <3yrs old leading to *dactylitis*. Occlusion may cause *mesenteric ischaemia*, mimicking an acute abdomen. *Acute chest syndrome* (p337) and *multi-organ failure* (ischaemia/infarction in multiple organ systems) are life-threatening complications. CNS infarction occurs in ~10% of children, leading to *stroke, seizures,* or *cognitive defects.* Transcranial Doppler ultrasonography (in <16yr-olds) indicates risk of impending stroke, and blood transfusions can prevent this by reducing HbS. Also *avascular necrosis* (eg of femoral head), *leg ulcers* (fig 8.41) and low-flow *priapism* (also seen in CML, may respond to hydration, α-agonists, eg phenylephrine, or aspiration of blood + irrigation with saline)

Aplastic crisis This is due to parvovirus B19, with sudden reduction in marrow production, especially RBCs. Usually self-limiting <2wks; transfusion may be needed.

Sequestration crisis Mainly affects children as in adults the spleen becomes atrophic. There is pooling of blood in the spleen ± liver, with organomegaly, severe anaemia, and shock. Urgent transfusion is needed.

Complications • Splenic infarction occurs before 2yrs old, due to microvascular occlusion, leading to functional asplenia and ↑susceptibility to infection (40% of childhood sickle deaths are caused this way). • Poor growth. • Renal infarction, papillary necrosis, CKD. • Gallstones. • Retinal disease. • Iron overload (see BOX 'A 7-year-old tells us what it's like to have sickle cell disease'). • Asthma/obstructive lung disease. • Pulmonary hypertension. • Cardiomyopathy. • Hepatotoxicity. • Osteoporosis.

Management of chronic disease ►Should be managed by a haematologist.
• Folic acid, iron-free multivitamin ± vitamin D and calcium.
• Hydroxycarbamide if frequent crises (↑production of fetal haemoglobin, HbF). Dose example: 20mg/kg/d if eGFR >60mL/min. Iron chelator if chronic transfusions and iron overload.
• Antibiotic (phenoxymethylpenicillin) prophylaxis and immunizations against encapsulated bacterial infections (p369).
• Febrile children risk septicaemia: repeated admission may be avoided by early-rescue outpatient antibiotics (eg ceftriaxone (eg 2 doses, 50mg/kg IV on days 0 and 1). Consider admission if Hb <50g/L, WCC <5 or >30 × 10⁹/L, T° >40°C, severe pain, volume depletion, lung infiltration. Seek expert advice.
• Bone marrow transplant can be curative but there are significant risks.

Prevention Genetic counselling; prenatal tests (*OHCS* pp274–5). Parental education can help prevent 90% of deaths from sequestration crises.

Managing sickle cell crises

- Give *prompt*, generous analgesia, eg IV opiates (p575). ►Most sickle patients will have a personalized analgesia plan—ask them! ►Seek expert help early.
- Crossmatch blood, check FBC and reticulocyte count.
- Do a septic screen: blood cultures, MSU ± CXR if T°↑ or chest signs.
- Rehydrate with IVI and keep warm. Give O_2 by mask if ↓P_aO_2 or O_2 sats <95%.
- Consider starting antibiotics empirically if T° >38°, unwell, or chest signs.
- Measure PCV, reticulocytes, liver, and spleen size twice daily.
- Give simple blood transfusion if Hb or reticulocytes fall sharply. This helps oxygenation, and is as good as exchange transfusion. Match blood for the blood group antigens Rh(C, D, E) and Kell, to prevent alloantibody formation.
- Exchange transfusion is reserved for those who are rapidly worsening: it is a process where blood is removed and donor blood is given in stages. Indications: severe chest crisis, suspected CNS event, or multiorgan failure—when the proportion of HbS should be reduced to <30%.

The acute chest syndrome Entails pulmonary infiltrates involving complete lung segments, causing pain, fever, tachypnoea, wheeze, and cough. Major cause of mortality. Incidence: ~0.1 episodes/patient/yr. 13% in the landmark Vichinsky study needed ventilation, 11% had CNS symptoms, and 9% of those over 20 years old died. Prodromal painful crisis occurs ~2.5 days before any abnormalities on CXR in 50% of patients. The chief causes of the infiltrates are fat embolism from bone marrow or infection with *Chlamydia*, *Mycoplasma*, or viruses. **R** O_2, analgesia, incentive spirometry, empirical antibiotics (cephalosporin + macrolide) until culture results known. Bronchodilators (eg salbutamol, p164) have proved to be effective in those with wheezing or obstructive pulmonary function at presentation. Blood transfusion (exchange if severe). *Take to ITU if* P_aO_2 *cannot be kept above 9.2kPa (70mmHg) when breathing air.*

Patient-controlled analgesia is a good option if supportive measures and oral analgesia do not control pain. Start with morphine 1mg/kg in 50mL 5% glucose (paediatric dose) and try a rate of 1mL/h, allowing the patient to deliver extra boluses of 1mL when needed. Check respiratory rate and GCS every ¼h + O_2 sats if chest/abdominal pain. Liaise with the local pain service.

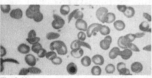
Fig 8.40 Sickle cell film: there are sickle cells, target cells, and a nucleated red cell.
© Prof. C Lawrence.

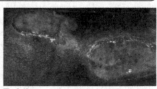
Fig 8.41 Leg ulcers in sickle cell disease.
© Prof. C Lawrence.

A 7-year-old tells us what it's like to have sickle cell disease

'I have been hospitalized over 50 times for complications from this disease. To keep it controlled I started having monthly transfusions. After repeated transfusions my body began to get too much iron so I had to start getting infusions. I was taking the medication desferal[6] which my mummy had to insert a needle in my belly hooked up to a pump which I had to carry on my back in my neat Spiderman backpack. I was hooked up to the machine for 10 hours a day 5 days a week but it was okay I still got to play!!! I suffered from pain crisis which makes my legs and back hurt like someone is hitting me with a hammer.

You may notice that I may move slow or look tired when it is time for my blood transfusion. That is because the transfusions are like a heartbeat for my body, without it I can't survive. When I'm in pain the only thing that helps is morphine... I tell my mummy when she's crying I WILL BE OK!!'

6 This was necessary until a once-daily oral iron chelator came along: deferasirox.

8 Haematology

The thalassaemias are genetic diseases of unbalanced Hb synthesis, with under-production (or no production) of one globin chain (see table 8.2 and BOX 'Structure of haemoglobin'). α thalassaemias and β thalassaemia are characterized by a reduction in α-globin and β-globin chains respectively. Unmatched globins precipitate, damaging RBC membranes, causing their destruction while in the marrow (ineffective erythropoiesis) and circulation (haemolysis). This results in a variable degree of microcytic anaemia and extramedullary haematopoiesis (RBCs made outside the marrow). They are common in the Mediterranean, Africa, and Asia.

The β thalassaemias Usually caused by point mutations in β-globin genes on chromosome 11, leading to ↓β chain production (β⁺) or its absence (β⁰). Various combinations of mutations are possible (eg β⁰/β⁰, β⁺/β⁺, or β⁺/β⁰).

Tests FBC, MCV, MCH (heterozygotes: 25–28pg; homozygotes: <25pg), film, iron studies, HbA₂, HbF, Hb electrophoresis, globin gene test, cardiac MRI.

β thalassaemia minor or trait (eg β/β⁺; heterozygous state): this is a carrier state, and is usually asymptomatic. Mild, well-tolerated anaemia (Hb >90g/L) which may worsen in pregnancy. MCV <75fL, HbA₂ >3.5%, slight ↑HbF.

β thalassaemia intermedia: describes an intermediate state with moderate anaemia but not requiring transfusions. There may be splenomegaly. There are a variety of causes including mild homozygous β thalassaemia mutations, eg β⁺/β⁺, or co-inheritance of β thalassaemia trait with another haemoglobinopathy, eg HbC thalassaemia (one parent has the HbC trait, and the other has β⁺). Sickle cell β⁺ thalassaemia produces a picture similar to sickle cell anaemia.

β thalassaemia major: denotes significant abnormalities in both β-globin genes, and presents in the 1st year, with severe anaemia and failure to thrive. Extramedullary haematopoiesis occurs in response to anaemia, causing characteristic head shape, eg skull bossing (figs 8.42, 8.43) and hepatosplenomegaly (also due to haemolysis). There is osteopenia (may respond to bisphosphonates). Skull x-ray shows a 'hair on end' sign due to ↑marrow activity. Lifelong blood transfusions are needed, with resulting iron overload/deposition. Thalassaemia major and intermedia are also associated with thrombotic risk. The film shows very hypochromic, microcytic cells + target cells + nucleated RBCs. ↑↑HbF, HbA₂ variable, HbA absent.

Treatment ▶Promote fitness; healthy diet. Folic acid supplements help.

- Regular (~2–4 weekly) lifelong transfusions to keep Hb >90g/L, to suppress the ineffective extramedullary haematopoiesis and to allow normal growth. ▶Iron overload is a big problem after ~10yrs causing hypothyroidism, hypocalcaemia, and hypogonadism, cardiac failure, and liver disease. Can be mitigated by iron chelators (desferrioxamine SC twice weekly. SE: pain, deafness, cataracts, retinal damage, ↑risk of *Yersinia* ± deferiprone PO if evidence of cardiac iron overload). Luspatercept is a promising new treatment that appears to reduce transfusion requirement by improving RBC maturation.[3]
- Splenectomy if hypersplenism persists with increasing transfusion requirements (p369)—this is best avoided until >5yrs old due to risk of infections.
- Hormonal replacement or treatment for endocrine complications, eg diabetes mellitus, hypothyroidism. Growth hormone treatment has had variable success.
- A histocompatible marrow transplant can offer the chance of a cure.

The α thalassaemias (fig 8.44) There are two separate α-globin genes on each chromosome 16 ∴ there are four genes (termed αα/αα). The α thalassaemias are mainly caused by gene deletions. If all four α genes are deleted (--/--), death is *in utero* (Bart's hydrops). Here, HbBarts (γ₄) is present, which is physiologically useless. HbH disease occurs if three genes are deleted (--/-α); there may be moderate anaemia and features of haemolysis: hepatosplenomegaly, leg ulcers, and jaundice. The blood film shows formation of β₄ tetramers (= HbH) due to excess β chains, HbBarts, HbA, and HbA₂. If two genes are deleted (--/αα or -α/-α), there is an asymptomatic carrier state (*minor*), with ↓MCV. With one gene deleted, the clinical state is normal.

Structure of haemoglobin

Table 8.2 The three main types of Hb in adult blood[7]

Type	Peptide chains	% in adult blood	% in fetal blood
HbA	$\alpha_2 \beta_2$	97	10–50
HbA2	$\alpha_2 \delta_2$	2.5	Trace
HbF	$\alpha_2 \gamma_2$	0.5	50–90

Adult haemoglobin (HbA) is a tetramer of 2 α- and 2 β-globin chains each containing a haem group. In the first year of life, adult haemoglobin replaces fetal haemoglobin (HbF).

It might be thought that because the molecular details of the thalassaemias are so well worked out they represent a perfect example of the reductionist principle at work: find out *exactly* what is happening *within* molecules, and you will be able to explain all the manifestations of a disease. But this is not so. We have to recognize that two people with the identical mutation at their β loci may have quite different diseases. Co-inheritance of other genes and conditions (eg α thalassaemia) is part of the explanation, as is the efficiency of production of fetal haemoglobin. The reasons lie beyond simple co-segregation of genes promoting the formation of fetal Hb. The rate of proteolysis of excess α-globin chains may also be important— as may mechanisms that have little to do with genetic or molecular events.

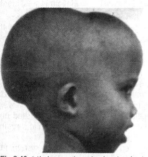

Fig 8.42 β thalassaemia major: bossing due to extramedullary haematopoiesis.

© Dr E van der Enden.

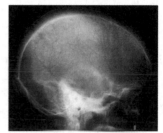

Fig 8.43 β thalassaemia major: skull x-ray.
© Crookston Collection.

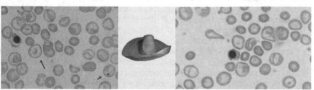

Fig 8.44 α thalassaemia showing target cells (also called Mexican hat cells)—arrow left panel. Note also the teardrop cell on the right panel, and the 2 normoblasts (nucleated red cells, one on each panel). The shorter arrow on the left panel points to a Howell–Jolly body. Note that the cells which are not target cells are rather small (microcytic). There is also poikilocytosis (*poikilos* is Greek for varied—so this simply means that the red blood cells are of varied shape).

Courtesy of Prof. Tangün and Dr Köroğlu.

7 Thalassaemia major and intermedia are characterized by microcytic anaemia and non-immune haemolysis. Hb electrophoresis ± globin gene testing are required to confirm the diagnosis. Hb Barts (gamma chain tetramers) or HbH (beta chain tetramers) are consistent with α thalassaemia; increased HbF or HbA₂ are consistent with a β thalassaemia syndrome but are non-specific.

Primary haemostasis refers to the initial steps in clot formation, which mostly rely on vessel wall and platelet function. Secondary haemostasis refers to the subsequent formation of the fibrin-based clot, which mostly relies on coagulation factors (p341). A bleeding disorder/tendency may be inherited or acquired and affect primary or secondary haemostasis. Evaluation of the patient with bleeding requires a detailed personal and family history, a thorough review of medications, physical examination, and laboratory testing.

History Ask about prior bleeding events and their severity (eg need for nasal packing or cautery), sites (mucocutaneous → platelet or vascular disorder (p342), deep tissues → coagulation disorder, recurrent epistaxis—think of von Willebrand disease (VWD) or HHT, timing (eg delayed bleeding after trauma/surgery suggests coagulation factor disorder or disorder of fibrinolysis), onset (since infancy/childhood in keeping with hereditary condition), easy bruising, history of IDA, menorrhagia (up to 10–30% may have an underlying bleeding disorder) or bleeding associated with pregnancy if female, prolonged bleeding after dental procedures/surgery, any prior medical conditions that may predispose to bleeding (eg liver disease, cancer, CKD, connective tissue disorders), any history of alcohol excess, family history, medications/herbal supplements/OTC (eg antiplatelets, vitamin E, garlic).

Bleeding score May be useful to quantify personal bleeding history. The International Society on Thrombosis and Haemostasis has an online bleeding assessment tool here: https://bleedingscore.certe.nl/

Signs Look for petechiae/purpura/bruises, telangiectasias, splenomegaly, joint hypermobility, murmurs (associated with acquired VWD), macroglossia (rarely occurs with amyloidosis, a cause of acquired coagulation factor deficiencies).

Tests FBC, film (is the platelet morphology normal?), coagulation screen (PT, APTT, INR, fibrinogen), U&E, LFTs for all, with further testing depending on the results of this initial screen. Tests for primary haemostasis include platelet count/morphology ± aggregation studies, VWF antigen and activity, factor VIII activity. Tests for secondary haemostasis include PT, APTT, thrombin time, factor assays. Newer tests of clotting function such as thromboelastography (TEG) are discussed on p775. Certain characteristic clotting screen abnormalities are highlighted in table 8.3.

- **Prothrombin time (PT)** Thromboplastin is added to test the *extrinsic system*. PT is expressed as a ratio compared to control (international normalized ratio (INR), normal range = 0.9–1.2). It tests for abnormalities in factors I, II, V, VII, X. Prolonged by: warfarin, vitamin K deficiency, liver disease, DIC.
- **Activated partial thromboplastin time (APTT)** A contact factor is added to test the *intrinsic system*. Tests for abnormalities in factors I, II, V, VIII, IX, X, XI, XII. Normal range 35–45s. Prolonged by: heparin treatment, haemophilia, DIC, liver disease.
- **Thrombin time** Thrombin is added to plasma to convert fibrinogen to fibrin. Normal range: 10–15s. Prolonged by: heparin treatment, DIC, dysfibrinogenaemia.
- **D-dimers** are a fibrin degradation product, released from cross-linked fibrin during fibrinolysis (p343). This occurs during DIC, or in the presence of venous thromboembolism—deep vein thrombosis (DVT) or pulmonary embolism (PE). D-dimers may also be raised in inflammation, eg with infection or malignancy.

Management Depends on the underlying cause and the degree of bleeding. If shocked, resuscitate (p770). If bleeding continues in the presence of a clotting disorder or a massive transfusion, discuss the need for fresh frozen plasma, cryoprecipitate, factor concentrates, or platelets with a haematologist. In ITP (p343), steroids ± IV immunoglobulin may be used. Especially in pregnancy (OHCS p99), consult an expert. Is there overdose of or need to reverse anticoagulants (p346)? In haemophiliac bleeds, *consult early* for coagulation factor replacement. ►*Never* give IM injections.

Table 8.3 Clotting screen abnormalities in coagulopathies

Disorder	INR	APTT	Thrombin time	Platelet count	Notes
Heparin	↑	↑↑	↑↑	↔	
DIC	↑↑	↑↑	↑↑	↓	↑D-dimer, p340
Liver disease	↑	↑	↔/↑	↔/↓	AST↑
Platelet defect	↔	↔	↔	↔	
Vit κ deficiency	↑↑	↑	↔	↔	
Haemophilia	↔	↑↑	↔	↔	See p342
von Willebrand's	↔	↑↑	↔	↔	See p698

Special tests may be available (factor assays: ►consult a haematologist).

Thrombocytopenia

Platelet count <150 000/microlitre but risk of spontaneous bleeding greatest with counts <10 000/microlitre, and surgical bleeding with counts <50 000/microlitre.

Causes Many: drug-induced, heparin-induced (HIT, p347), sepsis or cancer with DIC, liver disease, pregnancy (gestational, pre-eclampsia, etc.), ITP (p343), TTP, HUS, B_{12}/folate deficiency.

►If thrombocytopenia + thrombosis, consider DIC, HIT, antiphospholipid antibody syndrome or more rarely, paroxysmal nocturnal haemoglobinuria.

Evaluation As per p340—bleeding, past medical history, family history, medications, petechiae/purpura, lymphadenopathy, hepatosplenomegaly.

Tests FBC, film (pseudothrombocytopenia can occur with platelet clumping), coagulation screen, U&E, LFTs ± fibrinogen, haemolysis screen, HIV/HCV testing, ANA, antiphospholipid Abs, B_{12}/folate, bone marrow biopsy as appropriate.

Management Depends on the cause but urgent action (and haematology consult) needed if platelet count <50 000/microlitre, planned invasive procedure, if pregnant, suspected HIT, TTP, HUS, drug-induced thrombotic microangiopathy, acute leukaemia, or aplastic anaemia. Seek expert advice if considering stopping antiplatelets/anticoagulants or planning invasive procedure.

After injury, three processes halt bleeding: vasoconstriction, gap-plugging by platelets, and the coagulation cascade (fig 8.45). Disorders of haemostasis fall into these three groups. The pattern of bleeding is important—vascular and platelet disorders lead to prolonged bleeding from cuts, bleeding into the skin (eg easy bruising and purpura), and bleeding from mucous membranes (eg epistaxis, bleeding from gums, menorrhagia). Coagulation disorders cause delayed bleeding into joints and muscle.

1 **Vascular defects** Congenital Osler–Weber–Rendu syndrome (p694), connective tissue disease (eg Ehlers–Danlos syndrome, OHCS p846, pseudoxanthoma elasticum). **Acquired** Senile purpura, infection (eg meningococcal, measles, dengue fever), steroids, scurvy (perifollicular haemorrhages), Henoch–Schönlein purpura (p307).

2 **Platelet disorders** Decreased marrow production Aplastic anaemia (p348), megaloblastic anaemia, marrow infiltration (eg leukaemia, myeloma), marrow suppression (cytotoxic drugs, radiotherapy). **Excess destruction** *Immune:* immune thrombocytopenia (ITP, see BOX 'Immune thrombocytopenia'), other autoimmune causes, eg SLE, CLL, drugs, eg heparin, viruses; *Non-immune:* DIC (p350), thrombotic thrombocytopenic purpura (TTP), or HUS (p311), sequestration (in hypersplenism). **Poorly functioning platelets** Seen in myeloproliferative disease, NSAIDs, and ↑urea.

3 **Coagulation disorders** Congenital Haemophilia, von Willebrand disease. **Acquired** Anticoagulants, liver disease, DIC (p350), vitamin K deficiency.

Haemophilia A Factor VIII deficiency; inherited in an X-linked recessive pattern in 1:10 000 male births. There is a high rate of new mutations (30% have no family history). **Presentation** depends on severity and is often early in life or after surgery/ trauma—with bleeds into joints leading to crippling arthropathy, and into muscles causing haematomas (↑pressure can lead to nerve palsies and compartment syndrome). ICH is relatively rare but can be life-threatening. **Diagnose** by ↑APTT and ↓factor VIII assay (<40%). **Management** Seek expert advice. Avoid NSAIDs and IM injections (fig 8.46). *Minor bleeding:* pressure and elevation of the part. Desmopressin (0.3mcg/kg/12h IVI over 20min) raises factor VIII levels, and may be sufficient. *Major bleeds* (eg haemarthrosis): ↑factor VIII levels to 50% of normal, eg with recombinant factor VIII. *Life-threatening bleeds* (eg obstructing airway) need levels of 100%. **Genetic counselling** OHCS p274.

Haemophilia B (Christmas disease) Factor IX deficiency (inherited, X-linked recessive); behaves clinically like haemophilia A. *Treat* with recombinant factor IX.

Von Willebrand disease (VWD) Most common inherited haemostatic disorder (up to 1% prevalence). Von Willebrand factor (VWF) has three roles in clotting: 1 To bring platelets into contact with exposed subendothelium. 2 To make platelets bind to each other. 3 To bind to factor VIII, protecting it from destruction in the circulation. There are >22 types of VWD; the commonest are: **Type I** (60–80%) ↓Levels of VWF. Symptoms are mild. Autosomal dominant. **Type II** (20–30%) Abnormal VWF, with lack of high-molecular-weight multimers. Usually autosomal dominant inheritance. Bleeding tendency varies. **Type III** (1–5%) Undetectable VWF levels (autosomal recessive with gene deletions). VWF antigen is lacking and there is ↓factor VIII. Symptoms can be severe. *Signs* bruising, epistaxis, menorrhagia, ↑bleeding post-tooth extraction. **Tests** ↑APTT, ↓factor VIIIC (clotting activity), VWF ↓Ag and activity (functional assay); ↑INR and platelets. *R* Get expert help. Desmopressin is used in mild bleeding, VWF-containing factor VIII concentrate for surgery or major bleeds. Avoid NSAIDs. ↑Risk of postpartum haemorrhage.

Acquired haemophilia often presents with large mucosal bleeds. Caused by suddenly appearing autoantibodies that interfere with factor VIII. **Tests** ↑APTT; ↑VIII autoantibody; factor VIII activity <50%. *R* Steroids.

Liver disease Produces a complicated bleeding disorder with ↓synthesis of clotting factors, ↓absorption of vitamin K, and abnormalities of platelet function.

Malabsorption Leads to less uptake of vitamin K (needed for synthesis of factors II, VII, IX, and X). *Treat* with IV vitamin K (10mg). In acute haemorrhage, use human prothrombin complex or fresh frozen plasma.

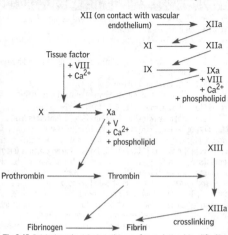

Extrinsic System Intrinsic System

XII (on contact with vascular
endothelium) ⟶ XIIa

XI ⟶ XIIa

Tissue factor
+ VIII
+ Ca²⁺

IX ⟶ IXa
+ VIII
+ Ca²⁺
+ phospholipid

X ⟶ Xa
+ V
+ Ca²⁺
+ phospholipid

XIII

Prothrombin ⟶ Thrombin

XIIIa
crosslinking

Fibrinogen ⟶ Fibrin

Fig 8.45 Intrinsic and extrinsic pathways of coagulation (simplified!).

8 Haematology

Fig 8.46 Mild haemo-
philia after an IM injec-
tion. ►Give vaccines
etc. SC!

© Crookston
Collection 53.

Fibrinolysis

The fibrinolytic system works by generating plasmin, which causes fibrin dissol-ution. The process starts with the release of tissue plasminogen activator (t-PA) from endothelial cells, a process stimulated by fibrin formation. t-PA converts inactive plas-minogen to plasmin which can then cleave fibrin, as well as several other factors. t-PA and plasminogen both bind fibrin thus localizing fibrinolysis to the area of the clot.

Fibrinolytic agents activate this system and can be utilized in order to break down pathological thrombi, eg acute ischaemic stroke, DVT, PE, and central ret-inal venous or arterial thrombosis. In all cases the risk of adverse effects of thrombolysis (eg haemorrhage) must be outweighed by the potential benefits. Streptokinase, a streptococcal exotoxin that binds and activates plasminogen, was the first licensed agent but risks anaphylaxis on repeat dosing. Alteplase is recombinant t-PA. Newer agents include tenecteplase and reteplase.

Immune thrombocytopenia (ITP)

Primary ITP is caused by antiplatelet autoantibodies and autoreactive cytotoxic T cells. There is both platelet destruction and underproduction. It is acute (usu-ally in children, 2wks after infection with sudden self-limiting purpura) or chronic (seen mainly in women). Chronic ITP runs a fluctuating course of bleeding, pur-pura, epistaxis, and menorrhagia. There is no splenomegaly. In secondary ITP, there is an underlying associated condition (eg SLE, HIV) and causes of drug-induced ITP include vancomycin, carbamazepine, etc. **Tests** ↑Megakaryocytes in marrow. Rule out other causes of ↓platelets. **℞** None if mild. If symptomatic or platelets <20 × 10⁹/L, prednisolone 1mg/kg/d and reduce after remission; aim to keep platelets >30 × 10⁹/L—takes a few days to work. Platelet transfusions are not used (except during splenectomy or life-threatening haemorrhage) as these are quickly destroyed by the autoantibodies. IV immunoglobulin may temporarily raise the platelet count, eg for surgery, pregnancy. If relapse or poor response to initial treatment, choices include B-cell depletion with rituximab or splenectomy (wait 12mths before considering as may spontaneously remit). Eltrombopag/avatrombopag and romiplostim are also licensed as second-line therapies that stimulate proliferation and differentiation of megakaryocytes. Vaccine-induced ITP (IVITT) is a rare side effect of certain adenoviral-vectored COVID-19 vaccines that can present with thrombosis (esp. CVST) or thrombocytopenia.

8 Haematology

▶Blood should only be given if strictly necessary *and there is no alternative*. Outcomes may be *worse* after an inappropriate transfusion.
* Know and use local procedures to ensure that the right blood gets to the right patient at the right time.
* Take blood for crossmatching from only one patient at a time. Label immediately. This minimizes risk of wrong labelling of samples.
* When giving blood, monitor T°, pulse, RR, and BP every ½h.
* Use a dedicated line where practicable (or dedicated lumen of multilumen line).

Products[4] **Red cells** (Packed to make haematocrit ~70%.) Use to correct anaemia or blood loss. 1u ↑Hb by 10–15g/L. In anaemia, transfuse until Hb ~80g/L. **Platelets** (p348.) Usually only needed if bleeding or count is <20 × 10⁹/L. 1u should ↑ platelet count by >20 × 10⁹/L. Failure to do so suggests refractory cause: discuss with haematologist. If surgery is planned, get advice if count is <100 × 10⁹/L. **Fresh frozen plasma (FFP)** Use to correct clotting defects: eg DIC (p350); as part of massive transfusion protocol to prevent dilutional coagulopathy; liver disease; thrombotic thrombocytopenic purpura (p311). It is expensive and carries all the risks of blood transfusion. Do not use as a simple volume expander. *Human albumin solution* is produced as 4.5% or 20% protein solution and is used to replace protein. 20% albumin can be used temporarily in the hypoproteinaemic patient (eg liver disease; nephrosis) who is fluid overloaded, without giving an excessive salt load. Also used as replacement in abdominal paracentesis (p749). **Others** Prothrombin complex concentrate (contains factors II, VII, IX, X; for rapid reversal of anticoagulants eg warfarin) Cryoprecipitate (a source of fibrinogen); coagulation concentrates (self-injected in haemophilia); immunoglobulins.

Irradiated blood products To prevent graft-vs-host disease (GVHD) in an immunocompromised host, eg severe T-lymphocyte immunodeficiency syndromes, recipients of allogeneic haemopoietic stem cell transplantation, Hodgkin's lymphoma, those treated with purine analogue drugs (eg fludarabine). Check with Haematology if unsure.

CMV-negative blood Required if pregnant, immunosuppressed, eg bone marrow, stem cell, solid organ recipients, HIV-positive patients.

Complications of transfusion ▶Management of acute reactions[4] see BOX 'Transfusion reactions' and table 84.
* **Early (within 24h)** Acute haemolytic reactions (eg ABO or Rh incompatibility); anaphylaxis (may be due to anti-IgA antibodies in IgA-deficient individuals that react with IgA in the transfusion or due to allergies to another constituent in the transfused product); bacterial contamination (sepsis); febrile reactions (eg from release of cytokines from WBCs in a product that has not been leukoreduced); allergic reactions (itch, urticaria, mild fever); transfusion-associated circulatory overload (TACO; may occur if RBCs given too rapidly or if underlying cardiac disease); transfusion-related acute lung injury (TRALI, ie ARDS due to antileucocyte antibodies in donor plasma; can be life-threatening). TACO more likely than TRALI if no fever, hypertension, diuretic response, cardiac history, older age or large transfusion volume.
* **Delayed (after 24h)** Infections (eg viruses: hepatitis B/C; HIV; bacteria; protozoa; prions); delayed haemolytic reactions, iron overload (treatment, p338); GVHD; post-transfusion purpura—rare but potentially lethal fall in platelet count 5–7d post-transfusion requiring specialist treatment with IVIG and platelet transfusions.

Massive blood transfusion This is defined as replacement of an individual's entire blood volume (>10u) within 24h. Complications: ↓platelets; ↓Ca²⁺; ↓clotting factors; ↑K⁺; hypothermia. ▶For emergency management, see p774. Seek early & ongoing support from haematologist & blood bank who should advise on products and monitoring. In acute haemorrhage, use crossmatched blood if possible, but if not, use 'universal donor' group O Rh–ve blood, changing to crossmatched blood as soon as possible.

Transfusing patients with heart failure Give each unit over 3–4h with furosemide (eg 40mg slow IV/PO; don't mix with blood) with alternate units. Check for ↑JVP and basal lung crackles; consider CVP line.

Acute transfusion reactions

All UK blood products are now leucocyte-depleted (white cells <5 × 10⁶/L) to reduce the incidence of complications such as alloimmunization to HLA class I antigens and febrile transfusion reactions. Consider an acute transfusion reaction if adverse symptoms/signs within 24h though many happen within the first 15 minutes. Initially **STOP** transfusion. Ensure IV access, correct product for patient, examine for fever, hypo/hypertension, respiratory distress, urticaria, angioedema. ►Get senior help in all cases. Significant ↓BP suggestive of acute haemolytic reaction, TRALI, and sepsis. Remember isolated fever may be related to a pre-existing diagnosis of sepsis (get history, look at temperature trend).

Table 8.4 Management of transfusion reactions

Acute haemolytic reaction (eg ABO incompatibility) Agitation, ↑T° (rapid onset), ↓BP, flushing, abdominal/chest pain, oozing venepuncture sites, DIC	**STOP** transfusion. Check identity and name on unit; tell haematologist; send unit + FBC, U&E, clotting, cultures, & urine (haemoglobinuria) to lab. Keep IV line open with crystalloids. Treat DIC (p350)
Anaphylaxis Bronchospasm, cyanosis, ↓BP, soft tissue swelling	**STOP** the transfusion. Maintain airway and give oxygen. Adrenaline, antihistamines, pressors. Contact anaesthetist. ►See p776
Bacterial contamination (transfusion-associated sepsis) ↑T° (rapid onset), ↓BP, and rigors	**STOP** the transfusion. Check identity against name on unit; tell haematologist and send unit + FBC, U&E, clotting, cultures & urine to lab. Start broad-spectrum antibiotics
Transfusion-related lung injury (TRALI) (See p344.) Dyspnoea, cough, fever; CXR 'white out'	**STOP** the transfusion. Give 100% O₂. ►Treat as ARDS, p178. Donor should be removed from donor panel
Non-haemolytic febrile transfusion reaction Dx of exclusion. More common with PLTs. Shivering and fever usually ½–1h after starting transfusion	**SLOW** or **STOP** the transfusion. Give an antipyretic, eg paracetamol 1g. Monitor closely. If recurrent, use WBC filter
Urticarial transfusion reaction Common (1–3%) Urticaria and itch	**SLOW** or **STOP** the transfusion; chlorphenamine 10mg slow IV/IM. Monitor closely
Transfusion-associated circulatory overload (TACO) Dyspnoea, hypoxia, tachycardia, ↑JVP, and basal crepitations. No fever	**SLOW** or **STOP** the transfusion. Give oxygen and a diuretic, eg furosemide 40mg IV initially. Consider CVP line

Blood transfusion and Jehovah's Witnesses

Adult human beings (with mental 'capacity', see p566) have an absolute right to refuse any medical treatment, even if to do so seems illogical or could result in their death. To treat patients despite such a refusal would amount to battery under common law, or could even amount to a degrading act or torture, against which the European Convention on Human Rights gives absolute, inalienable protection.

The biblical verse *'no soul of you shall eat blood'* (Leviticus 17:12) is one of several that have been interpreted by some religious groups to extend to acceptance of blood products in a medical context. Jehovah's Witnesses, for example, may refuse potentially vital blood transfusions on such grounds. These views must be respected, but complex issues arise if the patient is a child, or an adult who may not be able to give or withhold consent in an informed way. In an immediately life-threatening situation where further delay may cause harm, treatment such as blood products may be given in the child's best interest, but the team should always involve senior paediatricians and hospital ethicists where practical. If the requirement is less immediate, then the clinicians should seek further legal advice, which might involve approaching the Courts.

8 Haematology

8 Haematology

Main indications (See p573 if need to stop/hold prior to procedure.)
- **Therapeutic**   Venous thromboembolic disease (VTE)—DVT/PE, ACS.
- **Prophylactic**   Prevention of DVT/PE in high-risk patients (p371), eg post-op.
                      Prevention of stroke, eg in chronic AF or prosthetic heart valves.

Heparin 1 **Low-molecular-weight heparin (LMWH)** Eg dalteparin, enoxaparin, tinzaparin. The preferred option in the prevention and initial treatment of VTE. LMWH is also the anticoagulant of choice in malignancy and pregnancy. Inactivates factor Xa (but not thrombin). $t\frac{1}{2}$ is 2- to 4-fold longer than standard heparin, and response is more predictable: only needs to be given once or twice daily SC, and laboratory monitoring is usually not required except in pregnancy, kidney failure, or extremes of body weight. See BNF for doses and for adjustments (accumulates in CKD).

2 **Unfractionated heparin (UFH)** Used where close monitoring of therapeutic anti-coagulation is required, eg perioperatively. IV or SC. Binds antithrombin (an endogenous inhibitor of coagulation), increasing its ability to inhibit thrombin, factor Xa, and IXa. Rapid onset and has a short $t\frac{1}{2}$. Monitor and adjust dose with APTT (p340).

SE **for both** ↑Bleeding (eg at operative site, gastrointestinal, intracranial), heparin-induced thrombocytopenia (HIT, see BOX), osteoporosis with long-term use. HIT and osteoporosis are less common with LMWH than UFH. Beware hyperkalaemia.

CI Bleeding disorders, platelets <50 × 10⁹/L, previous HIT, peptic ulcer, cerebral haemorrhage, severe hypertension, neurosurgery. ►However, always check with someone senior if truly contraindicated in the individual context.

DOACs (Direct oral anticoagulants.) Rivaroxaban, apixaban, and edoxaban (factor Xa inhibitors), and dabigatran (a direct thrombin inhibitor). ►Generally first-line agents now as they are at least as effective as warfarin with lower bleeding/mortality rates, no regular monitoring required, and fewer drug interactions (notable exceptions include metal valves, valvular AF, or APLS). Do a bi-annual U&E to monitor kidney function (apixaban preferable in advanced CKD as it is less dependent on kidney function for clearance than other DOACs). CI Severe kidney/liver impairment; active bleeding; lesion at risk of bleeding; ↓clotting factors.

Warfarin Used PO OD as long-term anticoagulation. The therapeutic range is narrow, varying with the condition being treated (see BOX 'Warfarin guidelines and target levels for INR')—and effects are reflected in the INR. Warfarin inhibits the reductase enzyme responsible for regenerating the active form of vitamin K, producing a state analogous to vitamin K deficiency. CI Peptic ulcer, bleeding disorders, severe hypertension, pregnancy (teratogenic, see OHCS p844). Use with caution in elderly and those with past GI bleeds. ►Interactions: p741.

Beginning therapeutic anticoagulation (Follow local guidelines, and see BNF.) For treatment of VTE, LMWH or UFH are typically used initially. Treatment doses of FXa inhibitors can also be used. When transitioning to a DOAC, switch from heparin (ie do not co-administer DOAC and heparin). If transitioning to warfarin, give heparin in combination (as early as day 1) and continue until INR is in target therapeutic range on 2 consecutive days (see BOX 'Warfarin dosage'). If starting warfarin, check INR on day 3 (it takes 48–72h for anticoagulant effect to develop). Adjust subsequent doses according to the INR (see table 8.5).

Antidotes If UFH/LMWH overdose: stop infusion. If there is bleeding, protamine sulfate counteracts heparin: discuss with a haematologist. Warfarin: see BOX 'Warfarin dosage' and table 8.6. DOACs: stop anticoagulant, assess severity and timing of last dose, baseline coag/FBC/U&E, plasma drug levels if available, localization and management of specific bleeding site, 5g IV bolus dose idarucizumab (humanized monoclonal antibody fragment that binds dabigatran) indicated for dabigatran reversal if emergency surgery planned, life-threatening or uncontrolled bleeding. Andexanet alfa, a 'decoy' recombinant FXa molecule, is an FDA-approved reversal agent for FXa inhibitors in similar circumstances that has not yet been approved in Europe (↑ thrombotic risk). Consider haemodialysis and prothrombin complex concentrate (PCC) if idarucizumab and andexanet alfa not available, respectively.

Warfarin guidelines and target levels for INR

- Pulmonary embolism and DVT. Aim for INR of 2–3; 3.5 if recurrent PE or DVT whilst anticoagulated.
- Atrial fibrillation: for stroke prevention (p126). Target INR 2–3.
- Prosthetic metallic heart valves: for stroke prevention. Target INR 2–3 if aortic valve or 2.5–3.5 if mitral valve.

Duration of anticoagulation in DVT/PE First episodes of DVT or PE require at least 3 months of anticoagulation. Consider extending this to 6 months in patients with more extensive, life-threatening clot at presentation, for those with transient but persistent risk factors (eg prolonged immobility) or if evidence of persistent clot at 3 months. For those with recurrent unprovoked emboli or underlying thrombophilia (p370), consider bleeding risks against benefits of indefinite treatment.

Warfarin dosage and what to do when the INR is much too high

Below is a rough guide to warfarin dosing for target INR of 2–3. An INR needs to be measured on alternate days until stable, then weekly or less often.

Table 8.5 Suggested dosing for day 3 of warfarin loading

INR	<2	2	2.5	2.9	3.3	3.6	4.1
3rd dose	5mg	5mg	4mg	3mg	2mg	0.5mg	0mg
Maintenance	≥6mg	5.5mg	4.5mg	4mg	3.5mg	3mg	*

*Miss a dose; give 1–2mg the next day; if INR >4.5, miss 2 doses.

Table 8.6 When the INR is much too high (see also *BNF*)

INR 5–8, no bleed	Withhold 1–2 doses. Restart warfarin at a lower maintenance dose once INR <5
INR 5–8, minor bleed*	Stop warfarin and admit for urgent IV vitamin K (give slowly). Restart warfarin when INR <5
INR >8, no bleed	Stop warfarin and seek haematology advice
INR >8, minor bleed*	Stop warfarin and admit for urgent IV vitamin K. Check INR daily—repeat vitamin K if INR too high after 24h. Restart warfarin at a lower dose when INR <5
Any major bleed (including intracranial haemorrhage)	Stop warfarin. Give prothrombin complex concentrate 50 units/kg (if unavailable, give FFP 15mL/kg ≈ 1L for a 70kg man) and 5–10mg vitamin K IV. Discuss with haematologist

* Minor bleeding includes epistaxis.

Vitamin K may take several hours to work and can cause prolonged resistance when restarting warfarin, so should be avoided if possible when long-term anticoagulation is needed. Prothrombin complex concentrate contains a concentrate of factors II, VII, IX, and X and provides a more complete and rapid reversal of warfarin than FFP.

Heparin-induced thrombocytopenia (HIT)

Potentially life-threatening complication resulting from exposure to LMWH or UFH. Autoantibodies to platelet factor 4 complexed with heparin develop and cause thrombocytopenia and thrombosis by peripheral platelet consumption and activation, respectively. **Risk factors** UFH > LMWH, post-op, higher heparin doses, female sex. **Presentation** ↓Platelets, thrombosis (in 50%; venous > arterial). **Management** Calculate the 4 Ts (severity of thrombocytopenia, timing of platelet count drop, presence of thrombosis, and absence of other causes of thrombocytopenia) score to estimate the likelihood of HIT. If the score = 0–3, then there is a low probability of HIT—heparin should not be held, antibody testing should not be done, and other causes of thrombocytopenia should be considered (p343). If the score is >3, heparin should be stopped, a non-heparin anticoagulant (eg argatroban, bivalirudin) should be given, and HIT antibody should be sent. For patients with confirmed HIT, non-heparin anticoagulation is continued; the duration depends on whether or not there has been a thrombotic event.

Bone marrow is responsible for haematopoiesis. In adults, this normally takes place in the central skeleton (vertebrae, sternum, ribs, skull) and proximal long bones. In some anaemias (eg thalassaemia), increased demand induces haematopoiesis beyond the marrow (extramedullary haematopoiesis), in liver and spleen, causing organomegaly. All blood cells arise from an early pluripotent stem cell, which divides asymmetrically to produce another stem cell and a progenitor cell committed to a lineage (fig 847). Committed progenitors further differentiate into myeloid or lymphocyte lineages, releasing their progeny into the blood.

Pancytopenia Reduction in all the major cell lines: red cells, white cells, and platelets. Causes are due to: **1 ↓Marrow production** Aplastic anaemia (see BOX), infiltration (eg acute leukaemia, myelodysplasia, myeloma, lymphoma, solid tumours, TB), megaloblastic anaemia, myelofibrosis (p362). **2 ↑Peripheral destruction** Hypersplenism.

Agranulocytosis Implies that granulocytes (WBCs with neutrophil, basophil, or eosinophil granules) have stopped being made, leaving the patient at risk of fatal infections. Many drugs can be the culprit: eg carbimazole, procainamide, sulfonamides, gold, clozapine, dapsone. ►When starting drugs known to cause agranulocytosis, warn patients to report *any* fever. Neutropenia (WCC $\leq 0.5 \times 10^9$/L) may declare itself initially as a sore throat. Stop the drug, commence neutropenic regimen, & consider granulocyte colony stimulating factor (G-CSF) if indicated (p350).

Marrow support Red cells survive for ~120d, platelets for ~8d, and neutrophils for 1–2d, so early problems are mainly from neutropenia and thrombocytopenia.

1 **Red cell transfusion** Transfusing 1U should raise Hb by ~10–15g/L (p344). Transfusion may drop the platelet count (you may need to give platelets before or after).

2 **Platelets** Traumatic bleeds, purpura, and easy bruising occur if platelets $<50 \times 10^9$/L. Spontaneous bleeding may occur if platelets $<20 \times 10^9$/L, with intracranial haemorrhage rarely. Platelets are stored at room temperature (22°C; not in the fridge). In marrow transplant or if severely immunosuppressed, platelets may need irradiation before use to prevent transfusion-associated GVHD. Platelets must be ABO compatible. They are not used in ITP (p343). Indications: • Platelets $<20 \times 10^9$/L. • Haemorrhage (eg DIC, p350). • Before invasive procedures (eg biopsy, lumbar puncture) to increase count to $>50 \times 10^9$/L. 4U of platelets should raise the count to $>40 \times 10^9$/L in adults; check dose needed with lab.

3 **Neutrophils** Use neutropenic regimen if the count $<0.5 \times 10^9$/L (p350).

Bone marrow biopsy Gives diagnostic information where there are abnormalities in the peripheral blood; it is also an important staging test in the lymphoproliferative disorders. Ideally take an aspirate *and* trephine usually from the posterior iliac crest (aspirates can be taken from the anterior iliac crest or sternum). The aspirate provides a film which is examined by microscope. The trephine is a core of bone which allows assessment of bone marrow cellularity, architecture, and the presence of infiltrative disease (eg neoplasia). Coagulation disorders may need to be corrected pre-biopsy. Apply pressure afterwards (lie on that side for 1–2h if platelets are low).

Aplastic anaemia

This is a rare (~5 cases per million/year) stem cell disorder in which bone marrow stops making cells, leading to pancytopenia. Presents with features of anaemia (↓Hb), infection (↓WCC), or bleeding (↓platelets). **Causes** Most cases are autoimmune, triggered by drugs (eg cytotoxic agents, carbimazole, sulfonamides), viruses (eg parvovirus, hepatitis), or irradiation. May also be inherited, eg Fanconi anaemia (p331). **Tests** Bone marrow biopsy is diagnostic (profoundly hypocellular). **Treatment** Mainly supportive in asymptomatic patients. Treat the underlying cause where possible. Transfuse blood products as required and initiate neutropenic regimen if count $<0.5 \times 10^9$/L (p350). The treatment of choice in young patients with severe disease is allogeneic marrow transplantation from an HLA-matched sibling, which can be curative. Otherwise, immunosuppression with ciclosporin and antithymocyte globulin ± eltrombopag may be effective, although it is not curative in most. Eltrombopag is first line for refractory disease.

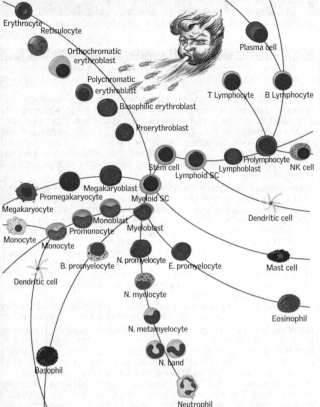

Fig 8.47 *Haematopoiesis and Sod's law.* When we contemplate a diagram like this (of seemingly galactic complexity) we, being doctors, think 'What can go wrong?' With a sinking feeling we realize that every arc is an opportunity for multiple disasters. Perhaps, using our own ingenuity, we might occasionally complete these pathways without Sod intervening (Sod's law states that if something can go wrong, it will—here Sod's tubercular breath is seen blowing the red cell line off course—TB is a famous cause of leukoerythroblastic anaemia). When we realize that *every day* each of us makes 175 billion red cells, 70 billion granulocytes, and 175 billion platelets we sense that Sod is smiling to himself with especial relish. *Anything* can go wrong. *Everything* can go wrong. This latter we call *aplastic anaemia.* *Agranulocytosis* is when the Southerly arcs go wrong; thrombocytopenia when the West-pointing arcs go wrong. To the East we have the *lymphocytes* and their B- and T-cell complexities. *Anaemia* lies in the North of this diagram. And as for bleeding—how could our predecessors bear to waste a single drop of this stuff on purpose? Our minds are reeling at 175 billion red cells per day—but this is just when the system is idling. When we bleed, throughput can rise by an order of magnitude—if Sod is turning a blind eye are there sufficient haematinics (eg iron, B$_{12}$, and folate) to allow maximum haemopoiesis?

Figure © Aria Rad.

Leukaemia divides into four main types depending on the cell line involved (table 8.7).

Table 8.7 Principal subtypes of leukaemia

	Lymphoid	Myeloid
Acute	Acute lymphoblastic leukaemia (ALL)	Acute myeloid leukaemia (AML)
Chronic	Chronic lymphocytic leukaemia (CLL)	Chronic myeloid leukaemia (CML)

These patients (esp. AML) fall ill suddenly and deteriorate fast, eg with: ▶infection (beware neutropenia, see BOX 'Neutropenia'), ▶bleeding (℞: platelets), and ▶hyperviscosity (p368) and thus, early involvement of their haematologist is essential. Take non-specific confusion/drowsiness or just 'I feel a bit ill today' *seriously*: do blood cultures, FBC, U&E, LFT, Ca²⁺, glucose, and clotting. Consider CNS bleeding—CT if in doubt. With any new patient, find out the agreed aim of treatment: cure; prolonging disease-free survival; or palliation with minimal toxicity? Direct your efforts accordingly; get help if lack of clarity here.

Neutropenic sepsis regimen (For when T° >38°C + neutrophil count ≤0.5 × 10⁹/L.)ˢ ▶Close liaison with a microbiologist and haematologist is vital. Abide by infection control procedures! Use a *risk-assessment tool* (eg see BOX 'ISTH DIC score').
• Full barrier nursing in a side room if possible. Hand-washing is vital. Look for infection (mouth, axillae, perineum, heart, spine, IVI hardware (eg CVC)). Take swabs.
• Check: FBC, platelets, INR, U&E, LFT, LDH, CRP. Take cultures (blood ×3—peripherally ± Hickman line; urine, sputum, stool if diarrhoea); CXR if clinically indicated. Consider CT abdomen to look for neutropenic enterocolitis (typhlitis) if abdo pain.
• Examine oral cavity, dentition, and peri-anal region; fissures, haemorrhoids, skin excoriation. Oral hygiene (eg hydrogen peroxide mouth washes/2h) and *Candida* prophylaxis are important (p242).
• Check vital signs 4hrly. High-calorie diet; avoid paracetamol/antipyretics as they may mask signs of sepsis. Vases containing flowers pose a *Pseudomonas* risk.

Use of antibiotics in neutropenia ▶Treat within 60min of neutropenic fever presentation. If T° >38°C (or T° >37.5°C on two occasions >1h apart) or the patient is septic, start empiric combination therapy according to local guidelines—eg piperacillin–tazobactam—p382. If signs of severe sepsis/shock (eg hypotension), add an aminoglycoside (eg gentamicin) and MRSA coverage (eg vancomycin). Consider also the addition of vancomycin, if Gram +ve organisms suspected, eg Hickman line or skin/soft tissue sepsis. If fever persists despite antibiotics, think of CMV, fungi (eg *Candida*; *Aspergillus*, p404) and central line infection. Consider treatment for *Pneumocystis* (p396, eg co-trimoxazole, though may worsen neutropenia). Remember TB. G-CSF use can be considered—consult haematologist.

Other dangers •**Tumour lysis syndrome** Results in ↑K⁺, ↑urate, and AKI. See p525.
• **Hyperviscosity** (p368). If WCC is >100 × 10⁹/L WBC thrombi may form in brain, lung, and heart (leukostasis). Avoid transfusing before lowering WCC, eg with hydroxycarbamide or leukapheresis, as viscosity rises (↑risk of leukostasis).
• DIC The release of procoagulants into the circulation causes widespread activation of coagulation, consuming clotting factors and platelets and causing ↑risk of bleeding. Fibrin strands fill small vessels, haemolysing passing RBCs. Fibrinolysis is also activated. *Causes:* malignancy, sepsis, trauma, obstetric events. *Signs:* (fig 8.48) Bruising, bleeding anywhere (eg venepuncture sites), AKI. *Tests:* (See BOX.) ↓platelets; ↑PT; ↑APTT; ↓fibrinogen (correlates with severity); ↑↑fibrin degradation products (D-dimers). Film: broken RBCs (schistocytes). ℞ Treat the cause. Replace platelets if <20 × 10⁹/L (or <50 × 10⁹/L if serious bleeding), cryoprecipitate to replace fibrinogen, FFP to replace coagulation factors. Heparin is controversial. The use of all-transretinoic acid (ATRA) has significantly reduced the risk of DIC in acute promyelocytic leukaemia (the commonest leukaemia associated with DIC).
• **Preventing sepsis** Give fluoroquinolone (eg ciprofloxacin) before neutropenia gets serious. Granulocyte colony stimulating factor (G-CSF) can increase the production of WBCs (granulocytes) from bone marrow, but should not be given routinely in chemotherapy. Herpes, pneumocystis, and CMV prophylaxis has a role.

Neutropenia: definitions and causes

Neutropenia refers to an absolute neutrophil count (ANC) <1.5 × 10⁹/L. Mild neutropenia (ANC >1.0 × 10⁹/L) in adults is most commonly attributable to benign ethnic neutropenia (BEN), drugs, infections (especially viral), nutritional deficiencies, rheumatological disorders, and haematologic conditions (eg MDS). Severe isolated neutropenia (ANC <0.5 × 10⁹/L) is usually caused by drugs (eg carbimazole, clozapine, sulfasalazine, various antibiotics/AEDs), and less commonly infections/sepsis. Neutropenia may also occur in the context of pancytopenia due to bone marrow infiltration/replacement (eg acute or chronic leukaemias), bone marrow failure (eg aplastic anaemia, cytotoxic drugs, nutritional deficiencies, alcohol excess, viral infection), excess destruction/sequestration (eg DIC, hypersplenism due to portal hypertension, etc.), or congenital conditions (eg Wiskott–Aldrich syndrome).

ISTH DIC score

The DIC score was developed by the International Society of Thrombosis and Hemostasis (ISTH) as diagnostic criteria for overt DIC:

• Platelet count, cells × 10⁹/L	>100	0
	50–100	1
	<50	2
• ↑↑Fibrin degradation products (D-dimers)	No increase	0
	Moderate increase	2
	Severe increase	3
• Prolonged PT, seconds	<3	0
	3–6	1
	≥6	2
• Fibrinogen level, g/L	≥1	0
	<1	1

<5: not suggestive of overt DIC, may be non-overt DIC; repeat within next 1–2 days and manage clinically as appropriate.
≥5: compatible with overt DIC; treat for DIC as appropriate and repeat scoring daily.

8 Haematology

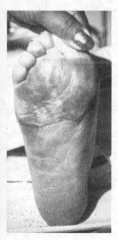

Fig 8.48 The appearance of disseminated intravascular coagulation (DIC) on the sole.
Courtesy of the Crookston Collection.

A malignancy of lymphoid cells, affecting B- or T-lymphocyte cell lineages, arresting maturation and promoting uncontrolled proliferation of immature blast cells, with marrow failure and tissue infiltration. Ionizing radiation (eg x-rays) during pregnancy, and Down syndrome are important associations. It is the commonest cancer of childhood, and represents about 15% of leukaemias in adults. CNS involvement is common.

Classification Surface markers are used to classify ALL into: precursor B-cell ALL, T-cell ALL, B-cell ALL. WHO classification depends on characterization of cytogenetic and molecular features. Cytogenetic features are characterized by chromosome analysis and fluorescence *in situ* hybridization (FISH), while a variety of molecular techniques are used for mutation analysis and gene expression studies (figs 8.49–8.52).

Signs and symptoms (fig 8.53) Due to:
• Marrow failure: anaemia (↓Hb), infection (↓WCC), and bleeding (↓platelets).
• Infiltration: hepato- and splenomegaly, lymphadenopathy—superficial or mediastinal, orchidomegaly, CNS involvement—eg cranial nerve palsies, meningism.

Common infections Especially chest, mouth, perianal, and skin. Bacterial septicaemia, zoster, CMV, measles, candidiasis, *Pneumocystis* pneumonia (p396).

Tests FBC (WCC usually high), PT, APTT, fibrinogen, LFTS, U&E. Immunophenotyping of blood or bone marrow to identify blast cells. DNA analysis is required to detect chromosomal abnormalities, eg BCR–ABL fusion gene indicative of t(9:22) 'Philadelphia chromosome'. CXR and CT scan to look for mediastinal and abdominal lymphadenopathy. Lumbar puncture should be performed to look for CNS involvement.

Treatment ►Educate and motivate patient to promote engagement with therapy.
• **Support** Blood/platelet transfusion, IV fluids, allopurinol (prevents tumour lysis syndrome). Insert a subcutaneous port system/Hickman line for IV access.
• **Infections** These are dangerous, due to neutropenia caused by the disease and treatment: give immediate IV antibiotics. Start the neutropenic sepsis regimen (p350) and give prophylactic antivirals, antifungals, and antibiotics.
• **Chemotherapy** Prolonged chemotherapy is required for cure, eg UKALL regimen-based clinical trials that can take up to 2 years. Depends on age and the presence/absence of the Philadelphia chromosome (Ph+ p356: BCR–ABL gene fusion due to translocation of chromosomes 9 and 22):
  • *Remission induction:* eg vincristine, prednisolone, L-asparaginase + daunorubicin. A BCR–ABL1 tyrosine kinase inhibitor (eg imatinib, p356) should be combined with steroids and chemotherapy if it is a Ph+ ALL.
  • *Consolidation:* high-medium-dose therapy in 'blocks' over several weeks.
  • *CNS prophylaxis:* intrathecal (or high-dose IV) methotrexate ± CNS irradiation.
  • *Maintenance:* prolonged chemotherapy, eg mercaptopurine (daily), methotrexate (weekly), and vincristine + prednisolone (monthly) for 2yrs. Relapse can occur in blood, CNS, or testis (examine these sites at follow-up). More details: OHCS p242.
• **Matched related allogeneic marrow transplantations** Once in 1st remission is the best option in standard-risk younger adults.

Haematological remission Means no evidence of leukaemia in the blood, a normal or recovering blood count, and <5% blasts in a normal regenerating marrow.

Prognosis Cure rates for children are 70–90%; for adults only 40% (higher when imatinib/rituximab, p356, are used). Poor prognosis if: age ≥40, male, Philadelphia chromosome, presentation with CNS signs, ↓Hb, WCC >100 × 10⁹/L, or B-cell ALL. PCR is used to detect minimal residual disease, undetectable by standard means. Prognosis in relapsed Ph-negative ALL is poor (but improvable by marrow transplant).

Personalized treatment ►Aim to tailor therapy to the exact gene defect, and according to individual metabolism. New treatments for relapsed disease include blinatumomab and inotuzumab. CAR-T cells have shown excellent responses in ALL. Clinical trials are an option for patients with relapsed/refractory disease. Biomarkers, eg thiopurine methyltransferase, can predict toxicity from thiopurines.

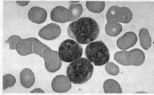

Fig 8.49 Blood film in ALL, L1 subtype. Small blasts with scanty cytoplasm.

Courtesy of Prof. Christine Lawrence.

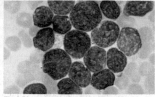

Fig 8.50 Bone marrow in ALL, L1 subtype.

Courtesy of Prof. Christine Lawrence.

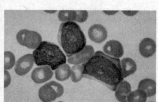

Fig 8.51 Blood film in ALL, L2 subtype. Larger blast cells with greater morphological variation and more abundant cytoplasm.

Courtesy of Prof. Christine Lawrence.

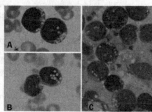

Fig 8.52 ALL L3. Blasts with vacuolated basophilic cytoplasm. (a, b) Blood films. (c) Lymph node.

Courtesy of Prof. Tangün and Dr Köroğlu.

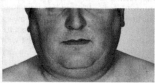

Fig 8.53 Bilateral parotid infiltration in ALL. (Enlarged salivary glands are also seen in mumps, HIV, bulimia, myxoedema, etc., p586.)

Neoplastic proliferation of blast cells derived from marrow myeloid elements. It progresses rapidly (5-year survival is now 55% for patients <60 and 17% for patients >60 after ℞).[6]

Incidence The commonest acute leukaemia of adults (1/10 000/yr; increases with age). The median age at presentation is 65–70 years. AML can be a long-term complication of chemotherapy, eg for lymphoma. Also associated with myelodysplastic states (see BOX 'Myelodysplastic syndromes'), prior radiation, and syndromes, eg Down's.

Morphological classification Four types based on WHO histological classification, cytogenetics, and molecular genetics:

1 AML with recurrent genetic abnormalities.
2 AML multilineage dysplasia (eg 2° to pre-existing myelodysplastic syndrome).
3 AML, therapy related (in those previously treated with cytotoxic drugs).
4 AML, other (not fitting above-listed).

Signs and symptoms • **Marrow failure** Anaemia, infection, or bleeding. DIC occurs in acute promyelocytic leukaemia, a subtype of AML, where there is release of thromboplastin (p350). • **Infiltration** Hepatomegaly, splenomegaly, gum hypertrophy (fig 8.54), skin involvement. CNS involvement at presentation is rare.

Diagnosis WCC is often ↑, but can be normal or even low. Blast cells may be few in the peripheral blood, so diagnosis depends on bone marrow biopsy, immunophenotyping, and molecular methods. On biopsy, AML is differentiated from ALL by Auer rods (figs 8.55–8.57). Cytogenetic analysis (eg type of mutation) guides treatment recommendations and prognosis. ≥3 cytogenetic abnormalities associated with worse prognosis.

Complications • Predisposition to infection by both the disease and the treatment; may be bacterial, fungal, or viral—prophylaxis is given for each during therapy. Be alert to septicaemia (p350): common organisms present oddly and rare organisms can infect commonly (particularly the fungi *Candida* and *Aspergillus*). Be aware that AML itself causes fever. • Chemotherapy causes ↑plasma urate levels (from tumour lysis)—so give allopurinol with chemotherapy, and keep well hydrated with IV fluids. • Leukostasis (p350) may occur if ↑↑WCC. This is associated with a very high blast count. Manifestations include respiratory compromise, altered mental status, visual changes, and headache. ℞ IV fluids, rapid initiation of chemotherapy, leukapheresis, or radiotherapy.

Treatment • **Supportive care** As for ALL.
• **Chemotherapy** Very intensive, resulting in long periods of marrow suppression with neutropenia and platelets ↓. The main drugs used include daunorubicin and cytarabine, with ~5 cycles given in 1-week blocks to get a remission (RAS mutations occur in ~20% of patients with AML and enhance sensitivity to cytarabine).
• **Bone marrow transplant (BMT)** Pluripotent haematopoietic stem cells are collected from the marrow. *Allogeneic* transplants from HLA-matched donors (held on international databases) are indicated in refractory or relapsing disease. The idea is to destroy leukaemic cells and the immune system by, eg cyclophosphamide + total body irradiation, then repopulate the marrow with donor cells infused IV. Ciclosporin ± methotrexate are used to reduce the effect of the new marrow attacking the patient's body (graft vs host disease (GVHD)).
  • *Complications:* GVHD (may help explain the curative effect of BMT); opportunistic infections; relapse of leukaemia; infertility.
  • *Prognosis:* lower relapse rates ~60% long-term survivors, but significant mortality of ~10%. Autologous BMT (where stem cells are taken from the patient themselves) is used in intermediate-prognosis disease, although some studies suggest better survival rates with intensive chemotherapy regimens.
  • *Autologous mobilized peripheral blood stem cell transplantation* may offer faster haemopoietic recovery and less morbidity.
• Supportive care, or lower-dose chemotherapy for disease control, may be more appropriate in elderly patients, where intensive therapies have poorer outcomes.

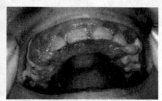

Fig 8.54 Gum hypertrophy in AML.
Courtesy of Prof. Christine Lawrence.

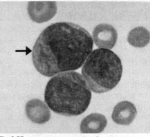

Fig 8.55 Auer rods (crystals of coalesced granules) found in AML myeloblast cells.
Courtesy of Prof. Christine Lawrence.

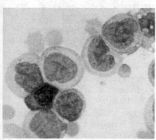

Fig 8.56 AML with monoblasts and myeloblasts on the peripheral blood film.
Courtesy of Prof. Christine Lawrence.

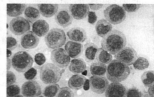

Fig 8.57 Marrow in AML: multiple monoblasts.
Courtesy of Prof. Christine Lawrence.

Myelodysplastic syndromes (MDS, myelodysplasia)

These are a heterogeneous group of clonal disorders characterized by inadequate and dysmorphic haematopoiesis that manifest as marrow failure with risk of life-threatening infection and bleeding (median survival varies from 6 months to 6 years according to disease type). Incidence increases with age. Mostly primary, but can develop secondary to chemotherapy or radiotherapy. 30% transform to acute leukaemia. **Tests** Pancytopenia (p348), with ↓reticulocyte count, ↑MCV. Marrow cellularity is usually increased due to ineffective haematopoiesis. Ring sideroblasts may also be seen in the marrow (fig 8.25, p327).

Differential diagnosis ACD, marrow infiltration, drug toxicity (eg alcohol, chemotherapy), viral infections (HIV), vitamin deficiency (B₁₂/folate deficiency).

Treatment
* Depends on age, performance status, and prognostic scoring systems.
* Multiple transfusions of red cells or platelets as needed. Chelation therapy may be needed for iron overload.
* Erythropoietin may lower transfusion requirement. G-CSF if recurrent infections.
* Allogeneic stem cell transplantation is one option (curative but often inappropriate owing to age-related comorbidities—most are >70yrs old).
* Low-intensity treatments that are not curative but may improve quality of life in symptomatic disease include thalidomide analogues (eg lenalidomide) or hypomethylating agents (eg azacitidine and decitabine).

Chronic myeloid leukaemia (CML)

CML is characterized by an uncontrolled clonal proliferation of myeloid cells (fig 8.58). It accounts for 15% of leukaemias. It is a myeloproliferative disorder (p362) having features in common with these diseases, eg splenomegaly. It occurs most often between 40–60yrs, with a slight male predominance, and is rare in childhood. ↑Risk associated with prior radiation exposure.

Philadelphia chromosome (Ph.) Present in >80% of those with CML. It is a hybrid chromosome comprising reciprocal translocation between the long arm of chromosome 9 and the long arm of chromosome 22—t(9;22)—forming a fusion gene BCR/ABL on chromosome 22, which has tyrosine kinase activity. Those without Ph have a worse prognosis. Some patients have a masked translocation—cytogenetics do not show the Ph, but the rearrangement is detectable by molecular techniques.

Symptoms Mostly chronic and insidious: ↓weight, tiredness, fever, sweats. There may be features of gout (due to purine breakdown), bleeding (platelet dysfunction), and abdominal discomfort (splenic enlargement). ~30% are detected by chance.

Signs Splenomegaly (>75%)—often massive. Hepatomegaly, anaemia, bruising (fig 8.59).

Tests ↑↑WBC (often >10 × 10⁹/L) with whole spectrum of myeloid cells, ie ↑neutrophils, monocytes, basophils, eosinophils. ↓Hb or ↔, platelets variable. ↑Urate, ↑B₁₂. Bone marrow hypercellular. Cytogenetic analysis of blood or bone marrow for Ph.

Natural history 5-year survival is 90%. There are three phases: *chronic*, lasting months or years of few, if any, symptoms. • *Accelerated phase*, defined as 10–19% blast cells in peripheral blood or bone marrow as per WHO with increasing symptoms and spleen size. • *Blast transformation*, with features of acute leukaemia ± death. **Treatment** See BOX.

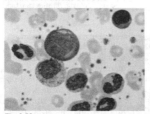

Fig 8.58 CML: numerous granulocytic cells at different stages of differentiation.
Courtesy of Prof. Christine Lawrence.

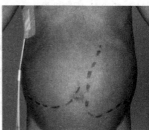

Fig 8.59 Hepatosplenomegaly in CML.

Treating CML

CML is the first example of a cancer where knowledge of the genotype has led to a specifically targeted drug—*imatinib*, a BCR–ABL tyrosine kinase inhibitor. This has transformed therapy over the last 10yrs. Side effects are usually mild: nausea, cramps, oedema, rash, headache, arthralgia. May cause myelosuppression.

More potent 2nd-generation BCR–ABL inhibitors: *dasatinib, nilotinib, bosutinib,* and *ponatinib*. Dasatinib and nilotinib allow more patients to achieve deeper, more rapid responses associated with improved outcomes, but are only indicated in chronic- or accelerated-phase patients who are intolerant or resistant to imatinib according to NICE. *Hydroxycarbamide* is also used.

Those with lymphoblastic transformation may benefit from treatment as for ALL. Treatment of myeloblastic transformation with chemotherapy rarely achieves lasting remission, and allogeneic transplantation offers the best hope.

Stem cell transplantation: allogeneic transplantation from an HLA-matched sibling or unrelated donor offers the only cure, but carries significant morbidity and mortality. Guidelines suggest that this approach should be only rarely used 1st line in young patients (where mortality rates are lower). Other patients should be offered a BCR–ABL inhibitor. Patients are then reviewed annually to decide whether to continue, to offer combination therapy or stem cell transplantation.

CLL is the commonest leukaemia (>25%; incidence: ~5/100 000/yr). ♂:♀ ≈ 2:1. The median age at diagnosis is 65 years. The hallmark is progressive accumulation of a malignant clone of functionally incompetent B cells. Mutations, trisomies, and deletions (eg del17p13) influence risk (table 8.8).

Table 8.8 Staging and survival in CLL

Rai stage:	0	Lymphocytosis alone	Median survival >13yrs
	I	Lymphocytosis + lymphadenopathy	8yrs
	II	Lymphocytosis + spleno- or hepatomegaly	5yrs
	III	Lymphocytosis + anaemia (Hb <110g/L)	2yrs
	IV	Lymphocytosis + platelets <100 × 10⁹/L	1yr

Symptoms Often none, presenting as a surprise finding on a routine FBC. Patients may be anaemic or infection-prone, or have ↓weight, sweats, anorexia if severe.

Signs Enlarged, rubbery, non-tender nodes (fig 8.60). Splenomegaly, hepatomegaly.

Tests ↑Lymphocytes—may be marked (fig 8.61). Later: autoimmune haemolysis (p334), marrow infiltration: ↓Hb, ↓neutrophils, ↓platelets.

Complications 1 Autoimmune haemolysis. 2 ↑Bacterial infections due to hypogammaglobulinaemia (= ↓IGG), especially encapsulated organisms. 3 Severe T cell immunosuppression with increased susceptibility to viral (eg herpes zoster) and fungal infections. 4 Marrow failure. 5 ↑Risk of secondary malignancies. 6 Risk of transformation to more aggressive disease (consider if rapidly enlarging nodes, rapid increase in LDH, B symptoms).

Treatment Depends on age/fitness and the presence of certain mutations. Many patients can be managed on a 'watch and wait' basis safely for several years. Consider treatment if symptomatic. Options include FCR (fludarabine + *cyclophosphamide* + rituximab), ibrutinib (Bruton tyrosine kinase inhibitor; SE: myelosuppression, AF, and bleeding) monotherapy, venetoclax (BCL-2 inhibitor; SE: tumour lysis syndrome, myelosuppression) + obinutuzumab, and BR (bendamustine + rituximab). Steroids and IV immunoglobulin help autoimmune haemolysis (seen after treatment with fludarabine). *Radiotherapy* helps lymphadenopathy and splenomegaly. *Stem-cell transplantation* may have a role in carefully selected patients. **Supportive care** Transfusions, IV human immunoglobulin if recurrent infection ± antimicrobial prophylaxis

Natural history ⅓ never progress (or even *regress*), ⅓ progress slowly, and ⅓ progress actively. CD23 and β₂-microglobulin correlate with bulk of disease and rates of progression. Death is often due to infection or transformation to aggressive lymphoma (Richter's syndrome).

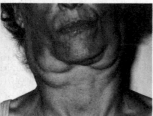

Fig 8.60 Bilateral cervical lymphadenopathy in CLL.

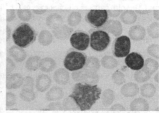

Fig 8.61 CLL: many lymphocytes and a 'smear' cell: a fragile cell damaged in preparation.
Courtesy of Prof. Christine Lawrence.

Lymphomas are disorders caused by malignant proliferations of lymphocytes. These accumulate in the lymph nodes causing lymphadenopathy, but may also be found in peripheral blood or infiltrate organs. Lymphomas are histologically divided into Hodgkin's and non-Hodgkin's types. In Hodgkin's lymphoma,[8] characteristic cells with mirror-image nuclei are found, called Reed–Sternberg cells (figs 8.62–8.64).

Incidence Two peaks: young adults (HL is the commonest malignancy in 15–24yr-olds) and elderly. ♂:♀ ≈ 2:1. ↑Incidence in industrialized countries. **Risk factors** An affected sibling; EBV (p401); SLE; post-transplantation.

Symptoms Often presents with enlarged, non-tender, 'rubbery' superficial lymph nodes (60–70% cervical, fig 8.65; also axillary or inguinal). Node size may fluctuate, and they can become matted. 25% have constitutional upset, eg fever, weight loss (> 10% in 6 months), night sweats, pruritus, and lethargy. There may be alcohol-induced lymph node pain. Mediastinal lymph node involvement can cause mass effect, eg bronchial or SVC obstruction (p524), or direct extension, eg causing pleural effusions.

Signs Lymphadenopathy. Also, cachexia, anaemia, spleno- or hepatomegaly.

Tests Tissue diagnosis Lymph node excision biopsy if possible (supraclavicular > cervical/axillary > inguinal; send for pathology, immunohistochemisty/flow cytometry). Image-guided needle biopsy, laparotomy, or mediastinoscopy may be needed. **Bloods** FBC, film, ESR, LFT, LDH, urate, Ca^{2+}. ↑ESR or ↓Hb indicate a worse prognosis. LDH ↑ as it is released during cell turnover. **Imaging** CXR, CT/PET of thorax, abdo, and pelvis.

Staging (Ann Arbor system.) Influences treatment and prognosis. Done by imaging ± marrow biopsy if B symptoms, or stage III–IV disease.
 I Confined to single lymph node region.
 II Involvement of two or more nodal areas on the same side of the diaphragm.
 III Involvement of nodes on both sides of the diaphragm.
 IV Spread beyond the lymph nodes, eg liver or bone marrow.

Each stage is either 'A'—no systemic symptoms other than pruritus; or 'B'—presence of B symptoms: weight loss >10% in last 6 months, unexplained fever >38°C, or night sweats (needing change of clothes). 'B' indicates worse disease. Localized extranodal extension does not advance the stage, but is indicated by subscripted 'E', eg I-A_E.

Chemoradiotherapy Radiotherapy + short courses of chemotherapy for stages I-A and II-A (eg with ≤3 areas involved). Longer courses of chemotherapy for II-A with >3 areas involved through to IV-B. 'ABVD': **A**driamycin® (doxorubicin), **B**leomycin, **V**inblastine, **D**acarbazine cures ~80% of patients. More intensive regimens are used if poor prognosis or advanced disease.[9] In relapsed disease: high-dose chemotherapy followed by autologous stem cell transplantation. Brentuximab vedotin + doxorubicin, vinblastine, and dacarbazine (BV + AVD) is a promising new combination chemotherapy.[7] **Complications of treatment** See pp518–21. *Radiotherapy* may ↑ risk of second malignancies (related to dose and field, with long latency and ↑ risk over time), solid tumours (especially lung and breast, also melanoma, sarcoma, stomach, and thyroid cancers), ischaemic heart disease, valvular heart or pericardial disease, hypothyroidism, and lung fibrosis due to the radiation field. *Chemotherapy* SE include myelosuppression, nausea, alopecia, infection, AML (p354), non-Hodgkin's lymphoma, and infertility may be due to both chemo- and radiotherapy—see p523.

5-year survival Depends on stage and grade (table 8.9): >95% in I-A lymphocyte-predominant disease; <40% with IV-B lymphocyte-depleted. There are competing risks in terms of overall survival between minimizing the risk of a recurrence and also preventing treatment-related complications such as secondary malignancy and cardiovascular disease.

Emergency presentations Infection; SVC obstruction—↑JVP, sensation of fullness in the head, dyspnoea, blackouts, facial oedema (seek expert help; see p524).

---

8 Thomas Hodgkin (1798–1866); rediscovered by Samuel Wilks (1824–1911) who magnanimously gave the disease Hodgkin's name.
9 Eg BEACOPP (bleomycin/etoposide/doxorubicin/cyclophosphamide/vincristine/procarbazine/prednisone). In IIB, III, or IV, BEACOPP gives better initial control, but 7yr event-free survival is similar: 78% vs 71%.

Table 8.9 HL subtypes

Classification (% of cases)	Prognosis
Nodular sclerosing (70%)	Good
Mixed cellularity* (20–25%)	Good
Lymphocyte rich (5%)	Good
Lymphocyte depleted* (<1%)	Poor

NB: nodular lymphocyte predominant Hodgkin's is recognized as a separate entity, behaving as an indolent B-cell lymphoma.
* Higher incidence and worse prognosis if HIV +ve.

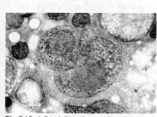

Fig 8.62 A Reed–Sternberg cell with two nuclei, characteristic of Hodgkin's lymphoma.
Courtesy of Prof. Christine Lawrence.

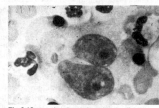

Fig 8.63 Another Reed–Sternberg cell.
Courtesy of the Crookston Collection.

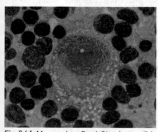

Fig 8.64 Mononuclear Reed–Sternberg cell in a lymph node.
© Prof. Tangün and Dr Köroğlu.

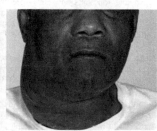

Fig 8.65 Cervical lymphadenopathy in Hodgkin's disease.

Quality of life, lymphoma, and the role of expressive writing

Being treated for Hodgkin's lymphoma is arduous. Our job is often to give encouragement—the more this is personalized for our individual patient the better.

One method is to encourage our patients to write about their experiences. In one study this gave clear-cut benefits in lymphoma patients. Participants report positive responses to writing, and half said that writing changed their thoughts about their illness in a positive way (this increased on subsequent follow-up). Textual analysis identifies themes related to experiences of positive change, transformation, and self-affirmation through reflection. These techniques are akin to those used in post-traumatic stress—and remind us that some of our treatments are as destabilizing to our patients as any shipwreck or earthquake. 'I can whine, I can complain, I can moan, and bitch, about all of the above, but I won't... The true feat isn't escaping death, rather, learning how to live.'

Sometimes narrating lymphoma experiences reveals bitterness, loss of control, and a feeling that life has been rendered void. Here our role is to receive these negatives and to try to keep the channels of communication open, as dialogue is the only validated means of filling these voids. The need to enhance support networks and bolster social ties may trump all our pharmacological imperatives.

This includes all lymphomas without Reed–Sternberg cells (p358)—a diverse group. They can be classified as B-cell or T- and NK-cell derived. However, most are derived from B-cell lines; diffuse large B-cell lymphoma (DLBCL) is commonest. Not all centre on nodes (extranodal tissues generating lymphoma include mucosa-associated lymphoid tissue, eg gastric MALT, later in this topic). Incidence has doubled since 1970 (to 2:10 000). The median age at diagnosis is 67 years.

Causes Immunodeficiency—drugs; prior radiotherapy or chemotherapy; viruses or bacteria—HIV (usually high-grade lymphoma from EBV transformed cells, p401; EBV is also associated with endemic Burkitt's lymphoma, DLBCL, NK-T-cell lymphoma, etc.); HTLV-1 (adult T-cell leukaemia/lymphoma) p401; *Helicobacter pylori* (marginal zone lymphoma); toxins; autoimmune condition; congenital.

Signs and symptoms • Superficial lymphadenopathy (75% at presentation).
• Extranodal disease (50%). **Gut** (Commonest.) 1 *Gastric MALT* is caused by *H. pylori*, and may regress with its eradication (p248). Symptoms: as for gastric Ca (p610), with systemic features (see below). MALT usually involves the antrum, is multifocal, and metastasizes late. 2 *Non-malt gastric lymphomas* (60%) are usually diffuse large-cell B lymphomas—high-grade and not responding well to *H. pylori* eradication. 3 *Small-bowel lymphomas*, eg IPSID (immunoproliferative small intestine disease, p364), or EATCL (enteropathy/coeliac-associated intra-epithelial T-cell lymphoma)—presents with diarrhoea, vomiting, abdominal pain, and ↓weight. Poor prognosis. **Skin** (2nd commonest—see fig 8.66.) Eg clonal T cells in mycosis fungoides (accounts for ~50%—p588). **Oropharynx** Waldeyer's ring lymphoma causes sore throat/obstructed breathing. **Other possible sites** Bone, CNS, and lung.
• Systemic features: low-grade-NHL—none/mild symptoms, lymphadenopathy; high-grade-NHL—weight loss, night sweats, fevers.
• Pancytopenia from marrow involvement—anaemia, infection, bleeding (↓platelets).

Tests Blood FBC, U&E, LFT. ↑ LDH ≈ worse prognosis, reflecting ↑cell turnover. *Marrow and node biopsy* for classification (complex, based on the WHO system of high or low grade). **Staging** Ann Arbor system (p358)—PET-CT of chest, abdomen, pelvis. Send *cytology* of any effusion; LP for CSF cytology if CNS signs.

Diagnosis/management This is multidisciplinary, synthesizing details from clinical evaluation, histology, immunology, molecular genetics, and imaging. *Generally:*
• Low-grade lymphomas are indolent, often incurable, and widely disseminated. Include: follicular lymphoma (2nd most common NHL—20%), marginal zone lymphoma/MALT, lymphocytic lymphoma (closely related to CLL and treated similarly), lymphoplasmacytoid lymphoma (produces IgM = Waldenström's macroglobulinaemia, p364). See fig 8.67.
• High-grade lymphomas are more aggressive, *but often curable.* There is often rapidly enlarging lymphadenopathy with systemic symptoms. Include: Burkitt's lymphoma (childhood disease with characteristic jaw lymphadenopathy; figs 8.68, 8.69), lymphoblastic lymphomas (like ALL), diffuse large B-cell lymphoma (most common subtype NHL—25%).

Treatment Huge range of options, depending on disease subtype. **Low grade** If symptomless, none may be needed (see BOX). Radiotherapy may be curative in localized disease. Chlorambucil is used in diffuse disease. Remission may be maintained by using interferon alfa or rituximab (see later in paragraph). Bendamustine is effective both with rituximab and as a monotherapy in rituximab-refractory patients. **High grade** (eg large B-cell lymphoma, DLBCL), '**R-CHOP**' regimen: **R**ituximab, **C**yclophosphamide, **H**ydroxydaunorubicin, vincristine (**O**ncovin®) and **P**rednisolone. Granulocyte colony-stimulating factors (G-CSFs) help neutropenia—eg filgrastim or lenograstim (at low doses it may be cost-effective).

Survival Histology is important. Prognosis is worse if, at presentation: • Age >60yrs. • Systemic symptoms. • Bulky disease (abdominal mass >10cm). • ↑LDH. • Disseminated disease. Typical 5yr survival for treated patients: ~30% for high-grade and >50% for low-grade lymphomas, but the picture is very variable.

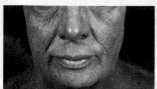

Fig 8.66 Cutaneous T-cell lymphoma, which has caused severe erythroderma (Sézary syndrome) in a Caucasian woman.
Courtesy of Prof. Christine Lawrence.

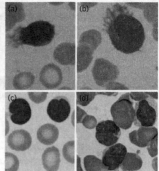

Fig 8.67 (a, b) Villous lymphocytes (splenic marginal zone lymphoma). (c) 'Buttock cells' with cleaved nuclei (follicular lymphoma). (d) Sézary cells with convoluted nuclei.
Courtesy of Prof. Tangün & Dr Köroğlu.

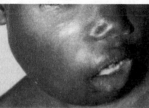

Fig 8.68 Burkitt's lymphoma, with characteristic jaw lymphadenopathy.
Courtesy of Dr Tom D Thacher.

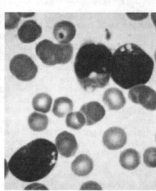

Fig 8.69 Burkitt's lymphoma, with three basophilic vacuolated lymphoma cells.
From the *New England Journal of Medicine*, Bain, B, 'Diagnosis from the blood smear', 353(5), 498. Copyright © 2005 Massachusetts Medical Society. Reprinted with permission from Massachusetts Medical Society.

Indications for treatment in indolent lymphoma
- Cytopenias secondary to BM infiltration.
- Threatened end-organ function.
- Symptoms attributable to disease.
- Bulk at presentation.
- Steady progression during a period of observation >6 months.
- Presentation with concurrent histologic transformation.
- Massive splenomegaly.

The myeloproliferative disorders

Caused by clonal proliferation of haematopoietic myeloid stem cells in the bone marrow. These cells retain the ability to differentiate into RBCs, WBCs, or platelets, causing an excess of one or more of these cell types (table 8.10).

Table 8.10 Classification of myeloproliferative disorders

By proliferating cell type	
RBC	→ Polycythaemia vera (PRV)
WBC	→ Chronic myeloid leukaemia (CML, p356)
Platelets	→ Essential thrombocythaemia
Fibroblasts	→ Myelofibrosis

Polycythaemia Refers to ↑Hb >16.5 g/dL in men or >16.0 g/dL in women and/or Hct >49% in men or >48% in women (see BOX 'Investigating polycythaemia'). **Relative polycythaemia** (↓plasma volume, normal RBC mass) may be acute (due to volume depletion) or chronic (associated with obesity, HTN, & ↑ alcohol/tobacco intake). **Absolute polycythaemia** (↑RBC mass) is classically measured by dilution of infused autologous radioactive chromium (^{51}Cr)-labelled RBCs. Causes are primary (*polycythaemia vera*) or secondary due to hypoxia (eg high altitudes, chronic lung disease, cyanotic congenital heart disease, heavy smoking) or inappropriately ↑erythropoietin secretion (eg RCC, HCC).

Polycythaemia vera The malignant proliferation of a clone derived from one pluripotent stem cell. A mutation in JAK2 (JAK2 V617F) is present in >95%. The erythroid progenitor offspring are unusual in not needing erythropoietin to avoid apoptosis. There is excess proliferation of RBCs, WBCs, and platelets, leading to hyperviscosity and thrombosis. Commoner if >60yrs old. **Presentation** May be asymptomatic and detected on FBC, or present with vague symptoms due to hyperviscosity (p368): headaches, dizziness, tinnitus, visual disturbance. Itching after a hot bath, and erythromelalgia, a burning sensation in fingers and toes, are characteristic. Signs: facial plethora and splenomegaly (in 60%). Gout may occur due to ↑urate from RBC turnover. Features of arterial (cardiac, cerebral, peripheral) or venous (DVT, cerebral, hepatic) thrombosis may be present. **Investigations** • FBC: ↑RCC, ↑Hb, ↑HCT, ↑PCV, often also ↑WBC and ↑platelets. • ↑B$_{12}$. • Marrow shows hypercellularity with erythroid hyperplasia. • Cytogenetics as required to differentiate from CML. • ↓Serum erythropoietin. • Raised red cell mass on ^{51}Cr studies and splenomegaly, in the setting of a normal P_aO_2, is diagnostic. **Treatment** Aim to keep HCT <0.45 to ↓ risk of thrombosis. In younger patients at low risk, this is done by venesection. If higher risk (age >60yrs, previous thrombosis), hydroxycarbamide (=hydroxyurea) is used. Interferon alfa is preferred in women of childbearing age. Ruxolitinib is 2nd line. Aspirin 75mg daily is also given. **Prognosis** Variable, many remain well for years. Thrombosis and haemorrhage (due to defective platelets) are the main complications. Transition to myelofibrosis occurs in ~30% or acute leukaemia in ~5%. Monitor FBC every 3 months.

Essential thrombocythaemia (fig 8.70) A clonal proliferation of megakaryocytes leads to persistently ↑platelets, often >1000 × 10^9/L, with abnormal function, causing bleeding or arterial and venous thrombosis, and microvascular occlusion—hypertension, ulceration, headache, atypical chest pain, erythromelalgia. Exclude reactive causes of thrombocytosis (see BOX 'Causes of thrombocytosis'). **Treatment** Aspirin 75mg OD. Hydroxycarbamide in high-risk patients.

Myelofibrosis There is hyperplasia of megakaryocytes which produce platelet-derived growth factor, leading to intense marrow fibrosis and haematopoiesis in the spleen/liver → massive hepatosplenomegaly. **Presentation** Hypermetabolic symptoms: night sweats, fever, weight loss; abdo discomfort due to splenomegaly; bone marrow failure (↓Hb, infections, bleeding). **Film** Leukoerythroblastic cells (nucleated red cells, p320); characteristic teardrop RBCs (fig 8.71). ↓Hb. Bone marrow trephine for diagnosis (fig 8.72). **Treatment** Marrow support (p348). Allogeneic stem cell transplant may be curative in young people. Ruxolitinib, fedratinib, or hydroxycarbamide if transplant ineligible and symptomatic **Prognosis** Median survival 4–5yrs.

Investigating polycythaemia

- Initial investigations should include history, physical examination, pulse oximetry, FBC, peripheral blood smear.
- Check if any evidence of volume depletion and thus, if Hb corrects with fluid repletion.
- If polycythaemia vera suspected from presentation (eg tinnitus, itching, erythromelalgia, etc.), send JAK2 V617F mutation screen.
- If not, check serum EPO.
- Is ↑EPO in keeping with known cardiorespiratory disease? If not, check carboxyhaemoglobin. ↑Carboxyhaemoglobin suggests secondary polycythaemia due to carbon monoxide toxicity from cigarette smoking or other exposure.
- If carboxyhaemoglobin is normal and no other clear explanation (eg post-transplant erythrocytosis complicates 10–20% of renal allograft), consider CT/MRI abdomen/pelvis to rule out EPO-secreting tumour.
- Seek Haematology advice.

Causes of thrombocytosis

↑Platelets >450 × 10⁹/L may be a reactive phenomenon, seen with many conditions including:

- Bleeding.
- Malignancy.
- Post-surgery.
- Infection.
- Trauma.
- Iron deficiency.
- Chronic inflammation, eg collagen disorders, IBD, coeliac disease.

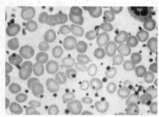

Fig 8.70 Essential thrombocythaemia: many platelets seen.

© Prof. Christine Lawrence.

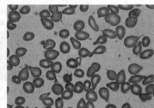

Fig 8.71 Teardrop cells, in myelofibrosis.

© Dr Nivaldo Medeiros.

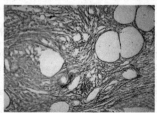

Fig 8.72 Marrow trephine in myelofibrosis: the streaming effect is caused by intense fibrosis. Other causes of marrow fibrosis: any myeloproliferative disorder, lymphoma, secondary carcinoma, TB, leukaemia, and irradiation.

© Prof. Christine Lawrence.

Paraproteinaemia

Paraproteinaemia denotes the presence in the circulation of immunoglobulins produced by a single clone of plasma cells. The paraprotein is recognized as a monoclonal band (M band) on serum electrophoresis.[10] There are six major categories:

1 **Multiple myeloma** See p366. Smouldering (asymptomatic) multiple myeloma refers to the presence of IgG or IgA >3g/dL or urinary monoclonal protein >500mg/24h and/or marrow plasma cells 10–60%, AND no end-organ damage (lytic lesions, anaemia, kidney disease, or hypercalcaemia) or other myeloma-defining events, and no amyloidosis

2 **Waldenström's macroglobulinaemia** This is a lymphoplasmacytoid lymphoma producing a monoclonal IgM paraprotein. Hyperviscosity is common (p368), with CNS and ocular symptoms. Lymphadenopathy and splenomegaly are also seen. ↑ESR, with IgM paraprotein on serum electrophoresis. ℞ None if asymptomatic. Combination chemotherapy (eg bendamustine + rituximab) may be used if symptomatic. Plasmapheresis[10] for hyperviscosity (p368).

3 **Primary amyloidosis** See 'Amyloidosis' (below).

4 **Monoclonal gammopathy of uncertain significance** See BOX p365.

5 **Paraproteinaemia in lymphoma or leukaemia** Eg seen in 5% of CLL.

6 **Heavy chain disease** Neoplastic cells produce free Ig heavy chains. α-chain disease is most important, causing malabsorption from infiltration of bowel wall (immunoproliferative small intestine disease—IPSID). It may progress to lymphoma.

Amyloidosis

This is a group of disorders characterized by extracellular deposits of a protein in abnormal fibrillar form, resistant to degradation. The following are the systemic forms of amyloidosis. Amyloid deposition is also a feature of Alzheimer's disease, type 2 diabetes mellitus, and haemodialysis-related amyloidosis.

AL amyloid (primary amyloidosis) Insidious multisystemic debilitating disease. Proliferation of plasma cell clone → amyloidogenic monoclonal immunoglobulins → fibrillar light chain protein deposition → organ failure → death. Associations: myeloma (15%); Waldenström's; lymphoma. Organs involved:
• Kidneys: glomerular lesions—proteinuria and nephrotic syndrome.
• Heart: restrictive cardiomyopathy (looks 'sparkling' on echo), arrhythmias, angina.
• Nerves: peripheral and autonomic neuropathy; carpal tunnel syndrome.
• Gut: macroglossia, malabsorption, haemorrhage, obstruction, hepatomegaly. Autonomic neuropathy & delayed gastric emptying can lead to nausea/↓weight.
• Vascular: purpura, especially periorbital—a characteristic feature (fig 8.73).

Diagnosis often suspected late due to non-specific symptoms. Send serum free light chain assay, serum & urine electrophoresis ± cardiac MRI, serum amyloid protein P (SAP) scan. Gold standard is tissue biopsy of kidney, fat pad, or bone marrow. Positive Congo red staining with apple-green birefringence under polarized light microscopy.

℞ Supportive care, nutrition, physiotherapy, disease education. First line; proteasome inhibitor, eg bortezomib, with cyclophosphamide and dexamethasone (CyBorD). Anti-CD138 monoclonal antibodies, eg daratumumab effective in clinical trials. Aim for disease reduction followed by high-dose melphalan with autologous stem cell transplantation.

Prognosis Median survival is 1–2 years. Patients with myeloma and amyloidosis have a shorter survival than those with myeloma alone.

AA amyloid (secondary amyloidosis) Rare nowadays. Here amyloid is derived from serum amyloid A, an acute phase protein, reflecting chronic inflammation in rheumatoid arthritis, UC/Crohn's, familial Mediterranean fever, and chronic infections—TB, bronchiectasis, osteomyelitis. It affects kidneys, liver, and spleen (fig 8.74), and may present with proteinuria, nephrotic syndrome, or hepatosplenomegaly. Macroglossia is not seen; cardiac involvement is rare (ventricular hypertrophy and murmurs). ℞ Manage the underlying condition optimally.

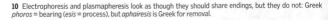

10 Electrophoresis and plasmapheresis look as though they should share endings, but they do not: Greek *phoros* = bearing (*esis* = process), but *aphairesis* is Greek for removal.

Monoclonal gammopathy of uncertain significance (MGUS)

MGUS is a common (3% > 50yrs) but asymptomatic premalignant clonal plasma cell or lymphoplasmacytic proliferative disorder. There is a paraprotein in the serum (<3g/dL) but no myeloma, 1° amyloid, macroglobulinaemia, or lymphoma, with no bone lesions, no Bence Jones protein, and a low concentration of paraprotein, with <10% plasma cells in the marrow. **Types** Non-IgM MGUS is most common and may progress to myeloma, IgM MGUS (may progress to Waldenström macroglobulinemia), and light chain MGUS (LC-MGUS; may progress to light chain multiple myeloma, AL amyloidosis). **Tests** FBC, U&E, Ca²⁺, serum & urine electrophoresis, serum free light chain (SFL) ratio, Ig levels, skeletal survey. **Natural history** Progress to more advanced disease at a rate of 1%/year. IgM MGUS > non-IgM MGUS. **Monitoring for progression** Follow-up initially at 3–6 months to recheck labs and ask if any red flag symptoms/signs have developed (eg bone pain, 'B' symptoms, lymphadenopathy, etc.). If asymptomatic and low-risk labs (eg IgG type, serum monoclonal protein <1.5g/dL or normal SFL ratio), only annual follow-up necessary. Check with Haematology if in doubt. Be aware that MGUS is also associated with increased risk of osteoporosis and VTE. Consider DEXA.

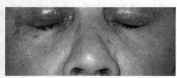

Fig 8.73 Periorbital purpura in amyloidosis.
© Prof. Christine Lawrence.

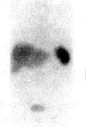

Fig 8.74 Areas of amyloid deposition in liver and spleen in amyloidosis (isotope scan).

Reproduced from Warrell *et al.*, *Oxford Textbook of Medicine*, 2010, with permission from Oxford University Press.

8 Haematology

PCDs are due to an abnormal proliferation of a single clone of plasma or lympho-plasmacytic cells leading to secretion of immunoglobulin (Ig) or an Ig fragment, causing the dysfunction of many organs (esp. kidney). The Ig is seen as a mono-clonal band, or paraprotein, on serum or urine electrophoresis.

Classification Based on Ig product—IgG in ~⅔; IgA in ~⅓; a very few are IgM or IgD. Other Ig levels are low ('immunoparesis', causing ↑susceptibility to infection). In ~⅔, urine contains Bence Jones proteins, which are free Ig light chains of kappa (κ) or lambda (λ) type, filtered by the kidney.

Incidence 5/100 000. Peak age: 70yrs. ♂:♀ ≈ 1:1. Afro-Caribbeans:Caucasians ≈ 2:1.

Clinical features • *Osteolytic bone lesions* cause backache, pathological fractures, & vertebral collapse. ▶Do serum electrophoresis on all >50yrs with new back pain.
• *Hypercalcaemia* may be symptomatic (p668). Lesions are due to ↑osteoclast acti-vation, from signalling by myeloma cells.
• *Anaemia, neutropenia, or thrombocytopenia* may result from marrow infiltration by plasma cells, leading to symptoms of anaemia, infection, and bleeding.
• *Recurrent bacterial infections* due to immunoparesis, and also because of neutro-penia due to the disease and from chemotherapy.
• *Kidney disease* seen in ~20% at diagnosis (p310, p364). Multiple causes but often due to light chain cast nephropathy ('myeloma kidney'). Light chains have a toxic/inflammatory effect on the proximal tubule, but main effect is due to precipitation in the distal loop of Henle. Deposits may rarely be AL-amyloid (causing nephrotic syndrome, see p364) or else monoclonal Ig can disrupt glomeruli to cause mono-clonal Ig deposition disease. May also be related to ↑Ca², contrast, or meds.
• *Neuropathy* sensory ± motor—uncommon at the time of diagnosis and mostly due to amyloidosis.

Tests Bloods FBC: normocytic normochromic anaemia. Film: rouleaux (p320). Persistently ↑ESR (p368). ↑Urea and creatinine, ↑Ca²⁺ (in ~40%). Alk phos usually ↔ unless healing fracture. **Bone marrow biopsy** See figs 8.75–8.78. **Screening test** Serum & urine electrophoresis, serum free light chain ratio, β₂-microglobulin (prognostic), LDH. **Imaging** Skeletal survey: x-rays of chest; all of spine; skull; pelvis may show lytic 'punched-out' lesions, eg pepper-pot skull, vertebral collapse, frac-tures, or osteoporosis. CT or MRI may be useful to detect lesions not seen on x-ray. **Diagnostic criteria** See BOX 'Myeloma diagnosis'.

Treatment Supportive • Analgesia for bone pain (avoid NSAIDs due to risk of AKI). Give all patients a bisphosphonate (sodium clodronate, zoledronic acid, or pamidronate disodium), as they reduce fracture rates and bone pain, and increase survival. Local radiotherapy can help rapidly in focal disease. Orthopaedic proced-ures (vertebroplasty or kyphoplasty) may be helpful in vertebral collapse. • Anaemia should be corrected with *transfusion*, and erythropoietin may be used. • AKI: re-hydrate, and ensure adequate fluid intake of 3L/day to prevent cast nephropathy. Dialysis may be needed in AKI. • Infections: treat rapidly with broad-spectrum anti-biotics until culture results are known. Regular IV *immunoglobulin infusions* may be needed if recurrent.

Chemotherapy Induction therapy with, eg lenalidomide, bortezomib, and dexa-methasone. In suitably fit patients this may be followed by autologous stem-cell transplantation. In those unsuitable for transplantation, induction therapy is typic-ally continued for 12–18 months, or until serum paraprotein levels have plateaued. Treatment is then typically held until (inevitably) paraprotein levels start to rise again, at which point further chemotherapy or stem cell transplantation may be considered. NB: lenalidomide is a teratogenic immunomodulator which has multiple SE, notably neutropenia and thromboembolism: monitor for sepsis and consider as-pirin or anticoagulation if risk ↑, eg hyperviscosity or other comorbidities.

Prognosis Worse if: >2 osteolytic lesions, β₂-microglobulin >5.5mg/L, Hb <11g/L; albumin <30g/L. Risk stratification increasingly based upon detection of specific cytogenetic abnormalities associated with high risk of progression. Causes of death: infection, AKI.

Myeloma diagnosis

Diagnostic criteria: ≥ 10% marrow plasma cells or extramedullary plasmacytoma and at least one of the following:
1 Evidence of end-organ damage from myeloma:
  • Hypercalcaemia.
  • Renal insufficiency.
  • Anaemia.
  • Bone lesions: do skeletal survey ± whole-body MRI and PET-CT.
2 Myeloma-defining biomarkers: >60% bone marrow plasma cells, serum free light ratio >100, or >1 focal lesion on MRI.

Causes of bone pain/tenderness

• Trauma/fracture (steroids ↑ risk).
• Myeloma and other primary malignancy, eg plasmacytoma or sarcoma.
• Secondaries (eg from breast, lung, etc.).
• Osteonecrosis, eg from microemboli.
• Osteomyelitis/periostitis (eg syphilis).
• Hydatid cyst (bone is a rare site).
• Osteosclerosis, eg from hepatitis C.
• Paget's disease of bone.
• Sickle cell anaemia.
• Renal osteodystrophy.
• CREST syndrome/Sjögren's syndrome.
• Hyperparathyroidism.

Tests PSA, ESR, Ca²⁺, LFT, electrophoresis.
Treatment Treat the cause; bisphosphonates & NSAIDs may control symptoms.

Complications of myeloma

• **Hypercalcaemia (p668)** This occurs with active disease, eg at presentation or relapse. Rehydrate vigorously with IV fluids 4–6L/d (careful fluid balance). IV bisphosphonates, eg zoledronic acid or pamidronate disodium, are useful for treating hypercalcaemia acutely.
• **Spinal cord compression (p462)** Occurs in 5% of those with myeloma. Urgent MRI if suspected. Treatment is with dexamethasone 8–16mg/24h PO and local radiotherapy.
• **Hyperviscosity (p368)** occurs particularly with IgM, IgA, IgG3. Causes reduced cognition, disturbed vision, and bleeding. It is treated with plasmapheresis to remove light chains.
• **AKI** is treated with rehydration. Urgent dialysis may be needed.

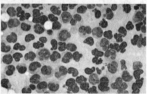

Fig 8.75 Myeloma bone marrow: many plasma cells with abnormal forms.
Courtesy of Prof. Christine Lawrence.

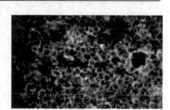

Fig 8.76 Marrow section in myeloma, stained with IgG kappa monoclonal antibody.
Courtesy of Prof. Christine Lawrence.

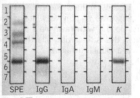

Fig 8.77 An IgG kappa paraprotein monoclonal band (immunofixation electrophoresis; a control sample has run on the left).
Courtesy of Prof. Christine Lawrence.

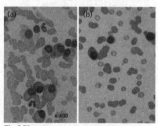

Fig 8.78 Plasma cells in myeloma. (a) Marrow smear. (b) Peripheral smear. Note rouleaux formation of red cells (p320, p366).
Courtesy of Prof. Tangun & Dr Köroğlu.

Erythrocyte sedimentation rate (ESR)

The ESR is a sensitive but non-specific indicator of the presence of disease. It measures how far RBCs fall through a column of anticoagulated blood in 1h. If certain proteins cover red cells, these cause RBCs to stick to each other in columns (the same phenomenon as rouleaux, p320) so they fall faster.

Causes of a raised ESR Any inflammation (eg infection, rheumatoid arthritis, malignancy, myocardial infarction), anaemia, and macrocytosis.

Caveats • ESR ↑ with age. The Westergren method is a rough guide to calculate the upper limit of normal in older patients: ♂: ESR = age ÷ 2; ♀: ESR = (age + 10) ÷ 2.
• Some conditions *lower* the ESR, eg polycythaemia (due to ↑red cell concentration), microcytosis, and sickle cell anaemia. Even a slightly raised ESR in these patients should prompt one to ask: *'What else is the matter?'*

Management • In those with a slightly raised ESR, the best plan is probably to wait a month and repeat the test. • If the ESR is markedly raised (>100mm/h), this can have a 90% predictive value for disease, so such patients should be thoroughly investigated, even in the presence of non-specific symptoms. Take a full history, examine carefully, and consider these tests: FBC, plasma electrophoresis, U&E, PSA, chest and abdominal imaging, ± biopsy of bone marrow or temporal artery.

Plasma viscosity (PV)

Normal range: 1.50–1.72mPa/s. In many labs, this has replaced the ESR, as it is less affected by anaemia and simpler to automate. PV is affected by the concentration of large plasma proteins and ↑ in the same conditions as the ESR—both PV and ESR ↑ in chronic inflammation and are less affected by acute changes (unlike CRP, p678).

Hyperviscosity syndrome

Symptoms Lethargy; confusion; ↓cognition; CNS disturbance; chest pain; abdominal pain (and sometimes spontaneous GI or GU bleeding); syncope; visual disturbance (eg ↓vision, amaurosis fugax, retinopathy—eg engorged retinal veins, haemorrhages, exudates; and a blurred disc as seen in fig 8.79). The visual symptoms are like 'looking through a watery car windscreen'.

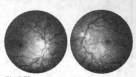

Fig 8.79 Hyperviscosity syndrome.

Causes of high blood viscosity Very high red cell count (haematocrit >50, eg polycythaemia vera), white cell count (>100 × 10⁹/L, eg leukaemia), or plasma components—usually immunoglobulins, in myeloma or Waldenström's macroglobulinaemia (p364, as IgM is larger and so ↑ viscosity more than the same amount of IgG). Drugs: eg diuretics, IV Ig, erythropoietin, chemotherapy, radio-contrast media.

Treatment Urgent treatment is needed which depends on the cause. Venesection is done in polycythaemia. Leukapheresis in leukaemias to remove white cells. Plasmapheresis in myeloma and Waldenström's: blood is withdrawn via a plasma exchange machine, the supernatant plasma from this is discarded, and the RBCs returned to the patient after being resuspended in a suitable medium.

The spleen and splenectomy

The spleen plays a vital immunological role by acting as a reservoir for lymphocytes, and in dealing with bacteraemias.

Causes of splenomegaly (See also p596.) *Massive* (enlarged to the RIF): CML, myelofibrosis, malaria (hyperreactive malarial splenomegaly), visceral leishmaniasis, 'tropical splenomegaly' (idiopathic—Africa, south-east Asia), and Gaucher's syndrome. *Moderate:* • Infection (eg EBV, endocarditis, TB, malaria, leishmaniasis, schistosomiasis). • Portal hypertension (liver cirrhosis). • Haematological (haemolytic anaemia, leukaemia especially CML, lymphoma). • Connective tissue disease (RA, SLE). • Others: sarcoidosis, primary antibody deficiency (*OHCS* p244), idiopathic.

When is a mass in the left upper quadrant a spleen? (Main differential: enlarged left kidney.) The spleen: • Is dull to percussion. • Enlarges towards the RIF. • Moves down on inspiration. • You may feel a medial notch. • 'You can't get above it' (ie the top margin disappears under the ribs).

Tests Image the spleen with abdominal USS or CT. Hunt for the cause of enlargement: look for lymphadenopathy and liver disease, eg: FBC, ESR, LFT ± liver, marrow, or lymph node biopsy.

Complications Symptoms of anaemia, infection, or bleeding can occur as a result of hypersplenism: cells become trapped in the spleen's reticuloendothelial system causing pancytopenia. Splenectomy may be required if severe.

Splenectomy Main indications: splenic trauma, hypersplenism, autoimmune haemolysis: in refractory ITP (p343), warm autoimmune haemolytic anaemia (p334), or congenital haemolytic anaemias. Mobilize early post-splenectomy as transient ↑platelets predisposes to thrombi. A characteristic blood film is seen following splenectomy, with Howell–Jolly bodies, Pappenheimer bodies, and target cells (p320).

▶*The main problem post-splenectomy is lifelong increased risk from infection.* The spleen contains macrophages which filter and phagocytose bacteria. Post-splenectomy infection is caused most commonly by encapsulated organisms: *Streptococcus pneumoniae, Haemophilus influenzae,* and *Neisseria meningitidis.* Reduce this risk by giving:

1 Immunizations:
  • Pneumococcal vaccine (p169), at least 2 weeks pre-op to ensure good response, or as soon as possible after emergency splenectomy, eg after trauma. Re-immunize every 5–10yrs. Avoid in pregnancy.
  • *Haemophilus influenzae* type b vaccine (Hib, see p387).
  • Meningococcal vaccination course, including Men B, Men C, and Men ACWY.
  • Annual influenza vaccine (p392).
2 Lifelong prophylactic oral antibiotics: phenoxymethylpenicillin (penicillin V) or erythromycin if penicillin allergic.
3 Pendants, bracelets, or patient-held cards to alert medical staff.
4 Advice to seek urgent medical attention if any signs of infection: will require admission for broad-spectrum antibiotics if infection develops.
5 If travelling abroad, warn of risk of severe malaria and advise meticulous prophylaxis, with nets, repellent, and medication.

The advice given here also applies to hyposplenic patients, eg in sickle cell anaemia or coeliac disease.

8 Haematology

8 Haematology

Thrombophilia is an inherited or, more commonly, acquired coagulopathy that predisposes to thrombosis, usually venous: DVT or PE. Determine if event was provoked or unprovoked. Special precautions are needed when there is an additional risk factor for thrombosis, eg *surgery, pregnancy* (see BOX for other risk factors). Only ~50% of patients with thrombosis and a +ve family history have an identifiable thrombophilia on routine tests: others may have abnormalities that are as yet unidentified.

Inherited
- **Activated protein c (APC) resistance/factor v Leiden** Chief cause of inherited thrombophilia. Present in ~5% of the population, although most will not develop thrombosis. Usually associated with a single point mutation in factor v (factor v Leiden), so that this clotting factor is not broken down by APC. Risk of DVT or PE is raised 5-fold if heterozygous for the mutation (50-fold if homozygous). Thrombotic risk is increased in pregnancy and those on oestrogens (*OHCS* p36, p121, & p155).
- **Prothrombin gene mutation** Causes high prothrombin levels and ↑thrombosis due to down-regulation of fibrinolysis, by thrombin-activated fibrinolysis inhibitor.
- **Protein c & s deficiency** These vitamin κ-dependent factors act together to cleave and so neutralize factors v & VIII. Heterozygotes deficient for either protein risk thrombosis. Skin necrosis also occurs (esp. if on warfarin). Homozygous deficiency for either protein causes neonatal purpura fulminans—fatal, if untreated.
- **Antithrombin deficiency** Antithrombin is a co-factor of heparin, and inhibits thrombin. Less common, affects 1:500. Heterozygotes' thrombotic risk is greater than protein c or s deficiency by ~4-fold. Homozygosity is incompatible with life.

Acquired Causes •Surgery • Cancer (Khorana score can help predict risk of VTE in cancer patients).[8] • Antiphospholipid syndrome (APLS: see BOX, p552) • Pregnancy. • Oestrogen-containing oral contraceptive pills/HRT (relative risk 2–4). • Any cause of thrombocytosis or polycythaemia may also cause thrombosis (p362).

Which tests? Ask the lab. Do FBC, film, clotting (PT, thrombin time, APTT, fibrinogen) ± APC resistance test, lupus anticoagulant and anticardiolipin antibodies, and assays for antithrombin and proteins c & s deficiency (± DNA analysis by PCR for the factor v Leiden mutation if APC resistance test is +ve, and for prothrombin gene mutation). ▶These tests should ideally be done when the patient is well, not pregnant, and off anticoagulation for 1 month.

Who? Test those with: • arterial thrombosis or MI at <50yrs old (eg for APL) • unprovoked VTE (ie at <40yrs with no risk factors) • VTE with oral contraceptives/ pregnancy • unexplained recurrent VTE • unusual site, eg mesenteric or portal vein thrombosis • recurrent fetal loss (≥3) • neonatal thrombosis.

Who not? Those already on lifelong anticoagulation, 1st-degree relatives of people with a history of DVT/PE or thrombophilia except in special circumstances. ▶There is often no benefit to testing (ie no change to management), it is expensive and may cause significant worry to patients: be sparing in requesting these tests.

Treatment Anticoagulate acute thrombosis (p346). If recurrence occurs with no other risk factors, consider lifelong anticoagulation. Recurrence whilst on treatment should be treated by increasing treatment intensity (eg ↑target INR to 3–4). In antithrombin deficiency, high doses of heparin may be needed; liaise with a haematologist. In protein c or s deficiency, monitor treatment closely as skin necrosis may occur with warfarin.

Prevention Lifelong anticoagulation is not needed in absence of VTE, but advise of ↑risk with oestrogen-containing oral contraceptive pill or HRT, and counsel as regards to the best form of contraception. Warn about other risk factors for VTE. Prophylaxis may be needed in pregnancy, eg in antiphospholipid syndrome (get expert help: aspirin and, sometimes, prophylactic heparin are used as warfarin is teratogenic, see *OHCS* p36). Prophylactic SC heparin may also be indicated in high-risk situations, eg pre-surgery.

Other risk factors for thrombosis

Arterial	Venous
• Smoking.	• Surgery.
• Hypertension.	• Trauma.
• Hyperlipidaemia.	• Immobility.
• Diabetes mellitus.	• Pregnancy, oestrogen-containing oral contraceptive pill, HRT.
	• Age.
	• Obesity.
	• Varicose veins.
	• Other conditions: heart failure, malignancy, inflammatory bowel disease, nephrotic syndrome, sickle cell anaemia, paroxysmal nocturnal haemoglobinuria (PNH)* (p334).

*PNH, HIT, and antiphospholipid antibody syndrome can cause both arterial and venous thrombi.

►If there are recurrent clots despite adequate anticoagulation, consider occult malignancy, HIT, or antiphospholipid antibody syndrome.

For thrombophilia in pregnancy, see *OHCS* p36; for anticoagulant use in pregnancy and thromboprophylaxis, see *OHCS* p36.

Antiphospholipid syndrome (APLS)

APLS is an autoimmune multisystem disorder characterized by arterial, venous, or small vessel thromboembolic events and/or pregnancy morbidity in the presence of persistent antiphospholipid antibodies. It can occur as a primary condition or in the setting of an underlying systemic autoimmune disease, particularly SLE. Other manifestations include thrombocytopenia, livedo reticularis, Libman–Sacks endocarditis, or renal disease.

The diagnosis requires at least one of two clinical criteria and at least one of three laboratory criteria to be met:

Clinical criteria
* One or more otherwise unexplained venous or arterial thrombotic events.
* Pregnancy morbidity including fetal death after 10 weeks' gestation, premature birth due to severe pre-eclampsia or placental insufficiency, or multiple embryonic losses (<10 weeks' gestation).

Laboratory criteria
* Lupus anticoagulant assay.
* IgG or IgM anticardiolipin antibody test.
* IgG or IgM anti-β_2 glycoprotein 1 antibody test.

►One or more of these antibodies must be present on two or more occasions at least 12 weeks apart.

Treatment
None for asymptomatic patients but pregnant patients may need low-dose aspirin or LMWH. Anticoagulation with warfarin for acute thromboembolism. Catastrophic APLS, a rare, life-threatening form of APLS characterized by disseminated intravascular thrombosis with multi-organ failure, is treated with anticoagulation, glucocorticoids, and, in severe cases, plasma exchange and/or IV immunoglobulin.

As well as being used in leukaemias and cancers, immunosuppression is required in organ and marrow transplants, and plays a role in the treatment of many diseases: rheumatoid arthritis, psoriasis, autoimmune hepatitis, asthma, SLE, vasculitis, and IBD, to name a few.

Prednisolone Steroids can be life-saving, but bear in mind:
- Long-term steroids (>3 weeks, or repeated courses) *must not* be stopped suddenly. ▶Risk of Addisonian crisis due to adrenal insufficiency, see p819. Plan a gradual taper over weeks (with the advice of an endocrinologist if needed).
- Certain conditions may be made worse by steroids, eg TB, hypertension, chickenpox, osteoporosis, diabetes: here careful monitoring is needed.
- Growth retardation may occur in young patients, and the elderly frequently get more SE from treatment.
- Interactions: efficacy is reduced by anti-epileptics (see later in topic) and rifampicin.
- Caution in pregnancy (may cause fetal growth retardation). See *BNF* for use in breastfeeding.

Side effects Multiple and serious (**table 8.11**): minimize these by using the lowest dose possible for the shortest period of time. Prescribe calcium and vitamin D supplements to reduce risk of osteoporosis (p674) or consider bisphosphonates. Before starting long-term treatment, explain *clearly* the potential SE to patients and ensure they are aware of the following:
- *Do not* stop steroids suddenly (p819).
- Consult a doctor if unwell; ↑ steroid dose (eg if requiring antibiotics or surgery).
- Carry a steroid card stating dose taken, and the indication.
- Avoid over-the-counter drugs, eg NSAIDs: aspirin and ibuprofen (↑risk of DU).
- Exercise and smoking cessation help to prevent osteoporosis.

Azathioprine SE Diarrhoea, abdominal pain, marrow suppression (anaemia, lymphopenia), pancreatitis, transaminitis. **Interactions** Mercaptopurine and azathioprine (which is metabolized to mercaptopurine) are metabolized by xanthine oxidase (XO). So toxicity results if full-dose azathioprine co-administered with XO inhibitors (eg allopurinol). **Monitoring** Local guidelines should be in place to guide; typically weekly FBC, U&E, creatine, LFT during initiation then 1–3-monthly once stable.

Ciclosporin, tacrolimus Calcineurin inhibitors with important roles in reducing rejection in organ and marrow transplant. The main SE is dose-related nephrotoxicity: check blood levels.
- Other SE: gum hyperplasia (ciclosporin), tremor, ↑BP (stop if ↑↑), oedema, paraesthesiae, confusion, seizures, hepatotoxicity, lymphoma, skin cancer—skin protection NB.
- Monitor U&E and creatinine every 2 weeks for the first 3 months, then monthly if dose >2.5mg/kg/d (every 2 months if less than this). ▶Check blood level and seek specialist advice if creatinine increasing. Also monitor LFT.
- Interactions are legion: potentiated by: ketoconazole, diltiazem, verapamil, the Pill, erythromycin, grapefruit juice. Efficacy is reduced by: barbiturates, carbamazepine, phenytoin, rifampicin. Concurrent NSAIDs augment hepatotoxicity—monitor LFT. Check with pharmacists if unsure regarding potential interaction.

Methotrexate An antimetabolite. Inhibits dihydrofolate reductase, which is involved in the synthesis of purines and pyrimidines. See p543.

Cyclophosphamide An alkylating agent. SE: marrow suppression (monitor FBC), nausea, infertility, teratogenic, haemorrhagic cystitis due to an irritative urinary metabolite. There is a slight ↑risk of later developing bladder cancer or leukaemia.

Rituximab Monoclonal antibody that targets the CD20 antigen and depletes B cells. **Pre-treatment** Screen for recent or recurrent infections. Check CXR, HBV/HCV/HIV, Ig levels. Vaccinate for pneumococcus and influenza prior to treatment. **Monitoring** B-cell depletion defined as CD19 levels <5 cells/microlitre. **Side effects** Infusion reactions, serum sickness, infections (eg reactivation of TB, HBV).

Table 8.11 Side effects of steroid use

System	Adverse reactions
Gastrointestinal	Pancreatitis
	Candidiasis
	Oesophageal ulceration
	Peptic ulceration
Musculoskeletal	Myopathy
	Osteoporosis
	Fractures
	Growth suppression
Endocrine	Adrenal suppression
	Hypertension, diabetes, Cushing's syndrome
CNS	Aggravated epilepsy
	Depression; psychosis
Eye	Cataracts; glaucoma
	Papilloedema
Immune	Increased susceptibility to and severity of infections, eg chickenpox

Steroids can also cause fever and ↑wcc; steroids only rarely cause leucopenia.

From *Frankenstein* to ciclosporin: unleashing immune control

Since the publication of Mary Shelley's *Frankenstein* in 1818, the concept of utilizing another person's organs to extend or enhance the life of another has captivated both the medical community and the general public. However, it wasn't until the late 19th century that this notion began to materialize in the real world. A key milestone was the discovery of the immunosuppressant effects of ciclosporin in the 1970s—the first of a new generation of immunosuppressive drugs called calcineurin inhibitors that could prevent organ rejection without the harmful toxicity of available products. Ciclosporin was first discovered in Norway in 1969 by Sandoz biologist Dr Hans Peter Frey from a soil sample collected in a plastic bag by a Sandoz employee on a trip (the company encouraged employees to collect such samples on business trips and holidays to search for new antibiotic drugs from fungal metabolites). Although initially investigated as an anti-fungal antibiotic, fellow Sandoz researcher Dr Jean Borel discovered the compound's promise in suppressing T-cells in the immune system. A purified form was synthesized in 1973, and further research, including trials on humans, revealed its potential for preventing organ rejection. While transplantation remains a significant medical procedure, and chronic rejection can be burdensome, ciclosporin played a crucial role in advancing medical science and turning a fantastical idea into reality.

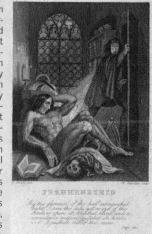

FRANKENSTEIN

By the glimmer of the half extinguished light, I saw the dull yellow eye of the creature open; it breathed hard, and a convulsive motion agitated its limbs.
... I rushed out of the room. Page 44.

London Published by H. Colburn and R. Bentley, 1831.

Fig 8.80 Victor Frankenstein observing the first stirrings of his creature.
Source: Engraving by W. Chevalier after Th. von Holst, 1831. Public Domain Mark. Source: Wellcome Collection.

9 Infectious diseases

Contents
What is life? 375
Infectious disease: an overview 376

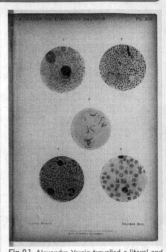

Fig 9.1 Alexandre Yersin travelled a literal and metaphorical half world away from the Pasteur Institute in Paris to work in French IndoChina in 1890. His medical fame was etched in a bamboo hut during the 1894 outbreak of plague in Hong Kong. He bribed morgue guards to acquire specimens from the dead and isolated the causative organism, later named *Yersinia pestis* in his honour. Yersin remained in IndoChina, directing Hanoi's first medical school, and establishing a medical laboratory in Nha Trang. He also delved into botany, introducing to the region the rubber tree, and the cinchona tree used to produce quinine. Of medicine, he said, 'I am very happy to treat those who come to me asking for advice, but I wouldn't like to make medicine my profession ... I consider medicine a calling, like priesthood.' He was the Ông Nam (fifth uncle) of many in Vietnam. Buried in his adopted home of Nha Trang, he remained to the last an eccentric, eclectic, and humble polymath. And so we too aspire to balance humanitarianism with forensic attention to detail in our approach to infectious disease.

La peste bubonique à Hong-Kong / A.E.J. Yersin.
Wellcome Collection.
Source: Wellcome Collection, Public Domain Mark.

We thank James Whitehorn, our Specialist Reader and Adam Komorowski, our Junior Reader for this chapter.

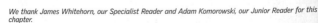

What is life?

By convention, life is anything which is organic and converts nutrients into progeny. Failure to meet this definition means non-living, dead, or dying. Life is a thing of dynamism, fragility, beauty, danger, and evanescence; gushing forth from a single source. But here the certainties end: what does it really take to be alive? Are viruses and prions living? How many branches are there on our tree? The harder we look, the more complexities we find. The Hillis plot is a circular phylogenetic tree, and a representation of humanity's place in nature. We are duly humbled by this challenge to our imagined self-importance, reminding us that we do not in reality occupy a privileged position in the hierarchy of the living, just a unique subunit RNA sequence (fig 9.2).

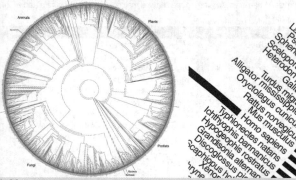

Fig 9.2 Tree of life based on subunit RNA sequences sampled from ~3000 species out of the 1.7 million species that are formally named. The image on the right is a close up of the 'animal' segment of the diagram (upper left quadrant) showing 'You are here'.
Copyright David M. Hillis, Derrick Zwickl, and Robin Gutell, University of Texas.
http://www.zo.utexas.edu/faculty/antisense/downloadfilesToL.html

Because micro-organisms kill our friends, we think of them as bad, '*I have no philosophy, nor piety, no art of reflection, no theory of compensation to meet things so hideous, so cruel, and so mad, they are just unspeakably horrible and irremediable to me and I stare at them with angry and almost blighted eyes.*' (Henry James, 1915, describing the death of Rupert Brooke from septicaemia.)

But this is a mistake. Kill off micro-organisms and the whole show fizzles out. Micro-organisms gave us the DNA and organelles needed for reading and digesting this page. Even killing a single pathogen might be a mistake: Sod's Law will probably ensure that something worse will come to inhabit the vacated ecospace. Prod one part of the system and events ripple out in an unending stream of unintended consequences, played out under the stars, which themselves are evolving, and which donate and receive our primordial elements.

Can we win against infectious diseases? No. But winning or losing is the wrong image: infectious diseases have made us who we are. All we can do is live with them. To help us do this in ways that are not too destructive we need robust public health surveillance, sound vector-control policies, political will, quarantine laws, openness, and cooperation. Most importantly, do not underestimate the importance of maintaining our infectious cohabitants in their apparent subordinate position. The speed and capacity for learning by ribonucleic malware and single-celled organisms is amazing. So do not inadvertently teach them. Preserve your precious warfare tactics. Expose them to antibiotic therapies only in a stand-off situation from which they cannot return to fight again.

It is not possible for any ID chapter to be constructed so that it has the right balance throughout the world. Many of our readers come from communities where malaria is the primary differential, and AIDS-related deaths are common. In contrast, it is chest, GU, and ENT infections which predominate in the UK; and AIDS is considered only where there is failure of either diagnosis or treatment of HIV, which are universally available and free at the point of care. Many of the diseases in this chapter cause multisystem pathology. For these infections, it may be helpful to classify by pathogen (table 9.1). However, infectious agents do not walk in the door and introduce themselves. Detective work may be necessary based on geography; or exposure: to vectors, animals, and contaminated water/food. And so other pages in this chapter have that as their (helpful) premise. When infection is organ specific, you may need to look elsewhere (table 9.2).

Table 9.1 Infectious disease by pathogen (illustrative, not exhaustive)

Bacteria	Viruses
Gram positive	**RNA viruses**
Staphylococci:	Picornavirus ('tiny RNA'):
• *Staph. aureus* (coagulase +ve)	• Rhinovirus
• *Staph. epidermidis* (coagulase −ve)	• Poliovirus
Streptococci:	Calicivirus ('cup'), eg Norwalk
• α-haemolytic, eg *Strep. pneumoniae*	Flavivirus ('yellow'):
• β-haemolytic, eg *Strep. pyogenes*	• Dengue • Zika • Yellow fever
Enterococci	Coronavirus ('crown'), eg SARS-COV-2 (COVID-19)
Clostridium species:	Rhabdovirus ('rod'), eg rabies
• *C. botulinum* (botulism)	Filovirus ('thread'), eg Ebola/Marburg
• *C. perfringens* (gas gangrene)	Paramyxovirus ('near mucus'), eg mumps
• *C. tetani* (tetanus)	**DNA viruses**
• *C. difficile* (diarrhoea)	Hepadnavirus ('liver DNA'): eg hepatitis B
Gram negative	Parvovirus ('small'): eg parvovirus B19
Neisseria:	Herpesvirus ('spreading')
• *N. meningitidis* (meningitis)	• HSV
• *N. gonorrhoeae* (gonorrhoea)	• EBV
Helicobacter pylori	• VZV
Escherichia coli	• CMV
Shigella species	**Fungi**
Salmonella species	*Candida*
Campylobacter jejuni	*Pneumocystis jirovecii*
Klebsiella pneumoniae	*Cryptococcus*
Pseudomonas aeruginosa	**Parasites**
Haemophilus influenzae	**Protozoa**
Bordetella pertussis (whooping cough)	*Entamoeba histolytica*
Vibrio cholerae (cholera)	*Giardia lamblia*
Yersinia pestis (plague)	*Cryptosporidium* species
Mycobacteria	*Toxoplasma gondii*
M. tuberculosis	*Plasmodium* species (malaria)
M. leprae	*Leishmania* species (leishmaniasis)
Intracellular bacteria	*Trypanosoma* species (trypanosomiasis)
Chlamydia	**Nematodes**
Rickettsia (rickettsial disease)	Soil-transmitted helminths
Coxiella burnetii	Filarial disease
Spirochaetes	**Trematodes**
Borrelia burgdorferi (Lyme disease)	*Schistosoma* (schistosomiasis), flukes
Treponema (syphilis, yaws)	**Cestodes**
Leptospira (Weil's disease)	Hydatid disease, tapeworm

Table 9.2 Infectious disease by organ system

System	Infection	Page
Respiratory	Pneumonia	pp168–171
	SARS-CoV-2 (COVID-19)	pp172-3
	Empyema—infected pleural effusion	p175
	Fungal infections of the lung	p174
GI	Peptic ulcer disease	p248
	Gastroenteritis	pp424–29
	Colitis, proctitis, diverticulitis, appendicitis	p255, p600, p620
	Viral hepatitis	p274
	Tropical liver disease	pp430–1
	Cholecystitis, cholangitis, gallbladder empyema	p626
	Peritonitis	p598
GU and gynaecology	Lower urinary tract infection, cystitis, pyelonephritis	pp292–3
	Cervicitis, vulvovaginitis	pp408–9
	Genital ulceration	pp408–9
	Genital warts	p402
	Pelvic inflammatory disease, endometritis	OHCS p134
Cardiovascular	Infective endocarditis	pp144–5
	Myocarditis	pp130–1
	Pericarditis	p132
Nervous system	Meningitis, encephalitis, subdural empyema	pp806–9
	Infective neuropathy	pp500–1
Skin and soft tissue	Skin ulcers, gangrene	pp652–3
	Tropical skin disease	pp436–7
	Surgical wound infection	p576, p580
Bone and joint	Osteomyelitis	OHCS p502
	Septic arthritis	p540
ENT	Pharyngitis, laryngitis, otitis media	OHCS p394
Eye	Tropical eye disease	pp434–5

The management of infectious disease includes prevention whenever possible. Tracing the source of disease and contacts are essential in the management of outbreaks. Notification to your local health protection team (see https://www.gov.uk/guidance/notifiable-diseases-and-causative-organisms-how-to-report) is a statutory duty in the UK for the following conditions (only clinical suspicion is required, accuracy of diagnosis is secondary):

* Acute encephalitis
* Acute infectious hepatitis
* Acute meningitis
* Acute poliomyelitis
* Anthrax
* Botulism
* Brucellosis
* Cholera
* Diphtheria
* Enteric fever
* Food poisoning
* HUS
* Infectious dysentery
* Invasive group A strep
* Legionnaire's disease
* Leprosy
* Malaria
* Measles
* Meningococcal sepsis
* Mumps
* Plague
* Rabies
* Rubella
* SARS
* SARS-CoV-2 (COVID-19)
* Scarlet fever
* Smallpox
* Tetanus
* Tuberculosis
* Typhus
* Viral haemorrhagic fever
* Whooping cough
* Yellow fever.

Infectious disease resources

The Hillis plot (**fig 9.2, p375**) tells us that ID chapters will always fail to be exhaustive. We therefore direct you to the following excellent resources:

* **Public Health England:** https://www.gov.uk/topic/health-protection/infectious-diseases
* **World Health Organization (WHO):** http://www.who.int/topics/en/
* **US Centers for Disease Control and Prevention:** http://www.cdc.gov
* **European Society of Clinical Microbiology and Infectious Diseases:** www.escid.org

Humans and bacteria are symbiotes, with each of us host to ten times as many bacterial cells as our own human cells. Our gut, skin, and mucosal linings are covered with bacteria. We rely on this for nutrition, functioning vitamin κ, anti-inflammatory effects, and immune system regulation.

Bacterial disease results from a breach of the measures that limit bacteria to their 'normal' roles: skin commensals moved into the bloodstream by a cannula, antibiotics altering the commensal microflora, immune system evasion or dysfunction allowing organisms to stray beyond their usual boundaries, and toxin production. When treating infections we should therefore remember to look beyond the offending organism and consider what factors may have aided pathogenesis: malnutrition, 'barrier' breach by cancer/plastic, or immunosuppression.

▶See 'Sepsis', p772.

Bacterial glossary

Bacteria Prokaryotic micro-organism without a membrane-bound nucleus.

Classification of bacteria By microscopy and culture of infected samples. Informs antibiotic choice. Includes:

- *Gram stain:* a staining technique. Bacteria with thick, exposed peptidoglycan layers will stain 'Gram positive' (purple/blue). Bacteria with a protected peptidoglycan layer will counterstain pink/red and are 'Gram negative' (fig 9.3).
- *Shape:* cocci = round; bacilli = rod-shaped; spirochaete = spiral.
- *Aerobes/anaerobes:* some bacteria cannot survive without oxygen (obligate aerobes), whilst others cannot grow in its presence (obligate anaerobes). Many more can survive in either environment (facultative anaerobes). Some types of infection are more likely to involve aerobic or anaerobic bacteria, eg GI infections are typically anaerobic.

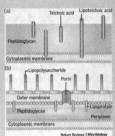

Fig 9.3 (a) Gram-positive versus (b) Gram-negative cell membranes.
Reprinted by permission from Macmillan Publishers Ltd: *Nature Reviews Microbiology*, Cabeen et al., 3(8), 601–610, copyright 2005.

Bacteraemia Bacteria circulating in the bloodstream.

Bactericidal Kills bacteria both in and out of the replication cycle.

Bacteriostatic Stops replication without killing existing bacteria.

Capsulate bacteria Bacteria with a thick outer capsule, eg *Haemophilus influenzae*, *Neisseria meningitidis*, and *Streptococcus pneumoniae*. These are destroyed in the spleen. Following splenectomy (or splenic infarction, eg sickle cell anaemia) there is an increased risk of infection by capsulate bacteria and prophylactic vaccination should be offered (p403).

Commensal An organism that lives in/on a host without causing harm.

Endotoxin A lipopolysaccharide complex found on the outer membrane of Gram-negative bacteria. Can elicit an inflammatory response. Activates complement via the alternative pathway.

Enterotoxin Exotoxin that targets the gut, eg *Clostridium difficile* toxin (p407).

Exotoxin Toxins secreted by bacteria acting at a site distant from bacterial growth. Production of an exotoxin can determine virulence, eg botulinum, tetanus, diphtheria, Shiga toxins.

Flagella A tail-like appendage that moves to propel the bacterium, eg *Helicobacter pylori*.

Nosocomial Acquired in a hospital/healthcare setting (pp406–7).

Obligate intracellular Bacteria that can only survive in host cells ∴ induce a cell-mediated immune response and will not grow on standard culture media.

Ziehl–Neelsen stain Mycolic acid in the cell wall of mycobacteria resists Gram staining but will appear red with acid-fast techniques (= acid-fast stain).

Antibiotics: action and resistance

The antibiotic revolution began in 1928 when an extraordinary series of fortuitous events (including a cancelled holiday and an unpredictable British summer) led to Alexander Fleming's observation that a contaminating *Penicillium* colony caused lysis of staphylococci. Mass production and the 'golden age' of antibiotics followed, with the introduction of a variety of drugs selectively toxic to bacterial, but not mammalian cells. This is achieved by:
- utilizing a target unique to bacteria, eg cell wall.
- selectively targeting bacterial-specific components, eg enzymes, ribosomes.
- preventing transport of the drug into human cells, eg metronidazole can only be transported into anaerobic bacteria.

The mechanism of action of different classes of antibiotic is shown in fig 9.4.

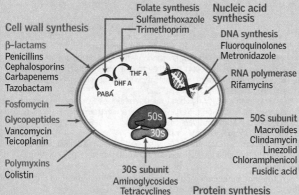

Fig 9.4 Classes of antibiotics and their bacterial cell targets.

This spectrum of available antibiotics revolutionized clinical practice and led to the declaration: '*It is time to close the book on infectious diseases, and declare the war against pestilence won*' (attributed in urban legend to Dr William H Stewart, US Surgeon General, 1965–1969). Such confidence failed to consider that the capacity for a prokaryotic micro-organism to develop resistance far outstrips the human capacity to develop new antibiotic drugs.

Antibiotic resistance can be:
- Intrinsic: due to inherent structural or functional characteristics, eg vancomycin cannot cross the outer membrane of Gram-negative organisms.
- Acquired: bacteria have been evolving to resist antibacterial agents for billions of years through mutation and/or the transfer of resistance properties. This evolutionary phenomenon is accelerated by selection pressure from antibiotic use (including agriculture, aquaculture, and horticulture) which provides a competitive advantage for mutated, resistant strains.

Resistance has emerged for all known antibiotics causing morbidity, mortality, and a huge cost burden worldwide.[1] Misadventure is evident. Quinolones are synthetic, resistance cannot be acquired in nature, and yet it is epidemic.

Which brings us back to Alexander Fleming who, within 2 years of the mass production of his 'miracle-mould', gave this sage warning in his Nobel lecture of 1945, '*Mr X has a sore throat. He buys some penicillin and gives himself, not enough to kill the streptococci, but enough to educate them to resist penicillin. He then infects his wife. Mrs X gets pneumonia and is treated with penicillin. As the streptococci are now resistant to penicillin the treatment fails. Mrs X dies. Who is primarily responsible for Mrs X's death? Why Mr X, whose negligent use of penicillin changed the nature of the microbe.*'

A guide to antibiotic prescribing
▶▶Give antibiotics immediately in patients with a systemic inflammatory response to infection. See 'Sepsis', p772.

Start smart
1 Do not prescribe[2] antibiotics in the absence of clinical evidence of bacterial infection, or for a self-limiting condition. Take time to discuss:
   * why an antibiotic is not the best option
   * alternative options, eg symptomatic treatment, delayed prescribing
   * the views and expectations of the patient
   * safety-netting advice: what the patient should do if their condition deteriorates.
2 Take microbiological samples *before* prescribing,[1] especially for:
   * hospital inpatients: review your prescription as soon as MC&S result is available
   * recurrent or persistent infection
   * non-severe infection: consider if your prescription can wait for MC&S results.
3 Follow local guidelines first, informed by local epidemiology and sensitivities.
4 Consider benefit and harm for each individual patient:
   * *Allergies:* clarify the patient's reaction—the true incidence of penicillin allergy in patients who report that they are allergic is <10%. In those with a confirmed penicillin allergy, cross-reactivity with 3rd-generation cephalosporins and carbapenems is possible but rare (<1%).
   * Dose adjust for kidney function (usually creatinine clearance) and weight (ideal body weight or ideal plus % excess weight in BMI extremes): follow local guidance.
   * Check for medication interactions.
   * In pregnancy and lactation, see p23.
5 Prescribe the shortest effective course. Most antibiotics have good oral availability. Use IV antibiotics in line with local or national (sepsis) guidelines.

Then focus
Review the clinical diagnosis and continuing need for antibiotics at 48h for all inpatients and all patients prescribed IV antibiotics:
* *Stop* antibiotics if there is no evidence of infection.
* Switch from IV to *oral* whenever possible.
* Change to a *narrower spectrum* antibiotic whenever possible.
* Continue regular clinical *review* whilst antibiotics are prescribed.

Antimicrobial stewardship

'This will be a post-antibiotic era. In terms of new replacement antibiotics, the pipeline is virtually dry... Prospects for turning this situation around look dim.'
Dr M Chan, Director-General of WHO, March 2012.

While overall antibiotic usage deceased by 15% in England between 2017 and 2021, severe antibiotic resistant infections increased to approximately 148 per day. 25 000 die in Europe every year from antibiotic-resistant bacteria, ~500 000/year develop multidrug-resistant TB. Cost is the only barrier to buying carbapenems over the counter in Egypt, India, and Pakistan. Antimicrobial resistance is a threat to public health, economic development, and security. It is estimated that antibiotic resistance will cause up to 10 million deaths by 2050 and lead to a $100 trillion global increase in healthcare costs.

Antimicrobial stewardship[2] is necessary in all healthcare settings:
* Monitoring, evaluation, and feedback on antimicrobial prescribing, bench-marked against up-to-date local and national guidelines.
* Evaluation of high/low levels of prescribing, and prescribing outside of guidelines.
* Review of patient safety events: avoidable infection, drug reactions, complications of antibiotic therapy, eg MRSA (p384), *C. difficile* (p255, p407).
* Education and decision support systems for antibiotic prescribers.
* Antibiotic pack sizes that correspond to appropriate course lengths.
* Regular review of antimicrobial policy, treatment, and prophylaxis guidelines.

1 Clinical diagnosis of low-severity community-acquired pneumonia is an exception, see also UTI, p292.

Inhibitors of cell wall synthesis

See **fig 9.4, p379**. The bacterial cell wall is unique in nature and therefore acts as a selective target for antibiotics. Antibiotics which act on the cell wall include:
* β-lactam antibiotics
* others: glycopeptides, polymyxins.

β-lactams: penicillins, cephalosporins, carbapenems, monobactam

Contain a β-lactam ring which inhibits the formation of peptidoglycan cross-links in the bacterial cell wall. Resistance occurs when the bacteria (eg staphylococci) produce a β-lactamase enzyme.

Penicillins: see **table 9.3, p382**. Include natural penicillins (penicillin G and V) and synthetic penicillins which are chemically modified to extend their spectrum of activity, eg amoxicillin, piperacillin.

In an attempt to overcome β-lactamase resistance, penicillins have been combined with β-lactamase inhibitors to create β-lactam-β-lactamase inhibitor combinations eg co-amoxiclav (amoxicillin + clavulanic acid), Tazocin® (piperacillin + tazobactam). Staphylococcal resistance is conventionally defined by stability to meticillin, an acid-labile and IV-only equivalent of flucloxacillin (see MRSA, p384).

Cephalosporins: see **table 9.4, p382**. Contain a β-lactam ring attached to a six-membered nuclear structure (five in penicillin), which allows synthetic modification at two sites (one in penicillin). This means that cephalosporins are the largest groups of available antibiotics. Classification into 'generations' is not standardized: as a rough rule, the higher the generation, the wider the spectrum.

Carbapenems: see **table 9.5, p382**. Broadest spectrum of all β-lactam antibiotics. Seek expert microbiology advice before use.

Monobactam: aztreonam is only active against Gram-negative species including *Neisseria meningitidis*, *Haemophilus influenzae*, *Pseudomonas*. Given IV/IM. Inhaled preparation for chronic pulmonary *Pseudomonas* (cystic fibrosis). Dose adjust for renal function. SE: N&V, GI bleed, rash, ↑LFTs, ↓plts, paraesthesia, seizures, bronchospasm.

Non-β-lactam cell wall inhibitors

See **fig 9.4, p379**, and **table 9.6, p382**. Glycopeptides, eg vancomycin, teicoplanin. Polymyxins, eg colistin. Fosfomycin (inhibits first step in cell wall synthesis).

Inhibitors of protein synthesis

See **fig 9.4, p379**, and **table 9.7, p383**. Includes:
* aminoglycosides
* macrolides
* tetracyclines and derivatives of tetracycline
* others: clindamycin, linezolid, chloramphenicol, fusidic acid.

Inhibitors of nucleic acid synthesis

See **fig 9.4, p379**, and **table 9.8, p383**. Includes:
* folate synthesis inhibitors: trimethoprim, co-trimoxazole
* fluoroquinolones
* others: metronidazole, rifampicin, fidaxomicin.

▶Nitrofurantoin is unique. Metabolites interfere with cell growth via ribosomes, DNA, RNA, and cell wall. Multiple sites of attack mean ↓resistance. Concentrates in the urine (but not if ↓GFR), used in uncomplicated UTI, not systemically active. SE: haemolysis, pulmonary fibrosis, hepatotoxicity.

▶Antibiotics for TB, see **pp390–1**.

9 Infectious diseases

Table 9.3 Penicillins

Antibiotic	Indications	Considerations
Benzylpenicillin (penicillin G, 'penicillin')	Gram +ve: streptococci (chest, throat, endocarditis, cellulitis), meningococcus, diphtheria, anthrax, leptospirosis	Give IV, poor oral absorption. Dose adjust for GFR. SE: allergy, rash, N&V, C. difficile, cholestasis
Phenoxymethyl-penicillin (penicillin v)	Throat, prophylaxis: splenectomy/hyposplenism, rheumatic fever	Oral bioavailability may vary
Ampicillin/amoxicillin	Extended penicillin spectrum includes enterobacteria (↓ activity against Gram +ve): sinusitis, chest, otitis media, UTI, H. pylori, Lyme disease	Ampicillin IV, amoxicillin PO. Dose adjust for GFR. SE: as per penicillin G, rash with EBV
Amoxicillin + clavulanic acid (co-amoxiclav)	Used if resistance to narrower-spectrum antibiotics: chest, pyelo-nephritis, cellulitis, bone	Dose adjust for GFR SE: as per amoxicillin
Piperacillin + tazobactam	Broad spectrum including Gram +ve, Gram –ve, Pseudomonas: neu-tropenic sepsis, hospital-acquired/complicated infection	Tazobactam ↓penetration of blood–brain barrier. Dose adjust for GFR. SE: as per penicillin G. Myelosuppression in prolonged use (rare)
Pivmecillinam	Gram –ve (not Pseudomonas or enterococcus): UTI	Risk of carnitine depletion SE: as per penicillin G
Flucloxacillin	β-lactamase resistant, Staphylococcus: skin, bone	Dose adjust for GFR. SE: allergy, rash, N&V, cholestasis

Table 9.4 Cephalosporins

Antibiotic	Indications	Considerations
Cefalexin (1st generation)	Gram +ve infection: UTI, pneumonia.	↓First-line use in UK due to risk of C. difficile
Cefuroxime (2nd generation)	Gram +ve and Gram –ve (Enterobacterales, H. influenzae): UTI, sinusitis, skin, wound	SE: allergy, rash, N&V, cholestasis, haemolysis
Cefotaxime, ceftriaxone, ceftazidime (3rd generation)	Broad spectrum (not Pseudomonas, Enterococcus spp., Bacteroides). Ceftazidime includes Pseudomonas but ↓activity against Gram +ve	Caution: false +ve urinary glucose and Coombs test
Cefepime (4th generation)	Gram +ve and Gram –ve (not MRSA)	Ceftriaxone precipitation in urinary/biliary tracts
Tazobactam/ceftolozane (5th generation)	Broad spectrum including Pseudomonas: complicated intra-abdominal and UTI, VAP	

Table 9.5 Carbapenems

Antibiotic	Indications	Considerations
Imipenem Meropenem Ertapenem	Broad spectrum (Gram +ve, Gram –ve, aerobes, anaerobes, ertapenem does not cover Pseudomonas): hospital-acquired/ventilator-associated/compli-cated infection, neutropenic sepsis	Dose adjust for GFR. Imipenem given with cilastatin to ↓renal metabolism SE: N&V, C. difficile, rash, eosino-philia, ↓plts, ↑LFTs, seizures

Table 9.6 Lipopeptides and polymyxins

Antibiotic	Indication	Considerations
Lipopeptides		
Vancomycin Teicoplanin	Complicated Gram +ve including MRSA. Oral for C. difficile (not absorbed)	Dose IV to trough serum concentration. SE: nephrotoxic (monitor creatinine, care with other nephrotoxics), ototoxic, ↓plts
Polymyxins		
Colistin, polymyxin B	Multi-resistant Gram –ve	Nephrotoxicity in ~50%. Inhaled colistin for ventilator-associated pneumonia

Table 9.7 Inhibitors of protein synthesis

Antibiotic	Indications	Considerations
Aminoglycosides		
Gentamicin Tobramycin Amikacin	Gram –ve infection (↓activity against most Gram +ve and anaerobes). Tobramycin has ↑activity against *Pseudomonas*. Amikacin has least resistance	SE: nephrotoxic (monitor drug levels and serum creatinine), vestibular toxicity, ototoxicity
Macrolides		
Azithromycin Clarithromycin Erythromycin	Gram +ve cocci (not entero-cocci and staphylococci), syphilis, chlamydia.	SE (↑ with erythromycin): GI, cholestasis, ↑QT. Cytochrome P450 inhibition (↓ with azithromycin): ↑warfarin, rhabdo-myolysis with statins, ↑calcineurin inhibitor levels
Tetracyclines and derivatives		
Doxycycline	Exacerbation COPD, chlamydia, MRSA, Lyme disease, mycoplasma, rickettsiae, brucella, anthrax, syphilis, malaria prophylaxis	CI: pregnancy, <8yrs (teeth/bones). SE: N&V, *C. difficile*, fatty liver, idio-pathic intracranial hypertension
Tigecycline	Gram +ve and Gram –ve including β-lactam-resistant strains	Dose adjust in liver dysfunction. SE: N&V, photosensitivity, ↑LFTs
Other		
Clindamycin	Gram +ve cocci (not entero-cocci), MRSA, anaerobes	↑Risk *C. difficile*
Linezolid	Gram +ve cocci, MRSA, VRE, anaerobes, mycobacteria	MAOI: check interactions, myelosuppression, optic neuropathy
Chloramphenicol	Gram +ve, Gram –ve, anaerobes, mycoplasma, chlamydia, con-junctivitis (topical)	Systemic use limited by myelosuppression
Fusidic acid	Staphylococci	SE: GI, ↑LFTs

Table 9.8 Inhibitors of nucleic acid synthesis

Antibiotic	Indications	Considerations
Folate synthesis inhibitors		
Trimethoprim	Gram –ve: UTI, prostatitis	Inhibits creatinine secretion: ↑serum creatinine without ↓GFR
Co-trimoxazole (sulfamethoxa-zole + trimetho-prim)	*Pneumocystis jirovecii*, MRSA, GI infection (eg *Shigella, E. coli*), protozoans (eg *Cyclospora*), listeria, nocardia	Synergistic action. Good oral ab-sorption and tissue/CSF penetration. SE: folate deficiency, ↑K+, rash, myelosuppression, haemolysis with G6PD deficiency
Fluoroquinolones		
Ciprofloxacin Levofloxacin Moxifloxacin	Broad including *Pseudomonas* (not moxifloxacin): UTI, prostatitis, atypical and hospital-acquired chest infection, infectious diarrhoea	SE: GI irritation, CNS effects (↓ seizure threshold, headache, drowsiness, mood change), per-ipheral neuropathy, tendinopathy (Achilles), ↑QT, *C. difficile*
Others		
Metronidazole	Anaerobic infection: intra-abdominal, pelvic, oral, soft-tissue. Bacterial vaginosis. *C. difficile*	Good oral absorption. Dose adjust for liver function. SE: Disulfiram reaction with alcohol, ↓ warfarin metabolism, peripheral neuropathy
Rifamycins: • Rifampicin • Rifabutin • Rifapentine	Mycobacteria (TB, non-TB myco-bacteria, leprosy), some staphylo-cocci, *Legionella*, meningococcal prophylaxis	SE: hepatitis (monitor LFTs), GI, CNS effects, myelosuppression, red secretions (urine, saliva, sweat, sputum, tears)
Fidaxomicin	Narrow Gram +ve: *C. difficile*	Poor systemic absorption, ↑cost

9 Infectious diseases

Gram-positive cocci
Staphylococci

Staphylococci are skin/nasal commensals in ~80% of adults. They can also cause infectious disease. This produces a diagnostic challenge: are the detected organisms causing infection or a contaminating commensal? The answer may lie in the presence or absence of coagulase, an enzyme which coagulates plasma.

Coagulase-negative staphylococci: eg *Staphylococcus epidermidis* are less virulent. Pathogenicity is likely only if there is underlying immune system dysfunction or foreign material (prosthetic valve/joint, IV line, PD catheter, pacemaker).

Staphylococcus aureus is coagulase positive. *Presentation:*

1 Toxin release causes disease distant from infection. Includes:
  * scalded skin syndrome—bullae and desquamation due to epidermolytic toxins (no mucosal disease, ↓skin loss compared to toxic epidermal necrolysis)
  * preformed toxin in food—sudden D&V (p424)
  * toxic shock—fever, confusion, rash, diarrhoea, ↓BP, AKI, multiorgan dysfunction. Tampon associated or occurs with (minor) local infection.

2 Local tissue destruction: impetigo, cellulitis, mastitis, septic arthritis, osteomyelitis, abscess, pneumonia, UTI.

3 Haematogenous spread: bacteraemia, endocarditis, 'metastatic' seeding.

Diagnosis: positive culture from relevant site of infection. *Treatment:* ▶▶Sepsis, see p772. Drain infected foci, antibiotic (topical/oral/IV) based on illness severity and risk factors. Consider local epidemiology of resistance. If systemic treatment indicated, use β-lactam whenever possible (may need to cover resistant strains until sensitivity available). Preformed toxin in food: supportive, antibiotics not usually indicated.

> ### Resistant *Staphylococcus aureus*: MRSA, VISA, VRSA
>
> *Staph. aureus* which produces β-lactamase, or an altered enzyme responsible for cell wall formation, will be resistant to β-lactam antibiotics (penicillins, cephalosporins, carbapenems, see p381). Resistance is usually defined by stability to meticillin, ie meticillin-resistant *Staph. aureus* (MRSA). Vancomycin resistance also exists and is classified by the amount of vancomycin needed to inhibit bacterial growth: vancomycin-intermediate *Staph. aureus* (VISA) and vancomycin-resistant *Staph. aureus* (VRSA). Resistant staphylococci cause ↑ morbidity and mortality compared to sensitive strains. Risk factors for colonization include: antibiotic exposure, hospital stay, surgery, nursing home residence. Treatment of infection (not colonization): vancomycin (for MRSA), teicoplanin. Oral agents with potential activity against MRSA include co-trimoxazole, doxycycline, linezolid. *Prevention:* surveillance, barrier precautions, hand-hygiene, decolonization (mupirocin 2%, chlorhexidine, tea tree oil), antimicrobial stewardship. See p380.

Streptococci

Classification based on Lancefield group persists in terminology (fig 9.5). Includes:
* *Streptococcus pyogenes* (β-haemolytic group A): colonizes throat, skin, anogenital tract. Range of infection: tonsillitis, pharyngitis, scarlet fever, impetigo, erysipelas, cellulitis, pneumonia, peripartum sepsis, necrotizing fasciitis. All can → streptococcal toxic shock = sudden-onset ↓BP, multiorgan failure. Post-infectious complications rare: rheumatic fever (p146), glomerulonephritis (p306). *Treatment:* penicillin.
* *Streptococcus agalactiae* (β-haemolytic group B): neonatal and puerperal infection, skin, soft tissue. Invasive disease (bacteraemia, endocarditis, osteomyelitis, septic arthritis, meningitis) usually has risk factors: DM, malignancy, chronic disease. *Treatment:* penicillin, macrolide, cephalosporin, chloramphenicol.
* *Streptococcus anginosus:* if found in blood culture look for an abscess—mouth, liver, lung, brain. *Treatment:* penicillin.
* *Streptococcus pneumoniae:* pneumonia (pp168–71), otitis media, meningitis, septicaemia. *Treatment:* penicillin. Vaccination: childhood, hyposplenism, >65yrs (p403).
* Viridans streptococci: commonest cause of oral/dental origin endocarditis (p144).
* *Streptococcus bovis:* bacteraemia→endocarditis. Look for colon/liver disease.

Enterococci

Gut commensal. Resistance to cephalosporins and quinolones leads to nosocomial colonization and infection. Most common is *Enterococcus faecalis*: if found in blood culture, assume endocarditis until proven otherwise. Treatment: intrinsic and acquired resistance including vancomycin-resistant enterococci (VRE). Seek expert help.

Gram-positive bacilli

Listeriosis

Caused by *Listeria monocytogenes* which lives in soil. Able to multiply at low temperatures. *Presentation:* most asymptomatic, or mild flu-like illness. In immunosuppressed (including elderly): gastroenteritis, local infection (abscess, osteomyelitis, septic arthritis, endocarditis, pneumonia), meningoencephalitis, life-threatening septicaemia. Listeria in pregnancy may cause mild disease in mother but transplacental infection→placentitis, amnionitis, preterm delivery, neonatal sepsis, intrauterine death. *Diagnosis:* culture: blood, placenta, amniotic fluid, CSF. PCR. Serology is non-specific. *Treatment:* ampicillin plus gentamicin (synergistic action) for systemic disease. Also co-trimoxazole (CNS disease), macrolides, tetracycline, rifampicin, vancomycin, carbapenem. ►Resistant to cephalosporins which are often 1st-line empirical treatment for meningitis so remember additional antimicrobial cover if listeria is a possibility.

Clostridia

* *Clostridium difficile*, see p255, p407.
* *Clostridium perfringens*:
  * Gastroenteritis, see p426.
  * Gas gangrene due to exotoxin production (alpha toxin most common). Previously *Clostridium welchii. Presentation:* sudden, severe pain due to myonecrosis, tissue crepitus, systemic shock. Most post surgery (GI, biliary), or following soft-tissue trauma/open fracture. If spontaneous, look for malignancy. *Treatment:* early recognition, surgical debridement, protein synthesis inhibitors, eg clindamycin inhibit toxins > penicillins. Hyperbaric O₂ unproven in trials (fig 9.4, table 9.7).
* *Clostridium botulinum*, see p432.
* *Clostridium tetani*, see p432.

Diphtheria

Caused by *Corynebacterium diphtheriae* toxin. Preventable with vaccine. *Presentation:* tonsillar pseudomembrane with fever, painful dysphagia, cervical lymphadenopathy (see *OHCS* p208). *Diagnosis:* culture, toxin detection, PCR *Treatment:* antitoxin within 48h. Benzylpenicillin/erythromycin. Airway support.

Actinomycosis

Due to *Actinomyces israelii*, a mucous membrane commensal. *Presentation:* subacute granulomatous/suppurative infection adjacent to mucous membrane. *Diagnosis:* culture. 'Sulfur' granules in pus/tissue are pathognomonic. *Treatment:* ampicillin, amoxicillin, or penicillin.

Nocardia

Rare cause of disease. *Presentation:* tropical skin abscess, lung/brain abscess, disseminated infection if immunosuppressed. *Treatment:* usually co-trimoxazole.

Anthrax See p420.

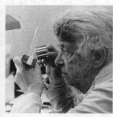

Fig 9.5 Streptococci are grouped by haemolytic pattern (α, β, or non-haemolytic), by Lancefield antigen (A–G), or by species. Rebecca Lancefield (1895–1981) is shown with her hand lens, typing streptococci with a variety of M protein-specific antibodies. Her lab became known as the 'Scotland Yard of Streptococcal Mysteries' after she found that the most grievous crimes of streptococci almost always involve M as a secret accomplice. Although she arrested M on many occasions, M outlived her, and still stalks our wards and clinics.

© Dr V Fischetti, Rockefeller University, NY.

9 Infectious diseases

Gram-negative cocci

Neisseria

Neisseria meningitidis (meningococcus) is an upper respiratory tract commensal in ~10% (~25% adolescents) adhering to non-ciliated epithelial cells in nasopharynx and tonsils. Person-to-person transmission via droplets or upper respiratory tract secretions. Most strains are harmless but induce immunity. Pathogenic, virulent strains are mostly encapsulated and have the potential to cause septicaemia and meningitis. Serogroups A, B, C, W, & Y account for nearly all invasive forms. ↓Group C following introduction of vaccination in UK. ↑ in serotype W in UK since 2009. Incubation 2–7d. Peak ages: <2yrs, ~18yrs. Risk factors: complement system defects, hyposplenism, HIV.

Presentation:
1 Meningitis (~50% cases). Main proliferation of bacteria is in CSF. Insidious onset with malaise, nausea, headache, vomiting. May be misdiagnosed as gastro-enteritis, URTI, or childhood viral illness. Later meningism: headache, vomiting, nuchal/back rigidity, photophobia, altered consciousness. Complications in up to 20%: sensorineural hearing loss, impaired vestibular function, epilepsy, diffuse brain injury.
2 Meningococcaemia. Symptoms/signs depends on amount of circulating bacteria. Mild disease presents with fever, macular rash (fig 9.6) but no signs of shock. High-grade meningococcaemia (~30% cases) causes pyrexia and septic shock within 6–12h due to rapidly escalating endotoxin levels: circulatory failure, coagulopathy with skin haemorrhage (fig 9.7), thrombosis of extremities/adrenals, AKI, ARDS. Meningism may be absent. Complications: amputation, skin necrosis, pericarditis, arthritis, ocular infection, pneumonia (especially serotypes Y and W), permanent adrenal insufficiency.

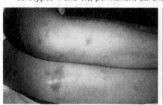

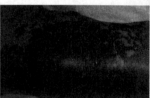

Fig 9.6 Macular lesions on legs.
Reproduced from Warrell *et al., Oxford Textbook of Medicine*, 2010, with permission from Oxford University Press.

Fig 9.7 Massive skin haemorrhage with fulminant meningococcal septicaemia.
Reproduced from Burge *et al., Oxford Handbook of Medical Dermatology*, 2016, with permission from Oxford University Press.

Diagnosis: ▶▶Start treatment immediately if meningitis/meningococcal sepsis is a possible diagnosis. Do not wait for confirmation: delay can be deadly. Intra- and extracellular diplococci on microscopy of CSF/blood/skin lesion. PCR of CSF/blood/skin lesion. *Treatment:* urgent antibiotic treatment: benzylpenicillin, ceftriaxone (pp806–7). Also cefotaxime, chloramphenicol, meropenem. *Prevention:* routine infant vaccination against capsular groups B and C in UK: duration of protection in group B unknown. Quadrivalent ACWY vaccine at age 14. Additional B, C, ACWY doses if vulnerable groups (p403). *Prophylaxis of contacts:* ciprofloxacin/ceftriaxone (single dose), or rifampicin 600mg BD for 48h; ACWY vaccination.

Neisseria gonorrhoeae: see p409.

Moraxella catarrhalis

Colonizes upper respiratory tract in children (↓ in adults). Resembles *Neisseria* commensal so may be overlooked. *Presentation:* pneumonia, exacerbation of COPD, up to 20% of acute otitis media, sinusitis. Bacteraemia is rare. *Diagnosis:* culture of sputum, ear effusion, sinusitis. Bacteraemia is rare. 'Hockey puck sign': colonies can be pushed along agar surface without disruption. *Treatment:* macrolide, cephalosporin.

Gram-negative bacilli

Enterobacterales

Enterobacterales family is large: >50 genera, >170 named species. In the clinical setting, 3 species make up 80–95% of isolates:

1 *Escherichia coli:* part of normal colonic flora. Pathogenic forms can cause:
Enterotoxigenic: a major cause of traveller's diarrhoea (pp424–5).
Enterohaemorrhagic: diarrhoea, haemorrhagic colitis, eg 0157:H7 (p427).
Enteropathogenic: infant diarrhoea in areas of poor sanitation.
Enteroinvasive: dysentery-like syndrome.
Enteroadherent: traveller's diarrhoea, chronic diarrhoea in children/HIV.
Extra-intestinal disease: usually commensal flora, pathogenic outside of the gut: UTI (pp292–3); nosocomia: pneumonia, meningitis, sepsis. Treat by susceptibility: trimethoprim, ampicillin, cephalosporin, ciprofloxacin, aminoglycoside.

2 *Klebsiella pneumoniae:* colonizes skin, nasopharynx, GI tract, hospitalized patients. Associated with antibiotic exposure, in-dwelling catheters, immunosuppression. Causes pneumonia (necrotizing disease and sepsis if immunosuppressed). Also UTI, nasopharyngeal inflammation. Treat according to susceptibility: aminoglycoside, cephalosporin, carbapenem, quinolone.

3 *Proteus mirabilis:* gut commensal. Causes UTI (pp292–3). Stone formation due to urease production: breaks down urea to produce ammonia, struvite stones then form in the presence of magnesium, calcium, and phosphate (pp630–1).

Other: *Salmonella, Shigella, Yersinia:* see enteric fever (p411), gastroenteritis (pp424–29), plague (p421).

Resistant Enterobacterales: ESBL, CPE

Widespread antibiotic use has led to the development of highly virulent, multiple resistant *E. coli* and *Klebsiella* species including:
• Extended-spectrum β-lactamase (ESBL) resistance to penicillins, cephalosporins. Treat by susceptibility: carbapenems, quinolones, aminoglycoside.
• Carbapenemase-producing Enterobacterales (CPE) resistant to carbapenems.

Prevention Antimicrobial stewardship (pp379–80), robust infection control (p407).

Pseudomonas aeruginosa

Environmental pathogen. Spread by contact/ingestion. *Presentation:* nosocomial infection. Infection of compromised tissue, eg wound, pneumonia with lung disease or ventilation, UTI with catheterization. Septicaemia if immunosuppressed. *Treatment:* ciprofloxacin, ceftazidime, piperacillin-tazobactam, aminoglycoside, colistin (not ertapenem). Combination may be needed. Impermeability of membrane and biofilm colonization ↑resistance. ↑Multidrug-resistance. ►Seek expert help.

Haemophilus influenzae

Divided into encapsulated, typeable forms (a–f); and unencapsulated, non-typeable forms. Upper respiratory tract carriage, transmitted by droplets. *H. influenzae b* (Hib) causes meningitis, epiglottitis, otitis media, pneumonia, cellulitis, septic arthritis, and bacteraemia. Fatal in ~5%. Routine immunization in childhood and splenectomy/hyposplenism (p403). Non-typeable forms cause pneumonia and sinusitis. *Treatment:* amoxicillin, macrolide, cephalosporin, chloramphenicol, rifampicin.

Whooping cough

Bordetella pertussis. Presentation: catarrhal phase 1–2wks, then paroxysmal coughing. 'Whoop' is a breath through partially closed vocal cords, seen mainly in children. Cough is prolonged ('100-day cough'). Infants have ↑complications/mortality. *Diagnosis:* PCR nasal/throat swab. Culture sensitivity 10–60%. *Treatment:* macrolides ↓infectivity, but may not alter disease course. Routine childhood vaccination. Vaccination in pregnancy ↑placental antibody transfer to protect neonate (p403).

Other

Burkholderia pseudomallei causing melioidosis in tropical water/soil. Causes pneumonia, pleural effusions, pulmonary abscess. Systemic abscess if haematogenous spread. *Treatment:* ceftazidime/meropenem. Co-trimoxazole eradication therapy. Also Brucellosis (p420), cholera (p426).

Tuberculosis (TB): presentation

Epidemiology

- 10 million new cases/yr of which 30% are unreported/undiagnosed (**fig 9.8**).
- 3.3% of new cases, and 18% of previously treated cases are drug resistant (p391).
- Co-infection with HIV in 9.5% of new cases. TB risk 19-fold higher if HIV positive.
- Leading cause of death worldwide, 1.5 million deaths/yr.
- Effective diagnosis and treatment saved 58 million lives between 2000 and 2018.
- UK ~8000/yr, ~12 per 100 000. 72% born outside UK, 70% in deprived areas, 29% with pulmonary disease wait >4 months from symptoms to treatment.

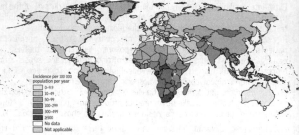

Incidence per 100 000
population per year
- 0–4.9
- 10–49
- 50–99
- 100–299
- 300–499
- ≥500
- No data
- Not applicable

Fig 9.8 Estimated TB incidence rate worldwide.

Reproduced with permission from World Health Organization, Global tuberculosis report 2022.
© World Health Organization 2022. http://www.who.int/tb/publications/global_report/en/

Pathophysiology

Caused by infection with *Mycobacterium tuberculosis*.

Active infection occurs when containment by the immune system (ie T cells/macrophages) is inadequate. It can arise from primary infection, or re-activation of previously latent disease. Transmission of TB is via inhalation of aerosol droplets containing bacterium. This means only pulmonary disease is communicable.

Latent TB is infection without disease due to persistent immune system containment (ie granuloma formation prevents bacteria growth and spread). Positive skin/blood testing (p390) shows evidence of infection but the patient is asymptomatic and non-infectious (normal sputum/CXR). ~2 billion persons worldwide (~⅓ of world's population) are estimated to have latent TB. Lifetime reactivation risk is 5–10%. Risk factors for reactivation: new infection (<2yrs), HIV, organ transplantation, immunosuppression (including corticosteroids), silicosis, illicit drug use, malnutrition, high-risk settings (homeless shelter, prison), low socio-economic status, haemodialysis.

Presentation

►TB, or not TB? That is the question. Maintain a high index of suspicion. TB can affect any organ in the body (**table 9.9**).

Table 9.9 UK TB case reports by site of disease.

Site of disease	% of cases in UK
Pulmonary	57
Extrathoracic lymph nodes	20
Intrathoracic lymph nodes	2
Pleural	9
Gastrointestinal	5
Spine	3
Other bone	1
Miliary	3
Meningitis	3
Genitourinary	2

Source data from: *Tuberculosis in England 2019 Report*, Public Health England. www.gov.uk/phe

- **Systemic features** Low-grade fever, anorexia, weight loss, malaise, night sweats, clubbing (bronchiectasis), erythema nodosum (p560).
- **Pulmonary TB** Cough (in ~50%, >2–3 weeks, dry then productive), pleurisy, haemoptysis (uncommon, seen with bronchiectasis ∴ not always active disease), pleural effusion. An aspergilloma/mycetoma (p174) may form in the cavities. Presentation varies and may be silent or atypical, especially with immunosuppression, eg HIV, post-transplantation.
- **Tuberculous lymphadenitis** (Usually) painless enlargement of cervical or supraclavicular lymph nodes. Axillary and inguinal node involvement less common. Coexisting systemic symptoms in 40–50%. Node is typically firm to touch and not acutely inflamed ('cold abscess'). Skin can adhere to the underlying mass with risk of rupture and sinus formation. Can occur with or without pulmonary disease. Investigate with fine-needle aspiration, AFB staining, and culture (p390).
- **Gastrointestinal TB** Most disease is ileocaecal. Causes colicky abdominal pain and vomiting. Bowel obstruction can occur due to bowel wall thickening, stricture formation, or inflammatory adhesions. Biopsy is required for diagnosis. Caseation necrosis and an absence of transmural cracks/fissures distinguish from Crohn's disease.
- **Spinal TB** Local pain and bony tenderness for weeks–months. Slow, insidious progression. May not present until deformity or neurological symptoms. Look for bony destruction, vertebral collapse, and soft tissue abscess (see Pott's vertebra, p694).
- **Miliary TB** Haematogenous dissemination leads to the formation of discrete foci (~2mm) of granulomatous tissue throughout the lung ('millet' seed appearance). CXR: fig 99. Dissemination throughout the body with meningeal involvement in ~25%. Sputum may be negative for AFB as spread is haematogenous. Have a low threshold for LP. Untreated mortality is assumed to be close to 100%. Do not delay treatment while test results are pending.
- **CNS TB** Haematogenous spread leading to foci of infection in brain and spinal cord. Foci can enlarge to form tuberculomas. Foci rupture leads to meningitis. ↑Risk with immune suppression, HIV, aged <3yrs. Headache, meningism, confusion, seizures, focal

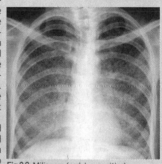

Fig 9.9 Miliary TB (nodular opacities).
© Dr Vijay Sadasivam, Radiologist, SKS Hosp, Salem, Tamil Nadu, India.

neurological deficit, and systemic symptoms. Needs LP and examination of CSF (leucocytosis, raised protein, CSF: plasma glucose <50%, AFB stain, PCR, and culture). Look for TB elsewhere (CXR, etc.), test for HIV. CT/MRI may show hydrocephalus, basal exudates. Tuberculomas are ring-enhancing. ►►All rapid diagnostic tests (p390) have ↓sensitivity, so treat on suspicion.
- **Genitourinary TB** Symptoms may be chronic, intermittent, or silent. Include dysuria, frequency, loin pain, haematuria, sterile pyuria (p292). Granuloma may cause fibrosis, strictures, infertility, and genital ulceration.
- **Cardiac TB** Usually involves the pericardium: pericarditis, pericardial effusion, and/or constrictive pericarditis (p132). Check chest imaging for other TB pathology, eg pulmonary disease, mediastinal lymph nodes. Pericardiectomy may be indicated for persistent constriction despite antituberculous treatment. Myocardial involvement (arrhythmias, heart failure, ventricular aneurysm, or outflow obstruction) is rare.
- **Skin** Lupus vulgaris = persistent, progressive, cutaneous TB: red-brown, 'apple-jelly' nodules. Scrofuloderma: skin lesion extended from underlying infection, eg lymph node, bone; causes ulceration and scarring.

9 Infectious diseases

Diagnostic tests for TB

Latent TB

Offer testing[3] to close contacts of those with pulmonary or laryngeal TB, those with immune dysfunction, healthcare workers, and high-risk populations, eg prison, homeless, vulnerable migrants.

* *Tuberculin skin testing (TST):* = Mantoux test. Intradermal injection of purified protein derivative (PPD) tuberculin. Size of skin induration is used to determine positivity depending on vaccination history and immune status (>5mm if risk factors, >15mm if no risk factors).
* *Interferon-gamma release assay (IGRA):* diagnose exposure to TB by measuring the release of interferon-gamma from T cells reacting to TB antigen. ↑Specificity compared to TST if history of BCG vaccination.

▶ Neither test can diagnose or exclude active disease (falsely negative in 20–25% of active disease): clinical evaluation is required.

▶ Immune-suppressed states reduce the sensitivity of both tests.

Active pulmonary TB

* *CXR:* fibronodular/linear opacities in upper lobe (typical), middle or lower lobes (atypical), cavitation, calcification, miliary disease (see fig 9.9, p389), effusion, lymphadenopathy.
* *Sputum smear:* sputum can be spontaneously produced or induced (with nebulized saline and precautions to prevent transmission). Three specimens are needed including an early-morning sample. It is stained for the presence of acid-fast bacilli (AFB). All mycobacteria are 'acid-fast' including *M. tuberculosis*. If AFB are seen, treatment should be commenced and the patient isolated (in hospital only if clinical indication, or public health reason for admission; or at home).
* *Sputum culture:* more sensitive than smear testing. Culture takes 1–3 weeks (liquid media) or 4–8 weeks (solid media). Can assess drug sensitivity.
* *Nucleic acid amplification test (NAAT):* direct detection of *M. tuberculosis* in sputum by DNA or RNA amplification. Rapid diagnosis (<8h). Can also detect drug resistance (p391).

Extrapulmonary TB

* Investigate for coexisting pulmonary disease alongside site-specific imaging.
* Obtain material from aspiration or biopsy (lymph node, pleura, bone, synovium, GI/GU tract) to enable AFB staining, histological examination (caseating granuloma) and/or culture.
* NAAT can be carried out on any sterile body fluid, eg CSF, pericardial fluid.

▶▶ Offer HIV test for all.

Treatment

Antibiotics used in the treatment[3] of TB are detailed in table 9.10.

Table 9.10 Antibiotics used in the treatment of sensitive TB

Antibiotic	Standard course for active disease	Notes
Rifampicin	2 months intensive 4 months continuation	Enzyme inducer: care with warfarin, calcineurin inhibitors, oestrogens, phenytoin; body secretions coloured orange-red (includes contact lens staining); altered liver function
Isoniazid	2 months intensive 4 months continuation	Inhibits formation of active pyridoxine (vit B_6) which causes a peripheral neuropathy (↑risk with DM, CKD, HIV, malnutrition) ∴ give with prophylactic pyridoxine; hepatitis
Pyrazinamide	2 months intensive	Idiosyncratic hepatotoxicity, ↓ dose if eGFR<30
Ethambutol	2 months intensive	Colour blindness, ↓visual acuity, optic neuritis. Check visual acuity at start of treatment, monitor for symptoms. Monthly visual check if treatment >2 months. Monitor levels if eGFR<30

Latent TB Balance the risk of development of active disease with the possible side effects of treatment. Consider treatment in all at ↑risk of active disease: HIV, transplantation, chemotherapy, biological agents, eg anti-TNFα (p261), diabetes, CKD including dialysis, silicosis, bariatric surgery, and recent close contact with pulmonary/laryngeal TB. Offer HIV, hepatitis B and C testing prior to treatment.

Treat with 3 months of isoniazid (with pyridoxine) and rifampicin OR 6 months of isoniazid (with pyridoxine).

If concerns about hepatotoxicity then 3 months of isoniazid and rifampicin may be preferred. In severe liver disease, seek specialist advice. If interactions with rifamycins are a concern (eg HIV, transplant) then 6 months of isoniazid may be preferred.

Active TB All forms of active TB are statutorily notifiable in the UK. This includes both clinical and culture diagnoses. Notification is via your local public health protection team (www.gov.uk/health-protection-team). Treatment is given under the care of a specialist TB clinician/service according to **table 9.10**. Exceptions include:
- Active CNS disease (including spinal cord involvement): continuation phase of treatment is extended from 4 to 10 months.
- CNS and pericardial disease: use adjunctive high-dose steroids (with weaning and withdrawal during the intensive treatment period).
- Drug-resistant TB.

Adherence is important for treatment to be effective and to prevent drug resistance. Directly observed therapy (DOT) should be considered if: previous treatment for TB, homelessness, drug/alcohol misuse, prison, psychiatric or cognitive disorder, multidrug-resistant disease, patient request.

Universal access to diagnosis and treatment of TB is part of social justice. WHO has developed an 'End TB' strategy aiming to reduce TB deaths by 90% by 2030, and TB incidence by 90% by 2035 (www.who.int/tb/strategy/en).

Drug-resistant TB

NAAT (p390) for drug resistance should be requested for all patients with risk factors for drug resistance: previous TB treatment, contact with drug-resistant disease, birth or residence in a country where ≥5% new cases are drug resistant (**fig 9.10**). Drug resistance may be:
- To any single agent in **table 9.10**.
- Multidrug-resistant TB (MDR-TB): resistant to rifampicin and isoniazid.
- Extensively drug-resistant TB (XDR-TB): resistant to rifampicin, isoniazid, one injectable agent (capreomycin, kanamycin or amikacin), and one fluoroquinolone.
►Seek expert advice for all drug-resistant cases

Test for resistance to 2nd-line drugs. Remember infection control measures.

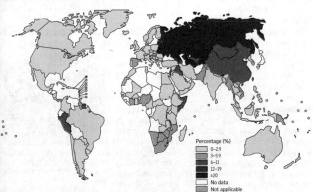

Percentage (%)
- 0–2.9
- 3–5.9
- 6–11
- 12–19
- ≥20
- No data
- Not applicable

Fig 9.10 Percentage of new TB cases with multidrug-resistant TB.

Reproduced with permission from World Health Organization, *Global tuberculosis report 2020*. © World Health Organization 2020. http://www.who.int/tb/publications/global_report/en/

Influenza is common throughout the world, affecting ∼5–10% of adults, and 20–30% of children each year. In most, it is a self-limiting illness. Complications can be life-threatening in the elderly, pregnant women, and those with chronic disease. There are ∼4 million cases of severe influenza and ∼500 000 deaths worldwide/yr.

Seasonal influenza
Acute viral infection of lungs and airways. Rapid person-to-person spread by aerosolized droplets and contact. Infectivity from 1d prior, to ∼7d after symptoms. Includes three subtypes of virus: A, B, and C. Type A influenza is subdivided according to combinations of virus surface proteins, eg A(H1N1), A(H3N2). Seasonal epidemics peak during the winter in temperate countries. Acquired immunity is specific to the virus subtype.

Presentation Incubation: 1–4d. Fever, dry cough, sore throat, coryzal symptoms, headache, malaise, myalgia, conjunctivitis, eye pain ± photophobia. Complications include pneumonia, exacerbation of chronic lung disease, croup, otitis media, D&V, myositis, encephalitis, Reye syndrome (encephalopathy + fatty degenerative liver failure).

Diagnosis Clinical: acute onset + cough + fever has positive predictive value >79%. Testing in outbreaks, complicated influenza, and public health surveillance. Includes: viral PCR, rapid antigen testing, viral culture of clinical samples (throat swab, nasal swab, nasopharyngeal washings, sputum).

Treatment
- *Uncomplicated influenza:* supportive. Antivirals only if high risk of complications (within 48h):
  - Chronic disease: lung, heart, kidney, liver, CNS, DM.
  - Immunosuppression: immunodeficiency, current or planned or within 6 months of immunosuppressive therapy, HIV.
  - Pregnancy. • >65yrs. • BMI >40. • <6 months old.
- *Complicated influenza* includes lower respiratory tract infection, exacerbation of any underlying medical condition, all needing hospital admission. Give antiviral⁴ inhibitors of influenza neuraminidase within 48h (see also BOX 'Hide and seek'):
  1 Oseltamivir: PO or NG. Adult dose: 75mg BD. 5d course. 1st line in UK.
  2 Zanamivir: inhaled (10mg BD, 5d course, confirm technique), nebulized, or IV (respiratory disease affecting nebulizer delivery, ITU). Used if: oseltamivir resistance (eg A(H1N1)), poor clinical response to oseltamivir, concerns re GI absorption of oseltamivir.

Retrospective observational data, and animal studies of oseltamivir and zanamivir show no evidence of harm in pregnancy. Supportive treatment for all. Extracorporeal membrane oxygenation (ECMO) has been used to support gas exchange in severe acute lung injury due to influenza.

Prevention
- *Post-exposure prophylaxis:* if high risk (see 'Treatment') AND not protected by vaccination: oseltamivir PO OD (inhaled zanamivir OD if oseltamivir resistance) for 10d.
- *Annual vaccination* in UK: all high risk (see 'Treatment'), children >2yrs, healthcare workers. See p403. Personal hygiene remains a key pillar of prevention (fig 9.11).

Pandemic influenza Seasonal influenza is subject to antigenic drift: small genetic changes during replication which can be accounted for in the annual vaccine. Antigenic shift is a major change in influenza A resulting in new haemagglutinin (H) and neuraminidase proteins (N) for which there is no pre-existing immunity in the population. Any non-human influenza viruses which transfer to humans are novel. If they also have, or develop, capacity for rapid human-to-human transmission, a pandemic results.

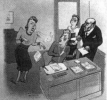

Fig 9.11 A woman coughing or sneezing without a handkerchief in an office with three other office workers.
Lithograph after H.M. Bateman.
Wellcome Collection, Public Domain Mark.

Sailing the choppy waters of pandemic disease

Pandemic respiratory disease is the stormy sea of clinical medicine. Like sailors, we know that choppy waters lie ahead, but we cannot predict their exact timing or nature. To prepare a boat for the tempestuous waters, the mast is key; without it the sails are unsupported and progress will flounder. The mast of pandemic influenza is a tall, vertical SPAR which produces maximum drive through the swell, and allows sailors to climb up high to see what lies on the horizon. When preparing for pandemic influenza, we must make for ourselves a SPAR framework fit for the storm ahead:

- **S**urveillance, planning, and communication: worldwide influenza virological surveillance has been conducted through the WHO for >50yrs. It offers a global alert mechanism for viruses with pandemic potential and defines methodologies for assessing antiviral susceptibility. Cooperation between international and national public health bodies is required for an understanding of clinical characteristics and disease spread. Communication to the individual (public and social media) is needed with advice about self-isolation, when and how to seek medical help, personal hygiene (fig 9.11).
- **P**rotect: vaccine development and production capacity (stockpiling), adequate personal protective equipment (apron, gloves, well-fitting mask), antiviral administration according to robust evidence and susceptibility.
- **A**nimals: limiting/eliminating the animal reservoir of virus by culling, restricting animal movement and trade, vaccination of livestock.
- **R**esearch: virus characteristics, disease severity predictors, epidemiological risk factors, antiviral development, targeting of treatment and vaccination, increased-spectrum vaccines with longer-lasting immunity, effective healthcare worker protection, evidence-based social distancing measures.

Hide and seek

In 2009, there was justifiable global concern about a 'swine flu' pandemic. Based on a Cochrane review in 2008, which showed reduced complications with oseltamivir, billions were spent stockpiling the drug worldwide.

In fact, the positive conclusion was driven mainly by data from an industry-funded summary of 10 trials, of which only two had been published.[5] Cochrane needed access to these missing data. The ensuing fight for information was to take 5 years. The offer of a secret contract, with secret terms, and secrecy about methods, was declined. These are not acceptable methods for meta-analysis. Inconsistencies began to arise in conclusions about effectiveness; being able to see *all* the data started to become increasingly important. But even the largest phase III trial of the drug had never been published. In December 2009, Cochrane could only declare that paucity of data undermined previous findings.

This battle for data became part of 'Alltrials': a campaign for transparency in clinical trials. ~50% of all clinical trials remain unpublished. The hunt goes on to find them. You can run your own drug trial, choose what to publish, and watch how the data become skewed at: www.alltrials.net/news/the-economist-publication-bias

After half a decade, the clinical study reports were released. These are normally used to provide authorities with a detailed trial report. 160 000 pages are not easy fodder for meta-analysis. And the conclusion: oseltamivir shortens symptoms by <1d and hospitalization is not reduced. Other complications were unreliably reported.

The WHO includes oseltamivir on its *WHO Model List of Essential Medicines* (22nd edition, 2021) which means it is considered efficacious, safe, cost-effective, and a minimum requirement for basic healthcare. Does this stand up to independent scrutiny? The evidence base is certainly tarnished. But a pandemic is not a RCT. And the threshold of evidence to reverse policy decisions may be different from the threshold needed to introduce them. If a new influenza pandemic looms, millions more will be thrown in, for now.

HIV is a retrovirus which infects and replicates in human lymphocytes (CD4 + T cells) and macrophages. This leads to progressive immune system dysfunction, opportunistic infection, and malignancy = acquired immunodeficiency syndrome (AIDS). The virus is transmitted via blood, sexual fluids, and breast milk. Virus subtypes include HIV1 (global epidemic) and HIV2 (less pathogenic, predominantly West Africa).

Epidemiology

~38 million adults and children are estimated to be living with HIV worldwide (fig 9.12), with 690 000 deaths/yr. Africa has most of the disease (~26 million), most of the mortality (440 000/yr), and ~1% of the world's wealth.

UK: estimated ~100 000 living with HIV (=1.7/1000). ~17% of those with HIV in UK are unaware of their infection.

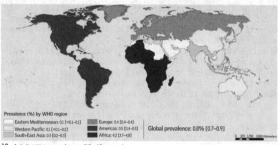

Prevalence (%) by WHO region

Eastern Mediterranean: 0.1 [<0.1–0.1]	Europe: 0.4 [0.4–0.4]	Global prevalence: 0.8% [0.7–0.9]
Western Pacific: 0.1 [<0.1–0.2]	Americas: 0.5 [0.4–0.5]	
South-East Asia: 0.3 [0.2–0.3]	Africa: 4.2 [3.7–4.8]	

Fig 9.12 Adult HIV prevalence (15–49 years).
Reproduced with permission from World Health Organization, 'Adult HIV prevalence (15–49 years), 2017 by WHO region'. ©World Health Organization 2018.
http://gamapserver.who.int/mapLibrary/Files/Maps/HIV_adult_prevalence_2017.png

Pathophysiology

HIV binds, via its GP120 envelope glycoprotein, to CD4 receptors on helper T cells, monocytes, and macrophages. These 'CD4 cells' migrate to lymphoid tissue where the virus replicates, producing billions of new virions. These are released, and in turn infect new CD4 cells. As infection progresses, depletion or impaired function of CD4 cells leads to ↓immune function. HIV is a retrovirus: it encodes reverse transcriptase, allowing DNA copies to be produced from viral RNA. This is error prone, meaning a significant mutation rate, which contributes to treatment resistance.

Prevention

Sexual transmission Consistent and correct use of (male and female) condoms ↓ transmission by ~90%. Serosorting (the restriction of unprotected sex depending on HIV status) is unsafe due to inaccuracies in HIV status (which is only as reliable as a person's last test) and failure to disclose. It does not consider transfer of treatment resistance, other STIs, or hepatitis.

Post-exposure prophylaxis (PEP) The short-term use of antiretroviral therapy (ART) after potential HIV exposure (sexual or occupational) should be considered an emergency method of HIV prevention. Can be given up to 72h (ideally <24h) after exposure. Not recommended if exposure is to a person on ART with a confirmed and sustained (>6 months) undetectable (<200 copies/mL) viral load. 1st-line PEP[6] in UK is Truvada® (tenofovir/emtricitabine) plus raltegravir for 28 days (refer to local guidelines). Test for HIV 8–12 weeks after exposure.

Pre-exposure prophylaxis (PrEP) ART in those at high risk of acquiring HIV including serodifferent relationships without suppression of viral load, condomless anal sex in MSM. Trials (PROUD, IPERGAY) show an 86% reduction in HIV incidence. PrEP has been commissioned in the UK since 2020. Results of a large-scale PrEP trial (IMPACT) awaited.

Vertical transmission All pregnant women living with HIV should have commenced ART by 24wks. Caesarean delivery indicated if viral load >50 copies/mL (and if safe and available). Neonatal PEP is given from birth–4wks old with formula-feeding.

Presentation
With symptoms of early HIV infection
• *Primary HIV infection* is symptomatic in ~80%, typically 2–4 weeks after infection (= seroconversion illness, acute retroviral syndrome). Maintain a high index of suspicion. Offer HIV testing to anyone (regardless of risk) presenting with flu-like symptoms and an erythematous/maculopapular rash. Consider primary HIV as a differential in any combination of fever, rash, myalgia, pharyngitis, mucosal ulceration, lymphadenopathy, and headache/aseptic meningitis. Diagnosis of primary HIV is a unique opportunity to prevent transmission (↑viral load and genital shedding). HIV antibody testing may be negative but HIV RNA levels are high—seek expert help regarding viral load testing (see HIV testing later in topic).
• *Persistent generalized lymphadenopathy* = swollen/enlarged lymph nodes >1cm in two or more non-contiguous sites (not inguinal) persisting for >3 months. Due to follicular hyperplasia caused by HIV infection. Exclude TB, infection, and malignancy.
In the asymptomatic, latent phase of chronic HIV infection
In the UK there is universal testing in sexual health clinics, antenatal services, drug dependency programmes, and in patients with TB/hepatitis B/hepatitis C/lymphoma. Where HIV prevalence is >2/1000 universal testing by GPs and medical admissions units should be considered. Any request for a HIV test should be met.
With complications of immune system dysfunction See pp396–9.

HIV testing
The prognosis for patients with HIV in the UK is much better than for many other serious illnesses for which doctors routinely test. HIV testing[6] should not be viewed differently. Any doctor can consent for a HIV test: explain the benefits of testing and detail how results will be given. Written consent is unnecessary. Arrange follow-up with a local HIV/GUM service within 2wks (preferably <48h) for patients testing positive for the first time.
• **ELISA for HIV antibody and antigen (p24)** 4th-generation assays test for HIV antibody and p24 antigen. This reduces the 'window period' (time of false-negative testing between infection and the production of measurable antigen/antibody) to average ~10 days. Diagnosis in UK is confirmed by a confirmatory assay.
• **Rapid point-of-care testing** Immunoassay kit which gives a rapid result from a finger-prick or mouth swab. Only CE-marked kits should be used. Needs serological confirmation.
• **Viral load** Quantification of HIV RNA. Used to monitor response to ART. Not diagnostic due to possibility of a false-positive result ∴ care if used to test for symptomatic primary HIV in the 'window period'—confirmation of seroconversion is still required.
• **Nucleic acid testing/viral PCR** Qualitative test for the presence of viral RNA. Used to test for vertical transmission in neonates as placental transfer of maternal antibodies can affect ELISA antibody testing up to 18 months of age.
• **CD4 count** Cannot diagnose HIV. Used to monitor immune system function and disease progression in patients with HIV. <200 cells/microlitre is one of the defining criteria for AIDS.
►See www.aidsmap.com for available HIV testing and country-specific resources.

Needle-stick injury

Risk of HIV transmission from a single needle-stick exposure from a person with HIV not on ART is ~1 in 300 (lower than risks of hepatitis B and C transmission).

Prevent
• Use 'safer sharps' (incorporates a mechanism to minimize accidental injury).
• Do not recap unprotected medical sharps.
• When using sharps, ensure there is a disposal container nearby.

Manage
• Encourage the wound to bleed, ideally under running water (do not suck).
• Wash with soap and running water, do not scrub.
• Seek advice from occupational health/infection control (or A&E outside of working hours) regarding source testing and post-exposure prophylaxis (p394).

Complications of HIV infection

Complications of HIV can be divided into:
• Complications of immune dysfunction (opportunistic infection/malignancy).
• Complicating comorbidity.
• Complications of treatment, ie adverse drug effects (see pp398–9).

The differential diagnosis for symptoms presenting in a person living with HIV is given in table 9.11. This is not exhaustive. ▶▶Do not forget the usual differentials, the presentation may not relate to the patient's HIV status.

Table 9.11 Differential diagnoses in HIV

Presentation	Differential diagnosis
Fever	Intraoral abscess, sinusitis, pneumonia, TB, endocarditis, meningitis, encephalitis, pyomyositis, lymphoma, immune reconstitution after commencement of ART, any non-HIV cause
Lymphadenopathy	Persistent generalized lymphadenopathy (p395), TB, syphilis, histoplasmosis, cryptococcus, lymphoma, Kaposi's sarcoma, local infection
Rash	Drug reaction, herpes zoster, scabies, cutaneous cryptococcus or histoplasmosis, Kaposi's sarcoma, seborrhoeic dermatitis
Cough/SOB	Community-acquired pneumonia, *Pneumocystis jirovecii*, TB, bronchial compression (TB, lymphoma, Kaposi's sarcoma), pulmonary Kaposi's sarcoma (uncommon), cardiac failure (HIV cardiomyopathy, infective pericardial effusion, HIV vasculopathy)
Diarrhoea	*Salmonella*, *Shigella*, *Clostridium difficile*, amoebiasis, *Giardia*, *Cryptosporidia*, CMV, HIV enteropathy is a diagnosis of exclusion
Abdominal pain	TB, CMV colitis, pancreatitis (CMV, TB, or secondary to ART)
Dysphagia	Candidiasis, HSV
↑Liver enzymes	Viral hepatitis (A, B, C, CMV, HSV, EBV), drug-induced liver injury (anti-TB or ART), HIV cholangiopathy, lymphoma, congestion due to cardiac disease (pericardial effusion?)
AKI	Pre-renal due to sepsis/dehydration, interstitial nephritis secondary to medication, HIV-associated nephropathy (proteinuria, CKD)
Headache/seizures/focal neurology	Meningitis (bacterial, TB, cryptococcal, syphilis), empyema, space-occupying lesion (toxoplasmosis, lymphoma, tuberculoma), adverse drug reaction, HIV encephalopathy, progressive multifocal leukoencephalopathy (PML), stroke (HIV vasculopathy). See p513
Eye disease	Herpes zoster, CMV retinitis (p434)
Peripheral neuropathy	ART, CMV, HIV neuropathy, nutritional deficiency

Complicating comorbidity

• **Cardiovascular disease** ↑Risk of CVD. Includes individuals where risk traditionally lower: young, normotensive, no DM, non-obese. Contributing factors: dyslipidaemia due to ART, accelerated pro-atherosclerotic inflammation by HIV. Management of CV risk factors though no data to guide lipid/BP targets.
• **Bone disease** ↑Risk of low bone mineral density and fragility fractures in HIV. Contributing factors: side effect of ART, increased prevalence of risk factors, eg poor nutrition, smoking, alcohol, low vitamin D levels. Risk assess and consider bisphosphonate.
• **TB** All patients with TB and HIV need ART (as soon as TB treatment tolerated and within 2 weeks if CD4 <100 cells/microlitre). Seek expert advice and refer to local guidelines. Consider Truvada® plus efavirenz as 1st line in UK (serum levels of integrase inhibitors are decreased by rifampicin). See ART, pp398–9, TB, pp390–1.
• **Hepatitis B (HBV)** Co-infection requires an ART regimen including antivirals with anti-HBV activity, eg tenofovir plus emtricitabine (not lamivudine or emtricitabine as a single agent due to potential for emergence of HBV resistance).
• **Hepatitis C (HCV)** Assess all for treatment. Pegylated interferon efficacy is less with lower CD4 count. Treat to CD4 >500 cells/microlitre with ART first.

Opportunistic disease

▶ART is part of the treatment regimen of all opportunistic infections (see pp398–9).

- ***Pneumocystis jirovecii*** ('Yee-row-vet-zee.') *Presentation:* progressive SOB on exertion, malaise, dry cough. Haemoptysis and pleuritic pain rare. *Examination:* ↑respiratory rate, often normal breath sounds. *Investigation:* SpO₂ (compare rest and exertion). CXR: classically perihilar infiltrates, but may be normal. Induced sputum or BAL with nucleic acid amplification (more sensitive than staining). *Treatment:* IV co-trimoxazole (convert to oral if favourable response). 21-day course. Steroids in moderate–severe disease (P_aO_2 <9.3kPa/SpO₂ <92%). 2nd line: pentamidine. *Prophylaxis:* co-trimoxazole if CD4 <200 cells/microlitre.

- ***Candidiasis*** Oral or oesophageal. Pain in the tongue, dysphagia, odynophagia. Diagnosed clinically or endoscopically. Treated with systemic '-azole', eg fluconazole.

- ***Cryptococcus neoformans*** Commonest systemic fungal infection in HIV (5–10% pre-ART). *Presentation:* meningitis: headache, fever, meningism variable. Associated skin (molluscum-like papules) and lung disease. *Investigation:* LP with manometry. CSF stain (India ink), CSF/blood cryptococcal antigen. *Treatment:* induction with single, high-dose liposomal amphotericin B (SE: renal tubular damage and AKI) plus 14d flucytosine (SE: haematological toxicity) and fluconazole. Maintenance fluconazole. Normalize ICP with LPS/shunt. Delay ART (risk of immune reconstitution).

- ***Toxoplasma gondii*** Toxoplasma abscesses are commonest cause of intracranial mass lesions when CD4 <200 cells/microlitre. *Presentation:* focal neurological signs ± seizures. Headache and vomiting if raised ICP. *Investigation:* ring-enhancing lesions on MRI (ΔΔ lymphoma) with associated oedema. CSF PCR for *T. gondii* is specific but only moderately sensitive. Blood serology is not diagnostic as most cases are a reactivation of previous infection. *Treatment:* consider in any brain mass lesion with CD4 <200 cell/microlitre. Pyrimethamine, sulfadiazine, folinic acid.

- ***Cytomegalovirus (CMV)*** Severe primary or reactivated disease (p401). *Presentation:* retinitis (blurred then loss of vision), encephalitis, GI disease (oesophagitis, colitis), hepatitis, bone marrow suppression, pneumonia. *Diagnosis:* serial CMV viral load, retinal lesions (p434), GI ulceration, 'owl's eye' inclusions on biopsy. *Treatment:* ganciclovir/valganciclovir. Side effects: rash, diarrhoea, bone myelosuppression.

- ***Cryptosporidium*** Common cause of chronic diarrhoea in HIV pre-ART. *Presentation:* acute or sub-acute non-bloody, watery diarrhoea. Also cholangitis, pancreatitis. *Investigation:* stool microscopy (multiple samples as oocyst excretion intermittent), PCR, enzyme immunoassay, direct fluorescent antibody. *Treatment:* supportive, ART.

Oncogenic disease

- **Lymphoma** Increased risk of non-Hodgkin's lymphoma in HIV. Includes: diffuse large B-cell lymphoma, Burkitt's lymphoma, primary CNS lymphoma. *Presentation:* dependent upon area of involvement. Includes lymphadenopathy, cytopenia, CNS symptoms. *Treatment:* combined ART and chemotherapy. Rituximab for non-CNS disease. Whole-brain radiotherapy for CNS disease if excess toxicity with chemotherapy.

- **Kaposi's sarcoma** Most common tumour in HIV and AIDS defining. Caused by Kaposi sarcoma herpes virus (human herpesvirus 8, p401). *Presentation:* cutaneous or mucosal lesions: patch, plaque, or nodular (fig 9.13). Visceral disease less common. *Investigation:* histological confirmation. *Treatment:* ART. Intralesional retinoids or vinblastine. Radiotherapy for cosmesis/pain. Chemotherapy (+ ART) in advanced disease.

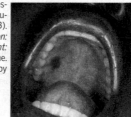

Fig 9.13 Palatal Kaposi's sarcoma.
Copyright D. A. Warrell.

▶ART[7] is recommended for everyone with HIV, regardless of CD4 count.

Strategic Timing of AntiRetroviral Treatment (START) study, 2015

4685 participants (215 sites, 35 countries) with HIV, CD4 >500 cells/microlitre, no previous ART. Randomized to:
• immediate ART
• deferred ART until CD4 <350 cells/microlitre or AIDS-defining illness.
▶Immediate initiation of ART reduced the risk of AIDS, serious non-AIDS events, or death by 57% (CI 38–70%) at 3 years.

Aims of ART To reduce the HIV viral load to a level undetectable by standard laboratory techniques leading to immunological recovery, reduced clinical progression, and reduced mortality. These aims should be met with the least possible side effects.

Mechanism of action (See fig 9.14.)

• *CCR5 antagonists* inhibit the entry of the virus into the cell by blocking the CCR5 co-receptor.
• *Nucleos(t)ide and non-nucleoside reverse transcriptase inhibitors (NRTIS, NNRTIS)* inhibit reverse transcriptase and the conversion of viral RNA into DNA.
• *Integrase strand transfer inhibitors (INSTIS)* inhibit integrase and prevent HIV DNA integrating into the nucleus.
• *Protease inhibitors (PIS)* inhibit protease, an enzyme involved in the maturation of virus particles.
• *Pharmacokinetic enhancers/boosters* increase the effectiveness of antiretroviral drugs allowing lower doses, eg cobicistat, ritonavir.

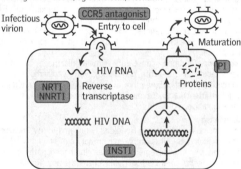

Fig 9.14 Mechanism of action of ART.

Starting treatment ▶Seek expert help.

1 Counselling: HIV transmission and sexual health, benefits of therapy (not cure), adherence (lifelong), resistance, side effects of treatment, necessary monitoring, disclosure to partner/family/friends, partner testing.
2 Screen for infections and malignancy (pp396–7). Includes TB, hepatitis B & C. Treat or offer prophylaxis with co-trimoxazole if CD4 <200 cells/microlitre. For latent TB see p391. Aim to start ART within 2 weeks of initiation of antimicrobial treatment for opportunistic or serious infection (seek expert advice if drug interactions or intracerebral disease).
3 Baseline tests: CD4, viral load, FBC, LFT, electrolytes, creatinine, pregnancy test, viral genotype for drug resistance.
4 Review usual medications for possible drug interactions. Advise the patient to check for drug interactions with any new medication.
▶See www.hiv-druginteractions.org

What to start

►Use local guidelines. ►Get expert help.

For a treatment-naïve patient consider two nucleoside reverse transcriptase inhibitors (= 'NRTI backbone') plus one of:
- ritonavir-boosted 'protease inhibitor
- non-nucleoside reverse transcriptase inhibitor
- integrase inhibitor.

1st-line drugs commonly used in the UK include:
- **NRTI backbone** Tenofovir & emtricitabine (combination tablet = Truvada®), abacavir & lamivudine (combination tablet = Kivexa®). Side effects: GI disturbance, anorexia, pancreatitis, hepatic dysfunction (severe lactic acidosis with hepatomegaly and hepatic steatosis reported, caution with hepatitis B/C), ↓bone mineral density. Avoid abacavir if high risk of CVD. Avoid tenofovir if eGFR <30.
- **Protease inhibitors** Atazanavir, darunavir. Side effects: hyperglycaemia, insulin resistance (mainly 1st-generation drugs), dyslipidaemia, jaundice, and hepatitis.
- **NNRTI** Rilpivirine (give with food, interaction with proton pump inhibitors), efavirenz (CNS toxicity, association with suicidality ∴ care in depression/anxiety, adverse lipid profile). Other side effects: rash, GI disturbance.
- **Integrase inhibitor** Dolutegravir, elvitegravir, raltegravir. Side effects: rash, GI disturbance, insomnia.

Monitor: adherence (see BOX 'Adherence'), adverse effects (LFTs, glucose), virological response (viral load). CD4 counts guide prophylaxis of opportunistic infection (values may not correlate with virological response, use viral load preferentially).

Adherence

↓Adherence to ART is associated with drug resistance, disease progression, and death. Adherence support should be integral to ART provision.

Assess Ask about adherence in a non-judgemental way. Do not blame. Explain the reasoning behind your questions. Is non-adherence due to practical problems or healthcare beliefs? Be ready to address both. What help would your patient like?

Intervene Normalize the situation—doubts and concerns about ART are common. Find time for discussion/information. Address concerns. Simplify the dosage regimen (single tablet regimens, eg Atripla®), offer a multicompartment medication system. Link the taking of medication to a regular daily activity. Discuss side effects: what are the risks/benefits to changing dose or ART regimen?

Resource-limited settings

In many resource-limited settings, universal access to ART remains an objective yet to be achieved. ~50% of those in need of treatment for HIV do not receive it. Interim prioritization of those with symptomatic HIV or CD4 count <350 cells/microlitre may be appropriate as these patients are at high risk of mortality and have most short-term benefit from ART.

Equality in the treatment of HIV requires:
- Effective, acceptable, and reliable methods to reduce HIV transmission, including treatment as prevention.
- Rapid, accurate, and low-cost diagnosis and monitoring.
- Standardization and simplification of ART regimens.
- Evidence-based ART to prevent the use of sub-standard protocols which compromise treatment and lead to the emergence of drug-resistant strains.
- Reduced ART costs and/or effective allocation of resources.

An HIV vaccine?

Vaccines are the most effective way to prevent infectious disease. They can also be therapeutic, clearing a virus after infection. HIV vaccines to date have failed to induce an immune response sufficient to confer protection. Research is ongoing into neutralizing HIV antibodies, peptides, genes, viral vectors, physiological 'boosters', and mechanisms to counter the mutational evolution of HIV. See www.hvtn.org

9 Infectious diseases

9 Infectious diseases

Herpes simplex virus (HSV) (human herpesvirus 1 and 2)

Includes HSV1 and HSV2. HSV1 infection in ⅔ of world's population (~3.7 billion <50yrs), and HSV2 in ~11% (~400 million). Viruses multiply in epithelial cells of mucosal surface producing vesicles or ulcers. Lifelong latent infection when virus enters sensory neurons at infection site. Can then reactivate, replicate, and infect surrounding tissue. Disseminated infection if impaired T-cell immunity: pneumonitis, hepatitis, colitis.

Presentation Primary infection: subclinical or sensory nerve (tingling) prodrome, then vesicles, shallow ulcers. Systemic symptoms possible: fever, malaise, lymphadenopathy, erythema multiforme. Heals 8–12d. Reactivation: usually less severe unless immunosuppressed. Anatomy of infection:
- Herpes labialis: cold sore lesion at lip border, predominantly HSV1.
- Genital herpes: predominantly HSV2 (p408).
- Gingivostomatitis: fever, sore throat followed by tender oropharyngeal vesicles.
- Keratoconjunctivitis: corneal dendritic ulcers. ►Avoid steroids. See *OHCS* p334.
- Herpetic whitlow: painful vesicles on distal phalanx due to inoculation through a break in the skin.
- Herpes encephalitis: most common treatable viral encephalitis. Transfer of virus from peripheral site to brain via neuronal transmission. Prodrome: fever, malaise, headache, nausea. Then encephalopathy: general/focal signs of cerebral dysfunction including psychiatric symptoms, seizure, focal neurology (temporal involvement in ~60%), memory loss. Predominantly HSV1 in immunocompetent patients.
- Secondary infection of eczematous skin—→eczema herpeticum. See *OHCS* p446.

Diagnosis Clinical diagnosis. Confirmation required in encephalitis, keratoconjunctivitis, or immunosuppression: viral PCR of CSF, swab, or vesicle scraping. Also culture, immunofluorescence, serology.

Treatment Supportive for most oral HSV in healthy adults. Aciclovir: ↓symptoms and viral shedding, will not prevent latent infection: consider if primary HSV, severe symptoms, immunocompromised, pregnancy. ►Empirical IV aciclovir as soon as HSV encephalitis suspected, mortality ~70% in untreated disease (p808).

Varicella zoster virus (VZV) (human herpesvirus 3)

Primary infection transmitted by respiratory droplets. Incubation 14–21d. Invades respiratory mucosa, replicates in lymph nodes. Disseminates via mononuclear cells to infect skin epithelial cells. Leads to virus containing vesicles = chicken pox. Virus then remains dormant in sensory nerve roots. Reactivation is dermatomal = shingles.

Presentation
- *Chicken pox:* prodrome 1–2d: fever, malaise, headache, abdominal pain. Then rash (fig 9.15): pruritic, erythematous macules→vesicles, crust in ~48h. Infectious 1–2d pre-, to 5d post-rash development (lesions scabbed). Complications ↑ in immunosuppression: encephalitis (cerebellar ataxia), VZV pneumonia, transverse myelitis, pericarditis, purpura fulminans/DIC.

Fig 9.15 Chicken pox (VZV).
© D A Warrell.

- *Shingles:* painful, hyperaesthetic area, then macular→vesicular rash in dermatomal distribution. Disseminated infection if immunosuppressed. Infectious until scabs appear. Chicken pox risk in non-immune contacts. Complications: post-herpetic neuralgia, Ramsay Hunt syndrome (p499).

Diagnosis Clinical diagnosis unless immunosuppressed: viral PCR, culture, immunofluorescence.

Treatment Oral aciclovir/valaciclovir for uncomplicated shingles/chicken pox in adults, aim to give within 72h of rash in shingles (↓risk post-herpetic neuralgia): give if within 24h of onset in chicken pox. IV aciclovir if pregnant, immunosuppressed, severe/disseminated disease (including ocular).

Prevention Chicken pox vaccination: not routine in children in UK. Shingles vaccination given at aged 70 to prevent reactivation. VZV immunoglobulin if non-immune exposure in immunosuppression, pregnancy, neonates.

Epstein-Barr virus (EBV) (human herpesvirus 4) Virus targets circulating B lymphocytes (lifelong latent infection) and squamous epithelial cells of oropharynx ('affectionately' termed the 'kissing disease').

Presentation Usually asymptomatic infection in childhood. Infectious mononucleosis in ~50% of primary infection in adults: sore throat, fever, anorexia, lymphadenopathy (esp. posterior triangle of neck), palatal petechiae, splenomegaly, hepatomegaly, jaundice. Malaise is prominent. Resolution of symptoms usually within 2 weeks. Chronic active infection and recurrence are rare. Oncogenicity: see BOX.

Diagnosis
- Blood film: lymphocytosis. Atypical lymphocytes (large, irregular nuclei) also occur in other viral infection (CMV, HIV, parvovirus, dengue), toxoplasmosis, typhus, leukaemia, lymphoma, drug reactions, lead poisoning.
- Heterophile antibody tests (eg Monospot®, Paul–Bunnell) detect non-EBV heterophile antibodies which are present in ~85% of sera. False +ve: pregnancy, autoimmune disease, lymphoma/leukaemia. ↑Sensitivity from 2nd week.
- Serology: IgM to EBV viral capsid antigen in acute infection. IgG if past infection. Consider if immunocompromised or negative antibody tests.
- Reverse transcriptase viral PCR.

Treatment Supportive. ►Seek expert help if severe disease/immunosuppression: observational data on the use of antivirals and steroids. Maculopapular rash with antibiotics, eg amoxicillin.

Cytomegalovirus (CMV) (human herpesvirus 5)

50–100% of adults are seropositive depending on socioeconomic and sexual risk. Latent infection: periodic, asymptomatic (but infectious) viral shedding in bodily fluids including blood transfusion, transplantation (CMV +ve donor to CMV –ve recipient).

Presentation Asymptomatic in most. Symptoms mimic infectious mononucleosis (see earlier in topic) or hepatitis. Severe disease in immunosuppressed (post-transplantation, HIV): oesophagitis, gastritis, colitis, retinitis (p434), pneumonitis, hepatitis. Infection in pregnancy is associated with congenital abnormality.

Diagnosis Primary infection in immunocompetent: IgM. Immunosuppressed: quantitative nucleic acid amplification testing (QNAT) in blood greater than a defined threshold, or rising titre. Invasive disease: tissue QNAT, histopathology.

Treatment Given in severe infection/immunosuppression. Ganciclovir, valganciclovir (↑oral bioavailability). Pre-emptive treatment in transplant patients based on QNAT results. Treatment in pregnancy remains unclear. Use CMV –ve, irradiated blood for transfusion if immunosuppressed and at risk: transplant, HIV, leukaemia.

Other herpes viruses
Human herpesvirus 6 (HHV6) Roseola infantum, febrile illness without rash.
Human herpesvirus 8 (HHV8) Oncogenic (see BOX), Castleman's disease.

Oncogenic viruses

~12% of human cancers are caused by viruses, >80% of these occur in low- and middle-income countries (**table 9.12**).

Common traits of oncoviruses:
- Virus is necessary but not sufficient to cause cancer.
- Cancers appear in context of chronic infection, taking years–decades to appear.
- Cancers are associated with immunosuppression and chronic inflammation.

Table 9.12 Oncogenic viruses

Virus	Cancers
EBV (HHV4)	Burkitt's lymphoma, Hodgkin's lymphoma, B-cell lymphoma in immunosuppression, gastric cancer, nasopharyngeal cancer, post-transplantation lymphoproliferative disease (PTLD)
HHV8	Kaposi's sarcoma (p396) and primary effusion lymphoma
HPV	Cancers of: cervix, anus, vulva, penis, head, neck, oropharynx (p402)
Hepatitis B and C	Hepatocellular carcinoma (p282)
HTLV-1	Human T-lymphotropic virus→adult T-cell leukaemia
MCV	Merkel cell polyomavirus→Merkel cell carcinoma

Respiratory tract viruses

Include rhinovirus, coronavirus (p172), adenovirus, respiratory syncytial virus (RSV). Transmission by direct contact, infected fomites, airborne droplets. **Presentation** Coryza, pharyngitis, croup, bronchiolitis, pneumonia. **Diagnosis** Clinical. Viral culture, antigen detection, PCR. **Treatment** None in uncomplicated disease/immunocompetent. Limited evidence for specific treatments in high-risk complicated disease, immunosuppression: cidofovir for adenovirus; aerosolized ribavirin, immunoglobulin, monoclonal antibody in RSV. For influenza see pp392–3.

Human papilloma virus (HPV)

>120 HPVs. Pathology:
• Skin warts, verrucas (HPV 1, 2). Treatment: none, topical salicylic acid, freezing.
• Anogenital warts (HPV 6, 11). Treatment: topical podophyllin, imiquimod; ablation.
• Cervical cancer (HPV 16, 18), other cancers (see p401).
Vaccination in UK: age 12–13 (♀ since 2008, ♂ since 2019). See p403.

Polyomavirus

~100% exposure. Disease only with immunosuppression: BK virus causes renal transplant nephropathy; JC virus causes progressive multifocal leucoencephalopathy.

Measles

Transmitted by respiratory droplets. Incubation 10–18d. Highly contagious: >95% population coverage needed for 'herd' immunity. ↑ cases in Europe since 2016. **Presentation** Prodrome (2–4d): fever, conjunctivitis, coryza, diarrhoea, Koplik spots (white spots on red buccal mucosa, fig 9.16). Then generalized, maculopapular rash, classically face/neck→trunk→limbs (fig 9.17). Complications:
• Secondary infection: bacterial pneumonia, otitis media, ocular herpes simplex, oral/GI candidiasis.

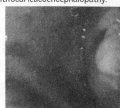
Fig 9.16 Koplik spots.
Courtesy of CDC.

• Acute demyelinating encephalitis: 1 in 1000, usually within 2wks of rash. Seizures, fever, irritability, headache, ↓conscious level.
• Subacute sclerosing panencephalitis: 5–10yrs after infection, disturbances in intellect, personality, seizures, motor dysfunction, decerebration. No treatment available.

Diagnosis Clinical. IgM. Antigen in saliva/urine. **Treatment** Prevent with vaccination. Human immunoglobulin within 3d of exposure in non-immune. Supportive. No benefit shown for dexamethasone in encephalitis.

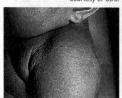
Fig 9.17 Measles rash.
Reproduced from Firth *et al.*, *Oxford Textbook of Medicine*, 2020, with permission from Oxford University Press.

Mumps

Respiratory droplet spread. Incubation 14–21d. Common cause of encephalitis pre-vaccination. **Presentation** Can be subclinical. Prodrome: fever, myalgia, headache. Infection and tender swelling of salivary glands: parotid > submandibular. Complications: meningoencephalitis, epididymoorchitis if pubertal/post-pubertal infection (warm, swollen, tender testes 4d–6wks after parotitis→subfertility in ~10%, infertility rare), oophoritis, pancreatitis, deafness. **Diagnosis** Clinical. If confirmation needed, eg meningitis/encephalitis: mumps specific IgM/IgA, PCR. **Treatment** Supportive.

Rubella (German measles)

Respiratory droplet spread. **Presentation** Usually mild/subclinical. Prodrome: fever, conjunctivitis, rhinorrhoea. Rash: generalized, pink, maculopapular. Lymphadenopathy: occipital, cervical, post-auricular. **Congenital infection** Up to 90% risk of fetal malformation in 1st trimester, sensorineural hearing loss/retinopathy in 2nd trimester. Offer IgM/IgG testing. Immunoglobulin may ↓viraemia but will not prevent infection.

▶Vaccinate *PRE*-pregnancy, **live** vaccines are contraindicated in pregnancy.

9 Infectious diseases

Passive immunity uses preformed antibody to protect against infection. It offers immediate but short-lived protection. Natural passive immunity occurs in the placental transfer of maternal antibodies to the fetus; acquired passive immunity includes treatment with immunoglobulin, eg hepatitis B, rabies, tetanus, varicella zoster.

Active immunity follows exposure to an antigen, which generates an adaptive immune response. Natural active immunity occurs following infection. Acquired active immunity is provided by vaccination. Routine vaccinations in the UK are shown in table 9.13. Additional vaccines are offered to specific vulnerable groups (table 9.14).

Immunosuppression is a contraindication to live vaccines due to the risk of disseminated disease. Includes immunodeficiency, immunosuppressive treatment, HIV. Inactivated vaccines can be given but the antibody response may be less: aim to give >2wks prior to immunosuppressive therapy when possible (or vaccinate whilst on treatment and considered repeat re-immunization when/if treatment complete).

Travel Travel advice (food/drink, insect repellent, malaria prophylaxis, condoms) is often more important than vaccination. Check routine vaccinations are up to date. Vaccination depends upon area of travel and planned activities: for up-to-date recommendations see http://www.fitfortravel.nhs.uk/destinations

Table 9.13 UK vaccination summary (*=live vaccine, † =HPV 6, 11, 16, 18, 31, 33, 45, 52, 58)

Vaccination	Age (m=months, y=years)								
	2m	3m	4m	12m	3–5y	12y	14y	>65y	70y
Diphtheria	+	+	+		+		+		
Tetanus	+	+	+		+		+		
Pertussis	+	+	+		+				
Poliomyelitis	+	+	+		+		+		
Haemophilus influenzae B (Hib)	+	+	+	+					
Hepatitis B	+	+	+						
Pneumococcal		+		+				+	
Rotavirus*	+	+							
Meningitis B	+		+	+					
Meningitis C				+					
Measles, mumps, rubella*				+	+				
Influenza					+			+	
HPV†						+			
Meningitis ACWY							+		
Varicella zoster*									+

Table 9.14 Additional vaccination of specific groups in UK (*=live vaccine)

Vaccination	Offered to
BCG*	Infants/children where TB incidence >40/100 000 or parent/grandparent born in country where incidence >40/100 000, TB contacts
Hib	Hyposplenism, complement disorders
Meningitis B, ACWY	Hyposplenism, complement disorders, high-risk travel
Influenza	Hyposplenism, DM, chronic heart disease, chronic respiratory disease, CKD, chronic liver disease, chronic neurological disease, immunosuppression, pregnancy
Pneumococcal	Hyposplenism, cochlear implants, complement disorders, DM, chronic heart disease, chronic respiratory disease, CKD, chronic liver disease, chronic neurological disease, immunosuppression
Hepatitis A, B	Chronic liver disease, haemophilia, CKD (hepatitis B only)
Pertussis	Pregnancy 16–32 weeks (neonatal protection)

Worldwide ↑ in fungal infection with new pathogenicity, ↑virulence, and new infective mechanisms. Incidence data limited by failures in recognition and diagnosis. Divided into superficial/cutaneous and systemic/invasive.

Superficial/cutaneous mycoses

- **Dermatophytosis** Dermatophyte fungi digest keratin. Cause infection of skin and
keratinized structures, eg hair, nails. *Presentation:* scale and pruritus. Skin lesion
may be annular with central healing, eg *ring worm*, *tinea corporis*. *Tinea pedis* affects up to 15% of healthy population: skin erosions and blisters in toe web spaces,
dry scale on soles. *Fungal nail disease* = onychomycosis/tinea unguium: discolouration, nail thickening. *Tinea capitis:* scalp scaling, alopecia.

- **Superficial candidiasis** Usually *Candida albicans* (fig
9.18), a commensal in mouth, vagina, and GI tract. Risk
factors: immunosuppression, antibiotic treatment.
Presentation: oropharyngeal—white patches on erythematous background (plaque type); sore, inflamed
areas (erythematous type). *GU*—soreness, white
patches/discharge (fig 9.19). *Skin*—usually in folds/
interdigital (fig 9.20).

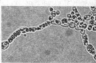

Fig 9.18 *Candida albicans.*
Courtesy of P-Y Guillaume.

- **Malassezia** Commensals of greasy skin. *Presentation: Pityriasis versicolor*—scaly
hypo/hyperpigmented rash with scaling (fig 9.21). *Seborrhoeic dermatitis*—
scaling of face, scalp (dandruff), anterior chest. *Malassezia folliculitis*—itchy, follicular rash on back and shoulders (ΔΔ acne). Can cause sepsis in neonates.

Diagnosis Clinical, microscopy of skin scrapings. **Treatment** All superficial mycoses: topical '-azole' antifungal or terbinafine 1–4wks. Also topical nystatin and
amphotericin in superficial candidiasis. Tinea capitis: griseofulvin, terbinafine,
itraconazole. Nail infection requires systemic treatment (terbinafine, itraconazole)
∴ confirm diagnosis, and caution re side effects including hepatotoxicity.

Systemic/invasive mycoses

- **Invasive candidiasis** Typically occurs in immunocompromised, comorbidity,
or ITU settings. Genetic susceptibility likely contributes. Estimated 250 000/yr
with 50 000 deaths. Candidaemia in ~7/1000 ICU patients. *Presentation:* risk factors for invasive fungal disease (p405), febrile with no microbiological evidence
of infection, new murmur, muscle tenderness, skin nodules. *Diagnosis:* (repeated)
blood/tissue culture. PCR. *Candida* in respiratory secretions alone is insufficient. *Treatment:* remove all possible catheters. Echinocandins (caspofungin,
anidulafungin, micafungin), fluconazole, amphotericin (liposomal for ↓renal toxicity). Consider fluconazole prophylaxis if risk factors for invasive disease (p399).
Consider empirical treatment if persistent fever, unresponsive to other therapy
(discuss with microbiologist, choice depends on local epidemiology, comorbidity).

- **Cryptococcus** See HIV, p396. Causes meningitis, pneumonia. *Presentation:* usually
immunosuppression, eg HIV, sarcoid, Hodgkin's, haematological malignancy, post-
transplant. History may be long, non-specific. Headache, confusion, ataxia, focal
neurological signs, fever, cough, pleuritic pain, SOB. *Diagnosis:* culture blood/CSF/
BAL, antigen testing in blood/CSF (Indian ink CSF stain less sensitive). *Treatment:*
amphotericin + flucytosine, fluconazole.

- **Histoplasmosis** Worldwide distribution of *Histoplasma*, ↑ in soil contaminated with bird/bat faeces. Illness depends on host immunity, estimated ~1%.
Presentation: flu-like symptoms, fever, malaise, cough, headache, myalgia, pneumonia, lung nodules/cavitation, pericarditis, mediastinal fibrosis/granuloma (ΔΔ
sarcoid, TB). *Diagnosis:* serology, antigen testing. *Treatment:* moderate–severe
lung disease or any CNS involvement: amphotericin, itraconazole.

- **Blastomycosis** *Blastomyces* in decomposing matter, mainly USA/Canada.
Presentation: fever, cough, night sweats, ARDS. ↑Risk of extrapulmonary disease
with immunosuppression: skin, bone, GU, CNS. *Diagnosis:* culture, antigen detection
(cross-reacts with histoplasmosis). *Treatment:* amphotericin, itraconazole.

►See also: Fungi and the lung, p174, *Pneumocystis jirovecii*, p396.

Invasive fungal infection

Invasion: fungus in normally sterile tissues.
Dissemination: infection of remote organs via haematogenous spread.
▶Suspect an invasive fungal infection in:
1 Any patient with risk factors (table 9.15).
2 Any systemically unwell patient who fails to respond to antibiotic therapy.
3 Any persistently febrile patient with no microbiological evidence of infection.

Table 9.15 Risk factors associated with invasive fungal infection.

Risk factor	Includes
Infection	HIV, CMV, TB, colonization/inadequate treatment of superficial fungal disease, broad-spectrum antibiotics, prior fungal infection
Malignancy	Neutropenia, mucositis, haematological malignancy
Critical illness	↑Mortality prediction score (eg APACHE), prolonged ITU admission, prolonged ventilation, severe trauma/pancreatitis
Catheter	Central venous catheter, urinary catheter, dialysis access, TPN
Transplantation	Immunosuppressant medication, recent rejection, graft-versus-host disease
Genetic	Hereditary chronic granulomatous disease, abnormalities in tumour necrosis factor/interleukins/cytokines
Surgical	Major surgery, GI perforation, anastomotic leak, length of transplant operation, delayed closure
Other comorbidity	Any disease managed with immunosuppressive therapy, burns

Source: data from Ramana KV *et al*, *Am J Infectious Diseases and Microbiology* 2013, 1(4);64–69.

Investigations
* Blood culture: three samples, different sites, same sitting, aim total 40–60mL blood.
* Microscopy + immunohistochemistry/fluorescence depending on site/risk.
* Other: antigen/antibody testing for general (eg mannan, galactomannan) and specific (eg cryptococcal) fungi; fungal metabolites; PCR: for typing/confirmation.
▶Seek expert advice on empirical treatment, agent depends on local epidemiology.

Facts of life for 'budding' mycologists

To the uninitiated, fungi are like bacteria, but their chitin cell walls and their knack of mitosis puts them in their own kingdom. They are larger than bacteria (eg 8μm across), and mostly reproduce by budding of germ tubes (fig 9.22), not by fission. Yeasts occur as single cells or as clusters. Hyphae often occur in a mass of cells (called moulds). A hyphal cell with cross-walls is called a mycelium. Some yeasts are dimorphic: single cells at 37°C but forming structures called mycelia, containing fruiting bodies (hyphae), at room temperature.

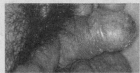
Fig 9.19 Candida of the glans.
Courtesy of P-Y Guillaume.

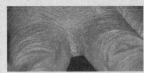
Fig 9.20 Web-space candida.
Courtesy of A Huntley.

Fig 9.21 Pityriasis versicolor.
Reproduced from Lewis-Jones (ed),
Paediatric Dermatology 2010, with permission
from Oxford University Press.

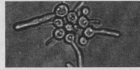
Fig 9.22 Germ tubes emerging from *Candida albicans* blastoconidia.
Courtesy of P-Y Guillaume.

9 Infectious diseases

9 Infectious diseases

Healthcare-associated, or nosocomial, infections include diseases which occur as a direct result of treatment or contact in a hospital or healthcare setting.

7–25% of hospital admissions are complicated by a nosocomial infection resulting in morbidity, mortality, and cost. The causal microbe may be benign in normal circumstances, but is able to cause disease when the patient:

1 Has been given broad-spectrum antibiotics (eg antibiotic-resistant organisms, *Clostridium difficile* colitis).
2 Is unwell/immunosuppressed (opportunistic infection).
3 Has compromised barriers (indwelling catheter/line, ventilation, surgery).

Healthcare-associated infection

Catheter-associated UTI

A catheter is inserted in ~20% of hospitalized patients. UTI is the most common infection acquired as a result of healthcare, accounting for 19% of all healthcare-associated infection. ~50% of UTIs are associated with a urethral catheter. Risk of infection is related to method of catheter insertion, duration of catheter, quality of catheter care, and patient susceptibility.

To reduce risk, only catheterize if necessary: Is there obstruction? Do you need precise urine output monitoring? Remove as soon as possible. See UTI, pp292–3.

Infections associated with intravascular access lines

Includes peripheral, central venous, and arterial catheters: tunnelled and non-tunnelled. >60% of bloodstream infections are associated with intravascular devices. Risk is higher with central catheters. Infection can result from introduction of microbes during insertion, access (eg when giving IV antibiotics), or from microbes elsewhere in the body seeding to the foreign material. Organisms include *Staphylococcus epidermidis* (p384), *Staphylococcus aureus* (including meticillin-resistant forms, ►MRSA see p384), *Candida* species (p404), and enterococci (p385).

Ensure that vascular access devices are used only when clinically indicated. Switch to oral treatment (fluid, medication, nutrition) as soon as clinically appropriate. Treatment includes removal/exchange of the device whenever possible.

Ventilator-associated pneumonia (VAP)

VAP affects up to 20% of patients admitted to intensive care units. Occurs as the endotracheal tube interferes with protective upper airway reflexes and facilitates microaspiration. Risks ↓ with non-invasive ventilation. In critical illness, the oropharynx becomes contaminated, commonly with Gram –ve bacteria, due to antibiotic exposure, altered host defences, and changes in mucosal adherence. Access to the airway occurs via folds in the endotracheal cuff and the bacterial biofilm is then propelled to the distal airways. Organisms include *Pseudomonas aeruginosa* (p387), Enterobacterales (p387), and *Staphylococcus aureus* (p384).

Clinical diagnosis has ↓sensitivity and ↓specificity. Suspect if new/persistent infiltrates on CXR plus two or more of: purulent sputum, leucocytosis (>12 × 10⁹/L), leucopenia (<4 × 10⁹/L), temperature >38.3°C.

Prevent by reducing colonization (silver-coated endotracheal tubes).

VAP prevention bundle includes:
• Nursing at 30–45° to ↓ aspiration risk.
• Wean off ventilator as soon as possible.
• Minimize ventilator circuit changes.
• Regular subglottic suction.

Surgical site infection

Affects 5% of patients undergoing surgical procedures, contributes to >⅓ of post-operative deaths. Common organisms include *Staphylococcus aureus* (p384), *Streptococcus pyogenes* (p384), and Enterobacterales when surgery involves entry to hollow viscera (p387). Prevention methods include hand hygiene, strict asepsis, MRSA screening and decolonization, hair removal, peri-operative normothermia, minimally disturbed low adherence/transparent dressings.

Clostridium difficile

Gram-positive anaerobic bacillus and most common healthcare-associated pathogen. Part of colonic flora in 2–5% of healthy adults, and 20–40% of hospitalized adults. Disease occurs when it converts to a vegetative (growth) state with production of enterotoxins A and B, causing colitis. Typically happens when inhibition by competing colonic flora is lost due to antibiotic exposure.

Presentation Watery diarrhoea, mild→fulminant colitis (pseudomembranes on endoscopy = 'pseudomembranous colitis'), ileus, toxic megacolon. Consider in diarrhoea with antibiotic use (usually >72h), especially if marked neutrophilia.

Diagnosis Immunoassay for glutamate dehydrogenase (common antigen) detects all strains of *C. difficile*. Detection of toxin (toxin immunoassay, toxin gene nucleic acid amplification) distinguishes infection from carriage.

Management SIGHT: Suspect, Isolate within 2h, Gloves and aprons, Hand wash with soap, Test immediately.
- Mild/moderate: metronidazole PO (local guidance may use vancomycin 1st line).
- Severe (WCC >15 × 10⁹/L or AKI or colitis or temperature >38.5°C): vancomycin PO (injection preparation can be given orally and may be cheaper than capsule) or fidaxomicin (↑cost).
- Non-responders: high-dose vancomycin + IV metronidazole, fidaxomicin, IV immunoglobulin (no RCT data). Surgical input if evidence of fulminant colitis.
- Recurrence: (weaning) vancomycin, fidaxomicin, faecal transplantation.

Management of healthcare-associated infection

Identify Screening (eg hospital admissions for MRSA, CPE) allows isolation and decolonization before harm. Be alert to new infections.

Protect Isolate multi-antibiotic-resistant microbes (eg MRSA), highly transmissible infections (eg norovirus), and high-risk groups including reverse barrier nursing (avoids transmission to, rather than from, patients, eg neutropenia). Patients with high-risk infections may need negative-pressure rooms (to prevent potentially infected air leaving the room), or in severe immunosuppression, positive-pressure rooms (to prevent potentially infected air entering the room). When many patients have the same nosocomial infection (eg norovirus) they may be barrier nursed together in dedicated bays.

Treat Refer to local guidelines, seek expert help. Initial antibiotic choice may differ for healthcare-associated infection.

Prevent Modify risk factors, eg nutrition, post-operative incentive spirometry to reduce pneumonia risk. Use/convert to narrow-spectrum antibiotics whenever possible. Remove catheters, intravascular access devices, and wean off ventilators as soon as clinically appropriate. Take measures to ↓ person-to-person transmission:

1 *Hand hygiene.* Wash hands before and after each patient contact (fig 9.23). Alcohol-based gels are helpful but soap is needed to kill *C. difficile* spores.

2 *Personal attire.* In the UK there is a bare-below-the-elbows policy. Long hair should be tied back. In areas where infection risk is particularly high (theatre, ICU), staff change into scrubs on arrival.

3 *Personal protective equipment (PPE).* Used for isolated patients and during procedures. Includes gloves, aprons, caps, respiratory protection/mask according to risk, eg FFP3 respirators in aerosolized infection.

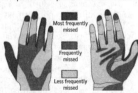

Fig 9.23 Areas commonly missed when washing hands.

Contains public sector information licensed under Open Government Licence v3.0, www.whatdotheyknow.com/request/21861/response/56086/attach/3/04072 Hand Hygiene 5 1.1.pdf

4 *Procedures.* Strict aseptic techniques for any procedure which breaches the body's defences including insertion/maintenance of invasive devices, IV infusions, wound care.

5 *Environment.* Should be clean and safe, with effective decontamination.

System interventions Up-to-date infection guidelines, audit, education, training.⁸

STIs[6] are common with increasing rates of diagnosis: ~×2 for *Chlamydia trachomatis*, *N. gonorrhoeae*, genital herpes, and syphilis since 2010. Prevalence highest in young adults (<25yrs) and MSM. For HIV, see pp394–99. For hepatitis B and C, see p274.

Taking a sexual history
- **Symptoms** ♂: urethral discharge, dysuria, genital skin problems, testicular pain/swelling, peri-anal or anal symptoms in MSM. ♀: vaginal discharge, vulval skin problems, abdominal pain, dyspareunia, unusual vaginal bleeding (post-coital, intermenstrual, consider referral for urgent colposcopy).
- **Exposure** Sexual contacts within last 3 months including sex of partner(s), type of contact (oral, vaginal, anal), insertive or receptive contact in contraceptive method (properly used?), type and duration of relationship, symptoms in partner(s), risk factors for HIV/hepatitis in partner(s), whether partner(s) can be contacted. STI history in all. Ask men whether they have ever had sex with another man.
- **Other** Last menstrual period, menstrual pattern, date of last cervical cytology (smear). Current contraceptive, concordance. Current/recent antimicrobial therapy. HPV vaccine history. There may be disclosure of non-consensual sex, or intimate partner violence. Do not be afraid to ask for help: *'Everything you tell me today is confidential unless you tell me something that worries me about your safety, at which point I may need to discuss this with another health professional in order to keep you safe.'*

Examination
♂: retract foreskin, inspect urethral meatus for discharge, scrotal contents/tenderness/swelling (stand patient up). ♀: vulval examination (lithotomy), speculum of vagina/cervix, bimanual examination for adnexal tenderness, abdomen/pelvis for masses. In all: genito-anal area, proctoscopy if anal symptoms, inguinal lymph nodes, oral mucosa if orogenital sex. Use a chaperone and document their name.

Urethritis/vaginal discharge See table 9.16.

Genital warts Caused by human papilloma virus (HPV). See p402.

Genital ulcer(s)
- **Genital herpes** HSV. *Presentation:* flu-like prodrome, then vesicles/papules around genitals, anus, throat. These burst, forming painful shallow ulcers. Also urethral discharge, dysuria, urinary retention, proctitis. *Diagnosis:* PCR. *Treatment:* analgesia, topical lidocaine. Antivirals within 5d: aciclovir, valaciclovir, famciclovir.
- **Syphilis** *Treponema pallidum. Presentation:*
  1 Primary: <90d after inoculation (median 3wk). Macule→papule→typically painless ulcer (chancre). Central slough, defined rolled edge. Highly infectious.
  2 Secondary: dissemination ~4–10wks after chancre. Rash (maculopapular in 50–75%, on palms/soles in 11–70%), mucous patches, condyloma lata (raised, pale plaques, often flexural), fever, headache, myalgia, lymphadenopathy, hepatitis.
  3 Tertiary: 20–40yrs after infection. *Neurosyphilis:* aseptic meningitis, focal neurological deficits, seizures, psychiatric symptoms, Argyll Robertson pupil (p68), tabes dorsalis (areflexia, extensor plantar reflex, dorsal column deficits, Charcot joints). *Gummatous syphilis:* destructive granulomata in skin, mucous membranes, bones, viscera. *Cardiovascular:* aortitis, aortic regurgitation/aneurysm. *Diagnosis:* PCR. Serology: non-specific (RPR, VDRL) sensitive in early infection then decline; specific (*T. pallidum* as antigen, eg TPHA, TPPA) reacts in early infection and persists. *Treatment:* parenteral benzylpenicillin (eg benzathine penicillin IM), duration depends on stage. Procaine benzylpenicillin boosted with probenecid in CSF disease.
- **Lymphogranuloma venerum** *Chlamydia trachomatis. Presentation:* mostly MSM in UK. Painless papule/ulcer→lymphadenopathy, fever, arthritis, pneumonitis. Direct transmission to rectal mucosa causes haemorrhagic proctitis: pain, rectal bleeding/discharge, tenesmus. *Diagnosis:* PCR. *Treatment:* doxycycline.
- **Tropical infections** Chancroid (*Haemophilus ducreyi*), granuloma inguinale (*Klebsiella granulomatis*). *Presentation:* both cause genital ulceration and lymphadenitis with spread of infection into overlying tissue (pseudobubo). *Diagnosis:* H. ducreyi PCR, Donovan bodies in tissue. *Treatment:* azithromycin.

Table 9.1b Overview of urethritis and vaginal discharge

STI	Presentation	Diagnosis	Treatment	Other
Chlamydia trachomatis	Often asymptomatic: detected on screening ♀: dyspareunia, dysuria, post-coital/inter-menstrual bleeding, ↑vaginal discharge ♂: dysuria, urethral discharge	Nucleic acid amplification test (NAAT) on: ♀: vulvo/vaginal swab—can be done by patient. Endocervical swabs and urine samples less sensitive ♂: first-pass urine Oral/anal swabs if oral/anal sex	100mg doxycycline BD for 7d. Alternative: azithromycin 1g PO (single dose) then 500mg BD for 2 days GUM: partner tracing, screening, treatment. Avoid sexual intercourse until treatment complete	Pharyngeal and rectal infection may be asymptomatic. Complications: ♀: pelvic inflammatory disease (PID), salpingitis, infertility, ectopic pregnancy, reactive arthritis, perihepatitis (Fitz-Hugh-Curtis syndrome) ♂: epididymo-orchitis, reactive arthritis Eye disease see p434
Neisseria gonorrhoeae	Urethral/vaginal discharge, dysuria Asymptomatic: 50% ♀, 10% ♂, most pharyngeal/rectal infection	Nucleic acid amplification test (NAAT) on: ♀: vaginal swab or endocervical swab. Urine samples less sensitive ♂: first-pass urine Culture (endocervical/urethral swab prior to antibiotics) for sensitivity	Ceftriaxone 1g IM. Ciprofloxacin 500mg PO if sensitive. Complicated disease: add doxycycline ± metronidazole. GUM: partner tracing, screening, treatment. Avoid sexual intercourse until treatment complete	↑Antibiotic resistance (36.4% ciprofloxacin resistance in UK) Complications: ♀: PID, salpingitis, infertility, ectopic pregnancy ♂: epididymitis, prostatitis, ↑HIV transmission, reactive arthritis; infective endocarditis, disseminated gonococcal infection
Non-gonococcal urethritis (NGU)	Urethral discomfort, dysuria, urethral discomfort Only assess symptomatic patients/visible discharge for urethritis	↑ Polymorphonuclear leucocytes on microscopy of urethral swab. Needs testing for chlamydia, gonorrhoea, and Mycoplasma genitalium. Exclude UTI	First episode as for Chlamydia trachomatis. Recurrent: metronidazole + azithromycin/moxifloxacin depending on first treatment	NGU refers to a pattern of infection rather than a cause. The main causes are Chlamydia trachomatis (11–50%) and Mycoplasma genitalium (6–50%)
Trichomonas vaginalis	♀: vaginal discharge (~70%), itch ♂: asymptomatic (~70%), discharge	NAAT, culture, microscopy (mobile trichomonads)	Metronidazole (2g single dose or 5-7d course). GUM: partner tracing, screening, treatment. Avoid sexual intercourse until treatment complete	Pregnancy: ↑risk of preterm delivery, low birth weight May enhance HIV transmission
Bacterial vaginosis	Thin, white, fishy-smelling vaginal discharge. No itch or soreness Asymptomatic in ~50%	Gram stain to examine vaginal flora (predominance/absence of lactobacilli), clue cells, vaginal pH >45	Oral or vaginal metronidazole, or vaginal clindamycin	Elevated vaginal pH alters vaginal flora: ↑anaerobic bacteria. Not sexually transmitted but associated with STI
Genital candidiasis	Genital itch, burning, cottage cheese-like discharge, dyspareunia	Microscopy and culture for Candida (p404)	-Azoles: pessary, eg clotrimazole, cream if vaginal symptoms, oral fluconazole if severe	Very common. No evidence for treatment of sexual partners. ↑Risk: pregnant, antibiotic therapy, DM, immunosuppressed

▶Exclude malaria in all travellers from the tropics (p412–15).
▶Exclude HIV in all (p394).
▶Most travellers have self-limiting illnesses potentially acquired in UK. Look for tropical infection[9] but remember usual differentials, including sepsis (qSOFA score).
▶Consider the need for early isolation and PPE.

History When Detailed geography of travel (table 9.17)[10] including setting (rural/urban). **When** Dates of travel, time of symptom onset, duration of symptoms (table 9.18).[10] **Risks and activities** Bites, diet, fresh-water exposure (schistosomiasis, leptospirosis), dust exposure, sexual activity, game parks (tick typhus, anthrax, trypanosomiasis), farms, caves (histoplasmosis, rabies, Ebola), unwell contacts. Higher risk in those visiting friends and relatives in lower-income countries.

Associated symptoms
• Respiratory: *S. pneumoniae*, *H. influenzae*, legionella, influenza, viral respiratory disease (SARS, MERS), TB, HIV-associated disease, melioidosis.
• Neurological: malaria, meningococcal meningitis, HIV, syphilis, Lyme disease, leptospirosis, brucellosis, tick-borne encephalitis, relapsing fever, trypanosomiasis.
• Gastrointestinal: traveller's diarrhoea, malaria, VHF, enteric fever, cholera, dengue.

Table 9.17 Differential diagnosis by geography

Area of travel	Common	Occasional	Rare but do not miss
Sub-Saharan Africa	Malaria (pp412–15) HIV (pp394–99) Rickettsiae (p418)	Schistosomiasis (p430) Amoebiasis (p428) Brucellosis (p420) Dengue (p416) Enteric fever (p411)	Other arbovirus (p416) Trypanosomiasis (p419) VHF (pp422–3) Visceral leishmaniasis (p419)
South-East Asia	Malaria (pp412–15) Chikungunya (p416) Dengue (p416) Enteric fever (p411)	Leptospirosis (p421) Melioidosis (p387)	Hanta virus (p422) Japanese encephalitis (p433) Rickettsiae (p418) Scrub typhus (p418)
South and Central Asia	Malaria (pp412–15) Dengue (p416) Enteric fever (p411)	Chikungunya (p416) Visceral leishmaniasis (p419)	VHF (CCHF) (pp422–3) Rickettsiae (p418) Japanese encephalitis (p433)
Middle East Mediterranean North Africa		Brucellosis (p420) Q-fever (p420) Zika (p417)	Visceral leishmaniasis (p419)
South America Caribbean	Malaria (pp412–15) Dengue (p416) Enteric fever (p411)	Brucellosis (p420) Leptospirosis (p421) Zika (p417)	Trypansomiasis (p419) Hanta virus (p422) Yellow fever (p416)
Eastern Europe		Lyme disease (p418)	Hanta virus (p422) Tick-borne encephalitis (p433)
Australia		Dengue (p416) Q fever (p420) Rickettsiae (p418)	Melioidosis (p387)
North America		Lyme disease (p418) Rickettsiae (p418)	Melioidosis (p387)

Table 9.18 Differential diagnosis according to incubation time

Incubation period	Infections
Short <10d	Dengue, chikungunya, gastroenteritis, relapsing fever, rickettsiae
Medium 10–21d	Malaria, HIV, brucellosis, enteric fever, leptospirosis, melioidosis, Q-fever, coccidioidomycosis, VHF, Chagas' disease, trypanosomiasis
Long >21d	Malaria, HIV, TB, viral hepatitis, brucellosis, schistosomiasis, amoebic liver abscess, trypanosomiasis, visceral leishmaniasis
Chronic fever <14d	TB, HIV plus opportunistic infection, pyogenic deep-seated abscess, infective endocarditis, brucellosis, enteric fever, fungal infection, schistosomiasis, visceral leishmaniasis, PE

9 Infectious diseases

Examination

Rash

- *Maculopapular:* dengue, chikungunya, EBV, HIV seroconversion, VHF.
- *Purpuric:* dengue, meningococcal infection, plague, DIC, VHF.
- *Ulcer/eschar:* Chagas', *Yersinia pestis*, Rickettsiae (fig 9.24), anthrax, tropical ulcer.

Jaundice Viral hepatitis, severe falciparum malaria, enteric fever, leptospirosis, relapsing fever, typhus, VHF, bartonellosis

Hepatosplenomegaly See table 9.28: viral hepatitis, HIV, enteric fever, brucellosis, leptospirosis, rickettsial infection, relapsing fever, schistosomiasis, amoebic liver abscess, trypanosomiasis, visceral leishmaniasis.

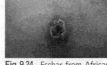

Fig 9.24 Eschar from African tick-bite fever.

Reproduced from Caplivski and Scheld, *Consultations in Infectious Disease* 2012, with permission from Oxford University Press.

Investigation

Directed by travel history and examination. In undifferentiated fever:
- Malaria film/rapid diagnostic testing (p413).
- HIV test (p395).
- FBC: lymphopenia in viral infection including HIV; eosinophilia in parasitic/fungal eg soil-transmitted helminths, filariasis, schistosomiasis, hydatid disease; ↓platelets in malaria, dengue, HIV, typhoid, severe sepsis.
- Blood culture ×2: prior to antibiotics, LFT. Consider: save serum, specific serology, or EDTA sample for PCR.

Support

- Local infectious diseases team (never underestimate the wisdom of your on-call microbiologist). Travel fever diagnostic website: www.fevertravel.ch
- Public Health England imported fever service: 0844 778 8990.
- National Travel Health Network and Centre (NaTHNaC)/TravelHealthPro: www.travelhealthpro.org.uk

---

Enteric fever: typhoid and paratyphoid

~20 million cases and 200 000 deaths per year worldwide, ~500/yr in UK mostly imported from India, Pakistan, and Bangladesh. Caused by related, Gram-negative strains of 'typhoidal' *Salmonella* spp.:
- Typhoid (~75–90%): *Salmonella typhi*.
- Paratyphoid (~10–25%, less severe): *Salmonella* serotype *Paratyphi* A > B > C.

The bacteria invade intestinal mucosa. Dissemination occurs without a primary diarrhoeal response. This distinguishes 'typhoidal' from D&V-inducing 'non-typhoidal' serovars of *Salmonella* (p424). Transmission is faecal–oral from contaminated water/food. Incubation 6–30d (most 10–20d). ~10 000 organisms are required to cause illness. Can be asymptomatic (but shed organism).

Symptoms Fatigue, headache, anorexia. Marked fever, 'stepwise' (rising through each day with progressive peaks) in <20%. Abdominal pain, relative bradycardia, cough, constipation. Rose spots in ~25% (salmon-coloured, 1–4cm, blanching, due to bacterial emboli to dermis). Diarrhoea ('pea-soup') and hepatosplenomegaly in 2nd week. Complicated disease in up to 10%: intestinal haemorrhage/perforation, myocarditis, hepatitis, pneumonia, DIC, CNS involvement (delirium, meningism, encephalitis, cerebellar signs, fits, coma), eye complications (corneal ulcer, uveitis, neuritis, thrombosis).

Diagnosis Isolation of *S. typhi* from: blood (take multiple cultures of 10–15mL in first 10d to ↑ sensitivity), bone marrow, intestinal secretions, or stool (↑sensitivity after 1st week). Serology has ↓sensitivity and specificity. (Widal test is −ve in ~30% of culture-proven cases.) ↑LFT. PCR (not routine).

Treatment Azithromycin ± IV ceftriaxone. >70% imported from Asia are resistant to fluoroquinolones. Fever takes median 5–7d to respond due to intracellular niche of organism. Antipyretics, fluid management, nutrition. CNS disease: dexamethasone 3mg/kg IV then 1mg/kg/6h for 8 doses (limited data).

Vaccine Ty21a (oral, live, CI: immunosuppression, pregnancy) or Vi (IM, capsular vaccine). ~50–80% effective for ~3yrs. Limited/no protection against paratyphoid.

Epidemiology
- 3.2 billion people at risk in 95 countries = half the world's population (**fig 9.25**).
- 228 million cases in 2018 with 405 000 deaths.
- Africa: 93% of malaria cases, 94% of deaths (most age <5yrs).
- Most common tropical disease imported into UK, ~2000 cases/yr.
- ~20% fever in travellers from Africa presenting to UK hospitals is due to malaria.
- *Plasmodium falciparum* is the most prevalent parasite in Africa and responsible for most malaria deaths worldwide (=~75% of malaria presenting in UK).
- *Plasmodium vivax* is the dominant parasite outside of sub-Saharan Africa.
- Preventable and treatable: incidence ↓ by 9% and deaths ↓ by 32% since 2010.
- Partial immunity widespread in endemic countries.

Malaria parasites
Malaria parasites belong to the genus *Plasmodium*. >100 species exist of which 5 cause human disease (**table 9.19**). Transmission occurs through the bite of an infected *Anopheles* mosquito. Only female mosquitoes transmit *Plasmodium* as only females require a blood meal for egg development. Transmission in the absence of a mosquito is rare: vertical (congenital transfer from mother to child), transfusion, organ transplantation, needle-sharing.

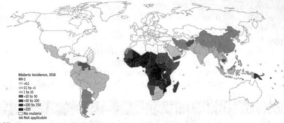

Malaria incidence, 2018
- 0
- <0.1
- 0.1 to <1
- 1 to 10
- >10 to 50
- >50 to 100
- >100 to 250
- >250
- No malaria
- Not applicable

Fig 9.25 Countries with malaria transmission.
Reproduced with permission from World Health Organization, *World malaria report 2018*. © World Health Organization 2018. https://www.who.int/publications/i/item/9789241565653

Table 9.19 Malaria species in humans

Species	Average incubation (range)	Persistent liver stage	Distribution
P. falciparum (fig 9.26)	12days (6 days–6 months)	No	Africa, India, South East Asia, Indonesia, Oceania, Central America, Middle East
P. vivax (fig 9.27)	14 days (days–years)	Yes	South Asia, South and Central America, Africa, Middle East
P. malariae (fig 9.28)	30 days (28 days–years)	No	Africa, South and Central America, South East Asia
P. ovale	11–16 days (years)	Yes	Africa
P. knowlesi	9–12 days	No	South East Asia

Reproduced from Detels *et al*., *Oxford Textbook of Global Public Health*, 2015, with permission from Oxford University Press.

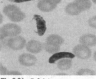

Fig 9.26 *P. falciparum* sausage-like gametocytes in RBC.
© S Upton, Kansas Univ

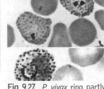

Fig 9.27 *P. vivax* ring partly hidden by Schuffner's dots. Stained and examined in the field by JML.

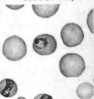

Fig 9.28 *P. malariae* ring and band forms from 2 specimens. © S Upton, Kansas Univ.

The life cycle of malaria is dependent on both humans and mosquitoes (**fig 9.29**). Sporozoites are transferred to a human host when an infected mosquito bites. These travel via the bloodstream to the liver where maturation occurs to form schizonts containing ~30 000 merozoite offspring. If a dormant stage exists (*vivax, ovale*, see **table 9.19**), and is inadequately treated, merozoites can be released from the liver weeks, months, or years later causing recurrent disease. The

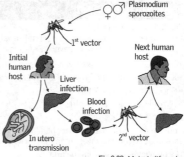

Fig 9.29 Malaria lifecycle.

rupture of schizonts releases merozoites which enter RBCs ('*What a fantastic niche!*'). In the RBC, merozoites form larger trophozoites and erythrocytic schizonts (poor prognostic indicator if seen on blood film). The rupture of erythrocytic schizonts produces the clinical manifestations of malaria.

Clinical features

►Consider in anyone with a fever who has previously visited a malarial area (fig 9.23), regardless of prophylaxis.

Presentation *P. falciparum* has a minimum incubation of 6 days and most commonly occurs within 3 months of return from an endemic area. Take a careful travel history: country, area of travel, date of return. Do not forget to ask about stopovers. Symptoms are non-specific: fever, headache, malaise, myalgia, diarrhoea, cough. Fever patterns are described but only occur if rupture of infected RBCs is synchronized: alternate day for *P. falciparum, P. vivax, P. ovale* ('*tertian*'); every 3rd day for *P. malariae* ('*quartan*'). ►Most patients have no specific fever pattern.

Examination Fever, hepatosplenomegaly, pallor; often unremarkable. If diagnosis is delayed or severe disease then may present with jaundice, confusion, seizures.

Diagnosis

Immediate blood testing is mandatory in the UK:
• Microscopy of thick and thin blood smear. Sensitive and specific in experienced hands.
• Rapid diagnostic test (RDT) detection of parasite antigen. Used for initial screen if expert microscopy is unavailable, eg out-of-hours. Used in addition to (not instead of) blood film.

Results should be available within 4h. ►If malaria is suspected but blood film is negative: repeat at 12–24h and after further 24h. Malaria is unlikely if three expert serial blood films are negative. ΔΔ: dengue, typhoid, hepatitis, meningitis/encephalitis, HIV, viral haemorrhagic fever. Care in pregnancy: thick films can be negative despite parasites in the placenta. Seek expert help.

If *P. falciparum* (or *P. knowlesi*) estimated % parasitized red cells should be given:
• >2% = ↑ chance of severe disease (indication for parenteral treatment see pp414–15).
• >10% = severe disease.

Other: FBC (anaemia, thrombocytopenia), creatinine and urine output (AKI), clotting (DIC), glucose (hypoglycaemia), ABG/lactate (acidosis), urinalysis (haemoglobinuria).

Malaria is notifiable to public health: www.gov.uk/health-protection-team

Errors to avoid

• Failure to consider diagnosis.
• Inadequate travel history.
• Belief prophylaxis prevents all malaria.
• Belief presents with a fever pattern.
• Non-specific symptoms not recognized.
• Delay in blood film/RDT.
• No serial blood film if first test negative.
• Inadequate treatment (pp414–15).
• Inappropriate treatment (pp414–15).
• Failure to anticipate/treat complications.

Based on Beeching et al., Returned travellers. In: *Principles and Practice of Travel Medicine*, 2013, John Wiley and Sons. Copyright © 2013 by Blackwell Publishing Ltd.

Falciparum malaria

Risk of deterioration ∴ admit to hospital. Treatment[11] depends upon whether the disease is **uncomplicated**, or **severe**. Features of severe disease are:

- Impaired consciousness/seizures (consider LP).
- AKI (oliguria <0.4mL/kg/h, creatinine >265µmol/L).
- Shock (BP <90/60) = 'Algid malaria'.
- Hypoglycaemia (<2.2mmol/L).
- Pulmonary oedema/ARDS.
- Hb <80g/L.
- Spontaneous bleeding/DIC.
- Acidosis (pH <7.3).
- Haemoglobinuria.
- Parasitaemia >10%.

Poor prognostic indicators: peripheral blood schizonts (p413), elevated serum lactate, ↑age, severe jaundice, organ dysfunction.

Uncomplicated falciparum malaria

Artemisinin combination therapies (ACT) achieve rapid clearance of parasites by combined action at different stages of the parasite cycle (p413):

1 Artemether-lumefantrine: 4 tablets (4×20/120mg) at 0, 4, 8, 24, 36, 48, and 60h. 1st line in UK (+ pregnant >13wks), with high-fat food to ↑ absorption. SE: vomiting. Redose if vomiting <2h post dose.

2 Dihydroartemisinin (DHA)-piperaquine: 4 tablets (4×40/320mg) OD for 3d (weight >60kg). Take >3h pre and post food to prevent excess peak levels. SE: ↑QT$_c$.

Options if ACT not available:

- Atovaquone-proguanil: 4 tablets OD for 3 days. Parasite clearance ~66% after 3d, GI SE in ~25%. Do not use for treatment if used for prophylaxis.
- Oral quinine sulfate 600mg TDS for 5–7d *plus* doxycycline 200mg OD (or clindamycin 450mg TDS if pregnant) for 7d. Parasite monitoring required. Can cause 'cinchonism': nausea, deafness, ringing in ears.

►Resistance to ACT is emerging in Asia.

►↑Failure rates with antifolate drugs mean Fansidar® is no longer used.

►Chloroquine is not used in the *treatment* of falciparum malaria.

Severe *P. falciparum* malaria

►Give urgent parenteral treatment. ***Artesunate is treatment of choice.*** Meta-analysis shows reduction in mortality of 39% (CI: 25–50%) compared to quinine, preventing 94 deaths for every 1000 adults treated.[12]

Artesunate regimen (adult)

2.4mg/kg IV at 0h, 12h, 24h and then daily for up to 5d. Converted to a full course of ACT (see uncomplicated falciparum malaria earlier in topic) when able to tolerate oral medication. Side effects: delayed haemolysis 7–21d post-treatment (usually self-limiting)—check Hb 14d post treatment. If artesunate is not available immediately, treatment should be started with quinine. It is safe to overlap/combine with artesunate when it is available.

Quinine regimen (adult)

Loading dose 20mg/kg over 4h. Then 10mg/kg every 8h for next 48h or until patient can swallow (dose every 12h if patient has renal failure or hepatic dysfunction or if IV needed >48h). Convert to 600mg PO TDS to total quinine course 5–7d. Give with 7d oral doxycycline (clarithromycin in children/pregnant ♀). Side effects: cinchonism (see earlier in topic), hyperinsulinaemia.

►Manage in a high dependency setting. ↑Capillary permeability so vulnerable to pulmonary oedema if over-filled. Lactate levels may reflect intravascular obstruction rather than circulating hypovolaemia. Monitor: blood glucose every 4h (2h if quinine infusion), Hb, clotting, electrolytes, creatinine. Daily parasite counts are sufficient NB: will fluctuate with the life cycle of the parasite (p413) and an increase in first 36h of treatment may not indicate treatment failure. Given the rapid action of artesunate, exchange transfusion is no longer considered to offer any additional benefit.

Pregnancy Little evidence on use/safety of artesunate. On balance of risk (pregnancy loss, pulmonary oedema, maternal mortality), artesunate should be given.

Non-falciparum malaria
P. vivax, P. ovale, P. malariae, P. knowlesi
* If mixed infection with falciparum, treat as falciparum.
* If severe/complicated non-falciparum disease, treat as severe falciparum.
* If uncomplicated disease, treat with ACT as uncomplicated falciparum.

Chloroquine can be used for susceptible non-falciparum disease. Dosing in adult: 620mg base at 0h, 310mg base at 6–8h, 310mg base on day 2 and 3. *But:*
* Do not use if *P. falciparum* cannot be excluded.
* Be aware that ACT may work more quickly on both fever and parasite count.
* Chloroquine resistance exists in *P. vivax* (Papua New Guinea, Indonesia).
►In addition to other treatment, *P. vivax* and *P. ovale* require eradication of liver hypnozoites with primaquine:
* *P. vivax:* adult 30mg (0.5mg/kg) daily for 14d.
* *P. ovale:* adult 15mg (0.25mg/kg) daily for 14d.
►Risk of haemolysis with primaquine in G6PD deficiency so screen prior to use. Seek expert advice for dosing/monitoring patients with G6PD deficiency, and in pregnancy.

Malaria prevention

Vector control for all people at risk of malaria. Includes:
* Source reduction by destruction of mosquito breeding sites (ie standing water).
* Long-lasting insecticidal nets. These should be provided free of charge and with equity of access. Nets last for ~3yrs, a lifespan of 5yrs could save ~$3.8bn. Insecticidal resistance is an increasing concern, should dual agents be used?
* Indoor residual spraying, effective for 3–6 months when >80% of houses included.
* Sterile male mosquito release. Estimated to initially require 20 males/human to be protected ∴ ~64 billion sterile mosquitoes worldwide.
* Genetic modification to develop mosquitoes that are not susceptible to malaria (and other) parasites. Requires modification that does not ↓ fertility or will not disperse in vector population. Requires acceptability, infrastructure, and money.

Chemoprophylaxis is the use of antimalarial drugs to prevent clinical disease. In high-transmission areas it is recommended for pregnant women (given at antenatal visits) and infants (given with routine vaccination).

Travellers from the UK to malaria areas should be given:
1 Bite prevention advice: insect repellents with 20–50% DEET (for all >2 months old including pregnant and breast-feeding women). Apply after sunscreen with SPF >30 as DEET may ↓ sunscreen efficacy.
2 Chemoprophylaxis (table 9.20) according to area of travel. See www.fitfortravel.nhs.uk/destinations.aspx

Table 9.20 Prophylactic regimen against malaria in adults (refer to *BNF*)

Area	Regimen	Notes
No drug resistance (non-*P. falciparum*)	Chloroquine 310mg base/ week *PLUS* proguanil 200mg OD	1wk before and 4wks after travel Chloroquine: GI disturbance, headache CI: epilepsy Proguanil: diarrhoea, anti-folate (care if possibility of pregnancy)
Chloroquine-resistant *P. falciparum*	Mefloquine 250mg/week *OR*	2–3wks prior and 4wks after travel Neuropsychiatric SE, dizziness
	Doxycycline 100mg OD *OR*	1–2d prior, 4wks after travel. SE: hepatic impairment, teratogenic
	Atovaquone-proguanil combination	1–2d prior, 1wk after travel. Expert advice if taking HIV ART

Vaccination (RTS,S) is being piloted for children by WHO within selected high-risk African nations. Results are awaited.

Malaria eradication is the permanent reduction of the incidence of malaria. Social, demographic, and economic factors, the available healthcare system, and investment all determine success. Parasitologic (as opposed to clinical) cure is required in order to eliminate asymptomatic transmission.

Mosquito-borne diseases[13] are transmitted by the bite of a mosquito infected with a virus, bacteria, or parasite. The mosquito acts as the disease vector. Mosquitoes are arthropods (see **table 9.21, p418**). Mosquito-borne diseases can therefore also be described as vector-borne or arthropod-borne disease. When a virus is transmitted by an arthropod it is termed an arbovirus (ARthropod-BOrne VIRUS).

▶**Malaria** See pp412–15.

Dengue

Most important arbovirus in humans. Dengue viruses (*Flaviviruses* DENV 1–4) are transmitted by day-biting *Aedes* mosquito. 120 countries (**fig 9.30**), 2.5 billion at risk. Symptoms in 100 million/yr. UK: ~500 imported cases/yr.

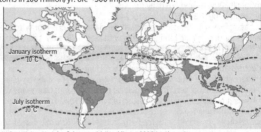

Fig 9.30 Countries at risk of dengue (dotted line = 10°C isotherm).
Reproduced from Johnson *et al.*, *Oxford Handbook of Expedition and Wilderness Medicine*, 2016, with permission from Oxford University Press.

Presentation Incubation 3–14d. Febrile phase: fever (up to 40°C), N&V, headache, retro-orbital pain, myalgia, arthralgia, +ve tourniquet test (inflate BP cuff to midway between systolic and diastolic for 5 min→≥10 petechiae/inch²). ▶*Warning signs/ critical phase* may occur 3–7d into illness and needs hospital admission: abdominal pain, persistent vomiting, fluid accumulation, mucosal bleeding, hepatomegaly, ↑haematocrit + ↓plts. ▶*Severe disease:* hypovolaemic shock, respiratory distress, severe bleeding, organ involvement (transaminases >1000, ↓GCS, other organ failure). **Diagnosis** PCR for virus/ELISA antigen² during viraemia (~1st 5d of fever). Serology (IgM, IgG) after 5d. Also ↓plts, ↓WCC, transaminitis. (ΔΔ: Chikungunya, Zika.) **Treatment** Supportive: prompt but careful fluid balance due to potential for plasma leak. IV crystalloid, to maintain effective circulation, only in severe disease. 20mL/kg over 15–30min if hypotensive shock. Monitor clinically and via haematocrit. Reduce IV fluid when stable. Beware: plasma leak maintains haematocrit unless bleeding. Consider transfusion if ↓haematocrit without clinical improvement. Avoid NSAIDs.

Chikungunya

Arbovirus (*Alphavirus*) transmitted by *Aedes* mosquito. Widespread: Asia, Africa, Europe, and Americas. Name derives from Kimakonde language meaning 'to become contorted' due to arthralgia. Blood-borne and vertical transmission possible, but rare. **Presentation** Incubation 1–12d. Fever. Polyarthralgia: bilateral, symmetrical, can be severe, persistent. Headache, myalgia, N&V, maculopapular rash. **Diagnosis²** Viral culture/PCR (~1st 8d), serology. **Treatment** Supportive. Analgesia.

Yellow fever

Arbovirus (*Flavivirus*) spread by *Aedes* mosquitoes in Africa, South America. **Presentation** Incubation ~3–6d. Viraemia ~3d with fever, headache, myalgia, anorexia, N&V, relative bradycardia (ΔΔ: enteric fever p411). ~15% have remission followed by severe symptoms ~48h later: epigastric pain, jaundice, AKI, cardiac instability, bleeding. Mortality 5–30%. **Diagnosis** Clinical and travel history. Virus/PCR in 1st 3d.² Serology: cross reacts with other flaviviruses, IgM can persist after vaccination. **Treatment** Supportive. Live vaccine, effective for life (certificate for 10yrs).

2 In UK testing done via Rare and Imported Pathogens Laboratory (RIPL): www.gov.uk/collections/rare-and-imported-pathogens-laboratory-ripl

Zika virus

Arbovirus (*Flavivirus*) transmitted by *Aedes* mosquito. First identified in Zika forest, Uganda, 1947. Human cases rare until outbreak in Pacific Islands (2007–2013), and Brazil (2015). Estimated 1.5 million cases in Brazil in 2016 peak. Fall to 30 000 cases in Americas in 2018. Estimated 1% transmission by sexual contact. Rare reported cases via blood products. **Presentation** Subclinical in ~80%. Mild illness in ~20%: fever, conjunctivitis, myalgia, rash. Rarely severe acute illness and Guillain–Barré syndrome. **Zika and birth defects** Evidence for causality between infection in first trimester and congenital abnormalities (congenital Zika syndrome, affecting 5–14%): microcephaly, intracranial calcification, eye pathology, congenital contractures. Small study evidence for ↑neonatal mortality.[14] **Diagnosis** PCR of viral RNA/ELISA in blood/body fluid. **Treatment** Vector control, avoid non-essential travel to high-risk areas in pregnancy (see www.travelhealthpro.org.uk), condoms to prevent sexual transmission. Vaccine trials ongoing (2020).

Lymphatic filariasis (elephantiasis)

>40 million affected and disfigured. 900 million at risk (80% in sub-Saharan Africa). Filarial parasites (nematodes) transmitted via mosquitoes which bite infected hosts and ingest microfilaria. These mature in the mosquito with infective larvae transferring to new hosts during feeding. Adult worms form nests in lymphatic vessels causing damage and lymphoedema. Transmission prevented by an annual dose of two drugs—7.7 billion treatments delivered by WHO since 2000.[13] Types of filarial worm:

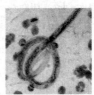

Fig 9.31 Blood smear of *W. bancrofti* (290 × 8.5✱m).
Courtesy of Prof S Upton, Kansas University.

• *Wuchereria bancrofti* (fig 9.31) ~90% of disease.
• *Brugia malaya* ~10%.
• *Brugia timori* possible cause of disease.

Presentation Asymptomatic infection ± subclinical lymphatic damage. Acute episodes of local inflammation: pain, fever. Chronic damage: lymphoedema (fig 9.32), hydrocele, chylocele, scrotal/penile swelling. CKD: proteinuria, haematuria. Immune hyperreactivity→tropical pulmonary eosinophilia (cough, wheeze, fibrosis, ↑eosinophil counts, ↑IgE). **Diagnosis** Microfilariae in blood smear (fig 9.31), antifilarial IgG, visualization of worms on USS/tissue sample. **Treatment** Lymphoedema care. Prevention in high-risk populations: albendazole plus either diethylcarbamazine (DEC) or ivermectin. DEC is contraindicated in onchocerciasis (p435), care with ↑circulating *Loa loa* (p435) due to risk of encephalopathy and renal failure. Household salt can be fortified with DEC.

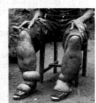

Fig 9.32 Lymphoedema.
CDC/Dr. Henry D. Pratt.
Photo Credit: J. McDowell.

West Nile and **Japanese encephalitis**, see 'Neurological disease', pp432–3.

The global advance of vector-borne disease?

Since 1990, five species of *Aedes* mosquito have become established in Europe. The adaptation of mosquitoes to a temperate environment, combined with future climate forecasts has led to models[15] that predict the UK will be suitable for:

• *Plasmodium falciparum* transmission by 2030–2080.
• *Plasmodium vivax* transmission by 2030.
• Chikungunya transmission in London by 2041.
• Dengue transmission after 2100.

Of course, modelling is not simple. Socio-economic development, urbanization, land-use change, migration, and globalization all come into play. Surveillance of mosquitoes at sea-ports, airports, and used-tyre companies remains uninteresting to date. But consider a time when a visit to South-East England offers an opportunity to explore the historical gems of our wonderful capital, and simultaneously becomes a pertinent question in your diagnostic sieve.

Vector-borne disease

Vector-borne diseases are infections transmitted by the bite of infected arthropod species including mosquitoes, ticks, flies, and bugs (**table 9.21**).

Table 9.21 Vector-borne disease

Vector/arthropod	Disease	Page
Mosquito *Anopheles*	Malaria	412–15
Aedes	Dengue, Chikungunya, yellow fever, Zika	416–17
Culex	Lymphatic filariasis, Japanese encephalitis, West Nile	417, 432–3
Ticks	Lyme disease, rickettsial disease, relapsing fever, tick-borne encephalitis, Crimean-Congo haemorrhagic fever	418–19, 422–3, 433
Bugs/flies	Leishmaniasis, trypanosomiasis, onchocerciasis, loiasis	419, 435
Snails	Schistosomiasis	430

Lyme disease (Lyme borreliosis)

Tick-borne multisystem disease due to spirochaete *Borrelia burgdorferi* (or related *Borrelia* spp.). ~All cases limited to northern hemisphere (mainly Europe and US). ~2000–3000 cases/yr in UK. Risk of infection from tick bite is 3–12% in Europe. **Presentation** ►≤75% remember tick bite. Needs attachment for 36–48h for transmission. Disease stages:

Fig 9.33 Erythema migrans: distinct advancing edge.

Reproduced from Lewis-Jones, *Paediatric Dermatology* 2010, with permission from Oxford University Press.

* *Early localized* (3–30d after bite): erythema migrans (**fig 9.33**), pain/pruritus, lymphadenopathy, ± constitutional symptoms: fever, malaise, headache. ⅓ do not see a rash.
* *Early disseminated* (wks–months): borrelial lymphocytoma = bluish-red plaque/nodule: check earlobes, nipples, genitals. Neuroborreliosis: lymphocytic meningitis, ataxia, amnesia, cranial nerve palsies, neuropathy (severe pain, worse at night), encephalomyelitis. Carditis: acute-onset 2nd/3rd-degree heart block, myocarditis.
* *Late disseminated* (months–yr): acrodermatitis chronic atrophicans = focal inflammation then atrophic skin; Lyme arthritis.

Diagnosis Clinical: erythema migrans with known exposure or evidence of infection. PCR, *Borrelia* culture (↓sensitivity: <20% for CSF).[3] Two-tier serology due to false-positive reaction with other spirochaete infection: ELISA + immunoblot. Sensitivity ↓ due to slow seroconversion: IgM 1–2wks (and may persist), IgG 4–6wks and background positivity 3–15%. **Treatment** Erythema migrans: doxycycline 100mg BD PO for 21d (CI: <9yrs, pregnancy). Alternatives: amoxicillin, azithromycin. Neuroborreliosis: ceftriaxone for 21d or doxycycline 200mg BD for 21d. Carditis: doxycycline or amoxicillin for 21d. Arthritis: doxycycline or ceftriaxone for 28d. ►**Jarisch–Herxheimer** Treatment reaction due to endotoxins (fever, sweating, malaise); observe 1st ~4h treatment, use cooling/antipyretics. Self-resolving 48h. **Prevention** Keep limbs covered; use insect repellent (DEET); inspect skin, remove ticks (use tweezers, hold close to head/mouth).

Rickettsial disease

Rickettsiae are obligate, intracellular coccobacillary forms between bacteria and viruses. Mammals and arthropods are natural hosts. ↑Risk with rural activities.

* *Spotted fevers:* eg Rocky Mountain spotted fever (Americas), rickettsialpox (ΔΔ chicken-pox).
* *Typhus:* scrub typhus in Asia-Pacific regions; endemic (flea-borne) typhus in tropical areas; epidemic (louse-borne) typhus in homeless populations, eg refugees.
* *Other emerging illnesses:* eg *Ehrlichia, Anaplasma*.

Presentation Incubation ~1–2wks. Fever, headache, malaise, rash (maculopapular, vesicular, or petechial), N&V, myalgia. Lymphadenopathy and an eschar at the site of the bite (scrub typhus). Fulminant, life-threatening infection possible with Rocky Mountain spotted fever, louse-borne typhus, scrub typhus. **Diagnosis** Clinical: fever + rash + travel to an endemic area. Serology, culture/PCR of blood/skin biopsy. **Treatment** Antibiotics in severe cases: doxycycline, azithromycin, chloramphenicol. Consider permethrin in louse-borne.

3 Specialist diagnostic service and advice in UK via Rare and Imported Pathogens Laboratory (**RIPL**): www.gov.uk/government/collections/rare-and-imported-pathogens-laboratory-ripl

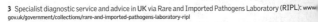

Leishmaniasis

Protozoan parasites of *Leishmania*[13] species, transmitted by infected female *phlebotomine* sandflies. 1 billion at risk. Risk factors: poverty, malnutrition, displacement, deforestation, dam building/irrigation. **Presentation**
- *Cutaneous*, most common form, ulceration (fig 9.58, p436).
- *Mucocutaneous* (fig 9.34): leads to tissue destruction of nose, mouth, throat. 90% occurs in Bolivia, Brazil, Peru.
- *Visceral leishmaniasis* (VL, kala-azar, 'black sickness') (fig 9.35): fever, weight loss, hepatosplenomegaly, anaemia. >95% mortality without treatment. Endemic in Indian subcontinent, East Africa. 90% of new cases occur in Bangladesh, Brazil, Ethiopia, India, South Sudan. 300 000 cases/yr, 20 000 deaths/yr. Post kala-azar is a complication of *Leishmania donovani* = a hypopigmented macular/nodular rash (ΔΔ leprosy), 6 months–1yr after apparent cure, can heal but is a reservoir for parasites and maintains transmission.

Fig 9.34 Mucocutaneous leishmaniasis.
Reproduced with permission from World Health Organization. © World Health Organization. http://www.who.int/leishmaniasis/mucocutaneous_leishmaniasis/en/

Diagnosis Clinical. Microscopy of tissue (skin, bone marrow) for parasite. Antibody detection in VL (indirect fluorescence, ELISA, western blot, direct agglutination test, immunochromatographic test) is limited due to: 1 Ab levels detectable after cure, cannot distinguish VL relapse/active infection. 2 Tests are +ve in many with no history of VL. 3 Serology may be –ve if HIV +ve. **Treatment** Liposomal amphotericin (single dose), oral miltefosine, pentavalent antimonials (resistance in India). 75% reduction in new cases due to WHO Kala-azar Elimination Programme.

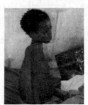

Fig 9.35 Visceral leishmaniasis.
Reproduced with permission from World Health Organization. © World Health Organization. http://www.who.int/leishmaniasis/visceral_leishmaniasis/en/

Human African trypanosomiasis (HAT, sleeping sickness)

Infection with *Trypanosoma* protozoan parasites,[16] transmitted by the tsetse fly in sub-Saharan Africa. 95% reduction in cases since 2000; <1000 cases in 2018. Includes:
- *Rhodesiense HAT*: incubation <21d, high fever, GI disturbance, lymphadenopathy, headache. Chancre at bite site in ~84%, maculopapular rash. Progresses to myopericarditis, arrhythmias, and neurological symptoms.
- *Gambiense HAT*: chronic disease in African population, presents years after infection (can present with acute febrile illness in travellers). Low-grade fever. Sleep disorder: reversal of sleep–wake cycle, uncontrollable sleep episodes. Weakness, abnormal gait, psychiatric symptoms.

Diagnosis ↓Hb, ↓plts, AKI, ↑LFTs, polyclonal ↑IgM. Microscopy of parasite (blood, lymph node, chancre, CSF). Serology and PCR if available. **Treatment** According to disease type and stage. Available from WHO. Includes suramin, melarsoprol, pentamidine, nifurtimox-eflornithine. Seek specialist advice—side effects from all.

Chagas' disease (American trypanosomiasis)

Life-threatening illness due to protozoan *Trypanosoma cruzi* transmitted by triatomine (kissing) bugs. Endemic in Latin America: ~6–7 million infected. **Presentation** *Acute phase* (~2 months): skin lesion (chagoma), fever, headache, myalgia, lymphadenopathy, unilateral conjunctivitis, periorbital oedema (Romaña's sign), myocarditis, meningoencephalitis. *Chronic phase* (yrs): cardiac: dilated cardiomyopathy; GI: mega-oesophagus (dysphagia, aspiration), mega-colon (abdominal distension, constipation); CNS symptoms. **Diagnosis** *Acute:* trypomastigotes in blood, CSF, node aspirate. *Chronic:* serology (Chagas' IgG ELISA). CXR for mega-oesophagus. **Treatment** Benznidazole, nifurtimox. ↓Effectiveness in chronic disease.

Relapsing fever

Caused by spirochaete *Borrelia recurrentis* (louse-borne, sub-Saharan Africa, refugee camps) or other *Borrelia* (tick-borne, worldwide). **Presentation** Intermittent fever 'crisis' due to antigenic variation (~3d fever, then afebrile ~7d), headache, myalgia, ↓BP. **Diagnosis** Spirochaetes on blood smear, false +ve serology for Lyme disease. **Treatment** Doxycycline/macrolides (single dose if louse-borne). Neuroborreliosis treatment if CNS disease (p418). Jarisch–Herxheimer reaction (p418) can mimic fever 'crisis'.

Anthrax (*Bacillus anthracis*)

Gram-positive, aerobic bacillus found in soil worldwide. Humans exposed via infected livestock or animal products, eg hide, wool, tusks. Infection via inhalation, ingestion, contamination of broken skin (includes IV drug use). Bacteria secrete exotoxins: oedema toxin and lethal toxin.

Presentation

• *Cutaneous (~95%):* itchy papule→vesicle→necrotic eschar. Oedema may be striking. Regional lymphadenopathy, malaise.

• *Inhalation:* fever, cough, myalgia, SOB, pleural effusion (haemorrhagic mediastinitis), stridor, death.

• *GI (rare):* fever, abdominal pain, ascites, mucosal ulcers, GI perforation.

Diagnosis Vesicular fluid culture (care, do not disseminate), blood culture, antibody ELISA, PCR. (NB: not pneumonic so sputum cultures are –ve.) **Treatment** Quinolone/doxycycline. Two agents if systemic disease, eg ciprofloxacin + clindamycin/linezolid (then narrow to susceptibility). Consider anti-anthrax monoclonal antibody/immunoglobulin as adjunct in inhalational disease.

Bartonella

• *B. henselae* (cat-scratch disease): from infected cat fleas. Low-grade fever, regional lymphadenopathy. Encephalitis rare. Skin lesions mimic Kaposi's sarcoma.

• *B. quintana* (trench fever): from human body louse. Fever, headache, bone pain.

• *B. bacilliformis* (bartonellosis): from infected sandflies in Andes mountains. Oroya fever = fever, headache, myalgia, haemolysis. Later nodular→vascular skin lesions.

Diagnosis Clinical, blood culture (fastidious ∴ needs prolonged culture), serology. **Treatment** Cat-scratch disease often self-limiting. Azithromycin, aminoglycoside.

Brucellosis

Most common zoonosis worldwide: 500 000 cases/yr. Gram –ve infection of cattle, swine, goats, sheep, dogs. Human infection via ingestion of infected meat/unpasteurized milk/cheese; or through inhalational/mucosal contact with animal body fluids (eg farmers, slaughterhouse workers, meat packers, hunters). ↑Risk in countries without animal health programmes. **Presentation** Acute (<1 month), sub-acute (1–6 months), or chronic (>6 months). Non-specific: fever, anorexia, sweats, weight loss, malaise (ΔΔ TB). Localized infection: septic arthritis, spondylitis, meningitis, endocarditis, orchitis, abscess. **Diagnosis** Culture with prolonged incubation due to slow doubling time.[17] Serology (four assays performed by Public Health England Brucella Reference Unit: 0151 529 4900). **Treatment** Doxycycline, rifampicin, aminoglycoside, co-trimoxazole. Needs prolonged course as intracellular with slow doubling time. Relapse usually due to inadequate dose/duration/adherence.

Coxiella burnetii (Q fever)

Q fever is derived from the label 'query' fever attributed to an unexplained disease in Australian abattoir workers. *C. burnetii* is now recognized as the pathogenic agent. Sheep, goats, cattle are main sources of infection (also cats, dogs, rabbits, ducks, ticks). Occurs worldwide. Spores can survive in soil, animal products, and water for months–yr. Transmitted by contact, inhalation of dust, or consumption of raw milk products. **Presentation** Incubation 3–30d. ~50% asymptomatic. Non-specific symptoms: fever (1–3wks), nausea, fatigue, headache. Pneumonia in 1–2%: typical or atypical, may have rapid progression. Also splenomegaly, granulomatous hepatitis, aseptic meningitis, encephalitis, osteomyelitis. Endocarditis is the most common form of chronic disease. **Diagnosis** *Coxiella* cannot be cultured using routine lab methods.[17] PCR is rapid. Serology can take 2–6wks to become positive and detects variation in lipopolysaccharide (LPS) coat. Phase II LPS appears before phase I LPS ∴ acute infection = IgM/IgG to phase II LPS, chronic infection = IgG to phase I LPS. Serology on paired sera 2–4wks apart provides best diagnostic evidence. **Treatment** Doxycycline. Also rifampicin, chloramphenicol, fluoroquinolone, macrolide. Hydroxychloroquine alkalinizes the phagosomes in which the bacteria resides and may ↑ bactericidal effect.

Leptospirosis (Weil's disease)

Pathogenic leptospire spirochaetes belonging to the subgroup *Leptospira interrogans*. >250 pathogenic serovars. Chronic renal infection of carrier animals: rodent, cattle, pigs. Spread by water/soil/food contaminated by infected animal urine. **Presentation** Incubation ~7d (2–30d). 1st (acute/septicaemic) phase: fever, non-specific flu-like symptoms. Mild/subclinical in ~90%. Followed by recovery or 2nd (immune/leptospiruric) phase: conjunctival suffusion, myalgia (↑CK), jaundice, meningitis, uveitis, AKI, pulmonary haemorrhage, ARDS, myo/pericarditis. (Weil's disease described in 1886: fever, jaundice splenomegaly, renal failure, CNS symptoms. Term now applied to all severe disease.) **Diagnosis** In UK[18] via National Leptospirosis Service (https://www.gov.uk/guidance/leptospira-reference-unit-services). Culture (blood/CSF) +ve during 1st phase. Serology. PCR. **Treatment** Mild: doxycycline, azithromycin. Severe: ceftriaxone, IV penicillin. Conflicting evidence of benefit for steroids in severe disease.

Yersinia pestis (plague)

Gram –ve, obligate intracellular pathogen transmitted by small animals and their fleas by bite, direct contact, inhalation, or ingestion (rare). ~300 cases/yr worldwide. **Presentation** Incubation: 3–7d. Flu-like symptoms, then one of three disease forms:

1 *Bubonic:* most common form. *Yersinia pestis* enters at bite and travels via lymphatics. Inflamed, painful lymph node is termed 'bubo' and can suppurate.
2 *Septicaemic:* direct spread without 'bubo', or advanced stage after 'bubo'.
3 *Pneumonic:* lung disease. Most virulent, least common. Usually from advanced bubonic form but can then transmit via droplets to other humans without fleas/animals.

Diagnosis Culture bubo fluid, blood, sputum. Rapid antigen testing available. **Treatment** Reduces mortality from 60% to <15%: streptomycin, tetracycline.[13]

Toxoplasmosis

Caused by protozoan *Toxoplasma gondii*. Found worldwide. Life cycle (**fig 9.36**). Infection is lifelong (~⅓ of population). HIV may cause reactivation (p396). **Presentation** Asymptomatic in ~90%. Self-limiting cervical lymphadenopathy, low-grade fever if normal immune system. Disseminated disease if immunosuppressed: cerebral abscess, encephalitis, choroidoretinitis, myocarditis, myositis, pneumonitis, hepatitis. Congenital infection: pregnancy loss, neurocognitive deficit, retinal damage. **Diagnosis** In UK via Toxoplasma Reference Laboratory (0179 228 5058). Serology: IgG = previous exposure (high avidity IgG suggests infection >3–5 months ago, used in pregnancy); IgM = acute infection, false +ve or chronic infection with persistent IgM; IgA in cord serum = congenital infection. PCR: blood/CSF/urine/amniotic fluid/aqueous/vitreous humour. **Treatment** If eye disease, immunosuppressed, or neonate: pyrimethamine + sulfadiazine + folinic acid. Corticosteroids for eye inflammation. Spiramycin reduces vertical transmission. Prophylaxis: co-trimoxazole.

Echinococcosis (hydatid disease) p431. *Rabies* p433. *Hanta virus* p422.

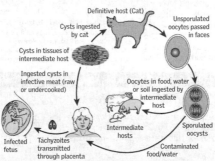

Fig 9.36 Oocysts in cat faeces can stay in the soil for months, where rats eat them. The rats get infected, and, under the direction of *Toxoplasma* in the amygdala, the rats lose their fear of cats, and so get eaten in turn. So the parasite ensure success by facilitating a jump from intermediate to definitive host. How does the parasite overwhelm the innate fear of cats? By causing a sexual attraction to normally aversive cat odour through limbic activity. From Fernando Monroy: www2.nau.edu/~fpm/research/res.html

Viral haemorrhagic fever (VHF)

Viral haemorrhagic fever (VHF) is a term used for severe, multi-organ disease in which the endothelium is damaged, and homeostasis is impaired. Haemorrhage complicates the disease course and can be life-threatening. VHF classification by viral subtype is shown in **table 9.22**.

Table 9.22 VHF classification (HF = haemorrhagic fever)

Virus family	Disease (virus subtype)	Details
Filovirus	Ebola	See Ebola, p423
	Marburg	See Marburg, p423
Arenavirus	Lassa fever (Lassa)	See Lassa, p423
	Argentinian HF (Junin)	South American VHFs are rare causes of infection in travellers. Incubation 2–16d. Resemble Lassa fever. Severe disease with bleeding in ~⅓. Supportive treatment. Live vaccine available for Junin virus
	Bolivian HF (Chapare, Machupo)	
	Brazilian HF (Sabia)	
	Venezuelan HF (Guanarito)	
Bunyavirus	Crimean-Congo HF	See CCHF, p423
	Hanta	Rodent host. Incubation 2d–8wk. Causes: 1 HF with renal syndrome: fever, headache, GI symptoms, and AKI. 2 Hanta virus pulmonary syndrome: bilateral interstitial pulmonary infiltrates, mortality 30–40%. Supportive treatment
	Rift valley fever	Endemic in Africa. 80% asymptomatic or self-limiting febrile illness. <2% CNS involvement/haemorrhagic
Flavivirus	Dengue	See p416
	Yellow fever	See p416

The Advisory Committee on Dangerous Pathogens (ACDP) classifies a pathogen as Group 4 (highest) when it causes severe human disease, with high risk of spread, and no effective prophylaxis or treatment. Ebola,[19] Marburg, Lassa, and Crimean-Congo haemorrhagic fever (CCHF) are all Hazard Group 4 haemorrhagic fever viruses, as was smallpox. They are largely confined to Africa (**fig 9.37**), with the exception of CCHF which occurs in the Middle East, Africa, Eastern Europe, and Asia.

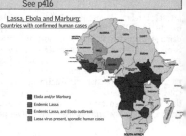

Lassa, Ebola and Marburg:
Countries with confirmed human cases

■ Ebola and/or Marburg
■ Endemic Lassa
■ Endemic Lassa, and Ebola outbreak
■ Lassa virus present, sporadic human cases

Fig 9.37 Lassa, Ebola, and Marburg risk in Africa.
Reproduced with permission from *Viral haemorrhagic fevers: origins, reservoirs, transmission and guidelines*, Crown copyright 2018. Contains public sector information licensed under the Open Government Licence v3.0.

Risk assessment for VHF in the UK

Assess for possible transmission *and* fever.
- Transmission:
  1 Travel to endemic area <21 days (rural for Lassa fever; caves/primates/antelopes/bats for Ebola/Marburg; tick/animal slaughter for CCHF).
  2 Travel to known outbreak (http://www.promedmail.org).
  3 Contact with infected specimen.
- Fever: >37.5°C in the past 24h.

If possible transmission *and* fever consider 'high possibility' (≠high probability), isolate, PPE (see BOX 'Equipment'). Inform local infectious disease team and contact the Imported Fever Service (0844 778 8990) for VHF investigation. ▶Bruising, bleeding, and uncontrolled D&V also need isolation and advice if relevant contact.

Ebola

Incubation 2–21d (usually 3–12d). Evidence for fruit bats as reservoir. Outbreaks with ↑mortality. Largest epidemic (2014–2016) due to Ebola virus (EVD, formally Zaire ebolavirus): 28 646 cases and 11 323 deaths in Guinea, Liberia, and Sierra Leone.

Cytokine activation→endothelial damage, oedema, coagulopathy, tissue necrosis, multi-organ failure. Transmission from index case via mucous membranes, or contact with body fluids (including burial contact), viral shedding in semen. **Presentation**

Equipment
• Double gloves
• Fluid-repellent gown
• Full-length plastic apron
• Head cover (surgical cap)
• Fluid-repellent footwear
• Full face shield
• Full-repellent respirator
• Meticulous removal.

* *Undifferentiated* (0–3d). Fever (>38°C axillary), myalgia, weakness, anorexia, headache, sore throat. May not look unwell.
* *GI* (4–10d). Epigastric/abdominal pain, liver tenderness, N&V, hiccups, diarrhoea, hypovolaemia.
* *Late organ stage* (>10d). Haemorrhagic: petechiae, ecchymoses, mucosal haemorrhage, GI bleeding, haemoptysis. Neurological: extreme weakness, confusion, agitation, bradypsychia, coma. Other: hypoglycaemia, electrolyte abnormalities, secondary infection, shock, DIC, multi-organ failure, death.
* *Post-infection:* arthralgia, hepatitis, orchitis, transverse myelitis, meningitis, uveitis, vision/hearing impairment, social isolation, psychological effects.

Diagnosis ►PPE (see BOX 'Equipment') if high possibility (see BOX 'Risk assessment'). ↓WCC, ↓plts, ↑AST > ALT. IgM (~day 3), IgG (~day 7), reverse transcriptase PCR on blood/urine/saliva/throat swab. ►Exclude malaria. **Treatment** Supportive: fluid resuscitation, correct electrolytes/coagulation/glucose, treat secondary infection, nutrition. Trace contacts, support family. Experimental and evolving therapies: anti-RNA agents, immunotherapy with blood/plasma from survivors, monoclonal antibodies (REGN-EB3, mAb114), Ebola vaccine (rVSV-ZEBOV, Ebola ça suffit! trial). **Ethics** Randomization versus compassionate use: is it ethical to withhold even potentially beneficial therapy to a control group with a life-threatening condition? Is observational data gained through the compassionate use of experimental therapy sufficient to guide clinical decisions? Where should resources be directed to improve outcome: drug development or basic healthcare provision, eg would the capacity to check K⁺ improve mortality?

Marburg, Lassa, and CCHF

Differentiating features are given in **table 9.23**.

Table 9.23 Differentiation between VHF

VHF	Clinical features
Marburg	Incubation typically 5–9d. Clinically identical disease course to Ebola. Ebola/Marburg suggested by liver tenderness
Lassa	~80% mild/asymptomatic. Haemorrhage in ~20%. Variable mortality in different epidemics 25–80%. Exudative pharyngitis. Convalescent hearing loss. Observational data shows response to ribavirin if given in first 6d
CCHF	Tick-borne. Sudden-onset prodrome. Haemorrhagic stage common, develops rapidly, but usually short-lived 2–3d. Ribavirin used in treatment (↓evidence).

Sacrifice

This book choses to celebrate Dr Ameyo Stella Adadevoh, a Nigerian physician whose diagnostic acumen protected a nation. On a post-take ward round in Lagos in 2014, she recognized the index case of Ebola virus in Nigeria despite never having seen the disease before. She isolated and treated the patient despite neither her hospital nor her country being ready to do so, and in the face of litigation threats. In order to save others, and for 'the greater public good' she sacrificed herself, dying from Ebola on 19 August 2014. Thus she protected Nigeria from a death toll far greater than 8 (including 4 other healthcare workers to whom we also pay our deepest respects). And so we go forward in the hope that when our own mortality salience is activated and we are not in the warm, comfortable bed of the octogenarian we all desire to become, our existential anxiety can be buffered by the memory of Dr Adadevoh who confers greater meaning to our doctoring lives: we did what we could to help the most.

9 Infectious diseases

Gastroenteritis = diarrhoea (± vomiting) due to enteric infection with viruses, bacteria, or parasites. Diarrhoea can be defined as:
• Acute diarrhoea: ≥3 episodes partially formed or watery stool/day for <14d.
• Dysentery: infectious gastroenteritis with bloody diarrhoea.
• Persistent diarrhoea: acutely starting diarrhoea lasting >14d.
• Traveller's diarrhoea: starting during, or shortly after, foreign travel.
• Food poisoning: disease (infection or toxin) caused by consumption of food/water.
▶Food poisoning is notifiable in the UK (www.gov.uk/health-protection-team).

Gastroenteritis can be classified according to infectious aetiology (table 9.24) or predominant clinical presentation (table 9.25, also see p255).

Table 9.24 Gastroenteritis by infectious aetiology

Infection	Organism	Incubation	Notes	Page
Virus ~50–60%	Norovirus	1d	Important cause of epidemic gastroenteritis. 600 000–1million cases/yr in UK	426
	Rotavirus	1–3d	Affects nearly all children by age 5yrs. Routine, childhood (live) vaccine in UK	426
	Astrovirus	4–5d	Often less severe than norovirus	
	Adenovirus	3–10d	Enteric adenovirus. Mainly children	
	Sapovirus	1–3d	Children. Not common in food-borne disease	
	CMV	~3–12wks	Usually asymptomatic. If immunosuppression: colitis, hepatitis, retinitis, pneumonia	397, 401
Bacteria ~30–40%	Salmonella (non-typhoidal)	12–72h	Under-cooked eggs, poultry, meat	427
	Campylobacter	2–5d	Under-cooked meat, cross-contamination, unpasteurized milk, water	427
	E. coli	1–10d (usually 3–4d)	Bloody diarrhoea if Shiga-toxin producing E. coli (STEC) eg 0157. Can cause HUS. Under-cooked beef, unpasteurized milk most common.	387, 425, 427
	Shigella	1–2d	S. sonnei most common. Deadly epidemics with S. dysenteriae in low-income countries	427
	Staphylococcus aureus	30min–6h	Unpasteurized milk/cheese, uncooked food. Multiplication leads to toxin production	384
	Clostridium perfringens	6–24h	Raw meat. Inadequately reheated food	426
	Clostridium difficile		Antibiotic-associated diarrhoea. Spore-forming therefore persists: wash your hands	407
	Listeria	3–70d	Cold meat, soft cheese, refrigerated pâté. Diarrhoea, fever, myalgia. ↑Severity in immunosuppression and pregnancy (bacteraemia, fetal loss)	385
	Vibrio cholerae	2h–5d	Human and aquatic reservoirs. Epidemics due to inadequate environmental management	426
	Yersinia enterocolitica	4–7d	Main source is undercooked pork. Most infection in young children	427
Parasites <2%	Giardia	1–3wks	Intestinal parasite. Cyst transfer via infected faeces, eg contaminated water. Malabsorption	428
	Cryptosporidium	1–12d	Transfer via infected faeces. Symptoms and ↑severity with immunosuppression, eg HIV	397, 428
	Entamoeba histolytica	2–4wks (can be years)	Asymptomatic carrier, intestinal disease and/or extra-intestinal disease (liver, skin, lung, brain)	428
	Cyclospora cayetanensis	~1wk	Transfer via infected faeces. May have relapsing course	429
	Trichinella	1–2d	Enteral at 1–2d. Parenteral at 2–8wks: larval migration, facial swelling, myocarditis, encephalitis	429
	Trichuriasis	~3months	Whipworm. Dysentery with heavy infection	429
	Intestinal flukes	4d—months	Eg Fasciolopsis buski	

Table 9.25 Gastroenteritis by clinical presentation

Diarrhoea without blood (enteritis)	Diarrhoea with blood (dysentery)
Norovirus	Shigellosis (bacillary dysentery)*
Rotavirus	Enterohaemorrhagic *E. coli*
Astrovirus	*Campylobacter* enterocolitis*
Enteric adenovirus	*Salmonella* enterocolitis*
Enterotoxigenic *E. coli*	*Clostridium difficile*
Enteropathogenic *E. coli*	*Yersinia* enterocolitis
Toxin-producing *Staph. aureus*	*Entamoeba histolytica* (amoebic dysentery)
Cholera	Trichuriasis (whipworm)
Clostridium perfringens	CMV
Giardia	
Cryptosporidium	
Cyclospora cayetanensis	

*Milder disease may present as diarrhoea without blood.

Traveller's diarrhoea

Diarrhoea affects 20–60% of travellers.[20,21] High-risk areas: South Asia, Central and South America, Africa. Major cause = enterotoxigenic *E. coli*.

Prevention Boil water, cook thoroughly, peel fruit and vegetables. Avoid ice, salads, shellfish. Drink with a straw. Hand washing with soap may ↓ risk.

Presentation Most diarrhoea is during first week of travel. Symptoms are often unreliable indicators of aetiology but the following may be indicative:
• Enterotoxigenic *E. coli*: watery diarrhoea preceded by cramps and nausea.
• *Giardia lamblia*: upper GI symptoms, eg bloating, belching.
• *Campylobacter jejuni* and *Shigella*: colitic symptoms, urgency, cramps.

Duration of diarrhoea: most <1wk, 10%>1wk, 5% >2wks, 1% >30d.

Treatment
• Oral rehydration. Clear fluid and oral rehydration salts. ►Home-made oral rehydration recipe: 6 teaspoons of sugar + half teaspoon salt in 1L clean water.
• Antimotility agents, eg loperamide, bismuth subsalicylates. Avoid if severe pain or bloody diarrhoea as may indicate invasive colitis.
• Antibiotics: usually not indicated. Balance risk (resistance, side effects, ↑ carriage non-typhoid salmonella, ↑ HUS in 0157:H7 *E. coli*.) and benefits. Considered if rapid cessation of diarrhoea needed and/or limited access to sanitation/healthcare. Reduce diarrhoea from ~3 to ~1.5 days. Choice depends on allergy, medication, and destination: azithromycin 500mg OD for 3d (risk of fluroquinolone resistance, particularly SE Asia), ciprofloxacin 500mg BD for 3d, or rifaximin 200mg TDS for 3d.
• Consider admission if severe dehydration/signs of shock.

Prophylaxis Not recommended as severe disease and long-term sequelae rare, risk of *C. difficile*. Consider in immunosuppressed (transplant, HIV, chemotherapy), GI pathology (IBD, ileostomy, short-bowel), ↑risk with dehydration (sickle cell, CKD). Care with interactions with usual medications.
• Ciprofloxacin 500mg OD (80–100% protection).
• Norfloxacin 400mg OD (75–95% protection).
• Rifaximin 200mg every 12–24h (72–77% protection).
• Bismuth subsalicylate 2 tablets QDS (62–65% protection, 1st line in US).

Persistent diarrhoea Investigate if >14d or dysentery: FBC, U&E, LFT, inflammatory markers, stool microscopy for ova/cysts/parasites (historically 3 samples but may not actually improve diagnostic yield, time intensive), molecular testing for (pre-defined) microbes. ΔΔ of persistent diarrhoea = *Giardia* (most common diagnosis, send PCR), *Entamoeba histolytica*, *Shigella*. Post-infectious irritable bowel syndrome is a diagnosis of exclusion (in up to 30%).

►Do not forget: malaria, HIV.

9 Infectious diseases

Diarrhoea without blood

Norovirus Single-stranded RNA virus. Highly infectious. Transmission by contact with infected people, environment, food (~10%). Most common cause of infectious GI disease, ~600 000 cases in England/yr. *Presentation:* 12–48h after exposure, lasting 24–72h: acute-onset vomiting, watery diarrhoea, cramps, nausea. Virus shed in stool even if asymptomatic. Numerous genotypes and unknown longevity of immunity ∴ repeat infection occurs. *Diagnosis:* clinical, stool sample reverse transcriptase PCR. *Treatment:* supportive, anti-motility agents, usually self-limiting.

Rotavirus Double-stranded RNA virus. Wheel-like appearance on EM ∴ 'rota'. Commonest cause of gastroenteritis in children (~50%). Most infected by 5yrs. *Presentation:* incubation ~2d. Watery diarrhoea and vomiting for 3–8d, fever, abdominal pain. *Diagnosis:* clinical, antigen in stool. *Treatment:* supportive. Routine vaccination in UK (p403). Virus shed in stool post vaccine ∴ careful hygiene if immunosuppressed and changing nappies. Live vaccine ∴ delay vaccination if *in utero* biological agents with active transfer across placenta (eg infliximab, adalimumab).

Enterotoxigenic *E. coli* Gram −ve facultative anaerobe. Disease due to heat-stable or heat-labile toxin which stimulates Na^+, Cl^-, and water efflux into gut lumen. ~20% of all infective diarrhoea, ~80% of traveller's diarrhoea. *Presentation:* incubation 1–3d. Watery diarrhoea, cramps. Lasts ~3–4d. *Diagnosis:* clinical, identification of toxin from stool culture. *Treatment:* supportive. See BOX 'Traveller's diarrhoea' (p425).

***Clostridium perfringens* (type A)** Gram +ve, anaerobe. Produces enterotoxin. Spores survive cooking and germinate during unrefrigerated storage. 2–30 outbreaks/yr in UK. *Presentation:* sudden-onset diarrhoea, cramps, usually lasts <24h. *Diagnosis:* stool toxin, quantification of faecal bacteria. *Treatment:* supportive. β-toxin of *C. perfringens* type C can cause a necrotizing enteritis with fulminant disease, pain, bloody diarrhoea, septic shock. β-toxin is sensitive to trypsin proteolysis so ↑ risk with trypsin inhibition by sweet potatoes, ascaris infection ∴ occurs in New Guinea ('pigbel'), central/south America, south-east Asia, China.

Cholera *Vibrio cholerae* is a Gram −ve, aerobic, 'comma-shaped' flagellated motile vibrating/swarming rod. Found in faecally contaminated water. Servovars 01 and 0139 cause disease. ~190 000 cases in 2014 (fig 9.38). Last indigenous case in UK in 1893. *Presentation:* incubation 2h–5d. ~75% asymptomatic but shed bacteria. Profuse (1L/h) diarrhoea ('rice-water' stool), vomiting, dehydration, metabolic acidosis, circulatory collapse, death. *Diagnosis:* clinical: death due to dehydration from watery diarrhoea age >5yrs, or any watery diarrhoea age >5yrs during known epidemic. Identification of serovars 01 or 0139 in stool. Rapid dipstick testing available but culture confirmation recommended. *Treatment:* ▶▶oral rehydration salts (WHO/UNICEF ORS sachet) will treat[13] up to 80%. Needs safe water. Adults may need 1L/h initially: offer 100mL/5min. NG if vomiting. IV fluids if severely dehydrated: Ringer's lactate or 0.9% saline *plus* ORS (beware ↓ K^+) up to 200mL/kg in first 24h. Antibiotics in severe dehydration to ↓ diarrhoea: doxycycline (single dose 300mg) or tetracycline (3d course) guided by local susceptibility (azithromycin in children/pregnancy). Zinc shortens illness in children (10–20mg/24h). *Prevention:* cholera loves filth: clean water (and clean politics) abolishes it. Oral cholera vaccines (56–94% efficacy in adults) dependent on logistics, cost, production capacity. Antibiotic prophylaxis breeds resistance.

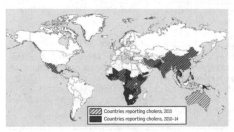

Fig 9.38 Cholera: areas reporting outbreaks 2010–2014.

Reproduced with permission from World Health Organization, *Countries reporting cholera, 2010–2015.* ©World Health Organization 2016. http://www.who.int/gho/epidemic_diseases/cholera/epidemics/en/

Legend within image: Countries reporting cholera, 2015 / Countries reporting cholera, 2010–14

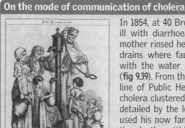

Fig 9.39 *Death's Dispensary,*
George Pinwell, 1866.
Image in the Public Domain.

In 1854, at 40 Broad St, London, a child became ill with diarrhoea, dying on 2 September. Her mother rinsed her soiled nappies into the house drains where faulty brickwork allowed mixing with the water supply of the Broad St pump (fig 9.39). From this confluence sprung the discipline of Public Health. The ensuing deaths from cholera clustered around the Broad St pump, as detailed by the local doctor, Dr John Snow. He used his now famous Voronoi diagram showing the deaths within a 'line of nearest pump' to motivate the parish vestry: 'In consequence of what I said, the handle of the pump was removed the following day', so inaugurating the control of cholera. These events illustrate a number of truths.

1 Knowledge of the microscopic cause of disease is not required for public health measures to succeed (*Vibrio cholerae* was identified by Robert Kock in 1883).
2 Even the most parochial are capable of life-saving action when assisted by a doctor in command of the facts.
3 Influential friends help. Snow remained largely unknown until the 1930s when *On the Mode of Communication of Cholera* was republished by Wade Hampton Frost, first professor of epidemiology at John Hopkins School.
4 Randomization (Broad St pump versus an alternative water supply) is king.

Diarrhoea with blood (dysentery)

Shigella **(sonnei, flexneri, dysenteriae, boydii)** Gram –ve anaerobe. *Presentation:* watery or bloody diarrhoea, pain, tenesmus, fever 1–2d after exposure. Lasts ~5–7d. ↑ in MSM. Complications: bacteraemia, reactive arthritis (~2% of *flexneri*), HUS (Shiga-toxin-producing *dysenteriae*). *Diagnosis:* stool culture. PCR/enzyme immunoassay. *Treatment:* supportive. Nutrition: green bananas (↑short-chain fatty acids in colon), zinc if age <6yrs, vitamin A. Antibiotics if systemically unwell, immunosuppressed. Guided by local susceptibilities (ciprofloxacin, azithromycin). Avoid antidiarrhoeal agents: risk of toxic dilatation.

Enterohaemorrhagic/Shiga-toxin producing *E. coli* **(STEC)**, eg 0157:H7 Gram –ve facultative anaerobe. Produces veratoxins which are 'Shiga-like' due to similarity with *Shigella dysenteriae*. *Presentation:* incubation 3–8d. Diarrhoea, haemorrhagic colitis. HUS in up to 10% (p311). *Diagnosis:* stool culture. PCR/enzyme immunoassay for Shiga toxin. **Treatment** Supportive. Do not give antibiotics: ↑ risk of HUS.

Campylobacter Gram –ve, spiral-shaped rod. *Presentation:* incubation 1–10d (usually 2–5d). Bloody diarrhoea, pain, fever, headache. Complications: bacteraemia, hepatitis, pancreatitis, miscarriage, reactive arthritis, Guillain–Barré. *Diagnosis:* stool culture. PCR/enzyme immunoassay. *Treatment:* supportive. Antibiotics only in invasive cases, refer to local susceptibilities (macrolide, doxycycline, quinolone).

Salmonella enterocolitis **(non-typhoidal)** Gram –ve, anaerobic, motile bacilli. *Presentation:* diarrhoea, cramps, fever, usually within 12–36h of exposure. Invasive infection (<10%) can cause bacteraemia/sepsis, meningitis, osteomyelitis, septic arthritis. *Diagnosis:* stool culture. PCR. *Treatment:* supportive. Meta-analysis shows no evidence of benefit for antibiotics in healthy people. Consider in severe/extraintestinal disease according to local susceptibilities (quinolone, macrolide).

Yersinia enterocolitica Gram –ve rod. *Presentation:* incubation 4–7d. Diarrhoea, fever, pain (may mimic appendicitis), vomiting. May last 1–3wk. Also erythema nodosum, reactive arthritis (~1 month after diarrhoea). *Diagnosis:* stool culture, agglutination titres. *Treatment:* antibiotics in severe disease depending on local susceptibilities (aminoglycosides, co-trimoxazole, quinolone).

►See also: *Staph. aureus* pre-formed toxin (p384), *GI parasites* (pp428–9), *Clostridium difficile* (p407).

Giardiasis

Giardia lamblia (fig 9.40) is a flagellate protozoan. Faecal–oral spread from infected drinking water/food/fomites. **Presentation** Asymptomatic in the majority. Incubation 1–3wks. Diarrhoea, flatulence, bloating, pain, malabsorption. Duration of symptoms typically ~2–6wks. Most common diagnosis if persistent traveller's diarrhoea (p425). **Diagnosis** Stool microscopy for cysts and trophozoites. Intermittent shedding so multiple samples (≥3) *may* ↑ sensitivity. Faecal immunoassay. PCR for diagnosis/subtype. Duodenal fluid aspirate analysis. **Treatment** Hygiene to prevent transmission. Metronidazole (treatment failure in up to 20%), tinidazole (single dose), albendazole (↓ side effects, simultaneous treatment of other parasites), nitazoxanide. Lactose-intolerance develops in 20–40%. No treatment for asymptomatic disease in endemic areas due to likelihood of re-infection.

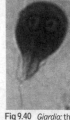

Fig 9.40 *Giardia:* the only diplomonad to trouble us.

Cryptosporidium

Apicomplexan protozoan (fig 9.41). Ingestion of oocytes in infected water. Asymptomatic or self-limiting diarrhoea in immunocompetent hosts. Chronic/severe diarrhoea with immunosuppression: HIV (p396), transplantation, hypogammaglobulinaemia, immunosuppressive therapy.

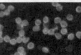

Fig 9.41 *Cryptosporidium* immunofluorescence.
© S Upton, Kansas Univ

Amoebiasis

Protozoan *Entamoeba histolytica* (fig 9.42) ~10% world's population, mortality ~100 000/yr. Faecal–oral spread. Boil water to destroy cysts.
Presentation
- Asymptomatic passage of cysts in ~90% ('luminal amoebiasis').
- Intestinal amoebiasis: dysentery (often insidious onset/relapsing), pain, colitis, appendicitis, toxic megacolon. Amoeboma = inflammatory abdominal mass, usually caecal/RIF ± obstruction.
- Extra-intestinal (invasive) disease. Amoebic liver abscess in ~1%. Single mass containing 'anchovy-sauce' pus. High swinging fever, RUQ pain/tenderness. LFT normal or ↑ (cholestatic). 50% have no history of amoebic dysentery. Also peritonitis (rupture of colonic abscess), pleuropulmonary abscess, cutaneous/genital lesions.

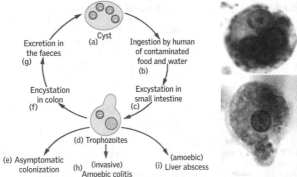

Fig 9.42 The lifecycle of *Entamoeba histolytica* is in two stages: cysts and trophozoites. Cysts (10–15μm across) typically contain four nuclei (upper right image). During excystation in the gut lumen nuclear division is followed by cytoplasmic division, giving rise to eight trophozoites. Trophozoites (10–50μm across) contain one nucleus with a central karyosome (lower right image). Trophozoites inhabit the caecum and colon. Re-encystation of the trophozoites occurs in the colon, and excretion of cysts in faeces perpetuates the lifecycle.

Left hand image from Hutson C *et al.*, 'Molecular-based diagnosis of Entamoeba histolytica infection', *Expert Reviews in Molecular Medicine*, 1(9): 1–11, 1999, reproduced with permission from Cambridge University Press. Upper and lower right images courtesy of Prof S Upton, Kansas University.

Diagnosis Microscopy of stool (cysts and trophozoites, fig 9.42), aspirate, or biopsy sample. Enzyme immunoassay: antigen detection as adjunct to microscopy, antibody detection in extra-intestinal disease. PCR can distinguish *E. histolytica* from morphologically identical but non-invasive *E. dispar*. **Treatment** Metronidazole/tinidazole for amoebic dysentery and invasive disease. Diloxanide furoate: luminal agent, 10d course to destroy gut cysts, given in asymptomatic gut carriers and symptomatic disease, in addition to other treatment. Abscess may require (image-guided) drainage.

Cyclospora

Coccidian protozoan *Cyclospora cayetanensis*. ~50 imported cases/yr in UK. **Presentation** Flu-like prodrome, watery diarrhoea, weight loss, marked fatigue, low-grade fever in ~25%. Self-limiting after 7–9wks in immunocompetent. **Diagnosis** Autofluorescent oocytes in stool (appear blue-green under UV fluorescence, fig 9.43), PCR. **Treatment** Co-trimoxazole.

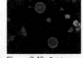

Fig 9.43 *Cyclospora* oocysts fluorescence.
CDC DPDx.

Nematodes (soil-transmitted helminths and *Trichinella*)

- Roundworm: *Ascaris lumbricoides* ~1 billion affected, *Trichinella spiralis* (contaminated meat source).
- Whipworm: *Trichuris trichiura*, 600–800 million affected.
- Hookworm: *Necator americanus*, *Ancylostoma duodenale* ~700 million affected.
- Threadworm: eg *Strongyloides stercoralis*, 30–100 million affected.

One of most common infections worldwide, affects poor and deprived (fig 9.44). Parasites live in intestines, producing 1000s egg/day in faeces. Humans infected by eggs (ascariasis, trichinosis) or larvae (*Ancylostoma*) in contaminated food; or via direct penetration of the skin (hookworm, *Strongyloides*). **Presentation** Diarrhoea, abdominal pain, blood/protein loss, impaired growth/cognitive development. Pruritus/urticaria if migration involves skin (*Strongyloides*, fig 9.44). Lung invasion (ascariasis, hookworm, *Strongyloides*) can lead to a Loeffler-like syndrome: cough, SOB, wheeze, haemoptysis, consolidation, eosinophilia. Other tissue invasion (trichinosis): myalgia, conjunctivitis, photophobia, meningitis, encephalitis, neuropathy. **Diagnosis** Clinical, eggs in stool sample (fig 9.45). Eosinophilia. *Strongyloides* serology/PCR. **Treatment** table 9.26.

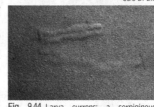

Fig 9.44 Larva currens: a serpiginous maculopapular rash pathognomonic of chronic strongyloidiasis. Oedema, an urticarial appearance, and speed of migration (>5cm/h) distinguish this from cutaneous larva migrans which is caused by animal (dog/cat) hookworm

Reproduced from Johnson *et al.*, *Oxford Handbook of Expedition and Wilderness Medicine*, 2016, with permission from Oxford University Press.

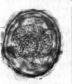

Fig 9.45 *Ascaris* eggs (45 ≈40μm) & ♂ worm (20cm).
Courtesy of Prof S Upton, Kansas University.

Table 9.26 Anthelmintic drugs

Drug	Mechanism	Indication
Mebendazole	Binds free beta-tubulin, causing ↓glucose uptake	Roundworm, whipworm, hookworm
Albendazole		Ascariasis, hookworm (*Strongyloides*)
Ivermectin	↑Cl⁻ permeability, hyperpolarization, paralysis	*Strongyloides*, ascariasis
Pyrantel pamoate	Depolarizing neuromuscular blockade causing spastic paralysis of worm	Single dose in threadworm, roundworm, hookworm
Piperazine	Binds GABA muscle receptors; flaccid paralysis	(Ascariasis), pregnancy
Praziquantel	Alters cell permeability, causing paralysis	Schistosomiasis, tapeworm

Taeniasis (tapeworm) Includes *Taenia solium* (pork, 2–8m, 50 000 eggs/worm), *Taenia saginata* (beef, 4–12m, 100 000 eggs/worm), *Taenia asiatica* (Asian, 4–8m, millions of eggs). **Presentation** No or mild GI symptoms, tapeworm segments (proglottids) through anus/in faeces. **Diagnosis** Eggs/proglottids in faeces. **Treatment** Praziquantel, niclosamide.

• See also *toxoplasmosis* (p421), *schistosomiasis* (p430), *cysticercosis* (p433).

9 Infectious diseases

Schistosomiasis (bilharzia)

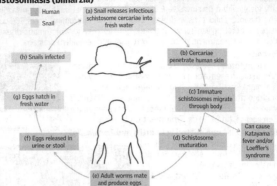

Fig 9.46 Schistosomiasis life cycle.
Reproduced from: Coltart C, CJM Whitty. Schistosomiasis in non-endemic countries. *Clin Med* 2015;15:67–9. https://doi.org/10.7861/clinmedicine.15-1-67. Copyright © 2015 Royal College of Physicians. Reproduced with permission.

Caused by blood-flukes (trematode worms) of the genus *Schistosoma* (table 9.27). 290 million people in 78 countries required treatment in 2018. The life cycle is shown in fig 9.46. Disease develops after contact with contaminated freshwater (swimming, washing). Symptoms are due to an immune complex response to the migrating parasite (Katayama syndrome), or chronic parasite egg deposition in body tissues.

Presentation ~50% asymptomatic or non-specific symptoms. Clinical syndromes:
• Larval penetration: pruritic papular rash ('swimmer's itch').
• Migration of schistosomules: Katayama syndrome 2–8wks after exposure: fever, urticaria, diarrhoea, cough, wheeze, hepatosplenomegaly, eosinophilia.
• Host response to egg deposition:
    • Intestinal disease: pain, diarrhoea, blood in stool, (granulomatous) hepatomegaly, splenomegaly. Heavy chronic infection can cause bowel perforation, hyperplasia, polyposis, liver fibrosis, portal hypertension→varices.
    • Urogenital disease: haematuria, dysuria, ureteric fibrosis→hydronephrosis, CKD, bladder fibrosis/cancer, genital lesions, vaginal bleeding, dyspareunia, vulva nodules, haemospermia, prostatitis.
    • Lung disease: pulmonary hypertension and cor pulmonale.
    • CNS disease: rare, acute lower limb paraplegia, transverse ('traveller's') myelitis.

Diagnosis Ova in urine (*S. haematobium*) or faeces (all other species) is specific, but sensitivity <50% if light infection. Serology for egg antigen becomes +ve once mature flukes lay eggs ∴ will be –ve in Katayama fever. Bowel/bladder histology. Chronic *S. haematobium*: bladder calcification on AXR, renal obstruction, hydronephrosis ± thick bladder wall on USS. **Treatment** Two doses of praziquantel 20mg/kg PO separated by 4h (30mg/kg in *S. japonica* and *S. mekongi*). Steroids for Katayama fever. If ↑eosinophils >3months after treatment look for other helminths (+ve serology can persist for years). **Prevention** Prophylactic praziquantel for at-risk groups.

Table 9.27 Parasite species and geographical distribution

Disease form	Species	Geography
Intestinal	*S. mansoni*	Africa, Middle East, Caribbean, Brazil, Venezuela, Suriname
	S. japonica	China, Indonesia, Philippines
	Other	*S. mekongi*: Cambodia, Laos; *S. guineensis/ intercalatum*: rainforests of central Africa
Urogenital	*S. haematobium*	Africa, Middle East, France

Echinococcosis (hydatid disease)

Zoonotic disease caused by tapeworms of the genus *Echinococcus*. Clinically important disease forms in humans are:

- Cystic echinococcosis (hydatid disease, hydatosis): *E. granulosus*. Found worldwide. Usual host is dog. Also goats, swine, horses, cattle, camels, yaks.
- Alveolar echinococcosis: *E. multilocularis*. Found in northern hemisphere. Usual hosts are foxes and rodents.

Human ingest parasite eggs via food/water contaminated by animal faeces, or by handing animals which are infected with the tapeworm. Disease is due to the development of cyst-like larvae in viscera, usually liver/lungs. **Presentation** Slow growing cysts may be asymptomatic for many years. Symptoms and signs depend on location:
- *Liver:* abdominal pain, nausea, hepatomegaly, obstructive jaundice, cholangitis, PUO.
- *Lung:* dyspnoea, chest pain, cough, haemoptysis.
- *cns:* space-occupying signs.
- *Bone:* an interesting osteolytic cause of knee pain, cord compression.
- Silent disease in breast, kidney, adrenals, bladder, heart, psoas.

Diagnosis USS/CT/MRI: avascular fluid-filled cysts ± calcification (ΔΔ benign cyst, TB, mycoses, abscess, neoplasm). Serology. Positive echinococcal antigen. **Treatment** Get help (including surgical). Depends on cyst type, location, size, and complications. Prolonged treatment (months/years) with albendazole. **PAIR:** **P**uncture, **A**spirate, **I**nject (hypertonic saline/chemicals), **R**e-aspirate. Beware spillage of cyst contents: praziquantel can be given peri-operatively.

***Fasciola hepatica* (common liver fluke)** Parasitic infection. ~2 million infected worldwide. Highest rates of infection in Bolivia and Peru. Infective larvae develop in aquatic snail hosts. Humans infected via contaminated water, waterplants, eg watercress, or by eating the undercooked liver of another host animal, eg sheep, goat. Disease caused by migration of parasite to bile ducts. **Presentation** *Acute phase* with migration from intestine through liver (2–4 months): abdominal pain, nausea, fever, urticarial rash, eosinophilia. *Chronic phase* with egg production in the bile ducts: cholecystitis, cholangitis, pancreatitis, cirrhosis. **Diagnosis** Serology in acute and chronic phase. Ova in stool/bile aspirate only in chronic phase. **Treatment** Triclabendazole as a single dose. Treat all suspected cases in endemic areas.

Other liver flukes: opisthorchiasis and clonorchiasis *Opisthorchis* and *clonorchis* are liver flukes acquired by eating contaminated fish, mainly in south-east Asia. Adult flukes lodge in the small bile ducts and gallbladder. **Presentation** Abdominal pain, GI disturbance, cholecystitis, cholangitis, cholangiocarcinoma. **Diagnosis** Ova in stool. **Treatment** Praziquantel.

Tropical liver disease

An overview of the differential diagnosis of tropical/imported liver disease is shown in **table 9.28**.

Table 9.28 Tropical liver disease by presentation[22]

Presentation	Differential diagnosis
Jaundice/hepatitis	Viral hepatitis, brucellosis, dengue, enteric fever, HIV, leptospirosis, malaria, rickettsial infection, sepsis, TB, viral haemorrhagic fever, yellow fever
Hepatomegaly	Amoebic/pyogenic liver abscess, echinococcosis, liver fluke, carcinoma
Massive hepatomegaly	Visceral leishmaniasis, tropical lymphoma, late-stage schistosomiasis
Fibrosis/cirrhosis	Chronic hepatitis, schistosomiasis, alcohol, non-alcoholic fatty liver disease

Consider liver toxicity: ackee fruit (Jamaica), aflatoxins (peanuts, corn, tropical countries without monitoring/regulation), death cap mushroom, iron, bush tea, methanol, copper, paraquat, pyrrolizidine alkaloids (herbal remedies).

Botulism

Neuroparalytic infection caused by neurotoxin from anaerobic, spore-forming *Clostridium botulinum* (rarely *C. butyricum*, *C. barattii*). Food-borne due to toxin production in poorly processed food (*botulus* is Latin for sausage), or wound botulism due to spore germination in wound (includes IV drug use). Toxin blocks release of acetylcholine at neuromuscular junction causing flaccid paralysis. **Presentation** Incubation up to 8d (usually 12–36h). Febrile, descending, flaccid paralysis: diplopia, ptosis, dysarthria, dysphagia, progressive paralysis of limbs, respiratory failure. Autonomic signs: dry mouth, fixed/dilated pupils, urinary/cardiac/GI dysfunction. ►*No sensory signs*. **Diagnosis** Clinical: do not delay treatment. Take samples (serum, faeces, wound swab) for later confirmation by culture/PCR. In UK contact GI Bacteria Reference Unit (020 8327 7887). **Treatment** Get help. Admit to ICU. Botulinum antitoxin (from Public Health England: 020 8200 4400). Benzylpenicillin and metronidazole if wound botulism.

Tetanus

Caused by anaerobic *Clostridium tetani* spores universally present in soil. Enters body via a breach in skin. Produces a neurotoxin (tetanospasmin) which disseminates via blood/lymphatics and interferes with neurotransmitter release causing unopposed muscle contraction and spasm (tetanus = 'to stretch'). ~4 cases/yr in England (2019). Maternal and neonatal tetanus important cause of preventable mortality in low–middle-income countries. **Presentation** Site of entry may be trivial/unnoticed. Incubation ~3–21d. Prodrome: fever, malaise, headache.

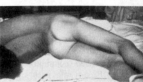

Fig 9.47 Spasm causing opisthotonus (arching of body with neck hyperextension). ΔΔ tetanus, rabies, cerebral malaria, neurosyphilis, acute cerebral injury, catatonia.
© Centers for Disease Control and Prevention.

Trismus (lockjaw, Greek 'trismos' = grinding). Risus sardonicus = a grin-like posture of hypertonic facial muscles. Opisthotonus (fig 9.47). Muscular spasms induced by movement, injections, noise, then spontaneous. Dysphagia. Autonomic dysfunction: arrhythmias ± fluctuating BP. Respiratory arrest. **Diagnosis** Clinical. Detection of tetanus toxin/isolation of *C. tetani*. **Treatment** ►►ICU: timely supportive care predicts outcome. Take blood for tetanus-toxin and anti-tetanus antibodies first. Tetanus immunoglobulin (TIG) IM (or equine antitetanus serum if not available). Wound debridement, metronidazole. Management of spasm: diazepam/lorazepam/midazolam (may need high doses IV), IV magnesium sulfate, baclofen (intrathecal administration needed for penetration of blood–brain barrier ∴ only with ICU ventilatory support), dantrolene, botulinum toxin A.[23] **Vaccination** Routine in UK (p403). Prophylaxis following injury: TIG if heavy contamination. If vaccination history unknown/incomplete: TIG plus dose of vaccine in a different site. Precautionary travel booster if >10yrs since last dose.

Poliomyelitis

A highly infectious picornavirus, transmitted via faeco–oral route or contaminated food/water. Replicates in intestine. Invades nervous system with destruction of anterior horn cells/brain stem→irreversible paralysis. Incidence ↓ by 99% since formation of Global Polio Eradication Initiative in 1988. 30 cases in 2022. Remains endemic in Afghanistan and Pakistan (2022).[13] **Presentation** Incubation 7–10d. Flu-like prodrome in ~25%. Pre-paralytic stage: fever, ↑HR, headache, vomiting, neck stiffness, tremor, limb pain. ~1 in 200 progress to paralytic stage: LMN/bulbar signs ± respiratory failure. ►*No sensory signs*. Post-polio syndrome in ~40% of survivors (up to 40yrs later): new progressive muscle weakness, myalgia, fatigue. **Diagnosis** Viral culture of stool (most sensitive, 2 samples >24h apart), pharyngeal swabs, blood, CSF. PCR can differentiate wild-type from vaccine. Paired serology. **Treatment** None. **Vaccination** Salk (inactivated, IM) or Sabin (live, oral). In previously endemic areas 200 million volunteers have vaccinated 3 billion children, meaning that 20 million people can walk today who would have otherwise been paralysed.

Rabies

Rhabdovirus transmitted through saliva or CNS tissue, usually from the bite of an infected mammal, eg bat (in UK), dog (95% of human transmissions), cat, fox. Disease is fatal once symptoms appear. Worldwide distribution. ~50 000 deaths/yr, most in Africa/Asia. **Presentation** Incubation ~9–90d. Prodrome: headache, malaise, odd behaviour, agitation, fever, paraesthesia at bite/wound site. Progresses to one of two disease forms:

- '*Furious rabies*': hyperactivity and terror (hydrophobia, aerophobia).
- '*Paralytic rabies*': flaccid paralysis in the bitten limb→coma→death.

Diagnosis Clinical: potential exposure + signs of myelitis/encephalitis (non-progressive disease and disease >3wks are negative indicators). Viral PCR (saliva, brain, nerve tissue) or CSF antibodies may offer later (postmortem) confirmation. **Treatment** If bitten, or lick to broken skin, wash (>15min) with soap and seek urgent help. Post-exposure prophylaxis: vaccination ± rabies immunoglobulin. Experimental treatments: ribavirin, interferon alfa, ketamine. Preventable and elimination feasible with pre-exposure vaccination of all at risk. Vaccination of dogs can ↓ human cases.

Japanese encephalitis virus

Flavivirus spread by *Culex* mosquito species. Endemic transmission (~3 billion at risk) and common cause of viral encephalitis in Asia and west Pacific. Severe disease is rare (1 in 250) but leads to neurological or psychiatric sequelae in up to 50%, mortality up to 30%. **Presentation** Incubation 5–15d. Most asymptomatic, or mild fever and headache only. Severe disease: high fever, headache, meningism, altered mental status, coma, seizures, spastic paralysis, death. **Diagnosis** Clinical in endemic area. Serum/CSF serology, PCR. **Treatment** Supportive. Vaccination.

West Nile virus

Mosquito-borne flavivirus with transmission in Europe, Middle East, Africa, Asia, Australia, and Americas. **Presentation** Incubation 2–14d. Asymptomatic in ~80%. West Nile fever in ~20%: fever, headache, N&v, lymphadenopathy. Neuroinvasive in ~1%: encephalitis, meningitis, flaccid paralysis, mortality ~10%. **Diagnosis** Serum/CSF IGM, viral PCR. **Treatment** Supportive. Human vaccine awaited (2023).

Neurocysticercosis

Most common helminthic disease of the CNS and most frequent cause of preventable epilepsy (~50% of epilepsy in endemic areas, fig 9.48). Caused by pork tapeworm *Taenia solium*. Consumption of infected pork leads to intestinal infection (taeniasis) and the shedding of *T. solium* eggs in stool. Invasive disease occurs when the shed eggs are ingested via faecal–oral transmission. Neurocysticercosis is due to larval cysts infecting the CNS. **Presentation** Determined by site and number of lesions (cysticerci) within the brain/spinal cord. Epilepsy in 70%. Focal neurology in ~20%: motor/sensory loss, language disturbance, involuntary movements. Also headache, visual loss, meningitis, hydrocephalus, cognitive impairment. **Diagnosis** CT/MRI imaging plus serology. **Treatment** Seizure control (↓evidence on drug choice, length of treatment, or prophylaxis). Neurosurgical advice if hydrocephalus/↑ICP. Albendazole for non-calcified lesions (better penetration of CNS than praziquantel). Beware inflammatory response provoked by treatment—consider dexamethasone.

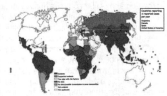

Fig 9.48 Endemicity (red) and suspected endemicity (orange) of *Taenia solium* 2015.
Reproduced with permission from WHO, *Endemicity of Taenia solium, 2015.* ©World Health Organization 2016. http://www.who.int/mediacentre/factsheets/Endemicity_Taenia_Solium_2015−1000x706.jpg?ua=1

Tick-borne encephalitis

Flavivirus spread by tick species endemic to Northern Eurasia. Growing incidence: ~10 000 cases/yr. First UK case in 2019. **Presentation** Incubation 7–28 days. Flu-like prodrome, progressing to meningism/encephalitis in ~30%, mortality ~1%. Long term sequelae in 10%. **Diagnosis** Serum/CSF serology. **Treatment** Supportive. Vaccination for at risk groups. Tick bite prevention.

Conjunctivitis

Common in tropical areas. Vision is normal. Differentiation is outlined in **table 9.29**.

Table 9.29 Common infectious causes of conjunctivitis

Cause	Secretions	Features	Treatment
Bacterial	Purulent	Red and swollen	Topical antibiotics for 5d
Viral	Watery	± Corneal lesion	Symptomatic
Trachoma (chlamydial)	Mucopurulent	Follicles and papillae on lid	Azithromycin PO or topical tetracycline

Reproduced from Brent *et al.*, *Oxford Handbook of Tropical Medicine*, 2014, with permission from Oxford University Press.

Trachoma

Leading infectious cause of blindness worldwide: visual impairment/blindness in 1.9 million, 136 million at risk. Prevalence in endemic areas 60–90% (Africa, Central and South America, Asia, Middle East). Caused by *Chlamydia trachomatis*. Human-to-human transmission with contact, or via flies which land on nose/eyes. **Presentation** Active infection causes purulent discharge and follicular inflammation of the eyelid (**fig 9.49a**)→scarring (**fig 9.49b**)→eyelids turn inwards (entropion) and irritate the cornea (trichiasis) (**fig 9.49c**)→visual loss. **Treatment** WHO public health strategy **SAFE**: **S**urgery to treat trichiasis, **A**ntibiotics (azithromycin: mass administration in endemic areas through International Trachoma Initiative), **F**acial cleanliness, **E**nvironmental improvement with access to water and sanitation.[13]

Immunosuppression and the eye

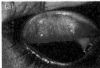 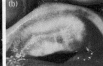 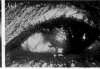

Fig 9.49 (a) Follicular trachoma. (b) Scarring. (c) Trichiasis.

Reproduced from Warrell *et al.*, *Oxford Textbook of Medicine*, 2010, with permission from Oxford University Press.

Herpes zoster ophthalmicus

Due to reactivation of latent varicella zoster virus (p400) in the ophthalmic branch of the trigeminal nerve. ↑ Risk of reactivation and ocular complications in immunosuppression: HIV, post-transplantation. *Presentation:* vesiculomacular skin rash and dysaesthesia in ophthalmic division of the trigeminal nerve (**fig 9.50**). Hutchinson's sign = lesion at tip/side of nose indicates involvement of nasociliary branch of V1 and ↑chance of eye involvement. Complications: corneal opacification, uveitis, ocular nerve palsy, eyelid deformity, optic neuritis, post-herpetic neuralgia. Can be sight-threatening ∴ recognition and urgent treatment are required. *Diagnosis:* clinical. Antibody staining/PCR of skin scrapings. *Treatment:* oral famciclovir/valaciclovir or systemic aciclovir reduce complications if given within 72h of symptoms. Analgesia. If retinitis IV cidofovir ± intravitreal ganciclovir or foscarnet.

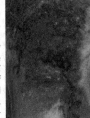

Fig 9.50 Herpes zoster ophthalmicus.

© MN Oxman, University of California.

CMV retinitis

Reactivation of CMV infection (p401). *Presentation:* floaters due to inflammatory cells in vitreous, flashing lights, scotomata, eye pain, visual loss. Peripheral lesions may be asymptomatic. Routine examination for those at risk (CD4 <100 cells/microlitre). *Diagnosis:* clinical. Fundoscopy: granular white dots, haemorrhage (**fig 9.51**).

Fig 9.51 CMV retinitis (mozzarella pizza fundus).

© Prof Trobe.

Can progress to an arcuate/triangular zone of infection, or can be linear following vessels/nerve fibres. *Treatment:* intravitreous ganciclovir ± oral valganciclovir. Also foscarnet, cidofovir. ART if underlying HIV (p398).

Ocular toxoplasmosis

Causes posterior uveitis. *Presentation:* blurred vision/floaters. *Diagnosis:* clinical. Fundoscopy (fig 9.52): focus of choroiditis, chorioretinal scar from previous infection, overlying vitreal haze due to inflammatory response. Multiple/bilateral/extensive lesions if ↑ immunosuppression. Serology. Ocular fluid PCR. *Treatment:* atovaquone (↓toxicity), sulfadiazine, and pyrimethamine.

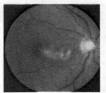

Fig 9.52 Retinal toxoplasmosis.
© Prof Trobe.

Filarial infection

Onchocerciasis ('river blindness')

Caused by filarial worm *Onchocerca volvulus* and endosymbiotic *Wolbachia* bacteria. Transmitted by the bite of infected black flies which breed in fast-flowing rivers and streams. Second most common infectious cause of blindness worldwide: predominantly sub-Saharan Africa, Brazil, Venezuela, Yemen. *Presentation:* a nodule forms at the site of the bite where larvae mature to adult worms. The female adult can release up to 1000 microfilariae/day causing:
• Skin disease: pruritis, altered pigmentation, lichenification, loss of elasticity.
• Eye disease: keratitis, uveitis, cataract, fixed pupil, fundal degeneration, optic neuritis/atrophy, visual impairment/loss (fig 9.53).
• Impaired lymphatic function: lymphadenopathy, elephantiasis.

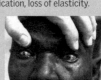

Fig 9.53 Bilateral sclerosing keratitis in onchocerciasis causing blindness.
Reproduced from Warrell *et al.*, *Oxford Textbook of Medicine*, 2010, with permission from Oxford University Press.

Diagnosis: visualization of microfilaria in eye or on skin snip biopsy: a fine shaving of clean skin is incubated in 0.9% saline to allow microfilariae to emerge for microscopic identification. Serology. *Treatment:* ivermectin 150mcg/kg, one dose every 3–12 months (depending on re-exposure risk). CI if coexisting *Loa loa* due to risk of fatal encephalitic reaction. 6wks of doxycycline for *Wolbachia*. No vaccine available.

Loiasis (African eye-worm)

Caused by parasitic worm *Loa loa*. Transmitted via bite of deerflies which breed in rainforests of west and central Africa. **Presentation** Recurrent pruritic lesions due to angioedema ('Calabar swellings'), myalgia, arthralgia. The adult worm can migrate through subcutaneous (fig 9.54) and subconjunctival (fig 9.55) tissue: 'Something's wiggling in my eye, doctor'. This eerie eye trip causes intense conjunctivitis, which heals if left alone. (Don't treat until transmigration in the eye is over: on detecting your therapy the worm tends to panic.) Also causes glomerulonephritis, and encephalitis. **Diagnosis** Microfilariae on blood smear, serology, PCR. Eosinophilia. **Treatment** Diethylcarbamazine (DEC) kills both microfilariae and adult worms. Risk of encephalopathy is related to microfilarial load: albendazole can be used to ↓ microfilarial load prior to DEC (response may be slow). Bite avoidance.

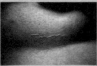

Fig 9.54 Migrating *Loa loa* in the skin.
Reproduced from Warrell *et al.*, *Oxford Textbook of Medicine*, 2010, with permission from Oxford University Press.

Fig 9.55 *Loa loa* crossing the conjunctiva
Reproduced from Warrell *et al.*, *Oxford Textbook of Medicine*, 2010, with permission from Oxford University Press.

►See also lymphatic filariasis p417.

9 Infectious diseases

Dermatoses occur in 8–23% of travellers and are the 3rd most common health problem in travellers after diarrhoea and fever. The differential of skin problems in travellers is outlined in fig 9.56.

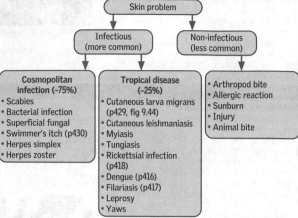

Fig 9.56 Skin problems in travellers.

Adapted from *Travel Medicine and Infectious Disease*, 7(3), O'Brien, BM, 'A practical approach to common skin problems in returning travellers', 125–46. Copyright 2009, with permission from Elsevier.

Scabies

Caused by microscopic mite *Sarcoptes scabiei*. Found worldwide, ~300 million cases/yr. Female mites burrow into the epidermis and deposit eggs. Symptoms due to an allergic reaction to the parasite. Transmission via direct and prolonged skin-to-skin contact. Epidemics linked to poverty, overcrowding, and poor water supply. **Presentation** Severe (nocturnal) pruritus, papular/scaly rash, burrows may be visible (fig 9.57). Severe crusted scabies if immunocompromised. Itch can lead to secondary bacterial infection. **Diagnosis** Clinical. Skin scraping for mite/eggs/faeces. **Treatment** Topical permethrin 5% or malathion 0.5%. Ivermectin in crusted scabies.

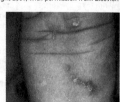

Fig 9.57 Scabies burrow.

Reproduced from Burge *et al.*, *Oxford Handbook of Medical Dermatology*, 2016, with permission from Oxford University Press.

Cutaneous leishmaniasis

Most common form of leishmaniasis. Estimated 0.6–1 million new cases/yr: Americas, Mediterranean basin, north Africa, Middle East, central Asia. **Presentation** Lesions develop at the bite site, beginning as an itchy papule; crusts fall off to leave a painless ulcer with a well-defined, raised border and a crusted base = 'Chiclero's ulcer' (fig 9.58). **Diagnosis** Skin biopsy + PCR. **Treatment** Most heal in ~2–15 months with scarring (disfiguring if extensive). 'New World' disease (South America) needs treating due to risk of mucocutaneous disease: pentavalent antimony, eg meglumine antimoniate, sodium stibogluconate. (See p419.)

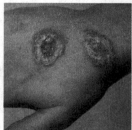

Fig 9.58 Cutaneous leishmaniasis with central crusting.

Reproduced from Lewis-Jones, *Paediatric Dermatology*, 2010, with permission from Oxford University Press.

Myiasis

Infection with fly larvae/maggot. Can affect living and necrotic tissue. In South and Central America the human botfly lays its eggs on mosquitoes which deposit them when they bite. In sub-Saharan Africa the tumbu fly lays its eggs on clothing which then transfer to skin. **Presentation** Painful swelling. May have sensation of movement within the lesion. May open to reveal larval breathing tubes (fig 9.59). **Diagnosis** Clinical. Identification of larvae in lesion. **Treatment** Petroleum or pork fat asphyxiate the maggot causing it to protrude further out of the skin enabling removal with tweezers. Care: backward-facing spines in botfly larvae may prevent complete removal unless done surgically. Ensure tetanus vaccination is up to date.

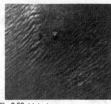

Fig 9.59 Myiasis.
Reproduced under Creative Commons CC0 1.0 Universal Public Domain from https://commons.wikimedia.org/wiki/File:Miasi s_human.jpg

Tungiasis

Infection of the skin by the sand/jigger flea *Tunga penetrans*. Acquired (usually walking barefoot) in sandy soil, rainforests, and banana plantations in South and Central America, sub-Saharan Africa, Asia, Caribbean. **Presentation** Painful, itchy papule on the feet. May be visible extrusion of eggs. Black crusting when flea dies. **Diagnosis** Clinical. **Treatment** Topical dimeticone, self-limiting.

Leprosy (Hansen's disease)

Caused by slow-growing, acid-fast *Mycobacterium leprae* which affects skin, nerves, and mucous membranes. Incubation 5–20yrs. Transmitted via droplets from nose/mouth during close and frequent contact. Classified as:
• Multibacillary ('lepromatous'): ↓immune response, ↑bacilli, +ve smear.
• Paucibacillary ('tuberculoid'): ↑immune response, granulomata with ↓bacilli, smears may be –ve.

Hypersensitivity reactive episodes occur: type 1 (erythema of skin lesions, neuritis), type 2 (erythema nodosum leprosum and organ/joint inflammation, eg neuritis, lymph-adenitis, arthralgias). Free multibacillary treatment via WHO since 1995: prevalence ↓ by 99% (5.2 million in 1985, 174 087 in 2022).[13] **Presentation** Hypopigmented skin lesions (fig 9.60, less well demarcated than vitiligo), sensory loss, thickened nerves, nodules, plaques, nasal congestion, epistaxis, muscle weakness, paralysis, neuropathic ulcers. Eye involvement: chronic iritis, scleritis, episcleritis, ↓corneal sensation (V nerve palsy), ↓blinking and lagophthalmos (VII nerve palsy), trauma from eyelashes (trichiasis). **Diagnosis** Clinical, +ve skin smear, skin biopsy. Serology unreliable. **Treatment** WHO multidrug therapy: rifampicin 600mg/month, dapsone 100mg OD, clofazimine 300mg/month and 50mg daily. Duration: 1yr for multibacillary, 6 months for paucibacillary. Treat type 1 and 2 reactions with steroids.

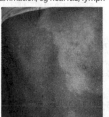

Fig 9.60 Leprosy: hypopigmented macules.
Courtesy of Prof Jayakar Thoma.

Yaws Chronic granulomatous disease caused by *Treponema pertenue*. Found in humid/rainforest areas in Africa, Asia, Latin American, Pacific. Associated with ↓socio-economic conditions. Transmission via direct contact. **Presentation** Primary disease = papilloma. If untreated will ulcerate (fig 9.61). Secondary disease: yellow skin lesions, dactylitis. CVS and CNS complications do not occur. **Diagnosis** Serology is indistinguishable from syphilis (*Treponema pallidum*). Dual-path platform (DPP) assay can distinguish between current and past infection. PCR. **Treatment** Single-dose azithromycin PO.

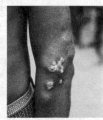

Fig 9.61 Ulcero-papillomatous yaws.
CDC/Dr. Peter Perine.

9 Infectious diseases

This chapter gives guidance on hundreds of pyrexia-causing infections; but what should you do if your patient has a fever that you cannot explain? Pyrexia of unknown origin (PUO)[24] has a differential of >200 diseases. 15–30% of these patients will eventually be given an infective diagnosis (depending on your corner of the globe). ~20% remain undiagnosed, but in most of these the fever will resolve within 4wks.

Diagnostic criteria
Pyrexia >3wks with no cause identified after evaluation in hospital for 3d or ≥3 out-patient visits.

Fever may also be undiagnosed in specific subgroups despite appropriate evaluation for 3d, including negative cultures at ≥2 days:
• **Nosocomial PUO** Patient hospitalized for >48h with no infection at admission.
• **Immunodeficient PUO** Pyrexia in patient with <500 neutrophils/microlitre.
• **HIV PUO** Pyrexia in HIV infection lasting 3d as an inpatient or >4wks as an outpatient.

History
Most PUO are due to common diseases with atypical presentation. Consider all details as potentially relevant. Include: travel (p410), diet, animal contact, changes in medication, recreational drug use, obstetric/sexual history, family history (table 9.30).

Examination
Confirm fever. Pattern of fever is rarely helpful (contrary to the textbooks, most malaria has no specific pattern). Full head-to-toe examination. Do not forget: mouth, genitals, skin, thyroid, lymphatic system, eyes/retina, temporal arteries (table 9.30).

Investigation
►Extent of investigation depends on immune status and how well the patient is.
• **Blood tests** FBC, U&E, LFT, CRP, ESR, electrophoresis, LDH, CK, ANA, ANCA, rheumatoid factor, HIV test, malaria smear, interferon-gamma release assay for TB (p390).
• **Microscopy and culture** Blood ×3, urine, sputum (including AFB), stool, CSF.
• **Imaging** CXR, abdominal/pelvic USS, venous Doppler. Consider: CT(PA), MRI, echo (TOE). Fluorodeoxyglucose-PET (FDG-PET) highlights areas of ↑glucose uptake including tumour and inflammation. It may aid/direct diagnosis in up to 50% of PUO.
• **Other** Hepatitis serology, CMV, EBV, autoimmune screen, cryoglobulins, toxoplasmosis, brucellosis, *Coxiella*, lymph node biopsy, endoscopy, temporal artery biopsy.

Table 9.30 PUO differential according to history and examination findings

History	Differential
Animal contact	Brucellosis, toxoplasmosis, *Bartonella*, leptospirosis, Q fever, psittacosis
Cough	TB, PE, Q fever, enteric fever, sarcoidosis, legionnaire's disease
Nasal symptoms	Sinusitis, GPA, relapsing fever, psittacosis
Confusion	TB, *Cryptococcus*, sarcoid, carcinomatosis, brucellosis, enteric fever
Arthralgia	SLE, infective endocarditis, Lyme disease, brucellosis, TB, IBD
Weight loss	Malignancy, vasculitis, TB, HIV, IBD, thyrotoxicosis
Family history	Familial Mediterranean fever
Drug history	Drug-induced fever (~7–10d after new drug)
Examination	**Differential**
Conjunctivitis	Leptospirosis, relapsing fever, spotted fever, trichinosis
Uveitis	TB, sarcoid, adult Still's disease, SLE, Behçet's disease
Mouth	Dental abscess, Behçet's disease, CMV, IBD
Lymphadenopathy	Lymphoma, TB, EBV, CMV, HIV, toxoplasmosis, brucellosis, *Bartonella*
Rash	HIV, EBV, SLE, vasculitis, Still's disease, endocarditis
Hepatomegaly	TB, EBV, malignancy, malaria, enteric fever, granulomatous hepatitis, Q fever, visceral leishmaniasis
Splenomegaly	Leukaemia, lymphoma, TB, brucellosis, infective endocarditis, CMV, EBV, rheumatoid arthritis, sarcoid, enteric fever, relapsing fever
Renal	Chronic pyelonephritis, perinephric abscess, renal tumour
Epididymo-orchitis	TB, lymphoma, EBV, brucellosis, leptospirosis

Listen to your patient You have two cultures to master: the host and the pathogen. Prolonged immersion in both may be needed.

Ask Do not expect to find apposite questions such as these in any other textbook:

1 *'Have you delivered any septic babies in the last year?'* Impress and cure your obstetrician friends who tell you that 'I'm so depressed about not being able to shake off this flu', and who have forgotten about transfer of brucellosis from baby to obstetrician.

2 *'Are your carp well at present?'* Mycobacterium marinum skin infection.

3 *'Where exactly did you get that sheep-skin rug?'* Anthrax from handling infected animal hides.

4 *'Who has been licking your face recently?'* Pasteurella multocida.

5 *'Did you have a stray pig living under your house when the monsoon started?'* Pigs + standing water + mosquitoes = Japanese encephalitis.

6 *'Has your pet hedgehog lost weight?'* Salmonella.

7 *'Did you develop your headache after you adopted your pet magpie?'* Zoonotic transmission of Cryptococcus neoformans causing meningitis.

8 *'Has your pet seal given you a nasty nip?'* Sealpox virus.

9 *'Was it windy when you visited the Grand Canyon?'* Valley fever from Coccidioides spores in Western US soil.

10 *'Did your goat miscarry last year?'* Coxiella burnetii.

11 *'Were you drunk when you fell in that rose bush?'* Sporotrichosis 'Rose gardener's disease'; disseminated disease with alcohol misuse disorder.

12 *'Can I see your pet lobster: he may be the cause of your bad hand?'* Lobsterman's hand, an erysipeloid infection from Erysipelothrix. Pet lobsters have a grand pedigree. Gérard de Nerval used to take his pet lobster for walks, on a blue silk lead, beside the Seine (**fig 9.62**). A lobster, he said, is, 'serious-minded and quiet, doesn't scratch or bark like a dog, and knows all of the secrets of the deep'. His lobster's mission was to combat the Philistinism chaining us all to mediocrity.

Fig 9.62 'Is your pet lobster well?' (Gérard de Nerval)

Ask also, 'Where have you been?' Though you will not be absolved of thought, even when the answer is, 'Southend'. It may be a question of amnesic stopovers. Or perhaps your patient is an airport baggage-handler, bitten by a hitch-hiking mosquito. And even when there has been no travel to the tropics, global warming and globalization are ensuring that the tropics are travelling to us. To the first writers of medical books, Paradise was just beyond the Far East, and the world was a disc surrounded by oceans of blue water. But the world moves on, tarnished, tawdry, and trashed; and Paradise is evolving with ever more serpents in the garden, beguiling us with an abundance of answers to our great questions.

Don't give up If the culture is negative, tests may need repeating. Perhaps the organism is 'fastidious' in its nutritional requirement or requires a longer incubation? Even if culture is achieved, it may be that the organism grown is flora not pathogen. If culture fails, look for antibodies or antigen. PCR is increasingly used for identification, but it is far from infallible; beware of inhibitors, contamination, and a primer that is not as unique as your patient.

Remember Sherlock: *'My mind,' he said, 'rebels at stagnation. Give me problems, give me work, give me the most abstruse cryptogram or the most intricate analysis, and I am in my own proper atmosphere. I can dispense then with artificial stimulants. But I abhor the dull routine of existence. I crave for mental exaltation. That is why I have chosen my own particular profession,—or rather created it, for I am the only one in the world.'*

The Sign of the Four, Arthur Conan Doyle, 1890.

No, Sherlock, you are not; you have infectious disease physicians for company.

10 Neurology

Contents

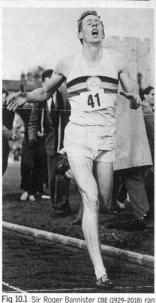

Fig 10.1 Sir Roger Bannister CBE (1929–2018) ran the first ever sub-4-minute mile on 6 May 1954 at the age of 25. At that time he was a medical student at Oxford University, and graduated the following year. He went on to become a prominent academic neurologist, conducting research into the autonomic nervous system, which he regarded as his greatest achievement. Autonomic activity and running are, of course, intimately linked, as Bannister reflected in a more poetic manner than the usual 'fight or flight' cliché: 'As a child I ran barefoot along damp, fresh sand by the seashore. The air there had a special quality... The sound of breakers shut out all others, and I was startled, almost frightened, by the tremendous excitement a few steps could create. It was an intense moment of discovery of a source of power and beauty that one previously hardly dreamt existed.' In 2014, Bannister spoke publicly of his sense of irony at being diagnosed with Parkinson's disease.
Photo by Keystone/Getty Images.

We thank Thomas Hughes and Marc Edwards, our Specialist Readers for this chapter.

It is the brain, more than any other organ, that marks *Homo sapiens* apart from other animals. Our ability to be self-aware, to think, and to reason has formed the basis of scientific inquiry and philosophical speculation for millennia, as we attempt to rationalize and define this cognitive capability. What is the mind? Less tangible than other aspects of our being, throughout time humans have looked to explanations from philosophy, folklore, religion, and now science. The concept of the sense of self and being that defines us all—whether it be called the ego, nous, or the soul—remains intriguing yet elusive to explain. Aristotle held that the psyche (Greek: ψυχή=*soul*) was not separate to its housing body, as one could not exist without the other. This view was directly contradicted by the 17th-century French philosopher René Descartes. He proposed the theory of 'mind–body dualism' in which the mind, located in the pineal gland, is an entirely separate entity to the material being, and controls the avatar of the physical body like a puppeteer.

These conflicting viewpoints well illustrate the spectrum of neurological disease and its blurred boundaries with psychiatry and psychology. Jean Martin Charcot (1825–1893), often credited as the father of neurology, appeared to be more interested in this crossover than neuronal dysfunction: he spent two decades of his career studying hysteria in Paris, initially attributing symptoms of crying, fainting, and temporary blindness to an organic, inherited cause, before revising his view in later life to conclude that this was a psychological disease. His controversial work in this field inspired his student Sigmund Freud's psychoanalytical theories, and illustrated the very real power of the conscious, or subconscious, to produce physical symptoms, a phenomenon familiar to all physicians. Perhaps reflecting our frustration with this challenging area as much as his limited success, we remember Charcot for his more tangible outputs, for example, in giving the inaugural description of, among other things, multiple sclerosis, Parkinson's disease, amyotrophic lateral sclerosis (ALS), Charcot–Marie–Tooth disease, and of course his eponymous misshapen joint resulting from proprioceptive loss.

However, both Aristotle and Charcot would have surely agreed with Descartes' proposition of 'cogito ergo sum': I think, therefore I am. Whether mind and brain are dual or one, they are inextricably linked and the very nature of awareness proves its existence.

This is an important first question to ask and depends on recognizing characteristic patterns of cognitive, cranial nerve, motor, and sensory deficits. Locating a focal lesion can be aided by features such as asymmetry (eg one pupil dilated, one upgoing plantar response) or a spinal level (effects may be symmetrical below the lesion). ▶Note that sometimes there is no single lesion, rather, a *general insult* causing a *falsely localizing sign*, eg abducens nerve palsy in ↑ICP. Other generalized causes of specific local effects are: trauma, encephalitis, anoxia, poisoning, or post-ictal states.

Motor deficits Establish if the pattern is consistent with an *upper (UMN)* or a *lower motor neuron (LMN)* lesion (table 10.1), then determine the level (table 10.2).

UMN Lesions are caused by damage anywhere along the corticospinal (= pyramidal) tracts: motor pathways from the precentral gyrus to the anterior horn cells in the cord (via the internal capsule and brainstem).[1,2] ▶UMN lesions can mimic LMN lesions acutely before spasticity and hyperreflexia develop. **LMN** Lesions are caused by damage anywhere from the anterior horn cells distally, including the nerve roots, plexuses, and peripheral nerves. ▶The chief differential for LMN weakness is a primary muscle disease (p506)—but unlike LMN weakness these typically exhibit symmetrical loss, with normal reflexes (or lost late), and have no sensory component.

Mixed LMN and UMN signs Can occur, eg in MND, ↓B₁₂, taboparesis (p462).

Table 10.1 Examination findings in upper versus lower motor neuron lesions

Exam	Upper motor neuron	Lower motor neuron
Inspection	Muscle wasting less prominent (disuse atrophy may be present)	*Muscle wasting ± fasciculation* (involuntary twitching)
Tone	Hypertonia/*spasticity*. *Velocity dependent*, ie the faster you move the patient's muscle, the greater the resistance, until it finally gives way (like a '*clasp-knife*')[2]	Hypotonia/*flaccidity*: the limb feels soft and floppy, providing little resistance to passive stretch
Power	Weakness affects muscle groups, typically in a '*pyramidal*' pattern: in the arm, extensors are predominantly affected; in the leg, flexors are weaker. Disability is *disproportionate* to the weakness (spasticity adds to it)	Weakness affects individual muscles (eg weakness of dorsiflexors in foot drop). The functional disability is *proportionate* to the weakness elicited on examination
Reflexes	*Hyperreflexia*: reflexes are brisk below the level of the lesion, ± *clonus* (elicited by rapidly dorsiflexing the foot; ≤3 rhythmic, downward beats of the foot are normal)	*Hyporeflexia*: reflexes are reduced (or absent) at the level of the lesion
Plantars	Plantars are *extensor* (+ve Babinski sign)	Plantars are flexor/absent

Sensory deficits It is important to test individual modalities and remember quirks of normal wiring: correctly interpreted, *the distribution* of sensory loss and the modality involved (pain, T°, touch, vibration, joint-position sense) will increase your confidence in localizing the lesion. Pain and T° sensations travel along small fibres in peripheral nerves and the *anterolateral (spinothalamic) tracts* in the contralateral cord and brainstem (p512), whereas joint-position and vibration sense travel in large fibres in peripheral nerves and the ipsilateral *dorsal columns* of the cord.

Also ask

What is the lesion? Are the cells diseased, dysfunctional, disconnected (after a stroke), or under- or overexcited (migraine; epilepsy)? Is there loss of a specific type of nerve cell, as in MND or subacute combined degeneration of the cord (↓B₁₂, p330)?

Why? Is there a systemic disease causing the neurology? Eg atrial fibrillation allowing an embolus to form, causing an infarct. Do a full systems examination and always beware the irregularly irregular pulse.

1 Most of the fibres of the corticospinal (= pyramidal) tract decussate at the medullary pyramids, hence the name and the contralateral nature of symptoms. *Extrapyramidal* denotes damage to the basal ganglia and presents as Parkinsonism (see p464, p490).
2 Whereas with *rigidity*, ↑tone is not velocity dependent but constant throughout the range of movement.

Table 10.2 From findings to neuroanatomy: localizing the lesion

Level of lesion	U/L	Signs
Cortex	UMN	May cause a particularly localized problem with, eg hand or foot movements, with normal or even ↓tone—but ↑reflexes more proximally in the arm or leg will point to this being an UMN rather than LMN lesion. Sensory loss may be confined to discriminative functions, eg stereognosis and two-point discrimination, and aphasia, visual field deficits, gaze deviation, and neglect may coexist (p495)
Internal capsule	UMN	Contralateral hemiparesis alone, or with generalized contralateral sensory loss. Lesions of the genu affect bulbar function
Brainstem	UMN	A cranial nerve palsy (III–XII) contralateral to a hemiplegia implicates the brainstem on the side of the cranial nerve palsy. Lateral brainstem lesions show both dissociated and crossed sensory loss with pain and T° loss on the side of the face ipsilateral to the lesion, and contralateral arm and leg sensory loss
Spinal cord	UMN	Paraparesis (both legs) or quadriparesis/tetraplegia (all limbs). A motor and reflex level (power is unaffected above the lesion, with LMN signs *at* the level of the lesion, and UMN signs *below* the lesion) suggests a cord lesion. A *sensory level* is the hallmark (albeit a rather unreliable one)—ie decreased sensation below the level of the lesion with normal sensation above. Hemi-cord lesions cause a *Brown-Séquard syndrome*: ipsilateral UMN signs below the lesion (corticospinal tract), ipsilateral dorsal column loss, and contralateral spinothalamic loss; caused by trauma, mass lesions, disc herniation, or myelitis. *Dissociated sensory loss* may occur, eg in *cervical cord lesions*—loss of fine touch and proprioception without loss of pain and temperature (or vice versa, eg syringomyelia, p512; or cord tumours)
Anterior horn cell	LMN	Distal weakness without sensory changes (p502)
Peripheral nerve	LMN	Most cause distal weakness, eg foot-drop; weak hand (note: although Guillain–Barré syndrome typically presents as distal weakness that ascends over time, some atypical forms of Guillain–Barré syndrome may present with proximal weakness due to nerve root involvement). Sensory loss is typically worse distally (may involve all sensory modalities or be selective, depending on nerve fibre size involved). Involvement of a single nerve (mononeuropathy) occurs with trauma or entrapment (carpal tunnel, p497); involvement of several nerves (mononeuritis multiplex) is seen, eg in DM or vasculitis. Sensory loss from individual nerve lesions will follow anatomical territories (dermatomes, p450), which are usually more sharply defined than those of root lesions
NMJ	LMN	Fatiguable weakness without sensory changes (p508)
Muscle	NA	Gradual-onset symmetrical weakness ± pain (p506)

Muscle weakness grading (MRC classification)

• Grade 0 No muscle contraction	• Grade 3 Active movement against gravity
• Grade 1 Flicker of contraction	• Grade 4 Active movement against resistance
• Grade 2 Some active movement	• Grade 5 Normal power (allowing for age)

It should be noted that this is an ordinal, not a ratio scale, so the categories do not represent equal increments of strength. Grade 4 covers a big range: 4–, 4, and 4+ denote movement against slight, moderate, and stronger resistance; avoid fudging descriptions—'strength 4/5 throughout' suggests a mild quadriparesis or myopathy. It is better to document 'poor effort' and the maximum grade for each muscle tested. ▶Distribution of weakness tells us more than grade of weakness, although sequential grading can help document improvement.

Drugs and the nervous system

The brain is a gland that secretes both thoughts and molecules: both products are modulated by neurotransmitter systems. Some target sites for drugs:

1 Precursor of the transmitter (eg levodopa).
2 Interference with the storage of transmitter in vesicles within the pre-synaptic neuron (eg tetrabenazine).
3 Binding to the post-synaptic receptor site (eg bromocriptine).
4 Binding to the receptor-modulating site (eg benzodiazepines).
5 Interference with the breakdown of neurotransmitter within the synaptic cleft (eg acetylcholinesterase inhibitors; monoamine oxidase inhibitors—MAOIs).
6 Reduce reuptake of transmitter from synaptic cleft into pre-synaptic cell (eg selective serotonin reuptake inhibitors—SSRIs, eg fluoxetine; or serotonin and noradrenaline reuptake inhibitors—SNRIs, eg mirtazapine).
7 Binding to pre-synaptic autoreceptors (eg pindolol, a β-blocker with partial 5HT auto receptor antagonist effects, can be used to augment antidepressant therapy).

Important neurotransmitters (and some associated drugs) are listed in **table 10.3**.

Storms on the sea of neurotransmission

The complex and subtle mixture of chemicals that bathes our hundreds of trillions of synapses has been likened to a 'sea' of neurotransmitters. If so, it is surely a seascape of exquisite beauty, no matter how disturbed cognition may become by the storms that whip the waves on the surface. A well-chosen prescription may offer a lifeboat from such storms, but before prescribing any drug that modulates neurotransmission, consider that you are about to release a blunt and poorly understood force into a delicate environment. • The drug (or a metabolite) must be able to pass through the blood–brain barrier to have an effect. • The consequences of any sedative effects may be severe. • There will be short- and long-term SE (eg tardive dyskinesia with neuroleptic drugs). • Most drugs affect many neurotransmitters, increasing therapeutic scope (and uncertainty), eg risperidone (blocks D_2, $5HT_2$, $α_1$ and $α_2$ receptors). • Metabolites of drugs may have equal or more important pharmacological effects resulting in clinically important interactions with drugs affecting, eg hepatic metabolism. • One neurotransmitter may have many effects, eg dopaminergic neurons go awry in Parkinson's disease, schizophrenia, and addiction to drugs and gambling, by affecting motor control, motivation, effort, reward, analgesia, stress, learning, attention, and cognition.

Table 10.3 Major neurotransmitters and associated drugs

Drugs increasing activity (≈ agonists)	Drugs decreasing activity (≈ antagonists)
Dopamine Acts on receptors D_{1-5}; affects mood and reward-seeking behaviour	
Pramipexole, ropinirole, levodopa, apomorphine (Parkinson's*) Cabergoline, bromocriptine (hyperprolactinaemia; acromegaly)	Chlorpromazine (schizophrenia, OHCS p704) Metoclopramide (nausea) *Inhibition of dopamine signalling may lead to drug induced parkinsonism*
Serotonin (5-hydroxytryptamine; 5HT) Many receptor types $5HT_{1-7}$; multiple effects	
Lithium (mood stabilizer) Sumatriptan (migraine) Buspirone (partial agonist; anxiety) Fluoxetine, sertraline (reuptake inhibitors; depression)	Ondansetron (nausea) Mirtazapine (depression) Olanzapine, clozapine (schizophrenia)
Amino acids Glutamate and aspartate act as excitatory transmitters on NMDA and non-NMDA receptors—relevant in epilepsy and CNS ischaemia. γ-aminobutyric acid (GABA) is mostly inhibitory	
Gabapentin, valproate (GABA agonists; epilepsy and neuropathic pain) Benzodiazepines (GABA agonists; sedation) Baclofen (GABA agonists; spasticity) Alcohol (GABA agonist)†	Memantine (glutamate antagonist; dementia) Lamotrigine, topiramate (glutamate antagonists, alongside NA channel blocking and other effects; epilepsy, bipolar disorder, migraine)
Acetylcholine Multiple receptors classed into muscarinic and nicotinic types. Peripheral agonists used in glaucoma (pilocarpine); myasthenia (anticholinesterases). Peripheral antagonists used in asthma (ipratropium); incontinence; to dry secretions pre-op; to dilate pupils; to ↑ heart rate (atropine). Centrally acting drugs include:	
Donepezil, galantamine, rivastigmine (acetylcholinesterase inhibitors; dementia)	Procyclidine, trihexyphenidyl (drug-induced parkinsonism)
Histamine and purines (eg ATP)	
	Cyclizine (antihistamine; nausea) Purinergic receptor blockers (emerging role in chronic pain)
Neuropeptides Multiple and growing list; includes opioids and substance P	
Exogenous opioids (wide-ranging analgesic and mood-related effects)	Aprepitant (↓chemotherapy-related nausea by blocking substance P receptors)
Noradrenaline, adrenaline (= norepinephrine, epinephrine) 4 receptor types: α_{1-2}, β_{1-2}. Noradrenaline is more specific for α-receptors but both transmitters affect all receptors. In the periphery, α-receptors drive arteriolar vasoconstriction and pupillary dilation; β_1 stimulation leads to ↑ pulse and myocardial contractility; β_2 stimulation leads to bronchodilatation, uterine relaxation, and arteriolar vasodilation. Centrally acting drugs include:	
Clonidine (refractory hypertension) Tricyclic antidepressants and venlafaxine (5HT and noradrenaline reuptake inhibitors; depression) MAOIs	

* Agonism at D_3 receptor agonists may cause pathological behavioural patterns, eg hypersexuality, pathological gambling or hobbying, and disorders of impulse control in people having no history of these.
† In chronic alcohol use, GABA receptors are downregulated; acamprosate, used in alcoholism, may help to maintain GABA signalling after alcohol withdrawal.

Knowledge of the anatomy of the arterial supply of the brain helps diagnosis and management of cerebrovascular disease (pp466–75). Always try to identify the area of brain that correlates with a patient's symptoms and identify the affected artery.

The circle of Willis (fig 10.2) An anastomotic ring at the base of the brain fed by the three arteries that supply the brain with blood: the internal carotids (anteriorly) and the basilar artery (posteriorly), formed by the joining of the vertebral arteries, which supply the brainstem). This arrangement may compensate for the effects of occlusion of a feeder vessel by allowing supply from unaffected vessels; however, the anatomy of the circle of Willis is variable and in many people it does not provide much protection.

Anterior circulation The *internal carotid arteries* supply the majority of blood to the anterior two-thirds of the cerebral hemispheres and the basal ganglia (via the lenticulostriate arteries). At worst, internal carotid artery occlusion causes fatal total infarction of these areas. More often, the picture is like middle cerebral artery occlusion. The *middle cerebral arteries* arise directly from the internal carotids and supply the lateral part of each hemisphere. Occlusion may cause contralateral hemiparesis, hemisensory loss (esp. face and arm), contralateral homonymous hemianopia due to involvement of the optic radiation, cognitive change including dysphasia with dominant hemisphere lesions, and visuospatial disturbance (eg cannot dress; gets lost) with non-dominant lesions. The *anterior cerebral arteries*, the other terminal branches of the internal carotids, supply the frontal and medial part of the cerebrum. Occlusion may cause a weak, numb contralateral leg ± similar, if milder, arm symptoms (unusually, shoulder much weaker than hand). The face is spared. Bilateral infarction is a rare cause of paraplegia and an even rarer cause of akinetic mutism.

Posterior (vertebrobasilar) circulation Supplies the cerebellum, brainstem, thalamus, and occipital lobes; occlusion causes signs relating to any or all: hemianopia; cortical blindness; diplopia; vertigo; nystagmus; ataxia; dysarthria; dysphasia; hemi-or quadriplegia; unilateral or bilateral sensory symptoms; hiccups; coma. In 80%, the basilar artery divides into the two *posterior cerebral arteries* (figs 10.2–10.4) that supply the occipital lobes, inferior temporal lobes, and the thalamus. Occlusion gives contralateral homonymous hemianopia (often with macular sparing), ± non-localizing symptoms such as disorientation, confusion, and memory loss. In 20%, a fetal origin is present, in which the bulk of the blood flow to the posterior cerebral artery comes from the anterior circulation, via the posterior communicating artery. Infarctions of the brainstem can produce various syndromes, eg *lateral medullary syndrome*, in which occlusion of one vertebral artery or the posterior inferior cerebellar artery causes infarction of the lateral medulla and the inferior cerebellar surface (→ vertigo, vomiting, dysphagia, nystagmus, ipsilateral ataxia, soft palate paralysis, ipsilateral Horner's syndrome, and a crossed pattern sensory loss—analgesia to pin-prick on ipsilateral face and contralateral trunk and limbs). *Locked-in syndrome* is caused by damage to the ventral pons due to basilar artery occlusion. Patients are unable to move, but retain full cognition and awareness, communicating by blinking, electronic boards, or special computers. Right-to-die legislation may be invoked... as one sufferer blinked: 'My life is dull, miserable, demeaning, undignified, and intolerable.' Locked-in syndrome is different from other right-to-die conditions because patients need someone to do the act for them.

Subclavian steal syndrome Subclavian artery stenosis proximal to the origin of the vertebral artery may cause blood to be *stolen* by retrograde flow down this vertebral artery down into the arm, causing brainstem ischaemia typically after use of the arm. Suspect if the BP in each arm differs by >20mmHg.

'Dizzy-plus' syndromes and arterial events
- SCA→dizzy.
- AICA→dizzy and deaf.
- PICA→dizzy and dysphagic and dysphonic.

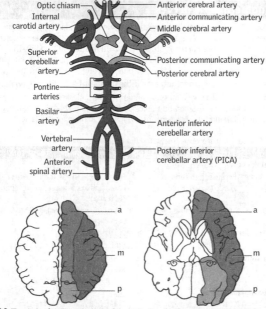

Optic chiasm — Anterior cerebral artery
Internal carotid artery — Anterior communicating artery
— Middle cerebral artery
Superior cerebellar artery — Posterior communicating artery
— Posterior cerebral artery
Pontine arteries
Basilar artery — Anterior inferior cerebellar artery
Vertebral artery — Posterior inferior cerebellar artery (PICA)
Anterior spinal artery

Fig 10.2 The circle of Willis at the base of the brain. See also **figs 10.19, 10.20** (and **fig 10.25** for veins).

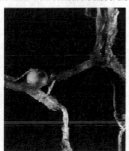

Fig 10.3 Berry aneurysm at junction of posterior communicating artery with internal carotid (p474). © Dr D Hamoundi.

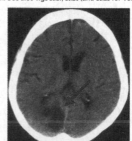

Fig 10.4 CT of stroke in posterior cerebral artery territory.
© J Trobe.

Thomas Willis

Thomas Willis (1621–1675) is one of those happy Oxford heroes who hold a bogus DM degree, awarded in 1646 for his Royalist sympathies while at Christ Church, the most loyally royal college in the University. He had a busy life inventing terms such as 'neurology' and 'reflex'. Not only has his name been given to his famous circle, but he was the first to describe myasthenia gravis, whooping cough, and the sweet taste of diabetic urine. He was the first person (few have followed him) to know the course of the spinal accessory nerve. He is unusual among Oxford neurologists in that he developed the practice of giving his lunch away to the poor. He also espoused iatrochemistry: a theory of medicine according to which all morbid conditions of the body can be explained by disturbances in the fermentations and effervescences of its humours.

Testing peripheral nerves

While there is some anatomical variation between individuals in ascribing particular nerve roots to muscles, **tables 10.4–10.6** represent a reasonable compromise. Dermatomes and sensory nerve roots are shown in **figs 10.5–10.9, pp450–1**.

Remember to test proximal muscle power: ask the patient to sit from lying, to pull you towards themselves, and to rise from squatting (if reasonably fit).

▶Observe walking—easy to forget, even if the complaint is of difficulty walking!

▶Don't be caught out by weakness secondary to musculoskeletal pathology—the traditional neurological examination relies on the musculoskeletal system being intact. Ruptured tendons and fractures may mimic focal neurological lesions.

Table 10.4 Assessment of peripheral nerve function in the lower limb

Nerve root	Muscle	Test by asking the patient to:
Femoral nerve		
L1, 2, 3	Iliopsoas (also supplied via L1, 2, & 3 spinal nerves)	Flex hip against resistance with knee flexed and lower leg supported: patient lies on back
L2, 3, 4	Quadriceps femoris	Extend at knee against resistance. Start with knee flexed
Obturator nerve		
L2, 3, 4	Hip adductors	Adduct leg against resistance
Inferior gluteal nerve		
L5, S1, S2	Gluteus maximus	Hip extension ('bury heel into the couch')—with knee in extension
Superior gluteal nerve		
L4, 5, S1	Gluteus medius and minimus	Abduction and internal hip rotation with leg flexed at hip and knee
Sciatic, common peroneal*, and tibial** nerves		
*L4, 5	Tibialis anterior	Dorsiflex ankle
*L5, S1	Extensor digitorum longus	Dorsiflex toes against resistance
*L5, S1	Extensor hallucis longus	Dorsiflex hallux against resistance
*L5, S1	Peroneus longus and brevis	Evert foot against resistance
*L5, S1	Extensor digitorum brevis	Dorsiflex proximal phalanges of toes
L5, S1, 2	Hamstrings (short head of biceps femoris is from the common peroneal nerve)	Flex knee against resistance
**L4, 5	Tibialis posterior	Invert plantarflexed foot
**S1, 2	Gastrocnemius	Plantarflex ankle or stand on tiptoe
**L5, S1, 2	Flexor digitorum longus	Flex terminal joints of toes
**S1, 2	Small muscles of foot	Make the sole of the foot into a cup

Table 10.5 Rapid screening tests for peripheral nerve roots

Shoulder	Abduction	C5	**Hip**	Flexion	L1–L2
	Adduction	C5–C7		Adduction	L2–3
Elbow	Flexion	C5–C6		Extension	L5–S1
	Extension	C7	**Knee**	Flexion	L5–S1
Wrist	Flexion	C7–8		Extension	L3–L4
	Extension	C7	**Ankle**	Dorsiflexion	L4
Fingers	Flexion	C8		Eversion	L5–S1
	Extension	C7		Plantarflexion	S1–S2
	Abduction	T1	**Toe**	Big toe extension	L5

* Wrist movement innervation differs in medial and lateral flexion/extension, and therefore is a poorer discriminator of peripheral nerve roots than, eg shoulder abduction

Table 10.6 Assessment of peripheral nerve function in the upper limb

Nerve root	Muscle	Test by asking the patient to:
C3, 4	Trapezius	Shrug shoulder (via accessory nerve)
C5, 6, 7	Serratus anterior	Push arm forward against resistance; look for scapula winging (p507) if weak
C5, 6	Pectoralis major (P major) clavicular head	Adduct arm from above horizontal, and push it forward
C6, 7, 8	P major sternocostal head	Adduct arm below horizontal
C5, 6	Supraspinatus	Abduct arm the first 15°
C5, 6	Infraspinatus	Externally rotate semi-flexed arm, elbow at side
C6, 7, 8	Latissimus dorsi	Adduct arm from horizontal position
C5, 6	Biceps	Flex supinated forearm
C5, 6	Deltoid	Abduct arm between 15° and 90°
Radial nerve (p496)		
C6, 7, 8	Triceps	Extend elbow against resistance
C5, 6	Brachioradialis	Flex elbow with forearm half way between pronation and supination
C5, 6	Extensor carpi radialis longus	Extend wrist to radial side
C6, 7	Supinator	Arm by side, resist hand pronation
C7, 8	Extensor digitorum	Keep fingers extended at MCP joint
C7, 8	Extensor carpi ulnaris	Extend wrist to ulnar side
C7, 8	Abductor pollicis longus	Abduct thumb at 90° to palm
C7, 8	Extensor pollicis brevis	Extend thumb at MCP joint
C7, 8	Extensor pollicis longus	Resist thumb flexion at IP joint
Median nerve (p498)		
C6, 7	Pronator teres	Keep arm pronated against resistance
C6, 7	Flexor carpi radialis	Flex wrist towards radial side
C7, 8, T1	Flexor digitorum superficialis	Resist extension at PIP joint (with proximal phalanx fixed by the examiner)
C7, 8	Flexor digitorum profundus I & II	Resist extension at index DIP joint of index finger
C7, 8, T1	Flexor pollicis longus	Resist thumb extension at interphalangeal joint (fix proximal phalanx)
C8, T1	Abductor pollicis brevis	Abduct thumb (nail at 90° to palm)
C8, T1	Opponens pollicis	Thumb touches base of 5th fingertip (nail parallel to palm)
C8, T1	1st lumbrical/interosseus (median and ulnar nerves)	Extend PIP joint against resistance with MCP joint held hyperextended
Ulnar nerve (p498)		
C7, 8, T1	Flexor carpi ulnaris	Flex wrist to ulnar side; observe tendon
C7, C8	Flexor digitorum profundus III & IV	Resist extension of distal phalanx of 5th finger while you fix its middle phalanx
C8, T1	Dorsal interossei	Finger abduction: cannot cross the middle over the index finger (tests index finger adduction too)
C8, T1	Palmar interossei	Finger adduction: pull apart a sheet of paper held between middle and ring finger DIP joints of both hands; the paper moves on the weaker side*
C8, T1	Adductor pollicis	Adduct thumb (nail at 90° to palm)
C8, T1	Abductor digiti minimi	Abduct little finger
C8, T1	Flexor digiti minimi	Flex little finger at MCP joint

*Metacarpophalangeal joint flexion may also be more on the affected side as flexor tendons are recruited—the basis of Froment's paper sign. Wartenberg's sign is persistent little finger abduction.

10 Neurology

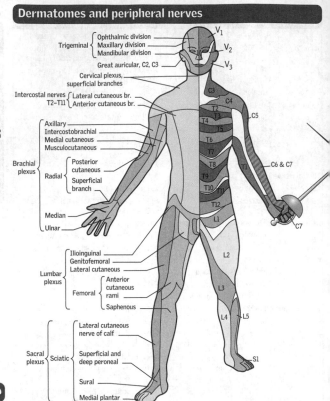

Trigeminal { Ophthalmic division — V₁
Maxillary division — V₂
Mandibular division — V₃

Great auricular, C2, C3

Cervical plexus, superficial branches

Intercostal nerves { Lateral cutaneous br.
T2–T11 { Anterior cutaneous br.

Brachial plexus {
Axillary
Intercostobrachial
Medial cutaneous
Musculocutaneous
Radial { Posterior cutaneous
Superficial branch
Median
Ulnar

Lumbar plexus {
Ilioinguinal
Genitofemoral
Lateral cutaneous
Femoral { Anterior cutaneous rami
Saphenous

Sacral plexus { Sciatic {
Lateral cutaneous nerve of calf
Superficial and deep peroneal
Sural
Medial plantar

C3, C4, C5, T1, T2, T3, T4, T5, T6, T7, T8, T9, T10, T11, T12, L1, L2, L3, L4, L5, S1, C6 & C7, C7

Fig 10.5 The white areas denote *terra incognita*: considerable inter-individual variation exists, and no single best option can be given.

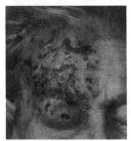

Fig 10.6 Pain in a dermatomal distribution suggests a problem with a cranial nerve or dorsal root ganglion (radiculopathy)—where the cell bodies of sensory fibres live. What is the dermatome? What is the lesion? See p400 for the answer.

Aim to keep a few key dermatomes up your sleeve (C5–T2)	
C3–4	Clavicles
C6–7	Lateral arm/forearm
T1	Medial side of arm
C6	Thumb
C7	Middle finger
C8	Little finger
T4	Nipples
T10	Umbilicus
L1	Inguinal ligament
L2–3	Anterior and inner leg
L5	Medial side of big toe
L5, S1–2	Posterior and outer leg
S1	Lateral margin of foot and little toe
S2–4	Perineum

Rough approximations!

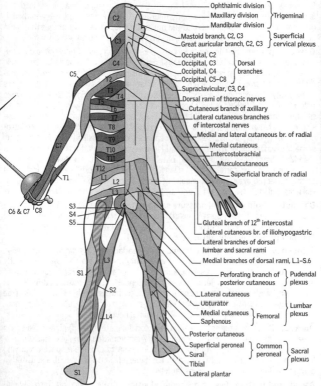

Ophthalmic division
Maxillary division   } Trigeminal
Mandibular division

Mastoid branch, C2, C3   } Superficial
Great auricular branch, C2, C3 } cervical plexus

Occipital, C2
Occipital, C3   } Dorsal
Occipital, C4   } branches
Occipital, C5–C8

Supraclavicular, C3, C4
Dorsal rami of thoracic nerves
Cutaneous branch of axillary
Lateral cutaneous branches
of intercostal nerves
Medial and lateral cutaneous br. of radial
Medial cutaneous
Intercostobrachial
Musculocutaneous
Superficial branch of radial

Gluteal branch of 12th intercostal
Lateral cutaneous br. of iliohypogastric
Lateral branches of dorsal
lumbar and sacral rami
Medial branches of dorsal rami, L1–S.6

Perforating branch of   } Pudendal
posterior cutaneous   } plexus

Lateral cutaneous
Obturator
Medial cutaneous   } Femoral   } Lumbar
Saphenous   } plexus

Posterior cutaneous
Superficial peroneal   } Common
Sural   } peroneal   } Sacral
Tibial   } plexus
Lateral plantar

Fig 10.7 Posterior view.

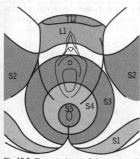

Fig 10.8 The anterior ⅓ of the scrotum is L1; the posterior ⅔ is S3. The penis is S2/3 (L1 at its root).

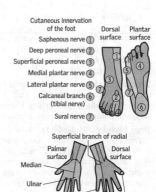

Cutaneous innervation
of the foot   Dorsal   Plantar
Saphenous nerve ①   surface surface
Deep peroneal nerve ②
Superficial peroneal nerve ③
Medial plantar nerve ④
Lateral plantar nerve ⑤
Calcaneal branch ⑥
(tibial nerve)
Sural nerve ⑦

Superficial branch of radial
Palmar   Dorsal
surface   surface
Median

Ulnar

Dorsal cutaneous branch of ulnar   Median
Fig 10.9 Feet and hands.

Every day, *thousands* of people visit the doctor complaining of headache. Headache is divided into *primary* (predominantly migraine, tension-type headache and the trigeminal autonomic cephalgias) and the much rarer *secondary* syndromes that must be excluded (space-occupying lesions, meningitis, subarachnoid haemorrhage).

Onset Rapid onset ►The key diagnosis to rule out here is: •*Subarachnoid haemorrhage* (SAH, p474): sudden-onset, 'worst ever' headache, often occipital, stiff neck, focal signs, ↓consciousness. Other differentials include: •*Reversible cerebral vasoconstriction syndrome:* often recurrent 'thunderclap' headaches mimicking SAH, triggers include physical exertion, sex, swimming, Valsalva, usually benign but beware stroke risk. •*Meningitis* (p806): fever, photophobia, stiff neck, purpuric rash, coma. Do an LP, start antibiotics. •*Encephalitis* (p808): fever, odd behaviour, fits, or reduced consciousness. Do an urgent MRI and LP •*Intracranial hypotension:* CSF leakage, eg iatrogenic after LP or epidural anaesthesia, or spontaneous (most likely spinal CSF leakage, sometimes after minor trauma or a sudden sneeze). Suspect if headaches worse on standing.; treat with epidural blood patch over leak, if conservative management with hydration and caffeine fails. •*Cervical artery dissection:* headache ipsilateral to the dissected artery that is usually progressive but can be rapid onset. Look for Horner's, pulsatile tinnitus, anterior (carotid) or posterior (vertebral) territory stroke.

Character Tight band/dull pressure sensation •*Tension-type headache:* the usual cause of bilateral, non-pulsatile headache ± scalp muscle tenderness, recognized as a separate condition but increasingly considered as mild/moderate migraine. **Throbbing/pulsatile/lateralizing** •*Migraine* (p454).

Frequency Continuous pain (chronic daily headache) •*Chronic migraine* (p454). •*Medication overuse headache* (see 'Drug history'). •*Hemicrania continua* (strictly unilateral, autonomic features, responds to indometacin). •*Sinusitis:* dull, constant ache over frontal or maxillary sinuses, with tenderness ± postnasal drip. Pain is worse on bending over. CT can confirm diagnosis but is rarely needed. **Pain-free most days** •*Migraine.* •*Trigeminal autonomic cephalgias* (see BOX 'Cluster headache'). •*Trigeminal neuralgia* (see BOX 'Trigeminal neuralgia').

Duration Chronic, progressive headaches can indicate ↑ICP. Typically worse on waking, lying, bending forward, or coughing. Also: vomiting, papilloedema, seizures, false localizing signs, or odd behaviour. Do imaging to exclude a space-occupying lesion, and consider idiopathic intracranial hypertension. ►LP is contraindicated in acute ↑ICP due to the risk of cerebellar herniation.

Associated features Eye pain ± reduced vision •*Acute glaucoma.* Typically elderly, long-sighted people. Constant pain develops rapidly around one eye, radiating to the forehead with markedly reduced vision, visual haloes, and a red, congested eye (p559). ►Seek expert help at once. If delay in treatment of >1h is likely, give eye drops (eg 0.5% timolol maleate ± 2% pilocarpine) and acetazolamide 500mg PO. **Jaw claudication, tender scalp with thickened, pulseless temporal arteries** •*Giant cell arteritis* (p554): subacute-onset headache with ESR >40mm/h. ►Exclude in all >50yrs old with a headache that has lasted a few weeks: prompt diagnosis and steroids avoid blindness.

Precipitating causes Head trauma Commonly causes localized pain but can be more generalized. It lasts ~2wks; often resistant to analgesia. Do CT to exclude subdural or extradural haemorrhage if drowsiness ± lucid interval, or focal signs (p476). **Also ask about** Analgesia, sex, food (eg chocolate, cheese, coffee).

Drug history •*Medication overuse headache:* culprits are mixed analgesics (paracetamol + codeine/opiates), ergotamine, and triptans ≥3d per week. This is a common reason for episodic headache becoming chronic daily headache. Analgesia must be withdrawn—aspirin or naproxen may mollify the rebound headache. A preventive may help once off other drugs (eg tricyclics, valproate, gabapentin; p500). Limit use of over-the-counter analgesia (no more than 6d per month).

Social history Ask about stress or recent life events; may not explain the pathology, but will help you appreciate the context in which symptoms are experienced.

Cluster headache and other trigeminal autonomic cephalgias

The trigeminal autonomic cephalgias (TACs) are a group of primary headache disorders that involve activation of the trigeminal and parasympathetic systems, characterized by short-lasting unilateral pain with variable ipsilateral cranial autonomic features. The cause of these is unknown.

Cluster headache The most common, and may be the most disabling of the primary headache disorders. σ:$\circ$ ≥5:1; onset at any age; commoner in smokers.

Symptoms: rapid-onset of excruciating pain around one eye that may become watery and bloodshot with lid swelling, lacrimation, facial flushing, rhinorrhoea, miosis ± ptosis (20% of attacks). Pain is strictly unilateral and almost always affects the same side. Agitation is typical during attacks, in contrast with migraine. It lasts 15–180min, occurs once or twice a day, and is often nocturnal. Clusters last 4–12wks and are followed by pain-free periods of months or even 1–2yrs before the next cluster. *Treatment: acute attack* 'Keep calm ... carry oxygen': give 100% O_2 for ~15min via non-rebreathable mask (not if COPD); sumatriptan SC 6mg at onset (or zolmitriptan nasal spray 5mg). *Preventives: avoid triggers*, eg alcohol. *Medication:* verapamil (360mg in three divided doses) is first line. Also consider: corticosteroids (short term only; many SE); topiramate; lithium (monitor carefully).

Paroxysmal hemicrania Shorter duration (2–30min) and more frequent attacks than cluster headache (up to 40/d). Like hemicrania continua (another TAC), it responds to indometacin treatment; a treatment trial is so easy so consider this!

Short-lasting unilateral neuralgiform headache with conjunctival injection and tearing (SUNCT) The longest name but the shortest duration (seconds–minutes) and the highest frequency (up to hundreds/day) of attacks.

Trigeminal neuralgia

Symptoms Paroxysms of intense, stabbing pain, lasting seconds, in the trigeminal nerve distribution. It is unilateral, typically affecting mandibular or maxillary divisions. The face screws up with pain (*hence tic douloureux*).

Triggers Washing affected area, shaving, eating, talking, dental prostheses.

Typical patient σ >50yrs old; in Asians $\circ$:σ ≈ 2:1.

Secondary causes Compression of the trigeminal root by anomalous or aneurysmal intracranial vessels or a tumour, chronic meningeal inflammation, MS, zoster, skull base malformation (eg Chiari).

MRI This is necessary to exclude secondary causes (~14% of cases).

R: Carbamazepine (start at 100mg/12h PO; max 400mg/6h; lamotrigine; phenytoin 200–400mg/24h PO; or gabapentin (p500). If drugs fail, surgery may be necessary. This may be directed at the peripheral nerve, the trigeminal ganglion, or the nerve root.

Microvascular decompression Anomalous vessels are separated from the trigeminal root. Stereotactic gamma knife surgery can work, but length of pain relief and the time to treatment response are limiting factors.

Facial pain ΔΔ: p61.

10 Neurology

15% of us suffer from migraines, ($♀:♂ \approx 3:1$); responsible for more disability than all other neurological conditions combined.

Symptoms **Prodrome** Premonitory symptoms hours/days before headache are present in the majority: tiredness, yawning, mood/concentration change. **Aura** Reversible neurological symptoms are present in a third, usually of gradual onset, resolves typically within an hour. Usually precede the headache, but may accompany it. • *Visual:* chaotic distorting, 'melting' and jumbling of lines, dots, or zigzags, scotomata or hemianopia. • *Somatosensory:* paraesthesiae spreading from fingers to face. • *Motor:* dysarthria and ataxia (migraine with brainstem aura), ophthalmoplegia, or hemiparesis. (▶Hemiplegic migraine is rare; misdiagnosed TIA/stroke is much more common.) • *Speech:* (8% of auras) dysphasia or paraphasia. • Isolated aura with no headache can occur. **Migraine headache** Unilateral, throbbing headache, typically aggravated by head movement or physical activity. Median duration is 24h. Accompanying neck pain, nausea, vomiting ± photophobia/phonophobia is common. There may be allodynia—all stimuli produce pain: 'I can't brush my hair, wear earrings or glasses, or shave, it's so painful.' **Postdrome** Occurs in 80%, symptoms similar to those listed in the prodrome, usually lasting <12h.

Partial triggers Seen in 50%: CHOCOLATE or: chocolate, hangovers, orgasms, cheese/caffeine, oral contraceptives, lie-ins, alcohol, travel, or exercise.

Diagnosis Clinical, based on the history. **Diagnostic criteria if no aura ≥5** headaches lasting 4–72h + nausea/vomiting (or photo/phonophobia) + any 2 of: • Unilateral • Pulsating • Impairs (or worsened by) routine activity.

Differentials Cluster or tension headache, cervical spondylosis, ↑BP, intracranial pathology, sinusitis/otitis media, dental caries. TIAs may mimic migraine aura.

Acute management Inadequate acute treatment is associated with progression to chronic migraine.[1] Triptans have strong evidence for effectiveness, and may be improved by combination with NSAIDs/paracetamol (the latter should be first tried alone in mild to moderate attacks). Evidence on stroke risk with triptan use is conflicting; use cautiously if there is a prior history of vascular events. Rescue IV therapy may be useful in emergency department presentations, eg metoclopramide 10mg.

Preventive management Can achieve ~50%↓ in attack frequency in most patients; consider after risks and benefits discussion. **Non-pharmacological therapies** Avoid identified triggers (a headache diary can help) and ensure analgesic rebound headache is not complicating matters (p452). Transcutaneous nerve stimulation may help. **Medications** 1st line: Propranolol 40–120mg/12h or topiramate 25–50mg/12h (teratogenic, can interfere with OCP efficacy). Amitriptyline 10–75mg nocte can be used, though this is off licence. Patients may be on previously recommended prophylactic agents (eg valproate, verapamil, pizotifen, pregabalin, or ACE-i/ARB): if achieving good control then continue as required. CGRP antagonists have been approved for migraine prevention for patients with at least 4 headache days per month who cannot tolerate or who have not achieved control with 2–3 previous preventive treatments (see BOX 'Stolen moments'). 12-weekly botulinum toxin type A injections are a last resort in chronic migraine.

Considerations in females Incidence of migraine (especially with aura) + ischaemic stroke is increased by use of a combined OCP. Use progesterone-only or non-hormonal contraception in migraine + aura, though a low-dose combined OCP can be used in those *without* aura. Further ↑risk: • Smoking. • Age >35yrs. • BP↑. • Obesity (body mass index >30). • Diabetes mellitus. • Hyperlipidaemia. • Family history of arteriopathy <45yrs. ▶Warn patients to stop OCP at once if they develop aura or worsening migraine; see OHCS p153. **Perimenstrual migraine** Consider NSAIDs or triptans on the days migraine is expected. **Pregnancy** Migraine often improves; if not, get help—worsening headaches in pregnancy are associated with a greater risk of pre-eclampsia and cardiovascular complications. Offer paracetamol 1st line. Triptans and NSAIDs can be used but discuss risks and benefits with patients first. Don't use aspirin if breastfeeding. Anti-emetic: metoclopramide (up to 5 days only) or promethazine. *Prophylaxis:* seek specialist advice.

Stolen moments

Decades after any hope of its safe return had been extinguished, along with the life of its former virtuoso owner, a stolen 1734 Stradivarius violin was recovered from a dusty Californian attic in 2015 and meticulously restored. Snatched by a former student after a lesson, the Totenberg Stradivarius (**fig 10.10**) spent 35 years of its life immured in darkness, ceding its rich velvet voice for uninterrupted silence. After a similar painstaking search, chronic migraine is finally giving up its secrets. There is renewed hope that precious moments callously stolen from migraineurs, relegated to silent darkness by piercing dissonance, might gradually be returned. The previously favoured theory of dilatation of meningeal arteries as the root

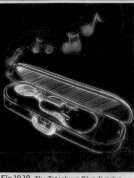

Fig 10.10 The Totenburg Stradivarius. Artwork by Gillian Turner.

cause has been largely disproved. Rather, neurogenic inflammation of trigeminal sensory neurons caused by cortical spreading depression modulates how pain is processed and also results in aura. The calcitonin gene-related peptide (CGRP), discovered in the 1980s, has been found to play a key role by mediating vasodilatation and pain transmission. IV monoclonal antibodies directed against CGRP or its receptor are approved for migraine prevention, and oral CGRP antagonists ('gepants') are effective for acute management and for prevention. They have not been studied in pregnancy, and should be avoided for now in people with recent ischaemic events, since CGRP has theoretical cardioprotective effects.

Causes of collapse ± loss of consciousness (LOC) are many; take a careful history (see BOX 'Blackout history').

Vasovagal (neurocardiogenic) syncope Occurs due to reflex bradycardia ± peripheral vasodilation provoked by emotion, pain, or standing too long (it cannot occur when lying down). Onset is over seconds (*not* instantaneous), and is often preceded by pre-syncopal symptoms, eg nausea, pallor, sweating, and narrowing of visual fields. Brief clonic jerking of the limbs may occur due to cerebral hypoperfusion, but there is no tonic/clonic sequence. Urinary incontinence is uncommon, and there is no tongue-biting. Unconsciousness usually lasts for <2min and recovery is rapid.

Situational syncope Symptoms as for vasovagal syncope but with a clear precipitant: *cough syncope* occurs after a paroxysm of coughing; *effort syncope* is brought on by exercise; there is usually a cardiac cause, eg aortic stenosis, HCM; *micturition syncope* happens during or after urination: mostly men, at night.

Carotid sinus syncope Hypersensitive baroreceptors cause excessive reflex bradycardia ± vasodilation on minimal stimulation (eg head-turning, shaving).

Epilepsy (p486) Features suggestive of this diagnosis include: attacks when asleep or lying down; aura; identifiable triggers (eg TV); altered breathing; cyanosis; typical tonic–clonic movements; incontinence of urine; tongue-biting; prolonged post-ictal drowsiness, confusion, amnesia, and transient focal paralysis (Todd's palsy).

Stokes–Adams attacks Transient arrhythmias (eg bradycardia due to complete heart block) cause ↓cardiac output and LOC. The patient falls to the ground (often with *no* warning except palpitations; injuries are common), and is pale, with a slow or absent pulse. Recovery is in seconds: the patient flushes, the pulse speeds up, and consciousness is regained. As with vasovagal syncope, anoxic clonic jerks may occur in prolonged LOC. Attacks may happen several times a day and in any posture.

Other causes Hypoglycaemia (p208) Tremor, hunger, and perspiration herald lightheadedness or LOC; rare in non-diabetics. **Orthostatic hypotension** Unsteadiness or LOC on standing from lying in those with inadequate vasomotor reflexes: the elderly; autonomic neuropathy (p501); antihypertensive medication; over-diuresis; multisystem atrophy (MSA; p490). **Anxiety** Hyperventilation, tremor, sweating, tachycardia, paraesthesiae, light-headedness, and no LOC suggest a panic attack. **Drop attacks** Sudden fall to the ground *without* LOC. Mostly benign and due to leg weakness but may also be caused by hydrocephalus, cataplexy, or narcolepsy. **Psychogenic** Pseudosyncope, non-epileptic seizures (p460), Münchausen's (p694).

Examination Cardiovascular, neurological. Measure BP lying and standing.

Investigation *ECG:* all with recurrent syncope (or falls) need cardiac assessment—urgently if associated with palpitations, arrhythmias, 3rd-degree AV block, or prolonged QT interval (p697) ± 24h ECG (arrhythmia, long QT, eg Romano–Ward, p88); U&E, FBC, Mg²⁺, Ca²⁺, glucose; tilt-table test;³ EEG, sleep EEG; echocardiogram; CT/MRI brain; ABG if practical (↓P_aCO_2 in attacks suggests hyperventilation as the cause).

▶While the cause is being elucidated, advise against driving (see p150).

Transient global amnesia

Characterized by a sudden onset of anterograde amnesia (the inability to form new memories) lasting up to 24h, with full recovery except for a 'blackout' of memory for the duration of the episode. The cause is uncertain, but hippocampal diffusion-weighted MRI lesions are common, suggesting a vascular mechanism. Triggers include physical exertion, sex, emotional events, and cold-water exposure. There is disorientation in time and place (but not person), often prompting repetitive questioning, but semantic memory is preserved.

Management Reassurance; there is no increased risk of stroke, episodes do not usually recur, and no driving restrictions apply. Frequent recurrences or occurrence on waking should prompt investigation for epileptic amnesia.

Blackout history

Talk to the patient *and* witnesses and let them tell you as much as possible without prompting or leading. Ask:

Before the attack
- Is there any warning?—Eg epileptic aura or pre-syncopal symptoms.
- In what circumstances do attacks occur?—Eg posture (standing/sitting/supine), exertion, if watching TV consider epilepsy.
- Can the patient prevent attacks?

During the attack
- Does the patient lose awareness?
- Does the patient injure themselves?
- Does the patient move? Are they stiff or floppy? (A tonic phase preceding clonic jerking points towards epilepsy.)
- Is there incontinence? (More common in epilepsy, but can occur with syncope.)
- Does their complexion change? (Pale/cyanosis suggests epilepsy; very pale suggests syncope or arrhythmia.)
- Does the patient bite the side of their tongue? (Suggests epilepsy.)
- Are there associated symptoms, eg palpitations, sweats, pallor, chest pain, dyspnoea (fig 10.11)?
- How long does the attack last?

After the attack
- How much does the patient remember about the attack?
- Is there muscle ache? (Suggests a tonic–clonic seizure.)
- Is the patient confused or sleepy? (Suggests epilepsy.)

Background to attacks
- When did they start?
- Are they getting more frequent?
- Is anyone else in the family getting them? Sudden arrhythmic death may leave no evidence at postmortem, or there may be hereditary cardiomyopathy (refer those with a relative who has had a sudden unexplained death <40yrs old).

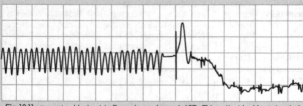

Fig 10.11 VT causing blackout in Brugada syndrome (p687). This patient had been treated with an implantable defibrillator (p128).

The dying of the light

People reporting that they have 'blacked out' may be inadvertently condemning themselves to the title of 'poor historian'; a lamentable part of the medical lexicon that ought to be expunged, not least because it is misaddressed (a historian records history). Why should we expect the storyteller to be able to clearly characterize the absence of something intangible? The light is extinguished for around a third of our lives, but even the most eloquent of us would be hard-pressed to begin to explain what we lose during the daily disconnect from our external world. The loss of light may be literal (amaurosis fugax, p469), metaphorical (transient amnesia), symbolic of independence (falls, p30), or all-encompassing (syncope, seizures).

3 Patient is subject to continuous ECG and BP monitoring while strapped to a table and moved rapidly from resting horizontal position to vertical. Induction of symptoms with inappropriate BP drop >30mmHg or bradycardia suggests neurally mediated syncope. Consider pacing.

10 Neurology

Is this vertigo? Complaints of 'dizzy spells' are very common and are used by patients to describe many different sensations. True vertigo is a *hallucination of movement*, often rotatory (table 10.7). In practice, simple 'spinning' is rare—the floor may tilt, sink, or rise. The key to diagnosis is to find out exactly what the patient means by 'dizzy': if this is not vertigo or if atypical symptoms are present consider other causes, eg if there is loss of awareness, think of epilepsy or syncope; if there is faintness, light-headedness, or palpitations, think of anaemia, dysrhythmia, anxiety, or hypotension.

Table 10.7 Causes of vertigo by time course and associated features

Cause	Duration	Characteristics
Benign positional paroxysmal vertigo (BPPV)	Recurrent episodes, seconds/ minutes	Provoked by changes in head position due to disruption of debris in the semicircular canal of the ears (canalithiasis). Fatiguable nystagmus on performing the Hallpike manoeuvre is diagnostic; Epley manoeuvres clear the debris (*OHCS* p405)
Posterior circulation TIA	Single or recurrent, minutes/ hours	See stroke, below. Requires urgent assessment and treatment; the risk of early recurrent stroke may even be greater than that for anterior circulation TIA
Ménière's disease	Recurrent episodes, minutes/ hours	Increased pressure in the endolymphatic system of the inner ear causes recurrent attacks of fluctuating (or permanent) sensorineural hearing loss, and tinnitus (with a sense of aural fullness ± falling to one side). *R:* bed rest and reassurance in acute attacks. An antihistamine (eg betahistine) is useful if prolonged, or buccal prochlorperazine if severe, for up to 7d
Migraine with brainstem aura	Recurrent episodes, minutes/ hours	History of migraine, migraine triggers (p454)
Vestibular neuronitis	Single episode, hours/ days	Viral/post-viral inflammation of the vestibular nerve; often preceded by upper respiratory viral infection. Abrupt onset of severe vertigo, nausea, vomiting ± prostration. Called 'labyrinthitis' when associated with hearing loss. Severe vertigo subsides in days, complete recovery takes 3–4wks. *R:* reassure. Sedate
Posterior circulation stroke	Single episode, days/ weeks	Usually accompanied by other symptoms (weakness, dysarthria, dysphagia, diplopia, nausea/vomiting, ataxia), but even isolated vertigo can be caused by ischaemia

Others MS; ototoxicity (aminoglycosides, loop diuretics, aspirin and cisplatin can cause deafness ± vertigo); trauma to petrous temporal bone; motion sickness (*mal de débarquement*); herpes zoster of the external auditory meatus; facial palsy ± deafness, tinnitus, and vertigo (Ramsay Hunt syndrome, see **p499**); alcohol intoxication.

Tinnitus

This ringing or buzzing in the ears is common, and may cause depression or insomnia. ▶Investigate unilateral tinnitus fully to exclude an acoustic neuroma (p459).
Causes Sensorineural hearing loss (leading to auditory cortex hyper-excitability), excess noise, head injury, ototoxic drugs, otitis media, Ménière's. If *pulsatile*, think of vascular causes (carotid stenosis/dissection, AV fistulae, and glomus jugulare tumours). **Management** Often a chronic condition; the goal is to lessen the impact and manage associations (depression, insomnia) rather than achieve a complete cure. *Behavioural therapies* such as 'tinnitus retraining training' and CBT can help reduce evoked annoyance. *Masking* may provide relief in conjunction: white noise (like an off-tuned radio) is given via a noise generator worn like a post-aural hearing aid, or by enhancing background noise (eg fans). *Drugs* are disappointing: misoprostol appears to help (small-scale trials only). If Ménière's disease is the cause, betahistine helps only a few.

Bedside tests Whisper test Simple but sensitive: whisper numbers in one ear while blocking the other. Make sure that failure to repeat the number is not from misunderstanding. Failure should prompt evaluation by an audiologist. **Tuning fork tests** (*Rinne:* bone conduction via the mastoid is louder than air conduction in conductive losses >20dB, and *Weber:* with the fork on the vertex, sound localizes to the affected ear with conductive loss, to the contralateral ear in sensorineural hearing loss, and to the midline if both ears are normal.) Designed for unilateral conductive losses and have poor sensitivity; these should not be used as screening tests.

Conductive deafness Causes Wax (remove, eg by syringing with warm water after softening with olive oil drops), otosclerosis, cholesteatoma, otitis media (*OHCS* p394).

Chronic sensorineural deafness Often due to accumulated noise exposure, presbycusis, or inherited disorders. **Presbycusis** Symmetrical reduction of acuity for high-frequency sounds starts before 30yrs old. We do not usually notice it until hearing of speech is affected. Hearing is most affected in the presence of background noise. Hearing aids are the usual treatment.

Sudden sensorineural deafness ▶Get an ENT opinion *today*. **Causes** Idiopathic (most cases); noise exposure; gentamicin/other toxin; mumps; acoustic neuroma; MS; stroke; vasculitis; TB. **Tests** ESR, FBC, LFT, pANCA, viral titres, and TB (see BOX 'Diagnostic tests for TB', p390); audiometry; MRI. **Management** All patients typically receive steroids, but there is no good evidence. Antivirals are no longer recommended.[2]

Acoustic neuroma (figs 10.12, 10.13) Doubly misnamed: it is a Schwannoma (not neuroma) arising from the vestibular (not auditory) nerve. They account for 80% of cerebellopontine angle tumours and often present with unilateral hearing loss/tinnitus, with vertigo occurring later. Growth rate is slow (usually 1–2 mm/year) and can be predicted by serial MRIs. With progression, ipsilateral Vth, VIth, IXth, and Xth nerves may be affected (also ipsilateral cerebellar signs). Signs of ↑ICP occur late, indicating a large tumour. Commoner in ♀ and neurofibromatosis (esp. NF2, p510).

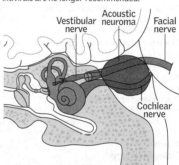

Fig 10.12 An acoustic neuroma (vestibular Schwannoma) growing dangerously near the facial nerve.

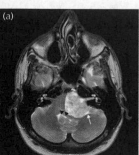

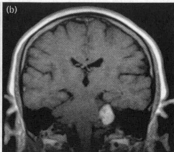

Fig 10.13 Large vestibular Schwannoma: axial T2W (a) and contrast-enhanced coronal MRI (b). Reproduced from Manji *et al.*, *Oxford Handbook of Neurology*, 2007 with permission from Oxford University Press.

10 Neurology

Unexplained changes in nervous system function without structural abnormalities make up at least a third of all outpatient neurological presentations, and are one of the biggest causes of disability. ♀:♂ ≥3:1. ►The presence of functional signs on examination does not rule out organic pathology, 'functional overlay' is common.

Presentation and diagnostic signs

Functional weakness History of leg dragging or dropping things, frequently unilateral and possibly more common on the non-dominant side. Typically increases with attention and decreases with distraction. Positive signs include obvious incongruence with functional ability (eg can stand on tip toes but no ankle plantar flexion on examination), collapsing or 'give-way' weakness (not specific, can occur in joint problems or pain), drift without pronation of a weak arm, Hoover's sign (see BOX 'Opening the floodgates') in a weak leg.

Functional sensory disturbances Sensory loss of one of more modalities is most common. Positive signs include precise midline splitting (eg of vibration sense across the forehead), inconsistent deficits when hand sensation is tested with the fingers interlocked behind the back, tubular visual field defects (tunnel vision of the same width regardless of distance, incompatible with the laws of physics), reported inaudible tuning fork test at the ipsilateral mastoid process for a reported unilateral hearing loss (transcranial attenuation of vibration is minimal so this should be perceived by the contralateral cochlea).

Functional gait disorders Commonly leg dragging, knee-buckling, excessive slowness, or bizarre gait not conforming to a usual pattern. A useful clue is the highly specific 'huffing and puffing' sign (excessive demonstration of effort).

Functional movement disorders Tremor is most common, and is typically variable, distractible, and associated with isometric contraction of antagonistic muscles in the limb. Functional myoclonus is also variable and distractible, with a predominantly axial location. Fixed dystonia at onset, and dystonia after peripheral trauma are likely to be functional in most cases.

Psychogenic non-epileptic seizures Suspect if seizures have a gradual onset, prolonged duration, and abrupt termination and are accompanied by closed eyes ± resistance to eye opening, rapid breathing, fluctuating motor activity, and episodes of motionless unresponsiveness. CNS exam, CT, MRI, and EEG are normal. It may coexist with true epilepsy.

Pathophysiology

'Conversion disorder' (psychological distress manifest in physical symptoms) is likely only to be a part of the cause, deficient inhibition and attentional dysregulation are also implicated. Functional MRI shows contrasting findings to feigned symptoms.

Diagnosis

Make a positive diagnosis based on suggestive signs as well as negative investigations. The delivery of the diagnosis is key; acknowledge that these are genuine symptoms, regardless of their incongruence with known neurological disease, cause distress and disability, and that they are potentially reversible with treatment.

Differential diagnosis

Any neurological disorder with an atypical presentation, psychiatric disorders, including somatic symptom disorder, depersonalization/derealization disorder, factious disorder (deliberately feigned to obtain care), Münchausen's (p694), and malingering (deliberately feigned for external benefit, eg medicolegal context).

Management

Avoid treatments directed at the symptomatology. The diagnosis alone with a follow-up visit to rediscuss can be therapeutic. Referral to psychiatry and cognitive behavioural therapy might be required for patients not showing signs of improvement, as well as identification and treatment of any comorbid psychiatric disorder.

Opening the floodgates

In 1935, the Hoover Dam (**fig 10.14**) on the Colorado River, an unprecedented triumph of engineering, began to nourish and power a parched Southwest USA. 6.6 million tonnes of steadfast concrete served the altogether unanticipated function of symbolizing perseverance amid the depths of the Great Depression. We are unequipped to understand disconnect between structure and function in the human body. The dualistic mind–brain rift deepened in the 20th century and functional disorders fell beyond the grasp of the organically rooted doctor. A naturalistic philosophy of medicine would even discount these as diseases entirely. What then do we say to the person who shudders without seizing, or who senses without feeling? Their account wouldn't satisfy any perception of 'health'. 'Draining the symptoms dry' is a good place to start.[3] Asking them to list all their symptoms saves rather than costs time. Demonstrate paradoxical findings to the patient, such as *Hoover's sign* (functional weakness of hip extension returns to normal during contralateral hip flexion against resistance). The understanding that structure may not be determining function can be therapeutic in itself.

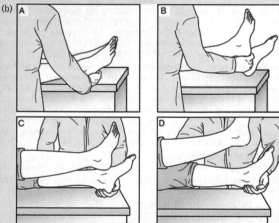

Fig 10.14 (a) The Hoover Dam, Bureau of Reclamation, public domain work of US government. (b) Hoover sign in a 23-year-old man who has a psychogenic left hemiparesis. A, Neurologist asks him to raise his left leg as she holds her hand under his right heel. B, Revealing his lack of effort, the patient exerts so little downward force with his right leg that she easily raises it. C, When she asks him to raise his right leg while cupping his left heel, the patient reveals his intact strength as he unconsciously forces his left 'paretic' leg downward. D, As if to carry the example to the extreme, the patient forces his left leg downward with enough force to allow her to use his left leg as a lever to raise his lower torso.

Source: (a) US Bureau of Reclamation. https://www.usbr.gov/lc/hooverdam/;
(b) Reproduced from Kaufman et al., *Kaufman's Clinical Neurology for Psychiatrists* (2022), with permission from Elsevier under the STM Agreement.

Acute bilateral leg weakness

It is crucial to establish a diagnosis quickly to avoid permanent disability. Look for specific patterns (see later in topic) and ask these questions to help elicit the diagnosis:

1 *Where is the lesion?* • Are the legs flaccid or spastic? (ie LMN or UMN?) • Is there sensory loss? A sensory *level* usually means spinal cord disease. • Is there loss of bowel or bladder control? (Lesion more likely to be in the conus medullaris or cauda equina.)

2 *What is the lesion?* • Was onset sudden or rapidly progressive? ►This is an emergency; it suggests cord compression or spinal stroke so get urgent help (see next paragraph). • Are there any signs of infection (eg tender spine, ↑T°, ↑WCC, ↑ESR, ↑CRP: extradural abscess)?

Cord compression (See also p524.) **Symptoms** Bilateral leg weakness (arm weakness—often less severe—suggests a cervical cord lesion, see p504) a sensory level ± preceding back pain (p538). Bladder (and anal) sphincter involvement is late and manifests as hesitancy, frequency, and, later, as painless retention. **Signs** Look for a motor, reflex, and sensory level, with normal findings above the level of the lesion, LMN signs at the level (especially in cervical lesions), and UMN signs *below* the level (but remember tone and reflexes are usually reduced in *acute* cord compression; *OHCS* p562). **Causes** Secondary malignancy (breast, lung, prostate, thyroid, kidney) in the spine is commonest. Rarer: infection (epidural abscess), cervical disc prolapse, haematoma (warfarin), intrinsic cord tumour, atlanto-axial subluxation, myeloma. ∆∆ Transverse myelitis, MS, carcinomatous meningitis, cord vasculitis (PAN, syphilis), spinal artery thrombosis or aneurysm, trauma, Guillain–Barré syndrome (p500). **Investigations** ►Do not delay imaging at any cost. Spinal x-rays are unreliable; MRI is the definitive modality. Biopsy or surgical exploration may be needed to identify the nature of any mass. Do a CXR (primary lung malignancy, lung secondaries, TB). Bloods: FBC, ESR, B₁₂, syphilis serology, U&E, LFT, PSA, serum electrophoresis. **Treatment** Give urgent dexamethasone in malignancy (p524) while considering more specific therapy, eg radiotherapy or chemotherapy ± decompressive laminectomy; which is most appropriate depends on tumour type, quality of life, and likely prognosis. Epidural abscesses must be surgically decompressed and antibiotics given.

Cauda equina and conus medullaris lesions The big difference between these lesions and those high up in the cord is that leg weakness is flaccid and areflexic, not spastic and hyperreflexic. **Causes** As above, plus congenital lumbar disc disease and lumbosacral nerve lesions. **Signs** *Conus medullaris lesions* feature mixed UMN/LMN signs, leg weakness, early urinary retention and constipation, back pain, sacral sensory disturbance, and erectile dysfunction. *Cauda equina lesions* feature back pain and radicular pain down the legs; asymmetrical, atrophic, areflexic paralysis of the legs; sensory loss in a root distribution; and ↓sphincter tone; do PR.

Other patterns of leg weakness

Unilateral foot drop DM, common peroneal nerve palsy, stroke, prolapsed disc, MS.

Weak legs with no sensory loss MND, polio, parasagittal meningioma (an exception to the rule that weak legs mean cord or distal lesion).

Chronic spastic paraparesis MS, cord primary malignancy/metastasis, MND, syringomyelia, subacute combined degeneration of the cord (p330), hereditary spastic paraparesis, taboparesis (tertiary syphilis, see p408), histiocytosis X, parasites (eg schistosomiasis).

Chronic flaccid paraparesis Peripheral neuropathy, myopathy.

Absent knee jerks and extensor plantars (Ie combined LMN or UMN signs.) Combined cervical and lumbar disc disease, conus medullaris lesions, MND, myeloradiculitis, Friedreich's ataxia, subacute combined degeneration of the cord, taboparesis.[4]

4 Tertiary syphilis (p408): in tabes dorsalis the afferent pathways from muscle spindles are lost, with reduced tone and tendon reflexes (without weakness). Later, additional involvement of the pyramidal tracts causes taboparesis—a spastic paraparesis with the peculiar combination of extensor plantars (from the taboparesis) and absent tendon reflexes (from the tabes dorsalis).

Gait disorders

Spastic Stiff, circumduction of legs ± scuffing of the toe of the shoes: UMN lesions.

Extrapyramidal Flexed posture, shuffling feet, slow to start, postural instability, eg Parkinson's disease.

Apraxic Pathognomonic 'gluing-to-the-floor' on attempting walking or a wide-based unsteady gait with a tendency to fall, like a novice on an ice-rink. Seen in normal pressure hydrocephalus and multi-infarct states.

Ataxic Wide-based; falls; cannot walk heel-to-toe. Caused by cerebellar lesions (eg MS, posterior fossa tumours, alcohol, phenytoin toxicity); proprioceptive sensory loss (eg sensory neuropathy, ↓B₁₂). Often worse in the dark or with eyes closed.

Myopathic Waddling gait, cannot climb steps or stand from sitting due to hip girdle weakness.

Functional Suspect if there is a bizarre gait not conforming to any pattern of organic gait disturbance and without any signs when examined on the couch (p460).

Tests Spinal x-rays; MRI; FBC; ESR; syphilis serology; serum B₁₂; U&E; LFT; PSA; serum electrophoresis; CXR; LP; EMG; muscle ± sural nerve biopsy.

Non-neurological considerations in paralysed patients

Avoid pressure sores by turning and review weight-bearing areas often. Use appropriate pressure-relieving mattresses/cushions. Prevent thrombosis in paralysed limbs by frequent passive movement, pressure stockings, and LMWH (p346). Bladder care is vital; catheterization is only one option (do not control incontinence by decreasing fluid intake). Bowel evacuation may be manual or aided by suppositories; increasing dietary fibre intake may help. Exercise of unaffected or partially paralysed limbs is important to avoid unnecessary loss of function.

These are characterized by impairment of the planning, control, or execution of movement. They can have multiple manifestations:

Tremor Note frequency, amplitude, and exacerbating factors (stress; fatigue).
• **Rest tremor** Abolished on voluntary movement. *Cause:* parkinsonism (p490).
• **Intention tremor** Irregular, large-amplitude, worse at the end of purposeful acts, eg finger-pointing or using a remote control. *Cause:* cerebellar damage (eg MS, stroke).
• **Postural tremor** Absent at rest, present on maintained posture (arms outstretched) and may persist (but is not worse) on movement. *Causes:* essential tremor (autosomal dominant; improves with alcohol), thyrotoxicosis, anxiety, β-agonists.
Re-emergent tremor Postural tremor developing after a delay of ~10s. *Causes:* Parkinson's disease (don't mistake for essential tremor).

Chorea Non-rhythmic, jerky, purposeless movements flowing from one place to another—eg facial grimacing, raising the shoulders, flexing/extending the fingers.
Causes Sydenham's chorea (rare complication of group A streptococcal infection).
Huntington's disease Incurable, progressive, autosomal dominant, neurodegenerative disorder presenting in middle age, often with prodromal phase of mild symptoms (irritability, depression, incoordination). Progresses to chorea, dementia ± fits (within ~15yrs of diagnosis). Atrophy and neuronal loss of striatum and cortex, due to expansion of CAG repeat on Chr. 4. *R* (p70). No treatment prevents progression, but trials for antisense oligonucleotides are underway. Counselling for patient and family. Worsened by levodopa.

Hemiballismus Large-amplitude, flinging hemichorea (affects proximal muscles) contralateral to a vascular lesion of the subthalamic nucleus (often elderly diabetics). Recovers spontaneously over months.

Athetosis Slow, sinuous, confluent, purposeless movements (especially digits, hands, face, tongue), often difficult to distinguish from chorea. **Causes** Commonest is cerebral palsy (*OHCS* p262). Most other 'athetoid' patterns may now be better classed as dystonias. **Pseudoathetosis** Caused by severe proprioceptive loss.

Tics Brief, repeated, stereotyped movements which patients may suppress for a while. Tics are common in children (and usually resolve). In Tourette's syndrome (p690), motor and vocal tics occur. Consider psychological support, clonazepam or clonidine if tics are severe (haloperidol may help but risks tardive dyskinesia).

Myoclonus Sudden involuntary focal or general jerks arising from cord, brainstem, or cerebral cortex, seen in metabolic problems, neurodegenerative disease (eg lysosomal storage enzyme defects), CJD (p483), and myoclonic epilepsies (infantile spasms, juvenile myoclonic epilepsy). **Benign essential myoclonus** Childhood onset with frequent generalized myoclonus, without progression. Often autosomal dominant. It may respond to valproate, clonazepam, or piracetam. **Asterixis ('metabolic flap')** Jerking (~1–2 jerks/s) of outstretched hands, worse with wrists extended, from loss of extensor tone—ie incoordination between flexors and extensors (= 'negative myoclonus'). **Causes** Liver or kidney failure, ↓Na⁺, ↑CO₂, gabapentin, thalamic stroke (consider if unilateral).

Tardive syndromes Delayed onset yet potentially irreversible symptoms occurring after chronic exposure to dopamine antagonists (eg antipsychotics, antiemetics). **Classification** •*Tardive dyskinesia:* orobuccolingual, truncal, or choreiform movements, eg vacuous chewing and grimacing movements. • *Tardive dystonia:* sustained, stereotyped muscle spasms of a twisting or turning character, eg retrocollis and back arching/opisthotonic posturing. • *Tardive akathisia:* sense of restlessness or unease ± repetitive, purposeless movements (stereotypies, eg pacing). • *Tardive myoclonus.* • *Tardive tourettism* (p690). • *Tardive tremor.* **Treating tardive dyskinesia** Gradually withdraw neuroleptics and wait 3–6 months. Tetrabenazine may help. Quetiapine, olanzapine, and clozapine are examples of atypical antipsychotics that are less likely to cause tardive syndromes.

Dystonia

Dystonia describes prolonged muscle contractions causing abnormal posture or repetitive movements.

Idiopathic generalized dystonia Childhood-onset dystonia often starting in one leg with ipsilateral progression over 5–10yrs. Autosomal dominant inheritance is common (DYT1 deletion). Exclude Wilson's disease and dopa-responsive dystonia (needs an L-dopa trial). Anticholinergics and muscle relaxants may help. Deep brain stimulation for refractory, disabling symptoms.

Focal dystonias Confined to one part of the body, eg *spasmodic torticollis* (head pulled to one side), *blepharospasm* (involuntary contraction of orbicularis oculi, OHCS p341), *writer's cramp*. Focal dystonias in adults are typically idiopathic, and rarely generalize. They are worsened by stress. Patients may develop a *geste antagoniste* to try to resist the dystonic posturing (eg a touch of the finger to the jaw in spasmodic torticollis). Injection of botulinum toxin into the overactive muscles is usually effective.

Acute dystonia May occur on starting many drugs, including neuroleptics and some anti-emetics (eg metoclopramide, cyclizine). There is torticollis (head pulled back), trismus (oromandibular spasm), and/or oculogyric crisis (eyes drawn up). You may mistake this for tetanus or meningitis, but such reactions rapidly disappear after a dose of an anticholinergic, see p827.

St Vitus' dance

Throughout the Middle Ages, Europe was plagued by epidemics of 'dancing mania', in which afflicted individuals were described to have danced wildly, displaying strange contortions and convulsions until they collapsed from exhaustion. If the afflicted touched a relic of St Vitus they were miraculously cured: observing this, Paracelsus, 16th-century Swiss-German physician and philosopher, described the phenomenon of *chorea Sancti Viti* ('St Vitus' dance'). There may have been an infectious component, although mass hysteria induced by religious cults that swept across medieval Europe seems a more likely cause. Chorea was subsequently used as a general term for large-amplitude involuntary movements before being further refined by physicians such as Sydenham (though he did not connect his eponymous chorea seen in rheumatic fever with an infectious trigger) and Charcot. Nowadays, a more frequent cause of involuntary movements with behavioural disturbance is NMDA-receptor antibody encephalitis, the impact of which was documented in Susannah Cahalan's excellent 2012 autobiography *Brain on Fire: My Month of Madness*. (See also BOX 'Sydenham's chorea', p147.)

Infarction or bleeding into the brain manifests with sudden-onset focal CNS signs. Incidence rates have fallen by 20% in the last two decades, but stroke remains the fourth leading cause of death and the largest cause of neurological disability in the UK.

Causes Ischaemic • Cardioembolic (AF; endocarditis; MI—see BOX 'Cardiac causes of stroke'). • Large artery disease; atherothromboembolism (eg from carotids) or thrombosis *in situ* • Small vessel occlusion/cerebral microangiopathy. **Haemorrhagic** (p468).
Rarer causes Haemodynamic; sudden BP drop by ≥40mmHg (most likely to affect the boundary zone between vascular beds), carotid artery dissection (spontaneous, or from neck trauma or connective tissue disorders), vasculitis, vasospasm (p474), neoplasm, venous sinus thrombosis (p478), Fabry disease (p316), CADASIL[5]

Modifiable risk factors ↑BP, smoking, DM, heart disease (valvular, ischaemic, AF), peripheral vascular disease, combined OCP, ↑lipids, ↑alcohol use, ↑clotting (p370).

Symptoms Ask about: • Exact time of onset of symptoms (use the time definitely last well for 'wake-up' strokes); crucial to determine if within the reperfusion therapy treatment window • Progression; usually sudden and maximal at onset, but exceptions include bleeds and certain TIAs (p469). • Features of *stroke mimics*: seizures with post-ictal paresis (Todd's palsy), aphasia, or neglect; sepsis; migraine; intracranial tumours; hypoglycaemia.

Signs Worst at onset. *Pointers to bleeding (unreliable!):* meningism, severe headache, coma. *Pointers to ischaemia:* carotid bruit, AF!, past TIA, IHD. **Cerebral infarcts** (50%) Depending on site there may be contralateral sensory loss or hemiplegia; dysphasia; homonymous hemianopia. **Brainstem infarcts** (25%) Varied; include quadriplegia, disturbances of gaze and vision, vertigo, locked-in syndrome (aware, but unable to respond). **Lacunar infarcts** (25%) Basal ganglia, internal capsule, thalamus, and pons. Five syndromes: ataxic hemiparesis, pure motor, pure sensory, sensorimotor, and dysarthria/clumsy hand. Cognition/consciousness are intact except in some thalamic strokes.

Acute investigation and management ▶ *'Time is brain.'*
▶**Protect the airway** This avoids hypoxia/aspiration. ▶Check glucose pre-hospital.
• **History and exam** Establish time of onset (see above), establish severity (NIHSS[6]).
• **CT/MRI** Without delay if: thrombolysis considered, risk of haemorrhage (↑GCS, signs of ↓ICP, severe headache, meningism, progressive symptoms, bleeding tendency or anticoagulated), or unusual presentation (eg fluctuating consciousness, fever). Diffusion-weighted MRI is most sensitive for an acute infarct (fig 10.15).
• **Urgent reperfusion treatment** Assess suitability for *thrombectomy* (see BOX 'Endovascular thrombectomy'). Consider IV *thrombolysis* in disabling stroke as soon as haemorrhage has been excluded, provided the onset of symptoms was ≤4.5h ago (the benefits outweigh the risks within this window, though best results are ≤90min), or for 'wake-up' stroke with imaging signs of hyperacuity. Alteplase is the agent of choice. ▶Always do CT 12–24h post-lysis to identify bleeding. Absolute CI to thrombolysis: • Resolved deficit • Any haemorrhage on CT. • Recent surgery, trauma, or artery or vein puncture at uncompressible site. • AVM/aneurysm or intracranial tumour (active). • Stroke or serious head injury in last 6 weeks. • GI or urinary tract haemorrhage in the last 21 days. • Anticoagulants (if INR >1.7 or aPTT >40s), or spontaneous INR >1.7 • Platelets <50 × 10⁹/L. • Endocarditis or CNS vasculitis.
• **Admit to an acute stroke unit** Multidisciplinary care improves outcomes (p470).
• **Maintain homeostasis** Blood glucose: keep between 4–11 mmol/L. Blood pressure: only treat within 24h if there is a hypertensive emergency (eg encephalopathy or aortic dissection) or thrombolysis is considered as treating BP may impair cerebral perfusion.
• **Screen swallow** 'Nil by mouth' until this is done (but keep hydrated).
• **Secondary prevention** To be commenced as soon as haemorrhagic stroke is excluded (p470).

5 Cerebral Autosomal Dominant Arteriopathy with Subcortical Infarcts & Leucoencephalopathy: the main genetic cause of stroke (there is also an autosomal recessive form).
6 The best-established deficit rating scale, used to select patients for reperfusion: www.nihstrokescale.org.

Endovascular thrombectomy: a new era in stroke therapy

Although early reperfusion with thrombolysis is extremely effective, only ¼ of those with large proximal intracranial vessel occlusion have a good outcome. Intra-arterial mechanical clot removal has revolutionized care in this group, with an unprecedented number needed to treat of <3 for improved outcomes (for anterior circulation events). CT angiography or MR angiography should be performed to assess suitability where thrombectomy is available (the main limiting factor is service provision, typically by interventional radiologists).

Who to refer Acute stroke with confirmed large vessel occlusion, no official severity cut-off especially if the occlusion is proximal, <6h of symptom onset (beneficial in anterior events 6–24h after careful selection with CT perfusion imaging).[4] **Procedure** A stent clot retriever is passed via the femoral artery. Usually under conscious sedation rather than general anaesthesia, but evidence is lacking. **Complications** In ~15%; vasospasm, arterial perforation/dissection, device misplacement.

Cardiac causes of stroke

Cardioembolic causes are the source of stroke in >30% of patients. The finding of infarcts in multiple arterial territories on imaging is particularly suggestive.

Non-valvular atrial fibrillation (p126) Associated with an overall risk of stroke of 4.5%/yr, and ischaemic strokes in AF carry a worse prognosis.

- **CHA₂DS₂VASC score** (p127) can be used to calculate risk of stroke in patients with AF. Offer anticoagulation in patients with a score of 2 or above. ►Take bleeding risk into account: calculate the risk of major bleeding using the HAS-BLED score. Caution and regular review of oral anticoagulants are required if the HAS-BLED score >3. ►Do not offer primary stroke prevention therapy in patients with AF if <65yrs and CHA₂DS₂VASC score is 0 for men or 1 for women.
- **Anticoagulation** (p346) commence within 48h after a minor or moderate stroke and 7 days after a major stroke, and immediately after TIA. Offer a direct oral anticoagulant (DOAC).

Other cardiac sources of emboli • Cardioversion. • Prosthetic valves. • Acute myocardial infarct with large left ventricular wall motion abnormalities on echocardiography. • Patent foramen ovale/septal defects (stroke cause by 'paradoxical emboli'). • Cardiac surgery. • Infective endocarditis (gives rise to septic emboli; 20% of those with endocarditis present with CNS signs).

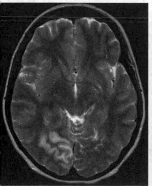
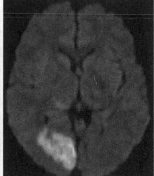

Fig 10.15 The T2-weighted (p730) image on the left shows oedema in the right occipital lobe. Differentials: infarct (right PCA), inflammation, or tumour. The diffusion-weighted image on the right shows restricted diffusion in the region, suggesting this is an infarct.

© Prof Peter Scally.

Bleeding within the brain parenchyma (versus intracranial haemorrhage, which refers to any bleeding within the cranial vault, p478, p476). ICH is the second most common form of stroke (accounting for 15%) and the most severe. The 1-month case fatality rate is 40% and <50% survive 1 year. Therapeutic nihilism is rife because of these harrowing statistics, but evidence in favour of aggressive management is amassing and undue care-limiting decisions in the early stages worsen outcomes.

▶ Offer full supportive care & postpone DNR orders until at least 24–48h in most cases.

Symptoms/signs Similar presentation to ischaemic stroke, but features of mass effect (headaches, vomiting, decreased level of consciousness, seizures) due to the haematoma are more suggestive of ICH.

Causes Traumatic ICH is by far the most common type and easily identified; the remainder in the absence of trauma or surgery are termed 'spontaneous'. • *Cerebral small vessel disease (85%)* rupture of small vessels damaged by hypertension or amyloid angiopathy (amyloid protein deposition in cortical arterioles) • *Underlying macrovascular or neoplastic cause (20%)* eg arteriovenous malformations, cavernomas (fig 10.16), aneurysms, venous thrombosis.

Diagnosis Acute evaluation as for ischaemic stroke (p466); the diagnosis is readily made on plain CT (fig 10.16). Perform vascular imaging (CT/MR angiography) when there is a suspicion of a macrovascular cause, + MRI and formal angiography if –ve.

Specific management General principles of acute management are the same as for ischaemic stroke, including multidisciplinary stroke unit care (p466), but consider:
• **Anticoagulation/antiplatelet therapy associated bleeds** Stop the offending agent in the short term. Reversal agents for anticoagulation should be administered as soon as possible (prothrombin complex concentrate for warfarin, specific reversal drugs for direct oral anticoagulants, eg andexanet alfa for factor Xa inhibitors, idarucizumab for dabigatran).
• **Acute BP lowering** IV antihypertensive treatment (eg labetalol, GTN) for all patients with systolic BP >150 and symptom onset <6h, targeting 130–140 mmHg.[5]
• **Referral for neurosurgery** Rapidly deteriorating patients with risk of brainstem compression from cerebellar ICH should be referred for urgent surgical evacuation/decompression. For patients with supratentorial ICH, early referral for craniotomy is recommended in some deteriorating, but not stable, patients. External ventricular drain insertion is offered for hydrocephalus, especially in the context of intraventricular extension/primary intraventricular haemorrhage.

Complications Haematoma expansion; seizures; perihaematomal oedema; hydrocephalus; hyperglycaemia; venous thromboembolism. Surveillance and early management is critical.

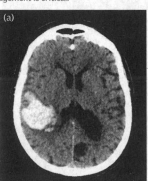
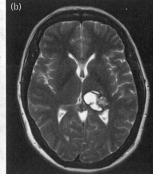

Fig 10.16 The axial plain CT (a) shows an acute large right temporoparietal primary ICH with some effacement of the right lateral ventricle. The T2-weighted MRI (b) shows a left thalamic cavernoma with intracapsular haemorrhage (secondary ICH). © Iain McGurgan

Temporary focal neurological symptoms caused by cerebral, retinal, or spinal cord ischaemia, without infarction. About 20% of stroke patients report a preceding TIA.

►Without intervention, 1 in 10 will go on to have a stroke within a week, so emergency investigation and management is imperative; all patients should be seen within 24 hours of onset of symptoms.

Symptoms/signs Abrupt onset of maximal symptoms specific to the arterial territory involved (p446); these should be the same as known stroke syndromes. TIAs usually last <1 hour. *Amaurosis fugax* occurs when the retinal artery is occluded, causing unilateral progressive vision loss 'like a curtain descending'. Attacks may be single or many; multiple highly stereotyped attacks ('crescendo' TIAs) suggest a critical intracranial stenosis (commonly the superior division of the MCA) or recurrent lacunar events due to disease of an internal capsule penetrating artery ('capsular warning syndrome').

Causes (As causes of ischaemic stroke, see p466.) Large-artery disease-induced TIAs have the highest risk of early stroke.

Differentials Over a half of TIA clinic referrals are mimics, but an overly dogmatic approach runs the risk of dismissing the not infrequent chameleons. Hypoglycaemia, migraine aura (p454), focal epilepsy (symptoms spread over seconds and often include twitching and jerking), hyperventilation, retinal bleeds can mimic TIA. *Global* events (eg syncope, dizziness, amnesia) are *not* typical of TIAs, but transient thalamic or brainstem ischaemia can cause loss of consciousness. Limb-shaking TIAs can occur in hemispheric hypoperfusion due to severe large artery stenosis. **Rare mimics of TIA** Malignant hypertension, MS (paroxysmal dysarthria), intracranial tumours, peripheral neuropathy, phaeochromocytoma, somatization.

Tests Routine CT is not recommended[5] in suspected TIA (where symptoms have resolved), unless there are clinical features suggesting ICH or another cause (head injury, headache, anticoagulation use, repetitive stereotyped events). Diffusion-weighted MRI ± vascular imaging (CT/MR angiography, or carotid Doppler if referral for endarterectomy is a possibility) are performed in the TIA clinic to confirm the diagnosis and establish the territory and cause if necessary. Blood tests and cardiac investigations as in the assessment of ischaemic stroke (p466).

Treatment Advise aspirin 300mg daily immediately in suspected cases (unless CT is required first to investigate for an alternative cause, as above) and refer urgently to the TIA clinic. Once the diagnosis is confirmed:
• **Antiplatelet drugs** Recent trial evidence supports acute dual antiplatelet therapy in TIA and minor stroke.[6] Commence aspirin & clopidogrel (both 75mg OD, in the place of aspirin 300mg if already started), switching to clopidogrel alone after 10–21 days.
• **Anticoagulation indications** Stop antiplatelet treatment and start anticoagulation if a cardioembolic source is confirmed (p467).
• **Urgent carotid endarterectomy** Perform within 2wks of first presentation if there is 70–99% stenosis,[7] the symptoms are referable to the carotid artery distribution, and operative risk is acceptable (higher risk in: ♀, >75yrs, ↑systolic BP, contralateral artery occluded; ipsilateral carotid syphon/external carotid stenosed). Do not stop aspirin preoperatively. Surgery is preferred to endovascular carotid artery angioplasty with stenting in those fit enough to tolerate due to higher peri-procedure stroke and mortality rates with stenting.
• **Commence other secondary prevention** (See p470.)

Driving Prohibited for at least 1 month, see p150.

Prognosis Risk of recurrent stroke in the 3 months after TIA is reduced by 80% with early initiation of secondary preventive treatment. Long-term risk of stroke or cardiovascular events following TIAs is dependent on the aetiology (worse for large-artery disease and cardioembolic TIA) underlying vascular risk factors.

7 Interventions for 50–69% stenoses can be justifiable; individualize risk and check local guidelines. In particular, check which criteria used to estimate degree of stenosis since NASCET (North American Symptomatic Carotid Endarterectomy Trial) criteria tend to include some more severe lesions in 50–69% range as compared to the ECST (European Carotid Surgery Trialists' Collaborative Group) criteria.

10 Neurology

More than 1 in 4 people with stroke have had a previous stroke or TIA.

Primary prevention (Ie before any TIA/stroke.)
Control risk factors (p466): look for and treat hypertension, DM, ↑lipids (p682), cardiac disease (see BOX 'Cardiac causes of stroke', p467) and help quit smoking (p85). Exercise helps (↑HDL, ↑glucose tolerance). Use *lifelong anticoagulation* in AF (see BOX 'Cardiac causes of stroke', p467) and prosthetic heart valves.

Secondary prevention (Ie preventing further strokes.) Accurate diagnosis of TIA/stroke subtype (see causes of ischaemic stroke, p466) is crucial for determining the best secondary prevention approach.

Perform further testing (See p466 for imaging.) Investigate promptly to identify the subtype and risk factors for further strokes. Look for:
• *Hypertension.* Check blood pressure and consider home or ambulatory measurement.
• *Cardiac source of emboli.* (See BOX 'Cardiac causes of stroke', p467.) 24h ECG to look for AF (p126), and more prolonged monitoring if this is negative and imaging is suggestive of a cardioembolic source. Echocardiogram may reveal an enlarged left atrium, mural thrombus due to AF, or a hypokinetic segment of cardiac muscle post-MI. It may also show valvular lesions in infective endocarditis, rheumatic heart disease, or atrial septal abnormalities (bubble study). Transoesophageal echo is more sensitive than transthoracic.
• *Carotid artery stenosis.* Do carotid Doppler US ± CT/MRI angiography (**fig 10.17**). Benefits and risks of revascularization should be individualized by an expert but generally most with ≥70% stenosis and life expectancy ≥5yrs will benefit while some (especially ♂) will benefit with 50–69% stenosis (p469).
• *Hypoglycaemia, hyperglycaemia, dyslipidaemia,* and *hyperhomocysteinaemia.*
• *Vasculitis.* ↑ESR, ANCA (p554). VDRL to look for active, untreated syphilis (p408).
• *Prothrombotic states,* eg thrombophilia (p370), antiphospholipid syndrome (p552).
• *Hyperviscosity,* eg polycythaemia (p362), sickle cell disease (p336).
• *Thrombocytopenia* and other bleeding disorders.
• *Genetic tests.* CADASIL (p466); Fabry disease (p316).

Commence secondary prevention treatment
• *Antihypertensive treatment.* Elevated BP is the strongest modifiable risk factor for stroke, and in stroke survivors, BP lowering reduces recurrent cerebrovascular events independently of the baseline BP. Initiate (or reinstate) antihypertensive therapy 24–48 hours after major stroke and immediately after minor stroke/TIA to target a BP of <130/<80mmHg.
• *Control modifiable risk factors.* (As 'Primary prevention'.)
• *Antiplatelet agents.* (See BOX 'Antiplatelets', and TIA treatment, p469.) If no primary haemorrhage on CT, give 2 weeks of aspirin 300mg, then switch to long-term clopidogrel monotherapy. If this is CI or not tolerated then give low dose aspirin plus slow-release dipyridamole (equally effective but dipyridamole has a poorer side effect profile).
• *Anticoagulation.* Commence in cardioembolic stroke; relative risk reduction of recurrent stroke of 60% (see BOX 'Cardiac causes of stroke', p467).
• *Cholesterol-lowering treatment.* Commence high-dose statin treatment (atorvastatin 80mg first line, if tolerated) regardless of baseline LDL.
• *Patent foramen ovale closure.* Percutaneous transcatheter device closure is more effective than medical therapy alone in cryptogenic cases (stroke with no established cause), at least in those aged ≤60yrs.[7]

Prognosis *Overall mortality:* 38 000/yr in the UK, 1 in 8 are fatal within 1 month. Age, stroke severity, and the aetiology (worst for cardioembolic and large artery) are the biggest predictors of prognosis. Avoid pressure ulcers (**fig 10.18**).

Antiplatelets: mechanism of action

Aspirin Inhibits COX-1, suppressing prostaglandin and thromboxane synthesis.

Clopidogrel A thienopyridine that inhibits platelet aggregation by modifying platelet ADP receptors, preventing further strokes and MIs.

Dipyridamole ↑cAMP and ↓thromboxane A2.

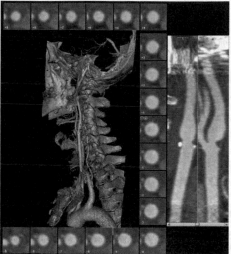

Fig 10.17 A digitally reformatted CT angiogram with magnified axial and coronal segments, showing a left internal carotid artery stenosis of 65% at the level of the carotid bifurcation.
© Iain McGurgan.

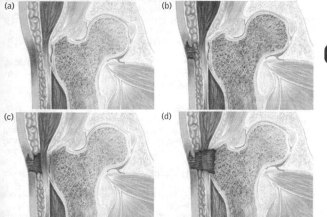

(a) (b)

(c) (d)

Fig 10.18 Categorization of pressure ulcers. (a) Stage 1: non-blanchable redness of intact skin, typically over a bony prominence. (b) Stage 2: partial-thickness loss of dermis presenting as a shallow open ulcer with a red/pink wound bed, without slough. May also present as an intact or open/ruptured serosanguinous blister. (c) Stage 3: full-thickness skin loss with visible subcutaneous fat. Bone, tendon, or muscle are not exposed. (d) Stage 4: full-thickness tissue loss with exposed bone, tendon, or muscle.

Images (a) to (d) reproduced from Gosney *et al. Managing older people in primary care*, 2009, with permission from Oxford University Press.

A large majority of people with stroke will survive the initial illness. Living with the long-term consequences of stroke exerts a great toll on survivors, their families, and healthcare systems. It is our role to ensure that this is a life worth living.

Principles of effective stroke rehabilitation
- Coordinated multidisciplinary care on a specialized stroke unit.
- Early commencement of dedicated stroke rehabilitation, beyond just the prevention of complications related to immobility.
- Input after discharge to consolidate inpatient gains and to help align the individual with their previous capability (early supported discharge/community rehab).
- The best outcomes are associated with high motivation among survivors and their families; preserving optimism to cultivate motivation and involving the carer/ spouse with all aspects of care-giving is key.
- Identify and quantify the level of impairment, set achievable goals that replicate the specific aims of the individual, and carefully monitor progress.

Prevention of complications
- Watch the patient swallow a small volume of water; if signs of *aspiration* (a cough or voice change) make NBM until formal assessment by a speech therapist. Use IV fluids, then semi-solids (eg jelly; avoid soups and crumbly food). Avoid early NG tube feeds; these may be needed to safeguard nutrition in those with swallowing problems that persist beyond the first 2–3d. If swallowing fails to recover, consider benefits of enteral feeding tube placement (p743). Speech therapists skilled in assessing swallowing difficulties are invaluable here.
- *Venous thromboembolism* prophylaxis for all stroke patients with limited mobility; thigh-length intermittent pneumatic compression at admission, plus low-molecular-weight heparin (except within 24h of thrombolysis, existing anticoagulation use, or ICH).
- Avoid further *injury:* minimize falls risk and take care when lifting the patient not to damage their shoulders.
- Ensure good *bladder and bowel* care through frequent toileting. Avoid early catheterization which may prevent return to continence.
- Position to minimize *spasticity* (occurs in ~40%). Get prompt physiotherapy. Splints and botulinum toxin injections are helpful for focal spasticity.
- Frequent monitoring, hygiene, and moisturizing for *pressure ulcer* prevention (fig 10.18, p471).
- Monitor mood: in pseudo-emotionalism/emotional lability (sobbing unprovoked by sorrow, from failure of cortical inhibition of the limbic system), an SSRI may help. Screen for and treat *post-stroke depression* early.

Rehabilitation interventions
- *Motor rehabilitation*. The majority of trials were neutral, but this could be a result of the challenges of delivering rehabilitation interventions in a standardized and blinded manner in trials.[8] Engage the patient in their own recovery by making physiotherapy fun. Swimming (a hemiplegic arm may be supported on a special float), music, and video games are all enjoyable and may ↑ recovery through promoting cerebral reorganization.
- *Cognitive rehabilitation*. Training can improve alertness and attention span for those with attention deficit.
- *Speech and language therapy*. Frequently used for aphasia and dysarthria, but there is a lack of supportive evidence.
- *Visual, sensory, continence impairment*. Interventions for improving sensory and visual impairment (eg compensatory techniques and prisms for field defects) and incontinence (eg bladder retraining, pelvic floor exercises) lack supportive evidence.

Tests. Asking to point to a named part of the body tests perceptual function. Copying matchstick patterns tests spatial ability. Copying a clock face tests for *constructional apraxia* (p70), miming actions such as brushing teeth for *ideomotor apraxia*, picking out and naming easy objects from a pile tests for *agnosia*.

End of life decisions. ►See p12.

Assessing dependence in daily life

Handicap entails inability to carry out social functions. 'A disadvantage for a given individual, resulting from an impairment or disability, that limits or prevents the fulfilment of a role.' Two people with the same *impairment* (eg paralysed arm) may have different *disabilities* (Barthel's Index of activities of daily living; eg one may be able to dress but the other cannot). Disabilities are likely to determine quality of future life. Treatment is often best aimed at reducing disability, not curing disease. For example, Velcro® fasteners in place of buttons may enable a person to dress.

Barthel's paradox

The more we contemplate Barthel's eulogy of independence, the more we see it as a mirage reflecting a greater truth about human affairs: ►there is no such thing as independence—only *interdependence*—and in fostering this interdependence lies our true vocation:

No man is an Island, intire of it selfe; every man is a peece of the Continent, a part of the maine; if a Clod bee washed away by the Sea, Europe is the lesse, as well as if a promontorie were, as well as if a Mannor of thy friends or of thine owne were. Any man's death diminishes me, because I am involved in mankinde; And therefore never send to know for whom the bell tolls: It tolls for thee.'

John Donne 1572-1631; *Meditation* XVII.

10 Neurology

Non-traumatic SAH is spontaneous bleeding into the subarachnoid space, often catastrophic (**table 10.8**) and accounts for 5–6% of stroke.

Incidence 8/100 000/yr (far higher in Japan and Finland); typical age: 35–65.

Symptoms Sudden-onset excruciating headache, typically occipital—like a 'thunderclap'. Vomiting, collapse, seizures, and coma often follow. Coma/drowsiness may last for days. Some patients report a preceding, 'sentinel' headache, perhaps due to a small warning leak from the offending aneurysm (~6%).

Signs Neck stiffness; Kernig's sign (takes 6h to develop); retinal, subhyaloid, and vitreous bleeds (= Terson's syndrome; ↑mortality ×5). Focal neurology at *presentation* may suggest site of aneurysm (eg pupil changes indicating a IIIrd nerve palsy with a posterior communicating artery aneurysm) or intracerebral haematoma. Later deficits suggest complications (see later in topic).

Causes • *Berry aneurysm rupture (80%).* Common sites: junctions of posterior communicating with the internal carotid (see **fig 10.3, p447**) or of the anterior communicating with the anterior cerebral artery, or bifurcation of the middle cerebral artery (**fig 10.19**). 15% are multiple. • *Arteriovenous malformations (15%).* • *Other causes:* encephalitis, vasculitis, tumour, amyloid angiopathy, idiopathic.

Risk factors Previous aneurysmal SAH (new aneurysms form, old ones get bigger), smoking, alcohol misuse, ↑BP, bleeding disorders, SBE (mycotic aneurysm), family history (3–5× ↑risk of SAH in close relatives). Polycystic kidneys, aortic coarctation, and Ehlers–Danlos syndrome (p143) are all associated with berry aneurysms.

Differentials Meningitis (p806), migraine (p454), intracerebral bleed, cortical vein thrombosis (p478), dissection of a carotid or vertebral artery, benign thunderclap headache (triggered by Valsalva manoeuvre, eg cough, coitus).

Tests • **Urgent** CT Detects >95% of SAH in the 1st 24h (**fig 10.20**), but sensitivity drops rapidly with elapsed time thereafter. • LP If CT −ve but the history is very suggestive of SAH (and no CI: p752). This needs to be done >12h after headache onset to allow breakdown of RBCs so that a positive sample is xanthochromic (yellow, due to bilirubin: differentiates between old blood from SAH vs a 'bloody tap').

Management ►Refer all proven SAH to neurosurgery immediately.
• *Re-examine CNS* often; chart BP, pupils, and GCS (p766). Repeat CT if deteriorating and monitor for vasospasm with CT/MR angiography or transcranial Doppler ultrasound.
• *Maintain cerebral perfusion* by keeping well hydrated, but aim for SBP <160mmHg.
• *Nimodipine* (60mg/4h PO for 3wks, or 1mg/h IVI) is a Ca²⁺ antagonist that reduces vasospasm and consequent morbidity from cerebral ischaemia.
• *Surgery:* endovascular coiling vs surgical clipping (requiring craniotomy): the decision depends on the accessibility and size of the aneurysm, though coiling is preferred where possible (fewer complications, better outcomes). Do catheter or CT angiography to identify single vs multiple aneurysms *before* intervening. Newer techniques such as balloon remodelling, flow diversion, and new embolic materials can be helpful in anatomically challenging aneurysms.

Complications *Rebleeding* is the commonest cause of death, and occurs in 10%, often in the 1st few days. *Cerebral ischaemia* due to vasospasm may cause a permanent CNS deficit, and is the commonest cause of morbidity. If this happens, surgery is not helpful at the time but may be so later. *Hydrocephalus*, due to blockage of arachnoid granulations, requires a ventricular or lumbar drain. *Hyponatraemia* is common, usually due to syndrome of inappropriate secretion of antidiuretic hormone (SIADH, p235), but should not be managed with fluid restriction as this can prompt vasospasm. Seek expert help.

Table 10.8 Mortality in subarachnoid haemorrhage, according to Hunt and Hess grade

Grade	Signs	Mortality: %
I	None	0
II	Neck stiffness and cranial nerve palsies	11
III	Drowsiness	37
IV	Drowsy with hemiplegia	71
V	Prolonged coma	100

Most mortality occurs in 1st month. 90% of survivors of the 1st month, survive >1 year.

Unruptured aneurysms: 'the time-bomb in my head'

Bear in mind the old adage: 'if it ain't broke, don't fix it'—usually, risks of *preventive* intervention outweigh any benefits, except perhaps in • young patients (more years at risk, and surgery is twice as hazardous if >45yrs old) who have • aneurysms >7mm in diameter, especially if located at the • junction of the internal carotid and the posterior communicating cerebral artery, or at the • rostral basilar artery bifurcation, and especially if there is • uncontrolled hypertension or a • past history of bleeds. Data from the 2003 International Study of Unruptured Intracranial Aneurysms (ISUIA) show that relative risk of rupture for an aneurysm 7–12mm across is 3.3 compared with aneurysms <7mm across; if the diameter is >12mm, the relative risk is 17.

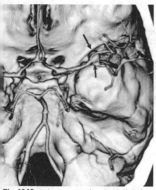

Fig 10.19 CT images can be manipulated to show only high-density structures such as bones and arteries containing contrast. Here is a middle cerebral artery aneurysm.

© Prof Peter Scally.

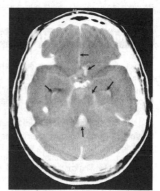

Fig 10.20 Blood from a ruptured aneurysm occupies the interhemispheric fissure (top arrow), a crescentic intracerebral area presumably near the aneurysm (2nd arrow), the basal cisterns, the lateral ventricles (temporal horns), and the 4th ventricle (bottom arrow). © Prof Peter Scally.

Subdural haematoma

►Consider this very treatable condition in all whose conscious level fluctuates, and also in those having an 'evolving stroke', especially if on anticoagulants. Bleeding is from bridging veins between cortex and venous sinuses (vulnerable to deceleration injury), resulting in accumulating haematoma between dura and arachnoid. This gradually raises ICP, shifting midline structures away from the side of the clot and, if untreated, leads to eventual tentorial herniation and coning. Most subdurals are from trauma but the trauma is *often forgotten as it was so minor or so long ago* (up to 9 months; chronic subdurals). It can also occur without trauma (eg ↓ICP; dural metastases). The elderly are most susceptible, as brain atrophy makes bridging veins vulnerable. *Other risk factors:* falls (epileptics, alcoholics); anticoagulation.

Symptoms Fluctuating level of consciousness (seen in 35%) ± insidious physical or intellectual slowing, sleepiness, headache, personality change, unsteadiness, and occasionally seizures.

Signs ↑ICP (p814), seizures. Localizing neurological symptoms (eg unequal pupils, hemiparesis) occur late, often >1 month after the injury.

Differentials Stroke, dementia, CNS masses (eg tumours, abscesses).

Imaging (fig 10.21) CT/MRI shows clot ± midline shift (but beware bilateral isodense clots). Look for crescent-shaped collection of blood over one hemisphere. The sickle shape differentiates subdural blood from extradural haemorrhage.

Management Reverse clotting abnormalities urgently. Surgical management depends on the size of the clot, its chronicity, and the clinical picture: generally those >10mm or with midline shift >5mm need evacuating (via craniotomy or burr hole washout). Address the cause of the trauma (eg falls, abuse).

Prognosis Often favourable, but mortality rates are as high as 50% in those requiring surgery for acute subdurals.

Extradural (epidural) haematoma

►Beware deteriorating consciousness after any head injury that initially produced no loss of consciousness or after initial drowsiness post injury seems to have resolved. This *lucid interval* pattern is typical of extradural bleeds.

Cause ►Suspect after any traumatic skull fracture. Often due to a fractured temporal or parietal bone causing laceration of the middle meningeal artery and vein, typically after trauma to a temple just lateral to the eye. Any tear in a dural venous sinus will also result in an extradural bleed. Blood accumulates between bone and dura.

Clinical features The lucid interval may last a few hours to a few days before a bleed declares itself by ↓GCS from rising ICP. Increasingly severe headache, vomiting, confusion, and seizures follow, ± hemiparesis with brisk reflexes and an upgoing plantar. If bleeding continues, the ipsilateral pupil dilates, coma deepens, bilateral limb weakness develops, and breathing becomes deep and irregular (brainstem compression). Death follows a period of coma and is due to respiratory arrest. Bradycardia and ↑BP are late signs.

Differentials Epilepsy, carotid dissection, carbon monoxide poisoning.

Tests CT (fig 10.22) shows a haematoma (often biconvex/lens-shaped; the blood forms a more rounded shape compared with the sickle-shaped subdural haematoma as the tough dural attachments to the skull keep it more localized). Skull x-ray may be normal or show fracture lines crossing the course of the middle meningeal vessels. ►*Lumbar puncture is contraindicated.*

Management Stabilize and transfer urgently (with skilled medical and nursing escorts) to a neurosurgical unit for clot evacuation ± ligation of the bleeding vessel. Care of the airway in an unconscious patient and measures to ↓ICP often require intubation and ventilation (+ mannitol IVI, p815).

Prognosis Excellent if diagnosis and operation early. Poor if coma, pupil abnormalities, or decerebrate rigidity are present pre-op.

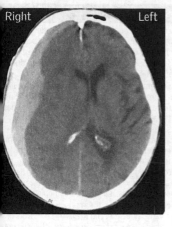

Fig 10.21 This image explains the cause as well as the pathology. On the patient's left, cerebral sulci are prominent and prior to this adverse event would have been even larger. The brain had shrunk within the skull as a result of atherosclerosis, and poor perfusion, leaving large subarachnoid spaces. A simple, quick rotation of the head is enough to tear a bridging vein, causing this *acute subdural haematoma*.

© Prof Peter Scally.

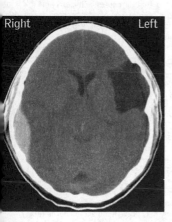

Fig 10.22 The blood (high attenuation, fusiform or biconvex collection) on the right side is limited anteriorly by the coronal suture and posteriorly by the lambdoid suture. This is therefore an *extradural haematoma*. The low-attenuation CSF density collection on the left is causing scalloping of the overlying bone. It is in the typical location of an arachnoid cyst; an incidental finding of a congenital abnormality.

© Prof Peter Scally.

Cerebral venous thrombosis (CVT)

Thrombosis of the cerebral sinuses or veins causes cerebral infarction, though much less commonly than arterial disease. Seizures are common and focal; they can complicate diagnosis and post-ictal drowsiness may impair GCS assessment. Although ~80% will make a good functional recovery, death is mainly due to transtentorial herniation from mass effect or oedema.[8] ♀:♂ ≥3:1.

Dural venous sinus thrombosis Most commonly sagittal sinus thrombosis (**figs 10.23**, 10.24; 47% of all CVT) or transverse sinus thrombosis (35%). Sagittal sinus thrombosis often coexists if other sinuses are thrombosed. Symptom onset is gradual (over days or weeks). Features are dependent on the sinus affected:
• **Sagittal sinus** Headache, vomiting, seizures, ↓vision, papilloedema.
• **Transverse sinus** Headache ± mastoid pain, focal CNS signs, seizures, papilloedema.
• **Sigmoid sinus** Cerebellar signs, lower cranial nerve palsies.
• **Inferior petrosal sinus** Vth and VIth cranial nerve palsies, with temporal and retro-orbital pain (Gradenigo's syndrome, suggesting otitis media is the cause).
• **Cavernous sinus** Often due to spread from facial pustules or folliculitis, causing headache, chemosis, oedematous eyelids, proptosis, painful ophthalmoplegia, fever.

Cortical vein thrombosis Usually occurs with a sinus thrombus as it extends into the cortical veins, causing infarction in a venous territory (**fig 10.25**). These infarcts give rise to stroke-like focal symptoms that develop over days. There are often seizures and an associated headache which may come on suddenly (thunderclap headache).

Causes Numerous, including anything that promotes a hypercoagulable state (p370). **Common causes** Pregnancy/puerperium, combined OCP, head injury, dehydration, blood dyscrasias, tumours (local invasion/pressure), extracranial malignancy (hypercoagulability), recent LP. **Other causes** Infection (meningitis, abscesses, otitis media, cerebral malaria, TB). Drugs (eg antifibrinolytics, androgens), SLE, vasculitis, Crohn's or UC.

Differential diagnosis Subarachnoid haemorrhage, meningitis, encephalitis, intracranial abscess, arterial infarction, idiopathic intracranial hypertension (p478).

Investigations Exclude subarachnoid haemorrhage (if thunderclap headache p474) and meningitis (p806). **Bloods** Thrombophilia screen. **Imaging** CT/MRI venography may show the absence of a sinus (**fig 10.23**), though an absent transverse sinus can be a normal variant. MRI T2-weighted gradient echo sequences can visualize thrombus directly (**fig 10.24**), and also identify haemorrhagic infarction. CT may be normal early, but show a filling defect at ~1wk (delta sign). LP (if no CI): raised opening pressure. CSF may be normal, or show RBCs and xanthochromia.

Management Anticoagulation with heparin or LMWH, and long-term prevention with a DOAC or warfarin (INR 2–3) for 3–6 months (up to 12 months if unprovoked CVT). If there is deterioration despite adequate anticoagulation, endovascular thrombolysis or mechanical thrombectomy may provide limited benefit (but not in those with large infarcts and impending herniation). ↑ICP requires prompt attention (p814); decompressive hemicraniectomy may prevent impending herniation.

Idiopathic intracranial hypertension

Think of this in those presenting with symptoms of ↑ICP (headache, vision loss, papilloedema)—*when no cause is found*. Most commonly seen in obese females in 3rd decade, who present with narrowed visual fields, blurred vision ± diplopia, VIth nerve palsy, and an enlarged blind spot, if papilloedema is present (it usually is). Opening pressure on LP is usually >25cmH$_2$O.

Associations Endocrine abnormalities (Cushing's syndrome, hypoparathyroidism, ↑↓TSH, SLE, CKD, PRV, IDA, drugs (tetracycline, steroids, nitrofurantoin, and oral contraceptives).

Management Weight loss, acetazolamide (avoid in pregnancy) or topiramate, loop diuretics. Consider ventriculoperitoneal shunt or optic nerve sheath fenestration if drugs fail and visual loss worsens. Venous sinus stenting is under investigation.

Prognosis R$_x$ can often be tapered/withdrawn. Permanent significant visual loss in 10%.

8 Predictors of poor prognosis include: GCS score on admission <9, deep CVT location, CNS infection, malignancy, intracranial haemorrhage, mental status abnormality, age >37 years, and ♂.

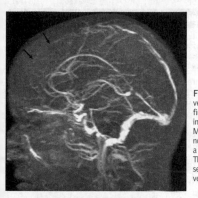

Fig 10.23 This magnetic resonance venogram (MRV) could look normal at first glance: the hardest thing to see in imaging is often that which is not there. Much of the superior sagittal sinus is not seen because it is filled with clot—a superior sagittal sinus thrombosis. The arrows point to where it should be seen. Posteriorly, the irregularity of the vessel indicates non-occlusive clot.

© Prof P. Scally.

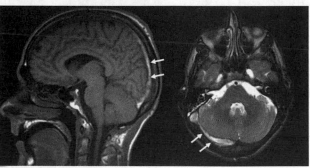

Fig 10.24 MRI showing thrombus (arrows) in the sagittal sinus (sagittal T1-weighted image, LEFT), and in the right transverse sinus (axial T2-weighted image, RIGHT). Often more than one sinus is involved.   © Prof David Werring.

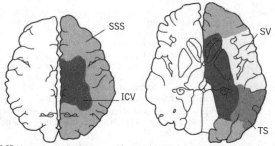

Fig 10.25 Venous territories (compare with arterial territories on p447). SSS—superior sagittal sinus; TS—transverse sinus; SV—Sylvian veins; ICV—internal cortical veins.

There is much greater variation in venous anatomy between individuals than there is in arterial anatomy, so this diagram is only a rough guide. The key point is to realize that infarction that crosses boundaries between arterial territories may be venous in origin.

Delirium (acute confusional state)

Delirium[9] affects up to 50% of inpatients >65yrs, and is associated with a longer admission, more complications, and higher mortality. ►Look for an underlying cause in *any* acute fluctuating, baffling behaviour change; it may be an early indication of treatable pathology (eg UTI).

Clinical features Globally impaired cognition, perception, and consciousness which develops over hours/days, characterized by a marked memory deficit, disordered or disorientated thinking, and reversal of the sleep–wake cycle. Some patients experience tactile or visual hallucinations. Delirium can be: • *hyperactive*, with restlessness, mood lability, agitation, or aggression • *hypoactive* in which the patient becomes slow and withdrawn or • *mixed*. ►Hypoactive and mixed delirium are much harder to recognize: it is crucial to compare current behaviour to the patient's baseline (see BOX).

Risk factors >65yrs, dementia/previous cognitive impairment, hip fracture, acute illness, psychological agitation (eg pain).

Causes
• Surgery/post-GA.
• Systemic infection: pneumonia, UTI, malaria, wounds, IV lines.
• Intracranial infection or head injury.
• Drugs/drug withdrawal: opiates, levodopa, sedatives, recreational.
• Alcohol withdrawal (2–5d post-admission; ↑LFTs, ↑MCV; history of alcohol abuse).
• Metabolic: uraemia, liver failure, Na+ or ↑↓glucose, ↓Hb, malnutrition (beriberi, p240).
• Hypoxia: respiratory or cardiac failure.
• Vascular: stroke, myocardial infarction.
• Nutritional: thiamine, nicotinic acid, or B_{12} deficiency.

Differentials Dementia (see BOX), anxiety, epilepsy: ►non-convulsive status epilepticus is an underdiagnosed cause of impaired cognition and odd behaviour: consider an EEG. Primary mental illness (eg schizophrenia) can also mimic delirium, but this is rare on the wards (especially if no past history).

Tests Look for the cause (eg UTI, pneumonia, MI): do FBC, U&E, LFT, blood glucose, ABG, septic screen (urine dipstick, CXR, blood cultures); also consider ECG, malaria films, LP, EEG, CT.

Management As well as identifying and treating the underlying cause, aim to:
• Reorientate the patient: explain where they are and who you are at each encounter. Hunt down hearing aids/glasses. Visible clocks/calendars may help.
• Encourage visits from friends and family.
• Monitor fluid balance and encourage oral intake. Be vigilant for constipation.
• Mobilize and encourage physical activity.
• Practise sleep hygiene: restrict daytime napping, minimize night-time disturbance.
• Avoid or remove catheters, IV cannulae, monitoring leads and other devices (they increase infection risk and may get pulled out).
• Watch out for infection and physical discomfort/distress.
• Review medication and discontinue any unnecessary agents. Only use sedation if the patient is a risk to their own/other patients' safety (never use physical restraints). Consider short-term haloperidol 0.5–2mg PO if they will take it, IM if not (p15). Wait 20min to judge effect—further doses can be given if needed.
  NB: avoid in those with Parkinson's disease or Lewy body dementia.

►Be aware that delirium may persist beyond the duration of the original illness by several weeks in the elderly. Do not assume this must be dementia—provide support and reassess 1–2 months later.

9 Delirium, from the Latin *de* (from) and *lira* (ridge between furrows), meaning 'out of one's furrow'.

Delirium vs dementia

One is often mistaken for the other, yet perhaps the interconnectedness of these two conditions is greater than we realize: not only is dementia the leading risk factor for delirium, but delirium itself confers a greater risk of subsequently developing dementia.[9] It is likely that this is due to a number of factors: delirium is a marker of vulnerability of the brain, and may also emphasize previously unrecognized dementia symptoms. Furthermore, there may be direct causation through the noxious insults incurred during an episode of delirium, which can lead to permanent neuronal damage.

In distinguishing the two conditions (not always an easy task), the presence of inattention, distractibility, and disorganized thinking will all point you towards delirium. But the fundamental question is 'Has there been an *acute* change from the patient's cognitive baseline?' Family or carer collateral reports are invaluable, but may not always be available. Document cognition in all patients >65yrs admitted to hospital (eg AMTS, **p61**, many admission proformas allow for this). This will then allow you to compare their admission score with subsequent assessments and track any improvements, deteriorations, or fluctuations in cognition throughout the admission.

A neurodegenerative syndrome with progressive decline in several cognitive domains. The initial presentation is usually of memory loss over months or years (►look for other causes if over days/weeks). Prevalence increases with age: 20% of people >80yrs are known to have dementia, yet probably only half of cases are diagnosed.

Diagnosis Is made by: *History* from the patient with a thorough collateral narrative—ask about the timeline of decline and the domains affected. Non-cognitive symptoms such as agitation, aggression, or apathy indicate late disease. *Cognitive testing:* use a validated dementia screen such as the AMTS (p61) or similar, plus short tests of executive function and language. Carry out a mental state examination to identify anxiety, depression, or hallucinations. *Examination* may identify a physical cause, risk factors (eg for vascular dementia), or parkinsonism. *Medication review* is important to exclude drug-induced cognitive impairment.

Investigations Look for reversible/organic causes: ↓TSH/↓B₁₂/↓folate (treat low-normals, p330), ↓thiamine (eg alcohol), ↓Ca²⁺. Check MSU, FBC, ESR, U&E, LFT, and glucose. An MRI (preferred to CT) can identify other reversible pathologies (eg subdural haematoma, p476; normal-pressure hydrocephalus[10]), as well as underlying vascular damage or structural pathology. Functional imaging (FDG, PET, SPECT) may help delineate subtypes where diagnosis is not clear. Consider EEG in: suspected delirium, frontotemporal dementia, CJD, or a seizure disorder. If clinically indicated then check autoantibodies, syphilis, HIV, CJD, or other rare causes (see later in topic).

Subtypes • **Alzheimer's disease (AD)** See p484. • **Vascular dementia** (~25%.) Cumulative effect of many small strokes: sudden onset and stepwise deterioration is characteristic (but often hard to recognize). Look for evidence of arteriopathy (↑BP, past strokes, focal CNS signs). ►Do not use acetylcholinesterase inhibitors or memantine in these patients. • **Lewy body dementia** (15–25%.) Fluctuating cognitive impairment, detailed visual hallucinations, and later, parkinsonism (p490). Histology is characterized by Lewy bodies (eosinophilic intracytoplasmic inclusion bodies) in brainstem and neocortex. ►Avoid using antipsychotics in Lewy body dementia (↑↑risk of SE, see p485). • **Frontotemporal dementia** Frontal and temporal atrophy with loss of >70% of spindle neurons. Patients display executive impairment; behavioural/personality change; disinhibition; hyperorality; stereotyped behaviour; and emotional unconcern. Episodic memory and spatial orientation are preserved until later stages. *Pick's disease* refers to the few frontotemporal dementia patients who have Pick inclusion bodies on histology (spherical clusters of tau-laden neurons).

Other causes Alcohol/drug abuse; repeated head trauma; pellagra (p240); Whipple's disease (p263); Huntington's (p464); CJD (BOX); Parkinson's (p490); HIV; cryptococcosis (p404); familial autosomal dominant Alzheimer's; CADASIL (p466).

Management ►Refer suspected or diagnosed dementia to integrated memory services for further assessment and management. **Medication** (p485). Avoid drugs that impair cognition (eg neuroleptics, sedatives, tricyclics). **Non-pharmacological interventions** Non-cognitive symptoms (eg agitation) may respond to measures such as aromatherapy, multisensory stimulation, massage, music, and animal-assisted therapy.

Other considerations • **Depression** Common. Try an SSRI (eg citalopram 10–20mg OD) or, if severe, mirtazapine (15–45mg at night if eGFR >40). Cognitive behavioural therapy can help with social withdrawal and catastrophic thinking. • **Capacity** Can the patient make decisions regarding medical or financial affairs? Wherever possible, allow them to. Suggest making an advanced directive or appointing a Lasting Power of Attorney in the early stages of the disease.

---

10 Dilated ventricles *without* enlarged sulci. *Signs:* gait apraxia, incontinence, dementia; CSF shunts help.

Creutzfeldt-Jakob disease (CJD)

The cause is a prion (PrPSC), a misfolded form of a normal protein (PrPC), that can transform other proteins into prion proteins (hence its infectivity). ↑PrPSC leads to spongiform changes (tiny cavities ± tubulovesicular structures) in the brain. Most cases are *sporadic* (incidence: 1–3/million/yr). *Variant* CJD (VCJD; ≈235 cases worldwide) is transmitted via contaminated CNS tissue affected by bovine spongiform encephalopathy. **Inherited forms** (eg Gerstmann–Sträussler–Scheinker syndrome, P102L mutation in PRNP gene with ataxia ± self-mutilation), the 'normal' protein is too unstable, readily transforming to PrPSC. **Iatrogenic causes** Contaminated surgical instruments, corneal transplants, growth hormone from human pituitaries, and blood (VCJD only). Prion protein resists sterilization. **Signs** ►CJD should be considered in all patients presenting with *rapidly progressive dementia*, especially if accompanied by myoclonus (present in 95%), depression, eye signs (diplopia, supranuclear palsies, complex visual disturbances, homonymous field defects, hallucinations, cortical blindness). **Tests** MRI; EEG (periodic sharp wave complexes); CSF markers (RT-QUIC is 92% sensitive and 100% specific,[10] 14-3-3 protein), MRI. **Treatment** None proven. Death occurs in ~6 months in sporadic CJD.

Who will care for the carers?

Our ageing population and improvements in medicine mean that we not only have an increasing number of people with dementia in the UK, but that those people are living longer with the disease in more advanced stages. Their needs become more complex and they become increasingly dependent. Currently, informal (mostly family) carers of people with dementia save the UK £11 billion a year. Yet this is not an easy task: most dementia sufferers display behavioural or psychological symptoms, which can be particularly distressing for the carer. Carer stress is inevitable and causes ↑morbidity and mortality. Ameliorate this with:

- *A care coordinator* (via Social Services or the local Old Age Community Mental Healthcare Team); vital to coordinate the various teams and services available:
  - Laundry services for soiled linen.
  - Car badge giving priority parking.
  - Help from occupational therapist, district nurses, and community psychiatric nurses.
  - Attendance allowance.
  - Respite care in hospital.
  - Council tax rebate (forms from local council office).
- *Day services* can be invaluable for stimulating patients and providing regular, much-needed breaks for carers.
- *Moral support*: support groups, telephone helplines, and charities can all ease the burden, eg UK Alzheimer's Disease Society.
- *Combatting challenging behaviour*: first rule out pain, infection, and depression. Then consider trazodone (50–300mg at night) or lorazepam (0.5–1mg/12–24h PO). Haloperidol (0.5–4mg) can be useful in the short term.

This leading cause of dementia is *the* big neuropsychiatric disorder of our times, dominating the care of the elderly and the lives of their families who give up work, friends, and ways of life to support relatives through the long final years as they exit into their '*worlds of preoccupied emptiness*'. Suspect AD in adults >40yrs with persistent,[11] progressive, and *global* cognitive impairment: visuospatial skill, memory, verbal abilities, and executive function (planning) are all affected, unlike other dementias which may affect certain domains but not others (identify which with neuropsychometric tests). There is also anosognosia—a lack of insight into the problems engendered by the disease, eg missed appointments, misunderstood conversations or plots of films, and mishandling of money. Later there may be irritability; mood disturbance (depression or euphoria); behavioural change (eg aggression, wandering, disinhibition); psychosis (hallucinations or delusions); agnosia (may not recognize self in the mirror). There is no standard natural history. Cognitive impairment is progressive, but non-cognitive symptoms may come and go over months. Eventually many patients become sedentary, taking little interest in anything.

Cause Environmental and genetic factors both play a role. Accumulation of β-amyloid peptide, a degradation product of amyloid precursor protein, results in progressive neuronal damage, neurofibrillary tangles, ↑numbers of amyloid plaques, and loss of the neurotransmitter acetylcholine (**fig 10.26**). Neuronal loss is selective—the hippocampus, amygdala, temporal neocortex, and subcortical nuclei are most vulnerable. Vascular effects are also important—95% of AD patients show evidence of vascular dementia.

Risk factors 1st-degree relative with AD; Down's syndrome (in which AD is inevitable, often <40yrs); homozygosity for apolipoprotein E (APOE) E4 allele; PICALM, CLI1 & CLU variants; vascular risk factors (↑BP, diabetes, dyslipidaemia, ↑homocysteine, AF); ↓physical/cognitive activity; depression; loneliness (↑risk × 2; simply living alone is not a risk factor); smoking.

Management ►See p482 for a general approach to management in dementia. • Refer to a specialist memory service. • Acetylcholinesterase inhibitors (see BOX 'Pharmacological treatment'). • BP control (in heart failure there is a 2× ↑risk of AD; extra risk halves with BP control).

Prevention in the context of AD's time course Changes in CSF β-amyloid are seen ~25yrs before onset of unequivocal symptoms (USY) and its deposition is detected 15yrs before USY. CSF tau protein and brain atrophy are also detected 15yrs before USY. Cerebral hypometabolism and impaired episodic memory occur 10yrs before USY. Global cognitive impairment occurs 5yrs before USY. Prevention will probably be most effective before any of this starts—though there is currently insufficient evidence to recommend any specific interventions. Ultimately, there is no simple relationship between brain structure, neurofibrillary tangles, and function.

Prognosis Mean survival = 7yrs from USY.

11 'Enduring' doesn't mean unfluctuating: cognition comes and goes, allowing poetic insights, as in Iris Murdoch's poignant self-diagnosis: 'I am sailing into the dark'.

There is overlap between Lewy body dementia, AD, and Parkinson's disease (PD), complicating treatment decisions: levodopa (p491) can precipitate delusions, and antipsychotic drugs worsen PD. Rivastigmine may help all three.

Acetylcholinesterase (ACHE) inhibitors Donepezil, rivastigmine, and galantamine are all modestly effective in treating AD and are recommended by NICE, though none should be used in mild disease and they should be discontinued if there is no worthwhile effect on symptoms. Doses:
- Donepezil: initially 5mg PO, eg doubled after 1 month.
- Rivastigmine: 1.5mg/12h initially, ↑ to 3–6mg/12h. Patches are also available.
- Galantamine: initially 4mg/12h, ↑ to 8–12mg/12h PO.

►The cholinergic effects of acetylcholinesterase inhibitors may exacerbate peptic ulcer disease and heart block. Ask about symptoms and do an ECG first.

Antiglutamatergic treatment Memantine (an NMDA antagonist, p445) is reasonably effective in late-stage AD, and is recommended in patients with severe disease or those with moderate disease in which ACHE inhibitors are not tolerated/CI. *Dose:* 5mg/24h initially, ↑ by 5mg/d weekly to 10mg/12h. *SE:* hallucinations, confusion, hypertonia, hypersexuality.

Amyloid-beta monoclonal antibodies Aducanumab (monthly IV infusion) was a promising development that has been controversially approved by the US FDA, but refused in Europe in view of weak supportive evidence in mild PET-confirmed AD. There is more promising recent evidence for lecanemab, but both are associated with amyloid-related imaging abnormalities (oedema or haemorrhage).

Antipsychotics Consider in severe, non-cognitive symptoms only (eg psychosis or extreme agitation). ►Possible increased risk of stroke/TIA so discuss risks and assess cerebrovascular risk factors. Avoid in mild-to-moderate: Lewy body dementia (risk of neuroleptic sensitivity reactions), AD, and vascular dementia.

Vitamin supplementation Trials of dietary and vitamin supplements have been mixed and disappointing. Perhaps the best evidence exists for vitamin E (2000IU OD) which may confer a modest benefit in delaying functional progression in mild-to-moderate AD, but with no effect on cognitive performance.

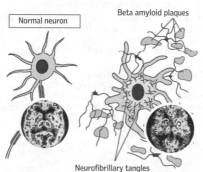

Fig 10.26 Normal neuron (left) and one exhibiting senile plaques and neurofibrillary tangles (right). The corresponding changes on functional neuroimaging are also shown.

Epilepsy is a recurrent tendency to spontaneous, intermittent, abnormal electrical activity in part of the brain, manifesting as *seizures*. *Convulsions* are the motor signs of electrical discharges.

Elements of a seizure Some patients may experience a preceding *prodrome* lasting hours or days in which there may be a change in mood or behaviour. An *aura* implies a focal seizure, often, but not necessarily, from the temporal lobe. It may be a strange feeling in the gut, an experience such as *déjà vu* or strange smells or flashing lights. *Post-ictally* there may be headache, confusion, and myalgia; or temporary weakness after a focal seizure in the motor cortex (Todd's palsy, p696), or dysphasia following a focal seizure in the temporal lobe.

Causes ⅔ are idiopathic. **Structural** Cortical scarring (eg head injury years before onset), developmental (eg dysembryoplastic neuroepithelial tumour or cortical dysgenesis), space-occupying lesion, stroke, hippocampal sclerosis (eg after a febrile convulsion), vascular malformations. **Others** Tuberous sclerosis, sarcoidosis, SLE, PAN, antibodies to voltage-gated potassium channels.

Diagnosis Can be difficult due to the heterogeneous nature of the disease (there are >40 different types of epilepsy). NICE estimate 5–30% of people with 'epilepsy' have been wrongly diagnosed. ▶All patients with a seizure must be referred for specialist assessment and investigation in <2wks.

Take a thorough history Including a detailed description from a witness. Ask specifically about tongue-biting and a slow recovery. If this is a first seizure, enquire about past funny turns/odd behaviour. Déjà vu and odd episodic feelings of fear may well be relevant. Are there any triggers (eg alcohol, stress, flickering lights/ TV)? Triggered attacks tend to recur.

Establish the type of seizure See BOX 'Seizure classification'. ▶Don't forget psychogenic non-epileptic seizures (p460).

Rule out provoking causes Most people would have a seizure given sufficient provocation (eg reflex anoxic seizures in faints) but would not be classed as epileptic: only 3–10% of provoked seizures recur; generally when the provocation is irreversible. *Causes:* trauma; stroke; haemorrhage; ↑ICP; alcohol or benzodiazepine withdrawal; metabolic disturbance (hypoxia, ↑↓Na^+, ↓Ca^{2+}, ↑↓glucose, uraemia, liver disease); infection (eg meningitis, encephalitis); ↑T°; drugs (tricyclics, cocaine). ▶Unprovoked seizures have a recurrence rate of 30–50%.

Investigations Look for provoking causes. Consider an EEG: it cannot exclude epilepsy and can be falsely +ve, so don't do one if simple syncope is the likely diagnosis. Only do *emergency* EEGs if non-convulsive status is the problem. Other tests: MRI (structural lesions); drug levels (if on anti-epileptics: is the patient adherent?); drugs screen; LP (eg if infection suspected).

Counselling After any 'fit', advise about dangers, eg swimming, driving, heights until the diagnosis is known; then give *individualized* counselling on employment, sport, insurance, and conception (*OHCS* p32). The patient must contact DVLA and avoid driving until seizure-free for >1yr, or >6mths for a one-off awake seizure (p151).

Seizure classification

Focal seizures Originating within networks linked to one hemisphere and often seen with underlying structural disease. Various subclasses include:
- **Without impairment of consciousness** (Previously described as 'simple'.) Awareness is unimpaired, with focal motor, sensory (olfactory, visual, etc.), autonomic, or psychic symptoms. No post-ictal symptoms.
- **With impairment of consciousness** (Previously described as 'complex'.) Awareness is impaired—either at seizure onset or following a simple partial aura. Most commonly arise from the temporal lobe, in which post-ictal confusion is a feature.
- **Evolving to a bilateral, convulsive seizure** (Previously described as 'secondary generalized'.) In ⅔ of patients with partial seizures, the electrical disturbance, which starts focally, spreads widely, causing a generalized seizure, which is typically convulsive.

Generalized seizures Originating at some point within, and rapidly engaging bilaterally distributed networks leading to simultaneous onset of widespread electrical discharge with no localizing features referable to a single hemisphere. Important subtypes include:
- **Absence seizures** Brief (≤10s) pauses, eg suddenly stops talking in mid-sentence, then carries on where left off. Presents in childhood.
- **Tonic-clonic seizures** Loss of consciousness. Limbs stiffen (tonic), then jerk (clonic). May have one without the other. Post-ictal confusion and drowsiness.
- **Myoclonic seizures** Sudden jerk of a limb, face, or trunk. The patient may be thrown suddenly to the ground, or have a violently disobedient limb: one patient described it as *'my flying-saucer epilepsy'*, as crockery which happened to be in the hand would take off.
- **Atonic (akinetic) seizures** Sudden loss of muscle tone causing a fall, no LOC.
- **Infantile spasms** (*OHCS* p232) Commonly associated with tuberous sclerosis.

NB: the classification of epileptic syndromes is separate to the classification of seizures, and is based on seizure type, age of onset, EEG findings, and other features such as family history.

10 Neurology

Localizing features of focal seizures

Temporal lobe • Automatisms—complex motor phenomena with impaired awareness, varying from primitive oral (lip smacking, chewing, swallowing) or manual movements (fumbling, fiddling, grabbing), to complex actions. • Dysphasia. •*Déjà vu* (when everything seems strangely familiar), or *jamais vu* (everything seems strangely unfamiliar). • Emotional disturbance, eg sudden terror, panic, anger, or elation, and derealization (out-of-body experiences). • Hallucinations of smell, taste, or sound. • Delusional behaviour. • Bizarre associations—eg 'Canned music at Tesco always makes me cry and then pass out'.

Frontal lobe • Motor features such as posturing or peddling movements of the legs. • Jacksonian march (a spreading focal motor seizure with retained awareness, often starting with the face or a thumb). • Motor arrest. • Subtle behavioural disturbances (often diagnosed as psychogenic). • Dysphasia or speech arrest. • Post-ictal Todd's palsy (p696).

Parietal lobe • Sensory disturbances—tingling, numbness, pain (rare). • Motor symptoms (due to spread to the pre-central gyrus).

Occipital lobe • Visual phenomena such as spots, lines, flashes.

Living with epilepsy creates many problems: inability to drive and drug side effects to name a few. Good management of the condition by an integrated specialized team is therefore of utmost importance.

Anti-seizure medications (ASMs) Should only be commenced by a *specialist*, after confirmed epilepsy diagnosis, ≥2 seizures (unless risk of recurrence is high, eg structural brain lesion, focal CNS deficit, or unequivocal epileptiform EEG), and following a detailed discussion of treatment options with the patient. ASM choice depends on seizure type and epilepsy syndrome, comorbidities, lifestyle, and patient preference.

• **Focal (partial) seizures** 1st line: carbamazepine or lamotrigine. 2nd line: levetiracetam, oxcarbazepine, or sodium valproate.[12]
• **Generalized tonic–clonic seizures** 1st line: sodium valproate[12] or lamotrigine. 2nd line: carbamazepine, clobazam, levetiracetam, or topiramate.
• **Absence seizures** 1st line: sodium valproate[12] or ethosuximide. 2nd line: lamotrigine.
• **Myoclonic seizures** 1st line: sodium valproate.[12] 2nd line: levetiracetam, or topiramate (but ↑SE). Avoid carbamazepine and oxcarbazepine—may worsen seizures.
• **Tonic or atonic seizures** Sodium valproate[12] or lamotrigine.

Treat with *one* drug and with *one* doctor in charge only. Slowly build up dose over 2–3 months (see BOX 'Anti-seizure medications (ASMs)') until seizures are controlled or maximum dosage is reached. If ineffective or not tolerated, switch to the next most appropriate drug. To switch drugs, introduce the new drug slowly, and only withdraw the 1st drug once established on the 2nd. Dual (adjunct) therapy is necessary in <10% of patients—consider if all appropriate drugs have been tried singly at the optimum dose.

Stopping ASMs May be done *under specialist supervision* if the patient has been seizure-free for >2yrs and after assessing risks and benefits for the individual (eg the need to drive). The dose must be decreased slowly: over at least 2–3 months, or >6 months for benzodiazepines and barbiturates.

Other interventions **Psychological therapies** Eg relaxation, CBT. May benefit some, but do not improve seizure frequency so only use as an adjunct to medication. **Surgical intervention** Can be considered if a single epileptogenic focus can be identified (such as hippocampal sclerosis or a small low-grade tumour). Neurosurgical resection offers up to 70% chance of seizure resolution, but carries the risk of causing focal neurological deficits. Alternatives: vagal nerve stimulation, deep brain stimulation (DBS).

Sudden unexpected death in epilepsy (SUDEP) More common in uncontrolled epilepsy, and may be related to nocturnal seizure-associated apnoea or asystole. Those with epilepsy have 3× ↑mortality. >700 epilepsy-related deaths are recorded/yr in the UK; up to 17% are SUDEPs. The charity SUDEP Action may be of some help to families.

---

12 Sodium valproate is associated with significantly ↑risk of birth and developmental defects in children born to exposed mothers. The rates of congenital abnormality (neural tube defects) are 10% and 30–40% of children born are found to have a degree of non-developmental disability. Use in women of childbearing potential with caution and only after counselling.

Anti-seizure medications (ASMs): typical adult doses and side effects

Carbamazepine (As slow-release.) Initially 100mg/12h, increase by 200mg/d every 2wks to max 1000mg/12h. *SE:* leucopenia, diplopia, blurred vision, impaired balance, drowsiness, mild generalized erythematous rash (check presence of HLAB1502 allele in Han Chinese populations due to risk of toxic epidermal necrolysis), SIADH (rare; see p665).

Lamotrigine As monotherapy, initially 25mg/d, ↑ by 50mg/d every 2wks up to 100mg/12h (max 250mg/12h). ►Halve monotherapy dose if on valproate; double if on carbamazepine or phenytoin (max 350mg/12h). *SE:* maculopapular rash—occurs in 10% (but 1/1000 develop *Stevens–Johnson syndrome* or *toxic epidermal necrolysis*) typically in 1st 8wks, especially if on valproate; warn patients to see a doctor at once if rash or flu symptoms develop; Other *SE:* diplopia, blurred vision, photosensitivity, tremor, agitation, vomiting, aplastic anaemia.

Levetiracetam Initially 250mg/24h, increase by 250mg/12h every 2wks up to max 1.5g/12h (if eGFR >80). *SE:* psychiatric side effects are common, eg depression, agitation. Other *SE:* D&V, dyspepsia, drowsiness, diplopia, blood dyscrasias.

Sodium valproate Initially 300mg/12h, increase by 100mg/12h every 3d up to max 30mg/kg (or 2.5g) daily. *SE:* teratogenic. Nausea is very common (take with food). Other *SE:* liver failure (watch LFT especially during 1st 6 months), pancreatitis, hair loss (grows back curly), oedema, ataxia, tremor, thrombocytopenia, encephalopathy (hyperammonaemia).

Phenytoin No longer 1st line due to toxicity (nystagmus, diplopia, tremor, dysarthria, ataxia) and *SE:* ↓intellect, depression, coarse facial features, acne, gum hypertrophy, polyneuropathy, blood dyscrasias. Blood levels required for dosage.
►Carbamazepine, phenytoin, and barbiturates are liver enzyme inducing.

Epilepsy and pregnancy

Epilepsy carries a 5% risk of fetal abnormalities, so good seizure control prior to conception and during pregnancy is vital. Yet some anti-epileptics are teratogenic: the patient must be given accurate information and counselling about contraception, conception, pregnancy, and breastfeeding in order to make informed decisions. In particular:
* Advise women of child-bearing age to take folic acid 5mg/d.
* Strictly avoid sodium valproate and polytherapy before conception and during pregnancy (lamotrigine is preferred but transition needs to be planned).
* Advise that most ASMs except carbamazepine and valproate are present in breast milk. Lamotrigine is not thought to be harmful to infants.
* Discuss contraceptive methods, bearing in mind that: enzyme-inducing ASMs make progesterone-only contraception unreliable, and oestrogen-containing contraceptives lower lamotrigine levels—an increased dose may be needed to achieve seizure control.

10 Neurology

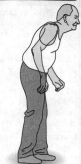

This is the extrapyramidal triad of:

1 *Tremor*. Worse at rest; often 'pill-rolling' of thumb over fingers (see p464).
2 *Hypertonia*. Rigidity + tremor gives 'cogwheel rigidity', felt by the examiner during rapid pronation/supination.
3 *Bradykinesia*. Slow to initiate movement; actions slow and decrease in amplitude with repetition, eg ↓blink rate, micrographia. Gait is festinant (shuffling, pitched forward, fig 10.27) with ↓arm-swing and freezing at obstacles or doors (due to poor *simultaneous* motor and cognitive function). Expressionless face.

Fig 10.27 'Marche à petit pas.'

Causes Parkinson's disease (PD) Loss of dopaminergic neurons in the substantia nigra, associated with Lewy bodies in the basal ganglia, brainstem, and cortex. Most cases are sporadic, though multiple genetic loci have been identified in familial cases. **Prevalence** ↑ with age: 3.5% at 85–89yrs. **Clinical features** The parkinsonian triad, plus non-motor symptoms such as: autonomic dysfunction (postural hypotension, constipation, urinary frequency/urgency, dribbling of saliva), sleep disturbance, and reduced sense of smell. Neuropsychiatric complications, such as depression, dementia, and psychosis, are common and debilitating. **Diagnosis** Is clinical and based on the core features of bradykinesia with resting tremor and/or hypertonia; cerebellar disease and frontotemporal dementia should be excluded; a clinical response to dopaminergic therapy is supportive. ►Signs are invariably worse on one side—if symmetrical look for other causes. If an alternative cause is suspected then consider MRI to rule out structural pathology. Functional neuroimaging (DaTscan™, PET) is playing an emerging role. **Treatment** Focuses on symptom control and does not slow disease progression (see BOX). Non-pharmacological options include deep brain stimulation (DBS, may help those who are partly dopamine responsive) and surgical ablation of overactive basal ganglia circuits (eg subthalamic nuclei).

Parkinson's plus syndromes Progressive supranuclear palsy (PSP, Steele–Richardson–Olszewski syndrome.) Early postural instability, vertical gaze palsy ± falls; rigidity of trunk > limbs; symmetrical onset; speech and swallowing problems; little tremor. **Multiple system atrophy** (MSA; Shy–Drager.) Early autonomic features, eg impotence/incontinence, postural ↓BP; cerebellar + pyramidal signs; rigidity > tremor. **Cortico-basal degeneration** (CBD.) Akinetic rigidity involving one limb; cortical sensory loss (eg astereognosis); apraxia (even autonomous interfering activity by affected limb—the 'alien limb' phenomenon). **Lewy body dementia** See p482.

Secondary causes Vascular parkinsonism (2.5–5% of parkinsonism, also called 'lower limb' parkinsonism). Eg diabetic/hypertensive patient with postural instability and falls (rather than tremor, bradykinesia, and festination). **Other secondary causes** Drugs (neuroleptics, metoclopramide, prochlorperazine, valproate), toxins (manganese), Wilson's disease (p281), trauma (dementia pugilistica), encephalitis, neurosyphilis.

Management Requires input of a multidisciplinary team (GP, neurologist, nurse specialist, social worker, carers, physio- and occupational therapist) to boost quality of life. Assess disability and cognition objectively and regularly, and monitor mood—depression is common. Involve palliative care services early on. Postural exercises and weight lifting may help. ►Don't forget the carers (p483): offer respite care.

A key decision is when to start supplementation of dopaminergic signalling with levodopa. The idea that levodopa should be 'rationed' according to the long-term needs of the patient on the basis that the efficacy is finite, requiring larger and more frequent dosing, is not well proven. There is increasing evidence that the choice and initial timing has little impact on the long-term outcome. However, worsening SE and response fluctuations with time (such as unpredictable freezing and pronounced end-of-dose reduced response: ~50% at 6yrs) supports starting only when PD seriously interferes with life: discuss pros and cons with the patient. ▶Do not withdraw medication suddenly—risks acute akinesia and neuroleptic malignant syndrome. Be aware of situations where malabsorption could also have this effect (eg abdominal surgery, gastroenteritis).

Levodopa Dopamine precursor, given combined with a dopa-decarboxylase inhibitor in co-beneldopa or co-careldopa. SE: dyskinesia, painful dystonia. Non-motor SE: psychosis; visual hallucinations, nausea and vomiting (give domperidone). Modified-release preparations should only be used in late disease.

Dopamine agonists (DAs) Ropinirole and pramipexole monotherapy can delay starting levodopa in early stages of PD, and allow lower doses of levodopa as PD progresses. Rotigotine transdermal patches are available as mono- or additive. SE: drowsiness, nausea, hallucinations, compulsive behaviour (gambling, hypersexuality, p445). Ergot-derived DAs (bromocriptine, pergolide, cabergoline) can cause fibrotic reactions, and are not favoured. Amantadine (weak DA) is used for drug-induced dyskinesias in late PD.

Apomorphine Potent DA agonist used with continuous SC infusion to even out end-of-dose effects, or as a rescue-pen for sudden 'off' freezing. SE: injection-site ulcers.

Anticholinergics (Eg benzhexol, orphenadrine.) Cause confusion in the elderly and have multiple SE—limit to younger patients (but not 1st line).

MAO-B inhibitors (Eg rasagiline, selegiline.) An alternative to dopamine agonists in early PD. SE include postural hypotension and atrial fibrillation.

COMT inhibitors (Eg entacapone, tolcapone, opicapone.) May help motor complications in late disease. Lessen the 'off' time in those with end-of-dose wearing off. Tolcapone has better efficacy, but may cause severe hepatic complications and requires close monitoring of LFT. Opicapone, unlike the others, is dosed once daily, does not cause harmless orange urine discolouration, and appears to cause less diarrhoea.

Inflammatory plaques of demyelination in the CNS *disseminated in space and time*; ie occurring at multiple sites, with ≥30d in between attacks. Demyelination heals poorly, eventually causing axonal loss; >80% of patients develop progressive disability. The exact cause of the disease remains unknown; it is most likely a combination of genetic and environmental factors. There is >30% concordance in identical twins, and unusual geographical distribution, with increasing incidence with latitude in some parts of the world (NB: adult migrants take their risk with them; children acquire the risk of where they settle)—leading to hypotheses of the roles of vitamin D and infection. *Mean age of onset* is 30yrs. ♀:♂ ≥3:1.

Presentation Usually monosymptomatic: ~20% present with unilateral optic neuritis (pain on eye movement and ↓rapid central vision). Corticospinal tract and bladder involvement are also common, and symptoms may worsen with heat (eg hot bath or exercise). Other symptoms/signs see table 10.9.

Diagnosis This is clinical, made by a consultant neurologist using established criteria (eg McDonald, see **table 10.10**) and after alternative diagnoses have been excluded. ►Early diagnosis and treatment reduce relapse rates and disability so refer to neurology as soon as MS is suspected.

Tests Depending on presenting symptoms, some patients may need extra supporting information to make a diagnosis (as per the McDonald criteria).

MRI Sensitive but not specific for plaque detection. It may also exclude other causes, eg cord compression.

CSF Oligoclonal bands of IgG on electrophoresis that are not present in serum suggest CNS inflammation. Delayed visual, auditory, and somatosensory *evoked potentials*.

Progression Most patients follow a relapsing–remitting course, with initial recovery in between relapses. With time, remission becomes incomplete, so disability accumulates (secondary progression). 10% of patients display steadily progressive disability in the absence of relapses (primary progressive MS), while a minority of patients experience no progressive disablement at all.

Poor prognostic signs Older ♂; motor signs at onset; many early relapses; many MRI lesions; axonal loss.

Pregnancy Does not alter the rate of progression: relapses may reduce during pregnancy and increase 3–6 months afterwards, but return to their previous rate thereafter.

Management As with all neurological conditions, requires the coordinated care of a multidisciplinary team and full involvement of the patient in all decisions.[11]

Lifestyle advice Regular exercise, stopping smoking and avoiding stress may help.

Disease-modifying drugs Should be offered to all patients with relapsing–remitting MS. First-line agents include interferon beta, glatiramer, oral dimethyl fumarate, diroximel fumarate, ozanimod or fingolimod for mild/moderate disease. The monoclonal antibodies ocrelizumab (acts against B cells), alemtuzumab (acts against T cells), and natalizumab (acts against α₄ integrin subunit that allows immune cells to cross the blood–brain barrier) are also approved, and are usually reserved for more aggressive cases.

Treating relapses ►First rule out infection, which can transiently worsen symptoms. Methylprednisolone, eg 0.5–1g/24h IV/PO for 3–5d shortens acute relapses; use sparingly (≤twice/yr; steroid SE, p373). It doesn't alter overall prognosis.

Symptom control *Spasticity:* offer baclofen or gabapentin. Tizanidine or dantrolene are 2nd line; if these fail consider benzodiazepines. *Tremor:* botulinum toxin type A injections improve arm tremor and functioning. *Urgency/frequency:* if post-micturition residual urine >100mL, teach intermittent self-catheterization; if <100mL, try tolterodine. *Fatigue:* amantadine, modafinil, SSRIs, CBT, and exercise may help.

Table 10.9 Clinical features of MS

Sensory	Dysaesthesia Pins and needles ↓Vibration sense Trigeminal neuralgia	**GI** Swallowing disorders; constipation. *Eye* Diplopia; hemianopia; optic neuritis; visual phenomena (eg on exercise); bilateral inter-nuclear ophthalmoplegia (p69); pupil defects
Motor	Spastic weakness Myelitis	*Cerebellum* Trunk and limb ataxia; intention tremor; scanning (ie monotonous) speech; falls
Sexual/GU	Erectile dysfunction Anorgasmia; urine re-tention; incontinence	*Cognitive/visuospatial decline* ▶A *big* cause of unemployment, accidents, amnesia, ↓mood, ↓executive functioning

NB ↑T°, malaise, nausea, vomiting, positional vertigo, seizures, aphasia, meningism, bilateral optic neuritis, CSF leucocytosis, and ↑CSF protein are rare in MS, and may suggest non-MS recurrent demyelinating disease, eg vasculitis or sarcoidosis.

Diagnostic criteria for MS

Table 10.10 McDonald criteria for diagnosing MS (2017)

Clinical presentation	Additional evidence needed for diagnosis
≥2 attacks (relapses) with ≥2 objective clinical lesions	None
≥2 attacks with 1 objective clinical lesion	MRI: spatially disseminated lesions, *or* 2nd attack at a new site
1 attack with ≥2 objective clinical lesions	Dissemination in time: • new lesion on repeat MRI after >3 months *or* • 2nd attack *or* • +ve CSF
1 attack with 1 objective clinical lesion (monosymptomatic presentation)	Dissemination in space: • MRI *or* +ve CSF if ≥2 MRI lesions consistent with MS • *and* dissemination in time (by MRI *or* a 2nd clinical attack)
Insidious neurological progression suggestive of primary progres-sive MS	Continued progression for ≥1yr + 2 of • MRI: characteristic brain lesion • MRI: 2 or more cord lesions • +ve CSF

▶A careful history may reveal past episodes, eg brief unexplained visual loss, and detailed examination may show more than 1 lesion.

Attacks must last >1h, with >30d between attacks.

Six MS eponyms

Devic's syndrome (= Neuromyelitis optica, NMO.) No longer considered an MS variant (p688). Transverse myelitis, (loss of motor, sensory, autonomic, reflex, and sphincter function below the level of a lesion), optic atrophy, and anti-aquaporin 4 antibodies.

Lhermitte's sign Neck flexion causes 'electric shocks' in trunk/limbs. (Also +ve in cervical spondylosis, cord tumours and ↓B₁₂.)

Uthoff's phenomenon Worsening of symptoms with heat, eg in bath.

Charles Bonnet syndrome (Rare.) ↓Acuity/temporary blindness ± complex visual hallucinations of faces, as well as animals, plants, and trees.

Pulfrich effect Unequal eye latencies, causing disorientation in traffic as straight trajectories seem curved and distances are misjudged on looking sideways.

Argyll Robertson pupil See p68.

10 Neurology

Signs
- **↑ICP** (See p814.) Headache worse on waking, lying down, bending forward, or with coughing (p452); vomiting; papilloedema (only in 50% of tumours); ↓GCS.
- **Seizures** Seen in ≤50%. Exclude SOL in all adult-onset seizures, especially if focal, or with a localizing aura or post-ictal weakness (Todd's palsy, p696).
- **Evolving focal neurology** See BOX for localizing signs. ↑ICP causes *false localizing signs*: VIth nerve palsy is commonest (p66) due to its long intracranial course.
- **Subtle personality change** Irritability, lack of application to tasks, lack of initiative, socially inappropriate behaviour.

Causes
Tumour (primary or metastatic, later in topic), aneurysm, abscess (25% multiple); chronic subdural haematoma, granuloma (p191, eg tuberculoma), cyst (eg cysticercosis).

Tumours 30% are metastatic (eg breast, lung, melanoma). *Primaries:* astrocytoma, glioblastoma multiforme, oligodendroglioma, ependymoma. Also meningioma, primary CNS lymphoma (eg as non-infectious manifestation of HIV), and cerebellar haemangioblastoma.

Differentials
Stroke, head injury, venous sinus thrombosis, vasculitis, MS, encephalitis, post-ictal, metabolic, or idiopathic intracranial hypertension.

Tests
CT ± MRI (good for posterior fossa masses). Consider biopsy. Avoid LP before imaging (risks *coning*, ie cerebellar tonsils herniate through the foramen magnum).

Tumour management
Benign Remove if possible but some may be inaccessible.

Malignant Excision of gliomas is hard as resection margins are rarely clear, but surgery does give a tissue diagnosis, it debulks pre-radiotherapy, and makes a cavity for inserting carmustine wafers (delivers local chemotherapy). If a tumour is inaccessible but causing hydrocephalus, a ventriculo-peritoneal shunt can help. Chemoradiotherapy is used post-op for gliomas or metastases, and as sole therapy if surgery is impossible. Oligodendroglioma with 1p/19q deletions is especially sensitive. In glioblastoma, temozolomide (alkylating agent) ↑ survival. Seizure prophylaxis (eg levetiracetam) is important, but often fails. Treat headache (eg codeine 60mg/4h PO).

Cerebral oedema Dexamethasone 4mg/8h PO; mannitol if ↑ICP acutely (p815). Plan meticulous palliative treatment (p530).

Prognosis
Poor but improving (<50% survival at 5yrs) for CNS primaries; 40% 20yr survival for cerebellar haemangioblastoma; benign tumours are curable by excision.

Third-ventricle colloid cysts
These congenital cysts declare themselves in adult life with amnesia, headache (often positional), obtundation (blunted consciousness), incontinence, dim vision, bilateral paraesthesiae, weak legs, and drop attacks.

R Excision or ventriculo-peritoneal shunting.

Localizing features

Temporal lobe • Dysphasia (p71). • Contralateral homonymous hemianopia (or upper quadrantanopia if only Meyer's loop affected). • Amnesia. • Many odd or seemingly inexplicable phenomena, p487.

Frontal lobe • Hemiparesis. • Personality change (indecent, indolent, indiscreet, facetious, tendency to pun). • Release phenomena such as the grasp reflex (fingers drawn across palm are grasped), significant only if unilateral. • Broca's dysphasia (p71), or more subtle difficulty with initiating and planning speech with intact repetition and no anomia—but loss of coherence. • Unilateral anosmia (loss of smell). • Perseveration (unable to switch from one line of thinking to another). • Executive dysfunction (unable to plan tasks). • ↓Verbal fluency.

Parietal lobe • Hemisensory loss. • ↓2-point discrimination. • Astereognosis (unable to recognize an object by touch alone). • Sensory inattention. • Dysphasia (p71). • Gerstmann's syndrome (p688).

Occipital lobe • Contralateral visual field defects. • Palinopsia (persisting images once the stimulus has left the field of view). • Polyopia (seeing multiple images).

Cerebellum Remember ᴅᴀɴɪsʜ: **D**ysdiadochokinesis (impaired *rapidly alternating* movements, p63) and **D**ysmetria (past-pointing); **A**taxia (limb/truncal—but if truncal ataxia is worse on eye closure, blame the dorsal columns); **N**ystagmus; **I**ntention tremor; **S**lurred speech (dysarthria); **H**ypotonia.

Cerebellopontine angle (Eg acoustic neuroma/vestibular Schwannoma; p459.) Ipsilateral deafness, nystagmus, ↓corneal reflex, facial weakness (rare), ipsilateral cerebellar signs (above), papilloedema, Vɪᴛʜ nerve palsy (p66).

Midbrain (Eg pineal tumours or midbrain infarction.) Failure of up or down gaze; light-near dissociated pupil responses (p68), nystagmus on convergent gaze.

Lesions of individual peripheral or cranial nerves. Causes are usually local, such as trauma, or entrapment (eg tumour), except for carpal tunnel syndrome (see BOX 'Carpal tunnel syndrome').

Median nerve C6–T1 The median nerve is the nerve of precision grip—muscles involved are easier to remember if you use your 'LOAF' (two Lumbricals, Opponens pollicis, Abductor pollicis brevis, and Flexor pollicis brevis). The clinical features depend on the location of the lesion: **At the wrist** (Eg see BOX 'Carpal tunnel syndrome'.) Weakness of abductor pollicis brevis and sensory loss over the radial 3½ fingers and palm. **Anterior interosseous nerve lesions** (Eg trauma.) Weakness of flexion of the distal phalanx of the thumb and index finger. **Proximal lesions** (Eg compression at the elbow.) May show combined defects.

Ulnar nerve C7–T1 Vulnerable to elbow trauma. **Signs** Weakness/wasting of medial (ulnar side) wrist flexors, interossei (cannot cross the fingers in the good luck sign), and medial two lumbricals (claw hand, more marked in wrist lesions with digitorum profundus intact); hypothenar eminence wasting, weak 5th digit abduction, and 4th and 5th DIP joint flexion; sensory loss over medial 1½ fingers and ulnar side of the hand. **Treatment** See BOX 'Managing ulnar mononeuropathies from entrapments'.

Radial nerve C5–T1 This nerve opens the fist. It may be damaged by compression against the humerus. **Signs** Test for wrist and finger drop with elbow flexed and arm pronated; sensory loss is variable—the dorsal aspect of the root of the thumb (the anatomical snuff box) is most reliably affected. Muscles involved: ('BEAST') Brachioradialis; Extensors; Abductor pollicis longus; Supinator; Triceps.

Brachial plexus Pain/paraesthesiae and weakness in the affected arm in a variable distribution. **Causes** Trauma, radiotherapy (eg for breast carcinoma), prolonged wearing of a heavy rucksack, cervical rib, thoracic outlet compression (also affects vasculature), or neuralgic amyotrophy (Parsonage–Turner syndrome: unilateral sudden, severe pain, followed over hours by profound weakness, resolving completely over days. May rarely involve the phrenic or lower cranial nerves).

Phrenic nerve C3–5 C3, 4, 5 keeps the diaphragm alive: lesions cause orthopnoea with a raised hemidiaphragm on CXR. **Causes** Lung cancer, TB, paraneoplastic syndromes, myeloma, thymoma, cervical spondylosis/trauma, thoracic surgery, infections (HZV, HIV, Lyme disease), muscular dystrophy.

Lateral cutaneous nerve of the thigh L2–L3 *Meralgia paraesthetica* is anterolateral burning thigh pain from entrapment under the inguinal ligament.

Sciatic nerve L4–S3 Damaged by pelvic tumours or fractures to pelvis or femur. Lesions affect the hamstrings and all muscles below the knee (foot drop), with loss of sensation below the knee laterally.

Common peroneal nerve L4–S1 Originates from sciatic nerve just above knee. Often damaged as it winds round the fibular head (trauma, sitting cross-legged). **Signs** Foot drop, weak ankle dorsiflexion/eversion, sensory loss over dorsal foot.

Tibial nerve L4–S3 Originates from sciatic nerve just above knee. Lesions lead to an inability to stand on tiptoe (plantarflexion), invert the foot, or flex the toes, with sensory loss over the sole.

Mononeuritis multiplex Describes the involvement of two or more peripheral nerves. Causes tend to be systemic: DM, connective tissue disorders (rheumatoid, SLE), vasculitis (granulomatosis with polyangiitis formerly Wegener's granulomatosis, PAN), and more rarely sarcoidosis, amyloid, leprosy. Electromyography (EMG) helps define the anatomic site of lesions.

Carpal tunnel syndrome: the commonest mononeuropathy

The median nerve and nine tendons compete for space within the wrist. Compression is common, especially in women who have narrower wrists but similar-sized tendons to men.

Clinical features Aching pain in the hand and arm (especially at night), and paraesthesiae in thumb, index, and middle fingers: relieved by dangling the hand over the edge of the bed and shaking it (remember 'wake and shake'). There may be sensory loss and weakness of abductor pollicis brevis ± wasting of the thenar eminence. Light touch, 2-point discrimination, and sweating may be impaired.

Causes Anything causing swelling or compression of the tunnel: myxoedema; prolonged flexion (eg in a Colles' splint); acromegaly; myeloma; local tumours (lipomas, ganglia); rheumatoid arthritis; amyloidosis; pregnancy; sarcoidosis.

Tests Neurophysiology helps by confirming the lesion's site and severity (and likelihood of improvement after surgery). Maximal wrist flexion for 1min (*Phalen's test*) may elicit symptoms, and tapping over the nerve at the wrist can induce tingling (*Tinel's test*) but both are rather non-specific.

Treatment Splinting, local steroid injection ± decompression surgery.

NB There is also *tarsal* tunnel syndrome: unilateral burning sole pain following tibial nerve compression.

Managing ulnar mononeuropathies from entrapments

The ulnar nerve asks for trouble in at least five places at the elbow, starting proximally at the arcade of Struthers (a musculofascial band ~8cm proximal to the medial epicondyle), and ending distally where it exits the flexor carpi ulnaris muscle in the forearm. Most often, compression occurs at the *epicondylar groove* or at the point where the nerve passes between the two heads of flexor carpi ulnaris (true *cubital tunnel syndrome*). Trauma can easily damage the nerve against its bony confines (the medial condyle of the humerus—the 'funny bone'). Normally, stretch and compression forces on the ulnar nerve at the elbow are moderated by its ability to glide in its groove. When normal excursion is restricted, irritation ensues. This may cause a vicious cycle of perineural scarring, consequent loss of excursion, and progressive symptoms—without antecedent trauma. Compressive ulnar neuropathies at the wrist (*Guyon's canal*—between the pisiform and hamate bones) are less common, but they can also result in disability.

Treatment centres on rest and avoiding pressure on the nerve, but if symptoms continue, night-time soft elbow splinting (to prevent flexion >60°) is warranted. A splint for the hand may help prevent permanent clawing of the fingers. For chronic neuropathy associated with weakness, or if splinting fails, a variety of *surgical procedures* have been tried. For moderately severe neuropathies, decompressions *in situ* may help, but often fail. Medial *epicondylectomies* are effective in ≤50% (but many will recur). Subcutaneous *nerve re-routing* (transposition) may be tried.

Bell's palsy (idiopathic facial nerve palsy)

Affects 15–40/100 000/yr, ♂ ≈ ♀. Risk possibly ↑ in diabetes, hypertension, and in pregnancy. The cause is unknown, but may not be the same in everyone. Reactivation of HSV type 1 in the geniculate ganglion (no. 14 in fig 10.28) and microvascular nerve ischaemia are possible causes.

Clinical features Abrupt onset (eg overnight or after a nap) with complete unilateral facial weakness at 24–72h; ipsilateral numbness or pain around the ear; ↓taste (ageusia); hypersensitivity to sounds (hyperacusis, from stapedius palsy). On examination the patients will be unable to wrinkle their forehead, confirming LMN pathology (see p66), or whistle (tests buccinator). **Other symptoms of VIIth palsy (from any cause)** • Unilateral sagging of the mouth. • Flattening of the ipsilateral nasolabial fold. • Drooling of saliva. • Food trapped between gum and cheek. • Speech difficulty. • Failure of eye closure may cause a watery or dry eye, ectropion (sagging and turning-out of the lower lid), injury from foreign bodies, or conjunctivitis.

Other causes of VIIth palsy Account for ~30% of facial palsies. Think of these if: rashes, bilateral symptoms, UMN signs, other cranial nerve involvement, or limb weakness. **Infective** Ramsay Hunt syndrome (see BOX), Lyme disease, meningitis, TB, viruses (HIV, polio). **Brainstem lesions** Stroke, tumour, MS. **Cerebellopontine angle tumours** Acoustic neuroma, meningioma. **Systemic disease** DM, sarcoidosis, Guillain–Barré. **Local disease** Orofacial granulomatosis, parotid tumours, otitis media or cholesteatoma, skull base trauma.

▶Lyme disease, Guillain–Barré, sarcoid, and trauma often cause bilateral weakness.

Tests If the presentation is typical of Bell's palsy, there are no associated neurological deficits, and no indications of an alternative cause, then blood tests and imaging need not be performed. If there is doubt, rule out the other causes: **Blood** ESR; glucose; ↑*Borrelia* antibodies in Lyme disease, ↑VZV antibodies in Ramsay Hunt syndrome (see BOX). CT/MRI Space-occupying lesions; stroke; MS. CSF (Rarely done) for infections.

Prognosis *Incomplete paralysis* without axonal degeneration usually recovers completely within a few weeks. Of those with *complete paralysis* ~80% make a full spontaneous recovery, but ~15% have axonal degeneration (~50% in pregnancy) in which case recovery is delayed, starting after ~3 months, and may be complicated by aberrant reconnections: *synkinesis*, eg eye blinking causes synchronous upturning of the mouth; misconnection of parasympathetic fibres (red in fig 10.28) can produce *crocodile tears* (gusto–lacrimal reflex) when eating stimulates unilateral lacrimation, not salivation.

Management Protect the eye • Dark glasses and artificial tears (eg hypromellose) if evidence of drying. • Encourage regular eyelid closure by pulling down the lid by hand. • Use tape to close the eyes at night. **Drugs** If given within 72h of onset, prednisolone (eg 60mg/d PO for 5d, tailing by 10mg/d) may speed recovery, with 95% making a full recovery. Antivirals (eg aciclovir) don't appear to help despite the possible role of HSV1 in the aetiology of some cases. Combination treatment with steroids is sometimes used in more severe cases, but there is no good evidence for this practice. There are little data to guide treatment if presenting after 72h of onset, but corticosteroids are widely used (though SE, p373). No advice on the use of steroids is universally agreed in pregnancy. **Surgery** Consider if eye closure remains a long-term problem (lagophthalmos) or ectropion is severe.

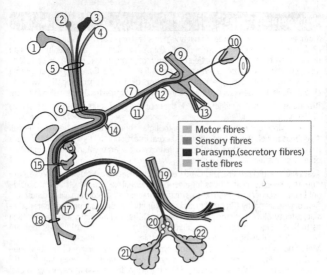

1 Facial nerve nucleus, deep in reticular formation of lower pons
2 Spinal nucleus of V
3 Superior salivary nuc.
4 Solitary tract
5 Porus acusticus internus
6 Meatal foramen
7 Large petrosal nerve
8 Sphenopalatine ganglion
9 Superior maxillary nerve
10 Lacrimal gland
11 Large deep petrosal nerve
12 Vidian nerve
13 Nose/palate gland nerves
14 Small petrosal nerve at geniculate ganglion
15 Stapedial nerve
16 Chorda tympani
17 Auricular branch
18 Stylomastoid foramen
19 Lingual nerve— and taste VII and general sensory from tongue (V³)
20 Submandibular ganglion (and gland, 21)
22 Sublingual gland

Fig 10.28 Facial nerve branches. The motor part moves the muscles of the face, scalp, and ears— also buccinator (puffs out the cheeks), platysma, stapedius, and the posterior belly of the digastric. It also contains the sympathetic motor fibres (vasodilator) of the submaxillary and sublingual glands (via the chorda tympani nerve). The sensory part contains the fibres of taste for the anterior ⅔ of the tongue and a few somatic sensory fibres from the middle ear region.

Ramsay Hunt syndrome

Latent varicella zoster virus reactivating in the geniculate ganglion of the VIIth cranial nerve. **Symptoms** Painful vesicular rash on the auditory canal ± on drum, pinna, tongue, palate, or iris (→hyphaema, ie blood under the cornea) with ipsilateral facial palsy, loss of taste, vertigo, tinnitus, deafness, dry mouth and eyes. The rash may be subtle or even absent ('*herpes sine herpete*' = herpes without herpes). **Incidence** ~5/100 000 (higher if >60yrs). **Diagnosis** Clinical, as antiviral treatment is thought to be most effective within the 1st 72h, while the virus is replicating. **℞** Antivirals (eg *aciclovir* 800mg PO 5 × daily for 7d) + *prednisolone*, as for Bell's palsy. **Prognosis** If treated within 72h, ~75% recover well; if not, ~⅓ make a good recovery, ⅓ a reasonable recovery, and ⅓ a poor recovery.

Motor and/or sensory disorder of multiple peripheral or cranial nerves: usually symmetrical, widespread, and often worse distally ('glove and stocking' distribution). They can be classified by: chronicity, function (*sensory, motor, autonomic, mixed*), or pathology (*demyelination, axonal degeneration, or both*). For example, Guillain–Barré syndrome (see below) is an acute, predominantly motor, demyelinating neuropathy, whereas chronic alcohol abuse leads to a chronic, initially sensory then mixed, axonal neuropathy.

Diagnosis The history is vital: be clear about the time course, the precise nature of the symptoms, and any preceding or associated events (eg D&V before Guillain–Barré syndrome; ↓weight in cancer; arthralgia from a connective tissue disease). Ask about travel, alcohol and drug use, sexual infections, and family history. If there is palpable nerve thickening think of leprosy or Charcot–Marie–Tooth. Examine other systems for clues to the cause, eg alcoholic liver disease.

Tests FBC, ESR, glucose, U&E, LFT, TSH, B₁₂, electrophoresis, ANA, ANCA, CXR, urinalysis, consider LP ± specific genetic tests for inherited neuropathies, lead level, antiganglioside antibodies. Nerve conduction studies distinguish demyelinating from axonal causes.

Sensory neuropathy (Eg DM, CKD, leprosy.) Numbness; pins and needles, paraesthesiae; affects 'glove and stocking' distribution. Difficulty handling small objects such as buttons. Signs of trauma (eg finger burns) or joint deformation may indicate sensory loss. Diabetic and alcoholic neuropathies are typically painful.

Motor neuropathy (Eg Guillain–Barré syndrome, lead poisoning, Charcot–Marie–Tooth syndrome.) Often progressive (may be rapid); weak or clumsy hands; difficulty in walking (falls, stumbling); difficulty in breathing (↓vital capacity). Signs: LMN lesion: wasting and weakness most marked in the distal muscles of hands and feet (foot or wrist drop). Reflexes are reduced or absent.

Cranial nerves Swallowing/speaking difficulty; diplopia.

Autonomic system See BOX.

Management *Treat the cause* (table 10.11). Involve physio and OT. Foot care and *shoe choice* are important in sensory neuropathies to minimize trauma. Splinting joints helps prevent contractures in prolonged paralysis. In Guillain–Barré and chronic inflammatory demyelinating polyradiculoneuropathy (CIDP: autoimmune demyelination of peripheral nerves), IV immunoglobulin helps. For vasculitic causes, steroids/immunosuppressants may help. Treat neuropathic pain with amitriptyline, duloxetine, gabapentin, or pregabalin.

Guillain–Barré syndrome

Incidence 1–2/100 000/yr.

Signs A few weeks after an infection a symmetrical ascending muscle weakness starts.

Triggers *Campylobacter jejuni*, CMV, mycoplasma, zoster, HIV, EBV, vaccinations. The trigger causes antibodies which attack nerves. In 40%, no cause is found. It may advance quickly, affecting all limbs at once, and can lead to paralysis. There is a progressive phase of up to 4 weeks, followed by recovery. Unlike other neuropathies, *proximal* muscles are more affected, eg trunk, respiratory, and cranial nerves (esp. VII). Pain is common (eg back, limb) but sensory signs may be absent (table 10.12).

Autonomic dysfunction Sweating, ↑pulse, BP changes, arrhythmias.

Nerve conduction studies Slow conduction. CSF ↑Protein (eg >5.5g/L), normal CSF white cell count. Respiratory involvement (the big danger) requires transfer to ITU. Do forced vital capacity (FVC) 4-hourly. ▶ *Ventilate sooner rather than later*, eg if FVC <1.5L, P_aO_2 <10kPa, P_aCO_2 >6kPa.

R IV immunoglobulin 0.4g/kg/24h for 5d. Plasma exchange is good too (?more SE). Steroids have no role.

Prognosis Good; ~85% make a complete or near-complete recovery. 10% are unable to walk alone at 1yr. *Complete paralysis is compatible with complete recovery.*

Mortality 10%. Variants include:

Chronic inflammatory demyelinating polyradiculopathy (CIDP) Characterized by a slower onset and recovery.

Miller Fisher syndrome Comprises of ophthalmoplegia, ataxia, and areflexia. Associated with anti-GQ1b antibodies in the serum.

Table 10.11 Causes of polyneuropathy

Metabolic	**Vasculitides**	**Malignancy**	**Inflammatory**
Diabetes mellitus Renal failure Hypothyroidism Hypoglycaemia Mitochondrial disorders	Polyarteritis nodosa Rheumatoid arthritis GPA	Paraneoplastic syndromes Polycythaemia rubra vera	Guillain–Barré syndrome Sarcoidosis; CIDP*
Infections	**Nutritional**	**Inherited syndromes**	**Drugs**
Leprosy HIV Syphilis Lyme disease	↓Vit B_1 ↓Vit B_{12}/folate ↓Vit B_6 ↓Vit E	Charcot–Marie–Tooth Refsum's syndrome Porphyria Leucodystrophy	Vincristine Cisplatin Isoniazid Nitrofurantoin Phenytoin Metronidazole
Others			
Paraproteinaemias, amyloidosis, lead, arsenic			

* Chronic inflammatory demyelinating polyradiculoneuropathy (CIDP): autoimmune demyelination of peripheral nerves (distal onset of weakness/sensory loss in limbs + nerve enlargement + ↑CSF protein).

Autonomic neuropathy

Sympathetic and parasympathetic neuropathies may be isolated or part of a generalized sensorimotor peripheral neuropathy.

Causes DM, amyloidosis, Guillain–Barré and Sjögren's syndromes, HIV, leprosy, SLE, toxic, genetic (eg porphyria), or paraneoplastic, eg paraneoplastic encephalomyeloneuropathies, and Lambert–Eaton myasthenic syndrome (LEMS, p508).

Signs Sympathetic: postural hypotension, ↓sweating, ejaculatory failure, Horner's syndrome (p48). **Parasympathetic:** constipation, nocturnal diarrhoea, urine retention, erectile dysfunction, Holmes–Adie pupil (p68).

Autonomic function tests
- BP: *postural drop* of ≳20/10mmHg is abnormal.
- ECG: a variation of <10bpm with respiration is abnormal (check R-R interval).
- **Cystometry:** bladder pressure studies.
- **Pupils:** instil 0.1% adrenaline (dilates if post-ganglionic sympathetic denervation, not if normal), 2.5% cocaine (dilates if normal; not if sympathetic denervation); 2.5% methacholine (constricts if parasympathetic lesion)—rarely used.
- **Paraneoplastic antibodies:** anti-HU, anti-YO, anti-RI, anti-amphiphysin, anti-CV2, anti-MA2. **Other Ab:** antiganglionic acetylcholine receptor antibody presence shows that the cause may be autoimmune autonomic ganglionopathy.

Primary autonomic failure Occurs alone (autoimmune autonomic ganglionopathy), as part of multisystem atrophy (MSA, p490), or with Parkinson's disease, typically in a middle-aged/elderly man. Onset: insidious; symptoms as listed previously.

Guillain-Barré polyneuritis (acute demyelinating polyneuropathy)

Table 10.12 Diagnostic criteria

Features required for	Features supporting diagnosis
• Progressive weakness of >1 limb • Areflexia	• Progression over days, up to 4wks • Near symmetry of symptoms
Features making diagnosis doubtful	• Sensory symptoms/signs only mild
• Sensory level • Marked, persistent asymmetry of weakness • Severe bowel and bladder dysfunction • CSF WCC >50	• CN involvement (eg bilateral facial weakness) • Recovery starts ~2wks after the period of progression has finished • Autonomic dysfunction • Absence of fever at onset • CSF protein ↑ with CSF WCC <10 × 10^6/L • Typical electrophysiological tests

MND is a cluster of neurodegenerative diseases affecting 6/100 000 (σ:φ ≈ 3:2), characterized by selective loss of neurons in motor cortex, cranial nerve nuclei, and anterior horn cells. Upper and lower motor neurons can be affected but there is *no* sensory loss or sphincter disturbance, thus distinguishing MND from MS and polyneuropathies. MND never affects eye movements, distinguishing it from myasthenia (p508). There are four clinical patterns:

1 *ALS/amyotrophic lateral sclerosis*. (Archetypal MND; up to 80%.) Loss of motor neurons in motor cortex *and* the anterior horn of the cord, so combined UMN + LMN signs (p442). Worse prognosis if: bulbar onset, ↑age, ↓FVC.

2 *Progressive bulbar palsy*. (10–20%.) Only affects cranial nerves IX–XII. See BOX 'Bulbar and corticobulbar ('pseudobulbar') palsy'.

3 *Progressive muscular atrophy*. (<10%.) Anterior horn cell lesion, so LMN signs only. Affects distal muscle groups before proximal. Better prognosis than ALS.

4 *Primary lateral sclerosis*. (Rare.) Loss of Betz cells in motor cortex: mainly UMN signs, marked spastic leg weakness and pseudobulbar palsy. No cognitive decline.

Presentation Think of MND in those >40yrs (median UK age at onset is 60) with stumbling spastic gait, foot-drop ± proximal myopathy, weak grip (door-handles don't turn) and shoulder abduction (hair-washing is hard), or aspiration pneumonia. Look for UMN signs: spasticity, brisk reflexes, ↑plantars; and LMN signs: wasting, fasciculation of tongue, abdomen, back, thigh. Is speech or swallowing affected (bulbar signs)? Fasciculation is not enough to diagnose an LMN lesion: look for weakness too. Frontotemporal dementia occurs in ~25%.

Diagnostic criteria (See BOX 'Revised El Escorial diagnostic criteria for ALS'). There is no diagnostic test. Brain/cord MRI helps exclude structural causes, LP helps exclude inflammatory ones, and neurophysiology can detect subclinical denervation and help exclude mimicking motor neuropathies.[13]

Prognosis Poor, <3yrs post onset in half of patients.

Management Adopt a multidisciplinary approach: neurologist, palliative nurse, hospice, physio, OT, speech therapist, dietician, social services—all orchestrated by the GP. Riluzole, an inhibitor of glutamate release and NMDA receptor antagonist, is the only medication shown to improve survival. Multiple other drugs that have shown promise in animal models have failed to prove benefit in clinical trials, including neurotrophic factors, anti-apoptotic agents, antioxidants, and immunomodulatory drugs. For supportive/symptomatic treatment: **Excess saliva** Advise on positioning, oral care, and suctioning. Try an antimuscarinic (eg propantheline) or glycopyrronium bromide (can be given SC). Botulinum toxin A may help. **Dysphagia** Blend food. Gastrostomy is an option—discuss early on. **Spasticity** Exercise, orthotics. See MS for drugs (p492). **Communication difficulty** Provide 'augmentative and alternative' communication equipment. **End of life care** ►Involve palliative care team from diagnosis (p528). Consider opioids to relieve breathlessness and discuss non-invasive ventilation (see BOX 'Finding middle ground').

---

13 If no UMN signs and distal arm muscles are affected in the distribution of individual nerves, suspect multifocal motor neuropathy with conduction block (diagnose on nerve conduction studies; ℞ IV Ig). Gynaecomastia, atrophic testes ± infertility suggests Kennedy syndrome (bulbospinal muscular atrophy).

Bulbar and corticobulbar ('pseudobulbar') palsy

Bulbar palsy denotes diseases of the nuclei of cranial nerves IX–XII in the medulla. **Signs** An *LMN lesion* of the tongue and muscles of talking and swallowing: flaccid, fasciculating tongue (like a sack of worms); jaw jerk is normal or absent, speech is quiet, hoarse, or nasal. **Causes** MND, Guillain–Barré, polio, myasthenia gravis, syringobulbia (p512), brainstem tumours, central pontine myelinolysis (p664).

Corticobulbar palsy *UMN lesion* of muscles of swallowing and talking due to bilateral lesions above the mid-pons, eg corticobulbar tracts (MS, MND, stroke, central pontine myelinolysis). It is commoner than bulbar palsy. **Signs** Slow tongue movements, with slow deliberate speech; ↑jaw jerk; ↑pharyngeal and palatal reflexes; pseudobulbar affect (PBA)—weeping unprovoked by sorrow or mood-incongruent giggling (emotional incontinence *without* mood change is also seen in MS, Wilson's, and Parkinson's disease, dementia, nitrous oxide use, and head injury). In some countries, dextromethorphan + quinidine is licensed for PBA.

Revised El Escorial diagnostic criteria for ALS

Definite Lower + upper motor neuron signs in 3 regions.

Probable Lower + upper motor neuron signs in 2 regions.

Probable with lab support Lower + upper motor neuron signs in 1 region, or upper motor neuron signs in ≥1 region + EMG shows acute denervation in ≥2 limbs.

Possible Lower + upper motor neuron signs in 1 region.

Suspected Upper or lower motor neuron signs only—in 1 or more regions.

Finding middle ground

The diagnosis of MND, with its unpredictable mélange of symptoms and signs, often comes stubbornly late. Late in the course of the pathophysiology perhaps, but agonisingly early in the journey of the person. Multiple visits to the GP, unnecessary investigation with unclear results (neuroimaging and electrophysiology can sometimes cause delays or muddy the waters), and well-meaning reassurance from loved ones may only quell for so long the suspicions of the individual. 'Breaking of bad news' may become more of a confirmation of the presupposed. The dichotomized portrayal of MND in popular culture may have already shaped their perception about what the diagnosis means. Ice buckets brimming with hope for a radical cure and Stephen Hawking's wondrous discoveries while defying his prognosis contrast starkly with coverage of court battles for assisted dying, which require emphasis of the most harrowing cases. The reality, as always, usually lies somewhere in between. Finding middle ground with the individual and their family will allow informed discussions about their wishes for end of life care. These conversations are crucial but not binding. The patient can change their mind at any point, and also refuse any life-prolonging treatment, knowing the consequence is death. Regardless of where they stand, our role is to let them know that we stand beside them, come what may.

Degeneration of the cervical spine with age is inevitable, and has a wide clinical spectrum, ranging from asymptomatic to progressive spastic quadriparesis and sensory loss due to compression of the cord (myelopathy).

Pathogenesis Degeneration of the annulus fibrosus (the tough coating of the intervertebral discs), combined with osteophyte formation on the adjacent vertebra leads to narrowing of the spinal canal and intervertebral foramina (figs 10.29, 10.30). As the neck flexes and extends, the cord is dragged over these protruding bony spurs anteriorly and indented by a thickened ligamentum flavum posteriorly.

Presenting complaint Neck stiffness (but common in anyone >50yrs old), crepitus on moving neck, stabbing or dull arm pain (brachialgia), forearm/wrist pain.

Signs Limited, painful neck movement ± crepitus (examine gently). Neck flexion may produce tingling down the spine (Lhermitte's sign, p493). NB: this does not distinguish between cord or roots (or both) involvement.

Root compression (radiculopathy) Pain/'electrical' sensations in arms or fingers at the level of the compression (table 10.13), with numbness, dull reflexes, LMN weakness, and eventual wasting of muscles innervated by the affected root. NB: UMN signs below level of the affected root suggests cord compression.

▶**Features of cord compression** Progressive symptoms (eg ↑weak, clumsy hands; gait disturbance); UMN leg signs (spastic weakness, ↑plantars); LMN arm signs (wasting, hyporeflexia); incontinence, hesitancy, and urgency are late features.

Which nerve root is affected? See table 10.13.

ΔΔ MS; nerve root neurofibroma; subacute combined degeneration of the cord (↓B₁₂); compression by bone or cord tumours.

Management ▶Urgent MRI and specialist referral guided by red flag symptoms (p538). Bear in mind that although these are stressed in virtually every set of guidelines, no two lists are alike and review of evidence suggests that the accuracy of these features is low. ▶Don't make referral decisions based upon the presence or absence of a single feature, but use these to inform your judgement. Otherwise: give analgesia (as per WHO ladder) and encourage gentle activity. Cervical collars may give respite during brief periods of increased pain, but restrict mobility, so may prolong symptoms: avoid where possible. If no improvement in 4–6 weeks then MRI and consider neurosurgical referral for: interlaminar cervical epidural injections, transforaminal injections or surgical decompression (via *anterior approach*, eg discectomy or *posterior approach*, eg laminectomy—**fig 10.31**, or laminoplasty—**fig 10.32**). There is no consensus or high-quality evidence to guide selection of approach or of patients, though interventions may be best reserved for those with progressive deterioration, myelopathy causing disabling neurologic deficits, or those at risk for deterioration (eg severe spinal cord compression on MRI).

Table 10.13 Clinical patterns of nerve root impingement

Typical motor and sensory deficits from individual root involvement (c5-8)		
Nerve root	**Motor and sensory deficit**	**Pain pattern**
C5 (C4/C5 disc)	Weak deltoid & supraspinatus; ↓supinator jerks; numb elbow	Pain in neck/shoulder that radiates down front of arm to elbow
C6 (C5/C6 disc)	Weak biceps & brachioradialis; ↓biceps jerks; numb thumb & index finger	Pain in shoulder radiating down arm below elbow*
C7 (C6/C7 disc)	Weak triceps & finger extension; ↓triceps jerks; numb middle finger	Pain in upper arm and dorsal forearm
C8 (C7/T1 disc)	Weak finger flexors & small muscles of the hand; numb 5th & ring finger	Pain in upper arm and medial forearm
►*Worrying symptoms:* night pain, ↓weight, fever.		

* Passive head turning may exacerbate c6 radicular pain but not carpal tunnel syndrome (Spurling's manoeuvre).

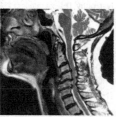

Fig 10.29 A T2-weighted MRI (∴ CSF looks bright). The cord is compressed between osteophytes anteriorly and the ligamentum flavum posteriorly.

© Prof P Scally.

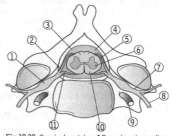

Fig 10.30 Cervical vertebra. **1** Dorsal root ganglion; **2** Dorsal root; **3** Dura mater; **4** Subarachnoid space; **5** Pia mater; **6** Grey matter; **7** Spinal nerve; **8** Ventral ramus; **9** Vertebral artery in the transverse foramen; **10** White matter; **11** Ventral spinal nerve.

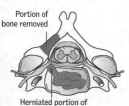

Portion of bone removed

Herniated portion of cervical disc to be removed

Fig 10.31 Laminectomy.

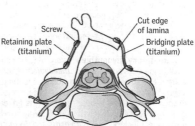

Screw

Retaining plate (titanium)

Cut edge of lamina

Bridging plate (titanium)

Fig 10.32 Laminoplasty (screws and plates).

Primary disorder of muscle with gradual-onset symmetrical weakness; it may be confused clinically with neuropathy. *In favour of myopathy:* • Gradual onset of symmetric *proximal* weakness—difficulty combing hair and climbing stairs (NB: weakness is also *distal* in myotonic dystrophy). • Specific muscle groups affected (ie *selective* weakness on first presentation). • Preserved tendon reflexes. • No paraesthesiae or bladder problems. • No fasciculation (suggests anterior horn cell or root disease).

Rapid onset suggests a toxic, drug, or metabolic myopathy (or a neuropathy). *Excess fatigability* (↑weakness with exercise) suggests myasthenia (p508). Spontaneous *pain* at rest and local tenderness occurs in inflammatory myopathies. Pain on exercise suggests ischaemia or metabolic myopathy (eg McArdle's disease). *Oddly firm* muscles (due to infiltrations with fat or connective tissue) suggest pseudohypertrophic muscular dystrophies (eg Duchenne's).

Tests ESR, CK, AST, and LDH may be raised. Do EMG and tests relevant to systemic causes (eg TSH, p210). Muscle biopsy and genetic testing may help reach a diagnosis.

Muscular dystrophies A group of genetic diseases (table 10.14) with progressive degeneration and weakness of specific muscle groups. The primary abnormality may be in the muscle membrane. There may be unusually firm muscles due to infiltration by fat or connective tissue, and marked variation in size of individual muscle fibres on histology. • **Duchenne's muscular dystrophy** The commonest (3/1000 male live births). Presents at ~4yrs old with clumsy walking, then difficulty in standing, and respiratory failure. Pseudohypertrophy is seen, especially in the calves. Serum creatine kinase ↑ >40-fold. There is no specific treatment. Some survive beyond 20yrs. Home ventilation improves prognosis. Genetic counselling is vital. • **Becker's muscular dystrophy** (~0.3/1000 ♂ births.) Presents similarly to Duchenne's but with milder symptoms, at a later age, and with a better prognosis. • **Facioscapulohumeral muscular dystrophy** (FSHD, Landouzy–Dejerine.) Almost as common as Duchenne's. Onset is ~12–14yrs old, with inability to puff out the cheeks and difficulty raising the arms above the head. *Signs:* weakness of face ('ironed out' expression), shoulders, and upper arms (often asymmetric with deltoids spared), foot-drop, scapular winging (fig 10.33), scoliosis, anterior axillary folds, and horizontal clavicles. ≤20% need a wheelchair by 40yrs.

Myotonic disorders Cause tonic muscle spasm (myotonia), and demonstrate long chains of central nuclei within muscle fibres on histology. The commonest is *myotonic dystrophy* which is, in fact, clinically and genetically heterogeneous, with two major forms (DM1 and DM2—see table 10.14), both showing abnormal trinucleotide repeat expansions in regulatory (non-coding) genetic regions. DM1 is the commoner, more severe, and typically presents between 20–40yrs old with *distal* weakness (hand/foot drop), weak sternomastoids, and myotonia. Facial weakness and muscle wasting give a long, haggard appearance. *Also:* cataracts, male frontal baldness, diabetes, testis/ovary atrophy, cardiomyopathy, and ↓cognition. Most DM1 patients die in late middle age of respiratory or cardiac complications. Mexiletine may help with disabling myotonia. Genetic counselling is important.

Inflammatory myopathies There may be spontaneous muscle pain at rest and local tenderness on palpation. *Inclusion body myositis* is the chief example if aged >50yrs. Weakness starts with quadriceps, finger flexors, or pharyngeal muscles. Ventral extremity muscle groups are more affected than dorsal or girdle groups. Response to therapy is poor and patients typically progress over a decade to require assistance with activities of daily living. Histology shows ringed vacuoles + intranuclear inclusions. *Polymyositis* and *dermatomyositis*, see p549.

Metabolic myopathies Eg *McArdle's disease* (glycogen storage disorder). Presents with muscle pain and weakness after exercise.

Acquired myopathies of late onset Often part of systemic disease—eg hyperthyroidism, malignancy, Cushing's, hypo- and hypercalcaemia.

Drug causes Alcohol; statins; steroids; chloroquine; zidovudine; vincristine; cocaine.

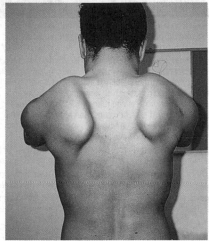

Fig 10.33 Winging of both scapulae in facioscapulohumeral muscular dystrophy, due to weakness of thoracoscapular muscles.

Reproduced from Donaghy, *Brain's Diseases of the Nervous System*, 12th edition, with permission from Oxford University Press.

Table 10.14 Genetics of some commoner congenital myopathies

Condition	Inheritance	Chr	Gene	Pathogenesis
Duchenne's muscular dystrophy	x-linked recessive	X	Dystrophin (stabilizes muscle fibres)	Partial deletions or duplications in dystrophin render *non*-functional
Becker's muscular dystrophy	x-linked recessive	X	Dystrophin	Partial deletions or duplications in dystrophin render *hypo*-functional
FSHD type 1	Autosomal dominant	4	DUX4 (transcriptional activator)	Partial deletion of D4Z4 repeating unit releases normal repression of DUX4 expression
FSHD type 2	Autosomal dominant	4	DUX4 (transcriptional activator)	Hypomethylation of D4Z4 releases normal repression of DUX4 expression
DM type 1	Autosomal dominant	19	DMPK (serine-threonine kinase)	Expansion of short repetitive sequences of nucleotides; in both forms this expanded sequence is transcribed into RNA which then misfolds and sequesters other RNA binding proteins
DM type 2	Autosomal dominant	3	ZNF9 (transcriptional regulator)	

Myasthenia gravis (MG)

MG is an acquired autoimmune disease mediated by antibodies to nicotinic acetylcholine receptors (ACHR) on the post-synaptic side of the neuromuscular junction (fig 10.34). Prevalence: 10/100 000. Bimodal age of onset: <40yrs (♀ > ♂) and >70 (♂ > ♀).

Presentation Slowly increasing or relapsing muscular fatigue. Muscle groups affected, in order: extraocular; bulbar (swallowing, chewing); face; neck; limb girdle; trunk. **Signs** Ptosis (observe after sustained upgaze), diplopia, myasthenic snarl on smiling, 'peek sign' of orbicularis fatigability (eyelids begin to separate after manual opposition to sustained closure). On counting to 50, the voice fades (dysphonia is a rare presentation). Tendon reflexes and sensation are normal. **Symptoms exacerbated by** Pregnancy, ↓K⁺, infection, medications (gentamicin, tetracycline, quinine, β-blockers), over-treatment, change of climate, emotion, exercise.

Differentials Polymyositis/other myopathies (p506); thyroid ophthalmopathy; Guillain–Barré syndrome (initial proximal weakness, p500); botulism (see BOX).

Associations Other autoimmune disease (screen TFTs); thymic abnormalities in ¾ patients: hyperplasia (85%), thymoma (15%). ½ patients with thymoma have MG.

Tests • **Antibodies** ↑Anti-ACHR antibodies in 90% (70% in MG variant confined to ocular muscles). If anti-ACHR −ve look for MuSK antibodies (muscle-specific tyrosine kinase; especially in ♀; predominantly ocular/facial/bulbar). • **EMG** Decremental muscle response to repetitive nerve stimulation ± ↑single-fibre jitter. • **Imaging** CT to exclude thymoma (68% 5yr survival). • **Other** Ptosis improves by >2mm after ice application to the eyelid for >2min—a neat, non-invasive test (but not diagnostic). The Tensilon® (edrophonium) test is no longer used: many false +ves and has risks.

Treatment • **Symptom control** Anticholinesterase, eg pyridostigmine (start at 30mg PO 4×daily; max 1.2g/d). Cholinergic SE: ↑salivation, lacrimation, sweats, vomiting, miosis, diarrhoea, colic (controllable with propantheline 15mg/8h).
• **Immunosuppression** Start at 5mg (ocular MG) or 10mg (generalized MG) on alternate days, ↑ by 5–10mg/3 doses up to 1mg/kg on each treatment day. ↓Dose on remission (may take months). Give osteoporosis prophylaxis. SE: weakness (hence low starting dose). Use alternative (azathioprine, ciclosporin, or mycophenolate mofetil) if a steroid dose of >15–20mg on alternate days is required.
• **Thymectomy** Has beneficial effects, even in patients without a thymoma: consider especially in younger patients with generalized anti-ACHR +ve MG, onset <5yrs previously and poor response to medical therapy. Improved symptom scores sustained over 3yrs, with reduced need for immunosuppression. Surgery also prevents local invasion if thymoma is present.

Myasthenic crisis Life-threatening weakness of respiratory muscles during a relapse. ▶Can be difficult to differentiate from cholinergic crisis (ie overtreatment—but this is rare, and usually only occurs in doses of pyridostigmine >960mg/d). Monitor forced vital capacity. *Ventilatory support* may be needed. Treat with plasmapheresis (removes ACHR antibodies from the circulation) or IVIG and identify and treat the trigger for the relapse (eg infection, medications).

Lambert–Eaton myasthenic syndrome (LEMS)

20 times less common than MG. LEMS can be paraneoplastic (50% are associated with malignancies, in particular small-cell lung cancer) or autoimmune. Unlike MG, antibodies are to voltage-gated Ca²⁺ channels on *pre*-synaptic membrane (fig 10.35; anti-P/Q type VGCC antibodies are +ve in 90%).

Clinical features •Gait difficulty before eye signs. •Autonomic involvement (dry mouth, constipation, impotence). •Hyporeflexia and weakness, which improve after exercise (in contrast with MG). •Diplopia and respiratory muscle involvement are rare. •EMG shows similar changes to MG except amplitude increases greatly post-exercise.

Treatment 3,4-diaminopyridine, ±pyridostigmine. IVIG or plasmapheresis in severe cases (get specialist help). ▶Do regular CXR/high-resolution CT as symptoms may precede the cancer by >4yrs.

How synapses work—the neuromuscular junction

1 Before transmission can occur, neurotransmitter must be packed into synaptic vesicles. At the neuromuscular junction (NMJ) this is acetylcholine (ACH). Each vesicle contains ~8000 ACH molecules.

2 When an action potential arrives at the pre-synaptic terminal, depolarization opens voltage-gated Ca^{2+} channels (VGCCs). In *Lambert–Eaton* syndrome, anti-P/Q type VGCC antibodies disrupt this stage of synaptic transmission.[14]

3 Influx of Ca^{2+} through the VGCCs triggers fusion of synaptic vesicles with the pre-synaptic membrane (a process that *botulinum toxin* interferes with), and neurotransmitter is released from the vesicles into the synaptic cleft.

4 Transmitter molecules cross the synaptic cleft by diffusion and bind to nicotinic receptors on the post-synaptic membrane, causing depolarization of the post-synaptic membrane (the end-plate potential). This change in the post-synaptic membrane triggers muscle contraction at the NMJ, or onward transmission of the action potential in neurons. In *myasthenia gravis*, antibodies block the post-synaptic ACH receptors, preventing the end-plate potential from becoming large enough to trigger muscle contraction—and muscle weakness ensues.

5 Transmitter action is terminated by enzymatic hydrolysis by membrane-bound acetylcholinesterase or circulating butylcholinesterase. Anticholinesterase treatments for myasthenia gravis, such as *pyridostigmine*, reduce the rate of degradation of ACH, increasing the chance that it will trigger an end-plate potential.

10 Neurology

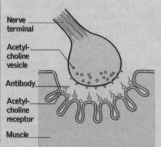

Nerve terminal
Acetylcholine vesicle
Antibody
Acetylcholine receptor
Muscle

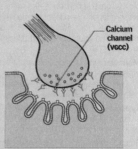

Calcium channel (VGCC)

Fig 10.34 Myasthenia gravis features *post-synaptic* ACHR antibodies. Tendon reflexes are normal because the synapses do not have time to become fatigued with such a brief muscle contraction. Ocular palsies are common (it's not exactly clear why).

Fig 10.35 Lambert–Eaton syndrome features pre-synaptic Ca^{2+}-channel antibodies. Depressed tendon reflexes are common because less transmitter is released, but reflexes may ↑ after maximum voluntary contraction due to a build of transmitter in the synaptic cleft (post-tetanic potentiation).

14 Disruption of pre-synaptic transmission affects release of ACH in autonomic nervous system as well as at neuromuscular junction, explaining the prominence of dysautonomia in LEMS unlike in MG.

Type 1 neurofibromatosis (NF1, von Recklinghausen's disease)

Autosomal dominant inheritance (gene locus 17q11.2). Expression of NF1 is variable, even within a family. **Prevalence** 1 in 2500, ♀:♂≈1:1; no racial predilection.

Signs *Café-au-lait spots:* flat, coffee-coloured patches of skin seen in 1st year of life (clearest in UV light), increasing in size and number with age. Adults have ≥6, >15mm across. They do *not* predispose to skin cancer. *Freckling:* typically in skin-folds (axillae, groin, neck base, and submammary area), and usually present by age 10. *Dermal neuro-fibromas:* small, violaceous nodules, gelatinous in texture, which appear at puberty, and may become papillomatous. They are not painful but may itch. Numbers increase with age. *Nodular neurofibromas* arise from nerve trunks. Firm and clearly demar-cated, they can give rise to paraesthesiae if pressed. *Lisch nodules* (fig 10.36) are tiny harmless regular brown/translucent mounds (hamartomas) on the iris (use a slit lamp) ≤2mm in diameter. They develop by 6yrs old in 90%. Also short stature and macrocephaly.

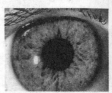

Fig 10.36 Multiple brown Lisch nodules on the iris.
© Jon Miles.

Complications Occur in 30%. Mild learning disability is common. *Local effects of neurofibromas:* nerve root compression (weakness, pain, paraesthesiae); GI—bleeds, obstruction; bone—cystic lesions, scoliosis, pseudarthrosis. ↑BP from renal artery stenosis or phaeochromocytoma. Plexiform neurofibromas (large, subcuta-neous swellings). *Malignancy* (5% patients with NF1): optic glioma, sarcomatous change in a neurofibroma. ↑Epilepsy risk (slight). *Rare association:* carcinoid syndrome (p266).

Management Multidisciplinary team with geneticist, neurologist, surgeon, and physiotherapist, orchestrated by a GP. Yearly cutaneous survey and measurement of BP. Dermal neurofibromas are unsightly, and catch on clothing; if troublesome, excise, but removing all lesions is unrealistic. Genetic counselling is vital (*OHCS* p274).

Type 2 neurofibromatosis (NF2)

Autosomal dominant inheritance, though 50% are *de novo*, with mosaicism in some (NF2 gene locus is 22q11). Rarer than NF1 with a prevalence of only 1 in 35 000.

Signs *Café-au-lait* spots are fewer than in NF1. *Bilateral vestibular Schwannomas* (= acoustic neuromas; p459) are characteristic, becoming symptomatic by ~20yrs old when sensorineural hearing loss is the 1st sign. There may be tinnitus and vertigo. The rate of tumour growth is unpredictable and variable. The tumours are benign but cause problems by pressing on local structures and by ↑ICP. They may be absent in mosaic NF2. *Juvenile posterior subcapsular lenticular opacity* (a form of cataract) occurs before other manifestations and can be useful in screening those at risk.

Complications Tender Schwannomas of cranial and peripheral nerves, and spinal nerve roots. Meningiomas (45% in NF2, often multiple). Glial tumours are less common. Consider NF2 in any young person presenting with one of these tumours in isolation.

Management Hearing tests yearly from puberty in affected families, with MRI brain if abnormality is detected. A normal MRI in the late teens is helpful in as-sessing risk to any offspring. A clear scan at 30yrs (unless a family history of late onset) indicates that the gene has not been inherited. Treatment of vestibular Schwannomas is neurosurgical and complicated by hearing loss/deterioration and facial palsy. Mean survival from diagnosis is ~15yrs.

Schwannomatosis Multiple tender cutaneous Schwannomas without the bilat-eral vestibular Schwannomas that are characteristic of NF2. Indistinguishable from mosaic NF2, where vestibular Schwannomas are also absent, except by genetic ana-lysis of tumour biopsies. There is typically a large tumour load, assessable only by whole-body MRI. Mutations in the tumour suppressor genes SMARCB1 and LZTR1 and spontaneous NF2 mutations have all been described. Life expectancy is normal.

Diagnostic criteria for neurofibromatosis

NF1 (von Recklinghausen's disease)

Diagnosis is made if 2 of the following are found:

1 ≥6 café-au-lait macules >5mm (pre-pubertal) or >15mm (post-pubertal).
2 ≥2 neurofibromas of any type or 1 plexiform.
3 Freckling in the axillary or inguinal regions.
4 Optic glioma.
5 ≥2 Lisch nodules.
6 Distinctive osseous lesion typical of NF1, eg sphenoid dysplasia.
7 First-degree relative with NF1 according to the above-listed criteria.

Differential diagnosis: McCune–Albright syndrome (OHCS p854), multiple lentigines, urticaria pigmentosa.

NF2

Diagnosis is made if either of the following are found:

1 Bilateral vestibular Schwannomas seen on MRI or CT.
2 First-degree relative with NF2, and either:
  (a) Unilateral vestibular Schwannoma; or
  (b) One of the following:
   • Neurofibroma
   • Meningioma
   • Glioma
   • Schwannoma
   • Juvenile cataract (NF2 type).

Differential diagnosis: NF1, Schwannomatosis.

Causes of café-au-lait spots Normal (eg up to 5); NF1 (↑melanocyte density vs 'normal' *café-au-lait* spots); NF2; rare syndromes: Gaucher's; McCune–Albright; Russell–Silver; tuberous sclerosis; Wiskott–Aldrich.

Syringomyelia

The presence of a CSF-filled tubular cavity (syrinx) in or close to the central canal of the cervical cord. *Mean age of onset:* 30yrs. *Prevalence:* 8/100 000. Symptoms may be static for years, but then worsen fast—eg on coughing or sneezing, as ↑pressure causes extension, eg into the brainstem (syringobulbia, see later in topic).

Causes *Typically,* blocked CSF circulation with ↓flow from basal posterior fossa to caudal space, eg Chiari malformation (see below); basal arachnoid fibrosis (postinfectious/ haemorrhagic); masses (cysts, tumours). *Less commonly,* a syrinx may develop after cord trauma, myelitis, or within spinal tumours (ependymoma or haemangioblastoma).

Signs *Dissociated sensory loss* (absent pain and T° sensation, with preserved light touch, vibration, and joint-position sense) due to pressure from the syrinx on the decussating spinothalamic fibres (fig 10.37) in a root distribution reflecting the location of the syrinx (eg for typical cervical cervical syrinx there is a cape-like distribution over the trunk and arms); *wasting/weakness* of hands ± *claw-hand* (then arms→shoulders→respiratory muscles). Anterior horn cells are also vulnerable. **Other signs** Horner's syndrome (can be bilateral and therefore more difficult to spot); UMN leg signs; body asymmetry, limb hemi-hypertrophy, or unilateral odo- or chiromegaly (enlarged hand or foot), perhaps from release of trophic factors via anterior horn cells; Charcot's joints in the shoulder/wrist due to lost joint proprioception (see fig 5.11, p207).

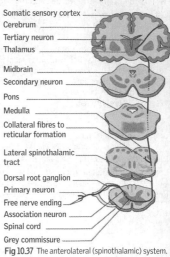

Somatic sensory cortex
Cerebrum
Tertiary neuron
Thalamus

Midbrain
Secondary neuron

Pons

Medulla
Collateral fibres to reticular formation

Lateral spinothalamic tract
Dorsal root ganglion
Primary neuron
Free nerve ending
Association neuron
Spinal cord
Grey commissure

Fig 10.37 The anterolateral (spinothalamic) system.

Syringobulbia (Brainstem involvement.) Nystagmus, tongue atrophy, dysphagia, pharyngeal/palatal weakness, vth nerve sensory loss.

MRI imaging How big is the syrinx? Any Chiari malformation/cord tumours?

Management Surgical treatment of Chiari malformations may reduce pain and progression, but depends on symptoms and is not essential. Drainage procedures with shunt insertion are used in cases of progressive deficits. Deterioration is usually gradual and obvious. Advise patients to avoid breath-holding during exercise to prevent Valsalva-induced sudden expansions.

Chiari malformations

A group of disorders (predominantly types I–IV) characterized by anatomical abnormalities of the cerebellum, brainstem, and/or posterior fossa causing herniation of the cerebellum ± medulla through the foramen magnum. This may cause infantile hydrocephalus with intellectual disability, optic atrophy, ocular palsies, and spastic paresis of the limbs. Spina bifida, syringomyelia, or focal cerebellar and brainstem signs may occur (p495). Type I, the most common and least severe, is characterized by downward displacement of abnormal cerebellar tonsils only. Often presents in early adulthood. In type II, the Arnold–Chiari malformation, there is also herniation of the vermis and brainstem associated with myelomeningocoele (a neural tube defect).

Management The diagnosis is made on MRI. Foramen magnum decompression surgery is undertaken depending on the degree of associated impairment. CSF flow studies can be helpful in equivocal cases.

HIV and AIDS (See p394.) Can have multiple neurological manifestations: these conditions are part of the differential diagnosis of meningitis, intracranial mass lesions, dementia, encephalomyelitis, cord problems, and peripheral neuropathies.

Acute infection May be associated with transient aseptic meningoencephalitis (typically self-limiting), myelopathy, and neuropathy.

Opportunistic infections Arise during low CD4 counts, which allow unusual or atypical organisms to infect the nervous system: • *Toxoplasma gondii* (p397) is the main CNS pathogen in AIDS, causing cerebral abscesses which present with focal signs, eg seizures, hemiparesis. CT/MRI shows ring-shaped contrast-enhancing lesions. Treat with pyrimethamine (+ folinic acid) + sulfadiazine or clindamycin for 6 months. Continue secondary prophylaxis until CD4 count >200. Pneumocystis prophylaxis also protects against toxoplasmosis. • *Cryptococcus neoformans* (fig 10.38) causes a chronic meningitis with fever and headache (neck stiffness may be absent). Cognition alters slowly, seizures and coma may follow. Treat with amphotericin followed by fluconazole. • *Cytomegalovirus* (CMV) can cause encephalopathy. • *Progressive multifocal leukoencephalopathy* (PML) is caused by the JC virus. There is progressive white matter inflammation. Mortality even with antiretroviral therapy (ART) is around 50% at 1yr. • Syphilis and TB may also cause meningitis.

Tumours Affecting the CNS include primary cerebral lymphoma (associated with EBV) and B-cell lymphoma. CSF JC virus PCR is useful in distinguishing PML from lymphoma.

Neuropathies Common in HIV, and may be a result of the disease itself or ART. Up to 30% of patients have peripheral neuropathy, which is painful and predominantly sensory. Others include polyradiculopathy, mononeuritis multiplex, and proximal myopathy.

HIV-associated neurocognitive disorders (HAND) While ART has decreased the incidence of CNS complications in HIV/AIDS, people are living longer with the disease and chronic complications such as HIV-associated dementia (HAD) are increasing. This occurs in 7–15%, late in the disease, and usually when the CD4 count is <200. Progressive behavioural changes are seen along with subcortical features: memory loss, poor attention, and bradykinesia. Various encephalopathies may also contribute to this, eg PML. A 'CNS escape syndrome' occurs rarely, in which deficits such as HAD occur due to HIV replication in the CSF despite successful suppression elsewhere.

Human T-cell lymphotropic virus (HTLV-1) Is another retrovirus with neurological manifestations, though much more rarely than HIV (~0.5%). It causes: *tropical spastic paraplegia*, a slowly progressing myelopathy, typically affecting the thoracic area. There may be paraesthesiae, sensory loss, and disorders of micturition. *Demyelinating polyneuropathy* and *ataxia* may also occur.

10 Neurology

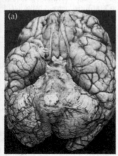
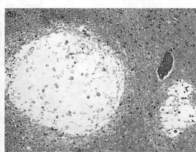

Fig 10.38 Cryptococcosis. (a) Chronic meningitis involving the basal leptomeninges with multiple small intraparenchymal cysts seen in the cerebral cortex. (b) Under the microscope we see these cysts as dilatation of the perivascular space to form cavities filled with colonies of cryptococci, which appear as round basophilic structures.

11 Oncology and palliative care

Contents

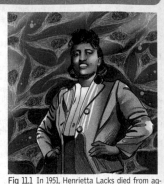

Fig 11.1 In 1951, Henrietta Lacks died from aggressive metastatic cervical cancer. Her family and friends mourned her. They remembered her for her stylish dress, her red nail varnish, and her love of spaghetti. They recalled that she would always open her door to those in need. They were saddened that they could no longer see her dance with one of her five children in her arms. But a small part of her was able to cheat death. An immortal part of a mortal woman. Taken to a laboratory without her consent, her cancer cells survived and reproduced to become the HeLa cell line: a mainstay of biological research leading to key discoveries in cancer, immunology, and infectious disease, to the tune of billions of dollars. But the HeLa cell line is not a story of success. It is the story of a Black woman, receiving care in a Black hospital where there was no legal requirement for consent. It is a story bound in immorality. Should the use of HeLa cell lines therefore stop in an attempt to make up for this injustice? Not according to her family, who advocate ongoing use provided that there can finally be an acknowledgement of this African American woman, her identity, and her life. And it remains beholden to us all to examine narratives of respect and race, to acknowledge the legacy of mistreatment of non-white patients in healthcare systems, and to understand that consent is not a legal waiver but a foundation for communication and equity in treatment and research.

Artwork by Gillian Turner.

We thank Matthew Wheater and Antonia Field-Smith, our Specialist Readers for this chapter.

Looking after people with cancer

Cancer will affect 50% of people born after 1960. More than a quarter of deaths in the UK are from cancer.[1] While many may not appreciate the poor prognosis attached to diagnoses such as liver failure or heart failure, 'cancer' has a widespread association with suffering and death. Yet 'cancer' is not a homogeneous disease but a group of conditions with prognoses ranging from very good (98% 10yr survival for testicular cancer) to extremely poor (21% 1yr survival for pancreatic cancer).[1]

Communication[2] is the first step on a cancer pathway. A range of feelings can surface upon receiving a cancer diagnosis: shock, numbness, denial, panic, anger, resignation ('I knew all along…'). Preconceptions may be deeply embedded leading to inappropriate despair or optimism. Without an understanding of your patient's starting point, you may fail to be effective in your guidance and support.

Tips for the discussion of a cancer diagnosis

1 Set the environment up carefully. Choose a quiet place where you will not be disturbed. Make sure family or friends are present according to your patient's wishes. Anticipate likely questions and be sure of your facts.
2 Find out what the patient already knows and believes (often a great deal). 'What are you worried about today?'
3 Give some warning: 'There is some bad news for us to address'.
4 Ascertain how much the person wants to know. 'Are you someone who likes to know all the details about your condition?' Although information is a priority for the majority of cancer patients, this may change with the individual, and the course of the disease. Some will seek information, some may need an alternative focus.
5 Share information about diagnosis and treatments. Specifically list supporting people (oncology multidisciplinary team) and institutions (hospices). Break information down into manageable chunks and check understanding for each.
6 Invite questions patients may feel they cannot ask. 'Is there anything else you want me to explain?' Do not hesitate to go over the same ground repeatedly. Allow denial, don't force the pace, give time. Listen to any concerns raised, encourage the airing of feelings. Empathize.
7 Address prognosis. Be honest. Doctors are often too optimistic. Survival rates are for the population, not the individual. Discuss prognosis in terms of days, weeks, months, or years. Encourage an appropriate level of hope (see BOX 'Spiritual pain', p531), refer to an expert.
8 Make a plan. The desire to be involved in decisions about treatment is variable: your patient's locus of control can be internal (desire control of their own destiny) or external (passive acceptance). Decision-making can be immediate, deferred, panicked, or rationally deliberated. Time may be required to facilitate any style of decision-making: your plan may be simply to come back and talk again.
9 Summarize, and offer availability. Record details of your conversation including the language used.
10 Follow through. ▶Leave your patient with the knowledge that you are with them, and that your unwritten contract will not be broken.

No rules guarantee success. Use whatever your patient gives you—closely observe both verbal and non-verbal cues. Getting to know your patient, seeking out the right expert for each stage of treatment, and making an agreed management plan, are all required.

For any situation which involves the communication of bad news, consider SPIKES:[3]
• **S**etting up the interview.
• Assess the patient's **P**erception of the situation.
• Obtain an **I**nvitation (asking the patient's permission to explain).
• Give **K**nowledge and information to the patient.
• Address the **E**motional response with **E**mpathy.
• **S**trategy and **S**ummary: aim for consensus with patient and family.

11 Oncology and palliative care

How cancers develop

Human life requires cells which are capable of dividing millions of times. These cells need to be able to adapt and change so that different tissues and organs can be formed. They need to command their own blood supply. Without extensive mechanisms to control cell growth and prevent the replication of abnormal cells, these requirements for life become the basis for the development of a cancer. Failure of cell control mechanisms causes cancer.

Cancer is a genetic disease. Genetic changes occur in cell growth, cell differentiation, and cell death pathways. Mutations can be inherited or acquired. Acquired or somatic errors occur due to age, exposure to carcinogens, and in unchecked rapid cell turnover. Mutations result in:
- 'Gain of function' *oncogenes* that have pathological activity in the absence of a relevant signal. For example, RAS is a protein involved in signal transduction. It is mutated in ~30% of human cancers. Oncogenes behave in a dominant manner: mutation to one allele results in unchecked activation.
- 'Loss of function' *tumour suppressor genes* no longer act as inhibitors of pro-malignant processes. In most cases, mutations to both alleles must occur for a cancer phenotype. This can occur either as two separate somatic events, or in the case of predisposition genes, the first 'hit' is inherited and the second occurs somatically. Tumours therefore occur earlier and more frequently in familial cancers. p53 is a tumour suppressor gene mutated in ~50% of human cancers.

Most cancers arise from multiple mutations. This is perhaps best represented in the stepwise accumulation of mutations in colorectal cancer (**fig 11.2**). An understanding of the molecular biology of cancer facilitates drug development (**fig 11.3**).

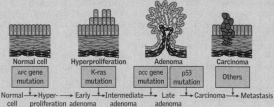

Fig 11.2 Cellular mutations and contributing genes in the development of colorectal cancer.

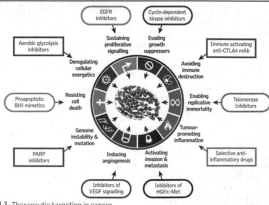

Fig 11.3 Therapeutic targeting in cancer.

Reprinted from *Cell*, 144(5), Hanahan *et al.*, Hallmarks of Cancer: the Next Generation, 646–74, 2011, with permission from Elsevier.

A variety of clinical signs and symptoms should alert you to the possible presence of malignancy. The following list is based on clinical features with a 3% positive predictive value for cancer.[4] It is by no means exhaustive and does not negate the value of clinical judgement. Urgent = within 2 weeks.

Lung
- Admit if: symptomatic superior vena caval obstruction (p524), stridor.
- Urgent referral if: >40yrs with unexplained haemoptysis, CXR suggestive of cancer.
- Urgent CXR if >40yrs and:
  - persistent/recurrent chest infection
  - finger clubbing
  - supraclavicular/cervical lymphadenopathy
  - thrombocytosis
  - two of: cough, fatigue, SOB, chest pain, weight loss, ↓appetite, smoker, asbestos.

Upper GI
- Urgent endoscopy if: dysphagia, or >55yrs with weight loss and upper abdominal pain/reflux/dyspepsia.
- Urgent referral if: >40yrs plus jaundice, or upper abdominal mass.
- Urgent CT of the pancreas if >60yrs plus weight loss plus any of: diarrhoea, back pain, abdominal pain, nausea, constipation, new-onset diabetes.
- Non-urgent endoscopy if:
  - >55yrs and one of: treatment-resistant dyspepsia, upper abdominal pain plus low Hb, ↑plts, or N&V plus upper GI symptoms/weight loss
  - haematemesis (if low-risk with no indications for urgent endoscopy).

Lower GI
PR examination and FBC in all.
- Urgent referral if: positive faecal occult blood, >40yrs with abdominal pain plus weight loss, >50yrs with unexplained rectal bleeding, >60yrs with iron-deficient anaemia or change in bowel habit.
- Consider urgent referral if: rectal/abdominal mass, anal ulceration, <50yrs with rectal bleeding plus lower GI symptoms or weight loss or iron-deficiency anaemia.
- Quantitative faecal immunochemical testing (FIT) if: >50yrs plus abdominal pain or weight loss, <60yrs with change in bowel habit or iron-deficiency anaemia, >60yrs and anaemia.

Gynaecological
- Urgent referral if: ascites, pelvic mass (fibroid excluded), >55yrs with post-menopausal bleeding.

Breast
- Urgent referral if: >30yrs with unexplained breast lump, >50yrs with symptoms or change to one nipple.
- Consider urgent referral if: skin changes, >30yrs with axillary lump.

Urology
- Urgent referral if:
  - irregular prostate on PR, abnormal age-specific PSA (p526)
  - >40yrs with unexplained visible haematuria, >60yrs with unexplained non-visible haematuria plus dysuria or ↑WCC
  - non-painful enlargement or change in shape/texture of testicle.

Central nervous system
- Urgent MRI in progressive, sub-acute loss of central neurological function.

▶Unexplained weight loss, ↓appetite, and DVT can be non-specific signs of cancer. Assess for any additional risk factors, symptoms, signs, and refer accordingly.
See also *haematology* (p350); *thyroid* (p592); *skin* (p588).

Chemotherapy[5] is the use of any chemical substance to treat disease, though use usually relates to the use of drugs in the treatment of cancer. Chemotherapy can be:
- *Untargeted:* cytotoxic (kills) rapidly dividing cells, given at intervals (cycles) to allow recovery of normal tissue.
- *Targeted:* act on molecular targets specific to cancer cells (biologic therapy), often cytostatic (block proliferation).

►*Chemotherapy should be prescribed and given only under expert guidance by people trained in its use.*

Untargeted chemotherapy
- **Single-agent** Rarely curative as genetically resistant cells are selected out.
- **Combination chemotherapy** Different mechanisms of action and side effect profiles reduce the likelihood of resistance and toxicity. The drugs used should have:
  - cytotoxic activity for that tumour, preferentially able to induce remission
  - different mechanisms of action, ideally additive or synergistic effects
  - non-overlapping toxicity to maximize benefit of full therapeutic doses
  - different mechanisms of resistance.
- **Adjuvant** After other initial treatment to reduce the risk of relapse, eg following surgical removal of cancer.
- **Neoadjuvant** Used to shrink tumours prior to surgical or radiological treatment. May allow later treatment to be more conservative.
- **Palliative** No curative aim, offers symptom relief, may prolong survival.

Classes of cytotoxic drugs include:
- **Alkylating agents** Anti-proliferative drugs that bind via alkyl groups to DNA leading to apoptotic cell death, eg cyclophosphamide, chlorambucil, busulfan.
- **Antimetabolites** Interfere with cell metabolism including DNA and protein synthesis, eg methotrexate, fluorouracil.
- **Antitumour antibiotics** Interrupt DNA function, eg dactinomycin, doxorubicin, mitomycin, bleomycin.
- **Topoisomerase inhibitors** Interrupt regulation of DNA winding, eg etoposide.
- **Vinca alkaloids and taxanes** 'Spindle poisons' which target mechanisms of cell division, eg vincristine, vinblastine, docetaxel.

Side effects
Due to cytotoxic effects on non-cancer cells. Greatest effect seen on dividing cells, ie gut, hair, bone marrow, gametes (see BOX 'Fertility', p523).
- **Vomiting** Prophylaxis is given with most cytotoxic regimens (p247).
- **Alopecia** May profoundly impact quality of life. Consider 'cold-cap', wig services.
- **Neutropenia** Most commonly seen 7–14d after chemotherapy. ►►Neutropenic sepsis is life-threatening and needs urgent assessment and empirical treatment (p350).

Extravasation of chemotherapy

Extravasation[6] = inadvertent infiltration of a drug into subcutaneous/subdermal tissue. **Presentation** Tingling, burning, pain, redness, swelling, no 'flashback'/resistance from cannula. **Management** Stop and disconnect infusion. Aspirate residual drug before cannula removed. Follow local policies: ask for the 'extravasation kit'. Drug-specific recommendations:
- DNA-binding drugs (anthracyclines, alkylating agents): dry cold compress to vasoconstrict and ↓ drug spread.
- Non-DNA-binding drugs (vinca alkaloids, taxanes, platin salts): dry warm compress to vasodilate and ↑ drug distribution.

Beau's lines

Beau's lines (fig 11.4) are horizontal depressions in the nail plate that run parallel to the nail bed. They result from an interruption of keratin synthesis and may be due to infection/trauma, systemic illness, or from medication (p75). Each line in this photo coincided with a round of chemotherapy.

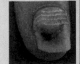

Fig 11.4 Beau's lines.

Targeted cancer treatments

A form of 'precision medicine' using the specific genetic/protein profile of a tumour. Utilizes tumorigenic pathways and control of immunity. The aim is that specificity confers efficacy and reduces adverse side effects.

Small molecule inhibitors
- Usually end with the stem '-ib'.
- Small size allows translocation through the cell membrane to cytoplasm.
- Interact with cytoplasmic domain of cell surface receptors and cell-signalling molecules.
- Interfere with enzymes, eg tyrosine kinase, epidermal/endothelial growth factors, matrix metalloproteinases, heat-shock and apoptotic proteins, specific mutations.
- An abnormal BCR-ABL fusion protein activates signal transduction pathways in *chronic myeloid leukaemia*. Imatinib binds to the BCR-ABL tyrosine kinase binding site and stabilizes it, preventing activation. This leads to ↓disease progression and ↑survival (>80% at 10 years).
- 50% of metastatic melanomas harbour a mutation that leads to BRAF gene activation leading to abnormal cell proliferation and survival via the mitogen-activated protein kinase (MAPK) pathway and MEK enzymes. MAPK pathway inhibition with combination BRAF plus MEK inhibition (eg dabrafenib+trametinib, vemurafenib+ cobimetinib, encorafenib+binimetinib) improves survival.
- Small molecule inhibitors may be less effective where tumorigenesis is driven by multiple pathways or complex genomic abnormalities, which are more common in advanced (blast) disease. Tumour resistance can also develop.

Antibody targeted therapies
- Usually end with the stem '-mab' (= monoclonal antibody).
- Immune system: alemtuzumab binds to CD52, marking B-cells for destruction in B-cell chronic lymphocytic leukaemia.
- Cell growth: trastuzumab targets human epidermal growth factor receptor 2 (HER2) in HER2-positive breast cancer.
- Monoclonal antibodies targeting epidermal growth factor receptor (EGFR) and vascular endothelial growth factor (VEGF) are used in the treatment of colon, lung, brain, kidney, and head and neck cancers.
- Antibody therapies can also be conjugated with chemotherapy (chemolabel) or radioactive particles (radiolabel) for added therapeutic efficacy.

Endocrine targets
- Anti-oestrogens: aromatase inhibitors (eg letrozole, anastrozole) and oestrogen receptor antagonists (eg tamoxifen, raloxifene) in breast cancer.
- Anti-androgens: androgen receptor inhibitors (eg enzalutamide and apalutamide) in prostate cancer.

Immunotherapy: immune-checkpoint inhibitors
- An immune checkpoint is the interaction between cellular proteins (eg cytotoxic T-lymphocyte-associated protein-4 (CTLA-4), programmed death-1 (PD-1), programmed death-ligand 1 (PDL-1)), and T-cells to prevent an immune response.
- Immune checkpoint expression by cancer cells prevents immune-mediated cell death.
- Inhibition of immune checkpoints therefore leads to cancer cell death.
- Immune-checkpoint inhibitors are now used therapeutically in >50 cancer subtypes. Examples include:
  - ipilimumab (blocks CTLA-4) in metastatic melanoma, renal cell carcinoma, non-small lung cell cancer, malignant pleural mesothelioma
  - pembrolizumab (activates PD1) in metastatic melanoma, non-small cell lung cancer, Hodgkin's lymphoma, urothelial carcinoma, head and neck cancers.
- Two in three cancer trials in 2020 were trials of T-cell modulators.
- Transient ↑tumour size due to immune cell recruitment = pseudo-progression.
- Inflammatory side effects occur as the physiological brake in the immune system is also lost, eg thyroiditis, enteritis, hepatitis, myocarditis, encephalitis, transplant rejection. May require (high-dose) steroids.

Radiotherapy[7] is used in more than 50% of all cancers. It is part of the treatment in 40% of those considered cured. It uses ionizing radiation to cause damage to DNA, preventing cell division and leading to cell death. The aim of radiotherapy treatment is to inactivate cancer cells whilst avoiding a severe reaction in normal tissue.

Radical treatment Given with curative intent. Total dose ranges from 40–70 gray (Gy) in up to 40 fractions. Some regimens involve several smaller fractions a day with a gap of 6–8h. Combined chemoradiation is used in some sites to increase response rate.

Palliative radiotherapy Aims to relieve symptoms, may not impact survival. Doses are smaller and given in fewer fractions to offer short-term tumour control with minimal side effects, eg brain metastases, spinal cord compression, visceral compression, haemoptysis, haematuria. Bone pain from metastases can be reduced or eliminated in 60%.

Early reactions
Occur ~2 weeks into treatment, peak ~2–4 weeks after treatment.
- **Tiredness** ~80%. Improves ~4 weeks after treatment completed but chronic in ~30%. Encourage patients to be as active as their condition allows.
- **Skin reactions** Include erythema, dry desquamation, moist desquamation, and ulceration. Aqueous cream can be used on unbroken areas.
- **Mucositis** All patients receiving head and neck treatment should have a dental check-up before therapy. Avoid smoking. Antiseptic mouthwashes may help. Soluble analgesic gargle can be tried. Treat oral thrush with fluconazole 50mg/24h PO, nystatin may exacerbate nausea.
- **Nausea and vomiting** Occur when stomach, liver, or brain treated. Treat with metoclopramide 10mg/8h PO (central and peripheral dopamine antagonist), domperidone 10mg/8h PO (peripheral dopamine antagonist), or ondansetron 4–8mg/8h PO/IV (serotonin 5HT$_3$ antagonist, can exacerbate constipation) (p530).
- **Diarrhoea** After abdominal or pelvic treatments. Maintain good hydration. Avoid high-fibre agents. Loperamide 2mg PO after loose stools (max 16mg/24h) may help.
- **Dysphagia** Following thoracic treatments. Speech and language input, nutrition.
- **Cystitis** After pelvic treatments. Oral fluid to maintain good urine output.

Late reactions Months–years after treatment.
- **CNS/PNS** *Somnolence:* 4–6wks after brain radiotherapy. Consider ↑steroid dose. *Spinal cord myelopathy:* progressive weakness. Needs MRI to exclude cord compression. *Brachial plexopathy:* numb, weak, painful arm after axillary radiotherapy.
- **Lung** *Pneumonitis* can occur 6–12wks after thoracic treatment causing dry cough ± dyspnoea. Bronchodilators and tapered steroids may help.
- **GI** *Xerostomia* = dry mouth due to reduced saliva. Dental care and nutrition important. Treat with water, saliva substitutes, salivary stimulants. *Benign strictures* of oesophagus or bowel. Treat with dilatation. Seek a specialist surgical opinion regarding *fistulae*. *Radiation proctitis* may be a problem after prostate irradiation.
- **GU** *Urinary frequency:* small fibrosed bladder after pelvic treatment. *Vaginal stenosis, dyspareunia, erectile dysfunction* can occur after pelvic radiotherapy. ↓*Fertility:* due to pelvic radiotherapy (p523).
- **Endocrine** *Panhypopituitarism* following radical treatment involving pituitary fossa. Check hormone profile in children: growth hormone replacement may be required. *Hypothyroidism* in ~50% after neck treatment: check TFTs annually.
- **Secondary cancers** Risk (2–4 per 10 000 person-years) is usually insignificant compared to recurrence/death from primary lesion. More important for younger patients after curative treatment. Women <35yrs receiving radiotherapy for Hodgkin's lymphoma should be offered breast screening from 8yrs after treatment.

▶↑Cancer survival may mean ↑numbers living with health effects or disability after treatment (~625 000 in the UK). Remember the emotional and physical impact of cancer extends beyond the prescribed course of radiotherapy/chemotherapy.

Methods of delivering radiotherapy

Conventional external beam radiotherapy (EBRT) The most common form of treatment. Delivers beams of ionizing radiation to the patient from an external linear accelerator.

Stereotactic radiotherapy A highly accurate form of EBRT used to target small lesions with great precision—most frequently in treating intracranial tumours. It is often referred to by the manufacturer's name, eg *Gamma Knife®*, *Truebeam®*.

Brachytherapy Involves a radiation source being placed within or close to a tumour, allowing a high local radiation dose. Implants may be placed within a cavity (eg uterus, post-surgical space) or within tissue (eg prostate, breast).

Radioisotope therapy Uses tumour-seeking radionuclides to target specific tissues. For example, ^{131}I (radioiodine) to ablate remaining thyroid tissue after thyroidectomy for thyroid cancer.

Interventional oncology

Interventional oncology refers to interventional radiology procedures used in the treatment or palliation of patients with cancer. Can be divided into disease-modifying and symptomatic procedures.

Disease-modifying interventional oncology

Intended to modify cancer progression and/or to improve prognosis. Includes:
- Image-guided ablation, eg radiofrequency ablation, cryoablation, irreversible electroporation.
- Embolization, eg transarterial embolization, chemoembolization.
- Image-guided radiation, eg brachytherapy: radiation source placed in/near the area to be treated; selective internal radiation therapy: radiation source administered in small beads via the bloodstream into organ affected by cancer.
- Isolated perfusion chemotherapy: uses occlusion techniques to protect normal tissue from high doses of chemotherapy.

Symptomatic interventional oncology

Provides relief from cancer-related symptoms, but does not modify the underlying disease process. The techniques (table 11.1) can offer significantly improved quality of life, reduce admissions, and increase time spent outside of hospital.

Table 11.1 Interventional techniques available for cancer symptom control

Clinical problem	Interventional treatment option
Ascites	Temporary/permanent image-guided ascitic drain
Pleural effusion	Temporary/permanent image-guided pleural drain
Superior vena cava obstruction (p524)	Superior vena cava stenting
Oesophageal obstruction	Oesophageal stenting
Large bowel obstruction	Colonic stenting
Tumour-related haemorrhage	Transarterial embolization
Jaundice	Biliary drainage and stenting
Renal tract obstruction	Nephrostomy, ureteric stenting
Bone metastases	Image-guided ablation

►Talk to your interventional radiologist.

Imaging

Imaging is essential in oncology for diagnosis, prognosis, and to inform and guide treatment. As well as plain radiographs, ultrasound scans, CT, and MRI, there is a wealth of more specialist imaging including:

PET-CT PET uses a non-specific radioactive tracer (FDG) which highlights areas of increased metabolism, cell proliferation, or hypoxia. It therefore accumulates in cancer cells >non-cancer cells. PET-CT is a powerful combination of anatomical (CT) and functional (PET) information allowing diagnosis, increased accuracy of staging, and assessment of treatment response.

Monoclonal antibodies Radiolabelled tumour antibodies specific to the tumour under investigation, eg prostate-specific membrane antigen, somatostatin (neuro-endocrine tumours), oestrogen receptor (breast). They can offer better specificity than standard PET images.

Bone scintigraphy (bone scan) Detects abnormal metabolic activity in bones including bone metastases.

Staging

Staging systems are used to describe the extent of a cancer. This is vital to determine the most appropriate treatment, to assess prognosis, and to identify relevant clinical trials. A cancer is always referred to by the stage given at diagnosis. The TNM system is most widely used and is based on the extent of tumour (T), spread to lymph nodes (N), and the presence of metastases (M) (table 11.2).

Table 11.2 TNM cancer staging

TX	Primary tumour cannot be measured	NX	Nodes cannot be assessed
T0	Primary tumour cannot be found	N0	No node involvement
Tis	Carcinoma *in situ* (abnormal cells present)	N1–3	Number/location of node metastases
T1–4	Size and/or extent of primary tumour (1 = small tumour/minimal invasion; 4 = large tumour/extensive invasion)	M0	No distant spread
		M1	Distant metastases

Other prefixes may also be used: c refers to clinical stage; p is the stage after pathological examination; y refers to stage after neoadjuvant therapy; r is used if a tumour is re-staged after a disease-free interval; a indicates stage at autopsy.

TNM staging may be converted to an overall, less detailed classification of cancer stage: 0–IV. Stage 0 refers to carcinoma *in situ*; stages I–III describe the size of cancer and/or nearby spread; stage IV indicates metastatic disease.

Some cancers may have alternative staging systems such as Duke's classification for colorectal cancer (p608). See also lung cancer (p182); breast cancer (p594); oesophageal cancer (p610); bladder cancer (p638).

Surgery

• **Prevention** Risk-reducing surgery, eg thyroidectomy in MEN (p217), colectomy in familial adenomatous polyposis.
• **Screening** Endoscopy, colposcopy.
• **Diagnosis and staging** Fine needle aspiration, core needle biopsy, vacuum-assisted biopsy, excisional/incisional biopsy, sentinel lymph node biopsy, endoscopy, diagnostic/staging laparoscopy, laparoscopic ultrasound.
• **Treatment** Resection of solid tumour (may be combined with chemo/radiotherapy, targeted therapy).
• **Reconstruction** eg following treatment for breast, head, and neck cancers.
• **Palliation** Bypass, stoma, stenting, pathological fractures.

The multidisciplinary team (MDT)

The care of all patients diagnosed with cancer is formally reviewed by a MDT. The aim of the MDT is to coordinate high-quality diagnosis, treatment, and care. The MDT should make a recommendation on the best initial treatment for cancer. Note: an MDT can only 'recommend'; the decision must be made in consultation with the patient. The MDT is made up of healthcare professionals with expertise in treating and supporting patients with cancer. Members should include, but are not limited to, the following:

• Lead clinician and lead nurse specialist.
• Radiologists (see BOX 'Interventional oncology', p521).
• Histopathologists.
• Expert surgeons, eg upper GI, colorectal, breast, plastics.
• Oncologists (medical and clinical).
• Palliative care physicians.
• Nominated member to support ongoing clinical trials.
• Patient representative.
• Administrative support.

Clinical trials

• **Advantages** Possibility of more effective treatment, close monitoring, direct access to a research team, reassurance from number of clinical encounters, gain from altruism.
• **Disadvantages** Possibility that therapy is no better or worse than standard, unknown toxicity, time-consuming, anxiety from number of clinical encounters.

You may look after patients who are participating in clinical trials. For many of these, you will not be familiar with the trial therapy or even know which therapy the patient is receiving: new therapy, standard therapy, or placebo.

►Contact the research team to discuss any clinical concerns or change in treatment. Contact details for the research team should be recorded in the clinical record. Look for, or ask the patient if they have a copy of, the 'Participant Information Sheet' which is mandatory for all UK research studies. Information on relevant trials is available:

• Cancer Research UK: www.cancerresearchuk.org/about-cancer/find-a-clinical-trial
• International Standard Randomised Controlled Trial Number (ISRCTN) registry: www.isrctn.com
• US National Library of Medicine database of international studies: www.clinicaltrials.gov
• EU Clinical Trials Register: www.clinicaltrialsregister.eu

Fertility

Cancer treatment may:
• Damage spermatogonia causing impaired spermatogenesis or male sterility.
• Hasten oocyte depletion leading to premature ovarian failure.

If cancer treatment carries a risk of infertility, fertility preservation techniques[8] should be discussed prior to treatment being given.

• **Men** Semen cryopreservation should be offered prior to treatment when there is risk of genetic damage in sperm. Intracytoplasmic sperm injection means that even a small amount of banked sperm can be used successfully in the future.
• **Women** Cryopreservation of:
  1 Embryos.
  2 Oocytes: if ethical objections to embryo preservation or no partner.
  3 Ovarian tissue: no ovarian stimulation required, experimental technique.
  Ovarian transposition (oophoropexy) may be possible prior to pelvic radiotherapy but protection is not guaranteed due to radiation scatter.

Emergencies[9,10] in oncology include:

Neutropenic sepsis
Temperature >38°C and neutrophil count <0.5 × 10⁹/L (or likely to fall to <0.5 within 48h). Suspect if unwell and within 6wks of chemotherapy. Localizing signs may be absent. Examine IV access sites. ▶▶Immediate treatment saves lives. Use local guidelines or treat empirically with piperacillin/tazobactam (p350).

Spinal cord compression
3–5% of cancer patients have spinal metastases. It is the first presentation of malignancy in up to 20% of metastatic cancers: lung, prostate, breast, myeloma, melanoma, kidney.

Causes Collapse or compression of a vertebral body due to metastases (common), or direct extension of tumour into vertebral column.

Signs and symptoms Back pain in ~95%. Ask about nocturnal pain and pain with movement/straining/sneezing. Urgent review if limb weakness, sensory loss, bowel/bladder dysfunction, unsteady gait. Have a high index of suspicion. Educate patients about symptoms requiring urgent presentation.

Management ▶▶Urgent treatment to preserve neurological function and relieve pain. Urgent (within 24h) MRI of the whole spine. Consider dexamethasone 10–16mg/24h PO (controlled trial data are limited) with gastroprotection (eg PPI), and blood glucose monitoring. If reduced mobility, consider thromboprophylaxis (compression stockings, LMWH). Radiotherapy is the commonest treatment and should be given within 24h of MRI diagnosis. Decompressive surgery ± radiotherapy may be appropriate and gives best functional outcome, depending on prognosis. Patients with loss of motor function for more than 48h are less likely to recover (p462).

Superior vena cava (SVC) syndrome
Reduced venous return from head, neck, and upper limbs. Due to extrinsic compression (most common), or venous thrombosis (consider if current/past central venous access). ▶▶SVC syndrome with airway compromise requires urgent treatment.

Causes >90% of SVC syndrome results from malignancy. Most common cancers are lung (~75%), lymphoma, metastatic (eg breast), thymoma, germ cell.

Signs and symptoms Diagnosis is made clinically. SOB, orthopnoea, stridor, plethora/cyanosis, oedema of face and arm, cough, headache, engorged neck veins (non-pulsatile ↑JVP), engorged chest wall veins. *Pemberton's test:*[1] elevation of the arms to the side of the head causes facial plethora/cyanosis.

Management Sit up. Assess for hypoxia (pulse oximetry, blood gas). Give oxygen if needed. Secure airway. Dexamethasone 16mg/24h or 10mg stat then 4mg/6h. CT to define the anatomy of the obstruction. Balloon venoplasty and SVC stenting provide most rapid relief of symptoms (see BOX 'Interventional oncology', p521). Radiotherapy/chemotherapy depend on the sensitivity of the underlying cancer.

Malignancy-associated hypercalcaemia
Most common metabolic abnormality in cancer patients: ~10–20% of patients with cancer, ~40% of myeloma. It is a poor prognostic sign: 75% mortality within 3 months. Calcium is highly protein bound and needs correcting to the serum albumin concentration. PTH levels should be suppressed (pp668–9).

Causes PTH-related protein produced by the tumour (p525), local osteolysis, eg myeloma, tumour production of calcitriol.

Signs and symptoms Weight loss, anorexia, nausea, polydipsia, polyuria, constipation, abdominal pain, volume depletion, weakness, confusion, seizure, coma.

Management Rehydration. Bisphosphonates (if eGFR ≥30), eg zoledronic acid IV, usually normalize calcium within 3 days and can be given as a repeated infusion. Calcitonin produces a more rapid (2h) but short-term effect and tolerance can develop. Denosumab if bisphosphonate resistant/contraindicated. Furosemide may exacerbate volume deletion. Long-term treatment is control of the malignancy.

---

1 Pemberton described this 'useful' sign of venous obstruction due to a goitre in 1946.

Brain metastases

~20% of patients with cancer. Most commonly lung, breast, colorectal, melanoma, kidney. Better prognosis with single lesion, breast cancer (p814).

Signs and symptoms Headache (~50% morning, coughing, bending), focal neurological signs (~30%), ataxia (~21%), seizure (~18%), nausea, vomiting, papilloedema.

Management Urgent CT/MRI. Dexamethasone 4–16mg/24h based on severity of mass effect symptoms. Analgesia. Seizure control. Surgery or stereotactic radiotherapy (p521). Whole brain radiotherapy does not ↑ survival and may ↓ quality of life due to SE.

Tumour lysis syndrome Chemotherapy for rapidly proliferating cancers (leukaemia, lymphoma, myeloma) causes tumour cell lysis releasing K^+(arrhythmias), phosphate, and nucleic acids, which are catabolized to uric acid. This precipitates in kidney tubules and causes vasoconstriction leading to kidney failure (p310).

Prevention Hydration. Rasburicase: oxidation of uric acid to soluble allantoin. Or allopurinol (febuxostat ↓data): block metabolism of hypo/xanthine to uric acid.

Paraneoplastic syndromes

Paraneoplastic syndromes[11] (table 11.3) are mediated by hormones, cytokines, or cross-reaction of tumour antibodies. They do not correlate with stage/prognosis and may predate other cancer symptoms.

Table 11.3 Examples of paraneoplastic syndromes

Paraneoplastic syndrome	Comment	Cancers	See
Hypercalcaemia	Parathyroid hormone-related protein secreted by tumour	Lung, oesophagus, skin, cervix, breast, kidney	p524
SIADH	Excessive antidiuretic hormone (ADH) secretion causing ↓Na⁺	Lung, pancreas, lymphomas, prostate	p665
Cushing's syndrome	Tumour secretes ACTH or CRF, causing adrenal to produce high levels of corticosteroid	Lung, pancreas, thymus, carcinoid	p218
Neuropathy	Antibody-mediated neuronal degeneration: peripheral, autonomic, cerebellar	Lung, breast, myeloma, Hodgkin's, GI	p500
Lambert–Eaton myasthenic syndrome	Antibody to voltage-gated ion channel on pre-synaptic membrane causes weakness (proximal leg most common)	Mostly lung. Also GI, breast, thymus	p508
Dermatomyositis & polymyositis	Inflammation of the muscles ± heliotrope rash	Lung, breast, ovary, GI	p549
Acanthosis nigricans	Velvety, hyperpigmented skin (usually flexural)	GI	p560
Pemphigus	Blisters to skin/mucous membranes	Lymphoma, thymus, Kaposi's sarcoma	
Hypertrophic osteoarthropathy	Periosteal bone formation, arthritis, finger clubbing	Lung	

Trousseau's sign

Trousseau (fig 11.5) was probably the first to discover a paraneoplastic syndrome. He noticed that many patients with migratory thrombophlebitis ('Trousseau's sign') developed gastric cancer. Unfortunately, he developed migratory thrombophlebitis himself and correctly predicted his own death from GI malignancy.

Fig 11.5 Armand Trousseau 1801–1867.
Wellcome Library, London. Armand Trousseau. Lithograph by JBA Lafosse, 1866, after P Petit.

Tumour markers[12] are specific molecules (usually glycoproteins) that may be found in higher concentrations in the serum, tissue, or urine in patients with certain cancers.

Tumour markers in diagnosis

▶*Tumour markers are insufficiently sensitive or specific to be diagnostic in isolation.*

• Tumour markers are ↑ in cancers but also in some benign conditions (**table 11.4**).

• Do not make opportunistic requests for panels of tumour markers in patients with non-specific symptoms: they are not helpful and lead to potentially unnecessary investigation. This includes PSA in females and CA-125 in males.

• In carefully selected patients, in whom cancer is suspected, highly raised levels of a tumour marker may be helpful:

  • α-fetoprotein (αFP) and human chorionic gonadotropin (hCG) in testicular/germ cell tumours.
  • CA-125 in ovarian cancer, in combination with USS and menopausal status.
  • αFP in those at high risk of hepatocellular carcinoma.
  • PSA >100ng/mL usually indicates metastatic prostate cancer.

• Measurement of hormones may offer clinical utility in the context of a specific clinical syndrome, eg insulin in insulinoma, glucagon in glucagonoma.

Tumour markers in monitoring

The main value of tumour markers is in monitoring patients known to have cancer. This includes the course of the disease, the effectiveness of treatment, and the detection of cancer recurrence. The following markers may be useful:

• αFP and hCG in testicular/germ cell tumours.

• CEA in colorectal cancer.

• CA-125 in ovarian cancer.

• Serum hormone concentrations after resection of hormone-secreting tumour.

• A cautious interpretation of PSA within the limits of its specificity and sensitivity.

Screening for cancer

The UK has well-established cancer screening programmes. Persons born female are offered mammography every 3yrs (50–70yrs) and cervical HPV tests every 3–5yrs (25–64yrs). Persons aged 60–74yrs are offered faecal occult blood testing every 2yrs. The aim of screening is to pick out those who need further investigation to rule out or diagnose a cancer, in the hope that earlier diagnosis and treatment results in better outcomes. All screening tests come with risk: anxiety, harm/discomfort from the test, cost, false-positive results leading to further invasive tests, false negatives conferring inappropriate reassurance when symptoms arise. When screening an asymptomatic population, the potential risks and benefits need to be weighed carefully and the Wilson criteria (p16) should be satisfied.

PSA and prostate cancer

Prostate cancer is the second most common cancer in persons born male. Most prostate cancer has a high prostate-specific antigen (PSA). The higher the PSA, the more likely cancer is. However, PSA is non-specific and also raised in benign prostatic disease, BMI <25, recent ejaculation, rectal examination, anal sex, prostatitis, and UTI. (Remember: 5α reductase inhibitors (finasteride, dutasteride) for benign prostatic hyperplasia cause ↓PSA). Approximately 76% of elevated PSA concentrations are not cancer. After a positive screening test, biopsy carries risk of bleeding, infection, and urinary retention, with ~1% requiring hospital admission.[13] ~1 in 800 avoid death from prostate cancer as a result of PSA screening. But screening also detects cancers that will not cause symptoms or shorten life. This 'overdiagnosis' is thought to occur in ~40% of positive screens with treatment risks including urinary incontinence, erectile dysfunction, and IHD. Population screening using PSA is not recommended due to this imbalance of risk versus benefit. Any patient >50yrs (or >45yrs if high risk) can, however, request PSA testing in primary care. This should be done only following shared decision-making using consistent, complete, and objective information.

▶Only request a test if you know how to interpret the result.

Table 11.4 Summary of tumour markers

Tumour marker	Relevant cancer	Use	Other associated cancers	Associated benign conditions
Alpha-fetoprotein (αFP)	Germ cell/testicular, Hepatocellular	Diagnosis, monitor treatment response, detect recurrence	Colorectal, gastric, hepatobiliary, lung	Cirrhosis; pregnancy; neural tube defects
Calcitonin	Medullary thyroid	Diagnosis, monitor treatment response, detect recurrence	None known	Thyroid C-cell hyperplasia (preneoplastic/carcinoma in situ: not considered entirely benign)
Cancer antigen (CA)-125	Ovarian	Monitor treatment response. Prognosis after chemotherapy	Breast, cervix, endometrium, hepatocellular, lung, non-Hodgkin's lymphoma, pancreas, medullary thyroid carcinoma, peritoneal	Liver disease, cystic fibrosis, pancreatitis, urinary retention, diabetes, heart failure, pregnancy, SLE, sarcoid, RA, diverticulitis, endometriosis, fibroids
CA-19-9	Pancreatic	Monitor treatment response	Colorectal, gastric, hepatocellular, oesophagus, ovary	Acute cholangitis, cholestasis, pancreatitis, diabetes, jaundice
CA-15-3	Breast	Monitor treatment response	Hepatocellular, pancreatic	Cirrhosis, benign breast disease
Carcinoembryonic antigen (CEA)	Colorectal	Monitor treatment response	Breast, gastric, lung, mesothelioma, oesophagus, pancreas	Smoking, chronic liver disease, chronic kidney disease, diverticulitis, jaundice, pregnancy
Human chorionic gonadotropin (hCG)	Germ cell/testicular, gestational trophoblastic	Diagnosis, monitor treatment response, prognosis	Lung	Pregnancy
Paraproteins	Myeloma	Diagnosis, monitor treatment, response detect recurrence	None known	None known
Thyroglobulin	Thyroid (follicular/papillary)	Monitor treatment response, detect recurrence	None known	None known

Source data from 'Serum tumour markers: how to order and interpret them', Sturgeon CM, Lai LC, Duffy MJ, 2012, BMJ Publishing Ltd.

Palliative care: principles and pain

*You matter because you are you and you matter to the last moment of your life.
We will do all we can to help you, not only to die peacefully, but to live until you die.*

Dame Cicely Saunders (1918-2005)

Palliative care is the active holistic care of individuals of all ages with serious health-related suffering due to severe illness, especially those near the end of life. It aims to improve the quality of life of patients, families, and caregivers. It combines management of pain and other symptoms, with psychological, social, and spiritual support.

►Palliative care is not just for the end of life and it is not just for cancer.

Palliative care should run in parallel with other treatments. Symptom control is important in any disease for improving quality of life and may prolong survival.[14]

Consider:
• physical
• psychological
• spiritual
• social.

Most hospitals have a dedicated palliative care team for help and advice (including out of hours). Referral is based on need, not diagnosis. Use their expertise.

►Each person comes with emotions, beliefs, experience, and people that are important to them. Include them all.

Assessment of pain

Pain is often the most feared sequela of a terminal diagnosis and yet it is not inevitable. Pain is a complex phenomenon. Pain is what the patient says it is. It is subjective, often multifactorial, and should always be acknowledged. While the aim is for the patient to be pain free, this may not be feasible for all, so do not promise it. However, control of pain is always possible, even when pain free is not achievable.

Do not assume a cause: detailed history and examination are needed to understand aetiology, which will guide treatment, eg pain from nerve infiltration/compression may respond better to agents other than opioids. Accurate assessment is essential for all patients, including those at the end of life. Severity, nature, functional deficit, and psychological state all contribute to the symptom burden.

Management of cancer pain

Modify the underlying pathology if possible, eg radio/chemotherapy, surgery. Use regular analgesia to relieve background pain with PRN doses for 'breakthrough' pain. Effective analgesia with opioids is possible for the majority using five principles:

1 *By the mouth*—give orally whenever possible.
2 *By the clock*—give at fixed intervals to offer continuous relief.
3 *By the ladder*—follow the WHO stepwise approach (see BOX 'The WHO analgesic ladder').
4 *For the individual*—there is no standard opioid dose, needs vary. Titrate carefully.
5 *Attention to detail*—communicate, set times carefully, warn of side effects.

The WHO analgesic ladder

Increase and decrease analgesia according to 3 steps on a 'ladder':[15]

1 Non-opioid, eg paracetamol, NSAID.
2 Opioid for mild to moderate pain, eg codeine.
3 Opioid for moderate to severe pain, eg morphine, diamorphine, oxycodone.

• Persisting/increasing pain and side effects inform the decision to step up and step down. Take one step at a time, aiming to achieve pain relief without toxicity (except in new, severe pain when step 2 may be omitted).
• Paracetamol (PO/PR/IV) should be continued at steps 2 and 3 if beneficial. Stop step 2 opioids if moving to step 3.
• Consider written instructions when initiating opioids.
• Ensure laxatives and anti-emetics are available when using strong opioids.
• Adjuvants at any step include: amitriptyline, pregabalin, corticosteroids, nerve block, transcutaneous electrical nerve stimulation (TENS), radiotherapy. Seek expert advice (oncology, palliative care, pain team) regarding non-drug options.

Opioids

The amount of opioid required varies and should be titrated on an individual basis. Oral morphine is first line for moderate/severe pain. If the oral route is unavailable, use sc morphine (tables 11.5, 11.6, 11.7, p532). Review regularly.

▶Ensure anti-emetics and laxatives are available for all patients on opioids.

Start low, go slow For an opioid-naïve patient with moderate to severe pain, start immediate-release oral morphine 5mg (2.5mg if frail, AKI/CKD, ↓BMI) every 4h, plus 2.5–5mg PRN (maximum hourly intervals). Onset is 20–30 minutes, peak effect 1h, lasts 3–4h. If pain is not controlled, ↑dose by 30–50% every 24h.

Convert to modified release When pain is controlled, calculate the total daily dose *including PRN* and divide into two 12h doses of a modified-release preparation (eg MST Continus® 12h). Transdermal preparations are available: seek expert help for dose, check adhesion, and rotate site.

Use a PRN dose for breakthrough pain 1/10th–1/6th of the total daily dose as an immediate-release preparation, eg Oramorph®, Sevredol®.

Side effects In >90% of patients. Drowsiness, nausea/vomiting (usually ↓ after 5 days), constipation, dry mouth. If difficulty tolerating morphine, or pain plus toxicity, consider an opioid switch (eg oxycodone) and ↓ equivalent dose by 25–30%.

Toxicity Sedation, ↓RR, visual hallucinations, myoclonic jerks, delirium. Be alert: recognize toxicity early so naloxone is avoided. Monitor oximetry, give oxygen if required. Consider ∆∆: intracranial bleed, kidney injury/failure, other sedatives. Seek help if remains opioid-toxic or in pain. ▶Naloxone is only indicated for life-threatening respiratory depression (p826). It can precipitate a pain crisis and (fatal) acute withdrawal in patients on regular opiates so use lower doses than for overdose, eg 80mcg every 2 minutes—check local guidelines.[16]

Kidney disease Accumulation of renally excreted opioids and metabolites. Monitor closely if eGFR <30. Fentanyl, alfentanil, and buprenorphine have predominantly hepatic metabolism and may be useful in kidney disease—seek expert advice.

Concerns Misconceptions are common: morphine is addictive; it's for the dying; if they use morphine now, it will not work when really needed. *Reassure patients that opioids are effective and safe when used appropriately.* Respiratory depression is rare when titrated correctly but opioids may get blamed if a patient deteriorates. It is illegal to drive if medication impairs ability to drive. Patients should consider whether their driving may be impaired, especially following dose adjustment. Risk of dependency is increased if use >3 months and for non-cancer pain.

Morphine-resistant pain Consider NSAIDs and adjuvants (p528). If neuropathic pain: amitriptyline, pregabalin, topical lidocaine if localized. Seek expert help if allodynia, sensory changes. Consider psychological and spiritual wellbeing (p531). Assess mood, consider talking therapies, antidepressants.

Rapid analgesia Most PRN medication takes time to have an effect. Seek expert help regarding rapid-release preparations (eg sublingual, intranasal, or buccal fentanyl). Pre-empt times of pain (eg dressing changes) and give in advance.

Table 11.5 Opioid dose equivalents: conversions are not exact, potency can vary. If in doubt, use a dose below your estimate. Refer to local guidelines first

Medication	Dose	Equivalent dose of oral morphine
Morphine sc/IV	5mg	10mg
Diamorphine sc/IV	5mg	15mg
Dihydrocodeine	30mg	3mg
Tramadol	50mg	5mg
Oxycodone PO	5mg	10mg
Oxycodone sc	5mg	20mg
Buprenorphine patch	10mcg/h	12mg/day
Alfentanil	1mg	30mg
Fentanyl patch	25mcg/h	60mg/day

Non-pain symptoms[17] include:

Nausea and vomiting

Causes Chemotherapy, constipation, hypercalcaemia, oral candidiasis, GI obstruction, drugs, pain, infection, kidney failure.

Treatment Reversible causes, eg constipation, pain, hypercalcaemia (p524), fluconazole for oral candidiasis. Select an anti-emetic based on the likely mechanism of nausea (table 11.6). If ↓oral absorption consider alternative routes (SC/IV/PR). Regular treatment often better than PRN, but make sure PRN doses are available. Consider antisecretory drugs (eg hyoscine butylbromide, octreotide) if bowel obstruction.

Table 11.6 Antiemetics

Medication	Dose	Considerations
Cyclizine	50mg/8h	Central action for intracranial pathology, mechanoreceptors for stretch, eg liver capsule, ureters, colic, bowel obstruction
Metoclopramide	10mg/8h	Prokinetic effects useful in gastroparesis, monitor for extrapyramidal side effects
Domperidone	10mg/8h	Peripheral action so no dystonic effects
Haloperidol	1.5mg/12–24h	Effective if drug or metabolically induced nausea, use lower doses IV/SC as twice as potent
Ondansetron	4–8mg/8h	Useful in chemo/radiotherapy-related nausea, may exacerbate constipation/headache
Levomepromazine	6.25mg/12–24h	Can sedate, but effective if anxiety contributing, use lower doses if SC as twice as potent

Constipation

Causes Common (but underrecognized and undertreated) side effect of opioids. Easier to prevent than treat: consider laxatives for all starting opioids. Also ↑Ca²⁺ (p524), dehydration, drugs, intra-abdominal disease. AXR may show faecal impaction.
Treatment Reversible causes. Fluid intake. Privacy and access to toilet.
• Stimulant (eg senna 2–4 tablets/bisacodyl 5–10mg) ± softener (eg sodium docusate 100mg BD).
• Osmotic laxative: eg macrogol (if able to tolerate required fluid intake).
• Rectal treatments: bisacodyl/glycerol suppositories, phosphate enema.
• Other: peripheral opioid antagonist, eg naloxegol: not first line as constipation rarely purely opioid induced. Avoid lactulose due to bloating and nausea.

Breathlessness

A distressing and frightening symptom, which can lead to hospital admission.
Causes Infection, effusion, anaemia, arrhythmia, thromboembolism. If stridor/superior vena cava syndrome, treat urgently (p524).
Treatment Reversible causes as appropriate. Thoracocentesis ± pleurodesis for effusion. Radiologically placed permanent drain for recurrent effusion (p521). If distressed, low-dose opioids to ↓ respiratory drive/sensation of breathlessness. If opioid naive, try 1.25mg of immediate-release morphine every 4–6h (convert to modified release if tolerated), or use appropriate breakthrough dose (p529). Physiotherapy/OT, non-drug interventions: fan, breathing exercises. Benzodiazepines may help if anxiety, eg lorazepam 500mcg SL, 4–6h. Oxygen only for symptomatic hypoxaemia.

Oral problems

Causes Poor oral hygiene, radiation, drugs (anticholinergics, chemotherapy, diuretics), infection (candidiasis, herpes simplex), opioids.
Treatment Oral candidiasis: topical miconazole, oral fluconazole 50–100mg OD (check for interactions). Nystatin may not be ineffective and can ↑ nausea. Herpes simplex: oral gan/aciclovir. Mouth care: frequent, small drinks, sugar-free chewing gum, saline (not alcohol) mouthwash, soft toothbrush. Salivary stimulants, eg pilocarpine eye drops 4%, 3 drops in the floor of mouth QDS. Ice may worsen dry mouth due to vasoconstriction. Severe mucositis may need admission and systemic opioid analgesia.

Insomnia

Causes Includes both physical and emotional fatigue. Common, complex, and often multifactorial. Poor sleep can ↑ symptom burden and ↓ quality of life.

Treatment Simple steps may make a big difference: appropriate room temperature, darkness and quiet during the night (request a side room for in-patients). Give prescribed glucocorticoids in the morning. Avoid waking patients for late medications and routine observations. Discuss and address psychosocial issues. Therapy input and goal setting. In some cases, zopiclone or benzodiazepines may be used to help rest and re-establish normal sleep–wake cycles (may exacerbate delirium).

Pruritus

Causes Systemic disease (renal failure, hepatitis, polycythaemia), cancer related (cholestasis, lymphoma, leukaemia, hepatoma, myeloma, paraneoplastic), primary skin disease, drug reaction (opioids, chemotherapy).

Treatment Underlying cause where possible: cholestasis (biliary stenting, colestyramine, sertraline, rifampicin), opioid induced (antihistamine, opioid switch), paraneoplastic (paroxetine). Topical emollients regularly and as a soap substitute. Emollients with menthol. Avoid topical antihistamines as risk of contact dermatitis.

Venepuncture

Consider whether venepuncture is really necessary. Only undertake if the results will change management.

Agitation See 'Care in the last days of life', p532.

Respiratory tract secretions See 'Care in the last days of life', p532.

Spiritual pain

The spiritual aspects of an illness concerns the human experiences of sickness (or 'dis-ease') and the search for meaning within it. Peter W Speck.

Spirituality is a means of experiencing life. It relates to the way in which people understand and live their lives. It is dynamic and includes experience, the seeking and expression of meaning, and the way in which people connect to the moment, to self, to others, and to the world. It is something greater than 'self'. It is distinct from faith and religion, which may or may not be part of spirituality. It may include orthodox and unorthodox beliefs. There is no single definition which encompasses all elements. Spiritual pain[18,19] or suffering is common when people are facing death. It can include feelings of hopelessness, guilt, isolation, meaninglessness, and confusion. Spiritual pain may derive from:
• The past: painful memories, guilt.
• The present: isolation, anger.
• The future: fear, hopelessness.

Reminiscence helps examine the past, provides context, and offers recognition. Anger should be acknowledged. Fear of the imagined future may not change, but may be reduced. The nature of hope may need to be modified. If hope for a cure is inappropriate, it should not be the main or only hope. Realistic hopes include discharge from hospital, seeing family members happy, being remembered. Making a will and dealing with unfinished business facilitate control and may allow a sense of completion.

►Seek to understand your patient's spirituality. Ask your patient, 'What is important to you today?' Recognize and reflect. Ask for help if needed. Remember the whole person: history, coping mechanisms, state of wellbeing. These will alter how disease affects the patient and how the patient responds to disease.

►Companionship is essential. A doctor may need to modify their role to simply accompany the dying patient. This is manageable within professional boundaries and is therapeutic. If you cannot do this, find someone who can: palliative care teams, Macmillan nurses, and chaplains (a listening ear for patients of all faiths and none) are valuable resources.

►Spiritual pain is exacerbated by physical symptoms. These must be addressed if spiritual support is to be effective.

11 Oncology and palliative care

Once it is recognized that a patient is likely to be entering the final days of life (p12), the foci of care should be relief of distressing symptoms,[20] safety, and comfort.

▶*The importance of clear and regular communication with dying patients, their families, and healthcare staff cannot be overemphasized.*[21]

An individualized plan should be made with your patient. Find out what and who are important to them. How much do they know and how much do they want to know? What matters most: being at home or feeling safe with staff available? Consider personal, social, religious, cultural issues. Be compassionate. Remember the person who existed before they became 'the patient'.

Prescribe as required subcutaneous end of life drugs before they are needed, in anticipation of symptoms (table 11.7).

Start a syringe pump when medications are needed regularly, if unable to swallow, or when rapid symptom control is needed (table 11.8). Practice is variable, drugs may be used outside of licensed indications. Defer to local guidelines. If pain relief is insufficient, review opioid dose and recalculate the PRN requirement (p529).

Review other conditions/interventions. Continue to treat reversible problems if beneficial to symptoms/comfort, eg urinary retention. Stop observations and blood tests (unless you are going to act on them). Rationalize medications: keep any that provide symptom benefit, eg analgesia, anti-epileptics.

Manage agitation. Look for reversible causes (pain, dehydration, urinary retention). Use an antipsychotic agent (eg haloperidol) to manage agitated delirium (tables 11.7, 11.8). Try a benzodiazepine such as midazolam if there is a large element of anxiety (but may ↑ delirium). *Opioids should not be used to sedate a dying patient.* Seek early advice from palliative care if agitation is escalating or a significant problem.

Manage excessive secretions. Noise is generated by turbulent air flow and pooling of saliva in the hypopharynx. This may be more distressing for relatives and staff than the patient. There is little evidence that pharmacological agents are beneficial, though they are commonly used. Repositioning and intermittent suctioning may help. If you think secretions are troublesome, consider a trial of an antisecretory drug (glycopyrronium or hyoscine butylbromide: see tables 11.7, 11.8).

Hydration. Many patients approaching the end of life have a poor appetite for food/fluid or are unable to eat/drink. Helping to take sips and good mouth care may suffice. Fluid via non-oral routes (NG, SC, IV) is given for symptomatic benefit; the effect on survival is unknown. Any potential benefit must be weighed against the risk of symptomatic fluid overload. Discuss the pros and cons of hydration and the uncertain effect on survival[21] with patients and families. Correct assumptions that the patient is dying faster because of dehydration or that thirst is causing suffering, especially if the dying phase is prolonged. Make decisions about fluids on a case-by-case basis. Review hydration status at least daily.

Anticipatory end of life medication

Table 11.7 Anticipatory ('just in case') injectable medications for symptoms at the end of life

Indication	Drug	Subcutaneous dose
Pain	Morphine	Opioid naïve: 2.5mg PRN every 1–2h Established on opioids: correct for SC potency (table 11.5) and usually 1/6th of daily dose (p529)
Agitation/anxiety	Midazolam	2.5–5mg SC every 1–2h
Agitation/delirium	Haloperidol	1–3mg every 4h
N&V	Haloperidol	0.5–1mg every 8h
Troublesome respiratory secretions	Glycopyrronium	200–400mcg SC every 4–8h

Plan for death. Ensure that a 'Do Not Attempt Resuscitation' order and treatment escalation plan are in place to avoid futile and distressing interventions. Discuss this with the patient and those who are important to them. Document clearly. Dying at home can usually be arranged at short notice with help from community teams. Hospice or nursing home care may also meet your patient's needs and wishes. Some patients feel safe in hospital and wish to die there.

Respond to changes in the clinical situation. Patients thought to be at the end of life occasionally improve. Acknowledge uncertainty and be ready to plan for different outcomes. Active treatment and palliative care can be given concurrently.

Syringe pumps

Syringe pumps (table 11.8) allow a continuous sc infusion of drugs over 24h, avoiding repeated injections when oral medication cannot be taken. Check compatibility: https://book.pallcare.info/index.php?op=plugin&src=sdrivers. Review daily: titrate doses guided by symptoms and SE. Do not forget anticipatory prescribing (table 11.7).

Table 11.8 Symptom control by sc infusion. Practice varies, defer to local guidelines first

Indication	Drug	Starting subcutaneous dose
Pain	Morphine	If opioid naïve: 5–15mg/24h. If on opioids: calculate daily dose (consider reducing by 25–30%) and convert (table 11.5) to sc morphine over 24h (sc morphine is twice as potent as oral) (p529). Seek palliative care advice
Anxiety	Midazolam	5–20mg/24h
Delirium	Haloperidol	1–5mg/24h
	Levomepromazine	25–100mg/24h (sedation at higher doses)
N&V	Cyclizine	100–150mg/24h
	Haloperidol	1–3mg/24h
	Levomepromazine	6.25–25mg/24h (sedation at higher doses)
Respiratory secretions	Hyoscine butylbromide	60–120mg/24h. Also used for bowel colic
	Glycopyrronium	600–1200mcg/24h
Seizures	Prophylaxis: midazolam 20–30mg/24h (may sedate). Dexamethasone, midazolam, levetiracetam, and sodium valproate can also be given sc	

On wanting to die

Assisted dying is the provision of life-ending drugs for terminally ill, mentally competent adults to administer with strict legal safeguards. It is distinct from euthanasia in which the doctor administers the lethal drug. Across the world, 200 million adults have legal access to medical help to assist with dying, though euthanasia and assisted suicide remain illegal in the UK.

Consider autonomy. Should competent patients have the right to determine their death? If their situation is unbearable, without prospect of improvement, it is a powerful argument. But bearable is subjective and prognosis is an inexact science. And beneficence is divided: is it merciful, or is it abandonment to end suffering through death? And what of consent? Consent is key, but complex. Can a law ensure informed consent? Not without a unique understanding of each patient and the means by which they experience life. A combination of law and medicine may offer false comfort, without full accountability by either. Protection of the vulnerable is a valid concern for doctors and society.

Requests to hasten death are complex and include personal, psychological, spiritual, social, and cultural factors. ~10% of terminally ill patients will consider euthanasia or assisted suicide. These wishes may or may not be fixed, and ~50% change their mind within 6 months. Discuss this. Ask your patient how they feel today and what they are afraid of feeling tomorrow. Listen. Answer questions. Offer palliative care. Palliative care is never futile. A wish to die is associated with the need for information, reassurance, and symptom control. Provide these, or find someone who can.

12 Rheumatology

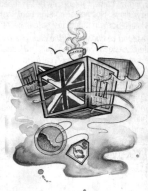

Fig 12.1 When William Pitt the Elder, British statesman, was struck by yet another attack of gout he was absent from Parliament in 1773 when its members were persuaded to levy a substantial tax on tea imports to the American colonies. The resulting Tea Act of 1773 was born. Colonists boarded ships of the East India Company in Boston Harbour and crates of tea were thrown overboard. In response, the British government sent troops to occupy Boston to control the colonists. The armed response to these occupying forces led to the American War of Independence. Thirteen colonies became independent from Britain. And so it is told that gout had a part to play in the beginning of the American Revolution!

Artwork by Gillian Turner.

A rapidly advancing specialty

Rheumatology originates from the Greek word 'rheuma' meaning that which 'flows as a river or stream'. The British Society of Rheumatology defines rheumatology as a 'multidisciplinary branch of medicine that deals with the investigation, diagnosis and management of patients with arthritis and other musculoskeletal conditions... incorporating over 200 disorders affecting joints, bones, muscles and soft tissues'. Rheumatological diseases affect over 10 million UK adults and 12 000 children. Osteoarthritis is the most common adult condition by far. Recent advances are mainly in the management of inflammatory disorders, owing to new discoveries about the immunology of these conditions and the development of biologic disease-modifying antirheumatic drugs (DMARDs).

We thank Kevin Davies, our Specialist Reader and Tom Weatherby, our Junior Reader for this chapter.

In the assessment of an arthritic presentation, pay particular attention to the distribution of joint involvement (including spine) and the presence of symmetry. Also look for disruption of joint anatomy, limitation of movement (by pain or contracture), joint effusions and peri-articular involvement (see p536 for a fuller assessment). Ask about, and examine for, *extra-articular features:* skin and nail (see p75) involvement (include scalp, hairline (particularly behind the ears), umbilicus, genitalia (where appropriate), and natal cleft—psoriasis can easily be missed); eye signs (see p558); lungs (eg fibrosis) (see p192); kidneys (see p310); heart; GI (eg mouth ulcers, diarrhoea); GU (eg urethritis, genital ulcers); and CNS (eg cognitive impairment, sleep pattern).

Three screening questions for musculoskeletal disease

1 Are you free of any pain or stiffness in your joints, muscles, or back?
2 Can you dress yourself without too much difficulty?
3 Can you manage walking up and down stairs?

If *yes* to all three, serious inflammatory muscle/joint disease is unlikely.

Presenting symptoms
- Pattern of involved joints.
- Symmetry (or not).
- Morning stiffness >30min (eg RA).
- Pain, swelling, loss of function, erythema, warmth.

Extra-articular features
- Rashes, photosensitivity (eg SLE).
- Raynaud's (SLE; systemic sclerosis; polymyositis and dermatomyositis).
- Dry eyes or mouth (Sjögren's).
- Red eyes, iritis (eg AS).
- Diarrhoea/urethritis (reactive arthritis).
- Nodules or nodes (eg RA; TB; gout).
- Mouth/genital ulcers (eg Behçet's, SLE).
- Weight loss (eg malignancy, any systemic inflammatory disease).
- Poor wound healing (eg RA, SLE, vasculitis).

Related diseases
- Crohn's/UC (in ankylosing spondylitis), preceding infections, psoriasis.
- HIV or other sexually transmitted disease.
- Inflammatory eye disease (eg uveitis).

Current and past drugs
- NSAIDs, DMARDs (p543).
- Biological agents (eg TNFα inhibitors).

Family history
- Arthritis, psoriasis, autoimmune disease.
- Hypermobility.

Social history
- Age.
- Occupation.
- Sexual history.
- Ethnicity (eg SLE is commoner in African Caribbeans and Asians).
- Ability to function (eg dressing, grooming, writing, walking).
- Domestic situation, social support, home adaptations.
- Smoking (may worsen RA).

Arthritides

The pattern of joint involvement can provide clues to the underlying cause (table 12.1).

Table 12.1 Patterns of presentation of arthritis

Monoarthritis	Oligoarthritis (≤5 joints)	Polyarthritis (>5 joints involved)	
		Symmetrical	Asymmetrical
Septic arthritis	Crystal arthritis	Symmetrical	Asymmetrical
Crystal arthritis (gout, CPPD)	Psoriatic arthritis	Rheumatoid arthritis	Reactive arthritis
Osteoarthritis	Reactive arthritis, eg *Yersinia, Salmonella, Campylobacter*	Osteoarthritis	Psoriatic arthritis
Trauma (haemarthrosis)	Ankylosing spondylitis	Viruses (eg hepatitis A, B, & C; mumps)	
	Osteoarthritis	Systemic conditions* (can be either)	

* Connective tissue disease (eg SLE and relapsing polychondritis), sarcoidosis, malignancy (eg leukaemia), endocarditis, haemochromatosis, sickle cell anaemia, familial Mediterranean fever, Behçet's.

▶▶Exclude septic arthritis in any acutely inflamed joint, as it can destroy a joint in under 24h (p540). Inflammation may be less overt if immunocompromised (eg from the many immunosuppressive drugs used in rheumatological conditions) or if there is underlying joint disease. Joint aspiration (p537) is the key investigation, and if you are unable to do it, find someone who can (ED or orthopaedics).

This aims to screen for rheumatological conditions primarily affecting mobility (as a consequence of underlying joint disease). It is based on the **GALS** locomotor screen (**G**ait, **A**rms, **L**egs, **S**pine).[1]

Essence 'Look, feel, and move' (active and passive). If a *joint looks normal* to you, *feels normal* to the patient, and has *full range of movement*, it usually is normal. Hypermobility is common in fibromyalgia and chronic fatigue. Look also for blue sclerae—common in Ehlers–Danlos syndrome and other hypermobility syndromes, even the benign ones. Make sure the patient is comfortable, and obtain their consent before examination. The GALS screening examination should be done in light underwear.

Spine *Observe from behind:* is muscle bulk normal (buttocks, shoulders)? Is the spine straight? Are paraspinal muscles symmetrical? Any swellings/deformities? *Observe from the side:* is cervical and lumbar lordosis normal? Any kyphosis? '*Touch your toes, please*': is lumbar spine flexion normal, eg Schober's test?[1] *Observe from in front:* '*Tilt your head*' (without moving the shoulders)—tests lateral neck flexion. Palpate for typical fibromyalgia tender points (see p556).

Arms '*Try putting your hands behind your head*'—tests functional shoulder movement. '*Arms out straight*'—tests elbow extension and forearm supination/pronation. Examine the hands: any deformity (fig 12.2), wasting, or swellings? *Squeeze across 2nd–5th metacarpophalangeal joints.* Pain may denote joint or tendon synovitis. '*Put your index finger on your thumb*'—tests pincer grip. Assess dexterity, eg fastening a button or picking up a coin.

Legs *Observe legs:* normal quadriceps bulk? Any swelling or deformity? *With patient lying supine:* any leg length discrepancy? *Internally/externally rotate each hip in flexion. Passively flex knee and hip to the full extent.* Is movement limited? Any crepitus? *Find any knee effusion* using the patella tap test. If there is fluid, consider aspirating and testing for crystals or infection. *With patient standing: observe feet*—any deformity? Are arches high or flat? Any callosities? These may indicate an abnormal gait of some chronicity. *Squeeze across metatarsophalangeal joints:* see as for arms. Also: although not in the GALS system, *palpate the heel and Achilles tendon* to identify plantar fasciitis and Achilles tendonitis often associated with seronegative rheumatological conditions. *Examine the patient's shoes* for signs of uneven wear.

Gait *Observe walking:* is the gait smooth? Good arm swing? Stride length OK? Normal heel strike and toe off? Can they turn quickly?

Range of joint movement Is noted in degrees, with anatomical position being the neutral position—eg elbow flexion 0°–150° normally, but with fixed flexion and limited movement, range may be reduced to 30°–90°. A valgus deformity deviates laterally (away from the midline, fig 12.3); a varus deformity points towards the midline.

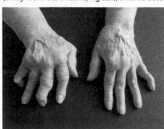

Fig 12.2 Swan-neck deformity.
Reproduced from Watts *et al.*, *Oxford Textbook of Rheumatology*, 2013, with permission from Oxford University Press.

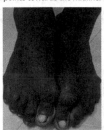

Fig 12.3 Hallux valgus.
Reproduced from Chakraborty U, *QJM*, 2021; 115:107, with permission from Association of Physicians of Great Britain and Ireland.

1 Schober's test: make a mark on the lumbar spine at the level of the posterior iliac spine. Measure out a line from 5cm below to 10cm above the mark. Ask to bend forward as far as they can. If the line does not lengthen by at least 5cm in flexion, there is reduced lumbar flexion, eg in ankylosing spondylitis.

Some important rheumatological investigations

Joint aspiration The most important investigation in any monoarthritic presentation (table 12.2, see also *OHCS* p512). Send synovial fluid for urgent white cell count, Gram stain, polarized light microscopy (for crystals, p544), and culture. Remember to alert the lab; many labs are not well set up to evaluate synovial fluid, especially out of hours. The risk of inducing septic arthritis, using sterile precautions, is <1:10 000.[2] Look for blood,[3] pus, and crystals (gout or CPPD crystal arthropathy; p544). ▶Do not attempt joint aspiration through inflamed and potentially infected skin (eg through a psoriatic plaque or overlying cellulitis).

Table 12.2 Synovial fluid in health and disease

	Appearance	Viscosity	WBC/mm³	Neutrophils
Normal	Clear, colourless	↔	≤200	None
Osteoarthritis	Clear, straw	↑	≤1000	≤50%
Haemorrhagic*	Bloody, xanthochromic	Varies	≤10 000	≤50%
Acutely inflamed				
• RA	Turbid, yellow	↓	1000–50 000	Varies
• Crystal	Turbid, yellow	↓	5000–50 000	~80%
Septic	Turbid, yellow	↓	10 000–100 000	>90%

* Eg trauma, tumour, or haemophilia.

Blood tests FBC, ESR, urate, U&E, CRP. Blood culture if infective pathology is suspected. Consider rheumatoid factor, anti-CCP, ANA, other autoantibodies (p550), and HLA B27 (p547)—as guided by presentation. Consider causes of reactive arthritis (p547), eg viral serology, urine *Chlamydia* PCR, hepatitis and HIV serology if risk factors are present.

Radiology Look for erosions, calcification, widening or loss of joint space, changes in underlying bone of affected joints (eg periarticular osteopenia, sclerotic areas, osteophytes). Characteristic x-ray features for various arthritides are shown in figs 12.4–12.6. Irregularity of the sacroiliac joints is seen in spondyloarthritis. Ultrasound and MRI are more sensitive in identifying effusions, synovitis, enthesitis, and infection than plain radiographs—discuss further investigations with a radiologist. Do a CXR for RA, vasculitis, TB, and sarcoid. Angiography or PET CT (if available) may be required for the evaluation of large vessel vasculitis (eg Takayasu's arteritis).

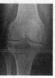
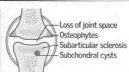

- Loss of joint space
- Osteophytes
- Subarticular sclerosis
- Subchondral cysts

Fig 12.4 x-ray features of osteoarthritis.
Courtesy of Dr DC Howlett.

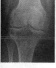

Fig 12.5 x-ray features of rheumatoid arthritis (MCPJ).
Courtesy of Dr DC Howlett.

- Juxta-articular osteopenia
- Soft tissue swelling
- Joint deformity
- Loss of joint space

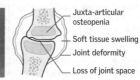

- Periarticular erosions
- Normal joint space
- Soft tissue swelling

Fig 12.6 x-ray features of gout (1st MTPJ).
Courtesy of Dr DC Howlett.

12 Rheumatology

Back pain is very common, and often self-limiting, but *be alert to sinister causes*, eg malignancy, infection, or inflammatory pathology.

Red flags for sinister causes of back pain	
►Aged <20yrs or >55yrs old	►Thoracic back pain
►Acute onset in elderly people	►Morning stiffness
►Constant or progressive pain resistant to simple analgesia	►Bilateral or alternating leg pain
►Nocturnal pain	►Neurological disturbance (incl. sciatica)
►Worse pain on being supine	►Sphincter disturbance
►Fever, night sweats, weight loss	►Current or recent infection
►History of malignancy	►Immunosuppression, eg steroids/HIV
►Abdominal mass	►Leg claudication or exercise-related leg weakness/numbness (spinal stenosis).

Examination

1 With the patient standing, gauge the extent and smoothness of lumbar forward/ lateral flexion and extension (see p536).

2 *Test for sacroiliitis:* palpate posteriorly down the length of the spine, including over spinous processes, paraspinal muscles, and the sacroiliac joints; examining for tenderness.

3 Neurological deficits (see BOX): test lower limb sensation, power, and deep tendon and plantar reflexes. Digital rectal examination for perianal tone and sensation.

4 Examine for nerve root pain (table 12.3): this is distributed in relevant dermatomes, and is worsened by coughing or bending forward. *Straight leg test* (L4, L5, S1): positive if raising the leg with the knee extended causes pain below the knee, which increases on foot dorsiflexion (Lasègue's sign). It suggests irritation to the sciatic nerve. The main cause is lumbar disc prolapse. Also *femoral stretch test* (L2–L4): pain in front of thigh on lifting the hip into extension with the patient lying face downwards and the knee flexed.

5 Signs of generalized disease—eg malignancy. Examine other systems (eg abdomen) as pain may be referred.

Causes Age determines the most likely causes:

15–30yrs: Prolapsed disc, trauma, fractures, ankylosing spondylitis (AS; p546), spondylolisthesis (a forward shift of one vertebra over another, which is congenital or due to trauma), pregnancy.

30–50yrs: Degenerative spinal disease, prolapsed disc, malignancy (primary or secondary from lung, breast, prostate, thyroid, or kidney ca).

>50yrs: Degenerative, osteoporotic vertebral collapse, Paget's (see p677), malignancy, myeloma (see p366), spinal stenosis, discitis.

Rarer Cauda equina tumours, psoas abscess, spinal infection (eg discitis, usually staphylococcal but also *Proteus*, *E. coli*, *S. typhi*, and TB—there are often no systemic signs, particularly in the elderly).

Investigations Arrange relevant tests if you suspect a specific cause, or if red flag symptoms: FBC, ESR, and CRP (myeloma, infection, tumour), U&E, ALP (Paget's), serum/ urine electrophoresis (myeloma), PSA. x-rays—imaging may not always be necessary but can exclude bony abnormalities and fractures. Correlation between radiographic abnormalities and clinical features can be poor. MRI is the imaging modality of choice and can detect disc prolapse, cord compression (fig 12.7), cancer, infection, or inflammation (eg sacroiliitis).

Management ►►Urgent neurosurgical referral if any neurological deficit (see BOX). For non-specific back pain, focus on *education* and *self-management*. Advise patients to continue normal activities and be active. Regular paracetamol ± NSAIDs ± codeine. Consider low-dose amitriptyline/duloxetine if these fail (not SSRIs for pain). Avoid the use of gabapentin and similar drugs if at all possible (these are best prescribed by pain specialists, have many side effects, and are often poorly tolerated). Offer *physiotherapy*, *acupuncture*, or an *exercise programme* if not improving. Address *psychosocial issues*, which may predispose to developing chronic pain and disability (see p557).

Neurosurgical emergencies

▶▶**Acute cauda equina compression** Alternating or bilateral root pain in legs, saddle anaesthesia (perianal), loss of anal tone on PR, bladder ± bowel incontinence.
▶▶**Acute cord compression** Bilateral pain, LMN signs (p442) at level of compression, UMN and sensory loss below, sphincter disturbance. Differential diagnosis: acute myelitis (eg in lupus (p552), MS (p492), or Devic's disease (p668)) can present in a similar way, and constitutes a neurological emergency. Urgent MRI + gadolinium, steroids.
Urgent specialist referral and treatment prevents irreversible loss, eg laminectomy for disc protrusions, radiotherapy for tumours, decompression for abscesses.
Causes (Same for both) bony metastasis (look for missing pedicle on x-ray), large disc protrusion, myeloma, cord or paraspinal tumour, TB (p388), abscess.

Table 12.3 Nerve root lesions

Nerve root	Pain	Weakness	Reflex affected
L2	Across upper thigh	Hip flexion and adduction	Nil
L3	Across lower thigh	Hip adduction, knee extension	Knee jerk
L4	Across knee to medial malleolus	Knee extension, foot inversion, and dorsiflexion	Knee jerk
L5	Lateral shin to dorsum of foot and great toe	Hip extension and abduction Knee flexion Foot and great toe dorsiflexion	Great toe jerk
S1	Posterior calf to lateral foot and little toe	Knee flexion Foot and toe plantar flexion Foot eversion	Ankle jerk

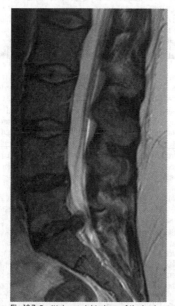

Fig 12.7 Sagittal T2-weighted MRI of the lumbar spine showing a herniated L5–S1 disc.
Courtesy of Norwich Radiology Department.

Osteoarthritis (OA)

Osteoarthritis is the most common joint condition worldwide, with a clinically significant impact on >10% of persons aged >60 years. It is usually primary (generalized), but may be secondary to inflammatory joint disease or other conditions (eg haemochromatosis, obesity, occupational). It also occurs in obesity, after trauma, due to occupational or sporting over-use, or as a consequence of congenital anatomical abnormality.

Signs and symptoms **Localized disease** (often knee or hip) Pain and crepitus on movement, with background ache at rest. Worse with prolonged activity. Joints may 'gel' (brief stiffness after rest, usually 10–15 minutes or so). Joints may feel unstable, with a perceived lack of power due to pain. **Generalized disease** 'Nodal OA' (typically DIP, PIP, CMC joints, and knees in postmenopausal females). There may be joint tenderness, derangement, and bony swelling (Heberden's at DIP and Bouchard's at PIP), reduced range of movement, and mild synovitis. First CMC arthritis may be very marked in some patients, in the absence of Heberden's and Bouchard's nodes. Such patients often have superadded knee and spinal disease. Assess effect of symptoms on occupation, family duties, hobbies, and lifestyle expectations.

Tests Plain radiographs show **L**oss: **L**oss of joint space, **O**steophytes, **S**ubarticular sclerosis and **S**ubchondral cysts (fig 12.4, p537).

Management **Core treatments** Exercise to improve local muscle strength and general aerobic fitness (irrespective of age, severity, or comorbidity). Weight loss if overweight.[4] **Analgesia** Regular paracetamol ± topical NSAIDs. If ineffective use codeine or short-term oral NSAID (+PPI)—see BOX. Topical capsaicin (derived from chillies) may help. Intra-articular steroid injections temporarily relieve pain in severe symptoms. Intra-articular hyaluronic acid injections (viscosupplementation) are not NICE approved. Glucosamine and chondroitin products are not recommended, although patients may try them if they wish (can be bought over the counter). **Nonpharmacological** Use a multidisciplinary approach, including physiotherapists and occupational therapists. Try heat or cold packs at the site of pain, walking aids, stretching/manipulation, or TENS. **Surgery** Joint replacement (hips, or knees) is the best way to deal with severe OA that has a substantial impact on quality of life.

▶▶ Septic arthritis

▶▶Consider septic arthritis in any acutely inflamed joint, as it can destroy a joint in under 24h and has a mortality rate up to 11%. Inflammation may be less overt if immunocompromised (eg from medication) or if there is underlying joint disease, or in the very elderly. The knee is affected in >50% cases.

Risk factors Pre-existing joint disease (especially rheumatoid arthritis); diabetes mellitus, immunosuppression, chronic renal failure, recent joint, dental, or other surgery, presence of indwelling catheters or lines, prosthetic joints (where infection is particularly difficult to treat), IV drug abuse, age >80yrs.

Investigations Urgent joint aspiration for synovial fluid microscopy and culture is the key investigation (p537), as x-ray and CRP can be normal. The main differential diagnoses are the crystal arthropathies (p544). Blood cultures are essential (prior to antibiotics). *Ask yourself* 'How did the organism get there?' Is there immunosuppression, or another focus of infection, eg from indwelling IV lines, infected skin, abscess (eg dental), meningococcal disease, or pneumonia (present in up to 50% of those with pneumococcal arthritis)?

▶▶**Treatment** If in doubt start empirical IV antibiotics (after aspiration). Common causative organisms are *Staph. aureus*, streptococci, *Neisseria gonococcus*, and Gram −ve bacilli. Follow local guidelines for antibiotic choice and microbiology for advice for all complex cases/immunosuppressed patients. Consider flucloxacillin 2g QDS IV (clindamycin if penicillin allergic); vancomycin IV plus 2nd- or 3rd-generation cephalosporin, eg cefuroxime if MRSA risk; 2nd- or 3rd-generation cephalosporin if Gram −ve organisms suspected. For suspected gonococcus or meningococcus, consider ceftriaxone. Antibiotics are required for a prolonged period, conventionally ~2 weeks IV, then if patient improving 2–4 weeks PO. Consider orthopaedic review for arthrocentesis, washout, and debridement; ▶▶always urgently refer patients with prosthetic joint involvement.

Prescribing NSAIDs: benefit vs risk profiling

Around 60% of patients will respond to any NSAID, but there is considerable variation in response and tolerance—if one isn't effective, try another. Mainly act as analgesics rather than modifying the disease process per se.

▶▶Individualized risk: benefit analysis for each patient (including indication, dose, proposed duration of use, and comorbidity) is crucial and needs careful and experienced thought. Follow local recommendations and national guidelines where available.

NSAID side effects ▶ The main serious side effects are GI bleeding (and ulcers and perforation), cardiovascular events (MI and stroke), and renal injury. The risks are dose related, starting with the first dose, so always aim to use the lowest possible dose for the shortest period of time. Risks increase considerably with age, polypharmacy, history of peptic ulcers, and renal impairment.

GI side effects NICE recommends co-prescription of PPI for any patient aged >45 years, and those with other risk factors for GI bleeding. Drug interactions can increase bleeding risks—avoid concomitant prescribing of anticoagulants, antiplatelet agents, SSRI, spironolactone, steroids, and bisphosphonates. Coxibs are slightly lower risk than non-selective NSAIDs.

Cardiovascular side effects NSAIDs—all are associated with a small increased risk of MI and stroke (independent of cardiovascular risk factor or duration of use).[5] Risks are higher in those with concomitant IHD risk factors, eg diabetes and hypertension. Coxibs and diclofenac are higher risk, and are contraindicated if prior history of MI, PVD, stroke, or heart failure. Naproxen has the lowest cardiovascular risk. Low-dose celecoxib may be considered for patients on low-dose aspirin (if NSAID is required) as it does not interact with it. Etoricoxib (60 or 90mg per day) is well tolerated by most patients, and requires only once-daily dosing due to its long half-life, but may cause hypertension and cannot be used coincidently with certain antibiotics (eg quinolones).

Renal risks Higher for patients already on diuretics, ACE, or ARB. Risks are also increased in the elderly, those with hypertension, and T2DM. Overall, naproxen (<1000mg/day) or ibuprofen (<1200mg/day) plus PPI may be the safest options.

Alternatives to NSAIDs Paracetamol, topical NSAIDs, opioids. Strengthening exercises may be more beneficial than mild oral analgesics.

Counselling patients Make sure patients understand about the drugs they are taking: *bleeding is more common in those who know less about their drugs.*[6]
• Only to take NSAIDs when they need them.
• Stop NSAIDs and seek urgent medical review if they develop abdominal pain or any symptoms of GI bleeding (eg report black stools ± faints immediately).
• Do not mix prescription NSAIDs with over-the-counter formulations: mixing NSAIDs can increase risks 20-fold.
• Smoking and alcohol increase risk profile of NSAIDs.

RA is a chronic systemic inflammatory disease, characterized by a symmetrical, deforming, peripheral polyarthritis. It increases the risk of cardiovascular disease by 2–3-fold. **Epidemiology** Prevalence is ~1% (↑ in smokers). ♀:♂ >2:1. Peak onset: 5th–6th decade. HLA DR4/DR1 linked (associated with ↑severity).

Presentation Typically Symmetrical swollen, painful, and stiff small joints of hands and feet, worse in the morning. This can fluctuate and larger joints may become involved. **Less common presentations** •Sudden-onset, widespread arthritis. •Recurring mono/polyarthritis of various joints (*palindromic RA*).[2] •Persistent monoarthritis (knee, shoulder, or hip). •Systemic illness with extra-articular symptoms, eg fatigue, fever, weight loss, pericarditis, and pleurisy, but initially few joint problems (commoner in ♂). •Polymyalgic onset—vague limb girdle aches. •Recurrent soft tissue problems (eg frozen shoulder, carpal tunnel syndrome, de Quervain's tenosynovitis).

Signs Early (Inflammation, no joint damage.) Swollen MCP, PIP, wrist, or MTP joints (often symmetrical). Look for tenosynovitis or bursitis. **Later** (Joint damage, deformity.) Ulnar deviation and subluxation of the wrist and fingers. Boutonnière and swan-neck deformities of fingers (fig 12.2, p536) or z-deformity of thumbs occur. Hand extensor tendons may rupture. Foot changes are similar. Larger joints can be involved. Atlanto-axial joint subluxation may threaten the spinal cord (rare).

Extra-articular manifestations Affect ~40% of RA patients. **Nodules** Elbows, lungs, cardiac, CNS, lymphadenopathy, vasculitis. **Lungs** Pleural disease, interstitial fibrosis, bronchiolitis obliterans, organizing pneumonia. **Cardiac** IHD, pericarditis, pericardial effusion; carpal tunnel syndrome; peripheral neuropathy; splenomegaly (seen in 5%; only 1% have Felty's syndrome: RA + splenomegaly + neutropenia, see p688). **Eye** Episcleritis, scleritis, scleromalacia, keratoconjunctivitis sicca (p558), osteoporosis; amyloidosis is rare (p364).

Investigations Rheumatoid factor (RhF) is positive in ~70% (p550). High titres associated with severe disease, erosions, and extra-articular disease. Anticyclic citrullinated peptide antibodies (anti-CCP) are highly specific (~98%) for RA with a reasonable sensitivity (70–80%); they may also predict disease progression. Anaemia of chronic disease, ↑platelets, ↑ESR, ↑CRP. *x-rays* show soft tissue swelling, juxta-articular osteopenia and ↓joint space. Later there may be bony erosions, subluxation, or complete carpal destruction (see fig 12.5 on p537). High-resolution ultrasound and MRI can identify synovitis more accurately, and have greater sensitivity in detecting bone erosions than conventional x-rays.[7]

Diagnostic criteria See table 12.4.

Management ▶Refer early to a rheumatologist.
• Disease activity is measured using the DAS28.[3] Treatment should be escalated until satisfactory control is achieved: 'treat to target'.
• Early use of DMARDs and biological agents improves long-term outcomes (see BOX 'Influencing inflammation in RA').
• Steroids rapidly reduce symptoms and inflammation. Avoid starting unless appropriately experienced. Useful for acute exacerbations, eg IM depot *methylprednisolone* 80–120mg. Intra-articular steroids have a rapid but short-term effect (*OHCS* pp512-15). Oral steroids (eg *prednisolone* 7.5mg/d) may control difficult symptoms, but side effects preclude routine long-term use.
• NSAIDs (p541) are good for symptom relief, but have no effect on disease progression. Paracetamol and weak opiates are rarely effective.
• Offer specialist physio- and occupational therapy, eg for aids and splints.
• Surgery may relieve pain, improve function, and prevent deformity.
• There is ↑risk of cardiovascular and cerebrovascular disease, as atherosclerosis is accelerated in RA.[8] Manage risk factors (p85). Smoking also ↑ symptoms of RA.

2 In rheumatological palindromes, arthritis lasting hours or days runs to and fro, visiting and revisiting three or more sites, typically knees, wrists, and MCP joints. It may presage RA, SLE, Whipple's, or Behçet's disease. Remissions are (initially) complete, leaving no radiological mark.

3 28-joint Disease Activity Score—assesses tenderness and swelling at 28 joints (MCPs, PIPs, wrists, elbows, shoulders, knees), ESR/CRP, and patient's self-reported symptom severity.

Table 12.4 Criteria for diagnosing RA[9]

	When to suspect RA? Those with ≥1 swollen joint and a suggestive clinical history, which is not better explained by another disease. Scores ≥6 are diagnostic		
A	Joint involvement (swelling or tenderness ± imaging evidence)		
	1 large joint = 0 2–10 large joints = 1 1–3 small* joints† = 2		
	4–10 small* joints† = 3 >10 joints (at least 1 small joint) = 5		
B	Serology (at least 1 test result needed)		
	Negative RF *and* negative anti-CCP = 0 Low +ve RF *or* low +ve anti-CCP = 2		
	High +ve RF *or* high +ve anti-CCP = 3		
C	Acute phase reactants (at least 1 test result needed)		
	Normal CRP and normal ESR = 0 Abnormal CRP or abnormal ESR = 1		
D	Duration of symptoms: <6 weeks = 0 ≥6 weeks = 1		

* = MCPJ, PIPJ, 2nd–5th MTPJ, wrists, and thumb IPJ; † = with or without involvement of large joints.

Influencing inflammation in RA

Over-produced cytokines and cellular processes erode cartilage and bone, and produce the systemic effects seen in RA.

Conventional disease-modifying antirheumatic drugs (DMARDs) Are 1st line and should ideally be started within 3 months of persistent symptoms. They can take 6–12 weeks for symptomatic benefit. Best results are often achieved with a combination of methotrexate, sulfasalazine, and hydroxychloroquine. Leflunomide is another option.
►*Immunosuppression* is a potentially fatal SE of treatment (especially in combination with methotrexate) which can result in pancytopenia, ↑susceptibility to infection (including atypical organisms), and neutropenic sepsis (p350). Regular FBC, LFT monitoring. *Other SE:* • ►►Methotrexate—pneumonitis (pre-treatment CXR), oral ulcers, hepatotoxicity, teratogenic. • Sulfasalazine—rash, ↓sperm count, oral ulcers, GI upset. • Leflunomide—teratogenicity (♂ and ♀), oral ulcers, ↑BP, hepatotoxicity. • Hydroxychloroquine—can cause retinopathy; pre-treatment and annual eye screen required.

Biological DMARDs Initiated by specialists, for patients with active disease despite adequate trial of at least 2 conventional DMARDs. Pre-treatment screening for TB, hepatitis B/C, HIV is essential.
1 *TNFα inhibitors:* eg infliximab (p261), etanercept, adalimumab, are approved by NICE as 1st-line agents. Where methotrexate is contraindicated, can be used as monotherapy. Clinical response can be striking, with improved function and health outcomes, although response may be inadequate/unsustained.
2 *B-cell depletion:* eg rituximab, used in combination with methotrexate and approved by NICE for severe active RA where DMARDs and a TNFα blocker have failed.
3 *IL-1 and IL-6 inhibition:* eg tocilizumab (IL-6 receptor blocker), approved by NICE in combination with methotrexate where TNFα blocker has failed (or is contraindicated). Monitor for hypercholesterolaemia and hepatotoxicity.
4 *Inhibition of T-cell co-stimulation:* eg abatacept—licensed for active RA where patients have not responded to DMARDs or TNFα blocker.

Targeted synthetic DMARDs *Janus kinase (JAK) inhibitors* Eg tofacitinib, baricitinib, upadacitinib, act to inhibit signalling through cytokine receptors. All are available in oral formulations. Approved by NICE in combination with methotrexate for severe (DAS28 >5.1) active RA where patients have not responded to DMARDs including at least 1 biological DMARD.

Side effects of biological and targeted synthetic DMARDs Serious infection, reactivation of TB (∴ screen and consider prophylaxis) and hepatitis B; worsening heart failure; hypersensitivity; injection-site reactions and blood disorders. ANA and reversible SLE-type illness may evolve. Data suggest there is no increased risk of solid organ tumours but skin cancers may be more common.[10] TNF inhibitors do not appear to be associated with a further increase in the already elevated lymphoma occurrence in RA.[11] JAK inhibitors have been associated with increased risk of cardiovascular disease compared with other DMARDs, therefore a careful risk-benefit assessment is required among those with vascular risk factors.[12]

Gout typically presents with an acute monoarthropathy with severe joint inflammation (fig 12.8). >50% occur at the MTP joint of the big toe (fig 12.12) (podagra). Other common joints are the ankle, foot, small joints of the hand, wrist, elbow, or knee. It can be polyarticular. It is caused by deposition of monosodium urate crystals in and near joints. Attacks may be precipitated by trauma, surgery, starvation, infection, or diuretics. It is associated with raised plasma urate. In the long term, urate deposits (= tophi, eg in pinna, tendons, joints; see fig 12.9) and renal disease (stones, interstitial nephritis) may occur. *Prevalence:* ~1%. ♂:♀ ≈ 4:1.

Differential diagnoses Exclude septic arthritis in any acute monoarthropathy (p540). Then consider reactive arthritis, haemarthrosis, CPPD (see following topic) and palindromic RA (p542).

Risk factors Reduced urate excretion Elderly, men, postmenopausal women, impaired renal function, hypertension, metabolic syndrome, diuretics, antihypertensives, aspirin. **Excess urate production** Dietary (alcohol, especially beer, sweeteners, red meat, seafood), genetic disorders, myelo- or lymphoproliferative disorders, psoriasis, tumour lysis syndrome, drugs (eg alcohol, warfarin, cytotoxics). **Associations** Cardiovascular disease, hypertension, diabetes mellitus, and chronic renal failure (p672). Gout is an independent risk factor for mortality from cardiovascular and renal disease. Screen for and treat CKD, hypertension, dyslipidaemia, diabetes.

Investigations Polarized light microscopy of synovial fluid shows *negatively bi-refringent* urate crystals (fig 12.10). Serum urate (SUA) is usually raised but may be normal. Radiographs show only soft tissue swelling in the early stages. Later, well-defined 'punched out' erosions are seen in juxta-articular bone (fig 12.6, p537). There is no sclerotic reaction, and joint spaces are preserved until late.

Treatment of acute gout High-dose NSAID (see BOX, p541) or use colchicine (500mcg BD) which is highly effective. NB: in renal impairment, NSAIDs and colchicine are problematic. Steroids (oral, IM, or intra-articular) may also be used. Rest and elevate joint. Ice packs and 'bed cages' can be effective.

Prevention Lose weight, avoid prolonged fasts, alcohol excess, purine-rich meats, and low-dose aspirin. **Prophylaxis** Start if >1 attack in 12 months, tophi, or renal stones. The aim is to ↓ attacks and prevent damage caused by crystal deposition. Use *allopurinol* and titrate from 100mg/24h, increasing every 4 weeks until plasma urate <0.3mmol/L (max 300mg/8h). SE: rash, fever, ↓WCC. Allopurinol may trigger an attack so wait 3 weeks after an acute episode, and cover with regular NSAID (for up to 6 weeks) or colchicine (0.5mg/12h PO for up to 6 months). Avoid stopping allopurinol in acute attacks once established. *Febuxostat* (80mg/24h) is an alternative if allopurinol is CI or not tolerated. It ↓ uric acid by inhibiting xanthine oxidase (SE: ↑LFTs) and is more effective at reducing serum urate than allopurinol (number of acute attacks the same). Uricosuric drugs ↑ urate excretion.

Calcium pyrophosphate deposition (CPPD)

- **Acute CPPD crystal arthritis** Acute monoarthropathy usually of larger joints in elderly. Usually spontaneous but can be provoked by illness, surgery, or trauma.
- **Chronic CPPD** Inflammatory RA-like (symmetrical) polyarthritis and synovitis.
- **Osteoarthritis** with CPPD chronic polyarticular osteoarthritis with superimposed acute CPP attacks.

Risk factors Old age, hyperparathyroidism (p216), haemochromatosis (p284), hypophosphataemia (p671).

Tests Polarized light microscopy of synovial fluid shows weakly positively birefringent crystals (fig 12.11). It is associated with soft tissue calcium deposition on x-ray.

Management Acute attacks: cool packs, rest, aspiration, and intra-articular steroids. NSAIDs (+PPI) ± colchicine 0.5–1.0mg/24h (used with caution) may prevent acute attacks. Methotrexate and hydroxychloroquine may be considered for chronic CPP inflammatory arthritis.

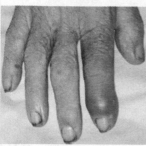

Fig 12.8 Acute monoarthritis in gout.

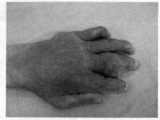

Fig 12.9 Tophi in gout.
Reproduced from Zang Y-S et al., *Rheumatology* 2012: 51(4):756, with permission from Oxford University Press, on behalf of British Society for Rheumatology.

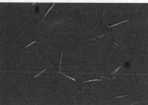

Fig 12.10 **N**eedle-shaped monosodium urate crystals found in gout, displaying **N**egative birefringence under polarized light.
Reproduced from Warrell et al., *Oxford Textbook of Medicine*, 2010, with permission from Oxford University Press.

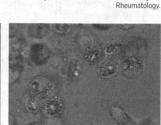

Fig 12.11 Rhomboid-shaped calcium pyrophosphate dihydrate crystals in **P**seudogout, showing **P**ositive birefringence in polarized light.
Image courtesy of Prof. Eliseo Pascual, Sección de Reumatología, Hospital General Universitario de Alicante.

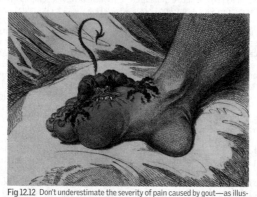

Fig 12.12 Don't underestimate the severity of pain caused by gout—as illustrated by satirical artist and gout sufferer James Gillray (1756–1815).
© Lordprice collection/Alamy Stock Photo.

The spondyloarthropathies (SPA) are a group of related chronic inflammatory conditions. They tend to affect the axial skeleton (but not always), with shared clinical features:

1 Seronegativity (rheumatoid factor −ve).
2 HLA B27 association—see BOX.
3 'Axial arthritis': pathology in spine (spondylo-) and sacroiliac joints.
4 Asymmetrical large-joint oligoarthritis (ie <5 joints) or monoarthritis.
5 Enthesitis: inflammation of the site of insertion of tendon or ligament into bone, eg plantar fasciitis, Achilles tendonitis, costochondritis.
6 Dactylitis: inflammation of an entire digit ('sausage digit'), due to soft tissue oedema, and tenosynovial and joint inflammation.
7 Extra-articular manifestations: eg iritis (anterior uveitis), psoriaform rashes (psoriatic arthritis), oral ulcers, aortic valve incompetence, IBD.

NB: Behçet's syndrome (p554) can also present with uveitis, skin lesions, and arthritis and is not always associated with gross oral or genital ulcerations.

Ankylosing spondylitis (AS) A chronic inflammatory disease of the spine and sacroiliac joints, of unknown aetiology (likely strong genetic/environmental interplay). **Prevalence** 0.25–1%. *Men present earlier:* ♂:♀ ~6:1 at 16yrs old, and ~2:1 at 30yrs old. ~90% are HLA B27 +ve (see BOX). **Symptoms and signs** The typical patient is a man <30yrs old with gradual onset of low back pain, worse during the night with spinal morning stiffness relieved by exercise. Pain radiates from sacroiliac joints to hips/buttocks, and usually improves towards the end of the day. There is progressive loss of spinal movement (all directions)—hence ↓thoracic expansion. See pp536–8 for tests of spine flexion and sacroiliitis. The disease course is variable; a few progress to kyphosis, neck hyperextension ('question mark' posture; fig 12.13), and spino-cranial ankylosis. Other features include *enthesitis*, especially Achilles tendonitis and plantar fasciitis. Anterior mechanical chest pain due to costochondritis. *Acute iritis* occurs in ~⅓ of patients and may lead to blindness if untreated (but may also have occurred many years before, so enquire directly). AS is also associated with osteoporosis (up to 60%), aortic valve incompetence (<3%), and pulmonary apical fibrosis. **Tests** Diagnosis is clinical, supported by imaging.[4] MRI allows detection of active inflammation (bone marrow oedema) as well as destructive changes such as erosions, sclerosis, and ankylosis. X-rays can show SI joint space narrowing or widening, sclerosis, erosions, and ankylosis/fusion. Vertebral syndesmophytes are characteristic (often T11–L1 initially): bony proliferations due to enthesitis between ligaments and vertebrae. These fuse with the vertebral body above, causing ankylosis. In later stages, calcification of ligaments with ankylosis lead to a 'bamboo spine' appearance. *Also:* FBC (normocytic anaemia), ↑ESR, ↑CRP. **Management** *Exercise*, not rest, for backache, including intense exercise regimens to maintain posture and mobility—ideally with a specialist physiotherapist. NSAIDs usually relieve symptoms within 48h, and may slow radiographic progression. *TNFα blockers* (eg etanercept, adalimumab) are indicated in severe active AS. *IL-17 inhibitors* (eg ixekizumab, secukinumab) are as effective, and are approved by NICE in patients with inadequate treatment response. They should be avoided in patients with coexisting IBD as they can exacerbate this. Local steroid injections provide temporary relief. Surgery includes hip replacement to improve pain and mobility if the hips are involved, and rarely spinal osteotomy. There is ↑risk of osteoporotic spinal fractures (consider bisphosphonates). **Prognosis** There is not always a clear relationship between the activity of arthritis and severity of underlying inflammation (as for all the spondyloarthritides). Prognosis is worse if ESR >30; onset <16yrs; early hip involvement or poor response to NSAIDs.

Enteropathic arthropathy Associations IBD, GI bypass, coeliac and Whipple's disease (p263). Arthropathy often improves with the treatment of bowel symptoms (beware NSAIDs). There is not always a clear relationship between the severity of bowel symptoms and the associated arthritis in all patients. Use DMARDs for resistant cases.

---

4 Sacroiliitis on imaging plus ≥1 SPA feature or HLA B27 positive plus ≥2 SPA features, if HLA B27 positive but only 0–1 SPA features, do an MRI.

Psoriatic arthritis (*OHCS* p444.) Occurs in 10–40% with psoriasis and can present before skin changes. Patterns are: • symmetrical polyarthritis (like RA) • DIP joints • asymmetrical oligoarthritis • spinal (similar to AS) • psoriatic arthritis mutilans (rare, ~3%, severe deformity). **Radiology** Erosive changes, with 'pencil-in-cup' deformity in severe cases. Associated with nail changes in 80%, synovitis (dactylitis), acneiform rashes, and palmo-plantar pustulosis. **Management** NSAIDs, sulfasalazine, methotrexate. *TNFα blockers* are also effective, and should be considered as first-line treatment in severe disease. In cases of severe disease and resistance to >1 anti-TNF treatment, switch to another biological DMARD, eg *IL-17 inhibitors* (p546), *IL-23 inhibitors* (eg risankizumab, guselkumab), or *JAK inhibitors* (p543).

Reactive arthritis A condition in which arthritis and other clinical manifestations occur as an autoimmune response to infection elsewhere in the body—typically GI or GU, although the preceding infection may have resolved or be asymptomatic by the time the arthritis presents. **Other clinical features** Iritis, keratoderma blennorrhagica (brown, raised plaques on soles and palms), circinate balanitis (painless penile ulceration secondary to *Chlamydia*), mouth ulcers, and enthesitis. Patients may present with a triad of urethritis, arthritis, and conjunctivitis (Reiter's syndrome). **Tests** ↑ESR & ↑CRP. Culture stool if diarrhoea. Infectious serology. Sexual health review. X-ray may show enthesitis with periosteal reaction. **Management** There is no specific cure. Splint affected joints acutely; treat with NSAIDs or local steroid injections. Consider sulfasalazine or methotrexate if symptoms >6 months. Treating the original infection may make little difference to the arthritis.

HLA B27 disease associations

The HLA system plays a key role in immunity and self-recognition. More than 100 HLA B27 disease associations have been made, yet the actual role of HLA B27 in triggering an inflammatory response is not fully understood. ~5% of the UK population are HLA B27 positive—most do not have any disease. The chance of an HLA B27-positive person developing spondyloarthritis or eye disease is 1 in 4.

Common associations include:
• **Ankylosing spondylitis** 85–95% of all those with AS are HLA B27 positive.
• **Acute anterior uveitis** 50–60% are HLA B27 positive.
• **Reactive arthritis** 60–85% are HLA B27 positive.
• **Enteropathic arthropathy** 50–60% are HLA B27 positive.
• **Psoriatic arthritis** 60–70% are HLA B27 positive.

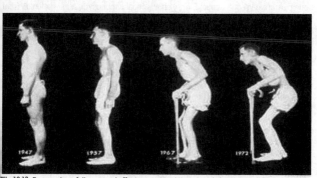

Fig 12.13 Progression of disease and effect on posture in severe ankylosing spondylitis.
Reproduced from *American Journal of Medicine* 1976:60;279–85 with permission from Elsevier/Alliance for Academic Internal Medicine.

Included under this heading are SLE (p552), systemic sclerosis, Sjögren's syndrome, idiopathic inflammatory myopathies (myositis—see following topic), mixed connective tissue disease, relapsing polychondritis, and undifferentiated connective tissue disease and overlap syndromes. They overlap with each other, affect many organ systems, and often require immunosuppressive therapies (p372). Consider as a differential in unwell patients with multi-organ involvement, especially if no infection.

Systemic sclerosis Features scleroderma (skin fibrosis), internal organ fibrosis, and microvascular abnormalities. Severe cases have a 40–50% mortality at 5 years. 90% are ANA positive and 30–40% have anticentromere antibodies (see BOX). Skin disease is limited or diffuse. *Limited* involves the face, hands, and feet (formally CREST syndrome). It is associated with anticentromere antibodies in 70–80%. Pulmonary hypertension is often present subclinically, and can become rapidly life-threatening, so should be looked for (R: sildenafil, bosentan). *Diffuse* can involve the whole body. Antitopoisomerase-1 (SCL-70) antibodies in 40% and anti-RNA polymerase in 20%. Prognosis is often poor. Control BP meticulously. Perform annual echocardiogram and spirometry. Both limited and diffuse have the potential for organ fibrosis: lung, cardiac, GI, and renal (p311) but this occurs later in limited subset.

Management Currently no cure. Immunosuppressive regimens, including IV cyclophosphamide, are used for organ involvement or progressive skin disease. Monitor BP and renal function. Regular ACE-i or A2RBs ↓ risk of renal crisis (p311). *Raynaud's phenomenon:* see later in topic.

Sjögren's syndrome A chronic inflammatory autoimmune disorder, which may be primary (♀:♂≈9:1, onset 4th–5th decade) or secondary, associated with connective tissue disease (eg RA, SLE, systemic sclerosis). There is lymphocytic infiltration and fibrosis of exocrine glands, especially lacrimal and salivary glands. **Features** ↓Tear production (dry eyes, keratoconjunctivitis sicca), ↓salivation (xerostomia—dry mouth, caries), parotid swelling. Other glands are affected causing vaginal dryness, dyspareunia, dry cough, and dysphagia. Systemic signs include polyarthritis/arthralgia, Raynaud's, lymphadenopathy, vasculitis, lung, liver, and kidney involvement, peripheral neuropathy, myositis, and fatigue. It is associated with other autoimmune diseases (eg thyroid disease, autoimmune hepatitis, PBC) and an ↑risk of non-Hodgkin's B-cell lymphoma. **Tests** Schirmer's test measures conjunctival dryness (<5mm in 5min is +ve). Rose Bengal staining may show keratitis (use a slit-lamp). Anti-Ro (SSA; in 40%) & anti-La (SSB; in 26%) antibodies may be present (in pregnancy, these cross the placenta and cause fetal congenital heart block in 5%). ANA is usually +ve (74%); rheumatoid factor is +ve in 38%. There may be hypergammaglobulinaemia. Biopsy shows focal lymphocytic aggregation. R Treat sicca symptoms: eg hypromellose (artificial tears), frequent drinks, sugar-free pastilles/gum. NSAIDs and hydroxychloroquine are used for arthralgia. Immunosuppressants may be indicated in severe systemic disease.

Mixed connective tissue disease Combines features of systemic sclerosis, SLE, and polymyositis and the presence of high titres of anti-U1-RNP antibodies.

Relapsing polychondritis Rare condition with recurrent episodes of cartilage inflammation and destruction. Affects pinna (floppy ears), nasal septum, larynx (stridor), tracheobronchial tree (infections), and joints. **Associations** Aortic valve disease, polyarthritis, and vasculitis. 30% have underlying rheumatic or autoimmune disease. Diagnosis is clinical. R Steroids, DMARDs, or CPAP/tracheostomy for airway involvement.

Raynaud's syndrome This is peripheral digital ischaemia due to paroxysmal vasospasm, precipitated by cold or emotion. Fingers or toes ache and change colour: pale (ischaemia) →blue (deoxygenation) →red (reactive hyperaemia). It may be idiopathic (Raynaud's *disease*—prevalence: 3–20%; ♀:♂ >1:1) or have an underlying cause (Raynaud's *phenomenon*; fig 12.14). **Tests** Exclude an underlying cause (see BOX 'Conditions in which Raynaud's phenomenon may be exhibited'). R Keep warm (eg hand warmers); stop smoking.[5] Nifedipine 5–20mg/8h PO helps, as may evening primrose oil, sildenafil, and epoprostenol (for severe attacks/digital gangrene). Relapse is common. Chemical or surgical (lumbar or digital) sympathectomy may help in those with severe disease.

5 Patient information on Raynaud's is available from www.raynauds.org.uk

Polymyositis and dermatomyositis

Rare conditions characterized by progressive symmetrical proximal muscle weakness and autoimmune-mediated *striated* muscle inflammation (myositis), associated with myalgia ± arthralgia. Muscle weakness may also cause dysphagia, dysphonia (ie poor phonation, *not* dysphasia), or respiratory weakness. The myositis (esp. in dermatomyositis) may be a paraneoplastic phenomenon, commonly from lung, pancreatic, ovarian, or bowel malignancy. Screen for cancers.

Dermatomyositis Myositis plus skin signs: • Macular rash (*shawl sign* is +ve if over back and shoulders). • Lilac-purple (*heliotrope*) rash on eyelids often with oedema (fig 12.27, p561). • Nailfold erythema (*dilated capillary loops*). • Gottron's *papules:* roughened red papules over the knuckles, also seen on elbows and knees (pathognomonic if ↑CK + muscle weakness). Malignancy in 30% cases.

Extramuscular signs In both conditions include fever, arthralgia, Raynaud's, interstitial lung fibrosis and myocardial involvement (myocarditis, arrhythmias).

Tests Muscle enzymes (ALT, AST, LDH, CK, & aldolase) ↑ in plasma; EMG shows characteristic fibrillation potentials; muscle biopsy confirms diagnosis (and excludes mimicking conditions). MRI shows muscle oedema in acute myositis. *Autoantibody associations:* (see BOX 'Plasma autoantibodies (Abs)', p550) anti-MI2, anti-J01—associated with acute onset and interstitial lung fibrosis that should be treated aggressively. The term *anti-synthetase syndrome* is often used. These patients often have *mechanic's hands*—with splitting of the skin around the nails, redness, and ragged cuticles (fig 12.30, p561).

Differential diagnoses Carcinomatous myopathy, inclusion-body myositis, muscular dystrophy, PMR, endocrine/metabolic myopathy (eg steroids), rhabdomyolysis, infection (eg HIV), drugs (penicillamine, colchicine, statins, or chloroquine).

Management Start prednisolone. Immunosuppressives (p372) and cytotoxics are used early in resistant cases. Hydroxychloroquine/topical tacrolimus for skin disease.

Conditions in which Raynaud's phenomenon may be exhibited

Connective tissue disorders Systemic sclerosis, SLE, rheumatoid arthritis, dermatomyositis/polymyositis.

Occupational Using vibrating tools.

Obstructive Thoracic outlet obstruction, Buerger's disease, atheroma.

Blood Thrombocytosis, cold agglutinin disease, polycythaemia rubra vera (p362), monoclonal gammopathies.

Drugs β-blockers.

Others Hypothyroidism.

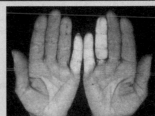

Fig 12.14 Raynaud's phenomenon in SLE.
Courtesy of the Crookston Collection.

Plasma autoantibodies (Abs): disease associations

▶Always interpret in the context of clinical findings: different antibodies have different disease associations.

Rheumatological Rheumatoid factor (RHF) positive in:

Sjögren's syndrome	≤100%	Mixed connective tissue disease	50%
Felty's syndrome	≤100%	SLE	≤40%
RA	70%	Systemic sclerosis	30%
Infection (SBE/IE; hepatitis)	≤50%	Normal	2–10%

Anticyclic citrullinated peptide Ab (anti-CCP):[6] rheumatoid arthritis (~96% specificity).

Antinuclear antibody (ANA) positive by immunofluorescence in:

SLE	>95%	Systemic sclerosis	96%
Autoimmune hepatitis	75%	RA	30%
Sjögren's syndrome	68%	Normal	0–2%

ANA titres are expressed according to dilutions at which antibodies can be detected, ie 1:160 means antibodies can still be detected after the serum has been diluted 160 times. Titres of 1:40 or 1:80 may not be significant. The pattern of staining may indicate the disease (although these are not specific):

- *Homogeneous* SLE.
- *Nucleolar* Systemic sclerosis.
- *Speckled* Mixed CT disease.
- *Centromere* Limited systemic sclerosis.

Anti-double-stranded DNA (dsDNA): SLE (60% sensitivity, but highly specific).

Antihistone Ab: drug-induced SLE (~100%).

Antiphospholipid Ab (eg anti-cardiolipin Ab): antiphospholipid syndrome, SLE.

Anticentromere Ab: limited systemic sclerosis.

Anti-extractable nuclear antigen (ENA) antibodies (usually with +ve ANA):

• Anti-RO (SSA)	SLE, Sjögren's syndrome, systemic sclerosis. Associated with congenital heart block.
• Anti-LA (SSB)	Sjögren's syndrome, SLE (15%).
• Anti-SM	SLE (20–30%).
• Anti-RNP	SLE, mixed connective tissue disease.
• Anti J0-1; anti-MI-2	Polymyositis, dermatomyositis.
• Anti-SCL70	Diffuse systemic sclerosis.

Gastrointestinal (For liver autoantibodies, see p280.)

Antimitochondrial Ab (AMA): primary biliary cholangitis (>95%), autoimmune hepatitis (30%), idiopathic cirrhosis (25–30%).

Anti-smooth muscle Ab (SMA): autoimmune hepatitis (70%), primary biliary cholangitis (50%), idiopathic cirrhosis (25–30%).

Gastric parietal cell Ab: pernicious anaemia (>90%), atrophic gastritis (40%), 'normal' (10%).

Intrinsic factor Ab: pernicious anaemia (50%).

α-gliadin Ab, antitissue transglutaminase, anti-endomysial Ab: coeliac disease.

Endocrine *Thyroid peroxidase Ab:* Hashimoto's thyroiditis (~87%), Graves' (>50%). *Islet cell Ab (ICA), glutamic acid decarboxylase (GAD) Ab:* type 1 diabetes mellitus (75%).

Renal *Glomerular basement membrane Ab (anti-GBM):* Goodpasture's disease (100%).

Antineutrophil cytoplasmic Ab (ANCA):

- *Cytoplasmic (cANCA)*, specific for *serine proteinase-3 (PR3 +ve)*. Granulomatosis with polyangiitis (Wegener's) (90%); also microscopic polyangiitis (30%), polyarteritis nodosa (11%).
- *Perinuclear (pANCA)*, specific for *myeloperoxidase (MPO +ve)*. Microscopic polyangiitis (45%), Churg–Strauss, pulmonary-renal vasculitides (Goodpasture's).

Unlike immune-complex vasculitis, in ANCA-associated vasculitis no complement consumption or immune complex deposition occurs (ie pauci-immune vasculitis).[13] ANCA may also be +ve in UC/Crohn's, sclerosing cholangitis, autoimmune hepatitis, Felty's, RA, SLE, or drugs (eg antithyroid, allopurinol, ciprofloxacin).

Neurological *Acetylcholine receptor Ab:* myasthenia gravis (90%) (see p508).

Anti-voltage-gated K⁺-channel Ab: limbic encephalitis.

Anti-voltage-gated Ca²⁺-channel Ab: Lambert–Eaton syndrome (see p508).

Anti-aquaporin 4: neuromyelitis optica (Devic's disease, p688).

---

6 Most centres now use anti-CCP antibodies for the initial workup of suspected RA.

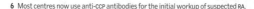

SLE is a multisystemic autoimmune disease. Autoantibodies are made against a variety of autoantigens (eg ANA) which form immune complexes. Inadequate clearance of immune complexes results in a host of immune responses which cause tissue inflammation and damage. Environmental triggers play a part (eg EBV, p401).

Prevalence ~0.2%. ♀:♂≈9:1, typically women of child-bearing age. Commoner in African Caribbeans, Asians, and if HLA B8, DR2, or DR3 +ve. ~10% of patients have a 1st- or 2nd-degree relative with SLE.

Clinical features See BOX. Remitting and relapsing illness of variable presentation and course. Features often non-specific (malaise, fatigue, myalgia, and fever) or organ-specific and caused by active inflammation or damage. Other features include lymphadenopathy, weight loss, alopecia, nail-fold infarcts, non-infective endocarditis (Libman–Sacks syndrome), Raynaud's (30%; see p548), stroke, and retinal exudates.

Immunology >95% are ANA +ve. A high anti-double-stranded DNA (dsDNA) antibody titre is highly specific, but only +ve in ~60% of cases. ENA (p550) may be +ve in 20–30% (anti-Ro, anti-La, anti-Sm, anti-RNP); 40% are RHF +ve; antiphospholipid antibodies (anticardiolipin or lupus anticoagulant) may also be +ve. SLE may be associated with other autoimmune conditions: Sjögren's (15–20%), autoimmune thyroid disease (5–10%). Antibodies to C1Q are associated with renal disease primarily in lupus, but can also occur in hypocomplementaemic urticarial vasculitis (HUVS).

Diagnosis See BOX. **Monitoring activity** *Three best tests:* **1** Anti-dsDNA antibody titres. **2** Complement: ↓C3, ↓C4 (denotes consumption of complement, hence ↓C3 and ↓C4, and ↑C3D and ↑C4D, their degradation products). **3** ESR. *Also:* BP, urine for casts or protein (lupus nephritis, below), FBC, U&E, LFTs, CRP (usually normal); ►think of SLE *whenever someone has a multisystem disorder and ↑ESR but CRP normal.* If ↑CRP, think instead of infection, serositis, or arthritis. Skin or renal biopsies may be diagnostic.

Drug-induced lupus Causes (>80 drugs) include isoniazid, hydralazine (if >50mg/24h in slow acetylators), procainamide, quinidine, chlorpromazine, minocycline, phenytoin, anti-TNF agents. It is associated with antihistone antibodies in >95% of cases. Skin and lung signs prevail (renal and CNS are rarely affected). The disease remits if the drug is stopped. Sulfonamides or the oral contraceptive pill may worsen idiopathic SLE.

Management Refer: complex cases should involve specialist SLE/nephritis clinics.
* **General measures** High-factor sunblock. Hydroxychloroquine, unless contraindicated, reduces disease activity and improves survival. Screen for comorbidities and medication toxicity. For skin flares, first trial topical steroids.
* **Maintenance** NSAIDs (unless renal disease) and hydroxychloroquine for joint and skin symptoms. Azathioprine, methotrexate, and mycophenolate as steroid-sparing agents. *Belimumab* (monoclonal antibody inhibitor of B-cell activating factor) is used as an add-on therapy for autoantibody-positive active disease. It has been associated with serious psychiatric events; assess psychiatric risk before starting.
* **Mild flares** (No serious organ damage.) Hydroxychloroquine or low-dose steroids.
* **Moderate flares** (Organ involvement.) May require DMARDs or mycophenolate.

►►**Severe flares** *If life- or organ-threatening,* eg haemolytic anaemia, nephritis, severe pericarditis or CNS disease; urgent high-dose steroids, mycophenolate, rituximab, cyclophosphamide. MDT vital for neuropsychiatric lupus (LP may be indicated).

Lupus nephritis (p310.) May require more intensive immunosuppression with steroids and cyclophosphamide or mycophenolate. Rituximab is now commonly used and its use with little or no additional steroid treatment is being evaluated. BP control vital (eg ACE-i). Renal replacement therapy (p302) may be needed if disease progresses; nephritis recurs in ~50% post-transplant, but is a rare cause of graft failure.

Prognosis ~80% survival at 15yrs. Increased long-term risk of CVD and osteoporosis.

Antiphospholipid syndrome Can be associated with SLE (20–30%). Antiphospholipid antibodies (anticardiolipin & lupus anticoagulant, anti-β₂ glycoprotein 1) cause **CLOTS: C**oagulation defect (arterial/venous), **L**ivedo reticularis (p555), **O**bstetric (recurrent miscarriage), **T**hrombocytopenia. Thrombotic tendency affects cerebral, renal, & other vessels. **Diagnosis** Persistent antiphospholipid antibodies with clinical features. ℞ Anticoagulation (no good evidence for DOACs); seek advice in pregnancy.

Systemic Lupus International Collaborating Clinics Classification

A favourite differential diagnosis, SLE mimics other illnesses, with wide variation in symptoms that may come and go unpredictably. Diagnose SLE[14] in an appropriate clinical setting if ≥4 criteria (at least 1 clinical and 1 laboratory) *or* biopsy-proven lupus nephritis with positive ANA or anti-DNA.

Clinical criteria

1 *Acute cutaneous lupus:* malar rash/butterfly. Fixed erythema, flat or raised, over the malar eminences, tending to spare the nasolabial folds (fig 12.15). Occurs in up to 50%. Bullous lupus, toxic epidermal necrolysis variant of SLE, maculopapular lupus rash, photosensitive lupus rash, or subacute cutaneous lupus (non-indurated psoriasiform and/or annular polycyclic lesions that resolve without scarring).

2 *Chronic cutaneous lupus:* discoid rash, erythematous raised patches with adherent keratotic scales and follicular plugging ± atrophic scarring (fig 12.16). Think of it as a three-stage rash affecting ears, cheeks, scalp, forehead, and chest: erythema→pigmented hyperkeratotic oedematous papules→atrophic depressed lesions.

3 *Non scarring alopecia* (in the absence of other causes).

4 *Oral/nasal ulcers* (in the absence of other causes).

5 *Synovitis* (involving two or more joints *or* two or more tender joints with >30 minutes of morning stiffness).

6 *Serositis:* (a) lung (pleurisy for >1 day, or pleural effusions, or pleural rub); (b) pericardial pain for >1 day, or pericardial effusion, or pericardial rub, or pericarditis on ECG.

7 *Urinalysis:* presence of proteinuria (>0.5g/d) *or* red cell casts.

8 *Neurological features:* seizures; psychosis; mononeuritis multiplex; myelitis; peripheral or cranial neuropathy; cerebritis/acute confusional state in absence of other causes.

9 *Haemolytic anaemia.*

10 *Leucopenia* (WCC <4): at least once, or lymphopenia (lymphocytes <1) at least once.

11 *Thrombocytopenia* (platelets <100): at least once.

Laboratory criteria

1 +ve ANA (+ve in >95%).

2 Anti-dsDNA.

3 Anti-Smith antibodies present.

4 Antiphospholipid Abs present.

5 Low complement (C3, C4).

6 +ve direct Coombs test.

Adapted from 'Derivation and validation of the Systemic Lupus International Collaborating Clinics classification criteria for systemic lupus erythematosus'. Petri M *et al.*, *Arthritis and Rheumatism*, vol 64, issue 8 (2012) 2677–2686.

12 Rheumatology

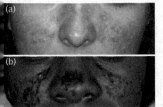

Fig 12.15 (a, b) Malar rash, with sparing of the nasolabial folds.

(a) Courtesy of David F. Fiorentino, MD, PhD; by kind permission of *Skin & Aging*. (b) Reproduced from Watts R, *et al.*, *Oxford Desk Reference: Rheumatology* (2009), with permission from Oxford University Press.

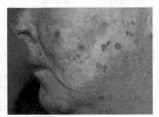

Fig 12.16 Discoid rash.

Courtesy of Amy McMichael, MD; by kind permission of *Skin & Aging*.

Vasculitis

Inflammatory disorders characterized by infiltrates and destruction of blood vessel walls, which can affect any organ system. Classification according to vessel size (table 12.5).

Symptoms See BOX 'Features of vasculitis'. ►A severe vasculitis flare is a medical emergency. If suspected, seek urgent help, as organ damage may occur rapidly (eg critical renal failure <24h). **Tests** ↑ESR/CRP. ANCA may be +ve. ↑Creatinine if renal failure. Urine: proteinuria, haematuria, casts on microscopy. Angiography ± biopsy may be diagnostic.

Giant cell arteritis (GCA) = temporal arteritis Common in the elderly—consider Takayasu's if under 55yrs. Associated with PMR in 50%. **Symptoms** Headache, temporal artery and scalp tenderness (eg when combing hair), tongue/jaw claudication, amaurosis fugax, or sudden unilateral blindness. Extracranial symptoms: malaise, dyspnoea, weight loss, morning stiffness, and unequal or weak pulses. ►The risk is irreversible bilateral visual loss, which can occur suddenly if not treated—ask an ophthalmologist. **Tests** ESR & CRP are ↑↑, ↑platelets, ↑ALP, ↓Hb. Temporal artery ultrasound (halo sign) is a non-invasive alternative to biopsy. ℞ Start prednisolone 60mg/d PO *immediately* or IV methylprednisolone if evolving visual loss or history of amaurosis fugax. **Prognosis** Typically a 2-year course, then complete remission. Reduce prednisolone once symptoms have resolved and ↓ESR; ↑ dose if symptoms recur. Main cause of death and morbidity in GCA is long-term steroid treatment so balance risks! Give PPI, bisphosphonate, calcium with colecalciferol, and consider aspirin.[7]

Takayasu's arteritis *(Aortic arch syndrome; pulseless disease.)* Systemic vasculitis affecting the aorta and its major branches. Granulomatous inflammation causes stenosis, thrombosis, and aneurysms. It often affects women aged 20–40yrs. The aortic arch is often affected, with cerebral, ophthalmological, and upper limb symptoms, eg dizziness, visual changes, weak arm pulses. Systemic features are common—eg fever, weight loss, and malaise. ↑BP is often a feature, due to renal artery stenosis. Complications include aortic valve regurgitation, aortic aneurysm, and dissection; ischaemic stroke (↑BP and thrombus); and ischaemic heart disease. **Diagnosis** ↑ESR and CRP; MRI/PET allows earlier diagnosis than standard angiography. ℞ Prednisolone (1mg/kg/d PO). Methotrexate or cyclophosphamide are used as steroid-sparing agents, with increasing use of biologic DMARDs for resistant cases: TNFα and IL-6 inhibitors have similar efficacy. BP control is essential to ↓ risk of stroke. Angioplasty ± stenting, or bypass surgery is performed for critical stenosis. **Prognosis** ~95% survival at 15 years.

Polyarteritis nodosa (PAN) PAN is a necrotizing vasculitis that causes aneurysms and thrombosis in medium-sized arteries, leading to infarction in affected organs with severe systemic symptoms. ♂:♀≈2:1. It may be associated with hepatitis B. **Symptoms** Systemic features, skin (rash, 'punched out' ulcers, nodules), renal (main cause of death, renal artery narrowing, glomerular ischaemia, insufficiency, HTN), cardiac, GI, GU, neuro involvement. Usually spares lungs. Coronary aneurysms occur in Kawasaki disease (OHCS p850). **Tests** Often ↑WCC, mild eosinophilia (in 30%), anaemia, ↑ESR, ↑CRP, ANCA −ve. Renal or mesenteric angiography (fig 12.17), or renal biopsy can be diagnostic. ℞ Control BP and refer. Steroids for mild cases and steroid-sparing agents if more severe. Hepatitis B should be treated (p274) after initial treatment with steroids.

Microscopic polyangiitis A necrotizing vasculitis affecting small- & medium-sized vessels. **Symptoms** Rapidly progressive glomerulonephritis usually features; pulmonary haemorrhage occurs in up to 30%; other features are rare. **Tests** pANCA (MPO) +ve (p550). ℞ Steroids plus, eg methotrexate. For maintenance: methotrexate, rituximab, or azathioprine.

Hypocomplementaemic urticarial vasculitis A lupus-like illness with urticaria and antibodies to complement (C1q), occasionally severe, with obstructive lung disease and nephritis. ℞ Hydroxychloroquine, antihistamines, or dapsone (check G6PD status first).

Behçet's disease Associated with HLA-B5, most common along the old Silk Road, from the Mediterranean to China. **Features** Recurrent oral and genital ulceration, uveitis, skin lesions (eg erythema nodosum); arthritis (non-erosive large joint); thrombophlebitis; myo/pericarditis; CNS involvement (pyramidal signs); and colitis. **Diagnosis** Mainly clinical. *Pathergy test:* needle prick leads to papule formation within 48h. ℞ Colchicine for orogenital ulceration; steroids, azathioprine/cyclophosphamide for systemic disease. Infliximab has a role in ocular disease unresponsive to topical steroids.

Table 12.5 Classification of vasculitides, Chapel Hill criteria (2012)[15]

May be primary or secondary to other diseases, eg SLE, RA, hepatitis B & C, HIV	
Large vessel	Giant cell arteritis, Takayasu's arteritis
Medium vessel	Polyarteritis nodosa, Kawasaki disease (OHCS p850)
Small vessel	ANCA-associated: microscopic polyangiitis; granulomatosis with polyangiitis (p700); and eosinophilic granulomatosis with polyangiitis (Churg–Strauss syndrome; 40–60% are ANCA positive) Immune complex vasculitis: Goodpasture's disease; cryoglobulinaemic vasculitis; IgA vasculitis (Henoch–Schönlein purpura)
Variable vessel	Behçet's syndrome, Cogan's syndrome

Features of vasculitis

The presentation of vasculitis will depend on the organs affected: often only overwhelming fatigue with ↑ESR/CRP. ▶▶*Consider vasculitis in any unidentified multisystem disorder.* If presentation does not fit clinically or serologically into a specific category consider malignancy-associated vasculitis.

Systemic Fever, malaise, weight loss, arthralgia, myalgia.

Skin Purpura, ulcers, livedo reticularis (fig 12.18), nailbed infarcts, digital gangrene.

Eyes Episcleritis, scleritis, visual loss.

ENT Epistaxis, nasal crusting, stridor, deafness.

Pulmonary Haemoptysis and dyspnoea (due to pulmonary haemorrhage).

Cardiac Angina or MI (due to coronary arteritis), heart failure, and pericarditis.

GI Pain or perforation (infarcted viscus), malabsorption (chronic ischaemia).

Renal Hypertension, haematuria, proteinuria, casts, and renal failure (renal cortical infarcts; glomerulonephritis in ANCA +ve vasculitis).

Neurological Stroke, fits, chorea, psychosis, confusion, impaired cognition, altered mood. Arteritis of the vasa nervorum (arterial supply to peripheral nerves) may cause mononeuritis multiplex or a sensorimotor polyneuropathy.

GU Orchitis—testicular pain or tenderness.

Polymyalgia rheumatica (PMR)

PMR is not a true vasculitis and its pathogenesis is unknown. PMR and GCA share the same demographic characteristics and, although separate conditions, the two frequently occur together. **Features** Age >50yrs; subacute onset (<2 weeks) of bilateral aching, tenderness, and morning stiffness in shoulders, hips, and proximal limb muscles ± fatigue, fever, ↓weight, anorexia, and depression. **Investigations** Bloods as GCA. Note CK levels are normal (helping to distinguish from myositis/myopathies). **℞** Prednisolone 15mg/d PO. Expect a dramatic response within 1 week and consider an alternative diagnosis if not. ↓ dose slowly, eg by 1mg/month (according to symptoms/ESR). NSAIDs are not effective. Inform patients to seek urgent review if symptoms of GCA develop.

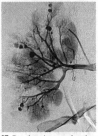

Fig 12.17 Renal angiogram showing multiple aneurysms in PAN.
Courtesy of Dr William Herring.

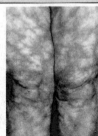

Fig 12.18 Livedo reticularis: pink–blue mottling caused by capillary dilatation and stasis in skin venules. Causes: physiological, cold, or vasculitis.

7 Low-dose aspirin has been shown to decrease the rate of visual loss and cerebrovascular accidents in GCA but there are also conflicting reports regarding its efficacy at preventing ischaemic events in GCA.

Fibromyalgia and chronic fatigue syndrome are part of a diffuse group of overlapping syndromes, sharing similar demographic and clinical characteristics, in which chronic symptoms of fatigue and widespread pain feature prominently. Their existence as discrete entities is controversial, especially in the absence of clear pathology, and some find such dysfunctional diagnoses frustrating. However, a correct diagnosis enables the doctor to give appropriate counselling and advise appropriate therapies, and allows the patient to begin to accept and deal with their symptoms.

Fibromyalgia

Fibromyalgia comprises up to 10% of new referrals to the rheumatology clinic.

Prevalence 0.5–5%, increases with age. ♀:♂≈6:1 but female bias is less prominent when criteria without tender points are used.

Risk factors BOX 'Risk factors'. Female sex, middle age (most common cause of generalized musculoskeletal pain in women aged 20–55yrs), low household income, divorced, coexistent hypermobility and autonomic dysfunction (eg postural ortho-static tachycardia syndrome). Other somatic syndromes such as chronic fatigue syndrome, irritable bowel syndrome (p264), and chronic headache syndromes (see OHCS p803) are associated. Also found in ~25% of patients with RA, AS, and SLE.

Features Diagnosis depends on pain that is *chronic* (>3 months) and widespread (involves left and right sides, above and below the waist, and the axial skeleton). Profound fatigue is almost universal. *Additional features:* morning stiffness (~80–90%), paraesthesiae (without underlying cause), headaches (migraine and tension), poor concentration, low mood, dysfunctional uterine bleeding in premenopausal women, and sleep disturbance (~70%, a non-restorative sleep pattern is typical). Widespread and severe tender points.

Investigations All normal. Diagnosis is clinical. Over-investigation can consolidate illness behaviour; but exclude other causes of pain and/or fatigue (eg RA; PMR, p555; vasculitis, p554; hypothyroidism, p214; myeloma, p366).

Management Multidisciplinary with optimal results coming from full engagement of the patient who should be encouraged to remain as active as they feel able, and ideally to continue to participate in the workforce. New symptoms should be fully reviewed to exclude an alternative diagnosis. Patients should be advised that there is no one specific treatment that is guaranteed to work, but any of the following may help: graded exercise programmes, including both aerobic and strength-based training. Pacing of activity is vital to avoid over-exertion and consequent pain and fatigue. Long-term *graded exercise programmes* improve functional capacity. Relaxation, rehabilitation, and physiotherapy may also help. *Cognitive behavioural therapy* (CBT) aims to help patients develop coping strategies and set achievable goals.

Pharmacotherapy Early initiation is helpful as it may increase adherence to exercise and cognitive behavioural techniques. Low-dose amitriptyline (eg 10–20mg at night) has been shown to help relieve pain and improve sleep. Pregabalin (150–300mg/12h PO) can be used if amitriptyline is ineffective. An SNRI (eg duloxetine) is a good choice for patients with comorbid anxiety and depression. Steroids or NSAIDs are not recommended because there is no inflammation (if it does respond, reconsider your diagnosis!).

Chronic fatigue syndrome (AKA myalgic encephalomyelitis)

Chronic fatigue syndrome is defined as persistent disabling fatigue lasting >6 months, affecting mental and physical function, present >50% of the time, plus ≥4 of: myalgia (~80%), polyarthralgia, ↓memory, unrefreshing sleep, fatigue after exertion >24h, persistent sore throat, tender cervical/axillary lymph nodes. Management principles are similar to fibromyalgia and include graded exercise and CBT. No pharmacological agents have yet been proved effective for chronic fatigue syndrome (see also OHCS p803).

Risk factors: yellow flags

Psychosocial risk factors for developing persisting chronic pain and long-term disability have been termed 'yellow flags':[16]

Belief that pain and activity are harmful.

Sickness behaviours such as extended rest.

Social withdrawal.

Emotional problems such as low mood, anxiety, or stress.

Problems or dissatisfaction at work.

Problems with claims for compensation or time off work.

Overprotective family or lack of support.

Inappropriate expectations of treatment, eg low active participation in treatment.

An existential approach to difficult symptoms

The manner in which management is discussed is almost as important as the management itself, which should focus on education of the patient *and their family* and on developing coping strategies. Such a diagnosis may be a relief or a disappointment to the patient. *Explain* that fibromyalgia is a relapsing and re-mitting condition, with no easy cures, and that they will continue to have good and bad days. *Reassure* them that there is no serious underlying pathology, that their joints are not being damaged, and that no further tests are necessary, but be sympathetic to the fact that they may have been seeking a physical cause for their symptoms. Take advice from the Danish philosopher Kierkegaard who wrote to a friend in 1835, *'What I really lack is to be clear in my mind what I am to do, not what I am to know... The thing is to understand myself... to find a truth which is true for me.'* Listen to the patient and accept their story. Then help them to focus on what they can *do* to improve their situation, and to move away from dwelling on finding a physical answer to their symptoms.

Pathogenesis of fibromyalgia

Fibromyalgia is likely to be a disorder of central pain processing. Two key features of the condition are *allodynia* (pain in response to a non-painful stimulus) and *hyperalgesia* (exaggerated perception of pain in response to a painful stimulus). Functional MRI supports this theory of central sensitization, with overactivation of pain-sensitive brain areas following pressure stimuli. This appears to be at least in part due to sensory neurotransmitter imbalance, possibly also explaining sleep/cognitive/mood abnormalities. Substance P, a neuropeptide linked to chronic pain, is increased in the CSF of patients with fibromyalgia, and levels of noradrenaline and serotonin metabolites are decreased. Antidepressants, especially those that have both serotonergic and noradrenergic activity (tricyclics and venlafaxine), seem to be most effective. Recent research has shown that serum from patients with fibromyalgia can adversely affect animals in an experimental model of the condition. The significance of these findings is currently being evaluated, but might ultimately result in the identification of new therapeutic targets and a shift towards the management of the condition as an autoinflammatory disease.

The eye is host to many diseases: the more you look, the more you'll see, and the more you'll enjoy, not least because the eye is as beautiful as its signs are legion.

Behçet's (p554.) Systemic inflammatory disorder, HLA B27 association. Causes a uveitis amongst other systemic manifestations. Cause unknown.

Granulomatous disorders Syphilis, TB, sarcoidosis, leprosy, brucellosis, and toxoplasmosis may inflame either the front chamber (anterior uveitis/iritis, table 12.6) or back chamber (posterior uveitis/choroiditis). Refer to an ophthalmologist.

Systemic inflammatory diseases May manifest as *iritis* in ankylosing spondylitis and reactive arthritis; *uveitis* in Behçet's; *conjunctivitis* (table 12.6) in reactive arthritis; *scleritis* or *episcleritis* in RA, vasculitis, and SLE. Scleritis in RA and granulomatosis with polyangiitis (Wegener's) may damage the eye. ▸▸Refer urgently if eye pain. GCA causes optic nerve ischaemia presenting as sudden blindness.

Keratoconjunctivitis sicca A reduction in tear formation, tested by the Schirmer filter paper test (<5mm in 5min). It causes a gritty feeling in the eyes, and a dry mouth (xerostomia from ↓saliva production). It is found on its own (Sjögren's syndrome), or with other diseases, eg SLE, RA, sarcoidosis. ℞ Artificial tears/saliva.

Hypertensive retinopathy ↑BP damages retinal vessels. Hardened arteries are shiny ('silver wiring'; fig 12.19) and 'nip' veins where they cross (AV nipping; fig 12.20). Narrowed arterioles may become blocked, causing localized retinal infarction, seen as cotton-wool spots. Leaks from these in severe hypertension manifest as hard exudates or macular oedema. Papilloedema (fig 12.21) or flame haemorrhages suggest accelerated hypertension (p108) requiring urgent treatment.

Vascular occlusion *Emboli* passing through the retinal vasculature may cause *retinal artery occlusion* (global or segmental retinal pallor) or *amaurosis fugax* (p469). Roth spots (small retinal infarcts) occur in infective endocarditis. In dermatomyositis, there is orbital oedema with retinopathy showing cotton-wool spots (micro-infarcts). *Retinal vein occlusion* is caused by ↑BP, age, or hyperviscosity (p368). Suspect in any acute fall in acuity. If it is the central vein, the fundus is like a stormy sunset (those angry red clouds are haemorrhages). In branch vein occlusion, changes are confined to a wedge of retina. Get expert help.

Haematological disorders *Retinal haemorrhages* occur in leukaemia; commashaped *conjunctival haemorrhages* and retinal new vessel formation may occur in sickle cell disease. *Optic atrophy* is seen in pernicious anaemia (and also MS).

Metabolic disease Diabetes mellitus: p204. Hyperthyroid exophthalmos: p213. Lens opacities are seen in hypoparathyroidism. Conjunctival and corneal calcification can occur in hypercalcaemia. In gout, conjunctival urate deposits may cause sore eyes.

Systemic infections Septicaemia may seed to the vitreous causing endophthalmitis. Syphilis can cause uveitis (+ pigmented retinopathy if congenital). Systemic fungal infections may affect the eye, eg in the immunocompromised or in IV drug users, requiring intravitreal antibiotics.

AIDS and HIV CMV retinitis (pizza-pie fundus—a mixture of cotton-wool spots, infiltrates, and haemorrhages, p434) may be asymptomatic but can cause sudden visual loss. If present, it implies AIDS (CD4 count <100 × 10⁶/L; p394). Cotton-wool spots on their own indicate HIV retinopathy and may occur in early disease. Kaposi's sarcoma may affect the lids (non-tender purple nodule) or conjunctiva (red fleshy mass).

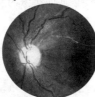
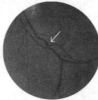
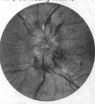

Fig 12.19 Silver wiring.
© Prof Jonathan Trobe.

Fig 12.20 AV nipping.
© Prof Jonathan Trobe.

Fig 12.21 Papilloedema.
© Prof Jonathan Trobe.

Table 12.6 Differential diagnosis of a red eye

	Conjunctiva	Iris	Pupil	Cornea	Anterior chamber	Intraocular pressure	Treatment	Appearance
Acute glaucoma	Both ciliary and conjunctival vessels injected. Entire eye is red See *OHCS* p331	Injected	Dilated, fixed, oval	Steamy, hazy	Very shallow	Very high	Refer IV acetazolamide + pilocarpine drops (miotic); peripheral iridotomy	
Anterior uveitis (iritis)	Redness most marked around cornea, which doesn't blanch on pressure. Usually unilateral *Causes:* AS, RA, Reiter's sarcoidosis, herpes simplex, herpes zoster, and Behçet's disease. NB: a similar scleral appearance but without papillary or anterior chamber involvement may be *scleritis* (eg RA, SLE, vasculitis)	Injected	Small, irregular due to adhesions between the anterior lens and the pupil margin	Normal	Turgid	Normal	Refer Steroid eye drops (eg 0.5% prednisolone) + mydriatic (eg cyclopentolate 0.5%)	
Conjunctivitis	Often bilateral Conjunctival vessels injected, greatest toward fornices, but blanching on pressure Mobile over sclera Purulent discharge	Normal	Normal	Normal	Normal	Normal	Most do not require treatment Consider chloramphenicol ointment or drops	
Subconjunctival haemorrhage	Bright red sclera with white rim around limbus. *Causes:* ↑BP, leptospirosis, bleeding disorders, trauma, snake venom, haemorrhagic fevers	Normal	Normal	Normal	Normal	Normal	Looks alarming but resolves spontaneously. Check BP if elderly; refer if traumatic; on warfarin?	

Images courtesy of Prof. Jonathan Trobe.

12 Rheumatology

Skin manifestations of systemic diseases

Erythema nodosum (fig 12.22) Painful, blue-red, raised lesions on shins (± thighs/arms). *Causes:* sarcoidosis, drugs (sulfonamides, contraceptive pill, dapsone), streptococcal infection. *Less common:* IBD, BCG vaccination, leptospirosis, *Mycobacterium* (TB, leprosy), *Yersinia*, or various viruses and fungi. Cause unknown in 30–50%.

Erythema multiforme (See *OHCS* p438) (fig 12.23) 'Target' lesions: symmetrical ± central blister, on palms/soles, limbs, and elsewhere. *Stevens–Johnson syndrome* (p696): a rare, severe variant with fever and mucosal involvement (mouth, genital, and eye ulcers), associated with a hypersensitivity reaction to drugs (NSAIDs, sulfonamides, anticonvulsants, allopurinol), or infections (herpes, *Mycoplasma*, orf). Also seen in collagen disorders. 50% of cases are idiopathic. Get expert help in severe disease.

Erythema migrans (fig 12.24) Presents as a small papule at the site of a tick bite which develops into a spreading large erythematous ring, with central fading. It lasts from 48h to 3 months and there may be multiple lesions in disseminated disease. *Cause:* the rash is pathognomonic of Lyme disease and occurs in ~80% of cases (p418).

Erythema marginatum Pink coalescent rings on trunk which come and go. It is seen in rheumatic fever (or rarely other causes, eg drugs). See fig 3.54, p147.

Pyoderma gangrenosum (fig 12.25) Recurring nodulo-pustular ulcers, ~10cm wide, with tender red/blue overhanging necrotic edge, purulent surface, and healing with cribriform scars on leg, abdomen, or face. *Associations:* IBD, autoimmune hepatitis, granulomatosis with polyangiitis (Wegener's), myeloma, neoplasia. ♀ > ♂. *Treatment:* get help. Oral steroids ± ciclosporin should be 1st-line therapy.[17]

Vitiligo (fig 12.26) *Vitellus* is Latin for *spotted calf:* typically white patches ± hyperpigmented borders. Sunlight makes them itch. *Associations:* autoimmune disorders; premature ovarian failure. Treat by camouflage cosmetics and sunscreens (± steroid creams ± dermabrasion). UK Vitiligo Society: 0800 018 2631.

Specific diseases and their skin manifestations

Crohn's Perianal/vulval/oral ulcers; erythema nodosum; pyoderma gangrenosum.

Dermatomyositis Gottron's papules (rough red papules on the knuckles/extensor surfaces); shawl sign; heliotrope rash on eyelids (fig 12.27). It may be associated with lung, bowel, ovarian, or pancreatic malignancy (p549).

Diabetes mellitus Ulcers, *necrobiosis lipoidica* (shiny yellowish area on shin ± telangiectasia; fig 12.28), *granuloma annulare* (*OHCS* p436), *acanthosis nigricans* (pigmented, rough thickening of axillary, neck, or groin skin with warty lesions; fig 12.29).

Coeliac disease Dermatitis herpetiformis Itchy blisters, in groups on knees, elbows, and scalp. The itch (which can drive patients to suicide) responds to *dapsone* 25–200mg/24h PO within 48h—and this may be used as a diagnostic test. The maintenance dose may be as little as 50mg/wk. A gluten-free diet should be adhered to, but in 30% dapsone will need to be continued. SE (dose-related): haemolysis (CI: anaemia, G6PD deficiency), hepatitis, agranulocytosis (monitor FBC and LFTs). There is an ↑ risk of small bowel lymphoma with coeliac disease *and* dermatitis herpetiformis—so surveillance is needed.

Hyperthyroidism Pretibial myxoedema Red oedematous swellings above lateral malleoli, progressing to thickened oedema of legs and feet, *thyroid acropachy*—clubbing + subperiosteal new bone in phalanges. **Other endocrinopathies** See p197.

Liver disease Palmar erythema; spider naevi; gynaecomastia; decrease in pubic hair; jaundice; bruising; scratch marks.

Malabsorption Dry pigmented skin, easy bruising, hair loss, leuconychia.

Neoplasia Acanthosis nigricans (See 'Diabetes mellitus' and fig 12.29.) Associated with gastric cancer. **Dermatomyositis** See earlier in topic. **Thrombophlebitis migrans** Successive crops of tender nodules affecting blood vessels throughout the body, associated with pancreatic cancer (especially body and tail). **Acquired ichthyosis** Dry scaly skin associated with lymphoma. **Skin metastases** Especially melanoma, and colonic, lung, breast, laryngeal/oral, or ovarian malignancy.

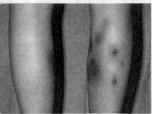

Fig 12.22 Erythema nodosum.

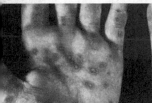

Fig 12.23 Erythema multiforme.
Courtesy of CDC/Dr. N.J. Fiumara.

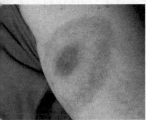

Fig 12.24 Erythema migrans.
Courtesy of CDC/James Gathany.

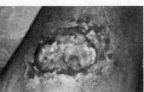

Fig 12.25 Pyoderma gangrenosum.
Reproduced from S.D. Lee, et al., *Inflammatory Bowel Diseases*, 2021, 28(2): 309–313, by permission of Oxford University Press, on behalf of Crohn's & Colitis Foundation.

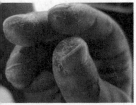

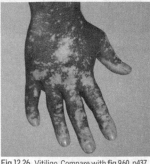

Fig 12.26 Vitiligo. Compare with fig 9.60, p437.

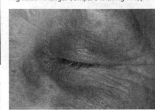

Fig 12.27 Heliotrope rash.
Courtesy of Nick Taylor, East Sussex Hospitals Trust.

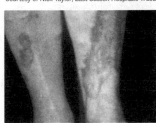

Fig 12.28 Necrobiosis lipoidica.
Reproduced from Warrell et al., *Oxford Textbook of Medicine*, 2010, with permission from Oxford University Press.

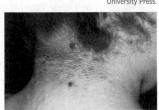

Fig 12.29 Acanthosis nigricans.
Reproduced from Lewis-Jones, *Paediatric Dermatology*, 2010, with permission from Oxford University Press.

Fig 12.30 Mechanic's hands.
Reproduced from Yin H et al., *Rheumatol Adv Pract*, 6(1), 2022, with permission from Oxford University Press, on behalf of British Society for Rheumatology.

13 Surgery

Contents

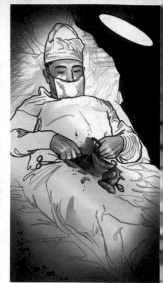

Fig 13.1 As a brutal polar winter rolled over Antarctica, heralding months of darkness and complete isolation, surgeon Leonid Rogozov fell ill with generalized abdominal pain. As blizzards swept down on their small camp of 12, so too his pain surged and descended on the right iliac fossa. The sole medic on the expedition, he made a rapid diagnosis and commenced conservative treatment, but the development of fever and vomiting signalled the inevitable. On 1 May 1961, scrubbed and semi-reclined, after briefing his team on how to ventilate him should he lose consciousness, he performed a successful auto-appendicectomy with a mirror, a couple of syringes of local anaesthetic, and surgical instruments stored outside in the snow.[1] And not a moment too soon, within only a day of perforation by his estimation as he examined the specimen he had excised. Whatever the situation, and regardless of the consequences, the maxim remains the same: the art of surgery lies in selecting the right operation at the right time for the right patient.

Artwork by Gillian Turner.

We thank Ruwan Weerakkody, our Specialist Reader and Christina Taylor, our Junior Reader for this chapter.

1	2	3
4	5	6
7	8	9

1 Right upper quadrant (RUQ) or hypochondrium.
2 Epigastrium.
3 Left upper quadrant (LUQ) or hypochondrium.
4 Right flank (merges posteriorly with right loin, p53).
5 Periumbilical or central area.
6 Left flank (merges posteriorly with left loin, p53).
7 Right iliac fossa (RIF).
8 Suprapubic area.
9 Left iliac fossa (LIF).

Fig 13.2 Abdominal areas.

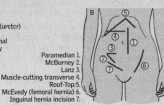

1. Kocher
2. Midline
3. Muscle splitting (ureter)
4. Pfannenstiel
5. Thoraco-abdominal (oesophagectomy) 9th or 10th ICS)

Paramedian 1.
McBurney 2.
Lanz 3.
Muscle-cutting transverse 4.
Roof-Top 5.
McEvedy (femoral hernia) 6.
Inguinal hernia incision 7.

Fig 13.3 Incisions.

-ectomy	Cutting something out.
-gram	A radiological image.
-pexy	Anchoring of a structure to keep it in position.
-plasty	Surgical refashioning in order to regain function/cosmesis.
-scopy	Procedure with instrumentation for looking into the body.
-stomy	An artificial union between a conduit and the outside or another conduit.
-tomy	Cutting something open to the outside world.
-tripsy	Fragmentation of an object.

angio-	Tube or vessel	**lith-**	Stone
appendic-	Appendix	**mast-**	Breast
chole-	Relating to gall/bile	**meso-**	Mesentery
colp-	Vagina	**nephr-**	Kidney
cyst-	Bladder	**orchid-**	Testicle
-doch-	Ducts	**oophor-**	Ovary
enter-	Small bowel	**phren-**	Diaphragm
eschar-	Dead tissue, eg from burn	**pyloro-**	Pyloric sphincter
gastr-	Stomach	**pyel-**	Renal pelvis
hepat-	Liver	**proct-**	Anal canal
hyster-	Uterus	**salping-**	Fallopian tube
lapar-	Abdomen	**splen-**	Spleen

abscess	A cavity containing pus. Remember: *if there is pus about, let it out*.
colic	Intermittent pain from over-contraction/obstruction of a hollow viscus.
cyst	Fluid-filled cavity lined by epi/endothelium.
fistula	An abnormal connection between two epithelial surfaces. Fistulae often close spontaneously, but will not in the presence of malignant tissue, distal obstruction, foreign bodies, chronic inflammation, and the formation of a muco-cutaneous junction (eg stoma).
hernia	The protrusion of a viscus/part of a viscus through a defect of the wall of its containing cavity into an abnormal position.
ileus	Used in this book as a term for adynamic bowel.
sinus	A blind-ending tract, typically lined by epithelial or granulation tissue, which opens to an epithelial surface.
stent	An artificial tube placed in a biological tube to keep it open.
stoma	(p582) An artificial union between conduits or a conduit and the outside.
ulcer	(p652) Interruption in the continuity of an epi/endothelial surface.
volvulus	(p603) Twisting of a structure around itself. Common GI sites include the sigmoid colon and caecum, and more rarely the stomach.

epi-	Upon	**pan-**	Whole	**peri-**	Around
end-	Inside	**para-**	Alongside	**sub-**	Beneath
mega-	Enlarged	**per-**	Going through	**trans-**	Across.

Aims To provide diagnostic and prognostic information. Ensures the patient understands the nature, aims, and expected outcome of surgery. Ensures that the right patient gets the right surgery. Have the symptoms and signs changed? If so, inform the surgeon.

• Assess/balance risks of anaesthesia, and maximize fitness. Comorbidities? Drugs? Smoker? Optimizing oxygenation *before* major surgery improves outcome.

• Obtain informed consent (p566).

• Check proposed anaesthesia/analgesia with anaesthetist.

Family history May be relevant, eg in malignant hyperpyrexia (p570); myotonic dystrophy (p506); porphyria; cholinesterase problems; sickle cell disease.

Drugs Any drug/plaster/antiseptic allergies? ►Inform the anaesthetist about *all* drugs even if 'over-the-counter'. ►Steroids: see p573; diabetes: see p572.

• **Antibiotics** Aminoglycosides may ↑ neuromuscular blockade.

• **Anti-seizure medications** Give as usual pre-op. Post-op, give drugs IV (or by NG tube) until able to take orally.

• **Antihypertensives** Check with the anaesthetist. Usually: continue *β-blockers* up to and including the day of surgery (precludes a labile cardiovascular response). *Calcium channel blockers* are also typically continued. The approach to *ACE-i and ARBs* is controversial, in general these are withheld on the morning of surgery, likewise for *diuretics* (beware hypokalaemia, dehydration, do U&E and bicarbonate).

• **Antithrombotics** See p573.

• **Contraceptive pill** See *BNF*. Stop 4wks before major/leg surgery; ensure alternative contraception is used. Restart 2wks after surgery, provided patient is mobile.

• **Digoxin** Continue up to and including morning of surgery. Check for toxicity on ECG, plasma K+ and Ca²⁺ (suxamethonium can ↑K⁺ and lead to ventricular arrhythmias in the fully digitalized).

• **HRT** As with contraceptive pill there may be ↑risk of DVT/PE.

• **Levodopa** Possible arrhythmias when patient under GA.

• **Lithium** Get expert help; may potentiate neuromuscular blockade and cause arrhythmias. See *OHCS* p716.

• **MAOIS** Get expert help as interactions may cause hypotensive/hypertensive crises.

• **SSRIs** May increase bleeding risk especially if combined with antiplatelet agents. Can also cause arrhythmia, hypertension, and hyperthermia (serotonin syndrome). This can occur as an interaction with common analgesics such as tramadol, and common anaesthetic drugs used to treat intra-operative hypotension (ephedrine and metaraminol).

• **Statins** May reduce perioperative vascular risk so should be continued, but *bile acid sequestrants* and *ezetimibe* might affect medication absorption and should not be given on the day of surgery.

• **Thyroid medication** See p592.

• **Tricyclics** These enhance adrenaline (epinephrine) and arrhythmias.

Preparation ►Starve patient; NBM ≥2h pre-op for clear fluids and ≥6h for solids. Is any bowel or skin preparation needed, or prophylactic antibiotics (p568)?

• Start DVT prophylaxis as indicated, eg graduated compression stockings (CI in peripheral arterial disease); LMWH (p346): eg moderate risk, 20mg ~2h pre-op then 20mg/24h; high risk (eg orthopaedic surgery), 40mg 12h pre-op then 40mg/24h; or heparin 5000U SC 2h pre-op, then every 8–12h SC for 7d or until ambulant.

• Ensure necessary premedications (p570), regular medications, analgesia, antiemetics, antibiotics are all prescribed as appropriate. Confirm NBM.

• Book any pre-, intra-, or post-operative X-rays or frozen sections.

• Book post-operative physiotherapy.

• If needed, site IV cannula, catheterize (p746), and/or insert a Ryle's tube (p743).

• Meta-analyses have shown no benefit to patients from mechanical bowel cleansing before colonic surgery—this is no longer considered good practice. There is also no evidence for the use of enemas prior to rectal surgery.

Pre-operative history, examination, and tests

It is the anaesthetist's responsibility to assess suitability for anaesthesia. The ward doctor assists with a good history and examination, should anticipate necessary tests, and can also reassure and inform the patient. The surgical team should consent the patient.

►The World Health Organization 'Surgical Safety Checklist' should be completed for every patient undergoing a surgical procedure, ensuring pre-operative preparation, intra-operative monitoring, and post-operative review.

History Assess past history of: MI,[1] diabetes, asthma, hypertension, valvular heart disease, epilepsy, jaundice. Existing illnesses, drugs, and allergies? Be alert to chronic lung disease, ↑BP, arrhythmias, and murmurs. Assess any specific risks, eg is the patient pregnant? Is the jaw/jaw immobile and teeth stable (intubation risk)? Has there been previous anaesthesia? Were there any complications (eg nausea, DVT)?

Examination Assess cardiorespiratory system, exercise tolerance. Is the neck unstable (eg arthritis complicating intubation)? ►Is DVT/PE prophylaxis needed (p578)? ►For 'unilateral' surgery, mark the correct arm/leg/kidney (surgeon).

Tests Be guided by the history and examination and local/NICE protocols.
* *U&E, FBC, and finger-prick blood glucose in most patients:* if Hb <100g/L tell anaesthetist. Investigate/treat as appropriate. U&E are particularly important if the patient is diabetic, on diuretics, a burns patient, has hepatic or renal disease, has an ileus, or is parenterally fed.
* *Crossmatch:* blood type is identified and units are allocated to the patient.
* *Group and save (G&S):* blood type is identified and held, pending crossmatch (if required). Contact your lab to discuss requirements—this decreases wastage and allows increased efficiency of blood stocks.
* *Specific blood tests:* LFT in jaundice, malignancy, or alcohol abuse. *Amylase* in acute abdominal pain. *Blood glucose* if diabetic (p572). *Drug levels* as appropriate (eg digoxin, lithium). *Clotting studies* in liver or renal disease, DIC (p350), massive blood loss, or if on valproate, warfarin, or heparin. HIV, HBsAg in high-risk patients, after counselling. *Sickle test* in those with a clinical suspicion or known family history. If known sickle cell disease/positive test: contact specialist. *Thyroid function tests* in those with thyroid disease.
* *CXR:* if known cardiorespiratory disease, pathology, or symptoms.
* *ECG:* if >55yrs old or poor exercise tolerance, or history of myocardial ischaemia, hypertension, valvular or other heart disease.
* *Echocardiogram:* may be performed if there is a suspicion of poor LV function.
* *Pulmonary function tests:* in known pulmonary disease/obesity.
* *Cervical spine x-ray/CT:* if history of rheumatoid arthritis/ankylosing spondylitis/Down's syndrome, to warn of difficult intubations: discuss with anaesthetist.
* *MRSA screen:* screen and decolonize nasal carriers according to local policy (eg nasal mupirocin ointment). Colonization is *not* a contraindication to surgery. Place patients last on the list to minimize transmission to others and cover with appropriate antibiotic prophylaxis, eg vancomycin or teicoplanin. Consider and document major blood-borne virus risk (HIV/HBV/HCV) according to local policies.

American Society of Anesthesiologists (ASA) classification

Class I Normally healthy patient.
Class II Mild systemic disease.
Class III Severe systemic disease that limits activity but is not incapacitating.
Class IV Incapacitating systemic disease which poses a constant threat to life.
Class V Moribund: not expected to survive 24h without the operation.
Class VI Declared brain-dead: organ removal for donor purposes.
You will see a space for an ASA number on most anaesthetic charts. It is a health index at the time of surgery. The suffix E is used in emergencies, eg ASA 2E.

---

1 If within the last 6 months, the perioperative risk of re-infarction (up to 40%) makes most elective surgery too risky. ECHO, and stress testing (+ exercise ECG or MUGA scan, p724) should be done.

In which of the following situations would you seek 'informed written consent' from a patient? 1 Feeling for a pulse. 2 Taking blood. 3 Inserting a central line. 4 Removing a section of small bowel during a laparotomy for division of adhesions. 5 Orchidectomy after a failed operation for testicular torsion. English law states that *any* intervention or treatment needs consent—ie all of the above—yet, for different reasons. In fact, *written* consent itself is not required by law, but it does constitute 'good medical practice' for more complex procedures. Sometimes actions and words can imply valid consent, eg by simply entering into conversation or holding out an arm. If the consequences are not clear and the patient has *capacity* to give consent, you should seek informed written consent as a record of your conversation. Remember, it is our responsibility to respect the legal and ethical rights of those we treat. We do this not only for the sake of the individual, but also for the sake of an enduring trust between the patient and doctor, remembering that it is the patient's right to refuse treatment (if a fully competent adult) even when this may result in their death.

For consent to be valid
- It can be given any time before the intervention/treatment is initiated. Earlier is better as this will give the patient time to think about the risks, benefits, and alternatives—they may even bring forward questions on issues that you had not considered relevant. Think of consent as an ongoing process throughout the patient's time with you, not just the moment of signing the form.
- The proposed treatment or test must be clearly understood by the patient, taking into account the benefits, risks (including complication rates if known, as well as the risks of proceeding without the procedure), additional procedures, alternative courses of action, and their consequences.
- It must be given *voluntarily*. This can be difficult to evaluate—eg when live organ donation is being considered—see BOX 'Special circumstances for consent' for other difficult situations.
- The doctor providing treatment or undertaking the test needs to ensure that the patient has given valid consent. The act of seeking consent is ultimately the responsibility of the doctor looking after the patient, though the task may be delegated to another health professional, as long as they are suitably trained and qualified.

Capacity Relates to the ability to: 1 understand 2 retain and 3 weigh up relevant information and 4 communicate the decision. Capacity is not a fixed state, but is specific to any given time and decision—a person may lack capacity to be involved in a particular complex decision but retain capacity to decide other aspects of their care, or recover capacity as they recover from acute illness. Therefore, do not label anyone as unable to make a decision unless you have taken all practicable steps to help them to do so without success—non-urgent decisions should always be deferred if there is a chance to recover capacity. When acting on behalf of a person who lacks capacity, do so in their best interests and involve family members or an appointed surrogate where clinical urgency allows.

When taking consent
- Does the patient currently have capacity for the decision in question?
- Are you the right person to be obtaining consent?
- Use words the patient understands and avoid jargon and abbreviations.
- Ensure that they believe your facts and can retain 'pros' and 'cons' long enough to inform their decision. Fact sheets/diagrams for individual operations help.
- Make sure their choice is free from pressure from others, and explain that they can withdraw consent at any time after the form is signed. Some patients may view the consent form as a contract from which they cannot *renege*.
- If the patient is illiterate, a witnessed mark does endorse valid consent. Similarly, if the patient is willing but physically unable to sign the consent form, then a witnessed entry into the medical notes stating so is valid.
- Remember to discuss further procedures that may become necessary during the proposed treatment. This avoids waking up to a nasty surprise (eg a missing testicle as in scenario 5 earlier in this topic).

13 Surgery

Special circumstances for consent

Consent is complex, but remember that it exists for the benefit of the patient *and* the doctor, giving you an opportunity to revisit expectations and involve the patient in their own care. There are some areas of treatment or investigation for which it may be advisable to seek specialist advice if it is not part of your regular practice[2]:

• Photography of a patient.
• Innovative or novel treatment.
• Living organ donation.
• Storage, use, or removal of human tissue (for any length of time).
• The storage, loss, or use of gametes.
• The use of patient records or tissue in research or teaching.
• In the presence of an advanced directive or living will, expressly refusing a particular treatment, investigation, or action.
• Consent if <16yrs (consent form 3 in NHS). In the UK, those >16yrs can give valid consent. Those <16yrs can give consent for a medical decision provided they understand what it involves—the concept of *Gillick* competence. It is still good practice to involve the parents in the decision, if the child is willing. If *<18yrs and refusing life-saving surgery*, talk to the parents and your senior; and seek legal advice if the intervention appears in their best interests. In Scotland, parents cannot authorize an intervention that a competent child has refused.
• Consent in the incapacitated (NHS consent form 4). No one (parents, relatives, or even members of a healthcare team) is able to give consent on behalf of an adult in England unless they have written power of attorney, but it is good practice to involve the family to try to best understand the likely wishes of the patient. The High Court may be required to give a ruling on the matters of lawfulness of a proposed procedure. In a patient lacking capacity it may advisable to involve an independent mental capacity advocate.

Exposing patients to our learning curves? The jury is still out ...

All surgeons get better over time (for a while), as they perform new techniques with increasing ease and confidence. When Wertheim (fig 13.4) did his first radical hysterectomies for cervical cancer, his first dozen patients died—but then one survived. He pressed ahead, and ultimately countless people owe their lives to his belief and to the sacrifice of those first 12. But had he tried to do this today, he would have been stopped. The UK's General Medical Council (GMC) and other august bodies tell us that we must protect the public by reporting doctors whose patients have low survival rates. The reason for this is partly ethical, and partly to preserve self-regulation.

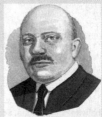

Fig 13.4 Ernst Wertheim.

We have the toughest codes of practice and disciplinary procedures of any group of workers. It is assumed that doctors are loyal to each other out of self-interest, and that this loyalty is bad. This has never been tested formally, and is not evidence based. We can imagine two clinical worlds: one of constant 'reportings' and recriminatory audits, and another of trust and teamwork. Both are imperfect, but we should not assume that the first world would be better for our patients.

When patients are sick with fear, they do not, perhaps, want to know everything. We may tell to protect ourselves. We may *not* tell to protect ourselves. Perhaps what we should do is, in our hearts, appeal to those 12 dead women-of-Wertheim—a jury as infallible as sacrificial—and try to hear their reply. And to those who complain that in doing so we are playing God, it is possible to reply with some humility that, whatever it is, it does not seem like play.

'It is amazing what little harm doctors do when one considers all the opportunities they have.' M. Twain.

2 If in any doubt, turn to: your senior/consultant; your employing organization; your legal defence organization; your national medical association; your local research ethics committee.

Prophylactic antibiotics in surgery

Prophylactic antibiotics are given to counter the risk of wound infection (see p578). Antibiotics are also given if infection elsewhere, although unlikely, would have severe consequences (eg when prostheses are involved). A single dose given before surgery has been shown to be just as good as more prolonged regimens in biliary and colorectal surgery. Additional doses may be given if high-risk/prolonged procedures, or if major blood loss. Time administration correctly (eg IV prophylaxis should be given 30min prior to surgery to maximize skin concentration; metronidazole PR is given 2h before).

- Use antibiotics which will kill anaerobes and coliforms.
- Consider use of peri-operative supplemental oxygen. This is a practical method of reducing the incidence of surgical wound infections.
- Practise strictly sterile surgical technique. (Ask for a hand with scrubbing up if you are not sure—theatre staff will be more than pleased to help!)

Antibiotic regimens ▶Adhere to local guidelines. *BNF* examples include:
- **Appendicectomy; colorectal resections and open biliary surgery** A single dose of IV cefuroxime 50mg/kg (max 1.5g) *or* gentamicin 1.5mg/kg + metronidazole 500mg *or* co-amoxiclav 1.2g alone.
- **Oesophageal or gastric surgery** 1 dose of IV gentamicin *or* cefuroxime *or* co-amoxiclav (doses as for appendicectomy).
- **Urological surgery** 1 dose of IV ciprofloxacin *or* flucloxacillin 1–2g + gentamicin. Add metronidazole if risk of anaerobes (eg amputations, gangrene, or diabetes).
- **Vascular surgery** 1 dose of PO cefuroxime 500mg + PO metronidazole 400mg *or* flucloxacillin 1–2g + gentamicin. Add metronidazole if risk of anaerobes (eg amputations, gangrene, or diabetes).
- **MRSA** For high-risk patients add IV teicoplanin or vancomycin to these regimens.

Minimally invasive and day case surgery

Laparoscopy was developed within gynaecology and is now in widespread use for diagnostic purposes and surgical procedures such as appendicectomy, fundoplication, splenectomy, adrenalectomy, hernia repair, colectomy, prostatectomy, and nephrectomy. As a rule of thumb, whatever can be done by laparotomy can also be done with the laparoscope. This does not mean that it *should* be done, but if the surgeon is adequately trained, and the patient feels better sooner, has less post-operative pain, can return to work earlier, and has fewer complications, then there are obvious advantages. Pre-procedure counselling should always discuss the complications of laparoscopic surgery (eg accidental damage to other intra-abdominal organs) as well as the risk of conversion to an open procedure.

Challenges of minimal access surgery The 2-dimensional visual representation and different surgical approach alters the normal appearance of familiar anatomy. Palpation is impossible and it may be harder to locate lesions prior to resection. As a result, pre-operative imaging may need to be more extensive. A new skill has to be learned and taught.

Day-case surgery Advances in surgical techniques as well as perioperative care mean better results for the patient (shorter waiting lists, fewer infections, fewer days off work, and ↑patient satisfaction). Many operations can now be performed as day cases. Theoretically any procedure is suitable, provided the time under general anaesthetic does not exceed ~1h. The use of regional anaesthesia helps to avoid the SE of nausea and disorientation that may accompany a general anaesthetic, thus facilitating discharge.

Bear in mind that the following groups of patients may not be suitable for day-case surgery: •Severe dementia. •Severe learning difficulties. •Living alone (and no helpers). •Children if supervision difficult—changes in expectation, delays, and pain relief can be problematic. •BMI >32 (p239). •ASA category ≥III (p565) thus potentially unstable comorbidities—discuss with the anaesthetist. •Infection at the site of the operation.

Sutures are central to the art of surgery. No single suture fits the bill for every occasion, and so suture selection (including size) depends on the job in hand (see tables 13.1, 13.2). In their broadest sense they are absorbable or non-absorbable, synthetic or natural, and their structure may be divided into monofilament, twisted, or braided. Monofilament sutures are quite slippery but minimize infection and produce less reaction. Braided sutures have plaited strands and provide secure knots, but they may allow infection to occur in surrounding tissue between their strands. Twisted sutures have 2 twisted strands and similar qualities to braided sutures. 'Plus' sutures (antimicrobial-infused synthetic absorbable sutures) are being increasingly used and are recommended by NICE[2] to prevent surgical site infection where absorbable sutures are envisaged. Sizes are denoted according to a scale running down from #5 (heavy braided suture). Most common modern sutures are smaller than size #0, hence rising numbers with a -0 suffix correspond to progressively finer grades of suture up to 11–0 (fine ophthalmic monofilaments). 3–0 or 4–0 are the best sizes for skin closure. Timing of suture removal depends on site and the general health of the patient. Face and neck sutures may be removed after 5d (earlier in children), scalp and back of neck after 5d, abdominal incisions and proximal limbs (including clips) after ~10d, distal extremities after 14d. In patients with poor wound healing, eg steroids, malignancy, infection, cachexia (p35), the elderly, or smokers, sutures may need ~14d.

Some commonly encountered suture materials

Absorbable

Table 13.1 Absorbable suture materials

Name	Material	Construction	Use
Monocryl®	Poliglecaprone	Monofilament	Subcuticular skin closure
PDS®	Polydioxanone	Monofilament	Closing abdominal wall
Vicryl®	Polyglactin	Braided multifilament	Tying pedicles; bowel anastomosis; subcutaneous closure
Dexon®	Polyglycolic acid	Braided multifilament	Very similar to Vicryl®

Non-absorbable

Table 13.2 Non-absorbable suture materials

Name	Material	Construction	Use
Ethilon®	Polyamide	Monofilament	Closing skin wounds
Prolene®	Polypropylene	Monofilament	Arterial anastomosis
Mersilk®N	Silk	Braided multifilament	Securing drains
Metal	Eg steel	Clips or monofilament	Skin wound/sternotomy closure

N = natural; other natural materials (eg cotton and catgut) are rarely used these days.

13 Surgery

Before anaesthesia, explain to the patient what will happen and where they will wake up, otherwise the recovery room or ITU will be frightening. Explain that they may feel ill on waking. Premedication is not routinely given, but may be considered in patients with severe anxiety or for paediatric surgery in selected patients.

Typical regimens might include

- **Anxiolytics** Benzodiazepines, eg lorazepam 2mg PO; temazepam 10–20mg PO. In children, use oral premeds as first choice, eg midazolam 0.5mg/kg (tastes bitter so often put in paracetamol suspension). Give oral premedication 2h before surgery (1h if IM route used).
- **Analgesics** Pre-emptive analgesia is not often used and effects are hard to determine. The aim is to dampen pain signals before they arrive. In children or anxious adults, local anaesthetic cream may be used on a few sites before inserting an IVI (the anaesthetist may prefer to site the cannula themselves!).
- **Anti-emetics** Post-operative nausea and vomiting is experienced by ~25% of all patients. 5HT$_3$ antagonists (eg ondansetron 4mg IV/IM) are the most effective agents; others, eg metoclopramide 10mg/8h IV/IM/PO, are also used—see p247.
- **Antacids** If the patient takes a PPI, this should be given on the morning of surgery.
- **Antisialagogues** Glycopyrronium (200–400mcg in adults, 4–8mcg/kg in children; given IV/IM 30–60min before induction) is sometimes used to decrease secretions that may cause respiratory obstruction in smaller airways.
- **Antibiotics** See p568.

Side effects of anaesthetic agents

- **Hyoscine, atropine** Anticholinergic, ∴ tachycardia, urinary retention, glaucoma, sedation (especially in the elderly).
- **Opioids** Respiratory depression, ↓cough reflex, nausea and vomiting, constipation.
- **Thiopental** (Induction agent.) Myocardial depression, hypotension.
- **Propofol** (Induction agent.) Respiratory/cardiac depression, pain on injection.
- **Volatile agents, eg isoflurane** Nausea and vomiting, cardiac depression, respiratory depression, vasodilation (see *BNF*).

The complications of anaesthesia are due to loss of

- **Pain sensation** Urinary retention, pressure necrosis, local nerve injuries (eg radial nerve palsy from arm hanging over the table edge).
- **Consciousness** Cannot communicate 'wrong leg/kidney'. NB: in some patients (eg 0.15%) *retained* consciousness is the problem. Awareness under GA sounds like a contradiction in terms, but remember that anaesthesia is a process rather than an event. Such awareness can lead to ill-defined, delayed neuroses and post-traumatic stress disorder (*OHCS* p718).
- **Muscle power** Corneal abrasion (∴ tape the eyes closed), no respiration, no cough (leads to pneumonia and atelectasis—partial lung collapse causing shunting ± impaired gas exchange: it starts minutes after induction, and may be related to the use of 100% O$_2$, supine position, surgery, age, and to loss of power).

Local/regional anaesthesia The use of regional or neuraxial nerve block can be an adjunct to a GA for analgesia, or serve as the sole mode of anaesthesia. Typically, long-acting local anaesthetics are used (eg bupivacaine or ropivacaine). See table 13.3 for doses and toxicity effects.

Drugs complicating anaesthesia ▶Inform anaesthetist. See p564 for lists of specific drugs, and actions to take.

Malignant hyperpyrexia This is a rare complication, precipitated by any volatile agent, eg sevoflurane, or suxamethonium. It exhibits autosomal dominant inheritance. There is a rapid rise in temperature (>1°C every 30min); masseter spasm may be an early sign. Complications include hypoxaemia, hypercarbia, hyperkalaemia, metabolic acidosis, and arrhythmias. ▶Get expert help immediately. Prompt treatment with dantrolene[3] (skeletal muscle relaxant), active cooling, and ITU care can reduce mortality significantly.

---

3 Give 1mg/kg every 5min IV—up to 10mg/kg in total (*OHCS* p673).

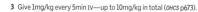

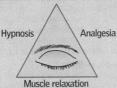

Fig 13.5 Principles of anaesthesia.

13 Surgery

The conduct of anaesthesia (fig 13.5) typically involves:
- **Induction** Either intravenous (eg propofol 1.5–2.5mg/kg IV over about 10s; thiopental is an alternative) or, if airway obstruction or difficult IV access, gaseous (eg sevoflurane ± nitrous oxide, mixed in O_2).
- **Airway control** Either a supraglottic airway device such as a laryngeal mask or i-gel® or endotracheal tube. The latter usually requires muscle relaxation with a depolarizing/non-depolarizing neuromuscular blocker (*OHCS* p664).
- **Maintenance of anaesthesia** Volatile agent + N_2O/O_2 mixture + high-dose opiates with mechanical ventilation, or total intravenous anaesthesia (TIVA, eg propofol 4–12mg/kg/h IVI).
- **Recovery** Change inspired gases to 100% oxygen only, then discontinue any anaesthetic infusions and reverse muscle paralysis. Extubate once spontaneously breathing, patient positioned in a semi-recumbent position and transferred to the recovery room, oxygen by facemask.
- For further details, see the *Anaesthesia* chapter in *OHCS* (p656).

⚠ Local anaesthetic toxicity and maximum doses

Anaesthetists are masters of the drug dose by weight! It is important to remember the maximum doses for local anaesthetics (3rd column, below), not least because we use them so frequently, but because the effects of overdose can be lethal. With this information, the maximal volume can be easily calculated = (1/concentration) × (maximum allowable dose) × (ideal body weight/10). A 1% concentration is equivalent to 10mg/mL.

Table 13.3 Maximum doses for local anaesthetic

Agent, % conc^n	Conc^n (mg/mL)	Maximum allowable dose	Approx. allowable volume for 70kg adult (mL)
Lidocaine 1%	10	3mg/kg	≤21 (1 × 3 × 7)
Lidocaine 1% + ad*	10	7mg/kg	≤49 (1 × 7 × 7)
Lidocaine 2%	20	3mg/kg	≤10.5 (0.5 × 3 × 7)
Bupivacaine 0.5%	5	2mg/kg	≤28 (2 × 2 × 7)
Bupivacaine 0.5% + ad*	5	3mg/kg	≤42 (2 × 3 × 7)
Ropivacaine 0.5%	5	3mg/kg	≤42 (2 × 3 × 7)

* A higher dose can be used when mixed with adrenaline. Local anaesthetic toxicity starts with peri-oral tingling and paraesthesiae, progressing to drowsiness, seizures, coma, and cardiorespiratory arrest. If suspected (the patient feels 'funny' and develops early signs) then stop administration immediately and commence ABC resuscitation as required. ►► Treatment is with lipid emulsion. Find out where this is stored in your hospital. Bupivacaine is the most cardiotoxic of the local anaesthetics, and is therefore not used in high doses, for example in a regional nerve block. Local anaesthetics are also basic, and so do not work well in acidic environments, eg abscesses.

Diabetic patients undergoing surgery

Over 10% of surgical patients have diabetes. This group face a greater risk of post-operative infection and cardiac complications; screen for the presence of asymptomatic cardiac and renal disease (p565) and be aware of possible 'silent' myocardial ischaemia. Tight glycaemic control is essential and improves outcome. Aim to achieve an HbA1c of <69mmol/mol (8.5%) prior to elective surgery.

Non-insulin-treated diabetes mellitus
- Give usual medications the night before surgery, except SGLT2 inhibitors (gliflozins) which should not be given the day before (risk of UTIs, AKI, and euglycaemic ketosis, check capillary blood ketones daily). GLP-1 receptor agonists and DPP4 inhibitors (gliptins) can be continued as usual.
- If on PM list, take normal medications with breakfast except for sulfonylureas (can cause prolonged hypoglycaemia when fasting), omit midday doses of metformin if taken three times daily. If on AM list, omit morning medication and take any missed drugs post-op with lunch, if eating and drinking. If not eating or drinking or diabetes control is poor, start a VRIII (see BOX) 2 hours prior to surgery.
- **Metformin and iodine IV contrast** If EGFR <60mL/min and contrast is to be used, omit metformin on the day of the procedure and for 48h after.

Insulin-treated diabetes mellitus
- Try to place the patient first on the list in order to minimize the fasting period.
- Give all usual insulin the night before surgery. Long-acting (basal) insulin is usually continued as normal times, at a dose of 80% when patients are on a VRIII.
- If on AM list, ensure no subcutaneous rapid-acting (bolus) or mixed insulin is given on the morning of surgery. If PM list, give 80% of the normal morning bolus insulin, or 50% the mixed insulin dose (NB: omit all mixed and rapid-acting insulin with VRIII).
- If eating and drinking post-operatively, resume the usual insulin with evening meal.
- If not eating or drinking post-op, start a VRIII 2h prior to surgery. When ready to eat, give normal dose of rapid acting or mixed insulin with the 1st meal and stop the VRIII 30–60min later.

Diet-controlled diabetes There are usually no problems; patients should be treated as if not diabetic (and do not need to be first on the list). Check capillary blood glucose peri-operatively, acceptable range is 6–10mmol/L. Avoid 5% glucose IVI.

How to write up a variable rate intravenous insulin infusion (VRIII)

The aim is to maintain glycaemia 6–10mmol/L, check 2-hourly. Prescribe 50 units of short-acting insulin in 50mL of 0.9% saline to infuse at the rate shown in table 13.4.

Table 13.4 A guide to VRIII according to blood glucose (NB: no one rate is suitable for all patients)

Capillary blood glucose (mmol/L)	IV soluble insulin (rate of infusion)
<6.0	Stop, treat hypoglycaemia, restart within 20min
6.1–8.0	1 unit/h
8.1–11.0	2 units/h
11.1–15.0	4 units/h
15.1–20.0	5 units/h
20.1–28.0	6 units/h; request diabetic review
>28.1	8 units/h; request urgent diabetic review

Fluids must be prescribed to run with the VRIII (through the same cannula via a non-return valve). Ideally use 0.45% sodium chloride with 5% glucose *and* either 0.15% potassium chloride (KCl) (=20mmol/L) or 0.3% KCl (=40mmol/L). Fluid should infuse at 83–125mL/h (ie 1L over 8–12 hours). Omit potassium if there is renal impairment or hyperkalaemia and slow the rate of infusion in heart failure.

Surgery in those on antithrombotic treatment

▶Inform the surgeon and anaesthetist. It is important to balance the thrombo-embolic risk from discontinuing anticoagulation (eg high in recent stroke or TIA, recent VTE, mitral valve prosthesis, AF with CHA₂DS₂-VASc score 7–9, see p127) with the procedural bleeding risk (high in any major operation lasting >45min).

DOACs See table 13.5. There is no evidence to support LMWH bridging or the use of reversal agent andexanet alfa in the setting of elective or emergency surgery.

Warfarin *Minor surgery* can be undertaken without stopping (if INR <3.5 it may be safe to proceed). In *major surgery*, stop warfarin for 5 days pre-op. Vitamin K ± PCC may be needed for emergency reversal of INR. Therapeutic LMWH bridging is neces-sary in high thromboembolic risk, start 3 days pre-op, stop 24h pre-op, and restart no sooner than 48h post-op in high bleeding risk.

Antiplatelets Avoid epidural, spinal, and regional blocks. *Aspirin* should probably be continued unless there is a major risk of bleeding. The bleeding effects reverse 5d after stopping—check local policy to see if cessation is required. Discuss stop-ping *clopidogrel* with the cardiologists/neurologists, there is little evidence to guide this, but it is often switched for aspirin 5 days pre-op. Premature discontinuation of clopidogrel in patients with drug-eluting stents can lead to stent thrombosis.

Table 13.5 Perioperative management of DOACs

DOAC, renal function	Procedural bleeding risk	Perioperative management
Dabigatran in those without renal impairment; Xa inhibitors in all	Low	Omit 1 day pre-op (ie last dose at least 36 hours prior), restart day 1 post-op
	High	Omit 2 days pre-op (ie last dose at least 60 hours prior), restart day 2–3 post-op
Dabigatran in those with CrCl <50mL/min	Low	Omit 2 days pre-op (ie last dose at least 60 hours prior), restart day 1 post-op
	High	Omit 4 days pre-op, restart day 2–3 post-op

Surgery in those on steroids

Patients on steroids may not be able to mount an appropriate adrenal response to meet the stress of surgery due to suppression of the hypothalamic–pituitary–adrenal (HPA) axis. Consider supplementation for any patient taking >5mg/d of prednisolone (or equivalent) for more than 4 weeks. Morning steroid dose should be taken pre-op.
• **Minor procedures under local anaesthetic** No supplementation required.
• **Moderate procedures** (Eg joint replacement.) Give 50mg IV hydrocortisone be-fore induction and 25mg IM every 8h for 24h. Resume normal dose thereafter.
• **Major surgery** Give 100mg IV hydrocortisone at induction, 200mg/24h infusion intra-op, and 50mg IM every 6h for 24h. After 24h, resume 2× normal PO dose for 48h.
The major risk with adrenal insufficiency is hypotension, so if this is encountered without an obvious cause, consider a stat dose of hydrocortisone. ▶See p819 for treatment of Addisonian crisis and *BNF* section 6.3 for steroid dose equivalents.

Jaundiced patients undergoing surgery

Obstructive jaundice is associated with ↑risk, and requires specific preoperative care.

Coagulopathy Vitamin K ↓ in obstruction (requires bile in order to be absorbed). Give IM vitamin K. FFP may be required in liver disease or active bleeding.

Sepsis ↑Risk of bacterial translocation. If cholangitis present, give antibiotics. Routine antibiotic prophylaxis for ERCP not recommended unless biliary decompres-sion is likely to be incomplete (malignant obstruction, primary sclerosing cholan-gitis), give oral ciprofloxacin or IV gentamicin (check local policy).

Renal failure ↑Risk of AKI post-op possibly due to ↑intestinal absorption of endo-toxin (normally limited by the detergent effect of bile) causing renal vasoconstriction. Lactulose or bile salts pre-op may help. Ensure adequate IV fluids pre- and post-op, and monitor urine output every 2h, measure and correct U&E daily.

Routine post-operative management varies widely according to the status of the patient and the complexity of the surgery. Use daily ward rounds to check pain management, examine exposed wounds and drains, check glycaemic control, review hydration and nutritional status, plan hospital discharge, and screen for the following general post-operative complications:

Pyrexia Mild pyrexia in the 1st 48h is often from tissue damage/necrosis, exposure to foreign materials, or even from blood transfusions, but still have a low threshold for infection screen. Consider evidence for peritonism, chest, urinary, wound, or cannula site infections, as well as possible DVT (also causes ↑T). Send blood for FBC, U&E, CRP, and cultures (±LFT). Dipstick the urine. Consider MSU, CXR, and abdominal ultrasound/CT depending on clinical findings.

Confusion May manifest as agitation, disorientation, and attempts to leave hospital, especially at night. More common in patients with existing cognitive impairment. Gently reassure the patient in well-lit surroundings. See p480 for a full workup. Common causes are:
• hypoxia (pneumonia, atelectasis, LVF, PE)   • infection
• drugs (opiates, sedatives, and many others)   • alcohol withdrawal (p276)
• urinary retention • liver/renal failure   • MI or stroke.

Occasionally, sedation is necessary to examine the patient; consider lorazepam 1mg PO/IM (antidote: flumazenil) or haloperidol 0.5–2mg IM. Reassure relatives that post-op confusion is common (seen in up to 40%) and reversible.

Dyspnoea or hypoxia Any previous lung disease? Sit patient up and give O_2, monitor peripheral O_2 sats by pulse oximetry (p154). Examine for evidence of: • Pneumonia, pulmonary collapse, or aspiration. • LVF (MI; fluid overload). • Pulmonary embolism (p186). • Pneumothorax (p186; due to CVP line, intercostal block, or mechanical ventilation). Tests FBC; ABG; CXR; ECG. Manage according to findings.

↓BP If severe, tilt bed head-down and give O_2. Check pulse and BP yourself; compare it with pre-op values. Post-op ↓BP is often from hypovolaemia resulting from inadequate fluid input, so check fluid chart and replace losses. Monitor urine output (may need catheterization). Hypovolaemia may also be caused by haemorrhage so review wounds, drains, and abdomen. If unstable, return to theatre for haemostasis. Beware cardiogenic and neurogenic causes and look for evidence of MI or PE. Consider sepsis and anaphylaxis. **Management** p770.

↑BP May be pain, urinary retention, idiopathic hypertension (eg missed medication), or inotropic drugs. Oral cardiac medications (including antihypertensives) should be continued throughout the perioperative period even if NBM. Treat the cause, consider increasing the regular medication, or if not absorbing orally try 50mg labetalol IV over 1min on a monitored bed (HDU/ICU/recovery room) (see p110).

↓Urine output (oliguria) Aim for output of >30mL/h in adults (or >0.5mL/kg/h). *Anuria* may reflect a blocked or mal-sited catheter (see p747) rather than AKI. Flush or replace catheter. *Oliguria* is usually due to too little replacement of lost fluid. Treat by increasing fluid input. ►Acute kidney injury may follow shock, drugs, transfusion, pancreatitis, or trauma (see p294 for classification and management of AKI).
• Review fluid chart and examine for signs of volume depletion.
• Urinary retention is also common, so examine for a palpable bladder.
• Establish normovolaemia; perform 3–4 crystalloid 'fluid challenges' of 250mL over 30min may also help; if urine output is still poor, seek senior help.
• Catheterize bladder (for accurate monitoring)—see p746; check U&E.
• If acute kidney injury is suspected, stop nephrotoxic drugs (eg NSAIDs) and refer to a nephrologist early.

Nausea/vomiting Any mechanical obstruction, ileus, or emetic drugs (opiates, digoxin, anaesthetics)? Consider AXR, NGT, and an anti-emetic (►*not* metoclopramide because of its prokinetic property). See p247 for choice of anti-emetics.

↓Na⁺ Pre-op level? Excess IV fluids may exacerbate the situation. Correct slowly (p664). SIADH (p665) can occur post-op from pain, opioids, and infections.

Talking about post-op complications ...

When asked to give your thoughts on the complications of an operation—maybe with an examiner or a patient—a good starting point is to divide them up accordingly (and for each of the following stratify as immediate, early, and late):
• **From the anaesthetic** (p570) Eg respiratory depression from prolonged GA/opiates.
• **From surgery in general** (p574) Eg wound infection, haemorrhage, neurovascular damage, DVT/PE.
• **From the specific procedure** Eg saphenous nerve damage in stripping of the long varicose vein.

Tailor the discussion towards the individual who, eg if an arteriopath, may have a significant risk of cardiac ischaemia during hypotensive episodes while under the anaesthetic.

Post-operative bleeding

Primary haemorrhage Continuous bleeding, starting during surgery. Replace blood loss. If severe, return to theatre for adequate haemostasis. Treat shock vigorously (pp770–788).

Reactive haemorrhage Haemostasis appears secure until BP rises and bleeding starts. Replace blood and re-explore wound.

Secondary haemorrhage (Caused by infection.) Occurs 1–2wks post-op.

Post-operative pain

Humans are the most exquisite devices ever made for experiencing pain. *Never forget how painful pain is*, nor how fear magnifies pain. Try not to let these sensations, so often interposed between the patient and recovery, be invisible to you as the patient bravely puts up with them.

Approach to management (See WHO pain ladder, p532.) Identify and treat the underlying pathology wherever possible. Explanation and reassurance contribute greatly to analgesia.
• Give *regular* doses rather than on an 'as-required' basis (*by the clock*).
• Choose the best route: PO, PR, IM, epidural, SC, or IV (*by the mouth*, where possible).
• Early use of opioid drugs for severe pain (*by the ladder*). Give with an anti-emetic, p247. Monitor for respiratory depression, constipation, cough suppression, urinary retention, ↓BP, and sedation (do not use in hepatic failure or head injury). Dependency is rarely a problem. *Naloxone* (eg 100–200mcg IV, followed by 100mcg increments, eg every 2min until responsive) may be needed to reverse the effects of excess opioids (p826).
• Allow the patient to be in charge. This promotes wellbeing, and does not lead to overuse. Patient-controlled continuous IV opiate delivery systems are useful.

Surgical drains in the post-operative period

The decision when to insert and remove drains may seem to be one of the great surgical enigmas—but there are basically three types to get a grip of:
  1 To drain the area of surgery and are often put under suction or −ve pressure (Redivac® uses a 'high vacuum'). These are removed when they stop draining. They protect against collection, haematoma, and seroma formation (in breast surgery this can cause overlying skin necrosis).
  2 To protect sites where leakage may occur in post-operative period, eg bowel anastomoses. These form a tract and are removed after about 1wk.
  3 To collect red blood cells from the site of the operation, which can then be autotransfused within 6h, protecting from the hazards of allotransfusion—it is used commonly in orthopaedics (eg Bellovac®).

'Shortening a drain' means withdrawing it (eg by 2cm/d) to allow the tract to seal, bit by bit. ▶Check the surgeon's wishes before altering a drain. ▶If a drain 'falls out' on the ward, avoid re-siting it because it is now covered in skin flora. Put a collecting bag over the wound and contact the surgical registrar.

Surgical site infections are the most preventable healthcare-associated infection, but are becoming the most common as the incidence of others are falling rapidly. The prevalence is probably underestimated, but rates of 10–20% are observed in elective GI surgery (up to 60% in emergency surgery). They are defined as infections that occur near the surgical incision within 30 days of the procedure, or within 90 days if prosthetic material is implanted.

Risk factors • Patient-related ↑Age, malnutrition (see p584), immunosuppression, obesity, metabolic disease (diabetes, uraemia, jaundice), smoking, bacterial colonization (eg meticillin-resistant *Staphylococcus aureus* (MRSA)), coexisting remote infection. • **Operation-related** Duration of pre-op hospitalization, type of surgery (see **table** 13.6), prolonged duration of surgery, presence of prosthesis/foreign body, high degree of tissue trauma, excessive use of electrosurgical cautery, inadequate prophylaxis (skin prep, hair removal, antibiotics, ventilation), post-op hypothermia.

Signs • Red, swollen, tender wound (may be discharging pus). • Fever. • Tachycardia.

Tests Observation is sufficient for the diagnosis of superficial surgical site infections. Imaging (CT or MRI) is necessary for deep or organ space infections. Swab the wound itself (not surrounding skin) and any discharging pus and send for microscopy, culture, and sensitivities. Negative cultures in an obviously infected wound can be a sign of an atypical infection (eg fungal or mycobacterial, consider if immunocompromised). Send blood for FBC (Hb, WCC) and cultures.

Prevention • Pre-op prophylaxis See p568. • **Post-op prophylaxis** Wound review daily, washing (sterile saline first 48h, then showering after 48h), change dressings using aseptic non-touch technique, negative-pressure wound therapy (VAC® therapy dressings).

Treatment ►Ensure there is IV access, give crystalloid fluid up to 1000mL if tachycardic or hypotensive. Give IV antibiotics if there are any systemic features. If there is no pre-existing infection, use anti-staphylococcals: flucloxacillin 1g + 500mg QDS. If the patient is immunosuppressed or very unwell, add in broad-spectrum cover to include anaerobic cover: metronidazole 500mg IV TDS and cefuroxime 1.5g IV + 500mg IV TDS (consult with microbiologist if in doubt). If there is real concern about MRSA infection, consult microbiology and consider adding IV vancomycin 500mg. If so, monitor drug plasma concentration. Open and aspirate/debride the wound if there is contained pus, and aim to excise all foreign bodies.

Complications Wound dehiscence (most are due to infection, p580), bacteraemia (common), and sepsis (less common unless the organism is resistant to antibiotic therapy or the patient is immunosuppressed).

Table 13.6 Classification of surgical procedures and wound infection risk

Category	Description	Infection risk before prophylactic antibiotics	Infection risk after prophylactic antibiotics	Microbiology
Clean	Incising uninfected skin without opening a viscus	<2%	<2%	Skin flora (eg *Staphylococcus aureus*, *Staphylococcus epidermidis*)
Clean-contaminated	Intra-operative breach of a viscus (but not colon)	Up to 30%	8–10%	Gram-negative rods and enterococci
Contaminated	Breach of a viscus + spillage or opening of colon	Up to 60%	15–20%	Polymicrobial
Dirty	The site is already contaminated with pus or faeces, or from exogenous contagion, eg trauma	>60%	25–40%	Polymicrobial

DVTs occur in 15–30% of surgical patients without prophylaxis. All hospital in-patients should be assessed for DVT/PE risk and offered prophylaxis if appropriate. 65% of below-knee DVTs are asymptomatic; these rarely embolize to the lung.

Risk factors •**Transient** (Do not necessarily require long-term anticoagulation.) Immobility, eg due to acute illness trauma, surgery with general anaesthesia (especially pelvic/orthopaedic), pregnancy, synthetic oestrogen. •**Persistent** Active cancer, inflammatory disorder, eg IBD, obesity, ↑age, thrombophilia (but not for routine testing).

Signs •Calf warmth/tenderness/swelling/erythema. •Mild fever. •Pitting oedema.

ΔΔ Cellulitis; ruptured Baker's cyst. Both may coexist with a DVT.

Tests ►Calculate Wells score (see table 13.7) before ordering *D-dimer* (see fig 13.6). D-dimer is sensitive but not specific for DVT (also ↑ in infection, pregnancy, malignancy, and post-op). In high-risk cases proceed directly to USS. Look for *underlying malignancy:* urine dip; FBC, LFT, Ca²⁺; CXR ± CT abdomen/pelvis (and mammography in ♀) if >40yrs.

Prevention • Stop the COCP 4wks pre-op. • Mobilize early. • LMWH, eg enoxaparin 40mg SC started the evening before surgery and continued once daily (caution if eGFR <30mL/min/1.73m²). • Graduated compression stockings ('thromboembolic deterrent (TED) stockings'; CI: ischaemia) and intermittent pneumatic compression devices ↓ risk of DVT by ~70% in surgical patients.

Treatment ►Start anticoagulation immediately after diagnosis of proximal DVT, and in distal DVT unless it is not extensive (<5cm) or there is a high bleeding risk (repeat imaging). Encourage mobilization. Start a DOAC (apixaban or rivaroxaban) or LMWH (eg enoxaparin 1.5mg/kg/24h SC if DOACs are unsuitable, for a minimum of 3 months (transient risk factor). In severe renal impairment (CrCl <15mL/min) use LMWH or unfractionated heparin (also preferred if ↑risk of bleeding; dose guided by anti-Xa or APTT, p346). Patients with persistent risk factors should receive LMWH for at least 6 months (then review). *Inferior vena caval filters* may be used in active bleeding or recent ICH, to minimize risk of PE, but have a high complication rate and should be removed as soon as no longer indicated. *Endovascular thrombolysis and/ or surgical thrombectomy* is usually reserved for severely symptomatic iliocaval DVT in selected patients—generally, young <65yrs, physically active patients, without underlying malignancy, or those with complications.

Complications PE (p186). *Post-phlebitic limb* can be seen in 10–30% and refers to long-term symptomatic deep venous incompetence due to scarring/valve damage, treated with compression stockings. ►*Phlegmasia cerulea dolens* is a rare limb & life-threatening complication usually associated with extensive iliofemoral DVT, often with underlying malignancy. Presents with severe pain, swelling, cyanosis with venous ischaemia. Requires aggressive treatment; unfractionated heparin ± thrombolysis/thrombectomy.

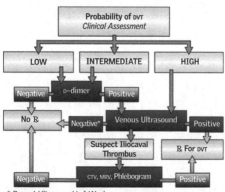

Fig 13.6 Diagnostic algorithm for suspected acute DVT.

Reproduced from Thompson MW et al., Oxford Textbook of Vascular Surgery (2016), with permission from Oxford University Press.

*Repeat Ultrasound in 1 Week

13 Surgery

Bilateral oedema Implies systemic disease with ↑venous pressure (eg right heart failure) or ↓intravascular oncotic pressure (any cause of ↓albumin, so test the urine for protein). It is *dependent* (distributed by gravity), which is why legs are affected early, but severe oedema extends above the legs. In the bed-bound, fluid moves to the new dependent area, causing a sacral pad. The exception is the local increase in venous pressure occurring in IVC obstruction: the swelling neither extends above the legs nor redistributes. **Causes** • Right heart failure (p134). • ↓Albumin (p678, eg renal or liver failure). • Venous insufficiency: acute, eg prolonged sitting, or chronic, with haemosiderin-pigmented, itchy, eczematous skin ± ulcers. • Vasodilators, eg *nifedipine, amlodipine.* •Pelvic mass (p53, p596). • Pregnancy—if ↑BP + proteinuria, diagnose pre-eclampsia (*OHCS* p50): find an obstetrician urgently. In all the above, both legs need not be affected to the same extent.

Unilateral oedema Pain ± redness implies DVT or inflammation, eg cellulitis or insect bites (any blisters?). Bone or muscle may be to blame, eg tumours; necrotizing fasciitis (p652); trauma (check for sensation, pulses, and severe pain esp. on passive movement: ▸a *compartment syndrome* needs prompt fasciotomy). Impaired mobility suggests trauma, arthritis, or a Baker's cyst (p686). *Non-pitting oedema* is oedema you cannot indent: see p35.

Nine questions to ask

1 Is it *both* legs?	4 Are they pregnant?	7 Are they mobile?
2 Any trauma?	5 Any pitting (p35)?	8 Past diseases/on drugs?
3 Any pain?	6 Any skin changes?	9 Any oedema elsewhere?

Tests ▸Look for proteinuria (+ hypoalbuminaemia ≈ nephrotic syndrome). CCF?

Treatment of leg oedema Treat the cause. Diuretics for all is not an answer. Elevating legs for dependent oedema (ankles higher than hips—do not just use footstools); raise the foot of the bed. Graduated support stockings may help (CI: ischaemia).

Pretest clinical probability scoring for DVT: the Wells score

In patients with symptoms in both legs, the more symptomatic leg is used.

Table 13.7 Wells score

Clinical features	Score
Active cancer (treatment within last 6 months or palliative)	1 point
Paralysis, paresis, or recent plaster immobilization of leg	1 point
Recently bedridden for >3d or major surgery in last 12wks	1 point
Local tenderness along distribution of deep venous system	1 point
Entire leg swollen	1 point
Calf swelling >3cm compared with asymptomatic leg (measured 10cm below tibial tuberosity)	1 point
Pitting oedema (greater in the symptomatic leg)	1 point
Collateral superficial veins (non-varicose)	1 point
Previously documented DVT	1 point
Alternative diagnosis at least as likely as DVT	–2 points
Pre-test probability of DVT	**Points**
Low risk (3–5%)	–2 to 0
Intermediate risk (17–33%)	1–2
High risk (50–85%)	3 or more

Reprinted from the *Lancet*, 350, Wells PS *et al.*, 'Value of assessment of pretest probability of deep-vein thrombosis in clinical management', 1795–8, Copyright 1997, with permission from Elsevier.

13 Surgery

Laparotomy Wound may break down from a few days to a few weeks post-op (incidence ≈ 3.5%). Particular risk in the elderly, malnourished (eg cancer; IBD, p584), if infection, uraemia, or haematoma is present, or in repeat laparotomies. Warning sign is a pink serous discharge. Always assume the defect involves the whole of the wound. Wound dehiscence may lead to a 'burst abdomen' with evisceration of bowel (mortality 15–30%). If you are on the ward when this happens, call your senior, put the viscera back into the abdomen, place a sterile dressing over the wound, and give IV antibiotics (eg piperacillin/tazobactam; see local guidelines). Allay anxiety, give parenteral pain control, set up an IVI, and return patient to theatre. *Incisional hernia* is a common late problem (20%), repairable by mesh insertion (if necessary).

Biliary surgery Early Iatrogenic bile duct injury; cholangitis; bile leakage; bleeding into the biliary tree (haemobilia—may lead to melaena or haematemesis); pancreatitis. Retained stones may be removed by ERCP (p726); if this is not available a 'T-tube' left in the bile duct at the time of closure allows free drainage to the exterior; unrelieved distal obstruction of the bile duct may result in fistula formation and chronic leakage of bile. If jaundiced, maintain a good urine output, monitor coagulation, and consider antibiotics. **Late** Bile duct stricture; post-cholecystectomy syndrome (symptoms arising from alterations in bile flow due to loss of the reservoir function of the gallbladder).

Thyroid surgery Early Recurrent (± superior) laryngeal nerve palsy (→hoarseness) can occur permanently in 0.5% and transiently in 1.5%—warn the patient that *their voice will be different* for a few days post-op because of intubation and local oedema (NB: pre-operative fibreoptic laryngoscopy should be performed to exclude pre-existing vocal cord dysfunction); thyroid storm (symptoms of severe hyperthyroidism—see p820); tracheal obstruction due to haematoma in the wound: ▶▶relieve by immediate removal of stitches or clips using the cutter/remover that should remain at the bedside; may require urgent surgery; hypoparathyroidism (p216); ▶check plasma Ca^{2+} daily; transient drops in serum concentration are common, permanent in 2.5%. **Late** Hypothyroidism; recurrent hyperthyroidism.

Mastectomy Arm lymphoedema in up to 20% of those undergoing axillary node sampling or dissection. The risk of lymphoedema increases with the level of axillary dissection: risk is lower with level 1 dissection (inferior to *pec. minor*) compared to level 3 dissection (superior to *pec. minor*, rarely done); skin necrosis.

Arterial surgery Bleeding; thrombosis; embolism; graft infection; MI; AV fistula formation. **Complications of aortic surgery** Gut ischaemia; renal failure; respiratory distress; trauma to ureters or anterior spinal artery (leading to paraplegia); ischaemic events from distal emboli from dislodged thrombus; aorto-enteric fistula.

Colonic surgery Early Sepsis; ileus; fistulae; anastomotic leak (11% for radical rectal surgery); haemorrhage; trauma to ureters or spleen. **Late** Adhesional obstruction (BOX).

Small bowel surgery Short gut syndrome (best defined *functionally*, as malabsorption due to insufficient residual small bowel; adults with ≤150cm at risk). Diarrhoea and malabsorption (particularly of fats) lead to a number of metabolic abnormalities including deficiency in vitamins A, D, E, K, and B_{12}, hyperoxaluria (causing renal stones), and bile salt depletion (causing gallstones). The management of short bowel syndrome is complex, aiming to correct metabolic abnormalities, optimize residual bowel function, and support nutrition (using parenteral route if necessary).

Tracheostomy Mediastinitis; surgical emphysema. Later: stenosis.

Splenectomy (p369) Acute gastric dilatation (a serious consequence of not using a NG tube, or to check that the one in place is working); thrombocytosis; sepsis. ▶Lifetime sepsis risk is partly preventable with pre-op vaccines, ie *Haemophilus* type B, meningococcal, and pneumococcal (p403 & p169), and prophylactic penicillin.

Genitourinary surgery Septicaemia (from instrumentation in the presence of infected urine)—consider a stat dose of gentamicin; urinoma—rupture of a ureter or renal pelvis leading to a mass of extravasated urine.

Gastrectomy See p614.

Prostatectomy See p634.

Haemorrhoidectomy See p624.

Adhesions—legacy of the laparotomy, bane of the surgeon

When re-operating on the abdomen, the struggle against adhesions tests the farthest and darkest boundaries of patience of the abdominal surgeon and the assistant. The skill and persistence required to gently and atraumatically tease apart these fibrous bands that restrict access and vision makes any progression, no matter how slight, cause for subdued celebration. Perseverance is the name of this game.

Surgical division of adhesions is known as *adhesiolysis*. Any surgical procedure that breaches the abdominal or pelvic cavities can predispose to the formation of adhesions, which are found in up to 90% of those with previous abdominal surgery. Handling of the serosal surface of the bowel causes inflammation, which over weeks to years can lead to the formation of fibrous bands that tether the bowel to itself or adjacent structures—though adhesions can also form secondary to infection, radiation injury, and inflammatory processes such as Crohn's disease. Their main sequelae are intestinal obstruction (the cause in ~60% of cases—see p602) and chronic abdominal or pelvic pain. Studies have shown that adhesiolysis may help relieve chronic pain, though for a small proportion of patients the pain never improves or even worsens after directed intervention.

As far as prevention is concerned, the best approach is to avoid operating; laparoscopy compared with laparotomy reduces the rate of local adhesions. Insertion of synthetic films (eg hyaluronic acid/carboxymethyl membrane) to prevent adhesions to the anterior abdominal wall reduces incidence, extent, and severity of adhesions, but not incidence of obstruction or operative re-intervention.

13 Surgery

A stoma (Greek = *mouth*) is an artificial union between a conduit and the outside world—eg a colostomy, in which faeces are made to pass through an opening in the abdominal wall when a loop of colon is brought out onto the skin. NB: a stoma can also be made between two internal conduits (eg a choledochojejunostomy).

Colostomies (Usually left iliac fossa and flush with the skin—**fig 13.9**.) May be temporary or permanent. Are they suitable for a laparoscopic operation?
• **Loop colostomy** A loop of colon is exteriorized and partially divided, forming two stomas that are joined together (the proximal end passes stool, the distal end passes mucus, see **fig 13.7**). A rod under the loop prevents retraction and may be removed after 7d. A loop colostomy is often temporary and performed to protect a distal anastomosis, eg after anterior resection.
• **End colostomy** The bowel is divided and the proximal end brought out as a stoma; the distal end may be: 1 *Resected*, eg abdominoperineal (AP) resection (inspect the perineum for absent anus when examining a stoma). 2 *Closed* and left in the abdomen (Hartmann's procedure). 3 *Exteriorized*, forming a 'mucous fistula'.
• **Paul–Mikulicz colostomy** A double-barrelled colostomy in which the colon is divided completely (eg to excise a section of bowel). Each end is exteriorized as two separate stomas.

Output Colostomies ideally pass 1–2 formed motions/day into an adherent plastic pouch. Some may be managed with irrigation, thus avoiding a pouch. **Incidence** 21 000 stomas/yr in UK (>50% are permanent). Most manage their stomas well. The cost for appliances is ~£2000/yr. If there is a skin reaction to the adhesive or pouch, a change of device may be all that is needed. Contact the stoma nurse.

Ileostomies (Usually right iliac fossa.) Protrude from the skin and emit frequent fluid motions which contain active enzymes (so the skin needs protecting—see fig 13.8). Loop ileostomies can be formed to defunction the colon as a temporary measure, eg during control of difficult perianal Crohn's disease. End ileostomy follows total or subtotal colectomy, eg for UC; subsequent formation of *ileal pouch-anal anastomosis* (pouch of ileum is joined to the upper anal canal) can allow for stoma reversal.

Alternative (non-stoma forming) surgery Low/ultra-low anterior resection All or part of the rectum is excised and the proximal colon anastomosed to the top of the anal canal (the lower the level of anastomosis, the higher the risk of complication). **Transanal endoscopic microsurgery** Allows excision of small tumours within the rectum with preservation of sphincter function.

Urostomies are fashioned after total cystectomy, bringing urine from the ureters to the abdominal wall via an *ileal conduit* that is usually incontinent. Formation of a catheterizable valvular mechanism may retain continence. Advances in urological surgery have seen an increase in continence-saving procedures such as orthotopic neobladder reconstruction, with good long-term continence rates.

When choosing a stoma site, avoid
• Bony prominences (eg anterior superior iliac spine, costal margins).
• The umbilicus.
• Old wounds/scars—there may be adhesions beneath.
• Skin folds and creases.
• The waistline.
• The site should be assessed pre-operatively by the stoma nurse, with the patient both lying and standing.

Complications of stomas

▶Liaise early with the stoma nurse, starting pre-operatively.

Early
- Haemorrhage at stoma site.
- Stoma ischaemia—colour progresses from dusky grey to black.
- High output (can lead to ↓K^+)—consider loperamide ± codeine to thicken output.
- Obstruction secondary to adhesions (p581).
- Stoma retraction.

Delayed
- Obstruction (failure at operation to close lateral space around stoma).
- Dermatitis around stoma site (worse with ileostomy).
- Stoma prolapse.
- Stomal intussusception.
- Stenosis.
- Parastomal hernia (risk increases with time). NB: prophylactic mesh insertion at the time of stoma formation reduces this risk.
- Fistulae.
- Psychological problems.

Psychological aspects of stoma care

The physical and psychological aspects of stoma care must not be undervalued. Be alert to any vicious cycle in which a skin reaction leads to leakage and precipitates a fear of going out, or a fear of eating. This in turn may lead to poor nutrition and further skin reactions, resulting in further leakage and depression. These cycles can be circumvented by the **stoma nurse**, who is *the* expert in fitting secure, odourless devices and providing patients with a wealth of physical and psychological support, both pre- and post-operatively (explaining what is going to happen, what the stoma will be like, and troubleshooting post-op problems). ▶*Early referral prevents problems.* Without input from the stoma nurse, a patient may reject their colostomy, never attend to it, and develop deep-seated psychological and psychiatric problems.

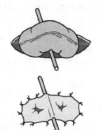

Fig 13.7 A loop colostomy with double-barrelled stoma and supporting ostomy rod.

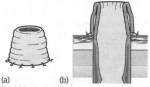

(a) (b)
Fig 13.8 An ileostomy sits proud, has prominent mucosal folds, and is often right-sided.

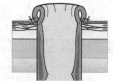

Fig 13.9 A colostomy sits flush with the skin and is typically sited in the left iliac fossa.

13 Surgery

Nutritional status might well fly under the radar more frequently on the surgical ward than elsewhere, where so much of the focus is dedicated to the intervention, but its importance ought to be elevated. Surgical patients are more likely to be malnourished at admission (40–50%), recover more slowly, and experience more complications.

Why are so many surgical patients malnourished?

1 Increased nutritional requirements (eg sepsis, burns, the surgery itself).
2 Increased nutritional losses (eg malabsorption, output from stoma).
3 Decreased intake (eg dysphagia, nausea, sedation, coma, prolonged periods nil by mouth, missed meals due to investigations, unappetizing food).

Identifying at-risk patients Assess nutritional state (using, eg Malnutrition Universal Screening Tool, p239) and weight on admission; reassess weekly thereafter. Involve dietitians early in those at risk.

• **History** Recent ↓weight (>20%, accounting for fluid balance); recent reduced intake; diet change (eg recent change in consistency of food); nausea, vomiting, pain, diarrhoea which might have led to reduced intake.

• **Examination** State of hydration (p658): dehydration can go hand-in-hand with malnutrition, and overhydration can mask malnutrition. Evidence of malnutrition: skin hanging off muscles (eg over biceps); no fat between fold of skin; hair rough and wiry; pressure sores; sores at corner of mouth. Calculate body mass index (BMI; p239); BMI <18.5kg/m² suggests malnourishment. Anthropomorphic indices, eg mid-arm circumference, skin fold measures, and grip strength are also used.

• **Investigations** Measuring albumin or prealbumin is generally unhelpful as they lack sensitivity and specificity (production is also decreased in systemic inflammation), but their trajectory can sometimes be helpful in monitoring recovery. Trace elements such as zinc, copper, selenium, and manganese, and vitamins A, D, & E should be checked at baseline in malnourished patients.

Enteral nutrition (Ie nutrition given into gastrointestinal tract.) If at all possible, give nutrition by mouth. An all-fluid diet can meet requirements (but get advice from dietitian). If danger of choking or aspiration (eg after stroke), consider texture-modified diet. Early post-op enteral nutrition has been shown to benefit patients (eg after GI surgery) and may reduce complications. **Tube feeding** Liquid nutrition via a tube: nasogastric typically placed without guidance (p743); nasojejunal tubes require endoscopic placement (used if gastric outlet obstruction, delayed gastric emptying, post-gastrectomy, or pancreatitis). Alternatively, gastric or jejunal tubes may be inserted radiologically or surgically (ie gastrostomy/jejunostomy). Use for nutritionally complete, commercially prepared feeds. Close liaison with a dietitian is essential. *Polymeric* feeds consist of undigested proteins, starches, and long-chain fatty acids. Typical requirements met with 2L/24h. *Pre-digested* feeds (peptide/semi-elemental/elemental) contain protein as short peptides or free amino acid, with fat as long- or medium-chain triglycerides, where the ratio can vary depending on the preparation.

Guidelines for success

• Use fine-bore (8Fr) nasogastric feeding tube when possible.
• Check position of nasogastric tube (pH testing) before starting feeding (p743); the positioning of a nasojejunal tube can be checked on abdominal x-ray.
• Initiate at a slow, continuous rate (distension, nausea, and vomiting less problematic) but patients may build up to shorter, bolus feeds, freeing them from pumps.
• Weigh at least weekly. Check blood glucose and plasma electrolytes (monitor for refeeding syndrome if previously malnourished).
• Treat underlying conditions vigorously, eg sepsis may impede +ve nitrogen balance.

Nil by mouth (NBM) before theatre, rules of thumb

• For *adult elective surgery* in healthy patients without GI comorbidity:
  • Water or clear fluids (eg black tea/coffee) are allowed up to 2h beforehand.
  • All other intake up to 6h beforehand.
• In *emergency surgery*, ≥6h NBM prior to theatre is best—but poor scheduling of an emergency list is not an excuse for starving patients for days.

If in doubt, liaise with the anaesthetist concerned.

Do not undertake parenteral feeding lightly: it has risks. Specialist advice is vital. It should only be considered if the patient is likely to become malnourished without it—this normally means that the gastrointestinal tract is not functioning (eg bowel obstruction), and is unlikely to function for at least 7d. Parenteral nutrition (PN) feeding may supplement other forms of nutrition (eg in short bowel syndrome or active Crohn's disease, when nutrition cannot be sufficiently absorbed in the gut) or it can be used alone (total parenteral nutrition—TPN). ►Even if there is GI disease, studies show that enteral nutrition is safer, cheaper, and at least as efficacious as parenteral nutrition in the perioperative period.[4]

Administration Nutrition must be given via a dedicated central venous line (or peripherally inserted central catheter—PICC line) or via a dedicated lumen of a multi-lumen catheter. Peripheral PN can also be administered in the short term, but only low-osmolarity formulas are suitable, and there is a risk of thrombophlebitis.

Complications and their prevention

►Liaise closely with line insertion team, nutrition team, and pharmacist. Review fluid balance at least twice daily, and weight + requirements for energy and electrolytes daily.

- **Sepsis** (Eg *Staphylococcus epidermidis* and *Staph. aureus*; *Candida*; *Pseudomonas*; infective endocarditis.) Look for spiking pyrexia and examine wound at tube insertion point. Stop PN, take line tip *and* peripheral cultures and give antibiotics via the line. If central venous line-related sepsis is suspected, the safest course of action is always to remove the line. Do not attempt to salvage a line when *Staph. aureus* or *Candida* infection has been identified. Avoid infection by maintaining meticulous sterility; do not use central venous lines for uses other than nutrition.
- **Thrombosis** Central vein thrombosis may occur, resulting in pulmonary embolus or superior vena caval obstruction (p524).
- **Metabolic imbalance** Electrolyte abnormalities—see BOX; deranged plasma glucose; hyperlipidaemia; deficiency syndromes (table 6.2, p240); acid–base disturbance (eg hypercapnia from excessive CO_2 production).
- **Mechanical** Pneumothorax; embolism of IV line tip.

Refeeding syndrome

►This is a life-threatening metabolic complication of refeeding via any route after a prolonged period of starvation. At-risk patients include those initiating artificial feeding (enteral or parenteral) after prolonged starvation, or with malignancy, anorexia nervosa, or alcoholism. As the body turns to fat and protein metabolism in the starved state, there is a drop in the level of circulating insulin (because of the paucity of dietary carbohydrates). The catabolic state also depletes intracellular stores of phosphate, although serum levels may remain normal (0.85–1.45mmol/L). When refeeding begins, the level of insulin rises in response to the carbohydrate load, and one of the consequences is to increase cellular uptake of phosphate.

A hypophosphataemic state (<0.50mmol/L) normally develops within 4d and is mostly responsible for the features of '*refeeding syndrome*', which include: rhabdomyolysis; red and white cell dysfunction; respiratory insufficiency; arrhythmias; cardiogenic shock; seizures; and sudden death.

Prevention Give high-dose Pabrinex® during re-feeding window. Identify at-risk patients, assess, and monitor closely during refeeding (check plasma glucose, creatinine and electrolytes including calcium, phosphate, and magnesium, and FBC daily until stable). Check LFT and lipid clearance three times a week until stable.

Treatment Is of the complicating features and includes parenteral phosphate administration (eg 18mmol/d) in addition to oral supplementation.

---

4 Enteral feeding promotes integrity of the gut mucosal barrier, thus preventing bacterial and endotoxin translocation across the gut wall, which can lead to multiple organ dysfunction and perpetuation of a systemic inflammatory response—even when the gut is not the primary source of pathology.

13 Surgery

▶Examine the regional lymph nodes as well as the lump. If the lump is a node, examine its area of drainage. Always examine the circulation and nerve supply distal to any lump.

History How long has it been there? Does it hurt? Any other symptoms, eg itch? Any other lumps? Is it getting bigger? Ever been abroad? Otherwise well?

Physical exam Remember the 6 **S**s: **s**ite, **s**ize, **s**hape, **s**moothness (consistency), **s**urface (contour/edge/colour), and **s**urroundings. **Other questions** Does it transilluminate (see next paragraph)? Is it fixed/tethered to skin or underlying structures (see BOX)? Is it fluctuant/compressible? Temperature? Tender? Pulsatile (US duplex may help)?

Transilluminable lumps After eliminating as much external light as possible, place a bright, thin 'pen' torch on the lump, from behind (or at least to the side), so the light is shining through the lump towards your eye. If the lump glows red it is said to transilluminate—a fluid-filled lump such as a hydrocele is a good example.

Lipomas These benign fatty lumps, occurring wherever fat can expand (ie *not* scalp or palms), have smooth, imprecise margins, a hint of fluctuance, and are not fixed to skin or deeper structures. Symptoms are only caused via pressure. Malignant change very rare (suspect if rapid growth/hardening/vascularization). Multiple scattered lipomas, which may be painful, occur in Dercum's disease, typically in postmenopausal women.

Sebaceous cysts Refer to either *epidermal* (fig 13.10) or *pilar cysts* (they are not of sebaceous origin and contain keratin, not sebum). They appear as firm, round, mobile subcutaneous nodules of varying size. Look for the characteristic central punctum. Infection is quite common, and foul pus exits through the punctum. They are common on the scalp, face, neck, and trunk. **Treatment** Excision of cyst and contents.

Lymph nodes Causes of enlargement: **Infection** Glandular fever; brucellosis; TB; HIV; toxoplasmosis; actinomycosis; syphilis. **Infiltration** Malignancy (carcinoma, lymphoma); sarcoidosis.

Cutaneous abscesses Staphylococci are the most common organisms. Haemolytic streptococci only common in hand infections. *Proteus* is a common cause of non-staphylococcal axillary abscesses. Below the waist, faecal organisms are common (aerobes and anaerobes). **Treatment** Incise and drain. *Boils (furuncles)* are abscesses involving a hair follicle and associated glands. A *carbuncle* is an area of subcutaneous necrosis which discharges itself on to the surface through multiple sinuses. Think of *hidradenitis suppurativa* if recurrent inguinal or axillary abscesses.

Rheumatoid nodules (fig 13.11) Collagenous granulomas which appear in established rheumatoid arthritis on the extensor aspects of joints—especially the elbows (fig 13.11).

Ganglia Degenerative cysts from an adjacent joint or synovial sheath commonly seen on the dorsum of the wrist or hand and dorsum of the foot. May transilluminate. 50% disappear spontaneously. Aspiration may be effective, especially when combined with instillation of steroid and hyaluronidase. For the rest, treatment of choice is excision rather than the traditional blow from your bible (the *Oxford Textbook of Surgery*)! See **fig 13.12**.

Fibromas These may occur anywhere in the body, but most commonly under the skin. These whitish, benign tumours contain collagen, fibroblasts, and fibrocytes.

Dermoid cysts Contain dermal structures and are found at the junction of embryonic cutaneous boundaries, eg in the midline or lateral to the eye. See **fig 13.13**.

Malignant tumours of connective tissue Fibrosarcomas, liposarcomas, leiomyosarcomas (smooth muscle), and rhabdomyosarcomas (striated muscle). These are staged using modified TNM system including tumour grade. Needle-core (Trucut®) biopsies of large tumours precede excision. Any lesion suspected of being a sarcoma should not be simply enucleated. ▶Refer to a specialist.

Neurofibromas See p510.

Keloids Caused by irregular hypertrophy of vascularized collagen forming raised edges at sites of previous scars that extend outside the scar (fig 13.14). Common in dark skin. Treatment can be difficult. Intralesional steroid injections are a mainstay.

In or under the skin?

Intradermal
- Sebaceous cyst
- Abscess
- Dermoid cyst
- Granuloma.

Subcutaneous
- Lipoma
- Ganglion
- Neuroma
- Lymph node.

If a lump is intradermal, you cannot draw the skin over it, while if the lump is subcutaneous, you should be able to manipulate it independently from the skin.

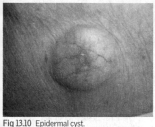

Fig 13.10 Epidermal cyst.
Copyright www.dermnetnz.org, reproduced with permission.

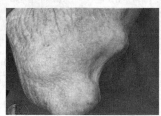

Fig 13.11 Rheumatoid nodule.
Copyright www.dermnetnz.org, reproduced with permission.

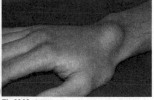

Fig 13.12 Ganglion.
Courtesy of John M Erikson, MD, Raleigh Hand Centre.

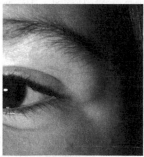

Fig 13.13 Dermoid cyst.
Reproduced from Lewis–Jones, *Paediatric Dermatology*, 2010, with permission from Oxford University Press.

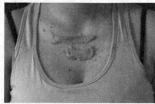

Fig 13.14 Keloid scar.
Courtesy of East Sussex Hospitals Trust.

13 Surgery

Malignant tumours

1 Malignant melanoma (See fig 13.15.) ♀:♂ ≈ 1.3:1. UK incidence: ≈20:100 000/yr (up ×4 in last 30yrs). Commonly affects younger patients ∴ early diagnosis is vital. Short periods of intense UV exposure is a major cause, particularly in the early years. May occur in pre-existing moles. If smooth, well-demarcated, and regular, it is unlikely to be a melanoma but diagnosis can be tricky. Most melanomas have features described by Glasgow 7-point checklist (table 13.8) and **ABCDE** criteria (BOX), but not all. ▶If in doubt, refer.

Table 13.8 Glasgow 7-point checklist (refer if ≥3 points, or with 1 point if suspicious)

Major (2 pts each)	Minor (1 pt each)	
• Change in size	• Inflammation	• Crusting or bleeding
• Change in shape	• Sensory change	
• Change in colour	• Diameter >7mm (▶unless growth is in the vertical plane)	

Superficial spreading melanomas (70%) grow slowly, metastasize later, and have better prognosis than *nodular melanomas* (10–15%) which invade deeply and metastasize early. Nodular lesions may be amelanotic in ∼5%. *Others: acral melanomas* occur on palms, soles, and subungual areas; *lentigo maligna melanoma* evolves from pre-existing lentigo maligna. Breslow thickness (depth in mm), tumour stage, and presence of ulceration are important prognostic factors. *R̶:* urgent excision can be curative. Systemic immunotherapy with nivolumab + ipilimumab (human monoclonal antibodies that block PD-1 and CTLA-4, respectively) improves survival in patients with metastatic melanoma with BRAF mutations, or in those without the mutation but with advanced disease who have already undergone surgery or radiation therapy.[3]

2 Squamous cell cancer Usually presents as an ulcerated lesion, with hard, raised edges, in sun-exposed sites. May begin in solar keratoses (see later in topic), or be found on the lips of smokers or in long-standing ulcers (=Marjolin's ulcer). Metastasis to lymph nodes is rare, local destruction may be extensive. *R̶:* excision + radiotherapy to treat recurrence/affected nodes. See fig 13.16. NB: the condition may be confused with a keratoacanthoma—a fast-growing, benign, self-limiting papule plugged with keratin.

3 Basal cell carcinoma (AKA *rodent ulcer.*) *Nodular:* typically a pearly nodule with rolled telangiectatic edge, on the face or a sun-exposed site. May have a central ulcer. See fig 13.17. Metastases are very rare. It slowly causes local destruction if left untreated. *Superficial:* lesions appear as red scaly plaques with a raised smooth edge, often on the trunk or shoulders. *Cause:* (most frequently) UV exposure. *R̶:* excision; cryotherapy; for superficial BCCs topical fluorouracil or imiquimod (see as for 'Solar keratoses').

Pre-malignant tumours

1 Solar (actinic) keratoses Appear on sun-exposed skin as crumbly, yellow-white crusts. Malignant change to squamous cell carcinoma may occur after several years. *Treatment:* cryotherapy; 5% fluorouracil cream or 5% imiquimod—work by causing: erythema → vesiculation → erosion → ulceration → necrosis → healing epithelialization, leaving healthy skin unharmed. Warn patients of expected inflammatory reaction. See *BNF* for dosing. Alternatively: diclofenac gel (3%, use thinly twice-daily for ≤90d).

2 Bowen's disease Slow-growing red/brown scaly plaque, eg on lower legs. *Histology:* full-thickness dysplasia (carcinoma *in situ*). It infrequently progresses to squamous cell cancer. Penile Bowen's disease is called Queyrat's erythroplasia. *Treatment:* cryotherapy, topical fluorouracil (see as for 'Solar keratoses') or photodynamic therapy.

3 See also Kaposi's sarcoma (p690); Paget's disease of the breast (p694).

Others • **Secondary carcinoma** Most common metastases to skin are from breast, kidney, or lung. Usually a firm nodule, most often on the scalp. See also acanthosis nigricans (p560). • **Mycosis fungoides** Cutaneous T-cell lymphoma usually confined to skin. Causes itchy, red plaques (Sézary syndrome variant also associated with erythroderma). • **Leucoplakia** This appears as white patches (which may fissure) on oral or genital mucosa (where it may itch). Frank carcinomatous change may occur. • **Leprosy** Suspect in any anaesthetic hypopigmented lesion (p437). • **Syphilis** Any genital ulcer is syphilis until proved otherwise. Secondary syphilis: papular rash—including, unusually, on the palms (p408).

ABCDE criteria for diagnosis of melanoma

Asymmetry.
Border—irregular.
Colour—non-uniform.
Diameter >6mm.
Evolution—change in size/shape/colour.

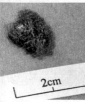

Fig 13.15 Melanoma.

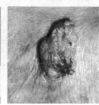

Fig 13.16 Squamous cell cancer.

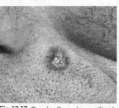

Fig 13.17 Basal cell carcinoma (BCC).

▶Don't biopsy lumps until tumours within the head and neck have been excluded by an ENT surgeon. Culture all biopsied lymph nodes for TB.

Diagnosis (See fig 13.18.) First, ask how long the lump has been present. If <3wks, self-limiting infection is the likely cause and extensive investigation is unwise. Next ask yourself where the lump is. Is it intradermal—eg sebaceous cyst with a central punctum (p586)? Is it a lipoma (p586)? If the lump is not intradermal, and is not of recent onset, you are about to start a diagnostic hunt over complicated terrain. 85% of neck swellings are *lymph nodes* (examine areas which they serve). Consider TB, viruses such as HIV or EBV (infectious mononucleosis), any chronic infection, or, if >20yrs, consider lymphoma (hepatosplenomegaly?) or metastases (eg from GI or bronchial or head and neck neoplasia), 8% are goitres (p592), and other diagnoses account for 7%.

Tests Do virology and TB tests (p390). US shows lump consistency: cystic, solid, complex, vascular. CT defines masses in relation to their anatomical neighbours. CXR may show malignancy or, in sarcoid, reveal bilateral hilar lymphadenopathy. Consider fine-needle aspiration (FNA).

Midline lumps • If patient is <20yrs old, likely diagnosis is *dermoid cyst* (p586). • If it moves *up* on tongue protrusion and is below the hyoid, likely to be a *thyroglossal cyst*, a fluid-filled sac resulting from incomplete closure of the thyroid's migration path. ℞: surgery; they are the commonest congenital cervical cystic lump. • If >20yrs old, it is probably a *thyroid isthmus* mass. • If it is bony hard, the diagnosis may be a *chondroma* (benign cartilaginous tumour).

Submandibular triangle (Bordered by the mental process, mandible, and the line between the two angles of the mandible.) • If <20yrs, self-limiting lymphadenopathy is likely. If >20yrs, exclude *malignant lymphadenopathy* (eg firm and non-tender). ▶Is TB likely? • If it is not a node, think of submandibular *salivary stone*, *sialadenitis*, or *tumour* (see BOX 'Salivary gland pathology').

Anterior triangle (Between midline, anterior border of sternocleidomastoid, and the line between the two angles of the mandible.) • *Branchial cysts* emerge under the anterior border of sternocleidomastoid where the upper third meets the middle third (age <20yrs). Due to non-disappearance of the cervical sinus (where 2nd branchial arch grows down over 3rd and 4th). Lined by squamous epithelium, their fluid contains cholesterol crystals. Treat by excision. There may be communication with the pharynx in the form of a fistula. • If lump in the superoposterior area of the anterior triangle, is it a *parotid tumour* (more likely if >40yrs)? • *Laryngoceles* are an uncommon cause of anterior triangle lumps. They are painless and may be made worse by blowing. These cysts are classified as external, internal, or mixed, and may be associated with laryngeal cancer. If pulsatile may be: • *carotid artery aneurysm* • *tortuous carotid artery*, or • *carotid body tumours* (chemodectoma). These are very rare, move from side to side but not up and down, and splay out the carotid bifurcation. They are usually firm and occasionally soft and pulsatile. They do not usually cause bruits. Diagnose by duplex USS (splaying at the carotid bifurcation) or CT/MR angiography. ℞: extirpation by vascular surgeon.

Posterior triangle (Behind sternocleidomastoid, in front of trapezius, above clavicle.) • *Cervical ribs* may intrude into this area. These are enlarged costal elements from C7 vertebra. The majority are asymptomatic but can cause Raynaud's syndrome by compressing subclavian artery and neurological symptoms (eg wasting of 1st dorsal interosseous) from pressure on lower trunk of the brachial plexus. • *Pharyngeal pouches* can protrude into the posterior triangle on swallowing (usually left-sided). • *Cystic hygromas* (usually infants) arise from jugular lymph sac. These macrocystic lymphatic malformations transilluminate brightly. Treat by surgery or hypertonic saline sclerosant injection. Recurrence can be troublesome. • *Pancoast's tumour* (see p694). • *Subclavian artery aneurysm* will be pulsatile.

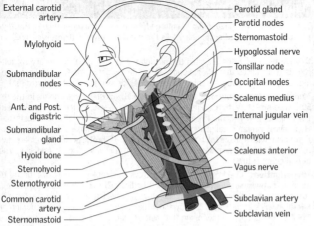

External carotid artery
Mylohyoid
Submandibular nodes
Ant. and Post. digastric
Submandibular gland
Hyoid bone
Sternohyoid
Sternothyroid
Common carotid artery
Sternomastoid

Parotid gland
Parotid nodes
Sternomastoid
Hypoglossal nerve
Tonsillar node
Occipital nodes
Scalenus medius
Internal jugular vein
Omohyoid
Scalenus anterior
Vagus nerve
Subclavian artery
Subclavian vein

Fig 13.18 Important structures in the head and neck.

Salivary gland pathology

There are three pairs of major salivary glands: parotid, submandibular, and sublingual (there are many minor glands). **History** Lumps; swelling related to food; pain. **Examination** Note external swelling; look for secretions; bimanual palpation for stones. Examine VIIth nerve and regional lymph nodes. **Cytology** Do FNA.

Acute swelling Think of mumps and HIV. *Recurrent unilateral pain and swelling* is likely to be from a stone. 80% are submandibular. The classical story is of pain and swelling on eating—with a red, tender, swollen, but uninfected gland. The stone may be seen on plain x-ray or by sialography (fig 13.19). Distal stones are removed via the mouth but deeper stones may require excision of the gland. *Chronic bilateral symptoms* may coexist with dry eyes and mouth and autoimmune disease, eg hypothyroidism, Mikulicz's or Sjögren's syndrome (p692 & p548)—also bulimia or alcohol excess. *Fixed swelling* may be from a tumour/ALL (fig 8.53, p353), sarcoid, amyloid, granulomatosis with polyangiitis, or be idiopathic.

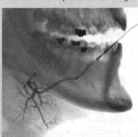

Fig 13.19 Normal sialogram of the submandibular gland. Wharton's (submandibular) duct opens into the mouth near the frenulum of the tongue.

Salivary gland tumours (table 13.9) '80% are in the parotid, 80% of these are pleomorphic adenomas, 80% of these are in the superficial lobe.' Deflection of the ear outwards is a classic sign. ▶Remove any salivary gland swelling for assessment if present for >1 month. VIIth nerve palsy means malignancy.

Table 13.9 Types of salivary gland tumours

Benign or malignant	Malignant	Malignant
Cystadenolymphoma	Mucoepidermoid	Squamous or adeno ca
Pleomorphic adenoma	Acinic cell	Adenoid cystic ca

Pleomorphic adenomas often present in middle age and grow slowly. Remove by superficial parotidectomy. Adenolymphomas (Warthin's tumour): usually older men; soft; treat by enucleation. Carcinomas: rapid growth; hard fixed mass; pain; facial palsy. Treatment: surgery + radiotherapy.

If the thyroid (figs 13.20–13.22) is enlarged (= goitre), ask yourself: 1 Is the thyroid diffusely enlarged or nodular? 2 Is the patient euthyroid, thyrotoxic (p212), or hypothyroid (p214)?

Diffuse goitre Causes Endemic (iodine deficiency); congenital; secondary to goitrogens (substances that ↓ iodine uptake); acute thyroiditis (de Quervain's); physiological (pregnancy/puberty); autoimmune (Graves' disease; Hashimoto's thyroiditis).

Nodular goitre • **Multinodular goitre (MNG)** The most common goitre in the UK. 50% who present with a single nodule actually have MNG. Patients are usually euthyroid, but may become hyperthyroid ('toxic'). MNG may be retro- or substernal. Hypothyroidism and malignancy within MNG are rare. Plummer's disease is hyperthyroidism with a single toxic nodule (uncommon). • **Fibrotic goitre** Eg Riedel's thyroiditis. • **Solitary thyroid nodule** Typically cyst, adenoma, discrete nodule in MNG or malignant (~10%).

Investigations Check TSH and USS (solid, cystic, complex, or part of a group of lumps). If abnormal consider: • T4, autoantibodies (p210, eg if Hashimoto's/Graves', suspected). • CXR with thoracic inlet view (tracheal goitres and metastases?). • Radionuclide scans (fig 13.21) may show malignant lesions as hypofunctioning or 'cold', whereas a hyperfunctioning 'hot' lesion suggests adenoma. • FNA (fine-needle aspiration) and cytology—will characterize lesion. ►A FNA finding of a follicular neoplasm can be challenging (15–30% malignant)—discuss with cytopathologist and perform molecular diagnostics where available; if any doubt, refer for surgery.

What should you do for incidentally discovered nodules on ultrasound?
• US-guided FNA is not indicated in purely cystic lesions, or in nodules <1cm across (which accounts for most; US can detect lumps <2mm; such 'incidentalomas' occur in 46% of routine autopsies).
• ►Perform US-guided FNA in all nodules where there are abnormal cervical lymph nodes, and in solid/mixed nodules ≥1cm with a past history of thyroid cancer or neck irradiation, or a family history of medullary cancer.

Thyroid cancer
1 **Papillary** (60%.) Often in younger patients. Spread: lymph nodes and lung (jugulodigastric node metastasis is the so-called lateral aberrant thyroid). R̶: total thyroidectomy to remove non-obvious tumour ± node excision ± radioiodine (^{131}I) to ablate residual cells. Give levothyroxine to suppress TSH. Prognosis: better if young and ♀.
2 **Follicular** (≤25%.) Occurs in middle-age and spreads early via blood (bone, lungs). Well-differentiated. R̶: total thyroidectomy + T4 suppression + radioiodine ablation.
3 **Medullary** (5%.) Sporadic (80%) or part of MEN syndrome (p217). May produce calcitonin which can be used as a tumour marker. They do not concentrate iodine. ►Perform a phaeochromocytoma screen pre-op. R̶: thyroidectomy + node clearance. External beam radiotherapy may prevent regional recurrence.
4 **Lymphoma** (5%.) ♀:♂≈3:1. May present with stridor or dysphagia. Do full staging pre-treatment (chemoradiotherapy). Assess histology for mucosa-associated lymphoid tissue (MALT) origin (associated with a good prognosis).
5 **Anaplastic** (Rare.) ♀:♂≈3:1. Elderly, poor response to any treatment. In the absence of unresectable disease, excision + radiotherapy may be tried.

Thyroid surgery Plays a significant role in the management of thyroid disease. Operations include partial lobectomy or lobectomy (for isolated nodules); and thyroidectomy (for cancers, MNG, or Graves'). **Indications** Pressure symptoms, relapse hyperthyroidism after >1 failed course of drug treatment, carcinoma, cosmetic reasons, symptomatic patients planning pregnancy. **Pre-operative management** Render euthyroid pre-op with antithyroid drugs (eg carbimazole up to 20mg/12h PO or propylthiouracil 200mg/12h PO but stop 10d prior to surgery as these increase vascularity). Propranolol up to 80mg/8h PO can be used to control tachycardia or tremor associated with hyperthyroidism (continue for 5d post-op). Check vocal cords by indirect laryngoscopy pre- and post-op (risk of recurrent laryngeal nerve injury). Check serum Ca^{2+} (and PTH if abnormal). **Complications** See p580.

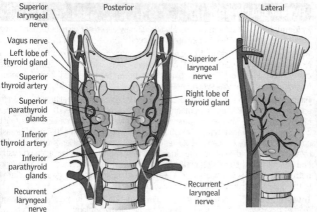

Fig 13.20 The anatomy of the region of the thyroid gland. The important structures that must be considered when operating on the thyroid gland include:
- Recurrent laryngeal nerve.
- Superior laryngeal nerve.
- Parathyroid glands.
- Trachea.
- Common carotid artery.
- Internal jugular vein (not depicted—see **fig 13.22**).

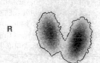

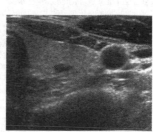

Fig 13.22 Transverse ultrasound of the left lobe of the thyroid showing a small low-reflectivity cyst within higher-reflectivity thyroid tissue. Note the proximity to the gland of the common carotid artery and internal jugular vein (the latter compressed slightly by pressure from the probe), both seen beneath the body of sternocleidomastoid muscle.

Image courtesy of Norwich Radiology Department.

Fig 13.21 Radionuclide study of the thyroid showing changes consistent with Graves' disease (see also *hot and cold nodules*, p210, and *nuclear medicine*, p722). There is increased uptake of the radionuclide trace diffusely throughout both lobes of the gland.

Image courtesy of Norwich Radiology Department.

13 Surgery

Epidemiology Affects 1 in 8 ♀; nearly 60 000 new cases per year in UK (incidence increasing). Rare in ♂ (~1% of all breast cancers).

Risk factors Risk is related to family history, age, and uninterrupted oestrogen exposure, hence: nulliparity; 1st pregnancy >30yrs old, early menarche; late menopause; HRT; obesity; BRCA genes; not breastfeeding; past breast cancer (metachronous rate ≈2%, synchronous rate ≈1%).

Pathology Non-invasive ductal carcinoma *in situ* (DCIS) is premalignant and seen as microcalcification on mammography (unifocal or widespread). Non-invasive lobular CIS is rarer and tends to be multifocal. Invasive ductal carcinoma is most common (~70%) whereas invasive lobular carcinoma accounts for 10–15% of breast cancers. Medullary cancers (~5%) tend to affect younger patients while colloid/mucoid (~2%) tend to affect the elderly. Others: papillary, tubular, adenoid-cystic and Paget's (p694). 60–70% of breast cancers are oestrogen receptor +ve, conveying better prognosis. ~30% over-express HER2 (growth factor receptor gene) associated with aggressive disease and poorer prognosis.

Investigations (See p80 for history and examination.) ►All lumps should undergo *'triple' assessment:* clinical examination + histology/cytology + mammography/ultrasound; see fig 13.23.

Staging Stage 1 Confined to breast, mobile. **Stage 2** Growth confined to breast, mobile, lymph nodes in ipsilateral axilla. **Stage 3** Tumour fixed to muscle (but not chest wall), ipsilateral lymph nodes matted and may be fixed, skin involvement larger than tumour. **Stage 4** Complete fixation of tumour to chest wall, distant metastases. Also TNM staging (p522) T1, <2cm, T2, 2–5cm, T3, >5cm, T4, fixity to chest wall or *peau d'orange*; N1, mobile ipsilateral nodes; N2, fixed nodes; M1, distant metastases.

Treating local disease (Stage 1–2.) • **Surgery** Removal of tumour by wide local excision (WLE) or mastectomy ± breast reconstruction + axillary node sampling/surgical clearance or sentinel node biopsy (see BOX 'Sentinel node biopsy'). • **Radiotherapy** Recommended for all patients with invasive cancer after WLE, and for patients at high risk for local recurrence after mastectomy (eg involvement of axillary lymph nodes). SE: pneumonitis, pericarditis, and rib fractures. • **Adjuvant systemic therapy** Improves survival and reduces recurrence in most groups of women (consider in all except excellent prognosis patients). In hormonal receptor (oestrogen and progesterone) +ve disease, give adjuvant endocrine therapy (aromatase inhibitors, eg anastrozole targeting peripheral oestrogen synthesis, ER blocker tamoxifen as second line). In human epidermal growth factor receptor 2 receptor (HER2) +ve disease, also give adjuvant anti-HER2 therapy with trastuzumab, in combination with chemotherapy if tumour >2cm or lymph node involvement. Note, endocrine therapy is only used if postmenopausal. If premenopausal and an ER+ve tumour, ovarian ablation (via surgery or radiotherapy) or GnRH analogues (eg goserelin) ↓ recurrence and ↑ survival. • **Support** Breast care nurses. •**Reconstruction options** Eg tissue expanders/implants/nipple tattoos, latissimus dorsi flap, TRAM (transverse rectus abdominis myocutaneous) flap.

Treating locally advanced disease (Stage 3.) Neoadjuvant chemotherapy (with addition of anti-HER2 therapy if +ve) is used prior to mastectomy + adjuvant therapy.

Treating metastatic disease (Stage 4.) Long-term survival is possible and median survival is >2yrs. Staging investigations should include CXR, bone scan, liver USS, CT/MRI or PET-CT (p722), + LFTs and Ca²⁺. Radiotherapy (p520) to painful bone lesions (*bisphosphonates*, p669, may ↓ pain and fracture risk). Tamoxifen is often used in ER +ve; if relapse after initial success, consider chemotherapy. Trastuzumab should be given for HER2 +ve tumours, in combination with chemotherapy. CNS surgery for solitary (or easily accessible) metastases may be possible; if not—radiotherapy. Get specialist help for arm lymphoedema (try decongestive methods first).

Preventing deaths • Promote awareness. • **Screening** 2-view mammography every 3yrs for women aged 50–71 in UK has ↓ breast cancer deaths by 30% in women >50yrs.

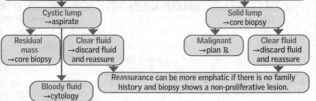

Fig 13.23 Triple assessment and investigation of a breast lump.

* US is more accurate at detecting invasive breast cancer, though mammography remains most accurate at detecting ductal carcinoma *in situ* (DCIS). MRI is used in the assessment of multifocal/bilateral disease and patients with cosmetic implants who are identified as high risk.

Sentinel node biopsy

Decreases needless axillary clearances in lymph node −ve patients.
- Patent blue dye and/or radiocolloid injected into periareolar area or tumour.
- A gamma probe/visual inspection is used to identify the sentinel node.
- The sentinel node is biopsied and sent for histology ± immunohistochemistry; further clearance only if sentinel node +ve.

Sentinel node identified in 90%. False −ve rates <5% for experienced surgeons.

Prognostic factors in breast cancer

Tumour size, grade, lymph node status, ER/PR status, presence of vascular invasion all help assess prognosis. Nottingham Prognostic Index (NPI) is widely used to predict survival and risk of relapse, and to help select appropriate adjuvant systemic therapy. $NPI = 0.2 \approx tumour\ size\ (cm) + histological\ grade + nodal\ status.$[5]

If treated with surgery alone, 10yr survival rates are: NPI <2.4: 95%; NPI 2.4–3.4: 85%; NPI 3.4–4.4: 70%; NPI 4.4–5.4: 50%; NPI >5.4: 20%.

Benign breast disease

Fibroadenoma Usually presents <30yrs but can occur up to menopause. Benign overgrowth of collagenous mesenchyme of one breast lobule. Firm, smooth, mobile lump, the 'breast mouse'. Painless. May be multiple. ⅓ regress, ⅓ stay the same, ⅓ get bigger. ℞: observation and reassurance, but if in doubt refer for USS (usually conclusive) ± FNA. Surgical excision if large.

Breast cysts Common >35yrs, esp. perimenopausal. Benign, fluid-filled rounded lump. Not fixed to surrounding tissue. Occasionally painful. ℞: diagnosis confirmed on aspiration (perform only if trained).

Infective mastitis/breast abscesses Infection of mammary duct often associated with lactation (usually *Staph. aureus*). Abscess presents as painful, hot swelling of breast segment. ℞: antibiotics. Open incision or percutaneous drainage if abscess.

Duct ectasia Typically around menopause. Ducts become blocked and secretions stagnate. Present with nipple discharge (green/brown/bloody) ± nipple retraction ± lump. Refer for confirmation of diagnosis. Usually no ℞ needed. Advise to stop smoking.

Fat necrosis Fibrosis and calcification after injury to breast tissue. Scarring results in a firm lump. Refer for triple assessment. No ℞ once diagnosis confirmed.

5 Nodal status is scored 1–3: 1 = node −ve; 2 = 1–3 nodes +ve; 3 = >3 nodes +ve for breast cancer. Histological grade is also scored 1–3.

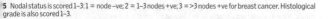

As with any mass (see p586), determine size, site, shape, and surface. Find out if it is pulsatile and if it is mobile. Examine supraclavicular and inguinal nodes. Is the lump ballotable (like bobbing an apple up and down in water)?

Right iliac fossa masses		
• Appendix mass/abscess	• Intussusception	• Transplanted kidney
• Caecal carcinoma	• TB mass	• Kidney malformation
• Crohn's disease	• Amoebic abscess	• Tumour in an
• Pelvic mass (see later in topic)	• Actinomycosis (p385)	undescended testis

Abdominal distension Flatus, fat, fluid, faeces, or fetus (p53)? Fluid may be outside the gut (ascites) or sequestered in bowel (obstruction; ileus). To demonstrate ascites, elicit signs of a fluid thrill and/or shifting dullness (p59).

Causes of ascites		Ascites with portal hypertension	
• Malignancy	• CCF; pericarditis	• Cirrhosis	• Portal nodes
• Infections—esp. TB	• Pancreatitis	• Budd–Chiari syndrome (p686)	
• ↓Albumin (eg nephrosis)	• Myxoedema	• IVC or portal vein thrombosis	

Tests Aspirate ascitic fluid (p748) for cytology, culture, and albumin;[6] US.

Left upper quadrant mass Is it spleen, stomach, kidney, colon, pancreas, or a rare cause (eg neurofibroma)? Pancreatic cysts may be true (congenital; cystadenomas; retention cysts of chronic pancreatitis; cystic fibrosis) or pseudocysts (fluid in lesser sac from acute pancreatitis).

Splenomegaly Causes are often said to be infective, haematological, neoplastic, etc., but grouping by associated feature is more useful clinically:

Splenomegaly with fever	With lymphadenopathy	With purpura
• Infection[HS] (malaria, SBE/IE, hepatitis;[HS] EBV,[HS] TB, CMV, HIV)	• Glandular fever[HS]	• Septicaemia; typhus
• Sarcoid; malignancy[HS]	• Leukaemias; lymphoma	• DIC; amyloid[HS]
	• Sjögren's syndrome	• Meningococcaemia
With arthritis	**With ascites**	**With a murmur**
• Sjögren's syndrome	• Carcinoma	• SBE/IE
• Rheumatoid arthritis; SLE	• Portal hypertension[HS]	• Rheumatic fever
• Infection, eg Lyme (p418)		• Hypereosinophilia
• Vasculitis/Behçet's (p554)		• Amyloid[HS] (p364)
With anaemia	**With ↓weight + CNS signs**	**Massive splenomegaly**
• Sickle cell;[HS] thalassaemia[HS]	• Cancer; lymphoma	• Malaria (hyper-reactivity after chronic exposure)
• Leishmaniasis;[HS] leukaemia[HS]	• TB; arsenic poisoning	• Myelofibrosis; CML[HS]
• Pernicious anaemia (p330)	• Paraproteinaemia[HS]	• Gaucher's syndrome[HS]
• POEMS syn. (p214)		• Leishmaniasis

[HS] =causes of hepatosplenomegaly.

Smooth hepatomegaly Hepatitis, CCF, sarcoidosis, early alcoholic cirrhosis (a small liver is typical later); tricuspid incompetence (→ pulsatile liver).

Craggy hepatomegaly Secondaries or 1° hepatoma. (Nodular cirrhosis typically causes a small, shrunken liver, not an enlarged craggy one.)

Pelvic masses Fibroids, fetus, bladder, ovarian cysts, or malignancies. *Is it truly pelvic?*—Yes, if by palpation you cannot get 'below it'.

Investigating lumps Check FBC (with film); CRP; U&E; LFT; Ca²⁺; tumour markers only as appropriate. Imaging by CT or US (transvaginal approach may be useful); MRI also has a role, eg in assessment of liver masses (p282). **Others** TB tests (p390). Biopsy to give a tissue diagnosis may be obtained using a fine needle guided by CT, US, or endoscopy.

6 Subtract fluid albumin from serum albumin to obtain serum–ascites albumin gradient (SAAG). Gradient <11g/L suggests malignancy, infections, or pancreatitis.

The first successful laparotomy...

In 1809, an American surgeon by the name of Ephraim McDowell performed an astonishing operation: the first successful elective laparotomy for an abdominal tumour. It was an ovariotomy for an ovarian mass in a 44-year-old who, prior to physical examination by McDowell, was believed to be gravid. Not only was this feat performed in the age before anaesthesia and antisepsis, but it was also performed on a table in the front room of McDowell's Kentucky home, at that time on the frontier of the West in the United States. His account of the operation makes fascinating reading. While the strength of his diagnostic convictions combined with his speed and skill at operating is to be admired (the operation took 25 minutes), there is an even more laudable part played in this story. The patient, Mrs Jane Todd-Crawford, was fully willing to be involved with what can only be described as experimental surgery in the face of uncertainty. She defied pain simply by reciting psalms and hymns, and was back at home within 4 weeks with no complications, ultimately living another 33 years. We would be well served in remembering the exceptional commitment of Mrs Todd-Crawford. In the rush and hurry of our daily tasks perhaps it is all too easy to forget that the undertaking of surgery today may be no less fear-provoking for patients than it was 200 years ago.

Someone who becomes acutely ill and in whom symptoms and signs are chiefly related to the abdomen has an acute abdomen. Prompt laparotomy is sometimes essential: *repeated examination is the key to making the decision.*

Clinical syndromes that usually require laparotomy

1 **Rupture of an organ/haemorrhage** (Spleen, aorta, ectopic pregnancy.) Shock is a leading sign—see table 13.10 for assessment of blood loss. Abdominal swelling may be seen. Any history of trauma (blunt trauma → spleen). *Delayed* rupture of the spleen may occur weeks after trauma. Peritonism may be mild.

2 **Peritonitis** (Visceral inflammation ± perforation, commonly, appendix, gall-bladder, peptic ulcer, diverticulum.) Signs: prostration, shock (tachycardia and often profound hypotension due to autonomic reaction), fever, lying still, +ve cough test (p58), tenderness (± rebound/percussion pain, p58), board-like abdominal rigidity, guarding, and no bowel sounds. Erect CXR may (60% of cases) show gas under the diaphragm (fig 13.25). NB: acute pancreatitis (p628) causes these signs, but does *not* require a laparotomy so don't be caught out and ►*always check serum amylase.*

Syndromes that may not require a laparotomy

Local peritonitis Eg diverticulitis, cholecystitis, salpingitis. If abscess formation is suspected (swelling, swinging fever, and ↑WCC) do US or CT. Drainage can be per-cutaneous (US or CT guided), or by laparotomy. Peritoneal inflammation can cause localized ileus with a 'sentinel loop' of intraluminal gas visible on plain AXR (p713).

Colic This is a regularly waxing and waning pain, caused by muscular spasm in a hollow viscus, eg gut, ureter, salpinx, uterus, bile duct, or gallbladder (in the latter, pain is often dull and constant). Colic, unlike peritonitis, causes restlessness and the patient may well be pacing around when you go to review!

Obstruction of the bowel See p602.

Tests U&E; FBC; amylase; LFT; CRP; lactate (is there mesenteric ischaemia?); urinalysis. ►►Urine and serum human chorionic gonadotropin (HCG) is vital to exclude ectopic pregnancy. Erect CXR (fig 13.25), AXR may show Rigler's sign (p712). Laparoscopy may avert open surgery. CT can be helpful provided it is readily available and causes no delay (pp716–17); US may identify perforation or free fluid (appropriate performer training is important).

Pre-op ►Don't rush to theatre. *Anaesthesia compounds shock,* so resuscitate prop-erly first (p770) unless blood being lost faster than can be replaced, eg ruptured ectopic pregnancy (OHCS p126), aneurysm leak (p646), trauma.

Plan Bed rest, keep NBM; assess volume status (BOX) and treat shock (p770); cross-match/group and save; analgesia (p570); arrange imaging; consider need for IVI, blood cultures, and antibiotics (eg piperacillin/tazobactam 4.5g/8h IV); ECG.

The medical acute abdomen IBD (p258) must be considered. Other causes:

►►Myocardial infarction	Pneumonia (p168)	Sickle cell crisis (p336)
Gastroenteritis or UTI	Thyroid storm (p820)	Phaeochromocytoma (p820)
Diabetes mellitus/DKA (p200)	Zoster (p400)	Malaria (p412)
Bornholm disease	Tuberculosis (p389)	Typhoid fever (p411)
Pneumococcal peritonitis	Porphyria (p684)	Cholera (p426)
Henoch–Schönlein (p307)	Narcotic addiction	*Yersinia enterocolitica* (p427)
Tabes dorsalis (p408)	PAN (p554)	Lead colic.

Hidden diagnoses ►►Mesenteric ischaemia (p617), ►►acute pancreatitis (p628), and ►►leaking AAA (p646) are the *Unterseeboote* of the acute abdomen—unsuspected, undetectable unless carefully looked for, and underestimatedly deadly. They may have non-specific symptoms and signs that are surprisingly mild, so always think of them when assessing the acute abdomen and hopefully you will 'spot' them! ►Finally: *always exclude pregnancy (± ectopic?).*

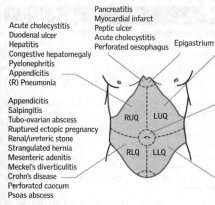

Acute cholecystitis
Duodenal ulcer
Hepatitis
Congestive hepatomegaly
Pyelonephritis
Appendicitis
(R) Pneumonia

Pancreatitis
Myocardial infarct
Peptic ulcer
Acute cholecystitis
Perforated oesophagus   Epigastrium

Ruptured spleen
Gastric ulcer
Aortic aneurysm
Perforated colon
Pyelonephritis
(L) Pneumonia

Appendicitis
Salpingitis
Tubo-ovarian abscess
Ruptured ectopic pregnancy
Renal/ureteric stone
Strangulated hernia
Mesenteric adenitis
Meckel's diverticulitis
Crohn's disease
Perforated caecum
Psoas abscess

RUQ   LUQ

RLQ   LLQ

Intestinal obstruction
Acute pancreatitis
Early appendicitis
Mesenteric thrombosis
Aortic aneurysm
Diverticulitis

Sigmoid diverticulitis
Salpingitis
Tubo-ovarian abscess
Ruptured ectopic pregnancy
Strangulated hernia
Perforated colon
Crohn's disease
Ulcerative colitis
Renal/ureteric stones

Fig 13.24 Causes of abdominal pain.

13 Surgery

Assessing hypovolaemia from blood loss

▶▶Treat suspected shock rather than wait for BP to fall. The most likely cause of shock in a surgical patient is hypovolaemia. Check urine output, GCS, and capillary refill (CR) as measures of renal, brain, and skin perfusion.

When there is any blood loss, assess the status of the following:

Table 13.10 Estimating blood loss based on patient's initial presentation[4]

Parameter	I: MILD	II: MODERATE	III: SEVERE	IV: CRITICAL
Blood loss	<750mL	750–1500mL	1500–2000mL	>2000mL
	<15%	15–30%	30–40%	>40%
Pulse	↔	↔ or ↑	↑	↑↑
BP	↔	↔	↔ or ↓	↓
Pulse pressure	↔ or ↑	↓	↓	↓
Respirations	↔	↔	↔ or ↑	↑
Urine output	↔	↔ or ↓	5–15mL/h	Negligible
Mental state	Slightly anxious	Anxious	↓GCS	↓GCS
Fluids/blood products	Monitor	Crystalloid	Crystalloid + blood	Massive transfusion protocol

Assumes a body mass of 70kg. An adaptation of 'Estimated blood loss based on initial presentation' table from the 9th edition of the *Advanced Trauma Life Support Manual*. Adapted with permission from the American College of Surgeons.

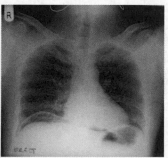

Fig 13.25 Erect CXR showing air beneath the right hemidiaphragm, indicating presence of a pneumoperitoneum. Causes:
• Bowel perforation (visible only in 75%) (fig 13.24).
• Gas-forming infection, eg *C. perfringens*.
• Iatrogenic, eg laparoscopic surgery (detectable on CXR up to 10d post-op).
• *Per vaginam* (eg sexual activity).
• Interposition of bowel between liver and diaphragm (Chilaiditi sign—not true free air).

Image courtesy of Mr P. Paraskeva.

13 Surgery

Incidence Most common surgical emergency (lifetime incidence = 6%). Can occur at any age, though highest incidence is between 10–20yrs.[7] It is rare before age 2 because the appendix is cone shaped with a larger lumen.

Pathogenesis Gut organisms invade the appendix wall after lumen obstruction by lymphoid hyperplasia, faecolith, or filarial worms. This leads to oedema, ischaemic necrosis, and perforation.

Presentation Classically periumbilical pain that moves to the RIF. Associated signs may include tachycardia, fever, peritonism with guarding, and rebound or percussion tenderness in RIF. Pain on right during PR examination suggests an inflamed, low-lying pelvic appendix. Anorexia is an important feature; vomiting is rarely prominent—*pain normally precedes vomiting* in the surgical abdomen. Constipation is usual, though diarrhoea may occur. **Additional signs** *Rovsing's sign* (pain > in RIF than LIF when the LIF is pressed). *Psoas sign* (pain on extending hip if retrocaecal appendix). *Cope sign* (pain on flexion and internal rotation of right hip if appendix in close relation to obturator internus).

Investigations Blood tests may reveal neutrophil leucocytosis and elevated CRP. US may help, but the appendix is not always visualized. CT has high diagnostic accuracy and is useful if diagnosis is unclear: it reduces −ve appendicectomy rate.

Variations in the clinical picture
• Inflammation in a retrocaecal/retroperitoneal appendix (2.5%) may cause flank or RUQ pain; its only sign may be ↑tenderness on the right on PR.
• The child with vague abdominal pain who will not eat their favourite food.
• The shocked, confused octogenarian who is not in pain.
• Appendicitis occurs in ~1/1000 pregnancies. Mortality is higher, especially from 20wks' gestation. Perforation is more common, and increases fetal mortality. Pain is often less well localized (may be RUQ) and signs of peritonism less obvious.

Hints
• If a child is anxious, use their hand to press their tummy.
• Check for recent viral illnesses and lymphadenopathy—mesenteric adenitis?
• Don't *start* palpating in the RIF (makes it difficult to elicit pain elsewhere).
• Expect diagnosis to be wrong half the time. If diagnosis is uncertain, re-examine often. A normal appendix is removed in up to 20% of patients.

Treatment Prompt *appendicectomy* (fig 13.26). **Antibiotics** Broad-spectrum IV antibiotics starting 1h pre-op (p568), reduces wound infections. Give a longer course if perforated. **Laparoscopy** Has diagnostic and therapeutic advantages (if surgeon experienced), especially in women and the obese. It is not recommended in cases of suspected gangrenous perforation as the rate of abscess formation may be higher.

Complications
• *Perforation* is commoner if a faecolith is present and in young children, as the diagnosis is more often delayed.
• *Appendix mass* may result when an inflamed appendix becomes covered with omentum. US/CT may help with diagnosis. Some advocate early surgery. Alternatively, initial conservative management—NBM and antibiotics. If the mass resolves, some perform an interval (ie delayed) appendicectomy. Exclude a colonic tumour (laparotomy or colonoscopy), which can present as early as the 4th decade.
• *Appendix abscess* may result if an appendix mass fails to resolve but enlarges and the patient gets more unwell. Treatment usually involves drainage (surgical or percutaneous under US/CT guidance). Antibiotics alone may bring resolution.

---

7 There is a second peak between 60–70yrs; older adults may present later with atypical symptoms.

Explaining the patterns of abdominal pain

Internal organs and the visceral peritoneum have no somatic innervation, so the brain attributes the visceral (splanchnic) signals to a physical location whose dermatome corresponds to the same entry level in the spinal cord. Importantly, there is no laterality to the visceral unmyelinated c-fibre pain signals, which enter the cord bilaterally and at multiple levels. Division of the gut according to embryological origin is the important determinant here: see table 13.11.

Table 13.11 Somatic referral of abdominal pain

Gut	Division points	Somatic referral	Arterial supply
Fore	Proximal to 2nd part of duodenum	Epigastrium	Coeliac axis
Mid	Above to ⅔ along transverse colon	Periumbilical	Superior mesenteric
Hind	Distal to above	Suprapubic	Inferior mesenteric

Early inflammation irritates the structure and walls of the appendix, so a colicky pain is referred to the mid-abdomen—classically periumbilical. As the inflammation progresses and irritates the parietal peritoneum (especially on examination), the somatic, lateralized pain settles at McBurney's point, ⅔ of the way along from the umbilicus to the right anterior superior iliac spine.

These principles also help us understand patterns of *referred pain*. In pneumonia, the T9 dermatome is shared by the lung and the abdomen. Also, irritation of the underside of the diaphragm (sensory innervation is from above through the phrenic nerve, c3–5) by an inflamed gallbladder or a subphrenic abscess refers pain to the right shoulder: dermatomes c3–5.

ΔΔ

- Ectopic (►►do a pregnancy test!)
- UTI (test urine!)
- Mesenteric adenitis
- Cystitis
- Cholecystitis
- Diverticulitis
- Salpingitis/PID
- Dysmenorrhoea
- Crohn's disease
- Perforated ulcer
- Food poisoning
- Meckel's diverticulum.

13 Surgery

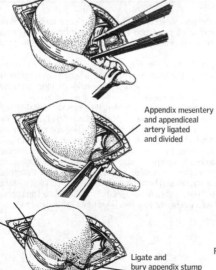

Appendix mesentery and appendiceal artery ligated and divided

Ligate and bury appendix stump with a purse-string suture

Fig 13.26 Appendicectomy.
Reproduced from McLatchie *et al.*, *Operative Surgery*, 2006, with permission from Oxford University Press.

Cardinal features of intestinal obstruction • *Vomiting*,[8] nausea, and anorexia. • *Colic* occurs early (↓ in long-standing obstruction). • *Constipation* may be absolute (ie no faeces or flatus passed) in distal obstruction; less pronounced if obstruction is high. • *Abdominal distension* ↑ as the obstruction progresses with active, 'tinkling' bowel sounds.

The key decisions

1 **Is it obstruction of the small or large bowel?** In small bowel obstruction, vomiting occurs early, distension is less, and pain is higher in the abdomen; in large bowel obstruction, absolute constipation (no gas in rectum on AXR) and distension are more prominent. The AXR plays a key role (fig 13.27 & p712).

2 **Is there an ileus or mechanical obstruction?** Ileus is functional obstruction from ↓bowel motility (see BOX 'Paralytic ileus or pseudo-obstruction?' & p712). Bowel sounds are absent; pain tends to be less.

3 **Is the obstructed bowel simple/closed loop/strangulated?** *Simple:* one obstructing point and no vascular compromise. *Closed loop:* obstruction at two points forming a loop of grossly distended bowel at risk of strangulation/perforation. *Strangulated:* blood supply is compromised and there is a higher risk of perforation. Look for more constant and *localized* pain/tenderness, ↑WCC. Peritonitis and systemic signs (SIRS) suggest perforation. ↑WCC, ↑lactate, ↑D-dimer suggest mesenteric ischaemia (p617).

Causes See table 13.12.

Table 13.12 Causes of bowel obstruction

Causes: small bowel	Causes: large bowel	Rarer causes
• Adhesions (p581)	• Colon ca (p608)	• Crohn's stricture
• Hernias (p604)	• Constipation (p256)	• Gallstone ileus (p626)
	• Diverticular stricture	• Intussusception
	• Volvulus	• TB (developing world)
	• Sigmoid (see BOX 'Sigmoid volvulus')	• Foreign body
	• Caecal	

Management

• **General principles** Cause, site, speed of onset, and completeness of obstruction determine definitive therapy: strangulation and large bowel obstruction require surgery; ileus and incomplete small bowel obstruction can be managed conservatively, at least initially.

• **Immediate action** ►'Drip and suck'—NG tube and IV fluids to rehydrate and correct electrolyte imbalance (p660). Being NBM does not give adequate rest for the bowel because it can produce up to 9L of fluid/d. Also: analgesia, blood tests (incl. amylase, FBC, U&E), AXR, erect CXR, catheterize to monitor fluid status.

• **Further imaging** CT to establish the cause of obstruction (may show dilated, fluid-filled bowel and a transition zone at the site of obstruction—figs 13.28, 13.29). Oral Gastrografin® prior to CT can help identify level of obstruction and may have mild therapeutic action against mechanical obstruction. Consider investigating the cause of large bowel obstruction by colonoscopy but beware risk of perforation.

• **Surgery** ►Strangulation needs emergency surgery. Closed loop obstruction may be managed with surgery or endoscopic decompression attempted. Endoscopic stenting may be used for obstructing large bowel malignancies either in palliation or as a bridge to surgery in acute obstruction (p608). Small bowel obstruction secondary to adhesions should rarely lead to surgery—see BOX 'Adhesions', p581.

8 Fermentation of the intestinal contents in established obstruction causes 'faeculent' vomiting. True 'faecal' vomiting is found when there is a colonic fistula with the proximal gut.

Paralytic ileus or pseudo-obstruction?

Paralytic ileus This is adynamic bowel due to the absence of normal peristaltic contractions. Contributing factors include abdominal surgery, pancreatitis (or any localized peritonitis), spinal injury, hypokalaemia, hyponatraemia, uraemia, peritoneal sepsis, and drugs (eg tricyclic antidepressants). *Treatment:* removal of inciting factors, bowel rest, bowel decompression (NG TUBE).

Pseudo-obstruction Resembles mechanical GI obstruction but with no obstructing lesion. *Acute* colonic pseudo-obstruction is called Ogilvie's syndrome (p694), and clinical features are similar to that of mechanical obstruction. Predisposing factors: electrolyte disturbance/uraemia; bedbound comorbid elderly patient; puerperium; pelvic surgery; trauma; cardiorespiratory/neurological disorders. *Treatment:* neostigmine or colonoscopic decompression are sometimes useful.

Sigmoid volvulus

Sigmoid volvulus occurs when the bowel twists on its mesentery, which can produce severe, rapid, strangulated obstruction (fig 13.27c). It tends to occur in the elderly, constipated, and comorbid patient, and is managed by insertion of a flatus tube or sigmoidoscopy. Sigmoid colectomy is sometimes required. ▶If not treated successfully, it can progress to perforation and fatal peritonitis.

13 Surgery

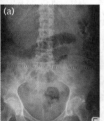
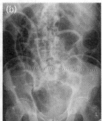
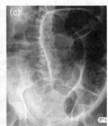

Fig 13.27 (a) Small bowel obstruction: AXR shows central gas shadows with *valvulae conniventes* that completely cross the lumen and no gas in the large bowel. (b) Large bowel obstruction: AXR shows peripheral gas shadows proximal to the blockage (eg in caecum) but not in the rectum. (c) Sigmoid volvulus: there is a characteristic AXR with an 'inverted-U' loop of bowel that looks a bit like a coffee bean.

Reproduced from Darby *et al.*, *Oxford Handbook of Medical Imaging*, 2011, with permission from Oxford University Press.

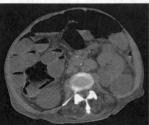
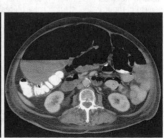

Fig 13.28 Unenhanced axial CT of the abdomen showing multiple loops of dilated, fluid-filled small bowel in a patient with small bowel obstruction.

Image courtesy of Norwich Radiology Dept.

Fig 13.29 Axial CT of the abdomen post-oral contrast showing dilated loops of fluid and air-filled large bowel (contrast medium is in the small bowel).

Image courtesy of Norwich Radiology Dept.

Definition The protrusion of a viscus or part of a viscus through a defect of the walls of its containing cavity into an abnormal position. See fig 13.30. **Terminology**
• *Irreducible:* contents cannot be pushed back into place (see p606 for technique).
• *Obstructed:* bowel contents cannot pass—features of intestinal obstruction (p602).
• *Strangulated:* ischaemia occurs—the patient requires urgent surgery.
• *Incarceration:* contents of the hernial sac are stuck inside by adhesions.

Care must be taken with reduction as it is possible to push an incarcerated hernia back into the abdominal cavity, giving the initial appearance of successful reduction.

Inguinal hernia The commonest type in both ♂ & ♀ (but ♂ >> ♀), p606.

Femoral hernia Bowel enters the femoral canal, presenting as a mass in the upper medial thigh where it points down the leg, unlike an inguinal hernia which points to the groin. They occur more often in ♀ especially in middle age and the elderly and are easy to miss. ►Always examine for this in elderly ♀ with small bowel obstruction. They are likely to be irreducible and to strangulate due to the rigidity of the canal's borders. **Anatomy** See fig 13.31. **Differential diagnosis** (See p643.) 1 Inguinal hernia. 2 Saphena varix. 3 An enlarged Cloquet's node (p607). 4 Lipoma. 5 Femoral aneurysm. 6 Psoas abscess. **Treatment** Surgical repair is recommended. *Herniotomy* is ligation and excision of the sac, *herniorrhaphy* is repair of the hernial defect.

Paraumbilical hernias Occur just above or below the umbilicus (vs true umbilical hernias, which present in infants). Risk factors are obesity and ascites. Omentum or bowel herniates through the defect. Surgical repair either by mesh or direct repair of the rectus sheath. Laparoscopic repair may be preferable for larger defects and in the obese patient.

Epigastric hernias Pass through linea alba above the umbilicus.

Incisional hernias Follow breakdown of muscle closure after surgery (11–20%). If obese, repair is not easy. Mesh repair has ↓recurrence but ↑infection over sutures.

Spigelian hernias Occur through the linea semilunaris at the lateral edge of the rectus sheath, below and lateral to the umbilicus.

Lumbar hernias Occur through the inferior or superior lumbar triangles in the posterior abdominal wall.

Richter's hernias Involve bowel wall only—not the whole lumen.

Maydl's hernias Involve a herniating 'double loop' of bowel. The strangulated portion may reside as a single loop *inside* the abdominal cavity.

Littré's hernias Hernial sacs containing strangulated Meckel's diverticulum.

Obturator hernias Occur through the obturator canal. Typically there is pain along the medial side of the thigh in a thin woman.

Sciatic hernias Pass through the lesser sciatic foramen (a way through various pelvic ligaments). GI obstruction + a gluteal mass suggests this rare possibility.

Sliding hernias Contain a partially extraperitoneal structure (eg caecum on the right, sigmoid colon on the left). The sac does not completely surround the contents.

Paediatric hernias Include: **Umbilical hernias** (3% of live births.) Are a result of a persistent defect in the transversalis fascia. Surgical repair rarely needed as most resolve by the age of 3yrs. **Indirect inguinal hernias** (~4% of all ♂ infants due to patent *processus vaginalis*—prematurity is a risk factor; uncommon in ♀ infants—consider testicular feminization.) Surgical repair is required. **Gastroschisis** Protrusion of the abdominal contents through a defect in the anterior abdominal wall to the right of the umbilicus. Prompt surgical repair required. **Exomphalos** Abdominal contents are found outside the abdomen, covered in a three-layer membrane consisting of peritoneum, Wharton's jelly, and amnion. Surgical repair less urgent because the bowel is protected by these membranes.

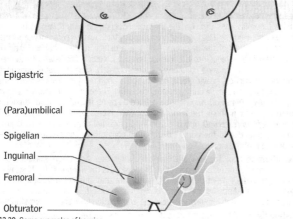

Epigastric

(Para)umbilical

Spigelian

Inguinal

Femoral

Obturator

Fig 13.30 Some examples of hernias.

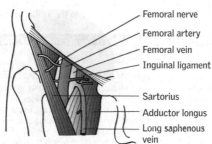

Femoral nerve

Femoral artery

Femoral vein

Inguinal ligament

Sartorius

Adductor longus

Long saphenous vein

Fig 13.31 The boundaries of the femoral canal are anteriorly the inguinal ligament; medially the lacunar ligament (and pubic bone); laterally the femoral vein (and iliopsoas); and posteriorly the pectineal ligament and pectineus. The canal contains fat and Cloquet's node. The neck of the hernia is felt inferior and lateral to the pubic tubercle (inguinal hernias are superior and medial to this point).

13 Surgery

Indirect hernias pass through the internal inguinal ring and, if large, out through the external ring (fig 13.32). *Direct* hernias push their way *directly* forward through the posterior wall of the inguinal canal, into a defect in the abdominal wall (Hesselbach's triangle; medial to the inferior epigastric vessels and lateral to the rectus abdominus). *Predisposing conditions:* males (♂:♀≈8:1), chronic cough, constipation, urinary obstruction, heavy lifting, ascites, past abdominal surgery (eg damage to the iliohypogastric nerve during appendicectomy). There are two landmarks to identify: *the deep (internal) ring* may be defined as being the mid-point of the inguinal ligament, ~1½ cm above the femoral pulse (which crosses the mid-inguinal point); *the superficial (external) ring* is a split in the external oblique aponeurosis just superior and medial to the pubic tubercle (the bony prominence forming the medial attachment of the inguinal ligament).

Examination Look for previous scars; feel the other side (more common on the right); examine the external genitalia. Then ask: • Is the lump visible? If so, ask the patient to reduce it—if they cannot, make sure that it is not a scrotal lump. Ask them to cough. Appears *above and medial to the pubic tubercle.* • If no lump is visible, feel for a cough impulse. • Repeat the examination with the patient standing.

Distinguishing direct from indirect hernias This is loved by examiners but is of little clinical use—not least because repair is the same for both (see 'Repairs' later in topic). The best way is to reduce the hernia and occlude the deep (internal) ring with two fingers. Ask the patient to cough or stand—if the hernia is restrained, it is indirect; if not, it is direct. The 'gold standard' for determining the type of inguinal hernia is at surgery: direct hernias arise medial to the inferior epigastric vessels; indirect hernias are lateral.

Indirect hernias	Direct hernias	Femoral hernias
• Common (80%)	• Less common (20%)	• More frequent in females
• Can strangulate.	• Reduce easily	• Frequently irreducible
	• Rarely strangulate.	• Frequently strangulate.

Irreducible hernias You may be called because a long-standing hernia is now irreducible and painful. It is always worth trying to reduce these yourself to prevent strangulation and necrosis (demanding prompt laparotomy). Learn how to do this from an expert, ie one of your patients who has been reducing their hernia for years. Then you will know how to act correctly when the emergency presents. Notice that such patients use the flat of the hand, directing the hernia from below, up towards the contralateral shoulder. Sometimes, as the hernia obstructs, reduction requires perseverance, which may be rewarded by a gurgle from the retreating bowel and a kiss from the attending spouse who had thought that surgery was inevitable.

Repairs Weight loss (if over-weight) and stop smoking pre-op. Warn that hernias may recur and patients should be counselled about possibility of chronic pain postoperatively. Mesh techniques (eg Lichtenstein repair) have replaced older methods. In mesh repairs, a polypropylene mesh reinforces the posterior wall. Recurrence rate is less than with other methods (eg <2% vs 10%). (CI: strangulated hernias, contamination with pus/bowel contents.) Local anaesthetic techniques and day-case 'ambulatory' surgery may halve the price of surgery. This is important because this is one of the most common operations (>100 000 per year in the UK). *Laparoscopic repair* gives similar recurrence rates. Methods include *transabdominal preperitoneal* (TAPP) in which the peritoneum is entered and the hernia repaired, and *totally extraperitoneal* (TEP), which decreases the risk of visceral injury. For benefits of laparoscopic surgery see p568.

Return to work Will depend upon surgical approach and patient—discuss this preoperatively. Rest for 4wks and convalescence over 8wks with open approaches, but laparoscopic repairs may allow return to manual work (and driving) after ≤2wks if all is well.

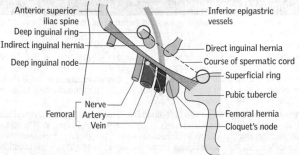

Fig 13.32 Anatomy of the inguinal canal. *Floor:* inguinal ligament and lacunar ligament medially. *Roof:* fibres of transversalis, internal oblique. *Anterior:* external oblique aponeurosis + internal oblique for the lateral ¼. *Posterior:* laterally, transversalis fascia; medially, conjoint tendon.

The contents of the inguinal canal in the male

- The external spermatic fascia (from external oblique), cremasteric fascia (from internal oblique and transverses abdominus), and internal spermatic fascia (from transversalis fascia) covering the cord.
- The spermatic cord:
  - Vas deferens, obliterated processus vaginalis, and lymphatics.
  - Arteries to the vas, cremaster, and testis.
  - The pampiniform plexus and the venous equivalent of the above.
  - The genital branch of the genitofemoral nerve and sympathetic nerves.
- The ilioinguinal nerve, which enters the inguinal canal via the anterior wall and runs anteriorly to the cord.

NB: in the female the round ligament of the uterus is in place of the male structures. A hydrocele of the canal of Nuck is the female equivalent of a hydrocele of the cord.

Colorectal carcinoma

This is the 4th most common cancer and 2nd most common cause of UK cancer death (17 000 deaths/yr). Usually adenocarcinoma. 86% of presentations are in those >60yrs old. Lifetime UK incidence: ♂ = 1:15; ♀ = 1:19.

Predisposing factors Neoplastic polyps (see BOX & p516); IBD (UC and Crohn's, p258); genetic predisposition (<8%), eg FAP and HNPCC; diet (low-fibre; ↑red and processed meat); ↑alcohol; smoking; previous cancer. **Prevention** While routine chemoprevention is not currently recommended due to gastrointestinal SE, aspirin ≥75mg/d reduces incidence and mortality.

Presentation Depends on site: **Left-sided** Bleeding/mucus PR; altered bowel habit or obstruction (25%); tenesmus; mass PR (60%). **Right-sided** ↓Weight; ↓Hb; abdominal pain; obstruction less likely. **Either** Abdominal mass; perforation; haemorrhage; fistula. See p517 for a guide to urgent referral criteria. See fig 13.33 for distribution.

Tests FBC (microcytic anaemia); faecal immunohistochemistry (see BOX); sigmoidoscopy or colonoscopy (figs 6.9 & 6.10, p245), which can be done 'virtually' by CT (fig 16.32, p727); LFT; liver MRI/US (metastases). CEA (p527) may be used to monitor disease and effectiveness of treatment. If family history of FAP, refer for DNA test once >15yrs old.

Spread Local, lymphatic, by blood (liver, lung, bone) or transcoelomic. The TNM system (Tumour, Node, Metastases, see BOX 'Staging', p522) is used to stage disease and is preferred to the older Dukes' classification. It is complex with several important subtypes, but in essence, stage 1 and 2 disease is localized to the more superficial bowel layers without nodal involvement or metastases. Lymph node involvement defines stage 3 disease whilst the presence of any metastases marks stage 4.

Surgery Aims to cure and may ↑ survival times by up to 50%. In elective surgery, anastomosis is typically achieved at the 1st operation. *Laparoscopic surgery* has revolutionized surgery for colon cancer. It is as safe as open surgery and there is no difference in overall survival or disease recurrence. • Right hemicolectomy for caecal, ascending, or proximal transverse colon tumours. • Left hemicolectomy for tumours in distal transverse or descending colon. • Sigmoid colectomy for sigmoid tumours. • Anterior resection for low sigmoid or high rectal tumours. • Abdominoperineal (AP) resection for tumours low in the rectum (≤8cm from anus): permanent colostomy and removal of rectum and anus. • Hartmann's procedure in emergency bowel obstruction, perforation, or palliation (p582). • Transanal endoscopic microsurgery allows local excision through a wide proctoscope for localized rectal disease. *Endoscopic stenting* should be considered for palliation in malignant obstruction and as a bridge to surgery in acute obstruction. Stenting ↓ need for colostomy, has less complications than emergency surgery, shortens intensive care and total hospital stays, and prevents unnecessary operations. Surgery with liver resection may be curative if single-lobe hepatic metastases and no extrahepatic spread.

Radiotherapy Mostly used in palliation for colonic cancer. It is occasionally used pre-op in rectal cancer to allow resection. Post-op radiotherapy is only used in patients with rectal tumours at high risk of local recurrence (negative resection margins are more difficult to achieve).

Chemotherapy Neoadjuvant chemotherapy is indicated only for locally advanced rectal cancer. Adjuvant chemotherapy for stage 3 disease has been shown to reduce disease recurrence by 30% and mortality by 25%. Benefits for stage 2 disease are more marginal and warrant an individualized approach. The FOLFOX regimen has become standard (fluorouracil, folinic acid, and oxaliplatin). Chemotherapy is also used in palliation of metastatic disease (most patients who present with metastases are not surgical candidates). **Biological therapies** Improve survival in selected patients when added to combination therapy in non-operable metastatic disease: bevacizumab (anti-VEGF) or cetuximab (anti-EGFR) in KRAS wild-type cancer, trastuzumab in HER2 overexpressors, larotrectinib or entrectinib (TRK inhibitors) in tropomyosin receptor kinase fusion-positive cancer.

Prognosis Survival is dependent on age and stage; for stage 1 disease, 5yr survival is ~90% but this drops to just 15% with diagnosis at stage 4, hence the imperative for effective screening (see BOX 'Polyps').

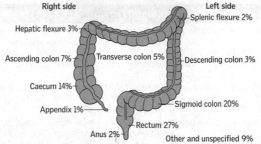

Fig 13.33 Distribution of colorectal carcinomas. These are averages: black females tend to have more proximal neoplasms. White males tend to have more distal neoplasms.

Polyps, the challenges of screening, and the NHS

Polyps are growths that appear above the mucosa and can be inflammatory, hamartomatous, or neoplastic. Left *in situ*, polyps carry a risk of malignant transformation that will relate to size and histology (tubular or villous adenomas, esp. if >2cm). Patients with polyps may have no symptoms and thus a colonoscopy is required to detect and remove. Colonoscopy allows the opportunity to detect colorectal cancer at an earlier stage when treatment may be more effective.

However, population-based colonoscopic screening is costly and the test does not appear to impact deaths from right-sided cancers (rarer and harder to detect, fig 13.33). An NHS one-off screening flexible sigmoidoscopy screen at age 55yrs has been abandoned in favour of the NHS Bowel Cancer Screening Programme (introduced in 2006). This offers colonoscopy to all men and women aged 60–74yrs (from age 50yrs in Scotland, and soon to be expanded in England, currently age 56yrs) who test positive for faecal occult blood (FOB) using a home faecal immunohistochemical test kit performed every 2yrs. The relative risk of death from colorectal cancer in patients undergoing screening is reduced by 16%. An increase in incidence rates since 2006 for people aged 60–69yrs was almost certainly due to earlier detection through the screening programme (10% of all cases are diagnosed by screening), but rates have again started to fall.

Carcinoma of the oesophagus

Incidence 2–8/100 000/yr UK; stable, as the decreasing incidence of squamous cell carcinoma (proximal) is balanced by a rapid increase in oesophageal adenocarcinoma (distal). **Risk factors** Diet, alcohol excess, smoking, achalasia, reflux oesophagitis ± Barrett's oesophagus (p251); obesity, hot drinks, nitrosamine exposure, Plummer–Vinson syndrome (p246). ♂:♀ ≈ 5:1.

Presentation Dysphagia; ↓weight; retrosternal chest pain. **Signs from the upper third of the oesophagus** Hoarseness; Horner's syndrome; cough (may be paroxysmal if aspiration pneumonia). ∆∆ See 'Dysphagia', p246.

Tests Oesophagoscopy with biopsy is the investigation of choice ± EUS, CT/MRI for staging (fig 13.34), or laparoscopy if significant infra-diaphragmatic component.

Treatment Survival rates are poor with or without treatment. Initial endoscopic resection can be performed for more superficial, localized disease, but combination with chemoradiotherapy (often neoadjuvant, ie pre-op, plus adjuvant, ie post-op) is necessary for more advanced disease. *Radical curative oesophagectomy* for thoracic oesophageal cancer incorporates thoracic oesophagectomy, cervical oesophagogastrostomy, lymph node dissection, and jejunostomy feeding tube placement. If surgery is *not* indicated, then chemoradiotherapy (carboplatin + paclitaxel) may be better than radiotherapy alone. Palliation in advanced disease aims to restore swallowing with chemo/radiotherapy, stenting, and laser use.

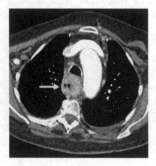

Fig 13.34 Axial CT of the chest after IV contrast medium showing concentric thickening of the oesophagus (arrow); the diagnosis here is oesophageal carcinoma. Loss of the fatty plane around the oesophagus suggests local invasion. Anterior to the oesophagus is the trachea and next to it is the arch of the aorta.

Image courtesy of Dr Stephen Golding.

13 Surgery

Incidence of adenocarcinoma at the gastro-oesophageal junction is increasing in the West, though incidence of distal and gastric body carcinoma has fallen sharply. It remains a tumour notable for its gloomy prognosis and non-specific presentation.

Incidence 10/100 000/yr in the UK, but there are unexplained wide geographical variations; it is especially common in Japan, as well as Eastern Europe, China, and South America. ♂:♀ ≈ 3:1. **Risk factors** Pernicious anaemia, blood group A, *H. pylori* (p248), atrophic gastritis, adenomatous polyps, obesity, smoking, diet (high nitrate, high salt, pickling, low vitamin C), nitrosamine exposure.

Pathology Lauren classification (microscopic): *intestinal* (glandular formation, more common in older males, better prognosis), *diffuse* (de novo formation from gastric mucous cells, 'signet ring' histology, ♂ = ♀ and affects younger individuals).

Presentation Symptoms Often non-specific. Dyspepsia (p55; age ≥55yrs with treatment-refractory symptoms demands investigation). ↓weight, vomiting, dysphagia, anaemia. *Signs* suggesting incurable disease: epigastric mass, hepatomegaly; jaundice, ascites (p596); large left supraclavicular (Virchow's) node (= Troisier's sign); acanthosis nigricans (p560). Most patients in the West present with locally advanced (inoperable) or metastatic disease. *Spread* is local, lymphatic, blood-borne, and transcoelomic, eg to ovaries (Krukenberg tumour).

Tests Gastroscopy + multiple ulcer edge biopsies. ►*Aim to biopsy all gastric ulcers as even malignant ulcers may appear to heal on drug treatment.* Endoscopic ultrasound (EUS) can evaluate depth of invasion; CT/MRI helps staging. Staging laparoscopy is recommended for locally advanced tumours. Cytology of peritoneal washings can help identify peritoneal metastases.

Treatment See p608 for a description of surgical resections. Early gastric cancers may be resectable endoscopically (endoscopic mucosal resection). Partial gastrectomy may suffice for more advanced distal tumours. If proximal, total gastrectomy may be needed. Stages T2 or higher are treated with neoadjuvant and adjuvant chemotherapy (eg epirubicin, cisplatin, and fluorouracil) which increases survival. Surgical palliation is often needed for obstruction, pain, or haemorrhage. In locally advanced and metastatic disease, chemotherapy increases quality of life and survival. Targeted therapies have an increasing role, eg trastuzumab for HER2-positive tumours.

5yr survival From 65% (T1-2, N0, M0) to 5% (M1). This has improved significantly, but still remains relatively poor as most patients present with advanced stage disease.

Bile duct and gallbladder cancers

All are rare, have an overall poor prognosis, and are difficult to diagnose. They account for ~3% of all GI cancers worldwide, but there is geographical variation (↑ in north-east Thailand, Japan, Korea, and Eastern Europe). Most are adenocarcinomas. Primary sclerosing cholangitis (p278) is the commonest predisposing factor in the West.

Presentation Varies according to location and may include obstructive jaundice, pruritus, abdominal pain, weight loss, and anorexia.

Investigations US, CT, and ERCP. MRI has a role for determining extent of invasion in bile duct cancers.

Treatment
* *Bile duct cancer:* surgical resection is the only potentially curative treatment yet ~80% present with inoperable disease. Palliation includes biliary stenting and chemotherapy.
* *Gallbladder cancer:* again, radical surgery is the only chance of cure. Patients with a calcified ('porcelain') gallbladder have an increased risk of cancer—prophylactic surgery should be considered. Palliative treatment of inoperable disease includes biliary stenting and chemotherapy.

13 Surgery

Epidemiology ≈3% of all malignancy; ~10 000 deaths/yr (UK). UK incidence is rising.

Typical patient ♂ >70yrs old.

Risk factors Smoking, alcohol, carcinogens, DM, chronic pancreatitis, obesity, and possibly a high-fat and red or processed meat diet. 10% have a genetic basis, more than previously thought (eg BRCA mutations, Peutz–Jeghers syndrome p694).

Pathology 95% ductal adenocarcinoma (metastasize early; present late). 60% arise in the pancreas head, 25% in the body, 15% tail. A few arise in the ampulla of Vater (ampullary tumour) or pancreatic islet cells (insulinoma, gastrinoma, glucagonomas, somatostatinomas (p217), VIPomas); both have a better prognosis.

Precursor lesions Pancreatic intraepithelial neoplasia (PanIN) is a precursor to invasive ductal adenocarcinoma and is extremely common in the elderly (>50% over 50yrs). Progression rates are estimated to be <1%, but p16 and KRAS2 gene mutations herald transformation (~95% established cases have mutations in both).

The patient Tumours in the head of the pancreas present with *painless obstructive jaundice*. 75% of tumours in the body and tail present with epigastric pain (radiates to back and relieved by sitting forward). Either may cause anorexia, weight loss, diabetes, or acute pancreatitis. **Rarer features** Thrombophlebitis migrans (eg an arm vein becomes swollen and red, then a leg vein); ↑Ca²⁺; marantic endocarditis; portal hypertension (splenic vein thrombosis); nephrosis (renal vein metastases). **Signs** Jaundice + palpable gallbladder (Courvoisier's 'law', p268); epigastric mass; hepatomegaly; splenomegaly; lymphadenopathy; ascites.

Tests Blood Cholestatic jaundice. ↑CA 19-9 (p527) is non-specific, but helps assess prognosis. **Imaging** US or CT can show a pancreatic mass ± dilated biliary tree ± hepatic metastases. They can guide biopsy and help staging prior to surgery/stent insertion. ERCP/MRCP (p726) show biliary tree anatomy and may localize the site of obstruction. EUS (endoscopic sonography) is an adjunct for diagnosis and staging.

Treatment Most ductal cancers present with metastatic disease; <20% are suitable for radical surgery. **Surgery** Resection (pancreatoduodenectomy: Whipple's, see fig 13.35) is a major undertaking best considered only where no distant metastases and where vascular invasion is still at a minimum. Post-op morbidity is high (mortality <5%); non-curative resection confers no survival benefit. **Laparoscopic excision** Tail lesions are easiest. **Post-op chemotherapy** Delays disease progression. **Palliation of jaundice** Endoscopic or percutaneous stent insertion may help jaundice and anorexia. Rarely, palliative bypass surgery is done for duodenal obstruction or unsuccessful ERCP. **Pain** Disabling pain may need big doses of opiates (p525), or radiotherapy. Coeliac plexus infiltration with alcohol may be done at the time of surgery, or percutaneously. Referral to a palliative care team is essential.

Prognosis Often dismal. Mean survival <6 months. 5yr survival: 3%. Overall 5yr survival after Whipple's procedure 5–14%. Prognosis is better if: tumour <3cm; no nodes involved; −ve resection margins at surgery; ampullary or islet cell tumours.

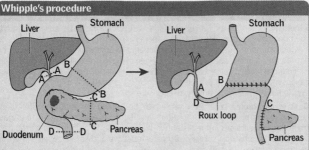

Whipple's procedure

Liver · Stomach · Liver · Stomach

B

A···A · A

C B · B

C · D

Duodenum D····D··C · Pancreas · Roux loop · Pancreas

Fig 13.35 Whipple's procedure may be used for removing masses in the head of the pancreas—typically from pancreatic carcinoma or, rarely, a carcinoid tumour.[5]

13 Surgery

▶Indications for gastric surgery include gastric cancer (p611) and perforated/ haemorrhaging peptic ulcers. Medical therapy (p248) for peptic ulcers has made elective surgery exceedingly rare/redundant. ▶▶*Emergency surgery* may be needed for haemorrhage or perforation. Haemorrhage is usually treated by under-running the bleeding ulcer base or excision of the ulcer. If the former is done, then a biopsy should be taken to exclude malignancy. Perforation is usually managed by excision of the hole for histology, then closure.

Gastric carcinoma Localized disease may be treated by curative gastrectomy. Lesions in the proximal third or extensive infiltrative disease require total gastrectomy, while lesions in the distal two-thirds can be treated with a partial gastrectomy. Laparoscopic surgery may be as effective and safe as open surgery in specialist centres.

Surgery
Billroth I Partial gastrectomy with simple gastroduodenal re-anastomosis.

Billroth II (aka Polya) gastrectomy (fig 13.36) Partial gastrectomy with gastrojejunal anastomosis. The duodenal stump is oversewn (leaving a blind afferent loop), and anastomosis is achieved by a longitudinal incision into the proximal jejunum.

Roux-en-Y (fig 13.37) Following total or subtotal gastrectomy, the proximal duodenal stump is oversewn, the proximal jejunum is divided from the distal duodenum and connects with the oesophagus (or proximal stomach after subtotal gastrectomy), while the distal duodenum is connected to the distal jejunum.

Lymph node clearance is a controversial area. RCTs and meta-analyses suggest there may be limited benefit and increased morbidity associated with extended lymph node resections (D_2 or D_3) over resection limited to the perigastric nodes (D_1).

Physical complications of gastrectomy
- **Abdominal fullness** Feeling of early satiety (± discomfort and distension) improving with time. Advise to take small, frequent meals.
- **Afferent loop syndrome** Post-gastrectomy (eg Billroth II), the afferent loop may fill with bile after a meal, causing upper abdominal pain and bilious vomiting. This is difficult to treat—but often improves with time.
- **Diarrhoea** May be disabling after vagotomy. Codeine phosphate may help.
- **Gastric tumour** A rare complication of any surgery which ↓ acid production.
- **↑Amylase** If with abdominal pain, this may indicate afferent loop obstruction after Billroth II surgery and requires emergency surgery.

Metabolic complications
- **Dumping syndrome** Fainting and sweating after eating due to food of high osmotic potential being dumped in the jejunum, causing oligaemia from rapid fluid shifts. 'Late dumping' is due to rebound hypoglycaemia and occurs 1–3h after meals. Both tend to improve with time but may be helped by eating less sugar, and more guar gum and pectin (slows glucose absorption). Acarbose may also help to reduce the early hyperglycaemic stimulus to insulin secretion.
- **Weight loss** Often due to poor calorie intake.
- **Bacterial overgrowth ± malabsorption** (Blind loop syndrome.) May occur.
- **Anaemia** Usually from lack of iron, hypochlorhydria, and stomach resection. B_{12} levels are frequently low but megaloblastic anaemia is rare.
- **Osteomalacia** There may be pseudofractures which look like metastases.

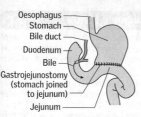

Oesophagus
Stomach
Bile duct
Duodenum
Bile
Gastrojejunostomy
(stomach joined
to jejunum)
Jejunum

Fig 13.36 Billroth II.

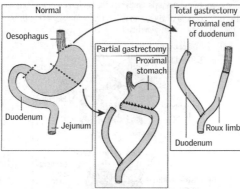

Fig 13.37 The Roux-en-Y reconstruction.

Theodor Billroth

Theodor Billroth was a surgeon of German–Austrian origin, whose name lives on as a set of operations on the stomach. He was a pioneer of abdominal surgery and the use of aseptic techniques, performing the first Billroth I procedure in 1881 for the resection of a pyloric gastric carcinoma. Among the many of his remarkable achievements is included the first laryngectomy. He was also a talented musician (a close friend of Brahms) and a dedicated educator with something of a realist's view of the world:

'The pleasure of a physician is little, the gratitude of patients is rare, and even rarer is material reward, but these things will never deter the student who feels the call within him.' Theodor Billroth (1829–94).

Fundoplication for gastro-oesophageal reflux

Laparoscopic fundoplication is the surgical procedure of choice when symptoms of GORD are refractory to medical therapy *and* there is severe reflux (confirmed by pH monitoring)—see p250. Symptoms may be complicated by a hiatus hernia, which is repaired during the procedure.

Surgery The defect in the diaphragm is repaired by tightening the crura. Reflux is prevented by wrapping the gastric fundus around the lower oesophageal sphincter—see fig 13.38. There are various types of procedure, eg Nissen (360° wrap), Toupet (270° posterior wrap), Watson (anterior hemi-fundoplication). Laparoscopic surgery is at least as effective at controlling reflux as open surgery but with a lower mortality and morbidity. Wound infections and respiratory complications are also more common in open surgery, though the incidence of dysphagia is similar for the two procedures—but see p568.

Complications Dysphagia (if the wrap is too tight), 'gas-bloat syndrome' (inability to belch/vomit), and new-onset diarrhoea.

13 Surgery

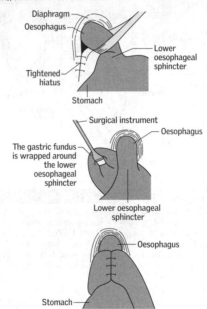

Fig 13.38 Laparoscopic Nissen fundoplication.

Oesophageal rupture

Causes • *Iatrogenic*, eg endoscopy/biopsy/dilatation (accounts for 85–90% of perforations). • *Trauma*, eg penetrating injury/ingestion of foreign body. • *Carcinoma*. • *Boerhaave syndrome*—rupture due to violent vomiting. • *Corrosive ingestion*.

Clinical features Odynophagia, tachypnoea, dyspnoea, fever, shock, surgical emphysema (a crackling sensation felt on palpating the skin over the chest or neck caused by air tracking from the lungs. ∆∆ Pneumothorax).

℞ Iatrogenic perforations are less prone to mediastinitis and sepsis and may be managed conservatively with NG tube, PPI, and antibiotics. Others require resuscitation, PPI, antibiotics, antifungals, and surgery (debridement of mediastinum and placement of T-tube for drainage and formation of a controlled oesophago-cutaneous fistula).

There are three main types of bowel ischaemia: ►AF with abdominal pain should always prompt thoughts of mesenteric ischaemia.

1 Acute mesenteric ischaemia Almost always involves the small bowel and may follow superior mesenteric artery (SMA; fig 13.39) thrombosis (~35%) or embolism (~35%), mesenteric vein thrombosis (~5%; younger patients with hypercoagulable states), or hypovolaemia (~20%; usually reflects poor cardiac output). Other causes include trauma, vasculitis (p554), radiotherapy, or strangulation (volvulus or hernia, p604). *Presentation* is a classical clinical triad: ►acute severe abdominal pain; no/minimal abdominal signs; rapid hypovolaemia→shock. Pain tends to be constant, central, or around the RIF. **Tests** There may be ↑Hb (due to plasma loss), ↑WCC, modestly raised plasma amylase, and a persistent metabolic acidosis (high lactate). Early on, the abdominal x-ray shows a 'gasless' abdomen. CT/MR may show evidence of ischaemia with CT/MR angiography or formal arteriography if doubt remains. Often the diagnosis is made on finding a nasty, necrotic bowel at laparotomy. **Treatment** The main life-threatening complications secondary to acute mesenteric ischaemia are **A** septic peritonitis and **B** progression of a systemic inflammatory response syndrome (SIRS) to multi-organ failure, mediated by bacterial translocation across the dying gut wall. Resuscitation with fluid, antibiotics (eg piperacillin/tazobactam, see table 9.3, p382), and, usually, LMWH/heparin are required. If arteriography is done, thrombolytics may be infused locally via the catheter. At surgery, dead bowel must be removed. Revascularization may be attempted on potentially viable bowel but it is a difficult process and often needs a 2nd laparotomy. **Prognosis** Poor for arterial thrombosis and non-occlusive disease (<40% survive), though not so bad for venous and embolic ischaemia.

2 Chronic mesenteric ischaemia (AKA intestinal angina.) The triad of severe, colicky post-prandial abdominal pain ('gut claudication'), ↓weight (eating hurts), and an upper abdominal bruit may be present ± PR bleeding, malabsorption, and N&V. Typically brought about through a combination of a low-flow state with atheroma (95% due to diffuse atherosclerotic disease in all three mesenteric arteries). It is rare and difficult to diagnose. **Tests** CT angiography and contrast-enhanced MR angiography are replacing traditional angiography. **Treatment** Once diagnosis is confirmed, surgery should be considered due to the ongoing risk of acute infarction. Percutaneous transluminal angioplasty and stent insertion has replaced open revascularization. It is associated with less post-operative morbidity and mortality, but has higher restenosis rates.

3 Chronic colonic ischaemia (AKA ischaemic colitis.) Usually follows low flow in the inferior mesenteric artery (IMA) territory and ranges from mild ischaemia to gangrenous colitis. **Presentation** Lower left-sided abdominal pain ± bloody diarrhoea. **Tests** CT may be helpful but lower GI endoscopy is 'gold-standard'. **Treatment** Usually conservative with fluid replacement and antibiotics. Most recover but subsequent development of ischaemic strictures is common. Gangrenous ischaemic colitis (presenting with peritonitis and hypovolaemic shock) requires prompt resuscitation followed by resection of the affected bowel and stoma formation. Mortality is high.

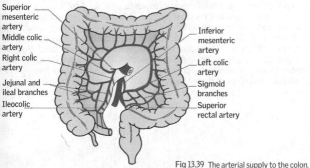

Fig 13.39 The arterial supply to the colon.

Severe obesity is increasing in prevalence worldwide and is associated with type 2 diabetes mellitus (T2DM); hypertension; ischaemic heart disease; sleep apnoea; osteoarthritis; and depression. Bariatric surgery has become very successful at weight reduction, symptom improvement, and improving quality of life. Surgery increases life expectancy by around 3 years (but may not prolong survival in high-risk men).

Indications According to NICE guidelines,⁶ weight-loss surgery in adults should be considered if *all* the following criteria are met:

1 BMI ≥40 (or ≥35 with significant comorbidities that could improve with ↓weight).
2 Failure of non-surgical management to achieve and maintain clinically beneficial weight loss for 6 months.
3 Fitness for surgery and anaesthesia.
4 Intensive management in tier 3 service (provides guidance on diet, physical activity, and psychosocial concerns, as well as lifelong medical monitoring).
5 The patient must be well informed and motivated.

If BMI ≥50, or in newly diagnosed T2DM with BMI ≥30, surgery is recommended as first-line treatment.

Comparison with medical therapy Surgery is more effective in achieving weight loss than non-surgical management and weight loss is more likely to be maintained in the longer term. Adverse events are more common following surgery, and vary from one procedure to another.

Procedures There are two main mechanisms causing weight loss: 1 Restriction of calorie intake by reducing stomach capacity. 2 Malabsorption of nutrients by reducing the length of functional small bowel. NB: this also affects the levels of circulating gut peptides (eg PYY and GLP-1), which are thought to play a role in the mechanism of satiety and weight loss. Choose surgical intervention jointly with patient:

- **Laparoscopic adjustable gastric banding (LAGB)** This restrictive technique creates a pre-stomach pouch by placing a silicone band around the top of the stomach, which serves as a new smaller stomach. The band can be adjusted by addition or removal of saline through a subcutaneous port (fig 13.40). LAGB is associated with improvements in comorbidities and quality of life. Weight loss is slower and less than with gastric bypass but there is lower mortality and fewer complications. Relatively non-invasive and band removal possible. *Complications:* pouch enlargement, band slip, band erosion, and port infection/breakage.

- **Sleeve gastrectomy** (fig 13.41) Involves division of the stomach vertically, reducing it in size by about 75%. The pyloric valve at the bottom of the stomach is left intact so function and digestion are unaltered. The procedure is not reversible and may be a first stage for progression to Roux-en-Y gastric bypass or duodenal switch in very obese patients where a single-stage procedure would be technically difficult or unsafe.

- **Roux-en-Y gastric bypass** (fig 13.42) Laparoscopic or open. A portion of the jejunum is attached to a small stomach pouch to allow food to bypass the distal stomach, duodenum, and proximal jejunum. It can be performed laparoscopically and works by both restriction and malabsorption. Mean excess weight loss at 5 years is 62.8%. Current evidence demonstrates greater weight loss, greater resolution of comorbidities, and lower reoperation rates compared to LAGB. *Complications:* micronutrient deficiency (requires vitamin supplementation and lifelong follow-up/blood tests), dumping syndrome, wound infection, hernias, malabsorption, diarrhoea, and a mortality of <0.5% (at experienced centres).

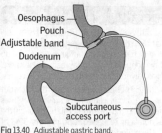

Fig 13.40 Adjustable gastric band.

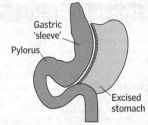

Fig 13.41 Vertical sleeve gastrectomy.

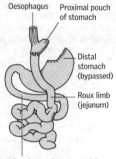

Fig 13.42 Gastric bypass.

13 Surgery

A GI *diverticulum* is an outpouching of the gut wall, usually at sites of entry of perforating arteries. *Diverticulosis* means that diverticula are present, and *diverticular disease* implies they are symptomatic. *Diverticulitis* refers to inflammation of a diverticulum. Diverticula can be acquired or congenital and may occur elsewhere, but the most important are acquired colonic diverticula, to which this topic refers.

Pathology Most within sigmoid colon with 95% of complications at this site, but right-sided and massive single diverticula can occur. High intraluminal pressures (due, perhaps, to lack of dietary fibre) force the mucosa to herniate through the muscle layers of the gut at weak points adjacent to penetrating vessels. 30% of Westerners have diverticulosis by age 60. The majority are asymptomatic.

Diagnosis Diverticula are a common incidental finding at colonoscopy (fig 6.13, p245). CT abdomen is best to confirm acute diverticulitis and can identify extent of disease and any complications (eg colovesical fistulae). AXR may identify obstruction or free air (perforation).

Diverticular disease Altered bowel habit ± left-sided colic relieved by defecation; nausea and flatulence. High-fibre diets do not help symptoms; try antispasmodics, eg mebeverine 135mg/8h PO. Surgical resection occasionally resorted to.

Diverticulitis Features above + pyrexia, ↑WCC, ↑CRP/ESR, a tender colon ± localized or generalized peritonism. Mild attacks can be treated at home with bowel rest (fluids only) ± antibiotics. If fluids and pain not tolerated, admit for analgesia, NBM, IV fluids, and IV antibiotics. Most attacks settle but complications include abscess formation (necessitating percutaneous CT-guided drainage), or perforation. ►Beware diverticulitis in immunocompromised patients (eg on steroids) who often have few symptoms and may present late.

Surgery The need for surgery is reflected by the degree of infective complications:

Stage 1	Pericolic or mesenteric abscess	Surgery rarely needed
Stage 2	Walled off or pelvic abscess	May resolve without surgery
Stage 3	Generalized purulent peritonitis	Surgery required
Stage 4	Generalized faecal peritonitis	Surgery required

Indications for elective surgery include stenosis, fistulae, or recurrent bleeding.

Complications ►►**Perforation** There is ileus, peritonitis ± shock. Mortality: 40%. Manage as for an acute abdomen. At laparotomy a Hartmann's procedure may be performed (p582). Primary anastomosis is possible in selected patients. Emergency laparoscopic management is an emerging alternative.

- *Haemorrhage* is usually sudden and painless. It is a common cause of big rectal bleeds (p621). Embolization (at angiography) or colonic resection only necessary if ongoing massive bleeding and colonoscopic haemostasis has been unsuccessful.
- *Fistulae:* enterocolic, colovaginal, or colovesical (pneumaturia ± intractable UTIs). Treatment is surgical, eg colonic resection.
- *Abscesses:* eg with swinging fever, leucocytosis, and localizing signs, eg boggy rectal mass (pelvic abscess—drain rectally). If no localizing signs, remember the aphorism: *pus somewhere, pus nowhere = pus under the diaphragm*. A subphrenic abscess is a horrible way to die, so do an urgent ultrasound. Antibiotics ± ultrasound/CT-guided drainage may be needed.
- *Post-infective strictures* may form in the sigmoid colon.

Rectal bleeding—an acute management plan

Causes Diverticulitis, colorectal cancer, haemorrhoids, IBD, perianal disease, angiodysplasia (submucosal arteriovenous malformations, typically elderly). Rarities: trauma, ischaemia colitis, radiation proctitis, aorto-enteric fistula.

An acute management plan For this common surgical event:

▸▸*ABC* resuscitation, if necessary.

▸▸*History and examination*.

▸▸*Blood tests:* FBC, U&E, LFT, clotting, CRP, group and save—await Hb result before crossmatching unless unstable and bleeding.

▸▸*Imaging:* may only need plain AXR, but if there are signs of perforation (eg sepsis, peritonism) or if there is cardiorespiratory comorbidity, then request an erect CXR.

▸▸*Fluid management:* insert 2 cannulae (≥18G) into the antecubital fossae. Insert a urinary catheter if there is a suspicion of haemodynamic compromise—there is no absolute indication, but remember that you are weighing up the risks and benefits. Give crystalloid as replacement and maintenance IV. Blood transfusion only if significant blood loss (**table 13.10**, p599).

▸▸*Clotting:* withhold ± reverse anticoagulation and antiplatelet agents (p347).

▸▸*Antibiotics:* may occasionally be required if there is evidence of sepsis or perforation, eg piperacillin/tazobactam 4.5g/8h IV.

▸▸*Keep bedbound:* the patient may feel the need to get out of bed to pass stool, but this could be another large bleed, resulting in collapse if they try to walk. ▸Don't allow them to mobilize and inform the nursing staff of this.

▸▸*Start a stool chart:* to monitor volume and frequency of motions. Send a sample for MC&S (×3 if known to have compromising comorbidity such as IBD).

▸▸*Diet:* keep on clear fluids so that they can have something, yet the colon will be as clear as possible if colonoscopy required.

▸▸*Interventions:* if bleeding not settling with conservative management. *Angiography* may allow localization of bleeding (eg sigmoid diverticulum or right-sided angiodysplasia) as well as therapeutic embolization; CT *angiography* is a non-invasive alternative (without interventional options); *colonoscopy* may permit endoscopic haemostasis.

▸▸*Surgery:* the main indication for this is unremitting, massive bleeding that is not controlled by other means.

Pruritus ani Itch occurs if the anus is moist/soiled; fissures, incontinence, poor hygiene, tight pants, threadworm, fistula, dermatoses, lichen sclerosis, anxiety, contact dermatitis (perfumed goods). Cause is often unknown. ℞ Avoid scratching, perianal hygiene, avoid foods which loosen stools. Soothing ointment, mild topical corticosteroid if peri-anal inflammation (max 2wks), oral antihistamine for nocturnal itch.

Fissure-in-ano Painful tear in the squamous lining of the lower anal canal—often, if chronic, with a 'sentinel pile' or mucosal tag at the external aspect. 90% are posterior (anterior ones follow parturition). ♂ > ♀. **Causes** Most are due to hard faeces. Spasm may constrict the inferior rectal artery, causing ischaemia, making healing difficult and perpetuating the problem. Rare causes (multiple ± lateral): syphilis; herpes; trauma; Crohn's; anal cancer; psoriasis. Groin nodes suggest a complicating factor (eg immunosuppression/HIV). ℞ 5% lidocaine ointment + GTN ointment (0.2–0.4%) or topical diltiazem (2%); dietary fibre, fluids, stool softener, and hygiene advice. Botulinum toxin injection (2nd line) and topical diltiazem (2%) are at least as effective as GTN with fewer side effects. If conservative measures fail, surgical options include *lateral partial internal sphincterotomy*.

Fistula-in-ano A track communicates between the skin and anal canal/rectum. Blockage of deep intramuscular gland ducts is thought to predispose to the formation of abscesses, which discharge to form the fistula. *Goodsall's rule* determines the path of the fistula track: if anterior, the track is in a straight line (radial); if posterior, the internal opening is *always* at the 6 o'clock position, taking a tortuous course. **Causes** Perianal sepsis, abscesses (see later in topic), Crohn's disease, TB, diverticular disease, rectal carcinoma, immunocompromise. **Tests** MRI; endoanal US scan. ℞ Fistulotomy + excision. High fistulae (involving continence muscles of anus) require 'seton suture' tightened over time to maintain continence; low fistulae are 'laid open' to heal by secondary intention—division of sphincters poses no risk to continence.

Anorectal abscesses Usually caused by gut organisms (rarely staphs or TB). ♂:♀≈1:8. Perianal (~45%), ischiorectal (≤30%), intersphincteric (>20%), supralevator (~5%) (fig 13.43). ℞ Incise & drain under GA. **Associations** DM, Crohn's, malignancy, fistulae.

Perianal haematoma (AKA thrombosed external pile—see p625.) Strictly, it is actually a clotted venous saccule. It appears as a 2–4mm 'dark blueberry' under the skin at the anal margin. It may be evacuated under LA or left to resolve spontaneously.

Pilonidal sinus Obstruction of natal cleft hair follicles ~6cm above the anus. Ingrowing of hair excites a foreign body reaction and may cause secondary tracks to open laterally ± abscesses, with foul-smelling discharge. (Barbers get these between fingers.) ♂:♀≈10:1. Obese Caucasians and those from Asia, the Middle East, and Mediterranean at ↑risk. ℞ Excision of the sinus tract ± primary closure. Consider pre-op antibiotics. Complex tracks can be laid open and packed individually, or skin flaps can be used to cover the defect. Offer hygiene and hair removal advice.

Rectal prolapse The mucosa (partial/type 1), or all layers (complete/type 2—more common), may protrude through the anus. Incontinence in 75%. It is due to a lax sphincter, prolonged straining, and related to chronic neurological and psychological disorders. ℞ *Abdominal approach*: fix rectum to sacrum (rectopexy) ± mesh insertion ± rectosigmoidectomy. Laparoscopic rectopexy is as effective as open repair. *Perineal approach*: Delorme's procedure (resect close to dentate line and suture mucosal boundaries), anal encirclement with a Thiersch wire.

Perianal warts Condylomata acuminata (viral warts) are treated with podophyllotoxin or imiquimod or cryotherapy/surgical excision. Giant condylomata acuminata of Buschke & Loewenstein may evolve into verrucous cancers (low grade, non-metastasizing). Condylomata lata secondary to syphilis is treated with penicillin.

Proctalgia fugax Idiopathic, intense, brief, stabbing/crampy rectal pain, often worse at night. The mainstay of treatment is reassurance. Inhaled salbutamol or topical GTN (0.2–0.4%) or topical diltiazem (2%) may help.

Anal ulcers Consider Crohn's, anal cancer, lymphogranuloma venerum, TB, syphilis.

Skin tags Seldom cause trouble but are easily excised.

Anal cancer

Incidence 1519 new cases of anal cancer in the UK annually (2018).

Risk factors Anoreceptive intercourse; HPV (HPV 16 associated with worse prognosis); HIV.

Histology Squamous cell (85%); rarely basaloid, melanoma, or adenocarcinoma. Anal margin tumours are usually well-differentiated, keratinizing lesions with a good prognosis. Anal canal tumours arise above dentate line, are poorly differentiated and non-keratinizing with a poorer prognosis.

Spread Tumours above the dentate line spread to pelvic lymph nodes; those below spread to the inguinal nodes.

Presentation Bleeding, pain, bowel habit change, pruritus ani, masses, stricture.

ΔΔ Perianal warts; leucoplakia; lichen sclerosis; Bowen's disease; Crohn's disease.

Tests Biopsy of the primary tumour, CT/MRI abdomen + pelvis and PET/CT for staging evaluation.

Treatment Chemo-irradiation (radiotherapy + fluorouracil + mitomycin/cisplatin) is usually preferred to anorectal excision & colostomy; 75% retain normal anal function.

13 Surgery

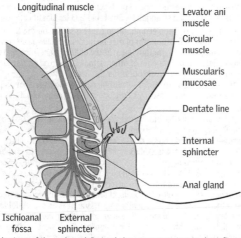

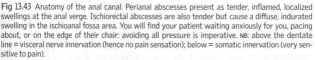

Fig 13.43 Anatomy of the anal canal. Perianal abscesses present as tender, inflamed, localized swellings at the anal verge. Ischiorectal abscesses are also tender but cause a diffuse, indurated swelling in the ischioanal fossa area. You will find your patient waiting anxiously for you, pacing about, or on the edge of their chair: avoiding all pressure is imperative. NB: above the dentate line = visceral nerve innervation (hence no pain sensation); below = somatic innervation (very sensitive to pain).

13 Surgery

Definition Haemorrhoids (≈*running blood* in Greek) are disrupted and dilated anal cushions. The anus is lined mainly by discontinuous masses of spongy vascular tissue—the anal cushions, which contribute to anal closure. Viewed from the lithotomy position, the three anal cushions are at 3, 7, and 11 o'clock (where the three major arteries that feed the vascular plexuses enter the anal canal). They are attached by smooth muscle and elastic tissue, but are prone to displacement and disruption, either singly or together. The effects of gravity (standing), increased anal tone (?stress), and the effects of straining at stool may make them become both bulky and loose, and so to protrude to form piles (Latin *pila*, meaning a ball). They are vulnerable to trauma (eg from hard stools) and bleed readily from the capillaries (bright red blood) of the underlying lamina propria. NB: piles are *not* varicose veins.

As there are no sensory fibres above the dentate line (squamomucosal junction), piles are not painful unless they thrombose when they protrude and are gripped by the anal sphincter, blocking venous return. See fig 13.44.

Differential diagnosis Perianal haematoma; anal fissure; abscess; tumour; proctalgia fugax. ►Never ascribe rectal bleeding to piles without examination or investigation.

Causes Constipation with prolonged straining is a key factor. In many the bowel habit may be normal. Congestion from a pelvic tumour, pregnancy, CCF, or portal hypertension are important in only a minority of cases. ►Elicit red flags in history.

Pathogenesis There is a vicious circle: vascular cushions protrude through a tight anus, become more congested, and hypertrophy to protrude again more readily. These protrusions may then strangulate. See table 13.13 for classification.

Symptoms Bright red rectal bleeding, often coating stools, on the tissue, or dripping into the pan after defecation. There may be mucous discharge and pruritus ani. Severe anaemia may occur. Symptoms such as weight loss, tenesmus, and change in bowel habit should prompt thoughts of other pathology. ►In all rectal bleeding do:
• An abdominal examination to rule out other diseases.
• PR exam: prolapsing piles are obvious. Internal haemorrhoids are not palpable.
• Colonoscopy/flexible sigmoidoscopy to exclude proximal pathology if ≥50 years old.

Treatment
1 **Medical** (1st degree.) ↑Fluid and fibre is key ± topical analgesics & stool softener (bulk forming). Topical steroids for short periods only.
2 **Non-operative** (2nd & 3rd degree, or 1st degree if medical therapy failed.) • *Rubber band ligation.* Cheap, but needs skill. Banding produces an ulcer to anchor the mucosa (SE: bleeding; infection; pain). It has the lowest recurrence rate. • *Sclerosants.* (1st or 2nd degree.) 2mL of 5% phenol in oil is injected into the pile above the dentate line, inducing fibrotic reaction. Recurrence higher (SE: impotence; prostatitis). • *Infra-red coagulation.* Applied to localized areas of piles, it works by coagulating vessels and tethering mucosa to subcutaneous tissue. It is as successful as banding and may be less painful. • *Bipolar diathermy and direct current electrotherapy.* Causes coagulation and fibrosis after local application of heat. Success rates are similar to those of infrared coagulation, and complication rates are low.

3 **Surgery** • *Excisional haemorrhoidectomy* is the most effective treatment (excision of piles ± ligation of vascular pedicles, as day-case surgery, needing ~2wks off work). Scalpel, electrocautery, or laser may be used. •*Stapled haemorrhoidopexy* (procedure for prolapsing haemorrhoids) may result in less pain, a shorter hospital stay, and quicker return to normal activity than conventional surgery. It is used when there is a large internal component, but has a higher recurrence and prolapse rate than excisional. *Surgical complications* include constipation; infection; stricture; bleeding.

Prolapsed, thrombosed piles Analgesia, ice packs, and stool softeners. Pain usually resolves in 2–3wks. Some advocate early surgery.

Table 13.13 Classification of haemorrhoids

1st degree	Remain in the rectum
2nd degree	Prolapse through the anus on defecation but spontaneously reduce
3rd degree	As for 2nd degree but require digital reduction
4th degree	Remain persistently prolapsed

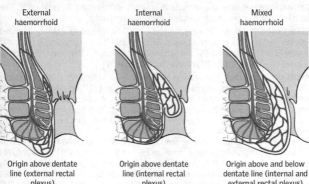

External
haemorrhoid

Internal
haemorrhoid

Mixed
haemorrhoid

Origin above dentate
line (external rectal
plexus)

Origin above dentate
line (internal rectal
plexus)

Origin above and below
dentate line (internal and
external rectal plexus)

Fig 13.44 Internal and external haemorrhoids.

Bile contains cholesterol, bile pigments (from broken down Hb), and phospholipids. If the concentrations vary, different stones may form. **Pigment stones** Small, friable, and irregular. **Causes** Haemolysis. **Cholesterol stones** Large, often solitary. **Causes** ♀, age, obesity (Admirand's triangle: ↑risk of stone if ↓lecithin, ↓bile salts, ↑cholesterol). **Mixed stones** Faceted (calcium salts, pigment, and cholesterol). **Gallstone prevalence** 8% of those over 40yrs. 90% remain asymptomatic. Risk factors for stones becoming symptomatic: smoking; parity.

Biliary colic Gallstones are symptomatic with cystic duct obstruction or if passed into the common bile duct (CBD[9]). RUQ pain (radiates → back) ± jaundice. ℞ Analgesia (see p628), rehydrate, NBM. Elective laparoscopic cholecystectomy (see BOX 'Early or delayed cholecystectomy?'). Do urinalysis, CXR, and ECG.

Acute cholecystitis follows stone or sludge impaction in the neck of the gallbladder (GB[9]), which may cause continuous epigastric or RUQ pain (referred to the right shoulder—see p601), vomiting, fever, local peritonism, or a GB mass. The main difference from *biliary colic* is the inflammatory component (local peritonism, fever, WCC↑; see table 13.14). If the stone moves to the CBD, obstructive jaundice and cholangitis may occur—see BOX 'Complications of gallstones'. *Murphy's sign*: lay 2 fingers over the RUQ; ask patient to breathe in. This causes pain & arrest of inspiration as an inflamed GB impinges on your fingers. It is only +ve if the same test in the LUQ does not cause pain. A *phlegmon* (RUQ mass of inflamed adherent omentum and bowel) may be palpable. **Tests** ↑WCC, US—a thick-walled, shrunken GB (also seen in chronic disease), pericholecystic fluid, stones, CBD (dilated if >6mm). Plain AXR only shows ~10% of gallstones; it may identify a 'porcelain' GB (associated risk of cancer). **Treatment** NBM, pain relief, IVI, and antibiotics, eg *co-amoxiclav* 625mg/8h IV. Laparoscopic cholecystectomy is the treatment of choice for all patients fit for GA. Open surgery is required if there is GB perforation. If elderly or high risk/unsuitable for surgery, consider percutaneous cholecystostomy; cholecystectomy can still be done later. Cholecystostomy is also the preferred treatment for acalculous cholecystitis.

Chronic cholecystitis Chronic inflammation ± colic. 'Flatulent dyspepsia': vague abdominal discomfort, distension, nausea, flatulence, and fat intolerance (fat stimulates cholecystokinin release and GB contraction). US to image stones and assess CBD diameter. MRCP (p726) is used to find CBD stones. ℞ Cholecystectomy. If US shows a dilated CBD with stones, ERCP (p726) + sphincterotomy before surgery. If symptoms persist post-surgery consider hiatus hernia/IBS/peptic ulcer/chronic pancreatitis/tumour.

Other presentations

- **Obstructive jaundice with CBD stones** (See p268.) If LFT worsening, ERCP with sphincterotomy ± biliary trawl, then cholecystectomy may be needed, or open surgery with CBD exploration. If CBD stones are suspected pre-operatively, they should be identified by MRCP (p726).
- **Cholangitis** (Bile duct infection.) Causing RUQ pain, jaundice, and rigors (Charcot's triad, see BOX 'Complications of gallstones'). Treat with, eg piperacillin/tazobactam 4.5g/8h IV.
- **Gallstone ileus** A stone erodes through the GB into the duodenum; it may then obstruct the terminal ileum. AXR shows: air in CBD (= pneumobilia), small bowel fluid levels, and a stone. Duodenal obstruction is rarer (Bouveret's syndrome).
- **Pancreatitis** See p628.
- **Mucocoele/empyema** Obstructed GB fills with mucus (secreted by GB wall)/pus.
- **Silent stones** Do elective surgery on those with sickle cell, immunosuppression (debatably diabetes) as well as all calcified/porcelain GBS.
- **Mirizzi's syndrome** A stone in the GB presses on the bile duct causing jaundice.
- **Gallbladder necrosis** Rare because of dual blood supply (hepatic artery via cystic artery, and from small branches of the hepatic artery in the GB fossa).
- **Other** Causes of cholecystitis and biliary symptoms other than gallstones are rare. Consider infection (typhoid, cryptosporidiosis, and brucellosis); cholecystokinin release; parenteral nutrition; anatomical abnormality; polyarteritis nodosa (p554).

9 Common abbreviations used in this section: CBD, common bile duct; GB, gallbladder.

Complications of gallstones

In the gallbladder & cystic duct
* Biliary colic
* Acute and chronic cholecystitis
* Mucocoele
* Empyema
* Carcinoma
* Mirizzi's syndrome.

In the bile ducts
* Obstructive jaundice
* Cholangitis
* Pancreatitis.

In the gut
* Gallstone ileus.

Table 13.14 Biliary colic, cholecystitis, or cholangitis?

	RUQ pain	Fever/↑WCC	Jaundice
Biliary colic	✓	X	X
Acute cholecystitis	✓	✓	X
Cholangitis	✓	✓	✓

Early or delayed cholecystectomy?

For acute cholecystitis Laparoscopic cholecystectomy for acute cholecystitis has traditionally been performed 6–12wks after the acute episode due to anticipated increased mortality and conversion to open procedure. Early laparoscopic cholecystectomy, within 7d of symptom onset, is now the treatment of choice. Early surgery reduces the duration of hospital admission compared with delayed surgery, but does not reduce mortality or complications. Up to one-quarter of people scheduled for delayed surgery may require urgent operations because of recurrent or worsening symptoms.

For biliary colic Patients with biliary colic due to gallstones waiting for an elective laparoscopic cholecystectomy may develop significant complications, such as acute pancreatitis (p628) during the waiting period. One high-bias trial found early laparoscopic cholecystectomy (within 24h of an acute episode) decreased potential complications that may develop during the wait for elective surgery.

This unpredictable disease (mortality ~12%) is characterized by self-perpetuating pancreatic enzyme-mediated autodigestion; oedema and fluid shifts cause hypovolaemia, as extracellular fluid is trapped in the gut, peritoneum, and retroperitoneum (worsened by vomiting). Although pancreatitis is mild in 80% of cases; 20% develop severe complicated and life-threatening disease: progression may be rapid from mild oedema to necrotizing pancreatitis. ~50% of cases that advance to necrosis are further complicated by infection.

Causes The one mnemonic we can all agree on: 'GET SMASHED'. **G**allstones (~40%), **E**thanol (~30%), **T**rauma (~1.5%), **S**teroids, **M**umps, **A**utoimmune (PAN), **S**corpion venom, **H**yperlipidaemia, hypothermia, hypercalcaemia, **E**RCP (~5%) and emboli, **D**rugs. Also pregnancy and neoplasia or no cause found (~10–30%).

Symptoms Gradual or sudden severe epigastric or central abdominal pain (radiates to back, sitting forward may relieve); vomiting prominent.

Signs ►May be subtle in serious disease. ↑HR, fever, jaundice, shock, ileus, rigid abdomen ± local/general tenderness, periumbilical bruising (Cullen's sign) or flanks (Grey Turner's sign) from blood vessel autodigestion and retroperitoneal haemorrhage.

Tests Raised serum *amylase* (>1000u/mL or around 3-fold upper limit of normal). The degree of elevation is not related to severity of disease. ►Amylase may be normal even in severe pancreatitis (levels starts to fall within 24–48h). Amylase is excreted renally so renal failure will ↑ levels. Cholecystitis, mesenteric infarction, and GI perforation can cause lesser rises. Serum *lipase* is more sensitive and specific for pancreatitis (especially when related to alcohol), and rises earlier and falls later. *ABG* to monitor oxygenation and acid–base status. *AXR:* no psoas shadow (↑retroperitoneal fluid), 'sentinel loop' of proximal jejunum from ileus (solitary air-filled dilatation). *Erect CXR* helps exclude other causes (eg perforation). *CT* is the standard choice of imaging to assess severity and for complications. *US* (if gallstones + ↑AST). *ERCP* if LFTs worsen. *CRP* >150mg/L at 36h after admission is a predictor of severe pancreatitis.

Management Severity assessment is essential (see BOX and table 13.15).
• Nil by mouth, consider nasojejunal feeding (decrease pancreatic stimulation). Set up IVI and give lots of crystalloid, to counter third-space sequestration, until vital signs are satisfactory and urine flow stays at >30mL/h. Insert a urinary catheter and consider CVP monitoring.
• Analgesia: pethidine 75–100mg/4h IM, or morphine (may cause Oddi's sphincter to contract more, but it is a better analgesic and not contraindicated).
• Hourly pulse, BP, and urine output; daily FBC, U&E, Ca²⁺, glucose, amylase, ABG.
• If worsening: ITU, O₂ if ↓PₐO₂. In suspected abscess formation or pancreatic necrosis (on CT), consider parenteral nutrition ± laparotomy & debridement ('necrosectomy'). Antibiotics may help in severe disease.
• ERCP + gallstone removal may be needed if there is progressive jaundice.
• Repeat imaging (usually CT) is performed in order to monitor progress.

ΔΔ Any acute abdomen (p598), myocardial infarct.

Early complications Shock, ARDS (p178), renal failure (►give lots of fluid!), DIC, sepsis, ↓Ca²⁺, ↑glucose (transient; 5% need insulin).

Late complications (>1wk.) *Pancreatic necrosis* and *pseudocyst* (fluid in lesser sac, fig 13.45), with fever, a mass ± persistent ↑amylase/LFT; may resolve or need drainage. *Abscesses* need draining. *Bleeding* from elastase eroding a major vessel (eg splenic artery); embolization may be life-saving. *Thrombosis* may occur in the splenic/ gastroduodenal arteries, or colic branches of the superior mesenteric artery, causing bowel necrosis. *Fistulae* normally close spontaneously. If purely pancreatic they do not irritate the skin. Some patients suffer *recurrent oedematous pancreatitis* so often that near-total pancreatectomy is contemplated. ►It can all be a miserable course.

Modified Glasgow criteria for predicting severity of pancreatitis

▶Three or more positive factors detected within 48h of onset suggest severe pancreatitis, and should prompt transfer to ITU/HDU. Mnemonic: **PANCREAS**.

Table 13.15 PANCREAS

PaO2	<8kPa
Age	>55yrs
Neutrophilia	WBC >15 × 10^9/L
Calcium	<2mmol/L
Renal function	Urea >16mmol/L
Enzymes	LDH >600IU/L; AST >200IU/L
Albumin	<32g/L (serum)
Sugar	Blood glucose >10mmol/L

Republished with permission of Royal College of Surgeons of England, from *Annals of the Royal College of Surgeons of England*, Moore E M, 82, 16–17, 2002. Permission conveyed through Copyright Clearance Center, Inc.

These criteria have been validated for pancreatitis caused by gallstones and alcohol; Ranson's criteria are valid for alcohol-induced pancreatitis, and can only be fully applied after 48h, which does have its disadvantages. Other criteria for assessing severity include the Acute Physiology and Chronic Health Examination (APACHE)-II, and the Bedside Index for Severity in Acute Pancreatitis (BISAP).

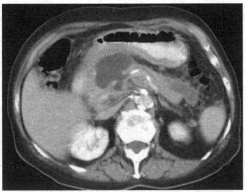

Fig 13.45 Axial CT of the abdomen (with IV and PO contrast media) showing a pancreatic pseudocyst occupying the lesser sac of the abdomen posterior to the stomach. It is called a 'pseudocyst' because it is not a true cyst, rather a collection of fluid in the lesser sac (ie not lined by epi/endothelium). It develops at ≥6wks. The cyst fluid is of low attenuation compared with the stomach contents because it has not been enhanced by the contrast media.
Image courtesy of Dr Stephen Golding.

Renal stones (calculi) consist of crystal aggregates. Stones form in collecting ducts and may be deposited anywhere from the renal pelvis to the urethra, though classically at: 1 Pelviureteric junction. 2 Pelvic brim. 3 Vesicoureteric junction.

Prevalence Common: lifetime incidence up to 15%. *Peak age:* 20–40yrs. ♂:♀≈3:1.

Types • Calcium oxalate (75%). • Magnesium ammonium phosphate (struvite/triple phosphate; 15%). • Also: urate (5%), hydroxyapatite (5%), brushite, cystine (1%), mixed.

Presentation Asymptomatic or: 1 *Pain:* excruciating spasms of renal colic 'loin to groin' (or genitals/inner thigh), with nausea/vomiting. Often cannot lie still (differentiates from peritonitis). *Obstruction of kidney:* felt in the loin, between rib 12 and lateral edge of lumbar muscles (like intercostal nerve irritation pain; the latter is not colicky, and is worsened by specific movements/pressure on a trigger spot). *Obstruction of mid-ureter:* may mimic appendicitis/diverticulitis. *Obstruction of lower ureter:* may lead to symptoms of bladder irritability and pain in scrotum, penile tip, or labia majora. *Obstruction in bladder or urethra:* causes pelvic pain, dysuria, strangury (desire but inability to void) ± interrupted flow. 2 *Infection* can coexist (↑risk if voiding impaired), eg UTI; pyelonephritis (fever, rigors, loin pain, nausea, vomiting); pyonephrosis (infected hydronephrosis) 3 *Haematuria*. 4 *Proteinuria.* 5 *Sterile pyuria.* 6 *Anuria.*

Examination Usually no tenderness on palpation. May be renal angle tenderness especially to percussion if there is retroperitoneal inflammation.

Tests FBC, U&E, Ca²⁺, PO₄³⁻, glucose, bicarbonate, urate. **Urine dipstick** Usually +ve for blood (90%). MSU MC&S. **Further tests for cause** Urine pH; 24h urine for: calcium, oxalate, urate, citrate, sodium, creatinine; stone biochemistry (sieve urine & send stone).

Imaging Non-contrast CT is investigation of choice for imaging stones (99% visible) & helps exclude differential causes of an acute abdomen. ►A ruptured abdominal aortic aneurysm may present similarly. 80% of stones are visible on KUB (kidneys + ureters + bladder) X-ray. Look along ureters for calcification over the transverse processes of the vertebral bodies. US an alternative for hydronephrosis or hydroureter.

Treatment Initially Analgesia, eg diclofenac 75mg IV/IM, or 100mg PR. (If CI: *opioids*) + IV fluids if unable to tolerate PO; antibiotics (eg piperacillin/tazobactam 4.5g/8h IV, or gentamicin) if infection. **Stones <5mm in lower ureter** ~90–95% pass spontaneously. ↑Fluid intake. **Stones >5mm/pain not resolving** *Medical expulsive therapy:* ►start at presentation; nifedipine 10mg/8h PO or α-blockers (tamsulosin 0.4mg/d) promote expulsion and reduce analgesia requirements. Most pass within 48h (>80% after ~30d). If not, try extracorporeal shockwave lithotripsy (ESWL) (if <1cm), or ureteroscopy using a basket. ESWL: US waves shatter stone. SE: renal injury, may also cause ↑BP and DM. *Percutaneous nephrolithotomy (PCNL):* keyhole surgery to remove stones, when large, multiple, or complex. Open surgery is rare.

►**Indications for urgent intervention** (*Delay kills glomeruli.*) Presence of infection *and* obstruction—a percutaneous nephrostomy or ureteric stent may be needed to relieve obstruction (p632); urosepsis; intractable pain or vomiting; impending AKI; obstruction in a solitary kidney; bilateral obstructing stones.

Prevention General Drink plenty. *Normal* dietary Ca²⁺ intake (low Ca²⁺ diets increase oxalate excretion). **Specifically** • *Calcium stones:* in hypercalciuria, a thiazide diuretic is used to ↓Ca²⁺ excretion. • *Oxalate:* ↓oxalate intake; pyridoxine may be used (p291). • *Struvite (phosphate mineral):* treat infection promptly. • *Urate:* allopurinol (100–300mg/24h PO). Urine alkalinization may also help, as urate is more soluble at pH>6 (eg with potassium citrate or sodium bicarbonate). • *Cystine:* vigorous hydration to keep urine output >3L/d and urinary alkalinization (as above-mentioned). Penicillamine is used to chelate cystine, given with pyridoxine to prevent vitamin B₆ deficiency.

Questions to address when confronted by a stone

What is its composition? (See table 13.16.)

Table 13.16 Types, causes, and x-ray appearance of renal stones

Type	Causative factors	Appearance on x-ray
Calcium oxalate (fig 13.46)	Metabolic or idiopathic	Spiky, radio-opaque
Calcium phosphate	Metabolic or idiopathic	Smooth, may be large, radio-opaque
Magnesium ammonium phosphate (fig 13.47)	UTI (*Proteus* causes alkaline urine and calcium precipitation and ammonium salt formation)	Large, horny, 'staghorn', radio-opaque
Urate (p672)	Hyperuricaemia	Smooth, brown, radiolucent
Cystine (fig 13.48)	Renal tubular defect	Yellow, crystalline, semi-opaque

Why has the patient got this stone now?
* *Diet:* chocolate, tea, rhubarb, strawberries, nuts, and spinach all ↑ oxalate levels.
* *Season:* variations in calcium and oxalate levels are thought to be mediated by vitamin D synthesis via sunlight on skin.
* *Work:* can the patient drink freely at work? Is there dehydration?
* *Medications:* precipitating drugs include: diuretics, antacids, acetazolamide, corticosteroids, theophylline, aspirin, allopurinol, vitamin C and D, indinavir.

Are there any predisposing factors? For example:
* *Recurrent UTIs* (in magnesium ammonium phosphate calculi).
* *Metabolic abnormalities:*
    * Hypercalciuria/hypercalcaemia (p668): hyperparathyroidism, neoplasia, sarcoidosis, hyperthyroidism, Addison's, Cushing's, lithium, vitamin D excess.
    * Hyperuricosuria/↑plasma urate: on its own, or with gout.
    * Hyperoxaluria.
    * Cystinuria (p317).
    * Renal tubular acidosis (pp312–13).
* *Urinary tract abnormalities:* eg pelviureteric junction obstruction, hydronephrosis (renal pelvis or calyces), calyceal diverticulum, horseshoe kidney, ureterocele, vesicoureteral reflux, ureteral stricture, medullary sponge kidney.[10]
* *Foreign bodies:* eg stents, catheters.

Is there a family history? ↑Risk of stones 3-fold. Specific diseases include x-linked nephrolithiasis and Dent's disease (proteinuria, hypercalciuria, and nephrocalcinosis).

▶**Is there infection above the stone?** Eg fever, loin tender, pyuria? This needs urgent intervention.

Fig 13.46 Calcium oxalate monohydrate.
Image courtesy of Dr Glen Austin.

Fig 13.47 Struvite stone.
Image courtesy of Dr Glen Austin.

Fig 13.48 Cystine stone.
Image courtesy of Dr Glen Austin.

10 Medullary sponge kidney is a typically asymptomatic developmental anomaly of the kidney mostly seen in adult females, where there is dilatation of the collecting ducts, which if severe leads to a sponge-like appearance of the renal medulla. *Complications/associations:* UTIs, nephrolithiasis, haematuria and hypercalciuria, hyperparathyroidism (if present, look for genetic markers of MEN type 2A, see p217).

▶Urinary tract obstruction is common and should be considered in any patient with impaired renal function. ▶▶Damage can be permanent if the obstruction is not treated promptly. Obstruction may occur anywhere from the renal calyces to the urethral meatus, and may be *partial* or *complete*, *unilateral* or *bilateral*. Obstructing lesions are *luminal* (stones, blood clot, sloughed papilla, tumour: renal, ureteric, or bladder), *mural* (eg congenital or acquired stricture, neuromuscular dysfunction, schistosomiasis), or *extra-mural* (abdominal or pelvic mass/tumour, retroperitoneal fibrosis, or iatrogenic—eg post surgery). Unilateral obstruction may be clinically silent (normal urine output and U&E) if the other kidney is functioning. ▶Bilateral obstruction or obstruction with infection requires urgent treatment. See p633.

Clinical features

- **Acute upper tract obstruction** Loin pain radiating to the groin. There may be superimposed infection ± loin tenderness, or an enlarged kidney.
- **Chronic upper tract obstruction** Flank pain, renal failure, superimposed infection. Polyuria may occur due to impaired urinary concentration.
- **Acute lower tract obstruction** Acute urinary retention typically presents with severe suprapubic pain ± acute confusion (elderly); often acute on chronic (hence preceded by chronic symptoms, see next bullet point). Clinically: distended, palpable bladder containing ~600mL, dull to percussion. Causes include prostatic obstruction (usual cause in older ♂), urethral strictures, anticholinergics, blood clots, eg from bladder lesion ('clot retention'), alcohol, constipation, post-op (pain/inflammation/anaesthetics), infection (p292), neurological (cauda equina syndrome, see p462).
- **Chronic lower tract obstruction** *Symptoms:* urinary frequency, hesitancy, poor stream, terminal dribbling, overflow incontinence. *Signs:* distended, palpable bladder (capacity may be >1.5L) ± large prostate on PR. Complications: UTI, urinary retention, renal failure (eg bilateral obstructive uropathy—see BOX 'Obstructive uropathy'). Causes include prostatic enlargement (common); pelvic malignancy; rectal surgery; DM; CNS disease, eg transverse myelitis/MS; zoster (S2–S4).

Tests **Blood** U&E, creatinine, FBC, and prostate-specific antigen (PSA, p526).[11] **Urine** Dipstick and MC&S. *Ultrasound* (p728) is the imaging modality of choice for investigating upper tract obstruction: if there is hydronephrosis or hydroureter (distension of the renal pelvis and calyces or ureter), arrange a CT scan. This will determine the level of obstruction. NB: in ~5% of cases of obstruction, no distension is seen on US. *Radionuclide imaging* enables functional assessment of the kidneys.

Treatment Upper tract obstruction Nephrostomy or ureteric stent. NB: stents may cause significant discomfort and patients should be warned of this and other risks (see BOX 'Problems of ureteric stenting'). α-blockers help reduce stent-related pain (↓ureteric spasm). Pyeloplasty, to widen the pelvi-ureteric junction (PUJ), may be performed for idiopathic PUJ obstruction.

Lower tract obstruction Insert a urethral or suprapubic catheter (p746) to relieve acute retention. In chronic obstruction only catheterize patient if there is pain, urinary infection, or renal impairment; intermittent self-catheterization is sometimes required (p747). If in clot retention the patient will require a 3-way catheter and bladder washout. If >1L residual check U&E and monitor for post-obstructive diuresis (see BOX 'Obstructive uropathy'). Monitor weight, fluid balance, and U&E closely. Treat the underlying cause if possible, eg if prostatic obstruction, start an α-blocker (see p634). After 2–3 days, trial without catheter (TWOC, p747) may work (especially if <75yrs old and <1L drained or retention was triggered by a passing event, eg GA).

---

11 Do venepuncture for PSA before PR, as PR can ↑ total PSA by ~1ng/mL (free PSA ↑ by 10%). It's difficult to know if acute retention raises PSA, but relieving obstruction does cause it to drop.

Problems of ureteric stenting (depend on site)

Common
- Stent-related pain
- Trigonal irritation
- Haematuria
- Fever
- Infection
- Tissue inflammation
- Encrustation
- Biofilm formation.

Rare
- Obstruction
- Kinking
- Ureteric rupture
- Stent misplacement
- Stent migration (especially if made of silicone)
- Tissue hyperplasia
- Forgotten stents.

Obstructive uropathy

In chronic urinary retention, an episode of *acute* retention may go unnoticed for days and, because of the patient's background symptoms, may only present when overflow incontinence becomes a nuisance—pain is not necessarily a feature.

After diagnosing acute-on-chronic retention and placing a catheter, the bladder residual can be as much as 1.5L of urine. Don't be surprised to be called by the biochemistry lab to be told that the serum creatinine is 1000μmol/L! The good news is that renal function usually returns to base-line after a few days (there may be mild background impairment). Ask for an urgent renal US (fig 13.49) and consider the following in the acute plan to ensure a safe course:

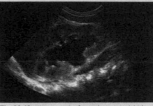

Fig 13.49 Ultrasound of an obstructed kidney showing hydronephrosis. Note dilatation of renal pelvis and ureter, and clubbed calyces.
Image courtesy of Norwich Radiology Department.

- **Hyperkalaemia** See p297.
- **Metabolic acidosis** On ABG there is likely to be a respiratory compensated meta-bolic acidosis. Concerns should prompt discussion with a renal specialist (a good idea anyway), in case haemodialysis is required (p302).
- **Post-obstructive diuresis** In the acute phase after relief of the obstruction, the kidneys produce *a lot* of urine—as much as a litre in the first hour. It is vital to provide resuscitation fluids and then match input with output. ►Fluid depletion rather than overload is the danger here.
- **Sodium- and bicarbonate-losing nephropathy** As the kidney undergoes diuresis, Na+ and bicarbonate are lost in the urine in large quantities. Replace 'in for out' (as mentioned above) with isotonic 1.26% sodium bicarbonate solution—this should be available from ITU. Some advocate using 0.9% saline, though the chloride load may exacerbate acidosis. Withhold any nephrotoxic drugs.
- **Infection** Treat infection, bearing in mind that the ↑WCC and ↑CRP may be part of the stress response. Send a sample of urine for MC&S.

Benign prostatic hyperplasia

Benign prostatic hyperplasia (BPH) Common (24% if aged 40–64yrs; 40% if older).
Pathology Benign nodular or diffuse proliferation of musculofibrous and glandular layers of the prostate. Inner (transitional) zone enlarges in contrast to peripheral layer expansion seen in prostate carcinoma. **Features** *Lower urinary tract symptoms* (LUTS) = nocturia, frequency, urgency, post-micturition dribbling, poor stream/flow, hesitancy, overflow incontinence, haematuria, bladder stones, UTI. **Management** Assess severity of symptoms and impact on life. PR exam. **Tests** MSU; U&E; ultrasound (large residual volume, hydronephrosis—fig 1349, p633), PSA (prior to PR exam; see also BOX 'Advice to asymptomatic men', p637), transrectal US ± biopsy. Then consider:

- **Lifestyle** Avoid caffeine, alcohol (to ↓ urgency/nocturia). Relax when voiding. Void twice in a row to aid emptying. Control urgency by practising distraction methods (eg breathing exercises). Train the bladder by 'holding on' to ↑ time between voiding.
- **Drugs** Useful in mild disease, and while awaiting surgery. • *α-blockers* are 1st line (eg tamsulosin 400mcg/d PO; also alfuzosin, doxazosin, terazosin). ↓Smooth muscle tone (prostate and bladder). SE: drowsiness; depression; dizziness; ↓BP; dry mouth; ejaculatory failure; extra-pyramidal signs; nasal congestion; ↑weight. • *5α-reductase inhibitors:* can be added, or used alone, eg finasteride 5mg/d PO (↓conversion of testosterone to the more potent androgen dihydrotestosterone). Excreted in semen, so use condoms; females should avoid handling. SE: impotence; ↓libido. ↓prostate size over 3–6mths and ↓ long-term retention risk.
- **Surgery**
  - *Transurethral resection of prostate* (TURP) ≤10% become impotent (see BOX). Crossmatch 2U. Beware bleeding, clot retention, and post-TURP syndrome: absorption of washout causing CNS & CVS disturbance. ~12% need redoing within 8yrs.
  - *Transurethral incision of the prostate* (TUIP) involves less destruction than TURP, and less risk to sexual function, gives similar benefit. Relieves pressure on the urethra. May be best surgical option for those with small glands <30g.
  - *Retropubic prostatectomy* is an open operation (if prostate very large).
  - *Transurethral laser-induced prostatectomy* (TULIP) may be as good as TURP.
  - *Robotic prostatectomy* is gaining popularity as a less traumatic and minimally invasive treatment option.

Advice for patients concerning transurethral prostatectomy (TURP)

Pre-op consent issues may centre on risks of the procedure, eg:

- Haematuria/haemorrhage
- Haematospermia
- Hypothermia
- Urethral trauma/stricture
- Post TURP syndrome (↓T°; ↓Na⁺)
- Infection; prostatitis
- Erectile dysfunction ~10%
- Incontinence ≤10%
- Clot retention near strictures
- Retrograde ejaculation (common).

Post-operative advice

- Avoid driving for 2wks after the operation.
- Avoid sex for 2wks after surgery. Then get back to normal. The amount ejaculated may be reduced (as it flows backwards into the bladder—harmless, but may cloud the urine). It means you may be infertile. Erections may be a problem after TURP, but do not expect this: in some men, erections improve. Rarely, orgasmic sensations are reduced.
- Expect to pass blood in the urine for the first 2wks. A small amount of blood colours the urine bright red. Do not be alarmed.
- At first you may need to urinate *more* frequently than before. Do not be despondent. In 6wks things should be much better—but the operation cannot be guaranteed to work (8% fail, and lasting incontinence is a problem in 6%; 12% may need repeat TURPS within 8yrs, compared with 1.8% of men undergoing open prostatectomy).
- If feverish, or if urination hurts, take a sample of urine to your doctor.

Causes Idiopathic retroperitoneal fibrosis (RPF), inflammatory aneurysms of the abdominal aorta, and perianeurysmal RPF. With idiopathic RPF there is an associated inflammatory response resulting in fibrinoid necrosis of the vasa vasorum, affecting the aorta and small and medium retroperitoneal vessels. The ureters get embedded in dense, fibrous tissue resulting in progressive bilateral ureteric obstruction. Secondary causes of RPF include malignancy, typically lymphoma.

Associations Drugs (eg β-blockers, bromocriptine, methysergide, methyldopa), autoimmune disease (eg thyroiditis, SLE, ANCA+ve vasculitis), smoking, asbestos.

Typical patient Middle-aged ♂ with vague loin, back, or abdominal pain, ↑BP.

Tests Blood ↑Urea and creatinine; ↑ESR; ↑CRP; anaemia. **Ultrasound** Dilated ureters (hydronephrosis). **CT/MRI** Periaortic mass (fig 13.50). Biopsy under imaging guidance is used to rule out malignancy.

Treatment Retrograde stent placement to relieve obstruction (removed after 12 months) ± ureterolysis (dissection of the ureters from the retroperitoneal tissue). Immunosuppression (in idiopathic RPF) with low-dose steroids has good long-term results.

13 Surgery

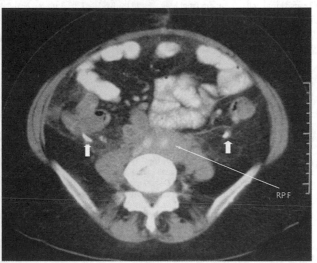

Fig 13.50 CT scan of retroperitoneal fibrosis (RPF), with subsequent obstruction and dilatation of the ureters (thick arrows).

Reproduced from Davison *et al.*, *Oxford Textbook of Nephrology*, 2005, with permission from Oxford University Press.

13 Surgery

Renal cell carcinoma (RCC) Arises from proximal renal tubular epithelium. **Epidemiology** Accounts for 90% of renal cancers; mean age 65yrs. ♂:♀≈2:1. 2% of haemodialysis patients develop RCC. **Features** 50% found incidentally. Haematuria, loin pain, abdominal mass, anorexia, malaise, weight loss, PUO—often in isolation. Rarely, invasion of left renal vein compresses left testicular vein causing a varicocele. Spread may be direct (renal vein), via lymph, or haematogenous (bone, liver, lung). 25% have metastases at presentation. **Tests** BP: ↑ from renin secretion. *Blood:* FBC (polycythaemia from erythropoietin secretion); ESR; U&E, ALP (bony mets?). *Urine:* RBCs; cytology. *Imaging:* US (p728); CT/MRI; CXR ('cannon ball' metastases). ℞ Radical nephrectomy (nephron-sparing surgery is as good for T1 tumours + preserves renal function). Cryotherapy and radiofrequency ablation is an option for patients unfit or unwilling to undergo surgery. RCC is generally radio- & chemoresistant, but adjuvant pembrolizumab (immune checkpoint inhibitor) is recommended for patients at high risk of post-op recurrence, and in those with unresectable or metastatic disease. Other options include: high-dose IL-2 and other T-cell activation therapies; anti-angiogenesis agents (eg pazopanib, sunitinib, axitinib, or bevacizumab); mTOR inhibitors, eg temsirolimus. The *Mayo prognostic risk score (SSIGN)* was developed to predict survival and uses information on tumour **s**tage, **si**ze, **g**rade, and **n**ecrosis. **Prognosis** 10yr survival ranges from 96.5% (scores 0–1) to 19.2% (scores ≥10).

Transitional cell carcinoma (TCC) May arise in the bladder (50%), ureter, or renal pelvis. **Epidemiology** Age >40yrs; ♂:♀≈4:1. **Risk factors** p638. **Presentation** Painless haematuria; frequency; urgency; dysuria; urinary tract obstruction. **Diagnosis** Urine cytology; IVU; cystoscopy + biopsy; CT/MRI. ℞ See 'Bladder tumours', p638. **Prognosis** Varies with clinical stage/histological grade: 10–80% 5yr survival.

Wilms' tumour (Nephroblastoma.) A childhood tumour of primitive renal tubules and mesenchymal cells. **Prevalence** 1:100 000—the chief abdominal malignancy in children. It presents with an abdominal mass and haematuria. ℞ OHCS p229.

Prostate cancer The commonest male malignancy. **Incidence** ↑ with age: 80% in men >80yrs (autopsy studies). **Associations** +ve family history (×2–3 ↑risk), ↑testosterone. Most are adenocarcinomas arising in peripheral prostate. Spread may be local (seminal vesicles, bladder, rectum) via lymph, or haematogenously (sclerotic bony lesions). **Symptoms** Asymptomatic or nocturia, hesitancy, poor stream, terminal dribbling, or obstruction. ↓Weight ± bone pain suggests mets. *Digital rectal exam (DRE) exam of prostate* may show hard, irregular prostate. **Diagnosis** ↑PSA (normal in 30% of small cancers); transrectal US & biopsy; bone scan; CT/MRI. **Staging** MRI. **Treatment** *Disease confined to prostate:* options depend on prognosis (see BOX 'Prognostic factors'), patient preference, and comorbidities. •*Radical prostatectomy* if <70yrs gives excellent disease-free survival (laparoscopic surgery is as good). The role of adjuvant hormonal therapy is being explored. •*Radical radiotherapy* (± neoadjuvant & adjuvant hormonal therapy) is an alternative curative option that compares favourably with surgery (no RCTs). It may be delivered as external beam or brachytherapy. •*Hormone therapy alone* temporarily delays tumour progression but refractory disease eventually develops. Consider in elderly, unfit patients with high-risk disease. •*Active surveillance*—particularly if >70yrs & low-risk. *Metastatic disease:* •*Hormonal drugs* may give benefit for 1–2yrs. LHRH agonists, eg 12-weekly goserelin (10.8mg SC) first stimulate, then inhibit pituitary gonadotropin. NB: risks tumour 'flare' when first used—start anti-androgen, eg cyproterone acetate, in susceptible patients. The LHRH antagonist degarelix is also used in advanced disease. **Symptomatic** ℞ Analgesia; treat hypercalcaemia; radiotherapy for bone mets/spinal cord compression. **Prognosis** 10% die in 6 months, 10% live >10yrs. **Screening** DRE of prostate; transrectal US; PSA (see BOX 'Advice to asymptomatic men').

Penile cancer **Epidemiology** Rare in UK, more common in the Far East and Africa, very rare in circumcised. Related to chronic irritation, viruses, smegma. **Presentation** Chronic fungating ulcer, bloody/purulent discharge, 50% spread to lymph at presentation. ℞ Radiotherapy & iridium wires if early; amputation & lymph node dissection if late.

Advice to asymptomatic men asking for a PSA blood test

- Many men over 50 consider a PSA test to detect prostatic cancer. *Is this wise?*
- The test is not very accurate, and we cannot say that those having the test will live longer—even if they turn out to have prostate cancer. Most men with prostate cancer die from an unrelated cause.
- If the test is falsely positive, you may needlessly have more tests, eg prostate sampling via the back passage (causes bleeding and infection in 1–5% of men).
- Only one in three of those with a high PSA level will have cancer.
- You may be worried needlessly if later tests put you in the clear.
- If a cancer is found, there's no way to tell *for sure* if it will impinge on health. You might end up having a bad effect from treatment that wasn't needed.
- There is much uncertainty on treating those who *do* turn out to have prostate cancer: options are radical surgery to remove the prostate (risks erectile dysfunction and incontinence), radiotherapy, or hormones.
- Screening via PSA has shown conflicting results. Some RCTs have shown no difference in the rate of death from prostate cancer, others have found reduced mortality, eg 1 death prevented per 1055 men invited for screening (if 37 cancers detected).
- ►Ultimately, you must decide for yourself what you want.

Prognostic factors in prostate cancer

A number of prognostic factors help determine if 'watchful waiting' or aggressive therapy should be advised: •Pre-treatment PSA level. •Tumour stage (as measured by the TNM system; p522). •Tumour grade—Gleason score. Gleason grading is from 1 to 5, with 5 being the highest grade, and carrying the poorest prognosis. Gleason grades are decided by analysing histology from two separate areas of tumour specimen, and adding them to get the total Gleason score for the tumour, from 2 to 10. Scores 8–10 suggest an aggressive tumour; 5–7: intermediate; 2–4: indolent.

Benign diseases of the penis

Balanitis Acute inflammation of the foreskin and glans. Associated with strep and staph infections. More common in diabetics. Often seen in young boys with tight foreskins. *R*: antibiotics, circumcision, hygiene advice.

Phimosis The foreskin occludes the meatus. In young boys this causes recurrent balanitis and ballooning, but time (+ trials of gentle retraction) may obviate the need for circumcision. In adulthood presents with painful intercourse, infection, ulceration, and is associated with balanitis xerotica obliterans.

Paraphimosis Occurs when a tight foreskin is retracted and becomes irreplaceable, preventing venous return leading to oedema and even ischaemia of the glans. Can occur if the foreskin is not replaced after catheterization. ►►*R*: ask patient to squeeze glans. Try applying a 50% glucose-soaked swab (oedema may follow osmotic gradient). Ice packs and lidocaine gel may also help. May require aspiration/dorsal slit/circumcision.

Prostatitis

May be acute or chronic. Usually those >35yrs. *Acute prostatitis* is caused mostly by *S. faecalis* and *E. coli*, also *Chlamydia* (and previously TB). **Features** UTIs, retention, pain, haematospermia, swollen/boggy prostate on DRE. *R*: analgesia; levofloxacin 500mg/24h PO for 28d. *Chronic prostatitis* may be bacterial or nonbacterial. Symptoms as for acute prostatitis, but present for >3 months. Nonbacterial chronic prostatitis does not respond to antibiotics. Anti-inflammatory drugs, α–blockers, and prostatic massage all have a place.

13 Surgery

>90% are transitional cell carcinomas (TCCs) in the UK. Adenocarcinomas and squamous cell carcinomas are rare in the West (the latter may follow schistosomiasis). UK incidence ≈ 1:6000/yr. ♂:♀≈5:2. Histology is important for prognosis: *grade 1*—differentiated; *grade 2*—intermediate; *grade 3*—poorly differentiated. 80% are confined to bladder mucosa, and only ~20% penetrate muscle (increasing mortality to 50% at 5yrs).

Presentation Painless haematuria; recurrent UTIs; voiding irritability.

Associations Smoking; aromatic amines (rubber industry); chronic cystitis; schistosomiasis (↑risk of squamous cell carcinoma); pelvic irradiation.

Tests
• Urine: microscopy/cytology (cancers may cause sterile pyuria).
• Cystoscopy with biopsy is diagnostic.
• CT urogram is both diagnostic and provides staging.
• Bimanual EUA helps assess spread.
• MRI or lymphangiography may show involved pelvic nodes.

Staging Is by TNM status according to depth of invasion (T), nodal involvement (N), and presence of metastatic disease (M).

Treating TCC of the bladder
• TIS/TA/T1 **(non-muscle invasive)** (80% of all patients.) Diathermy via transurethral cystoscopy/transurethral resection of bladder tumour (TURBT). Consider a regimen of intravesical *BCG* (which stimulates a non-specific immune response) for multiple small tumours or high-grade tumours. Alternative chemotherapeutic agents include mitomycin, epirubicin, and gemcitabine. 5yr survival ≈ 95%.
• T2-3 **(muscle invasive)** Radical cystectomy is the 'gold standard'. Radiotherapy gives worse 5yr survival rates than surgery, but preserves the bladder. 'Salvage' cystectomy can be performed if radiotherapy fails, but yields worse results than primary surgery. Post-op chemotherapy (eg M-VAC: methotrexate, vinblastine, doxorubicin, and cisplatin) is toxic but effective. Neoadjuvant chemotherapy with M-VAC or GC (gemcitabine and cisplatin) has improved survival compared to cystectomy or radiotherapy alone. Methods to preserve the bladder with transurethral resection or partial cystectomy + systemic chemotherapy have been tried, but long-term results are disappointing. If the bladder neck is not involved, orthotopic reconstruction rather than forming a urostoma is an option (both using ~40cm of the patient's ileum), but adequate tumour clearance must not be compromised. ►The patient should have all these options explained by a urologist and an oncologist.
• **More advanced or metastatic disease** Usually palliative chemo/radiotherapy. Chronic catheterization and urinary diversions may help to relieve pain.

Follow-up History, examination, and regular cystoscopy: • **High-risk tumours** Every 3 months for 2yrs, then every 6 months. • **Low-risk tumours** First follow-up cystoscopy after 9 months, then yearly.

Tumour spread Local → to pelvic structures; lymphatic → to iliac and para-aortic nodes; haematogenous → to liver and lungs.

Prognosis Overall prognosis for low-grade disease is very good, >80% 5-year survival. Overall prognosis for muscle invasive TCC is 40–50% (age dependent). Median survival for metastatic disease is 13 months (0% 5-year survival).

Complications Cystectomy can result in sexual and urinary malfunction. Massive bladder haemorrhage may complicate treatment or be a feature of disease treated palliatively. Determining the cause of bleeding is key. Consider alum solution bladder irrigation (if no renal failure) as 1st-line treatment for intractable haematuria in advanced malignancy: it is an inpatient procedure.

Is asymptomatic non-visible haematuria significant?

Dipstick tests are often done routinely for patients on admission. If non-visible (previously microscopic) haematuria is found, but the patient has no related symptoms, what does this mean? Before rushing into a barrage of investigations, consider:

- One study found that incidence of urogenital disease (eg bladder cancer) was no higher in those with asymptomatic microhaematuria than in those without.
- Asymptomatic non-visible haematuria is the sole presenting feature in only 4% of bladder cancers, and there is no evidence that these are less advanced than malignancies presenting with macroscopic haematuria.
- When monitoring those with treated bladder cancer for recurrence, non-visible haematuria tests have a sensitivity of only 31 in those with superficial bladder malignancy, in whom detection would be most useful.
- Although 80% of those with flank pain due to a renal stone have microscopic haematuria, so do 50% of those with flank pain but no stone.

The conclusion is not that urine dipstick testing is useless, but that results should not be interpreted in isolation. ►Unexplained non-visible haematuria in those >50yrs should be referred under the 2-week rule. Smokers and those with +ve family history for urothelial cancer may also be investigated differently from those with no risk factors. It is worth considering, that in a young, fit athlete, the diagnosis is more likely to be exercise-induced haematuria. Wise doctors work collaboratively with their patients. 'Shall we let sleeping dogs lie?' is a reasonable question for *some* patients.

►Think twice before inserting a urinary catheter.
►Carry out rectal examination to exclude faecal impaction.
►Is the bladder palpable after voiding (retention with overflow)?
►Is there neurological comorbidity: eg MS; Parkinson's disease; stroke; spinal trauma?

Incontinence in men Enlargement of the prostate is the major cause of incontinence: urge incontinence (see later in topic) or dribbling may result from partial retention of urine. TURP (p634) & other pelvic surgery may weaken the bladder sphincter and cause incontinence. Troublesome incontinence needs specialist assessment.

Incontinence in women Often under-reported with delays before seeking help.
- **Functional incontinence** Ie when physiological factors are relatively unimportant. The patient is 'caught short' and too slow in finding the toilet because of (eg) immobility, or unfamiliar surroundings.
- **Stress incontinence** Leakage from an incompetent sphincter, eg when intra-abdominal pressure rises (eg coughing, laughing). Increasing age and obesity are risk factors. The key to diagnosis is the loss of small (but often frequent) amounts of urine when coughing etc. Examine for pelvic floor weakness/prolapse/pelvic masses. Look for cough leak on standing and with full bladder. Stress incontinence is common in pregnancy and following birth. It occurs to some degree in ~50% of postmenopausal women. In elderly women, pelvic floor weakness, eg with uterine prolapse or urethrocele (*OHCS* p160), is a very common association.
- **Urge incontinence/overactive bladder syndrome** The urge to urinate is quickly followed by uncontrollable and sometimes complete emptying of the bladder as the detrusor muscle contracts. Urgency/leaking is precipitated by: arriving home (latchkey incontinence, a conditioned reflex); cold; the sound of running water; caffeine; and obesity. *Δ:* urodynamic studies. *Cause:* detrusor overactivity (see table 13.17), eg from central inhibitory pathway malfunction or sensitization of peripheral afferent terminals in the bladder; or a bladder muscle problem. Check for organic brain damage (eg stroke; Parkinson's; dementia). *Other causes:* urinary infection; diabetes; diuretics; atrophic vaginitis; urethritis.

In both sexes incontinence may result from confusion or sedation. Occasionally it may be purposeful (eg preventing admission to an old people's home) or due to anger.

Management ►Effective treatment can have a huge impact on quality of life.

Check for UTI; DM; diuretic use; faecal impaction; palpable bladder; GFR.
- **Stress incontinence** Pelvic floor exercises are 1st line (8 contractions ≈3/d for 3 months). Intravaginal electrical stimulation may also be effective, but is not acceptable to many women. A ring pessary may help uterine prolapse, eg while awaiting surgical repair. *Surgical options* (eg tension-free vaginal tape) aim to stabilize the mid-urethra. Urethral bulking also available. Medical options: duloxetine 40mg/12h PO (50% have ≥50% ↓ in incontinence episodes). SE = nausea.
- **Urge incontinence** The patient (or carer) should complete an 'incontinence' chart for 3d to define the pattern of incontinence. Examine for spinal cord and CNS signs (including cognitive test, p61); and for vaginitis (if postmenopausal). Vaginitis can be treated with topical oestrogen therapy for a limited period. Bladder training (may include pelvic floor exercises) and weight loss are important. Drugs may help reduce night-time incontinence (see BOX) but can be disappointing. Consider aids, eg absorbent pad. If ♂ consider a condom catheter.

►Do urodynamic assessment (cystometry & urine flow rate measurement) before any surgical intervention to exclude detrusor overactivity or sphincter dyssynergia.

Table 13.17 Managing detrusor overactivity in urge incontinence

Agents for detrusor overactivity	Notes
Antimuscarinics: eg tolterodine SR 4mg/24h; SE: dry mouth, eyes/skin, drowsiness, constipation, tachycardia, abdominal pain, urinary retention, sinusitis, oedema, ↑weight, glaucoma precipitation. Up to 4mg/12h may be needed (unlicensed)	Improves frequency & urgency. Alternatives: solifenacin 5mg/24h (max 10mg); oxybutynin, but more SE unless transdermal route or modified release used; trospium or fesoterodine (prefers M3 receptors). Avoid in myasthenia, and if glaucoma or UC are uncontrolled
Topical oestrogens	Postmenopausal urgency, frequency + nocturia may occasionally be improved by raising the bladder's sensory threshold. Systemic therapy worsens incontinence
β₃-adrenergic agonist: mirabegron 50mg/24h; SE: tachycardia; CI: severe hypertension; caution if renal/hepatic impairment	Consider if antimuscarinics are contraindicated or clinically ineffective, or if SE unacceptable
Intravesical botulinum toxin (Botox®)	Consider if above medications ineffective
Percutaneous posterior tibial nerve stimulation (PTNS). (A typical treatment consists of ×12 weekly 30min sessions)	Consider if drug treatment ineffective and Botox® not wanted. PTNS delivers neuromodulation to the S2–S4 junction of the sacral nerve plexus
Neuromodulation via transcutaneous electrical stimulation	Sacral nerve stimulation inhibits the reflex behaviour of involuntary detrusor contractions
Modulation of afferent input from bladder	Gabapentin (unlicensed)
Hypnosis, psychotherapy, bladder training*	(These all require good motivation)
Surgery (eg clam ileocystoplasty)	Reserved for troublesome or intractable symptoms. The bladder is bisected, opened like a clam, and 25cm of ileum is sewn in

NB: desmopressin nasal spray 20mcg nocte reduces urine production and ∴ nocturia in overactive bladder. Unsuitable if elderly (SE: fluid retention, heart failure, ↓Na⁺).

* Mind over bladder: • Void when you DON'T have urge; DON'T go to the bathroom when you do have urge. • Gradually extend the time between voiding. • Schedule your trips to toilet. • Stretch your bladder to normal capacity. • When urge comes, calm down and make it go using mind-over-bladder tricks.

Not all male urinary symptoms are prostate related!

Detrusor overactivity Men get this as well as women. Pressure-flow studies help diagnose this (as does detrusor thickness ≥2.9mm on US).

Primary bladder neck obstruction A condition in which the bladder neck does not open properly during voiding. Studies in men and women with voiding dysfunction show that it is common. The cause may be muscular or neurological dysfunction or fibrosis. *Diagnosis:* video-urodynamics, with simultaneous pressure-flow measurement, and visualization of the bladder neck during voiding. *Treatment:* watchful waiting; α-blockers (p634); surgery.

Urethral stricture This may follow trauma or infection (eg gonorrhoea)—and frequently leads to voiding symptoms, UTI, or retention. Malignancy is a rare cause. *Imaging:* retrograde urethrogram or antegrade cystourethrogram if the patient has an existing suprapubic catheter. *Internal urethrotomy* involves incising the stricture transurethrally using endoscopic equipment—to release scar tissue. *Stents* incorporate themselves into the wall of the urethra and keep the lumen open. They work best for short strictures in the bulbar urethra (anterior urethral anatomy, from proximal to distal: prostatic urethra→posterior or membranous urethra→bulbar urethra→penile or pendulous urethra→fossa navicularis→meatus).

▶Testicular lump = cancer until proved otherwise.
▶Acute, tender enlargement of testis = torsion (p644) until proved otherwise.

Diagnosing scrotal masses (fig 13.51)
1 Can you get above it? 2 Is it separate from the testis? 3 Cystic or solid?
• Cannot get above: inguinoscrotal hernia (p606) or hydrocele extending proximally.
• Separate and cystic: epididymal cyst.
• Separate and solid: epididymitis/varicocele.
• Testicular and cystic: hydrocele.
▶Testicular and solid—*tumour*, haematocele, granuloma (p190), orchitis, gumma (p408). US may help.

Epididymal cysts Usually develop in adulthood and contain clear or milky (spermatocele) fluid. They lie above and behind the testis. Remove if symptomatic.

Hydroceles (Fluid within the tunica vaginalis.) *Primary* (associated with a patent processus vaginalis, which typically resolves during the 1st year of life) or *secondary* to testis tumour/trauma/infection. Primary hydroceles are more common, larger, and usually in younger men. Can resolve spontaneously. ℞ Aspiration (may need repeating) or surgery: plicating the tunica vaginalis (Lord's repair)/inverting the sac (Jaboulay's repair). ▶Is the testis normal after aspiration? If any doubt, do US.

Epididymo-orchitis Causes *Chlamydia* (eg if <35yrs); *E. coli*; mumps; *N. gonorrhoeae*; TB. **Features** Sudden-onset tender swelling, dysuria, sweats/fever. Take '1st-catch' urine sample; look for urethral discharge. Consider STI screen. Warn of possible infertility and symptoms worsening before improving. ℞ If <35yrs; doxycycline 100mg/12h (covers chlamydia; treat sexual partners). If gonorrhoea suspected add ceftriaxone 500mg IM stat. If >35yrs (mostly non-STI), associated UTI is common so try ciprofloxacin 500mg/12h or ofloxacin 200mg/12h. Antibiotics should be used for 2–4wks. Also: analgesia, scrotal support, drainage of any abscess.

Varicocele Dilated veins of pampiniform plexus. Left side more commonly affected. Often visible as distended scrotal blood vessels that feel like 'a bag of worms'. Patient may complain of dull ache. Associated with subfertility, but repair (via surgery or embolization) seems to have little effect on subsequent pregnancy rates.

Haematocele Blood in tunica vaginalis, follows trauma, may need drainage/excision.

Testicular tumours The commonest malignancy in ♂ aged 15–44; 10% occur in undescended testes, even after orchidopexy. A contralateral tumour is found in 5%. **Types** Seminoma, 55% (30–65yrs); non-seminomatous germ cell tumour, 33% (NSGCT; previously teratoma; 20–30yrs); mixed germ cell tumour, 12%; lymphoma.

Signs Typically painless testis lump, found after trauma/infection ± haemospermia, secondary hydrocele, pain, dyspnoea (lung mets), abdominal mass (enlarged nodes), or effects of secreted hormones. 25% of seminomas & 50% of NSGCTs present with metastases. **Risk factors** Undescended testis; infant hernia; infertility.

Staging 1 No evidence of metastasis. 2 Infradiaphragmatic node involvement (spread via the para-aortic nodes *not* inguinal nodes). 3 Supradiaphragmatic node involvement. 4 Lung involvement (haematogenous).

Tests (Allow staging.) CXR, CT, excision biopsy. α-fetoprotein (FP) (eg >3IU/mL)[12] and β-human chorionic gonadotropin (p527) are useful tumour markers and help monitor treatment; check *before & during* ℞.

℞ Radical orchidectomy (inguinal incision; occlude the spermatic cord before mobilization to ↓ risk of intra-operative spread). Options are constantly updated (surgery, radiotherapy, chemotherapy). Seminomas are exquisitely radiosensitive. Stage 1 seminomas: orchidectomy + radiotherapy cures ~95%. Do close follow-up to detect relapse. Cure of NSGCT, even if metastases are present, is achieved by 3 cycles of bleomycin + etoposide + cisplatin. 5yr survival >90% in all groups.
▶Encourage regular self-examination (prevents late presentation).

12 αFP is *not* ↑ in pure seminoma; may also be ↑ in: hepatitis, cirrhosis, liver cancer, open neural tube defect.

Diagnosing groin lumps: lateral to medial thinking

- Psoas abscess (may present with back pain, limp, and swinging pyrexia).
- Neurinoma (Schwannoma) of the femoral nerve (usually painless mass).
- Femoral artery aneurysm (pulsatile mass).
- Saphena varix (like a hernia, it has a cough impulse).
- Lymph node (firm, distinct mass).
- Femoral hernia (usually below the inguinal ligament in the upper medial thigh).
- Inguinal hernia (usually originates above the inguinal ligament).
- Hydrocele or varicocele (cannot feel testis separate from mass).
- Also consider an undescended testis (cryptorchidism).

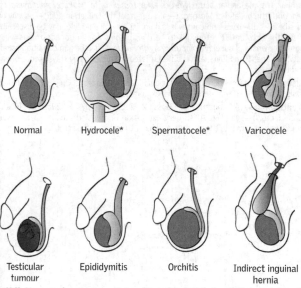

| Normal | Hydrocele* | Spermatocele* | Varicocele |

| Testicular tumour | Epididymitis | Orchitis | Indirect inguinal hernia |

Fig 13.51 Diagnosis of scrotal masses (*=transilluminates: position of pen torch shown in image).

►►Torsion of the testis

The aim is to recognize this condition before the cardinal signs and symptoms are fully manifest, as prompt surgery saves testes. If surgery is performed in <6h the salvage rate is 90–100%; if >24h it is 0–10%.

►*If in any doubt, surgery is required. If suspected refer immediately to urology.*

Presentation Symptoms Sudden onset of pain in one testis, which makes walking uncomfortable. Pain in the abdomen, nausea, and vomiting are common. **Signs** Inflammation of one testis—it is very tender, hot, and swollen. The testis may lie high and transversely. Torsion may occur at any age but is most common at 11–30yrs. With *intermittent torsion* the pain may have passed on presentation, but if it was severe, and the lie is horizontal, prophylactic fixing may be wise. **ΔΔ** The main one is epididymo-orchitis (p642) but with this the patient tends to be older, there may be symptoms of urinary infection, and more gradual onset of pain. Also consider tumour, trauma, and an acute hydrocele. NB: *torsion of testicular or epididymal appendage* (the hydatid of Morgagni—a remnant of the Müllerian duct)—usually occurs between 7–12yrs, and causes less pain. Its tiny blue nodule may be discernible under the scrotum. It is thought to be due to the surge in gonadotropins which signal the onset of puberty. *Idiopathic scrotal oedema* is a benign condition usually between ages 2 and 10yrs, and is differentiated from torsion by the absence of pain and tenderness.

Tests Doppler US may demonstrate lack of blood flow to testis. Only perform if diagnosis equivocal—do not delay surgical exploration.

Treatment ►Ask consent for possible orchidectomy + *bilateral* fixation (orchidopexy)—see p566. At surgery expose and untwist the testis. If its colour looks good, return it to the scrotum and fix *both* testes to the scrotum.

Incidence About 3% of boys are born with at least one undescended testis (30% of premature boys) but this drops to 1% after the first year of life. Unilateral is four times more common than bilateral. (If bilateral then should have genetic testing.)

- **Cryptorchidism** Complete absence of the testis from the scrotum (anorchism is absence of both testes).
- **Retractile testis** The genitalia are normally developed but there is an excessive cremasteric reflex. The testis is often found at the external inguinal ring. *R:* reassurance (examining while in a warm bath, for example, may help to distinguish from maldescended/ectopic testes).
- **Maldescended testis** May be found anywhere along the normal path of descent from abdomen to groin.
- **Ectopic testis** Most commonly found in the superior inguinal pouch (anterior to the external oblique aponeurosis) but may also be abdominal, perineal, penile, and in the femoral triangle.

Complications of maldescended and ectopic testis Infertility; ×40 increased risk of testicular cancer (risk remains after surgery but in cryptorchidism may be ↓ if orchidopexy performed before aged 10), increased risk of testicular trauma, increased risk of testicular torsion. Also associated with hernias (due to patent processus vaginalis in >90%, p605) and other urinary tract anomalies.

Treatment of maldescended and ectopic testis Restores (potential for) spermatogenesis; the increased risk of malignancy remains but becomes easier to diagnose.

Surgery Orchidopexy, usually dartos pouch procedure, is performed in infancy: testis and cord are mobilized following a groin incision, any processus vaginalis or hernial sac is removed and the testis is brought through a hole made in the dartos muscle into the resultant subcutaneous pouch where the muscle prevents retraction.

Hormonal Hormonal therapy, most commonly human chorionic gonadotropin (HCG), is sometimes attempted if an undescended testis is in the inguinal canal.

▸▸Aneurysms of arteries

An artery with a dilatation >50% of its original diameter has an aneurysm; remember this is an ongoing process. True aneurysms are abnormal dilatations that involve all layers of the arterial wall. False aneurysms (pseudoaneurysms) involve a collection of blood in the outer layer only (adventitia) which communicates with the lumen (eg after trauma). Aneurysms may be fusiform (eg most AAAs) or sac-like (eg Berry aneurysms; fig 10.19, p475).

Causes The most common cause is atherosclerotic degeneration (look out for vascular risk factors). Rarer causes include: infection (eg mycotic aneurysm in endocarditis; tertiary syphilis—especially thoracic aneurysms), trauma, connective tissue disorders (eg Marfan's, Ehlers–Danlos), inflammatory (eg Takayasu's aortitis, p554).

Common sites Aorta (infrarenal most common), iliac, femoral, and popliteal arteries.

Complications For AAA, rupture is the main complication. For popliteal aneurysms, it is thrombosis (presenting as an acutely ischaemic limb) or distal thromboembolism. Rarely: fistulae (aorto-caval/aorto-duodenal) or pressure on nearby structures.

Screening All ♂ at age 65yrs are invited for screening in UK (♂:♀≈8:1), decreases mortality from ruptured AAA.

Ruptured abdominal aortic aneurysm (AAA) Mortality is around 90% overall and 50% for someone reaching hospital. **Symptoms & signs** Intermittent or continuous abdominal pain (radiates to back, iliac fossae, or groins) collapse, an *expansile* abdominal mass (it expands and contracts, unlike swellings that are purely pulsatile, eg nodes overlying arteries). ▸Always consider a ruptured AAA in any male >65yrs with unexplained back/loin pain (don't dismiss as renal colic), syncope, or shock.

Unruptured AAA **Definition** >3cm diameter. **Prevalence** 3% of those >50yrs. ♂:♀ >3:1. Less common in diabetics. **Cause** Degeneration of elastic lamellae and smooth muscle loss. There is a genetic component. **Symptoms** Often none, they *may* cause abdominal/back pain, often discovered incidentally on abdominal examination (see BOX). **Monitoring** RCTs have failed to demonstrate benefit from early endovascular repair (EVAR, see later in paragraph) of aneurysms <5.5cm (where rupture rates are low). Risk of rupture below this size is <1%/yr, compared to ~15%/yr for aneurysms >6cm across. ~75% of aneurysms under monitoring will eventually need repair. Rupture is more likely if: • ↑BP. • Smoker. • ♀. • Positive family history. Modify risk factors if possible at diagnosis. **Elective repair** Reserve for aneurysms ≥5.5cm or expanding at >1cm/yr, or symptomatic aneurysms. **Stenting (EVAR)** Endovascular stent insertion via the femoral artery. Short-term morbidity and mortality is improved for EVAR vs open repair in randomized trials, but no differences in long-term outcomes. Risk of graft complications, eg failure of stent-graft to totally exclude blood flow to the aneurysm—'endoleak'. See fig 13.52. **Open repair** Operative mortality: ~5%; specific complications of open surgery include distal (lower limb) ischaemia/thromboembolism, visceral ischaemia, spinal cord ischaemia (rare).

Emergency management of a ruptured abdominal aneurysm

Mortality—treated: 41% and improving; untreated: ~100%.

▸▸Summon a vascular surgeon and an experienced anaesthetist; warn theatre.

▸▸Do an ECG, gain IV access with 2 large-bore cannulae and take blood for amylase, Hb, crossmatch (10–40u may eventually be needed). Catheterize the bladder. Treat shock with O Rh −ve blood (if not cross matched), but keep systolic BP ≤100mmHg to avoid rupturing a contained leak (NB: *raised* BP is common early on).

▸▸If the patient is in circulatory collapse (peri-arrest/requiring CPR), proceed straight to theatre if appropriate. Otherwise arrange immediate CT aortogram which allows planning of surgery or stenting.

▸▸Give prophylactic antibiotics, eg co-amoxiclav 625mg IV.

▸▸Current evidence suggests EVAR is associated with better outcomes in ruptured aneurysms than open graft insertion, and therefore is the first choice if anatomically suitable.

Blood splits the aortic media with sudden tearing chest pain (± radiation to back). As the dissection extends, branches of the aorta may occlude sequentially leading to hemiplegia (carotid artery), unequal arm pulses and BP, or acute limb ischaemia, paraplegia (anterior spinal artery), and anuria (renal arteries). Aortic valve incompetence, inferior MI, and cardiac arrest may develop if dissection moves proximally.

Type A (70%.) Dissections involving the ascending aorta or arch (proximal to the left subclavian artery origin) are an emergency (~30% mortality in the first 24h, >1% per hour). ▶▶Require immediate referral to cardiothoracics for consideration of surgical repair.

Type B (30%, not involving the ascending/arch.) These are initially treated conservatively if uncomplicated (strict BP control on HDU for the first 48h). Complications to monitor for are: visceral, spinal cord, or lower limb ischaemia; refractory pain or hypertension; evidence of aneurysmal dilatation of the aorta on imaging. 5yr mortality is ~50% and the challenge is selecting which patients require intervention. Usually treated with endovascular stenting. **Management** • Group & save. • ECG & CXR (expanded mediastinum is rare). • CT or transoesophageal echocardiography (TOE). Take to ITU; hypotensives: keep systolic at ~100–110mmHg: labetalol (p110) or esmolol (t½ is ultra-short) by IVI is helpful here (calcium-channel blockers may be used if β-blockers contraindicated). Acute operative mortality: <25%.

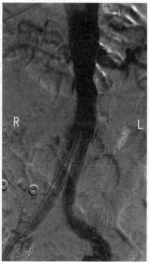

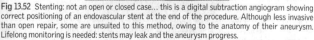

Fig 13.52 Stenting: not an open or closed case... this is a digital subtraction angiogram showing correct positioning of an endovascular stent at the end of the procedure. Although less invasive than open repair, some are unsuited to this method, owing to the anatomy of their aneurysm. Lifelong monitoring is needed: stents may leak and the aneurysm progress.

Image courtesy of Norwich Radiology Dept.

13 Surgery

Peripheral arterial disease (PAD)

Occurs due to atherosclerosis causing stenosis of arteries (fig 13.53) via a multifactorial process involving modifiable and non-modifiable risk factors. PAD exists on a spectrum: **asymptomatic or intermittent claudication** (= to limp, low risk of limb loss) to **critical limb ischaemia** (high risk of limb loss, requiring urgent intervention). The main risk, however, is cardiovascular morbidity/mortality: up to 50% of asymptomatic PAD or intermittent claudicants will suffer cardiovascular mortality, MI, or stroke at 5 years. In critical limb ischaemia: >25% mortality or limb loss at 1 year. ▶Cardiovascular risk factors should be identified and treated aggressively.

Symptoms Claudication: cramping pain in the calf, thigh, or buttock after walking for a given distance and relieved by rest (calf claudication suggests femoral disease while buttock claudication suggests iliac disease). Critical ischaemia: rest pain (eg burning pain at night relieved by hanging legs over side of bed), ulceration, gangrene (p652). Buttock claudication ± impotence imply Leriche's syndrome (p690). Young, heavy smokers are at risk from Buerger's disease (thromboangiitis obliterans, p686).

Fontaine classification for PAD 1 Asymptomatic. 2 Intermittent claudication. 3 Ischaemic rest pain. 4 Ulceration/gangrene (critical ischaemia).

Signs Absent femoral, popliteal, or foot pulses; cold, white leg(s); atrophic skin; punched out ulcers (often painful); postural/dependent colour change; Buerger's angle (angle that leg goes pale when raised off the couch) of <20° and capillary filling time >15s are found in critical limb ischaemia.

Tests Exclude DM, arteritis (ESR/CRP). FBC (anaemia, polycythaemia); U&E (renal disease); lipids (dyslipidaemia); ECG (cardiac ischaemia). Do thrombophilia screen and serum homocysteine if <50 years. **Ankle–brachial pressure index (ABPI)** Normal = 0.9–1.2; PAD = 0.5–0.9; critical limb ischaemia <0.5 or ankle systolic pressure <50mmHg. Beware falsely high results from incompressible calcified vessels in atherosclerosis.

Imaging Colour duplex US 1st line. If considering intervention MR/CT angiography for extent and location of stenoses and quality of distal vessels ('run-off').

℞ 1 **Risk factor modification** Quit smoking (vital). Treat hypertension and high cholesterol. Prescribe an antiplatelet (clopidogrel 1st line) for progression/vascular risk.
2 **Management of claudication** Most patients will improve or remain stable and therefore are treated conservatively. Supervised exercise programmes reduce symptoms by improving collateral blood flow (2h per wk for 3 months, the point of maximal pain). Vasoactive drugs, eg naftidrofuryl oxalate, offer modest benefit and are recommended only in those who do not wish to undergo revascularization and if exercise fails to improve symptoms.
3 **Management of critical limb ischaemia** Endovascular or open surgical intervention is required for limb salvage; if not suitable, amputation or palliation is required.

- **Percutaneous transluminal angioplasty (PTA)** is used 1st line for short lesions and in patients not fit for bypass surgery (often done under local anaesthetic). It will often require reintervention due to restenosis.
- **Surgical reconstruction** (bypass) is used for longer/more extensive occlusions in selected patients who are anaesthetically fit for major surgery. Procedures include femoral–popliteal bypass, femoral–femoral crossover, and aorto–bifemoral bypass grafts. Autologous vein grafts are superior to prosthetic grafts (eg Dacron® or PTFE) when the knee joint is crossed.
- **Amputation:** chronic critical limb ischaemia patients have an ≈ 25% risk of limb loss at 5 years (↑ in diabetes, p206). Amputation is indicated in three scenarios: 1 **dangerous:** saving life in uncontrollable diabetic sepsis/gangrene/necrotizing fasciitis; 2 **dead:** critical limb ischaemia with unreconstructable arterial disease; 3 **damn nuisance:** neuropathy or deformation with a non-functional limb. The principle is to chose a level of amputation that is likely to heal and preserves joints to help rehabilitation and prosthesis (if applicable). In a patient who is already bedbound and unlikely to mobilize, above-knee amputation is the default. Rehabilitation should be started early with a view to limb fitting. Gabapentin (regimen on p500) can be used to treat the gruelling complication of phantom limb pain.

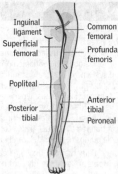

Fig 13.53 Leg arteries.

Acute limb ischaemia

▶▶Surgical emergency requiring revascularization within 4–6h to save the limb. May be due to thrombosis *in situ* (~40%), emboli (38%), graft/angioplasty occlusion (15%), or trauma. Thrombosis more likely in known 'vasculopaths'; emboli are sudden, eg in those without previous vessel disease; they can affect multiple sites, and there may be a bruit. Mortality: 22%. Amputation rate: 16%.

* **Symptoms and signs** The 6 'P's of acute ischaemia: **p**ale, **p**ulseless, **p**ainful, **p**aralysed, **p**araesthetic, and '**p**erishingly cold'. Onset of fixed mottling implies irreversibility. Emboli commonly arise from the heart (AF; mural thrombus) or aneurysms. ▶In patients with *known* PAD, sudden deterioration of symptoms with deep duskiness of the limb may indicate acute arterial occlusion. This appearance is due to extensive pre-existing collaterals and must not be misdiagnosed as gout/cellulitis.
* **Management** ▶Immediate management: 1 Heparin IV bolus 5000 units, IV fluids, ECG, cardiac enzymes (often associated with AF/MI), urinary catheter (risk of rhabdomyolysis). 2 Obtain urgent duplex scan or CTA. 3 Refer urgently to vascular surgeon. Definitive management (based on clinical status): *viable/marginally threatened limb* (preserved sensory and motor function) consider endovascular thrombolysis. *Imminently-threatened limb* (sensory loss, early motor loss) needs emergency thromboembolectomy. ▶Be aware of possible post-op reperfusion injury and subsequent compartment syndrome. *Irreversible* (insensate and paralysed limb with fixed mottling) amputation is the only surgical option (versus palliative care).

Long, tortuous, & dilated veins of the superficial venous system (see **fig 13.54**).

Pathology There are two systems of venous drainage in the lower limb: 1 *Deep veins* follow the arterial supply. Deep venous incompetence is often associated with previous DVT or proximal compression in the abdomen or pelvis. 2 *Superficial veins* (**fig 13.54**) drain into the deep system via perforators and at the saphenofemoral and saphenopopliteal junctions. Superficial venous valve incompetence results in reflux of blood from the deep system causing venous hypertension and dilatation of the superficial veins (varicose veins). **Risk factors** Prolonged standing, obesity, pregnancy, family history, and contraceptive pill. **Causes** Primary mechanical factors (in ~95%); secondary to obstruction (eg DVT, fetus, pelvic tumour), arteriovenous malformations, overactive muscle pumps (eg cyclists); rarely congenital valve absence.

Symptoms 'My legs are ugly.' Pain, cramps, tingling, heaviness, and restless legs. But studies show these symptoms are only slightly commoner in those with VVs.

Signs Oedema; eczema; ulcers; haemosiderin; haemorrhage; phlebitis; *atrophie blanche* (white scarring at the site of a previous, healed ulcer); lipodermatosclerosis (skin hardness from subcutaneous fibrosis caused by chronic inflammation and fat necrosis). On their own VVs don't cause DVTs (except possibly *proximally spreading thrombophlebitis* of the long saphenous vein).

Examination See p83.

Treatment ►NICE guidelines suggest that the criteria for specialist referral of patients with VVs should be: bleeding, pain, ulceration, superficial thrombophlebitis, or 'a severe impact on quality of life' (ie not for cosmetic reasons alone).

- *Treat any underlying cause.*
- *Education:* avoid prolonged standing and elevate leg(s) whenever possible; support stockings (compliance is a problem); lose weight; regular walks (calf muscle action aids venous return).
- *Compression stockings:* class II (safe if palpable pedal pulse or ABPI >0.8).
- *Endovascular treatment* (less pain and earlier return to activity than surgery).
  - *Endovenous ablation:* first line for those requiring intervention. A catheter is inserted into the incompetent vein and closed using heat energy either with radiofrequency or laser ablation.
  - *Injection sclerotherapy:* foam sclerotherapy is generally used for recurrent varicose veins below the knee and less commonly for main 'truncal' veins, eg LSV.
- *Surgical treatment:* there are several choices, depending on vein anatomy and surgical preference, eg saphenofemoral ligation (Trendelenburg procedure); multiple avulsions; stripping from groin to upper calf.
- *Post-op:* bandage legs tightly and elevate for 24h.

Saphena varix Dilatation in the saphenous vein at its confluence with the femoral vein (the SFJ). It transmits a cough impulse and may be mistaken for an inguinal or femoral hernia, but on closer inspection it may have a bluish tinge.

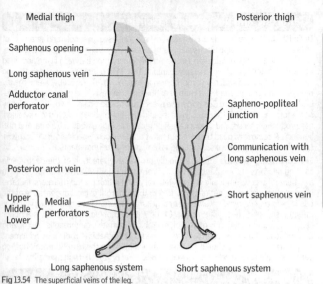

Medial thigh

Saphenous opening

Long saphenous vein

Adductor canal perforator

Posterior arch vein

Upper Middle Lower — Medial perforators

Long saphenous system

Posterior thigh

Sapheno-popliteal junction

Communication with long saphenous vein

Short saphenous vein

Short saphenous system

Fig 13.54 The superficial veins of the leg.

When do varicose veins become an illness?

Perhaps when they hurt? Or is this too simple? 'Certain illnesses are desirable: they provide a compensation for a functional disorder...' (Albert Camus); *this is known to be common with VVs.* Perhaps many opt for surgery as a displacement activity to confronting deeper problems. We adopt the sickness role when we want sympathy. Somatization is hard to manage; here is one approach to consider:
• Give time; don't dismiss these patients as 'just the "worried well".'
• Explore factors perpetuating illness behaviour (misinformation, social stressors).
• Agree a plan that makes sense to the patient's holistic view of themselves.
• Treat any underlying depression (drugs and cognitive therapy, *OHCS* p710).

Gangrene and necrotizing fasciitis

Definitions Gangrene is death of tissue from poor vascular supply and is a sign of critical ischaemia (see p648). Tissues are black and may slough. *Dry gangrene* is necrosis in the absence of infection. Note a line of demarcation between living and dead tissue.[13] ℞ restoration of blood supply ± amputation. *Wet gangrene* is tissue death and infection (associated with discharge) occurring together (p207, fig 5.10). ℞ ►emergency requiring immediate broad-spectrum IV antibiotics, analgesia, and prompt surgical debridement ± amputation. *Gas gangrene* is a subset of necrotizing myositis caused by spore-forming clostridial species. There is rapid onset of myonecrosis, muscle swelling, gas production, sepsis, and severe pain. Risk factors include diabetes, trauma, and malignancy. ℞ remove all dead tissue (eg amputation). Give benzylpenicillin ± clindamycin. Hyperbaric O_2 can improve survival and ↓ the number of debridements.

►►**Necrotizing fasciitis** This is a rapidly progressive infection of the deep fascia causing necrosis of subcutaneous tissue. Prompt recognition; always suspect this in a patient who is systemically very unwell (very high inflammatory markers, lactate) in spite of resuscitation, out of proportion to the apparent clinical appearance of the tissue. ►*In any atypical cellulitis, get early surgical help.* There is intense pain over affected skin and underlying muscle. Group A β-haemolytic streptococci is a major cause, although infection is often polymicrobial. Fournier's gangrene is necrotizing fasciitis localized to the scrotum and perineum. ℞ Immediate radical debridement ± amputation, patient should be taken immediately to theatre; IV antibiotics, eg benzylpenicillin and clindamycin (according to local protocol). High mortality.

Skin ulcers

Ulcers are abnormal breaks in an epithelial surface. Leg ulcers affect ~2%.

Causes May be multiple. For leg ulcers, venous disease accounts for 70%, mixed arterial and venous disease for 15%, and arterial disease alone for 2%. Other contributory factors include neuropathy (eg in DM), lymphoedema, malignancy (p588), infection (eg TB, syphilis), trauma (eg pressure sores: see fig 10.18, p471), pyoderma gangrenosum, drugs (eg nicorandil, hydroxycarbamide).

History Ask about number, pain, trauma. Explore comorbidities—eg VVs, peripheral arterial disease, diabetes, vasculitis. Length of history? Is the patient taking steroids? Are self-induced ulcers, *dermatitis artefacta*, a possibility? Has a biopsy been taken?

Examination Note features such as site, number, surface area, depth, edge, base, discharge, lymphadenopathy, sensation, and healing (see BOX and table 13.18). If in the legs, note features of venous insufficiency or arterial disease and, if possible, apply a BP cuff to perform ankle–brachial pressure index (ABPI). Ulcers on the sacrum, greater trochanter, or heel suggest *pressure sores* (OHCS p454), particularly if the patient is bed-bound with suboptimal nutrition.

Tests Skin and ulcer biopsy may be necessary—eg to assess for vasculitis (will need immunohistopathology) or malignant change in an established ulcer (Marjolin's ulcer = SCC presenting in chronic wound). If ulceration is the first sign of a suspected systemic disorder then further screening tests will be required.

Management Treat the cause(s) and focus on prevention. Optimize nutrition. Are there adverse risk factors (drug addiction, or risk factors for arteriopathy, eg smoking)? Get expert nursing care. Consider referral to specialist community nurse or leg ulcer/tissue viability clinic:
- 'Charing-Cross' 4-layer compression bandaging is better than standard bandages (use only if arterial pulses OK: ABPI (p648) should be >0.8). Negative pressure wound therapy (eg VAC®) helps heal diabetic ulcers.
- Surgery, larval therapy, and hydrogels are used to debride sloughy necrotic tissue (avoid hydrogels in diabetic ulcers due to ↑risk of wet gangrene).

►Routine use of antibiotics does not improve healing. Only use if there is infection (not colonization).

13 'The first sign of his approaching end was when one of my old aunts, while undressing him, removed a toe with one of his old socks.' Graham Greene, *A Sort of Life*, 1971, Simon & Schuster.

Features of skin ulceration to note on examination

Table 13.18 Differential diagnosis of lower limb ulcers

Type	Venous	Arterial	Neuropathic
Site	Above the medial malleolus ('gaiter' area, fig 13.55)	More distal; toes, pressure points	Arterial distribution, particularly pressure points
Hx	Previous DVT (post-phlebitic limb), varicose veins	Peripheral arterial disease, eg claudication, rest pain, gangrene	History of poor recent blood glucose control or peripheral neuropathy, recent trauma. Sensory impairment or neuropathic pain
Exam	Exudative, shallow, irregular edge. Venous hypertension-related superficial varicosities and skin changes (*lipodermatosclerosis* = induration, pigmentation, and inflammation of the skin)	'Punched out' ulcers. Absence of pedal pulses, pallor, cold foot, increased capillary refill time	Warm foot with pulses (pure neuropathic) *or* with coexisting arterial insufficiency; tend to be more aggressive, often presenting with deep tissue infection/ abscess/osteomyelitis
Pathology	Superficial and/or deep venous insufficiency	Chronic arterial insufficiency, ie ischaemia	Neuropathic 50% Neuro-ischaemic 50%
Imaging	Venous duplex	Arterial duplex	Arterial duplex/ABPI; HbA1c; monofilament test

Surface area Draw a map of the area to quantify and time any healing (a wound >4wks old is a chronic ulcer as distinguished from an acute wound).

Shape Oval, circular (cigarette burns), serpiginous (*Klebsiella granulomatis*, p408); unusual morphology can be secondary to mycobacterial infection, eg cutaneous tuberculosis or scrofuloderma (*tuberculosis colliquativa cutis*, where an infected lymph node ulcerates through to the skin).

Edge Shelved/sloping ≈ healing; punched-out ≈ ischaemic or syphilis; rolled/ everted ≈ malignant; undermined ≈ TB.

Base Any muscle, bone, or tendon destruction (malignancy; pressure sores; ischaemia)? There may be a grey-yellow slough, beneath which is a pale pink base. *Slough* is a mixture of fibrin, cell breakdown products, serous exudate, leucocytes, and bacteria—it need not imply infection, and can be part of the normal wound healing process. *Granulation tissue* is a deep pink gel-like matrix contained within a fibrous collagen network and is evidence of a healing wound.

Depth If not uncomfortable for the patient (eg in neuropathic ulceration), a probe can be used to gauge how deep the ulceration extends.

Discharge Culture before starting any antibiotics (which usually don't work). A watery discharge is said to favour TB; ▶bleeding can ≈ malignancy.

Associated lymphadenopathy Suggests infection or malignancy.

Position in phases of extension/healing Healing is

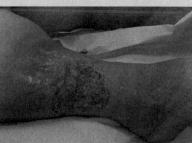

Fig 13.55 Venous ulcer in the gaiter area in an obese woman.
Reproduced from Burge *et al.*, *Oxford Handbook of Medical Dermatology*, 2016, with permission from Oxford University Press.

heralded by granulation, scar formation, and epithelialization. Inflamed margins ≈ extension.

Contents

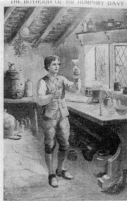

Fig 14.1 Sir Humphrey Davy (1778–1829) was a British chemist and inventor from Cornwall who is remembered for pioneering the field of electro-chemistry. By using electricity, he isolated several elements for the first time including potassium, sodium, calcium, strontium, barium, and magnesium. He also discovered the elemental nature of chlorine and iodine. Prior to this work, he had investigated inhaled nitrous oxide and described its potential analgesic and anaesthetic properties. Through extreme (and near-fatal) self-experimentation, he was the first to coin the name 'laughing gas'. His impression after first use was that 'Nothing exists but thoughts!... The world is composed of impressions, ideas, pleasures and pains!'

Humphrey Davy making his first experiment when a boy. Wellcome Collection. Attribution 4.0 International (CC BY 4.0). https://wellcomecollection.org/works/rude8b72

$Ca^{2+}Na^+$
K^+

On being normal in the society of numbers

Laboratory medicine reduces our patients to a few easy-to-handle numbers: this is the discipline's great attraction—and its greatest danger. The normal range (reference interval) is usually that which includes 95% of a given population (given a normal distribution, see p734). If variation is randomly distributed, 2.5% of our results will be 'too high', and 2.5% 'too low' on an average day, when dealing with apparently normal people. This statistical definition of normality is the simplest. Other definitions may be *normative*—ie stating what an upper or lower limit *should* be. The upper end of the reference interval for plasma cholesterol may be given as 6mmol/L because this is what biochemists state to be the *desired* maximum. 40% of people in some populations will have a plasma cholesterol >6mmol/L and thus may be at increased risk. The WHO definition of anaemia in pregnancy is an Hb of <110g/L, which makes 20% of mothers anaemic. This 'lax' criterion has the presumed benefit of triggering actions that result in fewer deaths from haemorrhage. So do not just ask 'What is the normal range?'—also enquire about who set the range, for what population, and for what reason.

We thank Yvelynne Kelly, our Specialist Reader for this chapter.

General principles

• Laboratory testing may contribute to four aspects of medicine:
  • Diagnosis (eg TSH in hypothyroidism).
  • Prognosis (eg clotting in liver failure).
  • Monitoring disease activity or progression (eg creatinine in chronic kidney disease).
  • Screening (eg phenylketonuria in newborn babies).

• Only do a test if the result will influence management. Make sure you look at the result.
• ►Always interpret laboratory results in the context of the patient's clinical picture.
• If a result does not fit with the clinical picture, trust clinical judgement and repeat the test. Could it be an artefact? The 'normal' range for a test (reference interval) is usually defined as the interval, symmetrical about the mean, containing 95% of results in a given population (p735). The more tests you run, the greater the probability of an 'abnormal' result of no significance (p735).
• Laboratory staff like to have contact with you. They are an excellent source of help and information for both requests and results.
• ►Involve the patient. Don't forget to explain to them where the test fits into their overall management plan.

Getting the best out of the lab—a laboratory decalogue

1 Interest someone from the laboratory in your patient's problem.
2 Fill in the request form fully.
3 Give clinical details, not your preferred diagnosis.
4 Ensure that the lab knows who to contact.
5 Label specimens as well as the request form.
6 Follow the hospital labelling routine for cross-matching.
7 Find out when analysers run, especially batched assays.
8 Talk with the lab before requesting an unusual test.
9 Be thoughtful: at 16:30h the routine results are being sorted.
10 Plot results graphically: abnormalities show sooner.

Artefacts and pitfalls in laboratory tests

• Do not take blood samples from an arm that has IV fluid running into it.
• Repeat any unexpected and inconsistent result before acting on it.
• For clotting time do not sample from a heparinized IV catheter.
• Serum K^+ is overestimated if the sample is old or haemolysed (this occurs if venepuncture is difficult).
• If using Vacutainer™ tubes, fill *plain* tubes first—otherwise, anticoagulant contamination from previous tubes can cause errors.
• Total calcium results are affected by albumin concentration (p668).
• INR may be overestimated if citrate bottles are underfilled.
• Drugs may cause *analytic* errors (eg prednisolone cross-reacts with cortisol). Be suspicious if results are unexpected.
• Food may affect result, eg bananas raise urinary HIAA (p266).

Ford Madox Ford 1915: *The Good Soldier*

Normal values can have hidden historical, social, and political desiderata—just like the normal values novelists ascribe to their characters: *'Conventions and traditions I suppose work blindly but surely for the preservation of the normal type; for the extinction of proud, resolute and unusual individuals... Society must go on, I suppose, and society can only exist if the normal, if the virtuous, and the slightly-deceitful flourish, and if the passionate, the headstrong, and the too-truthful are condemned to suicide and to madness. Yes, society must go on; it must breed, like rabbits. That is what we are here for... But, at any rate, there is always Leonora to cheer you up; I don't want to sadden you. Her husband is quite an economical person of so normal a figure that he can get quite a large proportion of his clothes ready-made. That is the great desideratum of life.'*

Oxford World's Classics, pp181–92

Volume depletion ↑Urea (disproportionate relative to smaller ↑ in creatinine),[1] ↑albumin (also useful to plot change in a patient's condition), ↑haematocrit (PCV); also ↓urine volume and ↓skin turgor.

Abnormal kidney function The pattern varies according to chronicity (table 14.1). **Causes** AKI (p294), CKD (p298). **Tubular dysfunction** Results from damage to tubules. Diagnosis is made by testing renal concentrating ability (p235). May be polyuric with ↑urinary glucose, amino acids, proteins (lysozyme, β₂-microglobulin) or phosphate. *Proximal tubular causes:* familial (eg cystinosis, Wilson's disease) or acquired (eg myeloma, carbonic anhydrase inhibitors, antiretroviral drugs). *Distal tubular causes:* Sjögren's syndrome, tubulointerstitial nephritis, nephrocalcinosis.

Table 14.1 Clinical, biochemical, and imaging differences between AKI and CKD

	AKI	CKD
History & exam	Usually acutely unwell	Better tolerance of biochemical abnormalities
Creatinine	Rapidly ↑ values	History of derangement
Bone profile	Usually normal Ca²⁺/PO₄³⁻	↓Ca²⁺ & ↑PO₄³⁻ due to secondary hyperparathyroidism
Hb	Usually normal	↓ due to EPO deficiency
Renal US	Often normal or shows ↑parenchymal echogenicity. Important to rule out hydronephrosis	Kidneys can be small or have cortical thinning and loss of corticomedullary differentiation Large kidneys in ADPKD

Thiazide and loop diuretics ↓Na⁺, ↓K⁺, ↑HCO₃⁻, ↑urea.

Bone disease See table 14.2 for typical biochemical patterns.

Table 14.2 Serum biomarkers in common diseases of bone

	Ca²⁺	PO₄³⁻	
Osteoporosis (p674)	Normal	Normal	Normal
Osteomalacia (p676)	↓	↓	↑
Paget's	Normal	Normal	↑↑
Myeloma	↑	↑, normal	Normal
Bone metastases	↑	↑, normal	↑
1° Hyperparathyroidism	↑	↓, normal	Normal, ↑
Hypoparathyroidism	↓	↑	Normal
CKD	↓	↑	Normal, ↑

Hepatocellular disease ↑Bilirubin, ↑↑AST, ALP ↑ slightly, ↓albumin. Also ↑clotting times. For details of the differences between AST and ALT, see p287.

Cholestasis ↑Bilirubin, ↑↑γGT, ↑↑ALP, ↑AST.

Excess alcohol intake Evidence of hepatocellular disease. Early evidence if ↑γGT, ↑MCV, and ethanol in blood before lunch.

Myocardial infarction ↑Troponin, ↑CK, ↑AST, ↑LDH (p114).

Addison's disease ↑K⁺, ↓Na⁺, ↑urea.

Cushing's syndrome May show ↓K⁺, ↑HCO₃⁻, ↑Na⁺.

Conn's syndrome May show ↓K⁺, ↑HCO₃⁻. Na⁺ ↔ or ↑. (Also hypertension.)

Diabetes mellitus ↑Glucose (↓HCO₃⁻ if acidotic).

Diabetes insipidus ↑Na⁺, ↑plasma osmolality, ↓urine osmolality. (Both hypercalcaemia and hypokalaemia may cause nephrogenic diabetes insipidus.)

Inappropriate ADH secretion (SIADH) (See p665.) ↓Na⁺ with ↓↔ urea and creatinine, ↓plasma osmolality. ↑Urine osmolality (>plasma osmolality), ↑urine Na⁺ (>20mmol/L).

Some immunodeficiency states Normal serum albumin but *low* total protein (because immunoglobulins are missing). Also makes crossmatching difficult because expected haemagglutinins are absent; OHCS p244).

Laboratory results: when to take action NOW

- On receiving a dangerous result, first check the name and date.
- Go to the bedside. If the patient is conscious, turn off any IVI (until fluid is checked: a mistake may have been made) and ask the patient how they are. *Any fits, faints, collapses, or unexpected symptoms?*
- Be sceptical of an unexpectedly, wildly abnormal result with a well patient. Compare with previous values. Could the specimens have got muddled up; whose is it? Is there an artefact? Was the sample taken from the 'drip' arm? Is a low calcium due to a low albumin (p668)? Perhaps the lab is using a new analyser with a faulty wash cycle? ▶*When in doubt, seek help and repeat the test.*

The following values are somewhat arbitrary and must be taken as a guide only. Many results less extreme than those listed will be just as dangerous if the patient is old, immunosuppressed, or has some other pathology such as pneumonia.

Plasma biochemistry

▶▶The main risks when plasma electrolytes are dangerously abnormal (table 14.3) are of cardiac arrhythmias and CNS events such as seizures. It's important to remember that a hypokalaemic cardiac arrest is more common than a hyperkalaemic one so you need to take this abnormality as seriously as the latter.

Table 14.3 Dangerous levels of the common serum electrolytes

Electrolyte	Lower limit	Upper limit	Relevant pages
Na^+	<120mmol/L	>155mmol/L	p664
K^+	<2.5mmol/L	>6.5mmol/L	p301, p666
Corrected Ca^{2+}	<2.0mmol/L	>3.5mmol/L	p668, p670
Glucose	<2.0mmol/L	>20mmol/L	p816, p818

Blood gases

- P_aO_2 <8.0kPa = *severe hypoxia*. Give O_2. See p158.
- pH <7.2 = *dangerous acidosis. See* p662 *to determine the cause.*

Haematology results

- Hb <70g/L with low mean cell volume (<75fL) or history of bleeding. This patient may need urgent transfusion—ask about symptoms, comorbidities, and baseline Hb. Check haematinics before transfusion. See p324.
- Platelets <40 × 10^9/L. May need a platelet transfusion; call a haematologist.
- *Plasmodium falciparum* seen on blood film. *Start antimalarials now.* See p414.
- ESR >30mm/h + headache. *Could this be giant cell arteritis?* See p554.

CSF results

▶▶Never delay treatment when bacterial meningitis is suspected.
- >1 neutrophil/mm³. *Is there meningitis: usually >1000 neutrophils?* See p806.
- Positive Gram stain. *Talk to a microbiologist; urgent blind therapy.* See p806.

Conflicting, equivocal, or inexplicable results ▶Get prompt help.

$Ca^{2+} Na^+$
K^+

1 Dehydration affects urea more than creatinine because in volume depletion a greater proportion of filtered urea is reabsorbed by the kidney. Creatinine is hardly reabsorbed at all.

Fluid requirement 25–30mL/kg/day which is ~2–2.5L in a normal person (~70kg) over 24h. Normal daily losses are through urine (1500mL), stool (200mL), and insensible losses (800mL). This requirement is normally met through food (1000mL) and drink (1500mL).

Intravenous fluids Given if sufficient fluids cannot be given orally. About 2–2.5L of fluid containing roughly 70mmol Na$^+$ and 70mmol K$^+$ per 24h are required.[1] The precise regimen depends on a combination of maintenance fluid requirements, existing deficits in volume status and/or electrolytes, ongoing losses, and kidney function.

►In a sick patient, don't forget to include additional sources of fluid loss when calculating daily fluid requirements, such as drains, fevers, or diarrhoea (see BOX 'Special cases'). Daily weighing helps to monitor overall fluid balance, as will fluid balance charts. Examine patients regularly to assess fluid balance (see BOX 'Assessing fluid balance').

Fluid compartments and types of IV fluid
For a 70kg man, *total bodily fluid* is ~42L (60% body weight). Of this, ⅔ is intracellular (28L) and ⅓ is extracellular (14L). Of the extracellular compartment, ⅓ is intravascular, ie blood (5L). Different types of IV fluid will equilibrate with the different fluid compartments depending on the osmotic content of the given fluid.

5% glucose (=Dextrose.) Initially behaves as an isotonic solution. Contains only a small amount of glucose (50g/L) and so provides little energy (~10% daily energy per litre). Eventually becomes hypotonic as the liver rapidly metabolizes all the glucose leaving only water, which rapidly equilibrates throughout all fluid compartments. It is, therefore, useless for fluid resuscitation (only $^1/_9$ will remain in the intravascular space), but suitable for maintaining water balance. Excess 5% glucose IV may lead to water overload and hyponatraemia (p664).

Hypertonic glucose (10%, 20%, or 50%) Small doses may be used in the treatment of hypoglycaemia (eg give 100mL 20% dextrose stat). It is irritant to veins, so care in its use is needed. Infusion sites should be inspected regularly, and flushed with 0.9% saline after use.

0.9% saline ('Normal saline (NS).') Although isotonic, it is considered to be an unbalanced crystalloid as the electrolyte composition (Na$^+$ and Cl$^-$ both 154mmol/L) differs from plasma. 0.9% saline will equilibrate rapidly throughout the extracellular compartment only, and takes longer to reach the intracellular compartment than 5% glucose. It is, therefore, appropriate for fluid resuscitation, as it will remain predominantly in the extracellular space (and thus ⅓ of the given volume in the intravascular space). However, with high-volume administration, there is a risk of hyperchloraemic acidosis since each litre of NS delivers around 50mmol more Cl$^-$ than a litre of plasma. It is superior to balanced solutions in cases of metabolic alkalosis, most of which are due to Cl$^-$ deficiency. Hypertonic and hypotonic saline solutions are also available, but are for specialist use only.

Hartmann's solution Balanced crystalloid—it contains Na$^+$ 131mmol, Cl$^-$ 111mmol, lactate 29mmol, K$^+$ 5mmol, HCO$_3^-$ 29mmol, and Ca^{2+} 2mmol per litre of fluid. It is generally preferred to 0.9% saline, particularly when large volume administration is required as it is more physiological. It prevents dilutional reduction of normal plasma components such as Ca^{2+} and K$^+$, and avoids hyperchloraemic acidosis. Potentially ↓ AKI and mortality in critically ill patients compared to 0.9% saline.[2]

Colloids (eg Gelofusine®.) Contain large molecules such as proteins that do not readily pass through the capillary membrane and thus remain in the intravascular space for extended periods. Here they increase the osmotic pressure causing fluid to move into the intravascular space and thus are often referred to as volume expanders. However, colloids are expensive and may cause anaphylactic reactions. They are not associated with any mortality benefit when compared to crystalloids.[3]

Isotonic sodium bicarbonate (1.26%) Prepare by adding 150mL of 8.4% NaHCO$_3$ to 850mL of 5% dextrose. Can be used as a buffered crystalloid for fluid resuscitation in cases of metabolic acidosis, eg due to GI, or renal losses.

Assessing fluid balance

Underfilled

* Tachycardia.
* Postural drop in BP (low BP is a late sign of hypovolaemia).
* ↓Capillary refill time.
* ↓Urine output.
* Cool peripheries.
* Dry mucous membranes.
* ↓Skin turgor.
* Sunken eyes.

Overfilled

* ↑JVP (p41).
* Pitting oedema of the sacrum, ankles, or even legs and abdomen.
* Tachypnoea.
* Bibasal crepitations.
* Pulmonary oedema on CXR (fig 16.3, p707).

See also p134 for signs of heart failure.

The JVP is a substitute marker of central venous pressure, and can help when assessing fluid balance is difficult. A CVP line may help to guide fluid management.

Special cases

Acute blood loss Resuscitate with Hartmann's or 0.9% saline via large-bore cannulae until blood is available.

Children Use glucose with sodium chloride for fluid maintenance: 100mL/kg for the first 10kg, 50mL/kg for the next 10kg, and 20mL/kg thereafter—all per 24h.

Elderly May be more prone to fluid overload, so use IV fluids with care (smaller fluid bolus).

GI losses (Diarrhoea, vomiting, NG tubes, etc.) Replace lost K⁺ as well as lost fluid volume.

Heart failure Use IV fluids with care to avoid fluid overload (p134).

Liver failure Patients often have a raised total body sodium, so use salt-poor albumin or blood preferentially for resuscitation, and avoid 0.9% saline for maintenance.

Acute pancreatitis Aggressive fluid resuscitation is required due to large amounts of sequestered 'third-space' fluid (p628).

Poor urine output Aim for >1mL/kg/h; the minimum is >0.5mL/kg/h. Give a fluid challenge, eg 500mL Hartmann's over 1h (or half this volume in heart failure or the elderly), and recheck the urine output. If not catheterized, exclude retention; if catheterized, ensure the catheter is not blocked!

Post-operative Check the operation notes for intra-operative losses, and ensure you chart and replace added losses from drains, etc.

Shock Resuscitate with balanced crystalloids via large-bore cannulae. Identify the cause of shock and treat accordingly (p770).

Transpiration losses (Fever, burns.) Beware the large amounts of fluid that can be lost unseen through transpiration. Severe burns in particular may require aggressive fluid resuscitation (p828).

Potassium in IV fluids

* Potassium ions can be given with 5% glucose or 0.9% saline, usually 20mmol/L or 40mmol/L.
* K⁺ may be retained in impaired kidney function, so beware giving too much IV.
* Gastrointestinal fluids are rich in K⁺, so increased fluid loss from the gut (eg diarrhoea, vomiting, high-output stoma, intestinal fistula) will need increased K⁺ replacement.

▶The maximum concentration of K⁺ that is safe to infuse via a peripheral line is 40mmol/L, at a maximum rate of 20mmol/h in a cardiac monitored patient. Fluid-restricted patients may require higher concentrations or faster rates in life-threatening hypokalaemia. Faster rates risk cardiac dysrhythmias and asystole, and higher concentrations thrombophlebitis, depending on the size of the vein, so give concentrated solutions >40mmol/L via a central venous catheter, and use ECG monitoring for rates >10mmol/h. For symptoms and signs of hyper- and hypokalaemia see p666.

14 Clinical chemistry

The kidney Controls the homeostasis of a number of serum electrolytes (including Na^+, K^+, Ca^{2+}, and PO_4^{3-}), helps to maintain acid–base balance, and is responsible for the excretion of many substances. It also makes erythropoietin and renin, and hydroxylates 25-hydroxy-vitamin D to 1,25-dihydroxy-vitamin D, the active form of vitamin D (see p668 for Ca^{2+} and PO_4^{3-} physiology). All of these functions can be affected in chronic kidney disease (p298) and can be used to monitor disease progression.

The renin–angiotensin–aldosterone system Plasma is filtered by the glomeruli, and Na^+, K^+, H^+, and water are reabsorbed from this filtrate under the control of the renin–angiotensin–aldosterone system. *Renin* is released from the juxtaglomerular apparatus (fig 7.13, p312) in response to low renal blood flow and raised sympathetic tone, and catalyses the conversion of *angiotensinogen* (a peptide made by the liver) to **angiotensin I**. This is then converted by angiotensin-converting enzyme (ACE), which is located throughout the vascular tree, to **angiotensin II**. The latter has several important actions including efferent renal arteriolar constriction (thus ↑perfusion pressure), peripheral vasoconstriction, and stimulation of the adrenal cortex to produce *aldosterone*, which activates the Na^+/K^+ pump in the distal renal tubule and increases insertion of ENaC into the luminal membrane, leading to re-absorption of Na^+ and water from the urine, in exchange for K^+ and H^+. Glucose spills over into the urine when the plasma concentration > renal threshold for re-absorption (≈10mmol/L, but this varies between people, and is ↓ in pregnancy).

Control of sodium Control is through the action of aldosterone on the distal convoluted tubule (DCT) and collecting duct to increase Na^+ reabsorption from the urine. Factors that increase urinary Na^+ excretion include ↑dietary Na^+ leading to ECFV expansion, ↑BP causing pressure natriuresis (eg in hypertensive emergencies), diuretics, tubulointerstitial disease, and ↓ mineralocorticoid activity or tubular responsiveness.

Control of potassium Most K^+ is intracellular, and thus serum K^+ levels are a poor reflection of total body potassium. This difference is created by the action of Na^+/K^+ ATPase, the activity of which is regulated by insulin, catecholamines, osmolality, and acid–base status. Both insulin and catecholamines stimulate K^+ uptake into cells by stimulating the Na^+/K^+ pump while acidosis (especially non-gap) and ↑osmolality promote K^+ efflux. K^+ is secreted in the collecting duct, stimulated by aldosterone and high tubular flow rates.

Serum osmolality A laboratory measurement of the number of osmoles per *kilogram* of solvent. It is approximated by *serum osmolarity* (the number of osmoles per *litre* of solution) using the equation $2(Na^+ + K^+)$ + Urea + Glucose, since these are the predominant serum electrolytes. Normal serum osmolality is 285–295mmol/L, which will always be a little less than the laboratory-measured osmolality—the *osmolar gap*. However, if the osmolar gap is greater than 10mmol/L, this indicates the presence of additional solutes: consider diabetes mellitus or high blood ethanol, methanol, mannitol, or ethylene glycol.

Control of water Control is mainly via serum Na^+ concentration, since water intake and loss are regulated to hold the extracellular concentration of Na^+ constant. Raised plasma osmolality (eg water losses from vomiting or ↑glucose in diabetes mellitus) causes thirst through the hypothalamic thirst centre and the release of antidiuretic hormone (ADH) from the posterior pituitary. ADH increases the passive water reabsorption from the renal collecting duct by opening water channels to allow water to flow from the hypotonic luminal fluid into the hypertonic renal interstitium. Low plasma osmolality inhibits ADH secretion, thus reducing renal water reabsorption.

Glomerular filtration rate (GFR) This is the volume of fluid filtered by the glomeruli per minute (units mL/min), and is one of the primary measures of disease progression in chronic kidney disease. It can be estimated in a number of different ways (see BOX).

Calculating GFR is useful because it is a more sensitive indication of the degree of kidney dysfunction than serum creatinine. Subjects with low muscle mass (eg the elderly, women) can have a 'normal' serum creatinine, despite a significant reduction in GFR. This can be important when prescribing nephrotoxic drugs, or drugs that are renally excreted, which may therefore accumulate to toxic levels in the serum.

A number of methods for estimating GFR exist, all relying on a calculation of the clearance of a substance that is renally filtered and then not reabsorbed in the renal tubule. For example, the rate of clearance of creatinine can be used as a marker for the rate of filtration of fluid and solutes in the glomerulus because it is only slightly reabsorbed from the renal tubule. The more of the filtered substance that is reabsorbed, however, the less accurate the estimate of GFR.

However, it must be emphasized that all GFR-estimating (eGFR) equations were developed in people with stable CKD and serum creatinine, and thus all equations are less accurate in situations where serum creatinine levels are changing rapidly (eg AKI), and in healthy people with normal renal function.

eGFR calculated with any creatinine-based equation will also be less accurate in people with other prominent determinants of serum creatinine (eg extremes of muscle mass or weight, patients with liver disease, children, or those with a high-protein diet).

CKD-EPI (Chronic Kidney Disease Epidemiology Collaboration) This provides an estimate of GFR from three simple parameters: *serum creatinine*, *age*, and *sex*. Consensus guidelines now recommend using the 2021 version of this formula to estimate GFR in most clinical scenarios.[4] Importantly, this updated version no longer includes a coefficient for race as this was shown to cause bias and contribute to healthcare inequities.

Cystatin C This is an endogenous low-molecular-weight protein that is filtered at the glomerulus and not reabsorbed but metabolized in the tubules. It can also be used to estimate GFR but not to directly measure clearance. Its accuracy is also influenced by non-eGFR determinants including sex, height, weight, lean and fat body mass, levels of inflammatory markers, and use of steroids. Combining creatinine and cystatin C measurements in the 2021 CKD-EPI creatinine-cystatin C equation is a very useful way to confirm eGFR measurements as it is more accurate than either alone. It is currently most often used in a specialist nephrology setting though, eg when evaluating potential living kidney transplant donors.

Older methods Use of the MDRD (Modification of Diet in Renal Disease Study Group) and Cockcroft–Gault equations are no longer recommended to estimate GFR as these were based on older techniques and derived from older populations with less obesity. The Cockcroft–Gault equation was developed prior to the use of standardized creatinine assays and has not been updated for use with creatinine values traceable to standardized reference materials.

Special scenarios If using eGFR to dose drugs in very large or very small patients, multiply the reported eGFR by the estimated body surface area (BSA) and divide by 1.73m², in order to obtain eGFR in units of mL/min. In the setting of rapidly changing creatinine values, an equation known as the kinetic eGFR may be useful to more accurately assess true GFR.

Creatinine clearance can also be calculated by measuring the excreted creatinine in a *24h urine collection* and comparing it with the serum creatinine concentration. Although difficult to collect accurately, it can be useful in helping to determine whether renal recovery is present for patients with severe AKI requiring RRT; given that estimated GFR calculations are not valid in this setting.[5]

GFR can also be measured by injection of a radioisotope followed by sequential blood sampling (*⁵¹Cr-EDTA*) or by an isotope scan (eg DTPA ⁹⁹Tc, p186). These methods allow a more accurate estimate of GFR than creatinine clearance, since smaller proportions of these substances are reabsorbed in the tubules. They also have the advantage of being able to provide split renal function.

Arterial blood pH is closely regulated in health to 7.40 ± 0.05 by various mechanisms including bicarbonate, other plasma buffers such as deoxygenated haemoglobin, and the kidney. Acid–base disorders needlessly confuse many people, but if a few simple rules are applied, then interpretation and diagnosis are easy. The key principle is that primary changes in HCO_3^- are *metabolic* and in CO_2 *respiratory*. See tables 14.4, 14.5.

A simple method

1 *Look at the pH*, is there an acidosis or alkalosis?
   • pH <7.35 is an acidosis; pH >7.45 is an alkalosis.
2 *Is the CO_2 abnormal?* (Normal range 4.7–6.0kPa.)
   If so, is the change in keeping with the pH?
   • CO_2 is an acidic gas—is CO_2 raised with an acidosis, lowered with an alkalosis? If so, it is in keeping with the pH and thus caused by a *respiratory* problem. If there is no change, or an opposite one, then the change is compensatory.
3 *Is the HCO_3^- abnormal?* (Normal concentration 22–28mmol/L.)
   If so, is the change in keeping with the pH?
   • HCO_3^- is alkaline—is HCO_3^- raised with an alkalosis, lowered with an acidosis? If so, the problem is a *metabolic* one.
4 *Is the P_aO_2 abnormal?* Interpret in the context of the FiO_2.

An example Your patient's blood gas shows: pH 7.05, CO_2 2.0kPa, HCO_3^- 8.0mmol/L. There is an *acidosis*. The CO_2 is low, and thus it is a compensatory change. The HCO_3^- is low and is thus the primary change, ie a *metabolic* acidosis.

The anion gap Estimates unmeasured plasma anions ('fixed' or organic acids such as phosphate, ketones, and lactate—hard to measure directly). It is calculated as the difference between plasma cations (Na^+ and K^+) and anions (Cl^- and HCO_3^-). Normal range: 10–18mmol/L. It is helpful in determining the cause of a metabolic acidosis.

Metabolic acidosis: ↓pH, ↓HCO_3^-

Causes of metabolic acidosis and an increased anion gap
Due to increased production, or reduced excretion, of fixed/organic acids. HCO_3^- decreases and unmeasured anions associated with the acids accumulate.
• Lactic acid (shock, infection, tissue ischaemia).
• Uraemia (AKI).
• Ketones (diabetes mellitus, alcohol).
• Drugs/toxins (salicylates, biguanides, ethylene glycol, methanol).

Causes of metabolic acidosis and a normal anion gap
Due to loss of bicarbonate or ingestion of H^+ ions (Cl^- is retained).
• Renal tubular acidosis.
• Diarrhoea.
• Drugs (acetazolamide).
• Addison's disease.
• Pancreatic fistula.
• Ammonium chloride ingestion.

Metabolic alkalosis: ↑pH, ↑HCO_3^-
• Protracted vomiting or nasogastric suction.
• Volume contraction.
• K^+ depletion (diuretics).
• Burns.
• Urinary acid loss (eg Bartter syndrome, Cushing's syndrome).
• Ingestion of base (eg antacids, milk-alkali syndrome).

Respiratory acidosis: ↓pH, ↑CO_2
• Type 2 respiratory failure due to any lung, neuromuscular, or physical cause (p158).
• Most commonly COPD. Look at the P_aO_2. It will probably be low. Is oxygen therapy required? Use controlled O_2 (Venturi connector) if COPD is the underlying cause, as too much oxygen may make matters worse (p159).
►►Beware exhaustion in asthma, pneumonia, and pulmonary oedema, which can present with this picture when close to respiratory arrest. A normal or high P_aCO_2 is worrying. These patients require urgent ITU review for ventilatory support.

Respiratory alkalosis: ↑pH, ↓CO_2
A result of hyperventilation of any cause.
• **CNS causes** Stroke; subarachnoid bleed; meningitis.
• **Hypoxia related** Altitude, anaemia, V/Q mismatch.
• **Pulmonary** CCF, pneumonia, pulmonary emboli.
• **Others** pregnancy, drugs, eg salicylates.

Terminology To aid understanding, we have used the terms acidosis and alkalosis, where a purist would sometimes have used acidaemia and alkalaemia. Technically acidaemia is the state of having a low blood pH, whereas acidosis refers to the processes which generate H^+, leading to the acidaemia.

Table 14.4 Determining the primary acid–base disorder and any compensation present

Acid–base disorder	pH	Primary disturbance	Compensation*
Metabolic acidosis	<7.4	Low HCO_3^-	Decrease pCO_2
Metabolic alkalosis	>7.4	High HCO_3^-	Increase pCO_2
Respiratory acidosis	<7.4	High pCO_2	Increase HCO_3^-
Respiratory alkalosis	>7.4	Low pCO_2	Decrease HCO_3^-

*Compensatory responses generally do not fully correct the arterial pH to 7.4. Hence a normal pH plus substantial derangement of serum HCO_3^- and pCO_2 indicates a mixed acid–base disorder with the exception of chronic respiratory acidosis/alkalosis, which sometimes fully compensate over time.

Table 14.5 Boston rules for acid–base interpretation

Acid–base disorder	Expected compensation
Metabolic acidosis	Expected $pCO_2 = (HCO_3^-/5) + 1$
Metabolic alkalosis	Expected $pCO_2 = 0.1$ kPa for each 1mmol/L change in HCO_3^-
Acute respiratory acidosis	1 mmol/L ↑ in HCO_3^- for each 1kPa ↑ in pCO_2
Acute respiratory alkalosis	2 mmol/L ↓ in HCO_3^- for each 1kPa ↓ in pCO_2
Chronic respiratory acidosis	4 mmol/L ↑ in HCO_3^- for each 1kPa ↑ in pCO_2
Chronic respiratory alkalosis	3 mmol/L ↓ in HCO_3^- for each 1kPa ↓ in pCO_2

Hypernatraemia

Excretion of concentrated urine requires: 1 Hypertonic medullary interstitium. 2 Intact ADH secretion and responsiveness. Problems with either can cause water loss. Thirst prevents hypernatraemia in cognitively intact patients with access to water, even if urinary concentrating mechanisms are defective. Hypernatraemia is always hyperosmolar and hypertonic.

Signs and symptoms Lethargy, thirst, weakness, irritability, confusion, coma, and fits, along with signs of dehydration (p658).

Causes Usually due to water loss in excess of Na^+ loss, in eg an elderly patient, that is not replaced because of impaired mental status or intubation.
• Non-renal water loss (eg NG drainage, vomiting, insensible losses, reduced water intake). Urine osmolality (UOsm) typically >600mOsmol/kg.
• Renal water loss (diabetes insipidus (p234). Suspect if large urine volume. This may follow head injury, or CNS surgery, especially pituitary. UOsm usually <300mOsmol/kg).
• Osmotic diuresis (from glucose, urea, mannitol, NG feeding, large volume saline administration). Daily solute excretion (UOsm × 24h urine output in litres) >1000mOsmol.

Management Give water orally or via NG tube if possible. If not, give hypotonic fluids 5% dextrose or 0.45% saline IV. Need to calculate free water deficit (Total body water × ((Na/140) − 1)), decide on the rate of correction (eg replace half in first 24h), and consider ongoing losses + maintenance. Correct underlying cause, eg DI.

Hyponatraemia

Plasma Na^+ concentration depends on the amount of both Na^+ and water in the plasma. Assessing volume status is the key to diagnosis (fig 14.2).

Signs and symptoms Look for anorexia, nausea, and malaise initially, followed by headache, irritability, confusion, weakness, ↓GCS, and seizures, depending on the severity and rate of change in serum Na^+. ↑Risk of falls in the elderly.[6]

Causes See fig 14.2. A common cause in older patients is a low solute intake due to a low-protein diet (eg 'tea & toast diet', beer potomania)—clues include a low plasma urea and plasma osmolality (POsm) > UOsm. Artefactual causes (POsm >295mOsmol/L) include: •blood sample was from a drip arm •high serum lipid/protein content cause over-dilution of the sample •hyperglycaemia.

Tests Send POsm & UOsm (↑UOsm reflects ADH activity), plasma & urine sodium (+ K^+, Cl^-), U&E, glucose, daily urine volume.

Management
• Correct the underlying cause. The presence of symptoms, the chronicity of the hyponatraemia, and volume status are all important. If chronic, do not ↑ Na^+ >8mmol/L in 24h.
• *Asymptomatic chronic hyponatraemia:* treatment depends on the underlying cause (see fig 14.2), eg volume repletion with crystalloids if deplete, diuretics if overload, fluid restrict if suspect SIADH. If urine (Na^+ + K^+) > serum Na^+, it is not physiologically possible to correct Na^+ using fluid restriction alone.
• ►►*Acute (<48h) or symptomatic hyponatraemia:* give 150mL 3% NaCl bolus over 20min, repeat up to twice if symptoms persist (eg seizures). Seek advice from Nephrology after initial bolus regarding further treatment.
• *Osmotic demyelination syndrome (ODS):* overly rapid correction of Na^+ can result in central pontine myelinolysis (or ODS); a catastrophic neurological injury resulting from demyelination of brainstem structures. Assess risk factors, eg female, ↓K^+, chronic ↓Na^+, alcoholism, malnourishment. If risk factors present, give desmopressin 2mcg SC TDS when starting 3% saline. This prevents rapid correction from a water diuresis due to 'switching off' of ADH activity by NaCl.
• *Vasopressor receptor antagonists* ('vaptans', eg tolvaptan) promote water excretion without loss of electrolytes, and appear to be effective in treating hypervolaemic and euvolaemic hyponatraemia but are expensive and risk of liver toxicity.[7]

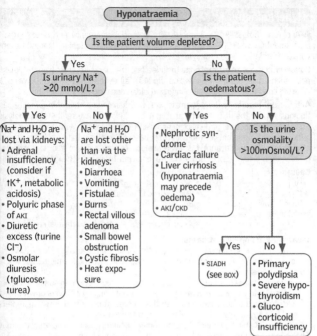

Fig 14.2 Hyponatraemia.

Syndrome of inappropriate ADH secretion (SIADH)

An important, but over-diagnosed, cause of hyponatraemia. Question this diagnosis if there is a coexisting electrolyte or acid–base disorder of any kind, if there is reduced GFR, or if there is no obvious drug, lung, CNS, or endocrine cause, which should be present in >90% cases of true SIADH.

Causes
- *Malignancy:* lung small-cell, pancreas, prostate, thymus, or lymphoma.
- *CNS disorders:* meningoencephalitis, abscess, stroke, subarachnoid or subdural haemorrhage, head injury, neurosurgery, Guillain–Barré, vasculitis, or SLE.
- *Chest disease:* TB, pneumonia, abscess, aspergillosis, small-cell lung cancer.
- *Drugs:* opiates, psychotropics, SSRIs, cytotoxics.
- *Other:* pain, nausea, exercise.

Diagnosis Low plasma osmolality (<275mOsmol/kg), urine osmolality >100mOsmol/kg, urine Na⁺ >30mmol/L in the presence of clinical euvolemia and absence of adrenal, thyroid, pituitary, or renal insufficiency. No recent use of diuretics.

Tests Normal electrolytes and acid–base, low urate, UOsm typically >POsm by 200mOsmol.

Treatment Treat the cause and restrict fluid (<800mL/day). Increase solute load (with salt or urea tabs), ± low-dose loop diuretic (blunts action of ADH by altering medullary concentration gradient for water). Vasopressin receptor antagonists ('vaptans', p664) can be used to treat SIADH but their utility is limited by concerns about hepatotoxicity, excessive thirst, cost, and the potential for overly rapid correction of the hyponatraemia.

▶▶A plasma potassium >6.5mmol/L is a potential emergency and needs urgent assessment (see p297). The worry is of myocardial hyperexcitability leading to ventricular fibrillation and cardiac arrest.

Concerning signs and symptoms Include a fast irregular pulse, chest pain, weakness, palpitations, and light-headedness. ECG (fig 14.3) Tall tented T waves, small P waves, a wide QRS complex (eventually becoming sinusoidal), and ventricular fibrillation.

Artefactual results If the patient is well, and has none of the above-mentioned findings, repeat the test urgently as it may be artefactual, caused by: • haemolysis (difficult venepuncture; patient clenched fist) • contamination with potassium EDTA anticoagulant in FBC bottles (do FBCs *after* U&Es) • thrombocythaemia (K⁺ leaks out of platelets during clotting) • delayed analysis (K⁺ leaks out of RBCs; a particular problem in a primary care setting due to long transit times to the lab).[8]

Causes
- Oliguric AKI.
- K⁺-sparing diuretics.
- Rhabdomyolysis (p315).
- Metabolic acidosis (DM).
- Excess K⁺ therapy.
- Addison's disease (p220).
- Massive blood transfusion.
- Burns.
- Drugs, eg ACE-i, suxamethonium.
- Artefactual result (see earlier 'Artefactual results').

Treatment in non-urgent cases
Treat the underlying cause; review medications. Dietician to advise re low-K⁺ diet.
- Loop diuretics may be helpful in fluid overload or for hyperkalaemic type IV RTA in diabetic patients.
- GI cation exchangers—polystyrene sulfonate resin (eg Calcium Resonium® 15g/8h PO) binds K⁺ in the gut, preventing absorption and bringing K⁺ levels down over a few days. Need to give laxatives with this to prevent constipation which impairs faecal K⁺ excretion. Short course only recommended.
- Newer oral K⁺ binding agents (eg patiromer, sodium zirconium cyclosilicate) may be used to treat mild chronic hyperkalaemia in advanced CKD.[9]
- Consider dialysis if severe kidney dysfunction.

Emergency treatment
▶▶If there is evidence of myocardial hyperexcitability, or K⁺ is >6.5mmol/L, get senior assistance, and treat as an emergency (p297).

Hypokalaemia

If K⁺ <2.5mmol/L, urgent treatment is required. Note that hypokalaemia exacerbates digoxin toxicity.

Signs and symptoms Muscle weakness, hypotonia, hyporeflexia, cramps, tetany, palpitations, light-headedness (arrhythmias), constipation.

ECG Small or inverted T waves, prominent U waves (after T wave), a long PR interval, and depressed ST segments.

Causes
- Diuretics.
- Vomiting and diarrhoea.
- Mg²⁺ deficiency.
- Pyloric stenosis.
- Intestinal fistula.
- Cushing's syndrome/steroids/ACTH.
- Conn's syndrome.
- Metabolic alkalosis.
- Diuretic/laxative abuse.
- Types I & II RTA (p312, p656).

Suspect Conn's syndrome if hypertensive, hypokalaemic alkalosis in someone not taking diuretics (p222).

Treatment Review medications. **If mild** (>2.5mmol/L, no symptoms.) Give oral K⁺ supplement (eg Sando-K® 2 tabs/8h; 20–80mmol/24h). Review K⁺ daily. If chronic, consider K⁺-sparing diuretic. **If severe** (<2.5mmol/L, and/or dangerous symptoms.) Give IV potassium cautiously, not more than 20mmol/h, and not more concentrated than 40mmol/L. Don't give K⁺ if oliguric. ▶▶*Never* give K⁺ as a fast stat bolus dose.

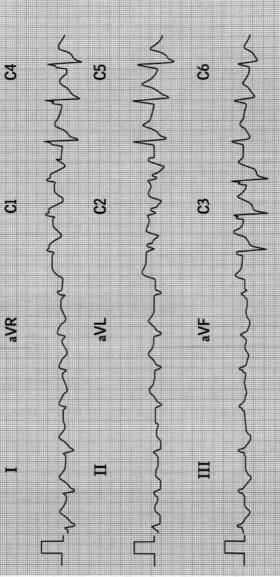

Fig 14.3 Hyperkalaemia—note the flattening of the P waves, prominent T waves, and widening of the QRS complex.

Calcium and phosphate physiology

Calcium and phosphate homeostasis is maintained through

Parathyroid hormone (PTH) Overall effect is $\uparrow Ca^{2+}$ & $\downarrow PO_4^{3-}$. Secretion by four parathyroid glands is triggered by $\downarrow$serum ionized Ca^{2+}; controlled by $-$ve feedback loop. *Actions are:* • $\uparrow$osteoclast activity releasing Ca^{2+} and PO_4^{3-} from bones • $\uparrow Ca^{2+}$ & $\downarrow PO_4^{3-}$ reabsorption in the kidney • $\uparrow$renal production of 1,25-dihydroxy-vitamin D_3.

Vitamin D and calcitriol Vit D is hydroxylated first in the liver to 25-hydroxy-vit D, and again in the kidney to 1,25-dihydroxy-vit D (calcitriol), the biologically active form, and 24,25-hydroxy-vit D (inactive). Calcitriol production is stimulated by $\downarrow Ca^{2+}$, $\downarrow PO_4^{3-}$, and $\uparrow$PTH. *Actions are:* • $\uparrow Ca^{2+}$ and $\uparrow PO_4^{3-}$ absorption from the gut • inhibition of PTH release • enhanced bone turnover • $\uparrow Ca^{2+}$ and $\uparrow PO_4^{3-}$ reabsorption in the kidney. Colecalciferol (vit D_3—from animal sources) and ergocalciferol (vit D_2—from vegetables) are biologically identical in their activity. Disordered regulation of calcitriol underlies familial normocalcaemic hypercalciuria, which is a major cause of calcium oxalate renal stone formation (p630).

Calcitonin Made in C cells of the thyroid, this causes $\downarrow Ca^{2+}$ and $\downarrow PO_4^{3-}$, but its physiological role is unclear. It can be used as a marker of recurrence or metastasis in medullary carcinoma of the thyroid.

Magnesium $\downarrow Mg^{2+}$ prevents PTH release, and may cause hypocalcaemia.

Plasma binding Labs usually measure total plasma Ca^{2+}. ~40% is bound to albumin, and the rest is free ionized Ca^{2+} which is the physiologically important amount (often available on blood gas analyser). Therefore, *correct total Ca^{2+} for albumin* as follows: add 0.1mmol/L to Ca^{2+} level for every 4g/L that albumin is below 40g/L, and a similar subtraction for raised albumin. However, many other factors affect binding (eg other proteins in myeloma, cirrhosis, individual variation) so be cautious in your interpretation. If in doubt over a high Ca^{2+}, take blood specimens uncuffed (remove tourniquet after needle in vein, but before taking blood sample), and with the patient fasted.

Hypercalcaemia

Signs and symptoms 'Bones, stones, groans, and psychic moans.' Abdominal pain; vomiting; constipation; polyuria; polydipsia; depression; anorexia; weight loss; lethargy; weakness; hypertension; confusion; pyrexia; renal stones; AKI; ectopic calcification (see cornea—see BOX); cardiac arrest. ECG $\downarrow$QT interval.

Causes (fig 14.4) Most commonly malignancy (eg from bone metastases, myeloma, PTH-related protein (PTHRP)) or primary hyperparathyroidism. Others include sarcoidosis, vit D intoxication, thyrotoxicosis, lithium, tertiary hyperparathyroidism, milk-alkali syndrome, and familial benign hypocalciuric hypercalcaemia (rare; defect in calcium-sensing receptor). HIV can cause both $\uparrow$ & $\downarrow Ca^{2+}$ (perhaps from PTH-related bone remodelling).[10]

Investigations The main distinction is malignancy vs 1° hyperparathyroidism. Pointers to malignancy are $\downarrow$albumin, $\downarrow Cl^-$, alkalosis, $\downarrow K^+$, $\uparrow PO_4^{3-}$, $\uparrow$ALP. $\uparrow$PTH indicates hyperparathyroidism. Also FBC, protein electrophoresis, serum ACE, vit D levels, TFTs, PTHRP, CXR, isotope bone scan, 24h urinary Ca^{2+} excretion (for familial hypocalciuric hypercalcaemia).

Causes of metastatic (ectopic) calcification: PARATHORMONE

Parathyroid hormone (PTH)$\uparrow$ (p216) and other causes of $\uparrow Ca^{2+}$, eg sarcoidosis; **A**myloidosis; **R**enal failure (relates to $\uparrow PO_4^{3-}$); **A**ddison's disease (adrenal calcification); **T**B nodes; **T**oxoplasmosis (CNS); **H**istoplasmosis (eg in lung); **O**verdose of vitamin D; **R**aynaud's-associated diseases (eg SLE; systemic sclerosis, p548; dermatomyositis); **M**uscle primaries/leiomyosarcomas; **O**ssifying metastases (osteosarcoma) or ovarian mets (to peritoneum); **N**ephrocalcinosis or calciphylaxis; **E**ndocrine tumours (eg gastrinoma).

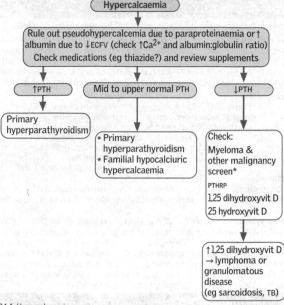

Fig 14.4 Hypercalcaemia.
* Most common primary: breast, kidney, lung, thyroid, prostate, ovary, colon.

Treating acute hypercalcaemia

Diagnose and treat the underlying cause. If Ca²⁺ >3mmol/L or symptomatic:

1 **Stop contributing medications** eg thiazide diuretic, Ca²⁺ supplements.

2 **Correct volume depletion** Give IV fluids (use balanced crystalloids unless acidotic in which case isotonic bicarbonate should be used).

3 **Bisphosphonates** These prevent bone resorption by inhibiting osteoclast activity. Zoledronic acid is preferred to reduce serum Ca²⁺ because it is superior to pamidronate in reversing hypercalcaemia related to malignancy. Usually, a single dose of 4mg IV (diluted to 100mL, over 15min) will normalize plasma Ca²⁺ within a week. If using pamidronate give 30mg in 300mL 0.9% saline over 3h via a largish vein. If impaired kidney function (GFR <30), use a reduced dose and/or slower infusion rate (2-4mg ZA over 30-60min, 30-45mg pamidronate over 4h) to minimize the risk of renal tubular toxicity which is related to the rate of infusion.

4 **Further management** Chemotherapy may help in malignancy. Steroids are used in sarcoidosis and myeloma, eg prednisolone 40-60mg/d. Calcitonin acts similarly to bisphosphonates, and has a quicker onset of action, but is not widely available (usual dose 4 units/kg SC BD). Denosumab is a monoclonal antibody that inhibits osteoclast formation and bone resorption. It may be an option for patients with hypercalcaemia refractory to bisphosphonates or where there are contraindications, particularly where the hypercalcaemia is malignancy related. Hyperparathyroidism may be treated with calcimimetics (cinacalcet). Dialysis may be indicated in cases of severe hypercalcaemia and oliguric AKI.

▶Apparent hypocalcaemia may be an artefact of hypoalbuminaemia (p668).

Signs and symptoms See BOX.[11] **Mild** Cramps, perioral numbness/paraesthesiae. **Severe** Carpopedal spasm (especially if brachial artery compressed, *Trousseau's sign*; see fig 14.5), laryngospasm, seizures. Neuromuscular excitability may also be demonstrated by tapping over parotid (facial nerve) causing facial muscles to twitch (*Chvostek's sign*; see fig 14.6). Cataract if chronic hypocalcaemia. **ECG** Long QT interval.

Causes	↓PTH	↔ or ↑ PTH
	• Primary hypoparathyroidism—surgical, autoimmune, storage disorder, eg haemochromatosis.	• Vitamin D deficiency.
		• Insufficient synthesis (CKD).
	• Dysregulation of PTH secretion, eg congenital, ↓Mg²⁺, sepsis.	• Altered protein binding (alkalosis).
		• Chelation or depletion (↑PO₄³⁻, tumour lysis syndrome, pancreatitis, coagulopathy).
		• Drugs (eg phenytoin, citrate).

Treatment
- **Mild symptoms** Give oral Ca^{2+} replacement & vitamin D (colecalciferol).
- **In CKD** See p298. Give the hormonally active version of vitamin D, alfacalcidol, eg 0.25–0.5mcg/24h PO.
- **Severe symptoms** Give 10mL of 10% calcium gluconate (2.25mmol) IV over 30min, and repeat as necessary ± IV infusion (eg 60mL of 10% calcium gluconate in 500mL of 5% dextrose —start at 0.5mg/kg/h).
- **Post-operative (eg parathyroidectomy)** Treat all patients with oral ± IV replacement if <1.90mmol/L or symptomatic. Symptomatic patients require IV bolus followed by infusion with frequent monitoring. Patients with known or likely hypoparathyroidism should also commence alfacalcidol 1mcg/24h PO.

Features of hypocalcaemia: SPASMODIC

Spasms (carpopedal spasms = Trousseau's sign).

Perioral paraesthesiae.

Anxious, irritable, irrational.

Seizures.

Muscle tone ↑ in smooth muscle—hence colic, wheeze, and dysphagia.

Orientation impaired (time, place, and person) and confusion.

Dermatitis (eg atopic/exfoliative).

Impetigo herpetiformis (↓Ca^{2+} and pustules in pregnancy—rare and serious).

Chvostek's sign; **c**horeoathetosis; **c**ataract; **c**ardiomyopathy (long QT interval on ECG).

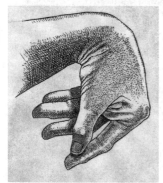

Fig 14.5 Trousseau's sign: on inflating the cuff, the wrist and fingers flex and draw together (carpopedal spasm).

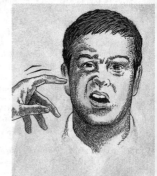

Fig 14.6 Chvostek's sign: the corner of the mouth twitches when the facial nerve is tapped over the parotid.

Phosphate

Hypophosphataemia Common and may herald the onset of refeeding syndrome in the malnourished patient. It can be particularly significant for mechanically ventilated patients where the resulting ATP loss can lead to diminution of respiratory muscle power and failure to wean from ventilation and to rehabilitate. **Causes** Vitamin D deficiency, alcohol withdrawal, refeeding syndrome (p585), inadequate oral intake, severe diabetic ketoacidosis, renal tubular dysfunction, and 1° hyperparathyroidism. **Signs and symptoms** Muscle weakness or rhabdomyolysis, red cell, white cell, and platelet dysfunction, and cardiac arrest or arrhythmias. **Treatment** Oral or parenteral phosphate supplementation, eg Phosphate Polyfusor® IVI (50mmol PO_4^{3-} in 500mL). Never give IV phosphate to a patient who is hypercalcaemic or oliguric.

Hyperphosphataemia Most commonly due to CKD, when it is treated with phosphate binders, eg sevelamer 800mg/8h PO with meals. Also catabolic states such as tumour lysis syndrome (p525) or rhabdomyolysis.

Magnesium

Magnesium is distributed 65% in bone and 35% in cells; plasma concentration tends to follow that of Ca^{2+} and K^+.

Hypomagnesaemia Causes paraesthesiae, ataxia, seizures, tetany, arrhythmias. Digitalis toxicity may be exacerbated. **Causes** Malabsorption syndromes, severe diarrhoea, ketoacidosis, alcohol abuse, total parenteral nutrition (monitor weekly), drugs (eg PPI, diuretics, aminoglycosides, amphotericin B), $\downarrow Ca^{2+}$, $\downarrow K^+$, and $\downarrow PO_4^{3-}$. **Treatment** If needed, give magnesium salts, PO or IV (eg Magnesium Verla® one sachet (5mmol Mg^{2+}) TDS PRN or 20mmol $MgSO_4$ IV in 100mL 0.9% saline over 1h, depending on the severity with frequent Mg^{2+} levels).

Hypermagnesaemia Rare because the kidney is able to increase the fractional excretion of Mg^{2+} to nearly 100%. **Causes** AKI, CKD with Mg^{2+} exogenous intake, or pre-eclampsia/eclampsia therapy. **Signs** If severe: neuromuscular depression, $\downarrow$BP, $\downarrow$pulse, hyporeflexia, CNS & respiratory depression, coma. **Treatment** Rarely requires treatment unless severe (>7mmol/L). In a patient with intact kidney function, consider forced saline diuresis and loop diuretics. Calcium gluconate will temporarily block the toxic effects of Mg^{2+}. If significant kidney dysfunction and the patient has severe symptoms, haemodialysis may be required.

Zinc

Zinc deficiency This may occur in parenteral nutrition or, rarely, from a poor diet (too few cereals and dairy products; anorexia nervosa; alcoholism). Rarely it is due to a genetic defect. **Symptoms** Alopecia, dermatitis (look for red, crusted skin lesions especially around nostrils and corners of mouth), night blindness, diarrhoea. **Diagnosis** Therapeutic trial of zinc (plasma levels are unreliable as they may be low, eg in infection or trauma, without deficiency).

Selenium

An essential element present in cereals, nuts, and meat. Low soil levels in some parts of Europe and China cause deficiency states. Required for the antioxidant glutathione peroxidase, which $\downarrow$ harmful free radicals. Selenium is also antithrombogenic, and is required for sperm motility proteins. Deficiency may increase risk of neoplasia and atheroma, and may lead to a cardiomyopathy or arthritis. Serum levels are a poor guide. Toxic symptoms may also be found with over-energetic replacement.

14 Clinical chemistry

Causes of hyperuricaemia High levels of urate in the blood (hyperuricaemia) may result from increased turnover (15%) or reduced excretion of urate (85%). Either may be drug induced.
• **Drugs** Cytotoxics, thiazides, loop diuretics, pyrazinamide.
• **Increased cell turnover** Lymphoma, leukaemia, psoriasis, haemolysis, muscle death (rhabdomyolysis, p315; tumour lysis syndrome, p525).
• **Reduced excretion** Primary gout (p544), chronic kidney disease, lead nephropathy, hyperparathyroidism, pre-eclampsia (OHCS p50).
• **Other** Hyperuricaemia may be associated with hypertension and hyperlipidaemia. Urate may be raised in disorders of purine synthesis such as the *Lesch–Nyhan syndrome* (OHCS p852).

Hyperuricaemia and kidney injury Advanced CKD from any cause may be associated with hyperuricaemia, and this may give rise to gout. Hyperuricaemia can also cause acute kidney injury (AKI) following cytotoxic treatment (tumour lysis syndrome, p525), and in muscle necrosis.

How urate causes AKI Urate is poorly soluble in water, so over-excretion can lead to crystal precipitation causing acute tubular injury. In the setting of tumour lysis syndrome, increased PO_4^{3-} levels combine with Ca^{2+} and deposit calcium phosphate in the kidney's tubules, also causing AKI. Uric acid precipitates readily in the setting of calcium phosphate crystals and calcium phosphate precipitates readily in the setting of uric acid crystals, thus worsening AKI. Increased urinary uric acid excretion is associated with a higher risk of uric acid stone formation, particularly in the setting of low urinary pH.

Prevention of AKI Before starting chemotherapy, ensure adequate hydration and initiate *allopurinol* (xanthine oxidase inhibitor) or *rasburicase* (recombinant urate oxidase), which prevent a sharp rise in urate following chemotherapy (p525). There is a remote risk of inducing xanthine nephropathy.

Treatment of tumour lysis syndrome (TLS) Use IV fluids to increase the urine output to prevent the precipitation of uric acid and calcium phosphate crystals in the tubules.[12] Rasburicase is currently the preferred drug for hyperuricaemia in TLS. Urinary alkalinization with isotonic bicarbonate to increase uric acid solubility is only recommended in those with metabolic acidosis as it may promote calcium phosphate deposition in the kidney, heart, and other organs. Dialysis may be required in severe AKI with life-threatening hyperkalaemia, hyperphosphataemia, and hyperuricaemia.

Gout See p544.

Urate renal stones Urate stones (fig 14.7) comprise 5–10% of all renal stones and are radiolucent.

Incidence ~5–10% in temperate climates (double if confirmed gout),[13] but up to 40% in hot, arid climates. ♂:♀≈4:1. But most urate stone formers have no detectable abnormalities in urate metabolism.

Risk factors Acidic or strongly concentrated urine; ↑urinary excretion of urate; chronic diarrhoea; distal small bowel disease or resection (regional enteritis); ileostomy; obesity; diabetes mellitus; chemotherapy for myeloproliferative disorders; inadequate caloric or fluid intake.

Tests Non-contrast CT; stone analysis.

Treatment Hydration to increase urine volume (aim >2L/d). Unlike most other renal calculi, existing uric acid stones can often be dissolved with urinary alkalinization. Potassium citrate or potassium bicarbonate at a dose titrated to alkalinize the urine to a pH of 6.5–7 dissolves some urate stones. If hyperuricosuria, consider dietary management ± allopurinol (xanthine oxidase inhibitor).

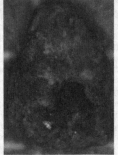

Fig 14.7 Urate stone.
© Dr G. Austin.

Osteoporosis is characterized by low bone mass, microarchitectural disruption, and skeletal fragility, resulting in decreased bone strength and an increased risk of fracture. It may be 1° (age related) or 2° to another condition or drugs. If trabecular bone is affected, crush fractures of vertebrae are common; if cortical bone is affected, long bone fractures are more likely, eg femoral neck: a major cause of death, loss of independence, and healthcare costs.

Prevalence (In those >50yrs): ♂ 4.4%, ♀ 19.6%.[14] Women tend to lose bone at a younger age and at a more rapid pace than men. Postmenopausal women are susceptible to 1° osteoporosis since osteoporosis is closely related to oestrogen deficiency. During the menopausal transition period, the drop of oestrogen leads to more bone resorption than formation, resulting in osteoporosis.

Risk factors Advancing age is the strongest risk factor for osteoporosis. Age-independent risk factors for 1° osteoporosis include parental history, alcohol >4 units daily, rheumatoid arthritis, BMI <19, prolonged immobility, and poor nutrition. See BOX 'Osteoporosis risk factors' for other risk factors, including for 2° osteoporosis.

Investigations *x-ray:* (low sensitivity/specificity, often with hindsight after a fracture). Bone densitometry (DEXA—see BOX 'DEXA bone densitometry'; table 14.6). *Bloods:* Ca^{2+}, PO_4^{3-}, and ALP normal. Check vitamin D. Consider specific investigations for 2° causes if suggestive history (eg 24h urine Ca^{2+}, coeliac screen, PTH, etc.).

Diagnosis A clinical diagnosis of osteoporosis may be made in the presence of a fragility fracture, particularly at the spine, hip, wrist, humerus, rib, and pelvis, without measurement of bone mineral density (BMD). In the absence of a fragility fracture, BMD assessment by DEXA scan (see BOX 'DEXA bone densitometry') is the standard test to diagnose osteoporosis, according to the WHO classification. A clinical diagnosis may be made when the FRAX (a WHO risk assessment tool) 10-year probability of major osteoporotic fracture is ≥20% or the 10-year probability of hip fracture is ≥3%.

Management

Lifestyle measures
• Quit smoking and reduce alcohol consumption.
• Weight-bearing exercise may increase bone mineral density.[15]
• Balance exercises such as tai chi reduce risk of falls.
• Calcium and vitamin D-rich diet (use supplements if diet is insufficient—see 'Pharmacological measures' later in this topic).
• Home-based fall-prevention programme, with visual assessment and a home visit.

Pharmacological measures (See BOX 'Indications for pharmacological treatment'.)
• *Calcium and vitamin D:* rarely used alone for prophylaxis, as questionable efficacy and some evidence of a small ↑CV risk. Offer if evidence of deficiency, eg calcium 1g/d + vit D 800u/d. Target serum 25-hydroxy-vitamin D level ≥75nmol/L.
• *Bisphosphonates:* preferred initial treatment, eg alendronic acid 10mg/d or 70mg/wk (not if eGFR <35). Use also for prevention in long-term steroid use. If intolerant, use risedronate or ibandronic acid. SE: photosensitivity; GI upset; oesophageal ulcers—stop if dysphagia or abdominal pain; rarely, jaw osteonecrosis.
• *Denosumab:* a monoclonal Ab to RANK ligand, given SC twice yearly ↓ reabsorption. Use in those intolerant of or unresponsive to other therapies (including IV bisphosphonates) and in those with impaired kidney function.
• *Hormone replacement therapy (HRT)* can prevent (not treat) osteoporosis in postmenopausal women but balance with risk of breast cancer, CVD, and VTE, and involve the patient in the decision. *Raloxifene* is a selective oestrogen receptor modulator (SERM) that acts similarly to HRT, but with ↓breast cancer risk. Usually used in those with an independent need for breast cancer prophylaxis. ↑ VTE risk.
• *Teriparatide* (recombinant PTH) is useful in those with severe osteoporosis, those intolerant of bisphosphonates, and in those who suffer further fractures despite treatment with other agents. Risk of ↑Ca^{2+}.

DEXA bone densitometry: WHO osteoporosis criteria

It is better to scan the hip than the lumbar spine. Bone mineral density (BMD; g/cm²) is compared with that of a young healthy adult. The 'T-score' is the number of standard deviations (SD, p735) the BMD is from the youthful average. Each decrease of 1 SD in BMD ≈2·6-fold ↑ in risk of hip fracture.

Table 14.6 Interpreting DEXA bone scan results

T-score >0	BMD is better than the reference
0 to −1	BMD is in the top 84%: no evidence of osteoporosis
−1 to −2.5	Osteopenia. Risk of later osteoporotic fracture. Offer lifestyle advice
−2.5 or worse	Osteoporosis. Offer lifestyle advice and treatment (p674). Repeat DEXA in 2yrs

The National Osteoporosis Foundation indications for DEXA*
- Women ≥65 years and men ≥70 years, regardless of clinical risk factors.
- Younger postmenopausal women, women in the menopausal transition, and men aged 50–69 years with clinical risk factors for fracture.
- Adults who have a fracture after age 50 years.
- Adults with a condition (eg rheumatoid arthritis) or taking a medication (eg glucocorticoids in a daily dose ≥5mg prednisone or equivalent for ≥3 months) associated with low bone mass or bone loss.[16]

*Recommendations vary by expert group.

Indications for pharmacological treatment

Recommended for postmenopausal females and males ≥50 years with:
- A history of fracture of vertebrae, hip, wrist, pelvis, or humerus.
- A T-score ≤−2.5 (DEXA) at the lumbar spine, femoral neck, or total hip.
- A T-score between −1 and −2.5 at the femoral neck or spine, and a 10-year probability of hip fracture ≥3% or a 10-year probability of any major osteoporosis-related fracture ≥20% (Fracture Risk Assessment Tool (FRAX)).

Osteoporosis risk factors: SHATTERED

Steroid use of >5mg/d of prednisolone.

Hyperthyroidism, hyperparathyroidism, hypercalciuria.

Alcohol and tobacco use ↑.

Thin (BMI <18.5).

Testosterone ↓ (eg anti-androgen ca prostate ℞).

Early menopause.

Renal or liver failure.

Erosive/inflammatory bone disease (eg myeloma or rheumatoid arthritis).

Dietary ↓Ca²⁺/malabsorption; diabetes mellitus type 1.

In osteomalacia, there is a normal amount of bone but its mineral content is low (there is excess uncalcified osteoid and cartilage). This is the reverse of osteoporosis in which mineralization is unchanged, but there is overall bone loss. Rickets is the result if this process occurs during the period of bone growth; osteomalacia is the result if it occurs after fusion of the epiphyses. Mineralization abnormalities occur as a result of inadequate Ca^{2+}, PO_4^{3-}, and/or ALP levels, or direct inhibition of the mineralization process.

Signs and symptoms

Rickets Growth retardation, hypotonia, apathy in infants. Once walking: knock-kneed, bow-legged, and deformities of the metaphyseal–epiphyseal junction (eg the rachitic rosary). Features of ↓Ca^{2+}—often mild (p670). Children with rickets are ill.

Osteomalacia Bone pain and tenderness; fractures (esp. femoral neck); proximal myopathy (waddling gait), due to ↓PO_4^{3-} and vitamin D deficiency per se.

Causes

Vitamin D deficiency The most common cause of osteomalacia in adults. Due to malabsorption (p262), poor diet, or lack of sunlight.

Renal osteodystrophy CKD leads to 1,25-dihydroxy-colecalciferol deficiency (1,25(OH)$_2$-vitamin D deficiency) due to impaired 1α hydroxylation in the kidney. See also *renal bone disease* (p308).

Drug induced Anti-epileptic drugs may induce liver enzymes, leading to an increased breakdown of 25-hydroxy-vitamin D.

Vitamin D resistance A number of mainly inherited conditions in which the osteomalacia responds to high doses of vitamin D (see 'Treatment' later in this topic).

Liver disease Due to reduced hydroxylation of vitamin D to 25-hydroxy-colecalciferol and malabsorption of vitamin D, eg in cirrhosis (p272).

Tumour-induced osteomalacia (Oncogenic hypophosphataemia.) Mediated by raised tumour production of phosphatonin fibroblast growth factor 23 (FGF-23) which causes hyperphosphaturia. ↓Serum PO_4^{3-} often causes myalgia and weakness.[17]

Investigations

Plasma Mildly ↓Ca^{2+} (but may be severe); ↓PO_4^{3-}; ↑ALP; PTH high; ↓25(OH)-vitamin D, except in vitamin D resistance. In CKD, ↓↓1,25(OH)$_2$-vitamin D (p308).

x-ray In osteomalacia, there is a loss of cortical bone; also, apparent partial fractures without displacement may be seen especially on the lateral border of the scapula, inferior femoral neck, and medial femoral shaft (Looser's zones; fig 14.8). Cupped, ragged metaphyseal surfaces are seen in rickets (fig 14.9).

Biopsy Bone biopsy is rarely needed but shows incomplete mineralization.

Treatment

• In severe vitamin D deficiency, give high-dose replacement (eg 50 000IU vitamin D$_2$ or D$_3$ orally once per week for 6–8 weeks), followed by a maintenance dose (eg vitamin D$_3$ 800IU daily) thereafter.

• If due to CKD or vitamin D resistance, give alfacalcidol (1α-hydroxy-vitamin D$_3$) 250ng–1mcg daily, or calcitriol (1,25-dihydroxy-vitamin D$_3$) 250ng–1mcg daily, and adjust dose according to plasma Ca^{2+}. ►► Alfacalcidol and calcitriol can cause hypercalcaemia.

• Monitor plasma Ca^{2+}, initially weekly, and if nausea/vomiting.

Vitamin D-resistant rickets Exists in two forms. Type I has low renal 1α-hydroxylase activity, and type II has end-organ resistance to 1,25-dihydroxy-vitamin D$_3$, due to a point mutation in the receptor. Both are treated with large doses of calcitriol.

x-linked hypophosphataemic rickets Dominantly inherited—due to a defect in kidney phosphate handling (due to mutations in the PHEX gene which encodes an endopeptidase). Rickets develops in early childhood and is associated with poor growth. Plasma PO_4^{3-} is low, ALP is high, and there is phosphaturia. Treatment is with high doses of oral phosphate, and calcitriol ± burosumab, a human anti-FGF23 monoclonal antibody.

Also called *osteitis deformans*, there is ↑bone turnover associated with ↑numbers of osteoblasts and osteoclasts with resultant remodelling, bone enlargement, deformity, and weakness. Rare in the under-40s. Incidence rises with age (3% over 55yrs old). Commoner in temperate climates, and those with Anglo-Saxon ancestry.

Clinical features Asymptomatic in ~70%. Deep, boring pain, and bony deformity and enlargement—typically of the pelvis, lumbar spine, skull, femur, and tibia (classically a bowed sabre tibia; fig 14.10). *Complications* include pathological fractures, osteoarthritis, ↑Ca²⁺, nerve compression due to bone overgrowth (eg deafness, root compression), high-output CCF (if >40% of skeleton involved), and osteosarcoma (<1% of those affected for >10yrs—suspect if sudden onset or worsening of bone pain).[18]

Radiology x-ray Localized enlargement of bone. Patchy cortical thickening with sclerosis, osteolysis, and deformity (eg *osteoporosis circumscripta* of the skull). Affinity for axial skeleton, long bones, and skull. Bone scan may reveal 'hot spots'.

Blood chemistry Ca²⁺ and PO₄³⁻ normal; ALP markedly raised.

Treatment If analgesia fails, bisphosphonates may be tried to reduce pain and/or deformity or fractures. If intolerant of bisphosphonates, consider calcitonin. Follow expert advice.

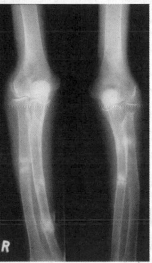

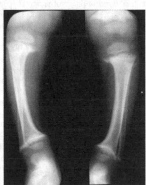

Fig 14.9 Rickets. Typical ragged metaphyseal surfaces are seen in the knee and ankle joints of a child with rickets, with bowing of the long bones.
Image courtesy of Dr Ian Maddison.

Fig 14.8 Osteomalacia. Cortical bone lucency and Looser's zones are seen in both forearms of a patient with osteomalacia.
Image courtesy of Dr Ian Maddison.

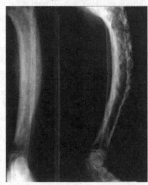

Fig 14.10 Paget's disease. The 'sabre tibia' seen in Paget's disease, with multiple sclerotic lesions.
Image courtesy of Dr Ian Maddison.

Plasma proteins

The plasma contains a number of proteins including albumin, immunoglobulins, α_1-antitrypsin, α_2-macroglobulin, caeruloplasmin, transferrin, low-density lipoprotein (LDL), fibrinogen, complement, and factor VIII. The most abundant is albumin (fig 14.11). Measure total protein, albumin, and the calculated ratio of albumin to globulins, termed the A/G ratio. The A/G ratio is calculated from measured total protein, measured albumin, and calculated globulin (total protein minus albumin). Because disease states affect the relative amounts of albumin and globulin, the A/G ratio may provide a clue as to the cause of the change in protein levels.

Albumin Synthesized in the liver; $t\frac{1}{2}\approx20d$. It binds bilirubin, free fatty acids, Ca^{2+}, and some drugs. **Low albumin** Results in oedema, and is caused by: • ↓*Synthesis:* liver disease, acute phase response (due to ↑vascular permeability—eg sepsis, trauma, surgery), malabsorption, malnutrition, malignancy. • ↑*Loss:* nephrotic syndrome, protein-losing enteropathy, burns. • *Haemodilution:* late pregnancy, artefact (eg from 'drip' arm). Also posture (↑5g/L if upright) and genetic variations. **High albumin** Causes are dehydration; artefact (eg stasis).

Immunoglobulins (Antibodies) are synthesized by B cells. Five isoforms Ig A, D, E, G, M exist in humans, and IgG is the most abundant circulating form. *Specific monoclonal band* in paraproteinaemia (p364). *Diffusely raised* in chronic infections, TB, bronchiectasis, liver cirrhosis, sarcoidosis, SLE, RA, Crohn's disease, 1° biliary cirrhosis, hepatitis, and parasitaemia. *Low* levels (ie hypogammaglobulinemia) may be congenital, sex-linked, and/or part of a combined immunodeficiency state. It may also be acquired, as in multiple myeloma, AL amyloidosis, chronic lymphocytic leukaemia, lymphoma, or the nephrotic syndrome.

Acute phase response The body responds to a variety of insults with, among other things, the synthesis by the liver of a number of proteins (normally present in serum in small quantities)—eg α_1-antitrypsin, fibrinogen, complement, haptoglobin, and CRP. A concomitant reduction in albumin level is characteristic of conditions such as infection, malignancy (especially α_2-fraction), trauma, surgery, and inflammatory disease. ↓↓α_1 globulin component is usually due to a deficiency of α_1-antitrypsin.

CRP So called because it binds to a polysaccharide (fraction C) in the cell wall of pneumococci. Levels help monitor inflammation/infection (normal <8mg/L). Like the ESR, it is raised in many inflammatory conditions, but changes more rapidly. It increases in hours and begins to fall within 2–3d of recovery; thus it can be used to follow disease activity (eg Crohn's disease) or the response to therapy (eg antibiotics). CRP values in mild inflammation 10–50mg/L; active bacterial infection 50–200mg/L; severe infection or trauma >200mg/L; see table 14.7.

Urinary proteins

Urinary protein loss >150mg/d is pathological (p290).

Albuminuria Usually caused by kidney disease (p290). **Moderately increased albuminuria** (formerly called 'microalbuminuria') Urinary protein loss between 30 and 300mg/d (so not detectable on normal dipstick) and may be seen with diabetes mellitus, ↑BP, SLE, and glomerulonephritis (see p310 for role in DM). Can also be quantified by measuring the urinary *albumin:creatinine ratio* (ACR), usually a first-in-the-morning spot urine sample. Moderately increased albuminuria refers to an ACR of 3–30mg/mmol whereas >30mg/mmol represents severely increased. This is a useful screening test in diabetics and subjects with reduced eGFR. When ACR is ≥70mg/mmol, measure urinary total protein rather than albumin using the protein:creatinine ratio (PCR).[19]

Bence Jones protein Consists of monoclonal free kappa or lambda light chains excreted in the urine by some patients with myeloma (p366). They are not detected by dipsticks and may occur with normal serum electrophoresis.

Haemoglobinuria Caused by intravascular haemolysis (p332).

Myoglobinuria Caused by rhabdomyolysis (p315).

Table 14.7 c-reactive protein (CRP)

Marked elevation	Normal-to-slight elevation
Bacterial infection	Viral infection
Abscess	Steroids/oestrogens
Crohn's disease	Ulcerative colitis
Connective tissue diseases (except SLE)	SLE
Neoplasia	Morbid obesity
Trauma	Atherosclerosis
Necrosis (eg MI)	

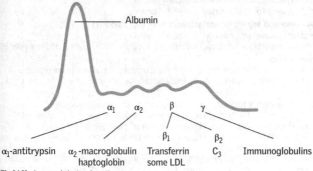

Fig 14.11 A normal electrophoretic scan.

14 Clinical chemistry

►Reference intervals vary between laboratories. See p736 for a guide to normal values.

Raised levels of specific enzymes can be a useful indicator of a disease. However, remember that most can be raised for other reasons too. Levels may be raised due to cellular damage, ↑cell turnover, cellular proliferation (malignancy), enzyme induction, and ↓clearance. The major causes of *raised enzymes:*

Alkaline phosphatase (Several distinguishable isoforms exist, eg liver and bone.)
- Liver disease (suggests cholestasis; also cirrhosis, abscess, hepatitis, or malignancy).
- Bone disease (isoenzyme distinguishable, reflects osteoblast activity) especially Paget's, growing children, healing fractures, bone metastases, osteomalacia, osteomyelitis, chronic kidney disease, and hyperparathyroidism.
- Congestive cardiac failure (moderately raised).
- Pregnancy (placenta makes its own isoenzyme).

Alanine and aspartate aminotransferase (ALT and AST)
- Liver disease (suggests hepatocyte damage).
- AST also ↑ in MI, skeletal muscle damage (especially crush injuries), and haemolysis.

α-amylase
- Acute pancreatitis (smaller rise in chronic pancreatitis as less tissue remaining).
- *Also:* severe uraemia, diabetic ketoacidosis, severe gastroenteritis, and peptic ulcer.

Creatine kinase (CK) ►A raised CK does not necessarily mean an MI.
- Myocardial infarction (p114; isoenzyme 'CK-MB'. Diagnostic if CK-MB >6% of total CK, or CK-MB mass >99th percentile of normal). CK returns to baseline within 48h (unlike troponin, which remains raised for ~10 days) ∴ useful for detecting re-infarction.
- Muscle damage (rhabdomyolysis, p315; prolonged running; haematoma; seizures; IM injection; defibrillation; bowel ischaemia; myxoedema; dermatomyositis, p549)—and *drugs* (eg statins).

Gamma-glutamyl transferase (GGT, γGT)
- Liver disease (particularly alcohol-induced damage, cholestasis, drugs).

Lactate dehydrogenase (LDH)
- Myocardial infarction (p114).
- Liver disease (suggests hepatocyte damage).
- Haemolysis (esp. sickle cell crisis), pulmonary embolism, and tumour necrosis.

Troponin
- Subtypes troponin T and troponin I are specific and sensitive biomarkers of myocardial injury.
- Cardiac damage or strain (MI, p114; pericarditis, myocarditis, PE, sepsis, CPR).
- Chronic kidney disease (stably elevated troponin levels possibly due to chronic myocardial injury rather than epicardial coronary disease; cTnI may be more specific for myocardial injury in patients with CKD than cTnT; serially measured troponins in the appropriate clinical context are helpful to make a diagnosis of MI in these patients).

Enzyme inducers and inhibitors

Hepatic drug metabolism is mainly by conjugation or oxidation. The oxidative pathways are catalysed by the family of cytochrome P450 isoenzymes, the most important of which is the CYP 3A4 isoenzyme. The cytochrome P450 pathway may be either induced or inhibited by a range of commonly used drugs and foods (table 14.8).

This can lead to important interactions or side effects. For example, phenytoin reduces the effectiveness of the contraceptive pill due to more rapid oestrogen metabolism, and ciprofloxacin retards the metabolism of methylxanthines (aminophylline) which leads to higher plasma levels and potentially more side effects. The *BNF* contains a list of the major interactions between drugs.

Table 14.8 Common inhibitors and inducers of cytochrome P450 isoenzymes

Enzyme inducers	Enzyme inhibitors	
Phenytoin	SSRIs	Amiodarone
Rifampicin	Ciprofloxacin	Diltiazem
Carbamazepine	Isoniazid	Verapamil
Alcohol	Macrolides	Omeprazole
St John's wort	HIV protease inhibitors	Grapefruit juice
Barbiturates	Imidazole and triazole antifungal agents	

14 Clinical chemistry

Lipids travel in blood packaged with proteins as lipoproteins. There are four classes: chylomicrons and VLDL (mainly triglyceride), LDL (mainly cholesterol), and HDL (mainly phospholipid) (for abbreviations see footnote[2]). The evidence that cholesterol is a major risk factor for cardiovascular disease (CVD) is undisputed ('4S' study,[20] WOSCOPS,[21] CARE study,[22] Heart Protection Study[23]) and indeed it may even be the 'green light' that allows other risk factors to act.[24] Half the UK population have a serum cholesterol level putting them at significant risk of CVD. HDL appears to correlate inversely with CVD.

Who to screen for hyperlipidaemia
►NB: full screening requires a fasting lipid profile. According to the ESC, routine screening should be considered in men >40 years old, and in women >50 years of age or postmenopausal.[25] Measure Lp(a) at least once in all adults to screen for this hereditary disorder as new treatments are emerging.

Those at risk of hyperlipidaemia •Family history of hyperlipidaemia. •Corneal arcus <50yrs old. •Xanthomata or xanthelasmata (fig 14.12).

Those at risk of CVD •Known CVD. •Family history of premature CVD (ie <60yrs old). •DM or impaired glucose tolerance. •Hypertension. •Smoker. •Diabetes •↑BMI. •CKD.

Types of hyperlipidaemia
Common primary hyperlipidaemia Accounts for 70% of hyperlipidaemia. ↑LDL only.

Familial primary hyperlipidaemias Multiple phenotypes exist (table 14.9). *Risk of ↑↑CVD*, although evidence suggests protection from CVD is achieved with lower doses of statin than for common primary hyperlipidaemia.[26] Refer to specialist.

Secondary hyperlipidaemia Causes include: Cushing's syndrome, hypothyroidism, nephrotic syndrome, or cholestasis. ↑LDL. Treat the cause first.

Mixed hyperlipidaemia Results in ↑ in both LDL and triglycerides. Caused by type 2 diabetes mellitus, metabolic syndrome, alcohol abuse, and CKD.

Management
Identify familial or 2° hyperlipidaemias, as Rx may differ. Give lifestyle advice; aim for BMI of 20–25; encourage a Mediterranean-style diet—↑fruit, vegetables, fish, unsaturated fats; and ↓red meat; ↑exercise. Top Rx priority are those with known CVD (there is no need to calculate their risk: *ipso facto* they already have high risk). Second Rx priority is primary prevention in patients with CKD or type 1 diabetes, and those with a 10yr risk of CVD (eg SCORE) >10%, *irrespective of baseline lipid levels*.

• **1st-line therapy** High-dose statins (eg atorvastatin 40mg or rosuvastatin 20mg) for secondary prevention or if ≥4.5mmol/L; otherwise maximally tolerated. ↓Cholesterol synthesis in the liver by inhibiting HMGCoA reductase. CI: porphyria, cholestasis, pregnancy. SE: myalgia ± myositis (stop if ↑↑CK ≥10-fold; if any myalgia, check CK; risk is 1 per 100 000 treatment-years),[27] abdominal pain, and ↑LFTs (stop if AST ≥100u/L). Cytochrome P450 inhibitors (p681) ↑ serum concentrations (200mL of grapefruit juice ↑ simvastatin concentration by 300%, and atorvastatin ↑ by 80%, but pravastatin is almost unchanged). Current guidelines suggest a target LDL-C <1.4 mmol/L if very high risk (ie established CVD) or <1.8 mmol/L if high risk (eg risk factors, diabetes, moderate CKD).

• **2nd-line therapy** Ezetimibe—a cholesterol absorption inhibitor, may be used in statin intolerance or combination with statins to achieve target reduction.

• **3rd-line therapy** Alirocumab—a monoclonal antibody against PCSK9 (acts to reduce hepatocyte LDL receptor expression), given by injection every 2 weeks or inclisiran—a small interfering RNA, that silences PCSK9, given every 6 months.

Hypertriglyceridaemia Statins are also 1st line. Consider fish oils (ie n-3 polyunsaturated fatty acids) if persistently high levels despite statins.

Xanthomata These yellow lipid deposits may be: *eruptive* (itchy nodules in crops in hypertriglyceridaemia); *tuberous* (plaques on elbows and knees); or *planar*—also called palmar (orange streaks in palmar creases), 'diagnostic' of remnant hyperlipidaemia; or in tendons (p38), eyelids (*xanthelasma*, see fig 14.12), or cornea (*arcus*, p39).

2 Abbreviations: (V)LDL = (very) low-density lipoprotein; IDL = intermediate-density lipoprotein; HDL = high-density lipoprotein; chol = cholesterol; trig = triglycerides.

Primary hyperlipidaemias

Table 14.9 Classification of primary hyperlipidaemias

Familial hyperchylomicronaemia (lipoprotein lipase deficiency or apoCII deficiency)[I]	Chol <6.5 Trig 10–30 Chylomicrons	↑	Eruptive xanthomata; lipaemia retinalis; hepatosplenomegaly
Familial hypercholesterolaemia[II] (LDL receptor defects)	Chol 7.5–16 Trig <2.3	↑LDL	Tendon xanthoma; corneal arcus; xanthelasma
Familial defective apolipoprotein B-100[IIa]	Chol 7.5–16 Trig <2.3	↑LDL	Tendon xanthoma; arcus; xanthelasma
Common hypercholesterolaemia[IIa]	Chol 6.5–9 Trig <2.3	↑LDL	*The commonest 1° lipidaemia;* may have xanthelasma or arcus
Familial combined hyperlipidaemia[IIb, IV, OR V]	Chol 6.5–10 Trig 2.3–12	↑LDL ↑VLDL ↓HDL	*Next commonest 1° lipidaemia;* xanthelasma; arcus
Dysbetalipoproteinaemia (remnant particle disease)[III]	Chol 9–14 Trig 9–14	↑IDL ↓HDL ↓LDL	Palmar striae; tuberoeruptive xanthoma
Familial hypertriglyceridaemia[IV]	Chol 6.5–12 Trig 3.0–6.0	↑VLDL	
Type V hyperlipoproteinaemia	Trig 10–30; chylomicrons found		Eruptive xanthomata; lipaemia retinalis; hepatosplenomegaly

Blue superscript numbers = WHO phenotype; chol/trig levels given in mmol/L.

Primary HDL abnormalities
- Hyperalphalipoproteinaemia: ↑HDL, chol >2.
- Hypoalphalipoproteinaemia (Tangier disease): ↓HDL, chol <0.92.

Primary LDL abnormalities
- Abetalipoproteinaemia (ABL): trig <0.3, chol <1.3, missing LDL, VLDL, and chylomicrons. Autosomal recessive disorder of fat malabsorption causing vitamin A & E deficiency, with retinitis pigmentosa, sensory neuropathy, ataxia, pes cavus, and acanthocytosis.
- Hypobetalipoproteinaemia: chol <1.5, ↓LDL, ↓IDL. Autosomal codominant disorder of apolipoprotein B metabolism. ↑Longevity in heterozygotes. Homozygotes present with a similar clinical picture to ABL.

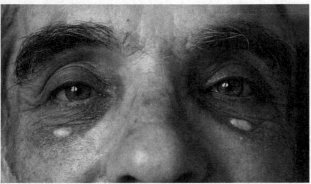

Fig 14.12 Xanthelasma. *Xanthos* is Greek for yellow, and *elasma* means plate. Xanthelasmata are lipid-laden yellow plaques, typically a few millimetres wide. They congregate around the lids, or just below the eyes, and signify hyperlipidaemia.

The porphyrias are a heterogeneous group of rare diseases caused by various errors of haem biosynthesis (produced when iron is chelated into protoporphyrin IXα), which may be genetic or acquired. Depending on the stage in haem biosynthesis that is faulty, there is accumulation of either porphyrinogens, which are unstable and oxidize to porphyrins, or their precursors, porphobilinogen and δ-aminolaevulinic acid. Porphyrin precursors are neurotoxic, while porphyrins themselves induce photosensitivity and the formation of toxic free radicals.

• Alcohol, lead, and iron deficiency cause abnormal porphyrin metabolism.
• Genetic counselling (*OHCS* p274) should be offered to all patients and their families.

Acute porphyrias Occur when the accumulation of porphyrinogen precursors predominates, and are characterized by acute neurovisceral crises, though some forms have additional photosensitive cutaneous manifestations.

Acute intermittent porphyria (see BOX 'The madness of King George') A low-penetrant autosomal dominant condition (porphobilinogen deaminase gene); 28% have no family history (*de novo* mutations). ~10% of those with the defective gene have neurovisceral symptoms. Attacks are intermittent, more common in women and those aged 18–40, and may be precipitated by drugs. Urine porphobilinogens are raised during attacks (the urine may go deep red on standing) and also, in ~50%, between attacks. Faecal porphyrin levels are normal. There is never cutaneous photosensitivity. It is the commonest form of porphyria—prevalence in UK: 1–2/100 000.

Variegate porphyria and hereditary coproporphyria Autosomal dominant, characterized by photosensitive blistering skin lesions and/or acute attacks. The former is prevalent in Afrikaners in South Africa. Porphobilinogen is high only during an attack, and other metabolites may be detected in faeces.

Triggers of an acute attack Include infection, starvation (including pre-operative 'nil-by-mouth'), reproductive hormones (pregnancy, premenstrual), smoking, anaesthesia, and cytochrome P450 enzyme inducers (alcohol, and other drugs—see BOX).

Features of an acute attack
• *Gastrointestinal:* abdominal pain, vomiting, constipation.
• *Neuropsychiatric:* peripheral neuropathy (weakness, hypotonia, pain, numbness), seizures (often associated with severe ↓Na⁺), psychosis (or other odd behaviour).
• *Cardiovascular:* hypertension, tachycardia, shock (due to sympathetic overactivity).
• *Other:* fever, ↓Na⁺, ↓K⁺, proteinuria, urinary porpholbilinogens, discoloured urine. Rare but serious complications include bulbar and respiratory paralysis.

▶▶Beware the 'acute abdomen' in acute intermittent porphyria: colic, vomiting, fever, and ↑WCC—so mimicking an acute surgical abdomen. Anaesthesia could be disastrous.

Treatment of an acute attack
• Remove precipitants (review medications; treat intercurrent illness/infection).
• IV fluids to correct electrolyte imbalance.
• High carbohydrate intake (eg Hycal®) by NG tube, or IV if necessary.
• IV haematin is 1st line (inhibits production of porphyrinogen precursors).
• Nausea controlled with prochlorperazine 12.5mg IM.
• Sedate if necessary with chlorpromazine 50–100mg PO/IM.
• Pain control with opiate or opioid analgesia (avoid oxycodone).
• Seizures can be controlled with diazepam (although this will prolong the attack).
• Treat tachycardia and hypertension with a β-blocker.

Non-acute porphyrias
Porphyria cutanea tarda (PCT), erythropoietic protoporphyria, and *congenital erythropoietic porphyria* are characterized by cutaneous photosensitivity alone, as there is no overproduction of porphyrinogen precursors, only porphyrins. PCT presents in adults with blistering skin lesions ± facial hypertrichosis and hyperpigmentation. Total plasma porphyrins and LFTs are ↑. Screen for associated disorders: hep C, HIV, iron overload, hepatocellular ca. ℞: phlebotomy, iron chelators, chloroquine, sunscreens.

Drugs to avoid in acute intermittent porphyria

There are many, many drugs that may precipitate an acute attack ± quadriplegia, and this is by no means an exhaustive list (see *BNF/Oxford Textbook of Medicine*).

▶▶For an up-to-date list of drugs considered safe in acute porphyria see https://www.wmic.wales.nhs.uk/specialist-services/drugs-in-porphyria/

- ACE-inhibitors
- Alcohol
- Amphetamines
- Anaesthetic agents (barbiturates, halothane)
- Antibiotics (cephalosporins, sulfonamides, macrolides, tetracyclines, rifampicin, trimethoprim, chloramphenicol, metronidazole)
- Anticonvulsants
- Antihistamines
- Benzodiazepines
- Ca^{2+}-channel blockers
- Diclofenac
- Furosemide
- Gold salts
- Lidocaine
- Metoclopramide
- Oral contraceptive pill & HRT
- Statins
- Sulfonylureas
- Tricyclic antidepressants.

The madness of King George

In the 1960s, Ida Macalpine and Richard Hunter, an unlikely duo of mother and son psychiatrists, published two papers in the *BMJ* stating categorically that King George III (1738–1820) (fig 14.13) had suffered from recurrent attacks of acute intermittent porphyria. During his life, King George was plagued by a constellation of episodic symptoms including mania, weakness, abdominal pain, and discoloured urine. However, in recent years, this porphyria theory has been strongly refuted with posthumous analysis of his own handwritten letters more consistent with the manic phase of psychiatric illnesses such as bipolar disorder. It is thought that the reported discoloured (blue) urine was related to gentian, a plant with deep blue flowers, that he was given as a medicine. The 'Madness of King George III' has been popularized in a number of plays, films, and TV series, including most recently in Netflix's *Queen Charlotte*.

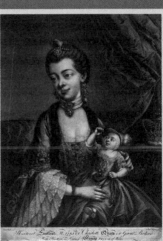

Fig 14.13 Queen Charlotte and George Prince of Wales as an infant seated on her lap.
Mezzotint by R. Houston after R. Pile (Pyle), ca. 1765. Wellcome Collection. Source: Wellcome Collection. Public Domain Mark.

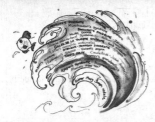

Fig 15.1 'No scientific discovery is named after its original discoverer' asserts Professor Stephen Stigler in 'Stigler's Law of Eponymy', and in doing so, names the sociologist RK Merton as its discoverer—deliberately making Stigler's law exemplify itself. Is the same true in medicine? At least six others described Alzheimer's disease before Alois Alzheimer in 1906, and tetralogy of Fallot (named after Étienne-Louis Fallot in 1888) was first described in 1672 by Niels Stenson. Not all medical eponyms obey Stigler's law. Forty years after it was first described, the French neurologist Jean-Marie Charcot (himself associated with at least 15 medical eponyms) attributed the name 'Parkinson's Disease' to the illness outlined in James Parkinson's 1817 essay 'The Shaking Palsy'. Monochromatic doctors may try to abolish eponyms by regimenting them to histologically driven disease titles. But classifications vary as facts emerge, and as a result the renaming of non-eponyms becomes essential. Eponyms, however, carry on forever, because they imply nothing about causes.

Artwork by Gillian Turner.

Alice in Wonderland syndrome Altered perception in size and shape of body parts or objects ± an impaired sense of passing time—as experienced by *Alice* in Lewis Carroll's novel. Seen in epilepsy, migraine, and cerebral lesions.[1,2]   *Alice Pleasance Liddell, 1865–1934*

Baker's cyst Fluid from a knee effusion escapes to form a popliteal cyst (often swollen and painful) in a sub-gastrocnemius bursa.[3] Usually secondary to degeneration. **ΔΔ** DVT (exclude if calf swelling); sarcoma. **Imaging** USS; MRI. **℞** None if asymptomatic. NSAIDs/ice if painful. Spontaneous resolution may take 10–20 months. Arthroscopy + cystectomy may be needed.   *William M Baker, 1838–1896 (British surgeon)*

Bazin's disease *(Erythema induratum)* Localized areas of fat necrosis that produce painful, firm nodules ± ulceration and an indurated rash, characteristically in ♀ adolescent calves. It is associated with TB. *Nodular vasculitis* is a variant unrelated to TB.[4]   *Pierre-Antoine-Ernest Bazin, 1807–1878 (French dermatologist)*

Bickerstaff's brainstem encephalitis Ophthalmoplegia, ataxia, areflexia, and extensor plantars ± tetraplegia ± coma. Variant form of the acute immune-mediated polyneuropathy, Guillain-Barré syndrome. *MRI:* hyperintense brainstem signals. GQ1b antibodies +ve.[5] Plasmapheresis/IV Ig may help.   *Edwin R Bickerstaff, 1920–2008 (British physician)*

Budd–Chiari syndrome Hepatic vein obstruction by thrombosis or tumour causes congestive ischaemia and hepatocyte damage. Abdominal pain, hepatomegaly, ascites, and ↑ALT occur. Portal hypertension occurs in chronic forms. **Causes** Include hypercoagulable states (combined OCP, pregnancy, malignancy, paroxysmal nocturnal haemoglobinuria, polycythaemia, thrombophilia), TB, liver, renal, or adrenal tumour. **Tests** USS + Dopplers, CT, or MRI. Angioplasty or a transjugular intrahepatic portosystemic shunt (TIPSS) may be needed. Anticoagulate (lifelong) unless there are varices. Consider liver transplant in fulminant hepatic necrosis or cirrhosis.[6]
   George Budd, 1808–1882 (British physician); Hans Chiari, 1851–1916 (Austrian pathologist)

Buerger's disease *(Thromboangiitis obliterans)* Non-atherosclerotic, smoking-related, inflammation and thrombosis of veins and mid-sized arteries causing thrombophlebitis and ischaemia (→ulcers, gangrene). **Cause** Unknown. Smoking cessation vital. Patients typically ♂ 20–45yrs (see BOX 'Poisoning your boss').   *Leo Buerger, 1879–1943 (US physician)*

Caplan's syndrome Multiple lung nodules in coal workers with RA, caused by an inflammatory reaction to anthracite (also associated with silica or asbestos exposure). CXR: bilateral peripheral nodules (0.5–5cm). **ΔΔ** TB.   *Anthony Caplan, 1907–1976 (British physician)*

Churg–Strauss syndrome *(Eosinophilic granulomatosis with polyangiitis)* A triad of adult-onset asthma, eosinophilia, and vasculitis (± vasospasm ± MI ± DVT), affecting lungs, ears/nose/throat, nerves, heart, and skin. Kidney involvement (22%) may vary from isolated haematuria and proteinuria to a rapidly progressive glomerulonephritis. 30–60% are ANCA +ve (usually MPO). **℞** Steroids; combined with either cyclophosphamide or rituximab if organ or life-threatening disease. Consider adding mepolizumab to steroids if non-severe disease.[7]   *Jacob Churg, 1910–2005; Lotte Strauss, 1913–1985 (US pathologists)*

Brugada syndrome

Note right bundle branch block and the unusual morphology of the raised ST segments in V1–V3 (fig 15.2; there are three ECG variants of this pattern). This is a predominantly autosomal dominant condition with faulty sodium channels that predispose to fatal arrhythmias (eg ventricular fibrillation), typically in young males (eg triggered by a fever). Asymptomatic patients with typical ECG features and no other clinical criteria are said to have the Brugada pattern. Patients with typical ECG features who have experienced sudden cardiac death, sustained ventricular tachyarrhythmia, or who have ≥1 of other associated clinical criteria, are said to have the Brugada syndrome. It is preventable by implanting a defibrillator in high-risk patients. ►*Consider primary electrical cardiac disease in all with unexplained syncope.* Mutations in the SCN5A gene (encodes the cardiac voltage-gated $Na_v1.5$ channel) are found in 15–20%. Other mutations have also been described. All first-degree relatives of patients with confirmed Brugada syndrome should undergo screening with clinical history and 12-lead ECG followed by targeted genetic testing.

Pedro & Josep Brugada, described 1992 (Spanish cardiologists)

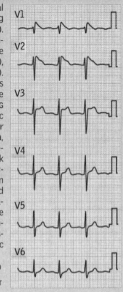

Fig 15.2 Note right bundle branch block and ST morphology in leads V1–V3.

Courtesy of Dr Shayashi.

Poisoning your boss

In 1931, Buerger's disease caused gangrene in the toes of Harvey Cushing (p218)—the most cantankerous (and greatest) neurosurgeon ever. He had to be wheeled to the operating theatre to carry on his brilliant art (and to continue terrifying his assistants).[8] He had to retire partially, whereupon his colleagues presented him with a magnificent silver cigarette box, containing 2000 cigarettes (to which he was addicted)—one for each brain tumour he had removed during his long career, so verifying the truth that although we owe everything to our teachers, we must eventually kill them to move out from under their shadow.[1]

1 *Der Vogel kämpft sich aus dem Ei. Das Ei ist die Welt. Wer geboren werden will, muss eine Welt zerstören.* [The bird struggles out of the egg. The egg is the world. Whoever will be born, must first destroy a world.] (Hermann Hesse. *Demian;* 1917.)

Devic's syndrome *(Neuromyelitis optica;* NMO) Inflammatory demyelination causes attacks of optic neuritis ± transverse myelitis[9] ± area postrema syndrome (hiccups or nausea and vomiting) ± narcolepsy. Abnormal CSF (pleocytosis and elevated protein levels) and serum anti-AQP4 antibody (in 73%) help distinguish it from MS[10] (table 15.1). *R̸* IV steroids; plasma exchange. Eculizumab and rituximab[11] help prevent relapses. **Prognosis** Variable; complete remission may occur.
Eugène Devic, 1858–1930 (French neurologist)

Dubin–Johnson syndrome There is defective hepatocyte excretion of conjugated bilirubin. Typically presents in late teens with intermittent jaundice ± hepatosplenomegaly (autosomal recessive). **Tests** ↑Bilirubin; ALT and AST are normal; bilirubinuria on dipstick; ↑ratio of urinary coproporphyrin I to III. Liver biopsy: diagnostic pigment granules.[12] *R̸* Usually none needed.
Isadore N Dubin, 1913–1981; Frank B Johnson, 1919–2005 (US pathologists)

Felty's syndrome A triad of rheumatoid arthritis + ↓WCC & splenomegaly (± hypersplenism, causing anaemia and ↓platelets), recurrent infections, skin ulcers, and lymphadenopathy. 95% are Rh factor +ve. Splenectomy may raise the WCC. *R̸* DMARDs (p543) ± *rituximab* if refractory.[14]
Augustus Roi Felty, 1895–1964 (US physician)

Foster Kennedy syndrome Optic atrophy of one eye due to optic nerve compression (most commonly from an olfactory groove meningioma), with papilloedema of the other eye secondary to ↑ICP. There is also central scotoma and anosmia.
Robert Foster Kennedy, 1884–1952 (British neurologist)

Friedreich's ataxia Expansions of the trinucleotide repeat GAA in the frataxin gene (recessive) causes degeneration of many nerve tracts: spinocerebellar tracts degenerate causing cerebellar ataxia, dysarthria, nystagmus, and dysdiadochokinesis. Loss of corticospinal tracts occurs (weakness and extensor plantar response) with peripheral nerve damage, so tendon reflexes are paradoxically depressed (differential diagnosis, p442). There is also dorsal column degeneration, with loss of positional and vibration sense. Pes cavus and scoliosis occur. Cardiomyopathy may cause CCF. Typical age at death: ~50yrs. *R̸* There is no cure. Treat CCF, arrhythmias, and DM.
Nikolaus Friedreich, 1825–1882 (German neurologist)

Froin's syndrome ↑CSF protein + xanthochromia with normal cell count—a sign of blockage in spinal CSF flow (eg from a spinal tumour). *Georges Froin, 1874–1932 (French physician)*

Gardner's syndrome A dominant variant of familial adenomatous polyposis, caused by mutations in the APC gene (5q21). There are multiple colon polyps (which inevitably become malignant; p516),[15] benign bone osteomas, epidermal cysts, dermoid tumours, fibromas, and neurofibromas. *Fundoscopy* reveals black spots (congenital hypertrophy of retinal pigment epithelium); this helps pre-symptomatic detection. **Presentation** Can present from 2–70yrs with colonic (eg bloody diarrhoea) or extracolonic symptoms. Prophylactic surgery (eg proctocolectomy) is the only curative treatment. Endoscopic polypectomy with long-term celecoxib therapy has been used to postpone prophylactic colectomy.[16]
Eldon J Gardner, 1909–1989 (US physician)

Gélineau's syndrome *(Narcolepsy)* The patient, usually a young man, succumbs to irresistible attacks of inappropriate sleep ± vivid hypnogogic hallucinations, cataplexy (sudden hypotonia), and sleep paralysis (paralysis of speech and movement, while fully alert, at sleep onset or on waking). **Hypothesis** Loss of hypothalamic orexin-secreting neurons, via autoimmune destruction.[17] There is a genetic predisposition, and 95% are +ve for HLA DR2. GSKS H1N1 'flu vaccination has also been associated with narcolepsy. *R̸* Stimulants (eg methylphenidate) may cause dependence ± psychosis. Modafinil may be better. SE: anxiety, aggression, dry mouth, euphoria, insomnia, ↑BP, dyskinesia, ↑ALP.
Jean-Baptiste-Édouard Gélineau, 1828–1906 (French physician)

Gerstmann's syndrome A constellation of symptoms suggesting a dominant parietal lesion: finger agnosia (inability to identify fingers), agraphia (inability to write), acalculia (inability to calculate), and left–right disorientation.
Josef Gerstmann, 1887–1969 (Austrian neurologist)

Devic's syndrome and multiple sclerosis

Table 15.1 Distinguishing Devic's syndrome from multiple sclerosis

	Devic's syndrome	Multiple sclerosis
Course	Monophasic or relapsing	Relapsing usually; see p492
Attack severity	Usually severe	Often mild
Respiratory failure	~30%, from cervical myelitis	Rare
MRI head	Usually normal	Many periventricular white-matter lesions
MRI cord lesions	Longitudinally extensive, central	Multiple, small, peripheral
CSF oligoclonal bands	Absent	Present
Permanent disability	Unusual, and attack related	In late progressive disease
Other autoimmunities	In ≤50% (eg Sjögren's)	Uncommon

Diagnostic criteria for Devic's

1 At least one core clinical characteristic: • optic neuritis • acute myelitis • area postrema syndrome (episode of unexplained hiccups or nausea/vomiting) • acute brainstem syndrome •symptomatic narcolepsy • symptomatic cerebral syndrome with NMOSD-typical brain lesions.
2 Positive test for AQP4-IgG*.
3 Exclusion of alternative diagnoses.
* There are additional MRI criteria if AQP4-IgG negative or unknown.

Cataplexy is highly specific for narcolepsy/Gélineau's syndrome

Daytime sleepiness has many causes, but if it occurs with cataplexy the diagnosis 'must' be narcolepsy. Cataplexy is bilateral loss of tone in antigravity muscles provoked by emotions such as laughter, startle, excitement, or anger. Associated phenomena include: falls, mouth opening, dysarthria, mutism, and phasic muscle jerking around the mouth. Most attacks are brief, but injury can occur (eg if several attacks per day). It is comparable to the atonia of rapid eye movement sleep *but without loss of awareness.* ΔΔ Bradycardia, migraine, atonic/akinetic epilepsy, delayed sleep phase syndrome, conversion disorder, malingering, and psychosis.

Don't confuse cata*plexy* with cata*lepsy*—a waxy flexibility where involuntary statue-like postures are effortlessly maintained (frozen) despite looking most uncomfortable.

Gilles de la Tourette syndrome Tonic, clonic, dystonic, or phonic tics: jerks, blinks, sniffs, nods, spitting, stuttering, irrepressible explosive obscene verbal ejaculations (coprolalia, in 20%) or gestures (coprophilia, 6%),[18] grunts, squeaks, burps, twirlings, and nipping others ± tantrums. There may be a witty, innovatory, phantasmagoric picture, with mimicry (echopraxia), antics, impishness, extravagance, audacity, dramatizations, surreal associations, uninhibited affect, speed, 'go', vivid imagery and memory, and hunger for stimuli. **The tic paradox** Tics are *voluntary*, but often *unwanted*: the desire to tic stems from the relief of the odd sensation that builds up prior to the tic and is relieved by it, 'like scratching a mosquito bite, tics lead to more tics'.[19] **Mean age of onset** 6yrs. ♂:♀≈4:1. **Pathogenesis** Unknown; multiple genetic loci implicated and neuroanatomical abnormalities reported on MRI. **Associations** Obsessive–compulsive disorder; attention deficit hyperactivity disorder. ℞ (None may be wanted.) Risperidone, aripiprazole, or tetrabenazine. Habit-reversal training.[20] Deep brain stimulation is rarely indicated, but may help.

Marquis Georges Albert Édouard Brutus Gilles de la Tourette, 1857–1904 (French neurologist)

Jervell and Lange-Nielsen syndrome Congenital, bilateral, autosomal recessive, sensorineural deafness, and long QT interval (p88, hence syncope, VT, *torsades*, ± sudden death—50% by age 15 if untreated). KCNQ1 or KCNE1 gene mutation causes K⁺ channelopathy. ℞ β-blocker, pacemaker, ICD, cochlear implants.[21]

Anton Jervell, 1901–1987; Fred Lange-Nielsen, 1919–1989 (Norwegian physicians)

Kaposi's sarcoma (KS) A spindle-cell tumour derived from capillary endothelial cells, caused by human herpes virus 8 (=Kaposi's sarcoma-associated herpes virus, KSHV). It presents as purple papules (½–1cm) or plaques on skin (fig 15.3) and mucosa (look in mouth, but any organ). It metastasizes to nodes. There are four types: 1 Classic, a rare disease of the elderly. 2 Endemic, a disease of children documented prior to HIV. 3 Iatrogenic KS due to immunosuppression, eg organ transplant recipients. 4 AIDS-associated KS. Usually presents with low CD4 count and can indicate failure of HAART (p398). However, ⅓ presents in HIV with near-normal CD4 counts and an undetectable viral load. Initiation of HAART with rapid immune system constitution can precipitate KS. Lung KS may present in HIV +ve men and women as dyspnoea and haemoptysis. Bowel KS may cause nausea, abdominal pain. **Rare sites** CNS, larynx, eye, glands, heart, breast, wounds, or biopsy sites. Δ Biopsy. ℞ Optimize HAART, local radiotherapy, surgical excision, intralesional therapy (vincristine, bleomycin), liposomal doxorubicin, paclitaxel. Current research includes mTOR inhibitors (eg sirolimus), molecularly targeted anti-angiogenic agents (eg pazopanib), and checkpoint inhibitor immunotherapy.

Moricz Kaposi, 1837–1902 (Hungarian dermatologist)

Klippel–Trénaunay syndrome A triad of port wine stain, varicose veins, and limb hypertrophy, due to vascular malformation. Usually sporadic (although AD inheritance has been reported).[22]

Maurice Klippel, 1858–1942; Paul Trénaunay, 1875–1938 (French physicians)

Korsakoff's syndrome Hypothalamic damage & cerebral atrophy due to thiamine (vitamin B₁) deficiency (eg in alcoholics). May accompany Wernicke's encephalopathy. There is ↓ability to acquire new memories, confabulation (invented memory, owing to retrograde amnesia), lack of insight, & apathy. ℞ See *Wernicke's*, p700; patients rarely recover.

Sergei Sergeievich Korsakoff, 1853–1900 (Russian neuropsychiatrist)

Langerhans cell histiocytosis *(Histiocytosis X)* A group of single- (73%, eg bone) or multisystem (27%) disorders, with infiltrating granulomas containing dendritic (Langerhans) cells (fig 15.4). ♂:♀≈1.5:1; at-risk organs are liver, lung, spleen, marrow. Pulmonary disease presents with pneumothorax or pulmonary hypertension. CXR/CT: nodules and cysts + honeycombing in upper and middle zones. Δ Biopsy (skin, lung). ℞ Local excision, steroids, cladribine or cytarabine ± lung transplantation. Radiotherapy for bone-only disease.[23]

Paul Langerhans, 1847–1888 (German pathologist)

Leriche's syndrome Absent femoral pulse, claudication/wasting of the buttock, a pale cold leg, and erectile dysfunction from aorto-iliac occlusive disease, eg a saddle embolus at the aortic bifurcation. Surgery may help.

René Leriche, 1879–1955 (French surgeon)

Löffler's eosinophilic endocarditis Restrictive cardiomyopathy + eosinophilia (eg 1.5 × 10⁹/L). It may be an early stage of tropical endomyocardial fibrosis (and overlaps with hypereosinophilic syndrome, p322) but is distinct from eosinophilic leukaemia. **Signs** Heart failure (75%) ± mitral regurgitation (49%) ± heart block. ℞ Suppress the eosinophilia (prednisolone ± azathioprine or mycophenolate mofetil), and then treat with heart failure management.

Wilhelm Löffler, 1887–1972 (Swiss physician)

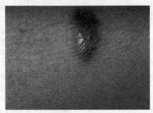

Fig 15.3 Kaposi's sarcoma.
Reproduced from *Oxford Handbook of Medical Dermatology*,
2010, with permission from Oxford University Press.

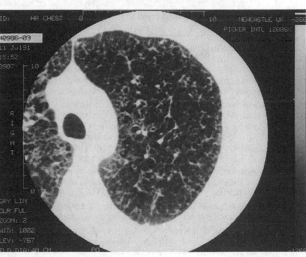

Fig 15.4 High-resolution CT of a 45-year-old smoking man with biopsy-proven Langerhans' cell histiocytosis, showing centrilobular nodules, cysts, and reticulation.
Reproduced from Firth J et al. *Oxford Textbook of Medicine* (2020),
with permission from Oxford University Press.

Adverse effects of alcohol on the CNS

- ↓Inhibitions (risk taking; ↑unsafe sex)
- Wernicke's encephalopathy
- Korsakoff's syndrome (p690)
- Hepatic encephalopathy
- Cerebral atrophy (dementia)
- Central pontine myelinolysis
- Cerebellar atrophy (eg falls)
- Stroke (ischaemic and haemorrhagic)
- Seizures
- Marchiafava–Bignami syndrome (p692).

ABC

Löffler's syndrome *(Pulmonary eosinophilia)* An allergic infiltration of the lungs by eosinophils. Allergens include: *Ascaris lumbricoides, Trichinella spiralis, Fasciola hepatica, Strongyloides, Ancylostoma, Toxocara, Clonorchis sinensis,* sulfonamides, hydralazine, and nitrofurantoin. Often symptomless with incidental CXR (diffuse fan-shaped shadows), or cough, fever, eosinophilia (in ~20%), & larval migrans (p429). ℞ Eradicate cause. Steroids (if idiopathic). *Wilhelm Löffler, 1887–1972 (Swiss physician)*

Lown–Ganong–Levine syndrome A pre-excitation syndrome, similar to Wolff–Parkinson–White (WPW, p129), characterized by a short PR interval (<0.12sec), a normal QRS complex (as opposed to the δ-waves of WPW), and risk of supraventricular tachycardia (but not AF/flutter). The cause is not completely understood, but may be due to paranodal fibres that bypass all or part of the atrioventricular node. The patient may complain of intermittent palpitations.[24]

Bernard Lown, 1921–2021 (US cardiologist); William F Ganong, 1924–2007 (US physiologist); Samuel A Levine, 1891–1966 (US cardiologist)

McArdle's glycogen storage disease (type v) Absence of muscle phosphorylase enzyme with resulting inability to convert glycogen into glucose (eg R50X mutation of PYGM gene; autosomal recessive). Fatigue & crises of cramps ± hyperthermia. Rhabdomyolysis/myoglobinuria follow exercise. **Tests** ↑↑CK. Muscle biopsy is diagnostic (necrosis and atrophy). ℞ Moderate aerobic exercise helps (by utilizing alternative fuel substrates).[25] Avoid heavy exertion and statins. Sucrose pre-exercise improves performance, as does a carbohydrate-rich diet. Low-dose creatine and ramipril (only if D/D ACE phenotype) may be of minimal benefit.[26] *Brian McArdle, 1911–2002 (British paediatrician)*

Marchiafava–Bignami syndrome Corpus callosum demyelination and necrosis, most often secondary to chronic alcoholism. Type A is characterized by coma, stupor, and pyramidal tract features involving the entire corpus callosum. In type B, symptoms are mild and the corpus callosum is partially affected.[27] Δ MRI. ℞ As for Wernicke's, p700 (see BOX 'Adverse effects of alcohol on the CNS').

Ettore Marchiafava, 1847–1935; Amico Bignami, 1862–1929 (Italian pathologists)

Meckel's diverticulum The distal ileum contains embryonic remnants of gastric and pancreatic tissue. There may be gastric acid secretion, causing GI pain & occult bleeding. Δ Radionucleotide scan; laparotomy. *Johann Friedrich Meckel, 1781–1833 (German anatomist)*

Meigs' syndrome A triad of: 1 benign ovarian tumour (fibroma) 2 pleural effusion (R > L) & 3 ascites. It resolves on tumour resection. *Joe Vincent Meigs, 1892–1963 (US gynaecologist)*

Ménétrier's disease Giant gastric mucosal folds up to 4cm high, in the fundus, with atrophy of the glands + ↑mucosal thickness + hypochlorhidria + protein-losing gastropathy (hence hypoalbuminaemia ± oedema). **Causes** CMV, *Strep, H. pylori.* There may be epigastric pain, vomiting, ± ↓weight. It is pre-malignant. ℞ Treat *H. pylori* or CMV if present; give high-dose PPI; if this fails, consider epidermal growth factor blockade with cetuximab or gastrectomy (eg if intractable symptoms or malignant change). Surgery if intractable symptoms or malignant change. *Pierre Eugène Ménétrier, 1859–1935 (French pathologist)*

Meyer–Betz syndrome *(Paroxysmal myoglobinuria)* Rare idiopathic condition causing necrosis of exercising muscles. There is muscle pain, weakness, and discoloured urine: pink→brown (as ↑myoglobin is excreted). DIC is associated. **Tests** ↑WCC, ↑LFT, ↑LDH, ↑CPK, ↑urine myoglobin. **Diagnosis** Muscle biopsy, ↑CPK, and ↑serum myoglobin. Exertion should be avoided. *Friedrich Meyer-Betz, described 1910 (German physician)*

Mikulicz's syndrome Benign persistent swelling of lacrimal and parotid (or submandibular) glands due to lymphocytic infiltration. Exclude other causes (sarcoidosis, TB, viral infection, lymphoproliferative disorders). It is thought to be an IgG4-related plasmacytic systemic disease.[29] *Johann Freiherr von Mikulicz-Radecki, 1850–1905 (Polish-Austrian surgeon)*

Milroy disease 1° congenital lymphoedema. Mutations in the VEGFR3 gene (dominant) cause lymphatic malfunction with lower leg swelling from birth (fig 15.5). Δ Lymphoscintigraphy; genetic testing. ℞ • Compression hosiery/bandages. • Encourage exercise. • Good skin hygiene. • Treat cellulitis actively.

William Forsyth Milroy, 1855–1942 (US physician)

ABC

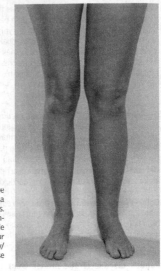

Fig 15.5 Milroy disease. Lymphoedema may be primary, as in Milroy or Meige disease, and is a feature in both Turner and Noonan syndromes. More commonly it is secondary to other conditions, eg cancer (after surgery, lymph node dissection, radiotherapy, or from direct tumour effect), cellulitis, varicose veins, or immobility/ dependency. Filariasis (p417) is a common cause in tropical regions.

ABC

Münchausen's syndrome Also known as factitious disorder imposed on self (FDIS), is a psychiatric disorder characterized by a person repeatedly and deliberately faking or exaggerating physical or psychological symptoms, often with the primary motivation of assuming the role of a patient. Individuals with Münchausen's syndrome may go to great lengths to fabricate illnesses, injuries, or conditions, and they may undergo unnecessary medical procedures, tests, or treatments, sometimes at different healthcare facilities. Münchausen-by-proxy entails injury to a dependent person by a carer (eg mother) to gain medical attention.

Karl Friedrich Hieronymus, Freiherr von Münchausen, 1720–1797 (German aristocrat).
Described by RAJ Asher in 1951[30]

Ogilvie's syndrome *(Acute colonic pseudo-obstruction)* Colonic obstruction in the absence of a mechanical cause, associated with recent severe illness or surgery. ℞ Correct U&E. Colonoscopy allows decompression, and excludes mechanical causes. Neostigmine is also effective, suggesting parasympathetic suppression is to blame.[31] Surgery is rarely needed (eg if perforation). *William Heneage Ogilvie, 1887–1971 (British surgeon)*

Ortner's cardiovocal syndrome Recurrent laryngeal nerve palsy from a large left atrium (eg from mitral stenosis) or aortic dissection.

Norbert Ortner, 1865–1935 (Austrian physician)

Osler–Weber–Rendu syndrome *(Hereditary telangiectasia)* Autosomal dominant (at least 5 possible gene mutations) telangiectasia of skin & mucous membranes (causing epistaxis and GI bleeds), see fig 15.7. Associated with pulmonary, hepatic, and cerebral arteriovenous malformations.

William Osler, 1849–1919 (Canadian); Frederick Weber, 1863–1962 (British);
Henri Rendu, 1844–1902 (French)—physicians

Paget's disease of the breast (PDB) Intra-epidermal spread of an intraduct cancer, which can look just like eczema. ▶Any red, scaly lesion at the nipple (fig 15.8) *must* suggest PDB: do a biopsy. ℞ Breast-conserving surgery + radiotherapy. Sentinel node biopsy should be performed. *Sir James Paget, 1814–1899 (British surgeon)*

Pancoast's syndrome Apical lung tumour invades the sympathetic plexus in the neck (→ipsilateral Horner's, p69) ± brachial plexus (→arm pain ± weakness) ± recurrent laryngeal nerve (→hoarse voice/bovine cough). *Henry Pancoast, 1875–1939 (US radiologist)*

Parinaud's syndrome *(Dorsal midbrain syndrome)* Upward gaze palsy + pseudo-Argyll Robertson pupils (p68) ± bilateral papilloedema. **Causes** Pineal or midbrain tumours; upper brainstem stroke; MS. *Henry Parinaud, 1844–1905 (French neuro-ophthalmologist)*

Peutz–Jeghers syndrome Dominant germline mutations of tumour suppressor gene STK11 (in 66–94%) cause mucocutaneous dark freckles on lips (fig 15.9), oral mucosa, palms and soles, + multiple GI polyps (hamartomas), causing obstruction, intussusception, or bleeds. There is a 15-fold ↑risk of developing GI cancer ∴ perform colonoscopy (from age 18yrs) and OGD (from age 25yrs) every 3yrs. NB: hamartomas are excessive focal overgrowths of normal cells in an organ composed of the same cell type.

Johannes LA Peutz, 1886–1957 (Dutch physician); Harold J Jeghers, 1904–1990 (US physician)

Peyronie's disease *(Penile angulation)* **Pathogenesis** A poorly understood connective tissue disorder most commonly attributed to repetitive microvascular trauma during sexual intercourse, resulting in penile curvature and painful erectile dysfunction (in 50%; p224). **Prevalence** 3–9%. **Typical age** >40yrs. **Associations** Dupuytren's (p75); atheroma; radical prostatectomy. **ΔΔ** Haemangioma. **Tests** Ultrasound/MRI. ℞ Oral pentoxifylline, intralesional verapamil, or collagenase clostridium histolyticum.[32] **Surgery** (If disease has persisted >12 months, is refractory to medical treatment, and is associated with a penile deformity compromising sexual function) tunica plication ± penile prostheses. Manage associated depression (seen in 48%). Penile rehabilitation can help (p224).[33] *Francois Gigot de la Peyronie, 1678–1747 (French surgeon)*

Pott's syndrome *(Spinal TB)* Rare in the West, this is usually from an extra-spinal source, eg lungs. **Features** Backache, and stiffness of *all* back movements. Fever, night sweats, and weight loss occur. Progressive bone destruction leads to vertebral collapse and gibbus (sharply angled spinal curvature). Abscess formation may lead to cord compression, causing paraplegia, and bowel/bladder dysfunction (p462). **X-rays** (fig 15.10) Narrow disc spaces and vertebral osteoporosis, leading to destruction with wedging of vertebrae. Lesions in the thoracic spine often lead to kyphosis. Abscess formation in the lumbar spine may track down to the psoas muscle, and erode through the skin. ℞ Anti-TB drugs (p390). *Sir Percival Pott, 1714–1788 (British surgeon)*

ABC

Who was Baron Münchausen?

Baron Karl Münchausen was an 18th-century German aristocrat and fabulist, whose tall tales became first a popular book, then a byword for circular logic, and finally a medical syndrome of self-delusion. He is famous for riding cannonballs, travelling to the moon, and pulling himself out of a swamp by his own hair. ▶▶In emergencies (we've all had that sinking feeling …), this method may save your life, eg in your final exams (fig 15.6):

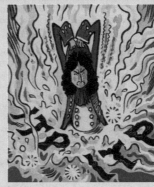

Fig 15.6 Münchausen during his finals.

Examiner: 'What is ITP?'

You: 'ITP is idiopathic thrombocytopenic purpura.' (You have scored 50% already.)

Examiner: 'And what is idiopathic thrombocytopenic purpura?'

You: 'It's when a cryptogenic cause of a low platelet count leads to purpura.'

You have deployed your skills with logical brilliance, without adding a single insight. For this Münchausen circularity you may be awarded 100%—unless your examiner is a philosopher, when the right answer would be 'What is ITP? I don't know'—and nor do you'—but don't try this too often. You see, you must never forget that medicine is marvellously scientific, and no one is popular who dares cast doubt on this article of faith.

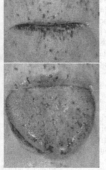

Fig 15.7 Telangiectasia in Osler–Weber–Rendu syndrome.
Reproduced from Cox and Roper, *Clinical Skills*, 2014, with permission from Oxford University Press.

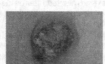

Fig 15.8 Paget's disease of the breast.

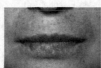

Fig 15.9 Perioral pigmentation, seen in Peutz–Jeghers syndrome.
Reproduced from Cox and Roper, *Clinical Skills*, 2014, with permission from Oxford University Press.

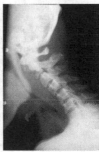

Fig 15.10 TB of axis: soft tissue swelling displaces the retropharyngeal air–tissue boundary forwards. There is an anterior defect in the vertebra, below the axis peg.
Courtesy of Dr Ian Maddison, myweb.lsbu.ac.uk.

ABC

Prinzmetal (vasospastic) angina Angina from coronary artery spasm, which may lead to MI, ventricular arrhythmias, or sudden death. Severe chest pain occurs usually at rest and often at night. Triggers include hyperventilation, cocaine and tobacco use. ECG: Transient ST segment changes. ℞ Establish the diagnosis. GTN treats angina. Use Ca²⁺-channel blockers (p106) and long-acting nitrates as prophylaxis.
Myron Prinzmetal, 1908–1987 (US cardiologist)

Refsum disease Phytanic acid accumulates in tissues and serum, due to PHYH or PEX7 gene mutation (recessive). This leads to anosmia (a universal finding) and early-onset retinitis pigmentosa, with variable combinations of neuropathy, deafness, ataxia, ichthyosis, and cardiomyopathy. **Tests** ↑Plasma phytanic acid. ℞ Restrict foods containing phytanic acid (animal fats, dairy products, green leafy vegetables); plasmapheresis is used for severe symptoms.[34]
Sigvald Bernhard Refsum, 1907–1991 (Norwegian physician)

Romano–Ward syndrome A dominant mutation in a K⁺ channel subunit causes long QT syndrome ± episodic VT, VF, *torsades*, ± sudden death. (Jervell and Lange-Nielsen syn is similar, p690.)
Cesarino Romano, 1924–2008 (Italian paediatrician); Owen C Ward, 1923–2021 (Irish paediatrician)

Rotor syndrome A rare, benign, autosomal recessive disorder. Primary non-haemolytic conjugated hyperbilirubinaemia, with almost normal hepatic histology (no pigmentation, in contrast to DJS, p688). Typically presents in childhood with mild jaundice. Cholescintigraphy reveals an 'absent' liver.
Arturo Belleza Rotor, 1907–1988 (Filipino physician)

Sister Mary Joseph nodule An umbilical metastatic nodule from an intra-abdominal malignancy (fig 15.11).
Sister Mary Joseph Dempsey, 1856–1939 (US catholic nun & Dr William Mayo's surgical assistant)

Stevens–Johnson syndrome (SJS) A severe cutaneous adverse reaction characterized by extensive necrosis and detachment of the epidermis. SJS and toxic epidermal necrolysis (TEN) exist as a continuum whereby in SJS <10% of body surface area is affected and in TEN >30% is affected. It is caused by a hypersensitivity reaction, usually to drugs (eg salicylates, sulfonamides, penicillin, barbiturates, carbamazepine, phenytoin), but is also seen with infections or cancer. There is ulceration of the skin and mucosal surfaces (fig 15.12). Typical target lesions develop, often on the palms or soles with blistering in the centre. There may be a prodromal phase with fever, malaise, arthralgia, myalgia ± vomiting and diarrhoea. ℞ Mild disease is usually self-limiting—remove any precipitant and give supportive care including wound care, fluid and electrolyte management, nutritional support, temperature management, pain control, infection prevention, and ocular care. Oral ciclosporin may be indicated. The role of steroids is controversial. Specialist multidisciplinary care. **Prognosis** Mortality ~5%. May be severe for the first 10d before resolving over 30d. Damage to the eyes may persist and blindness can result.
Albert M Stevens 1884–1945; Frank C Johnson, 1894–1934 (US paediatricians)

Sturge–Weber syndrome (SWS) Essential features: 1 Facial cutaneous capillary malformation (port wine stain; PWS) in the ophthalmic dermatome (V₁ ± V₂/V₃). 2 Clinical signs or radiologic evidence of a leptomeningeal vascular malformation. 75% of patients with unilateral involvement develop seizures by age 1 (95% if bilateral)—due (in part) to the increased metabolic demand of a developing brain in the setting of vascular compromise, somatic mosaic mutation in GNAQ gene. Early management of seizures is critical to minimize brain injury. Some patients have severe cognitive and neurologic deficits beyond simple seizure activity. Screen early for glaucoma (50%). EEG and MRI help establish early diagnosis and treatment in patients at risk for SWS. Treat the PWS early with pulsed dye laser.[36]
William A Sturge, 1850–1919; Frederick P Weber, 1863–1962 (British physicians)

Tietze's syndrome (*Idiopathic costochondritis*) Localized pain/tenderness at the costosternal junction, enhanced by motion, coughing, or sneezing. The 2nd rib is most often affected. The diagnostic key is *localized* tenderness which is marked (flinches on prodding). **Treatment** Simple analgesia, eg NSAIDs. Its importance is that it is a benign cause of what at first seems to be alarming, eg cardiac pain. In lengthy illness, local steroid injections may be used.
Alexander Tietze, 1864–1927 (German surgeon)

Todd's palsy Transient neurological deficit (paresis) after a seizure. There may be face, arm, or leg weakness, aphasia, or gaze palsy, lasting from ~30mins–36h. The aetiology is unclear.
Robert Bentley Todd, 1809–1860 (Irish physician)

Prinzmetal angina and vascular hyperreactivity

Coronary spasm causes Prinzmetal angina (now known as vasospastic angina) and also contributes to coronary heart disease in general, eg acute coronary syndrome (esp. in Japan). Coronary spasm can be induced by ergonovine, acetylcholine, and methacholine (the former is used diagnostically).[2] These cause vasodilatation by endothelium-derived nitric oxide when vascular endothelium is functioning normally, whereas they cause vasoconstriction if the endothelium is damaged. In the light of these facts, patients with coronary spasm are thought to have a disturbance in endothelial function as well as local hyperreactivity of the coronary arteries.

If full anti-anginal therapy does not reduce symptoms, stenting or intracoronary radiation (20Gy brachytherapy) to vasospastic segments may be tried. Prognosis is good (especially if non-smoker, no past MI, and no diabetes; progress to infarction is quite rare)[37]; β-blockers and large doses of aspirin are contraindicated.

Prinzmetal angina is associated with vascular hyper-reactivity/vasospastic disorders such as Raynaud's phenomenon and migraine. It is also associated with circle of Willis occlusion from intimal thickening (moyamoya disease).

Causes of a long QT interval

Many conditions and drugs (check *BNF*) cause a long QT interval. Brugada syndrome (p687) is similar, predisposing to sudden cardiac death.

Congenital Romano–Ward syndrome (autosomal dominant). Jervell and Lange-Nielsen syndrome (autosomal recessive) with associated deafness (p690).

Cardiac Myocardial infarction or ischaemia; mitral valve prolapse.

HIV May be a direct effect of the virus or from protease inhibitors.

Metabolic $\downarrow K^+$; $\downarrow Mg^{2+}$; $\downarrow Ca^{2+}$; starvation; hypothyroidism; hypothermia.

Toxic Organophosphates.

Anti-arrhythmic drugs Quinidine; amiodarone; procainamide; sotalol.

Antimicrobials Erythromycin; levofloxacin; pentamidine; halofantrine.

Antihistamines Terfenadine; astemizole.

Motility drugs Domperidone.

Psychoactive drugs Haloperidol; risperidone; tricyclics; SSRIs.

Connective tissue diseases Anti-RO/SSA antibodies (p550).

Herbalism Ask about Chinese folk remedies (may contain unknown amounts of arsenic). Cocaine, quinine, and artemisinins (and other antimalarials) are examples of herbalism-derived products that can prolong the QT interval.

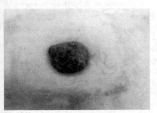

Fig 15.11 Sister Mary Joseph nodule.
Source: Hirata K, Narabayashi M, Murashima T, *et al.* (October 16, 2022) *Cureus* 14(10): e30344. doi:10.7759/cureus.30344, reproduced under Creative Commons Attribution License CC-BY 4.0.

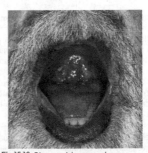

Fig 15.12 Stevens–Johnson syndrome.
Reproduced from Emberger *et al. Clinical Infectious Diseases* (2003) 37:1, with permission from Oxford University Press.

2 Since Prinzmetal angina is not a 'demand-induced' symptom, but a supply (vasospastic) abnormality, exercise tolerance tests don't help. The most sensitive and specific test is IV ergonovine; 50mcg at 5min intervals in a specialist lab until a +ve result or 400mcg is given. When positive, the symptoms and ↑ST should be present. Nitroglycerine rapidly reverses the effects of ergonovine if refractory spasm occurs.[38]

Vincent's angina *(Necrotizing ulcerative gingivitis)* Mouth infection with ulcerative gingivitis from *Borrelia vincentii* (a spirochaete) + fusiform bacilli, often affecting young ♂ smokers with poor oral hygiene. Try amoxicillin 500mg/8h and metronidazole 400mg/8h PO, + chlorhexidine mouthwash.

Jean Hyacinthe Vincent, 1862–1950 (French physician)

Von Hippel–Lindau syndrome A dominant germline mutation of a tumour suppressor gene. It predisposes to bilateral renal cysts and clear cell renal carcinoma (p316), retinal & cerebellar haemangioblastoma, and phaeochromocytoma. See figs 15.13, 15.14. It may present with visual impairment or cerebellar signs (eg unilateral ataxia).

Eugen von Hippel, 1867–1939 (German ophthalmologist); Arvid Lindau, 1892–1958 (Swedish pathologist)

Von Willebrand's disease (VWD) Von Willebrand's factor (VWF) has three roles in clotting: 1 To bring platelets into contact with exposed subendothelium. 2 To make platelets bind to each other. 3 To bind to factor VIII, protecting it from destruction in the circulation. There are >22 types of VWD; the commonest are:
• **Type I** (60–80%) ↓Levels of VWF. Symptoms are mild. Autosomal dominant.
• **Type II** (20–30%) Abnormal VWF, with lack of high-molecular-weight multimers. Usually autosomal dominant inheritance. Bleeding tendency varies. There are 4 subtypes.
• **Type III** (1–5%) Undetectable VWF levels (autosomal recessive with gene deletions). VWF antigen is lacking and there is ↓factor VIII. Symptoms can be severe.
Signs are of a platelet-type disorder (p340): bruising, epistaxis, menorrhagia, ↑bleeding post tooth extraction. *Tests* ↑APTT, ↑bleeding time, ↓factor VIIIC (clotting activity), VWF ↓Ag; ↔INR and platelets. *R* Get expert help. Desmopressin is used in mild bleeding, VWF-containing factor VIII concentrate for surgery or major bleeds. Avoid NSAIDs.

Erik Adolf von Willebrand, 1870–1949 (Finnish physician)

Wallenberg's lateral medullary syndrome This relatively common syndrome comprises lesions to multiple CNS nuclei, caused by posterior inferior cerebellar artery occlusion leading to brainstem infarction (fig 15.15). **Features** • Dysphagia, dysarthria (IX and X nuclei). • Vertigo, nausea, vomiting, nystagmus (vestibular nucleus). • Ipsilateral ataxia (inferior cerebellar peduncle). • Ipsilateral Horner's syndrome (descending sympathetic fibres). • Loss of pain and temperature sensation on the ipsilateral face (V nucleus) and contralateral limbs (spinothalamic tract). There is no limb weakness as the pyramidal tracts are unaffected.

In the rarer *medial medullary syndrome*, vertebral or anterior spinal artery occlusion causes ipsilateral tongue paralysis (XII nucleus) with contralateral limb weakness (pyramidal tract, sparing the face) and loss of position sense.

Adolf Wallenberg, 1862–1949 (German neurologist)

Waterhouse–Friderichsen's (WHF) syndrome Bilateral adrenal cortex haemorrhage, often occurring in rapidly deteriorating meningococcal sepsis, alongside widespread purpura, meningitis, coma, and DIC (fig 15.16). The meningococcal endotoxin acts as a potent initiator of inflammatory and coagulation cascades. Other causes include *H. influenzae*, pneumococcal, streptococcal, and staphylococcal sepsis. Adrenal failure causes shock, as normal vascular tone requires cortisol to set activity of α- and β-adrenergic receptors, and aldosterone is needed to maintain extracellular fluid volume. **Treatment** ▶▶Antibiotics, eg ceftriaxone (p806) and hydrocortisone 100mg IV bolus followed by 50mg IV every 6h for adrenal support. ICU admission.

Rupert Waterhouse, 1873–1958 (British physician); Carl Friderichsen, 1886–1979 (Danish paediatrician)

Weber's syndrome *(Superior alternating hemiplegia)* Ipsilateral oculomotor nerve palsy with contralateral hemiplegia, due to infarction of one-half of the midbrain, after occlusion of the paramedian branches of the basilar or posterior cerebral arteries.

Herman David Weber, 1823–1918 (German-born physician whose son described Sturge–Weber syndrome)

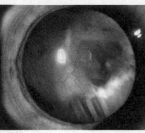

Fig 15.13 Von Hippel–Lindau syndrome showing retinal detachment.

Reproduced with permission from the National Eye Institute, National Institutes of Health.

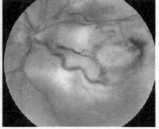

Fig 15.14 Von Hippel–Lindau syndrome showing a retinal tumour.

Reproduced with permission from the National Eye Institute, National Institutes of Health.

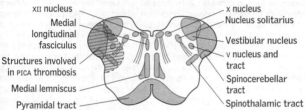

Fig 15.15 Cross section of the medulla showing structures involved in Wallenberg's lateral medullary syndrome (posterior inferior cerebellar artery occlusion).

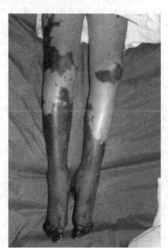

Fig 15.16 Meningococcal sepsis with purpura.

Wegener's granulomatosis This has been renamed *granulomatosis with polyangiitis* (GPA), in part because of concerns over the suitability of Friedrich Wegener, a member of the Nazi party during WWII, to be the source of an eponym. GPA is a multisystem disorder of unknown cause characterized by necrotizing granulomatous inflammation and vasculitis of small and medium vessels. It has a predilection for the upper respiratory tract, lungs, and kidneys. **Features** Upper airways disease is common, with nasal obstruction, ulcers, epistaxis, or destruction of the nasal septum causing a characteristic 'saddle-nose' deformity.[3] Sinusitis is often a feature. It can cause rapidly progressive glomerulonephritis with crescent formation, proteinuria, or haematuria. Pulmonary involvement may cause cough, haemoptysis (severe if pulmonary haemorrhage), or pleuritis. There may also be skin purpura or nodules, peripheral neuropathy, mononeuritis multiplex, arthritis/arthralgia, or ocular involvement, eg keratitis, conjunctivitis, scleritis, episcleritis, uveitis. **Tests** cANCA directed against PR3 is most specific and raised in the majority of patients (p550). Some patients express pANCA specific for MPO. ↑ESR/CRP. Urinalysis should be performed to look for proteinuria or haematuria. If these are present, consider a kidney biopsy. CXR may show nodules ± fluffy infiltrates of pulmonary haemorrhage. CT may reveal diffuse alveolar haemorrhage. Atypical cells from cytology of sputum/BAL can be confused with bronchial carcinoma.[39] **Treatment** Depends on the extent of disease. Organ- or life-threatening disease should be treated with an induction regimen of glucocorticoids in combination with either rituximab or cyclophosphamide. Rituximab, azathioprine, or mycophenolate mofetil are options for maintenance for 12–24 months after stable remission. Indications for plasma exchange are controversial but include patients presenting with severe kidney disease (eg creatinine >354μmol/L or need for dialysis) and those with pulmonary haemorrhage. Co-trimoxazole should be given as prophylaxis against *Pneumocystis jirovecii* and staphylococcal colonization.   *Friedrich Wegener, 1907–1990 (German pathologist)*

Wernicke's encephalopathy Thiamine (vitamin B_1) deficiency with a classical triad of 1 confusion 2 ataxia & 3 ophthalmoplegia (nystagmus, lateral rectus, or conjugate gaze palsies). There is inadequate dietary intake, ↓GI absorption, and impaired utilization of thiamine resulting in focal areas of brain damage, including periaqueductal punctate haemorrhages (mechanism unclear). Always consider this diagnosis in alcoholics: it may also present with memory disturbance, hypotension, hypothermia, or reduced consciousness.[40] **Recognized causes** Chronic alcoholism, eating disorders, malnutrition, prolonged vomiting, eg with chemotherapy, GI malignancy, or hyperemesis gravidarum. **Diagnosis** Primarily clinical. Red cell transketolase activity is decreased (rarely done). **Treatment** *Urgent* replacement to prevent irreversible Korsakoff's syndrome (p690). Give thiamine (Pabrinex®), 2 pairs of high-potency ampoules IV/IM/8h over 30mins for 2d, then 1 pair OD for a further 5d. Oral supplementation (100mg OD) should continue until no longer 'at risk' (+ give other B vitamins). Anaphylaxis is rare. If there is coexisting hypoglycaemia (often the case in this group of patients), make sure thiamine is given before glucose, as Wernicke's can be precipitated by glucose administration to a thiamine-deficient patient. **Prognosis** Untreated, death occurs in 20%, and Korsakoff's psychosis occurs in 85%—a quarter of whom will require long-term institutional care.   *Karl Wernicke, 1848–1905 (German neurologist)*

Willis–Ekbom disease *(Restless legs)* Criteria: 1 Compelling desire to move legs. 2 Worse at night. 3 Relieved by movement. 4 Unpleasant leg sensations (eg shootings or tinglings) worse at rest. **Mechanism** Endogenous opioid system fault causes altered central processing of pain. **Prevalence** 1–3%. ♀:♂≈2:1. **Associations** Iron deficiency, uraemia, pregnancy, DM, polyneuropathy, RA, COPD. **Exclude** Cramps, positional discomfort, and local leg pathology. ℞ Dopamine agonists are commonly used; also, anticonvulsants, opioids, and benzodiazepines.[13]

Thomas Willis, 1621–1675 (English physician); Karl Axel Ekbom, 1907–1977 (Swedish neurologist)

Zellweger syndrome *(Cerebrohepatorenal syndrome)* A rare recessive disorder characterized by absent peroxisomes (intracellular organelles required for many cellular activities including lipid metabolism). The syndrome has a similar molecular basis to infantile Refsum's disease, and although more severe, exhibits comparable biochemical abnormalities (p696). Clinical features include craniofacial abnormalities, severe hypotonia and intellectual disability, glaucoma, cataracts, hepatomegaly, and kidney cysts. A number of causative PEX gene mutations have been identified. Life expectancy is usually a few months only.   *Hans Zellweger, 1909–1990 (US paediatrician)*

Epilogue

25% of patients with rare diseases have to wait from 5–30 years for a diagnosis. 40% are misdiagnosed resulting in inappropriate drugs or psychological treatments—eg 20% of people with Ehlers–Danlos syndrome (p143) had to consult over 20 doctors before the diagnosis was made,[41] causing understandable loss of confidence in our profession. Lack of appropriate referral and rejection because of disease complexity are common problems. Let us cultivate our networks with each other and approach 'unexplained symptoms' with an open mind.

3 Common causes of a 'saddle-nose' deformity are trauma and iatrogenic (eg post-rhinoplasty). Rarer causes (popular with some finals examiners): GPA, relapsing polychondritis, syphilis, and leprosy.

16 Radiology

Contents

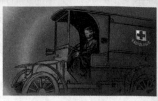

Fig 16.1 Marie Curie (1867–1934) was a Polish-born physicist and chemist and remains one of the most famous scientists of all time. She jointly won the Nobel Prize for Physics in 1903 (along with her husband Pierre, and Henri Becquerel) for her research on radioactivity and won the Nobel Prize for Chemistry in 1911 for her discovery of radium and polonium. Her research was instrumental in the development of x-rays and radiotherapy. During World War I, Curie also helped to equip ambulances with x-ray equipment (known as 'Little Curies'), which she herself drove to the front lines. It is estimated that one million wounded soldiers received x-rays because of her courage and resourcefulness.

Artwork by Gillian Turner.

We thank Aileen O'Shea, our Specialist Reader for this chapter.

Typical effective doses

Ionizing radiation (eg x-rays, CTs, and nuclear medicine studies) can be harmful and different tissues have varying sensitivity to radiation effects. The effective dose of an examination is calculated as the weighted sum of the doses to different body tissues. The weighting factor for each tissue depends on its sensitivity. The effective dose thus provides a single dose estimate related to the total radiation risk, no matter how the radiation dose is distributed around the body. This table is certainly not to be learnt; rather it serves as a reminder of the relative exposures to radiation that we prescribe in practice. ▶Remember that US and MRI don't involve any radiation dose—consider first if they could provide the answer to your clinical question.

Table 16.1 Radiation doses in common radiological investigations

Procedure	Typical effective dose (mSv)	CXR equivalents	Approx. equivalent period of background radiation
X-ray examinations			
Limbs and joints	<0.01	<1	<2 days
Chest (PA)	0.015	1	2.5 days
Abdomen	0.4	30	2 months
Lumbar spine	0.6	40	3 months
CT head	1.4	90	7.5 months
CT chest	6.6	440	3 years
CT abdo/pelvis	6.7	450	3 years
Radionuclide studies			
Lung ventilation	0.4	30	9 weeks
Lung perfusion	1	70	6 months
Bone	3	200	1.4 years
PET head	7	460	3.2 years
PET-CT	18	1200	8.1 years

Reproduced from iRefer, *Making the Best Use of Clinical Radiology*, 7th edition, © Royal College of Radiologists, 2012.

16 Radiology

Justifying exposure to ionizing radiation

The very nature of ionizing radiation that gives us vision into the human body also gives it lethal properties. In considering the decision to expose patients to radiation, the clinical benefits should outweigh the risks of genetic mutation and cancer induction. These risks can be hard to quantify (and estimates vary wildly—extrapolation of effects from doses associated with nuclear explosions are likely unreliable) but even with strict guidelines we still have a tendency to over-exposure in medical practice. Perhaps the best advice is to be certain of the importance of every dose of radiation that you sanction, and mindful of the comparative doses involved (table 16.1).

The responsibility lies with us not to rely too heavily on radiology. ▶Don't request examinations to comfort patients (or appease their consultants), to replace images already acquired elsewhere (or lost) simply to avoid medicolegal issues, or when the result will not affect management. To give an idea of relative doses, a CT of the abdomen and pelvis gives a typical effective dose of 500 times as much radiation as a CXR. This important factor also tells us about the preference of ultrasound over CT when investigating abdominal and pelvic complaints such as acute appendicitis, especially given the youthful demographics of this diagnosis.

▶Unwitting exposure of the unborn fetus to radiation is inexcusable at any stage of gestation—unless the mother's life is in immediate danger—and it is the responsibility of the referring clinician, as well as the radiographer and the radiologist, to ensure that this is avoided.

One of the most nerve-wracking moments that you can encounter as a recently qualified doctor is having to request an investigation from a seasoned consultant radiologist. What information do you need to give? How much? Who do you ask? Put yourself on the other side: what does the radiologist need to know to decide who needs what imaging and when? Keep the following in mind when requesting (never ordering!) an investigation:

Patient details Double check that you have selected the correct patient and account, prior to placing any electronic orders.

Clinical details Think of your clinical question, what answer are you hoping radiology will provide? It can:
• *Confirm* a suspected diagnosis.
• *'Exclude'* something important (though remember that exclusion is never 100%).
• *Define* the extent of a disease.
• *Monitor* the progress of a disease.
▶Don't forget to mention pertinent facts that may change the way the investigation is carried out: an agitated or confused patient may need sedation prior to an MRI of their head. A CT scan on a patient with an acutely raised creatinine may need to be done without contrast medium. Insertion of a drain on a patient with deranged clotting may need to wait while this is corrected. Include recent creatinine, Hb, and clotting on the form if appropriate. Don't forget to mention anticoagulants, eg warfarin, LMWH, and aspirin for intervention requests.

Investigation details What scan do you think is required, and how soon do you need it? Different clinical questions require different procedures. If you think the patient has a collection, would you like them to drain it? Always state whether intervention is required (eg US abdo ± drain insertion). Remember that the radiologist ultimately decides what imaging or procedure they undertake based on the information you have provided.

Tips
• Know your patient well, but keep your request brief and accurate.
• Know the clinical question and how the answer will change your management.
• Look up previous imaging before you go; asking for a CT on a patient who had one yesterday makes you look foolish and will not go down well.
• If in doubt, or if the investigation is very urgent, go down to the department in person. Regard this as an important opportunity: involving a radiologist will result in the best selection of imaging technique for your clinical question, will help expedite urgent requests, and should be of educational value for you.

If your request is turned down Don't be afraid to (politely) ask why. If you or your team still feel it is warranted, look back at the request; did you miss a relevant piece of information that would change the mind of the radiologist? If you still draw a blank, try speaking to a radiologist who specializes in that particular technique. Many teams have clinical radiology meetings; think about approaching someone who appreciates why you are asking that particular question. Alternatively, go back to your team; speak to your senior, who may have a better understanding of why the investigation is needed and be able to convey this to the radiologist.

▶Remember that there is a patient at the heart of this, and you are their advocate. If the results of an investigation will change their management then explain this to the radiologist. Moreover, don't forget to explain it to your patient. Being whisked off to the department for investigation and intervention can be particularly terrifying if you aren't expecting it.

Interpreting an image

You won't always be able to get an immediate radiologist's interpretation so it is important to know how to review an image. ►First make sure the image you are looking at is of your patient. Check its date. And remember:

- *Practice makes perfect*—always look at the image before checking the report, learning how to distinguish normal from abnormal.
- *Understand how the scan is done*—this makes interpretation easier and helps you appreciate which scan will give the answer you need. It also gives practical clues to the result—eg a routine CXR is performed in the postero-anterior (PA) direction (the source posterior to the patient to minimize the cardiac shadow).
- *Use a systematic approach*—so that you don't miss subtleties.
- *Understand your anatomy*—virtually all investigations yield a 2D image from a 3D structure. An understanding of anatomical relationships of the area in question will help reconstruct the images in your mind.
- *Orientation*—for axial cross-sectional imaging this is as if you are looking up at the supine patient ►*from the feet*. For images with non-conventional orientations (eg MRCP) look on the image for clue markings, or rely on your knowledge of anatomy—it can be tricky to visualize oblique sections!
- *Remember the patient*—an investigation is only one part of the clinical workup, don't rely solely on the investigation result for your management decisions. Go back to see the patient after looking at the investigation and reading the radiologist's report: you might notice something that you didn't before.

Presenting an image

Everyone has their own method for presenting, and the right way is *your own way*. As long as you cover everything systematically—because we all get 'hot-seat amnesia' at some point—the particulars will take care of themselves. Continue to polish your own method and remember a few extra tips for when an image is presented expectantly by your consultant/examiner and the floor is yours. A brief silence with a thoughtful expression as you analyse the image is fine, then:

- State the written details: name, date of birth, where and how the imaging was taken. Look for clues: weighting of an MRI, a '+ c' indicating that contrast medium has been used, the phase of the investigation (arterial/venous/portal), or even the name of the organ printed on an ultrasound.
- State the type, mode, and technical quality of investigation—not always easy!

Going through this list also gives you a bit of thinking time. Then:

- Start with life-threatening or very obvious abnormalities. *Then be systematic:*
- Is the patient's position adequate? Any lines, leads, or tubes? Note their position.
- Just like the bedside clues in a physical examination, there are clues in radiology examinations. Note oxygen masks, ECG leads, venous access, infusion apparatus, and invasive devices. Identifying what they are also helps you to look through what may otherwise appear to be a cluttered mess.
- Note any abnormalities and try to contextualize these with whatever you already know of the patient. The abnormality may be hiding in plain sight, but if struggling, step back and note any asymmetry or areas that just 'look different'.
- With cross-sectional imaging, scan through adjacent sections noting the anatomy of one organ system or structure at a time (this may mean going up and down through a CT abdomen multiple times).
- Giving a differential diagnosis is good practice, as not all findings are diagnostic.
- If there is additional clinical information that would help you to make a diagnosis, don't be afraid to ask. After all, we treat patients and not images!

Remember:	• x-ray = *radiodensity* (lucency/opacity);	• CT = *attenuation*,
	• US = *echogenicity*,	• MRI = *signal intensity*.

16 Radiology

Images are usually taken on inspiration with the x-ray source behind the patient (postero-anterior, PA). Mobile images may be antero-posterior (AP, fig 16.6, p711), magnifying heart size. If supine, distribution of air and fluid in lungs and pleural cavities is altered and the diaphragm is elevated.

Acclimatize yourself to the four cardinal elements of the chest radiograph (CXR), memorably (albeit slightly inaccurately) termed bone, air, fat, and 'water'/soft tissue. Each has its own radiographic density. ▶A border is only seen at an interface of two densities, eg heart (soft tissue) and lung (air); this 'silhouette' is lost if air in the lung is replaced by consolidation ('water'). The silhouette sign localizes pathology (eg middle lobe pneumonia or collapse causing loss of clarity of the right heart border; fig 16.2). When interpreting a CXR use a systematic approach that works for you.

Technical quality

- **Rotation** The sternal ends of the clavicles should symmetrically overlie the transverse processes of the 4th or 5th thoracic vertebrae. A rotated image can alter the position of structures, eg rotation to the right projects the aortic arch vessels over the right upper zone, appearing as though there is a mass.
- **Inspiration** There should be 5–7 ribs visible anteriorly (or 10 posteriorly). Hyperinflation can be abnormal, eg COPD. Poor inspiration can mimic cardiomegaly, as the heart is usually pulled down (hence elongated) with inspiration, and crowding of vessels at the lung bases can mimic consolidation or collapse. This is common in patients who are acutely unwell, particularly those in pain or unconscious. Take care in interpreting these images.
- **Exposure** An under-exposed image will be too white and an over-exposed image will be too black. Both cause a loss of definition and quality although some compensation can be made with standard viewing software.
- **Position** The entire lung margin should be visible.

Trachea Normally central or just to the right. Deviated by collapse (towards the lesion), expansion (away from the lesion), or patient rotation.

Mediastinum May be: *widened* by mediastinal fat; retrosternal thyroid; aortic aneurysm/unfolding; lymph node enlargement (sarcoidosis, lymphoma, metastases, TB); tumour (thymoma, teratoma); cysts (bronchogenic, pericardial); paravertebral mass (TB); *shifted* towards a collapsed lung or away from processes that add volume (eg a large mass or a tension pneumothorax).

There are three bulges normally visible on the left border of the mediastinum that help identify pathology if abnormal. From superior to inferior they are: 1 Aortic knuckle. 2 Pulmonary outflow tract. 3 Left ventricle.

Hila The left hilum is higher than the right or at the same level (not lower); they should be the same size and density. The hila may be: *pulled up or down* by fibrosis or collapse; *enlarged* by: pulmonary arterial hypertension; bronchogenic ca; lymph nodes. ▶Sarcoidosis, TB, and lymphoma can give *bilateral* hilar lymphadenopathy. *Calcified* due to: sarcoid; past TB; silicosis; histoplasmosis (p404).

Heart Normally less than half of the width of the thorax (cardiothoracic ratio <0.5). ⅓ should lie to the right of the vertebral column, ⅔ to the left. It may appear elongated if the chest is hyperinflated (COPD); or enlarged if the image is AP or if there is LV failure (fig 16.3), or a pericardial effusion. Are there metallic or calcified valves?

Diaphragm The right side is often slightly higher (due to the liver). **Causes of raised hemidiaphragm** Trouble above the diaphragm—lung volume loss or inflammation. Trouble with the diaphragm—stroke; phrenic nerve palsy (causes, p500; any mediastinal mass?). Trouble below the diaphragm—hepatomegaly; subphrenic abscess. NB: subpulmonic effusion (effusions having a similar contour to the diaphragm without a characteristic meniscus) and diaphragm rupture give apparent elevation. NB: bilateral palsies (polio, muscular dystrophy) cause hypoxia. ▶If this is a new finding, consider doing a decubitus CXR or US to look for pleural fluid. If absent and phrenic nerve palsy suspected, consider CT thorax to exclude a hilar or mediastinal mass.

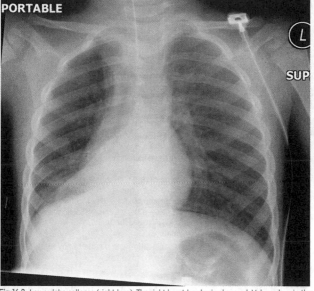

Fig 16.2 Lower lobe collapse (right lung). The right heart border is obscured. Volume loss in the right lower zone results in a hyperexpanded right upper lobe that is more radiolucent than the left upper lobe.

Courtesy of Dr Edmund Godfrey.

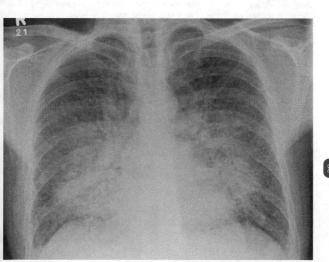

Fig 16.3 'Bat's wing', perihilar pulmonary oedema indicating heart failure and fluid overload.
Courtesy of Dr Edmund Godfrey.

The apex of the lower lobe rises up to the 4th rib posteriorly, so it is difficult to ascribe the true location of a lobe on a PA image without additional information from a lateral view. It may therefore be better to use the term 'zone' rather than lobe when localizing a lesion.

Opacification Lung opacities are described as nodular, reticular (network of fine lines, interstitial), or alveolar (fluffy). A single nodule may be called a space-occupying lesion (SOL).

Nodules (If >3cm across, the term pulmonary mass is used instead.)
• Neoplasia: metastases (often missed if small), lung cancer, hamartoma, adenoma.
• Infections: varicella pneumonia, septic emboli, abscess (eg as an SOL), hydatid.
• Granulomas: miliary TB, sarcoidosis (see GPA, p700), histoplasmosis.
• Pneumoconioses (except asbestosis), Caplan's syndrome (p686).

Reticular opacification = Lung parenchymal changes.
• Acute interstitial oedema.
• Infection: acute (viral, bacterial), chronic (TB, histoplasmosis).
• Fibrosis: usual interstitial pneumonia (UIP), non-specific interstitial pneumonia (NSIP), drugs (eg methotrexate, bleomycin, crack cocaine), connective tissue disorders (rheumatoid arthritis—p542, GPA—p700, SLE, PAN, systemic sclerosis—p548, sarcoidosis), industrial lung diseases (silicosis, asbestosis).
• Malignancy (lymphangitis carcinomatosa).

Alveolar opacification = Airspace opacification, can be due to any material filling the alveoli:
• Pus—pneumonia.
• Blood—haemorrhage, DIC (p350).
• Water—heart, renal (p298), or liver failure (p270), ARDS (p178), smoke inhalation, drugs (heroin), O₂ toxicity, near drowning.
• Cells—lymphoma, adenocarcinoma.
• Protein—alveolar proteinosis, ARDS, fat emboli (~7d post fracture).

'Ring' opacities Either airways seen end-on (bronchitis; bronchiectasis) or cavitating lesions, eg abscess (bacterial, fungal, amoebic), tumour, or pulmonary infarct (wedge-shaped with a pleural base).

Linear opacities Septal lines (Kerley B lines, ie interlobular lymphatics seen with fluid, tumour, or dusts); atelectasis; pleural plaques (asbestos exposure).

White-out of whole hemithorax (fig 16.4) Pneumonia, large pleural effusion, ARDS, post-pneumonectomy.

Gas outside the lungs Check for a pneumothorax (hard to spot if apical or in a supine image, can you see vascular markings right out to the periphery?), surgical emphysema (trauma, iatrogenic), and gas under the diaphragm (surgery, perforated viscus, trauma). **Pneumomediastinum** Air tracks along mediastinum, into the neck. Due to rupture of alveolar wall (eg asthma or pulmonary barotrauma) or bronchial or oesophageal trauma (can be iatrogenic, eg from endoscope). **Pneumopericardium** Rare (usually iatrogenic).

Bones Check the *clavicles* for fracture, *ribs* for fractures and lesions (eg metastases), *vertebral column* for degenerative disease, collapse, or destruction, and *shoulders* for dislocation, fracture, and arthritis.

An apparently normal CXR? Check for tracheal compression, absent breast shadow (mastectomy), double left heart border (left lower lobe collapse, fig 16.5), fluid level behind the heart (hiatus hernia, achalasia), and paravertebral abscess (TB).

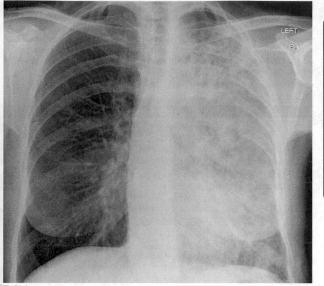

Fig 16.4 Opacification of the left hemithorax from consolidation.

Courtesy of Dr Edmund Godfrey.

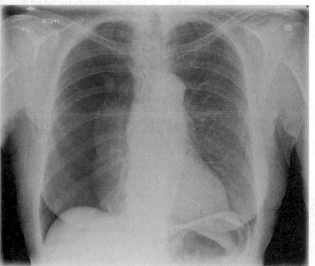

Fig 16.5 Large right-sided pneumothorax; note the trachea remains central, suggesting this is a simple pneumothorax, not a tension pneumothorax.

Courtesy of Dr Edmund Godfrey.

Chest x-ray—part 3

Confirming the position of various tubes, lines, and leads on a CXR can be a daunting task, as incorrect positioning can have deadly consequences: an NG tube which is misplaced can cause aspiration pneumonia, or a poorly positioned CVC can lead to fatal arrhythmias. However, this can be a straightforward task if you recall some basic anatomy (figs 16.6, 16.7; table 16.2).

▶If you are unsure, always ask a senior.

Table 16.2 Radiological confirmation of device placement

Line/tube/lead	Correct position for tip(s)
CVC (p758)	In the SVC or brachiocephalic vein
PICC	In the SVC or brachiocephalic vein
Tunnelled line, eg Hickman	At the junction of the SVC and right atrium
Endotracheal	3–5cm above the carina (in adult)
Nasogastric (p743)	10cm beyond the gastro-oesophageal junction
Chest drain (p750)	In the pleural space tracking either up (for pneumothorax) or down (for effusion)
Cardiac pacemaker/temporary pacing wire (p760)	Atrial lead—in the right appendage Ventricular lead—in the apex of the right ventricle

Normal anatomy

• The SVC begins at the right 1st anterior intercostal space.
• The right atrium lies at the level of the 3rd intercostal space.
• The carina should be visible at the level of T5–T7 thoracic vertebrae.
• The right atrial appendage sits at the level of the 3rd intercostal space.

Common bleeps from nursing staff

1 Central line not aspirating

• Is the tip in the right place (see earlier in topic) or has it gone up into the internal jugular, too far in (sitting against the tricuspid valve, does the patient have an arrhythmia?) or not far enough in (sitting against a venous valve)?
• Is the tip kinked, suggesting it may be in a side vessel or against the vessel wall?
• If the line looks appropriately positioned, consider flushing gently, could the line be blocked?

2 Patient not ventilating well

• Is the ET tube down the right main bronchus (causes left lung collapse, or rarely right pneumothorax)? Retract tube to correct position (see earlier in topic).
• Is the ET tube blocked? Most have a secondary port allowing ventilation even if the main hole is blocked, get anaesthetic assistance!

3 Chest drain not bubbling/swinging

• Is it correctly positioned (see earlier in topic)—if not in the pleural space, it cannot drain the air/fluid. Common problems include sitting in the soft tissue of the chest wall, or sitting above the effusion, below the pneumothorax, or in the oblique fissure.
• Is it blocked? If draining an effusion and correctly positioned, consider gently flushing with 10mL of sterile saline, then aspirating. If not successful, obtain senior advice.
• Has the effusion/pneumothorax resolved? Pneumothoraces can rapidly resolve with a correctly positioned drain.

4 Unable to aspirate from NG tube

• Is NG tube not far enough in/coiled in oesophagus? Tip is radio-opaque and should be visible below the diaphragm, if it is coiled it may lie in the pharynx or anywhere along the mediastinum.
• Is NG tube passing down the trachea and into the bronchus? The oesophagus is (generally speaking) a straight vertical line, if the tube veers off to left or right before it goes below the diaphragm, assume it is in the bronchus and replace it.

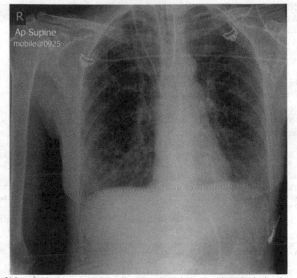

Fig 16.6 Image from ICU showing ET tube, CVC, and NG tube *in situ* with ECG leads placed across the chest.

Image courtesy of Dr Elen Thomson, Leeds Teaching Hospitals.

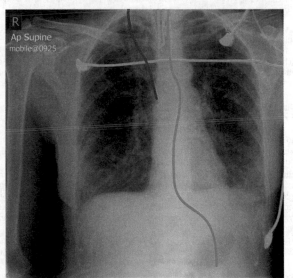

Fig 16.7 Knowing where lines and tubes should be placed is an essential skill. An ET tube (orange) should sit 3–5cm above the carina; this one is slightly high. The tip of the CVC (red, here a right internal jugular line) should lie in the SVC, as seen here, or just in the right atrium. The tip of the NG tube (green) must be seen below the diaphragm to ensure it is placed in the oesophagus, not the trachea. Do not confuse external leads (blue) with internal lines.

Plain abdominal x-ray

These are rarely diagnostic and involve a radiation dose equivalent to 50 CXRs. Royal College of Radiologists indications for AXR with acute abdominal symptoms:
• Suspicion of obstruction (or intussusception, eg in paediatrics).
• Acute flare of inflammatory bowel disease (eg to confirm/exclude megacolon).
• Constipation (specific circumstances, eg if obstruction suspected).
• Ingestion of a sharp or poisonous foreign body (eg lithium battery).
• Blunt or stab abdominal injury (in specific circumstances if patient is stable).

Bowel gas pattern is best assessed on supine images and free intraperitoneal gas (signifying perforation) is best seen on an erect CXR (fig 13.25, p599).

Gas patterns Look for: an abnormal quantity of gas in the stomach, small intestine, or colon. Decide whether you are looking at small or large bowel (fig 16.8; table 16.3).

Small bowel diameter is normally ~2.5cm, the colon ~5cm, the caecum up to 10cm. Dilated small bowel is seen in obstruction and paralytic ileus. Dilated large bowel (~6cm) is seen in both these, and also in 'toxic dilatation', and, in the elderly, in benign hypotonicity. Grossly dilated segments of bowel (coffee bean sign) are seen in sigmoid and caecal volvulae—fig 13.27c, p603. Loss of normal mucosal folds and bowel wall thickening are seen in inflammatory colitis (eg IBD)—fig 16.9. 'Thumb-printing' is protrusion of thickened mural folds into the lumen, seen in large bowel ischaemia and colitis.

Table 16.3 Radiological gas patterns in the bowel

Small bowel	Large bowel	Ileus
• Smaller calibre	• Larger calibre	• Both small and large bowel visible
• Central; multiple loops	• Peripheral	
• *Valvulae conniventes:* folds that go from wall to wall, all the way across the lumen; more regular and finer than haustra	• *Semilunar folds:* don't go all the way across the lumen, but may appear to do so if viewed from an angle	• There is no clear transition point that corresponds to an obstructing lesion
• Grey (contains air and fluid)	• Blacker (contains gas)	

Gas outside the lumen You must explain any gas outside the lumen of the gut. It could be: 1 Pneumoperitoneum; signs on the supine AXR include: gas on both sides of the bowel wall (Rigler's sign), a triangle of gas in the RUQ trapped beneath the falciform ligament, and a circle of gas beneath the anterior abdominal wall. Seen with bowel perforation but also after laparoscopic surgery. 2 Gas in the urinary tract—eg in the bladder from a fistula. 3 Gas in the biliary tree (see next paragraph), or rarely 4 Intramural gas, found in bowel necrosis.

Biliary tree Any stones ~10% visible on plain AXR. **Any gas** (Pneumobilia.) Caused by: •post-ERCP/sphincterotomy •post-surgery (eg Whipple's) •recent stone passage •anaerobic cholangitis (rare) •gallbladder–bowel fistula: gallstone migrates directly into the bowel (Rigler's triad is seen in 25%: pneumobilia, small bowel obstruction, an ectopic gallstone). **Calcification** ('Porcelain gallbladder'.) Chronic inflammation from gallstones (associated with gallbladder cancer).

Urinary tract Check for calculi (visible in 29–59% of cases) & normal anatomy: **Kidneys** Length equivalent to 2½–3½ vertebral bodies, slope inferolaterally. Right is lower than the left ('pushed down' by the liver). Their outline can usually be seen due to surrounding layer of perinephric fat. **Ureters** Pass near the tips of the lumbar transverse processes, cross the sacroiliac joints, down to the ischial spines, and turn medially to join the bladder.

Other soft tissues Look for size/position of: liver, spleen, and bladder. A big liver will push bowel to the left side of the abdomen. An enlarged spleen displaces bowel and stomach bubble to the right. A big bladder elevates these.

Medical devices Double-J and biliary stents, nephrostomy and gastrostomy tubes, intrauterine devices, laparoscopic clips, and peritoneal dialysis catheters can be seen.

Bones and joints Plain AXR is not ideal, but there may be important abnormalities. In the lumbar spine, look for scoliosis and degeneration (osteophytes, joint space narrowing) as well as bone metastases or sacroiliitis.

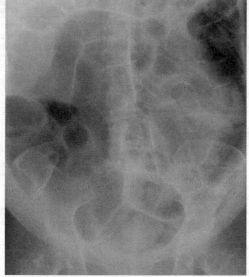

Fig 16.8 Multiple dilated air-filled loops of large and small bowel. This pattern is seen in ileus. Courtesy of Norwich Radiology Department.

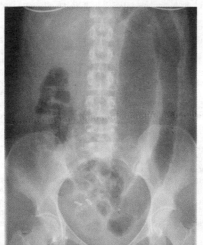

Fig 16.9 Abdominal image showing toxic megacolon associated with ulcerative colitis, note colon wall thickening and loss of mucosal folds.

Courtesy of Dr Edmund Godfrey.

Can give whole-body images in under one breath (thanks to continuous, helical data acquisition). Within a single slice (eg 0.5cm or 5mm thick), CT records the attenuation (= loss of energy from, eg absorption or reflection) of different tissues to ionizing radiation and calculates a mean value for a given volume of tissue (a 'voxel'). This value is represented in greyscale as a single point, called a pixel, in the final 2D image (or 3D 'reconstruction'—fig 16.13). The greyscale of the pixel is measured on the Hounsfield scale (fig 16.10) relative to the attenuation of water, 0 Hounsfield units (HU), and air, −1000HU. The human eye and display systems have a limited greyscale range, so different settings (levels and 'windows') are used to focus on differences in attenuation in ranges typical for tissues of different density, eg bone or lung (fig 16.11).

▶CTs are responsible for up to 40% of iatrogenic radiation in high-use settings, which could account for ~1% of all cancers: always balance benefits of CT vs other modalities with less or no radiation (ultrasound; MRI), particularly in the young or in those with chronic disease likely to undergo multiple imaging investigations. Discuss with a radiologist—there are several technical aspects of imaging that can limit radiation dose whilst still providing clinically useful information.

Advantages Fast, non-invasive, high temporal and spatial resolution, ability to differentiate overlying structures, less motion artefact than MRI, and compatible with implanted devices.

Disadvantages Radiation dose, suboptimal soft tissue imaging, not recommended in pregnancy unless medically necessary.

Imaging of choice for
• Staging and monitoring most malignant disease.
• Intracranial pathology, eg stroke, trauma, ↑ICP, and space-occupying lesions.
• Trauma.
• Pre-operative assessment of complex masses.
• Assessment of acute abdomen (figs 16.15, 16.16). NB ultrasound increasingly used (p720).
• Following abdominal surgery.

Contrast medium (p732) Enhance anatomical detail by use of a high- or low- (water)-attenuating medium to fill the lumen of a structure. *Give IV* to image vascular anatomy (fig 16.12) and vascular structures (including highly perfused tumours). Images acquired at different times ('phases') after injection will show the agent in arterial or venous structures or during 'washout' (= clearing). *Perfusion CT* maps cerebral blood flow by acquiring serial images after contrast administration then combines these into a colour-coded image of perfusion times (fig 16.14). It can help identify suitable candidates for thrombolysis or thrombectomy in acute stroke, enabling differentiation of salvageable ischaemic brain tissue (the penumbra) from the irrevocably damaged infarcted brain (the infarct core). Ensure IV cannulae secure and sufficient gauge to allow for rapid injection of agent as bolus— extravasation of contrast can cause significant tissue damage. *Give PO* eg 1–12h before imaging bowel. *Give PR* for examining distal colonic lumen.

Contrast-enhanced CTs may include a non-contrast series. Unenhanced imaging alone reduces radiation exposure and may be adequate for images of the brain, spine, lung, and musculoskeletal system or necessary in those with CKD (contrast is nephrotoxic). ▶If you are unsure as to whether contrast is required or what type of contrast is required, discuss this with radiology at the time of placing the request

Streak artefact Remember that the CT slice image is a matrix representation of the attenuation produced by rotating around the patient. High-attenuation items such as metal fillings, clips, and prostheses (and even bone) can cause interference.

CT combined with PET (See p722.) Combines the anatomical detail of CT with the metabolic information of PET, to aid assessment of, eg neoplastic lesions. Radiation doses are much higher than CT alone.

HOUNSFIELD SCALE (HU)

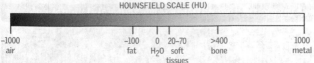

| −1000
air | | −100
fat | 0
H_2O | 20–70
soft
tissues | >400
bone | 1000
metal |

Fig 16.10 The Hounsfield scale.

Courtesy of Dr T Turmezei.

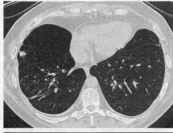

Fig 16.11 Axial high-resolution CT chest on a lung window algorithm; note solitary lesion in the right lung (in this case, from GPA).

Courtesy of Norwich Radiology Dept.

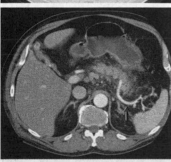

Fig 16.12 Axial CT of the abdomen after IV contrast (arterial phase). The tortuous splenic artery is enhanced (arrow)—so is the aorta, but not the inferior vena cava (compare to water in the stomach).

Courtesy of Norwich Radiology Dept.

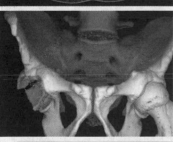

Fig 16.13 Surface rendered 3D CT reconstruction of the pelvis. The posterior aspect of the right acetabulum is fractured. The right femur has been digitally removed for better viewing.

Courtesy of Norwich Radiology Dept.

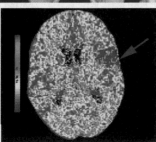

Fig 16.14 Cerebral perfusion CT showing ischaemia around the Sylvian fissure (arrow).

Courtesy of Dr C Cousens.

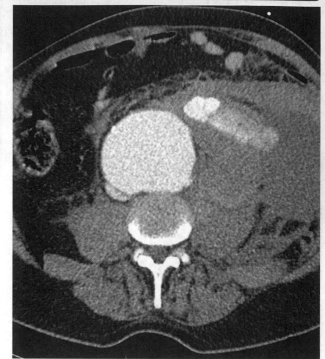

Fig 16.15 The history was of central abdominal pain with a non-peritonitic abdomen. The CT shows a leaking abdominal aortic aneurysm (AAA). Under fluoroscopic screening, this can be repaired using stents, inserted via femoral arterial puncture and deployed in the aneurysm (p646). This kind of endovascular aneurysm repair (EVAR) is commonly used in the treatment of leaking AAA as well as elective repair of intact but enlarging aneurysms.

The changing roles of surgeons and CT in the acutely unwell

In the days when general surgeons did their rounds towards the end of an on-call day, there would be wards of patients with undiagnosed abdominal pain having 'drip-and-suck' regimens (IVI and NG tube) while awaiting improvement or a change in their clinical condition that revealed the need for surgery. On opening up, the surgeon would try to deal with whatever pathology was found. With increased subspecialization and accurate emergency imaging (CT and US), patients are now matched to a team best equipped to deal with their condition. In this context, drip-and-suck is on the ebb, giving way to imaging, early intervention, rapid discharge, or onward referral. With increasing pressures to safeguard surgical beds for elective cases and on junior surgeons to polish their surgical logbooks in decreased training hours, can come attempts to deflect away from surgical teams the care of patients in whom imaging or clinical circumstances suggest no current requirement for an operation. But is this always appropriate? Do we expect on-call surgeons to be practitioners of medicine, assessing and managing patients with surgical pathology, even if a trip to the operating theatre is not currently called for, or simply technicians restricted to cutting?

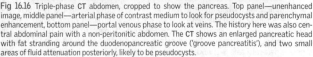

Fig 16.16 Triple-phase CT abdomen, cropped to show the pancreas. Top panel—unenhanced image, middle panel—arterial phase of contrast medium to look for pseudocysts and parenchymal enhancement, bottom panel—portal venous phase to look at veins. The history here was also central abdominal pain with a non-peritonitic abdomen. The CT shows an enlarged pancreatic head with fat stranding around the duodenopancreatic groove ('groove pancreatitis'), and two small areas of fluid attenuation posteriorly, likely to be pseudocysts.

Top panel courtesy of Dr Edmund Godfrey.

Magnetic resonance imaging (MRI)

1 A large proportion of the human body is fat or water (~80%).
2 Fat and water contain a large number of hydrogen nuclei (unpaired protons).
3 The spin of a positively charged hydrogen nucleus gives it magnetic polarity.

Thus ...
- Placing the human body in a magnetic field aligns its hydrogen nuclei either with (parallel) or against (anti-parallel) the field.
- A radiofrequency (RF) pulse at the resonant frequency flips a few nuclei away from their original alignment by an angle depending on the amount of energy they absorb.
- When the RF pulse stops, the nuclei flip back (or *relax*) into their original alignment, emitting the energy (called an *echo*) that was absorbed from the RF pulse.
- Measuring and plotting the energy of the returning signal according to location (provided the nuclei haven't moved) gives a picture of fat, tissue, and water as distributed throughout the body.
- The hydrogen nuclei in flowing blood move after receiving the RF pulses. The echo is not detected, and so the vessel lumen appears black (flow void).

Rather than radiodensity or attenuation, the correct descriptive terminology for the greyscale seen in MRI is signal intensity: high signal appears white and low signal black (table 16.4). Weighting is a quality of MRI that is dependent on the time between the RF pulses (repetition time, TR) and the time between an RF pulse and the echo (echo time, TE). MR images are most commonly T1-weighted (good for visualizing anatomy) or T2-weighted (good for visualizing disease) but can also be a mixture of both, called proton density (PD) weighting. FLAIR sequences produce heavily T2-weighted images. A good way to determine the weighting of an MR image is to look for water—eg in the aqueous humour of the eye, CSF, or synovial fluid (table 16.4; fig 16.17).

Table 16.4 MRI sequence characteristics

	T1-weighted	T2-weighted
TR	Short (<1000ms)	Long (>2000ms)
TE	Short (<30ms)	Long (>80ms)
Low signal	Water	Bone
	Flowing Hb	Flowing Hb
	Fresh Hb	DeoxyHb
	Haemosiderin	Haemosiderin
		Melanin
High signal	Bone marrow	Water
	Fat	Cholesterol
	Cholesterol	Fresh Hb
	Gadolinium (p732)	MetHb
	MetHb	

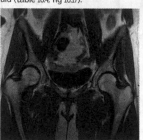

Fig 16.17 T1-weighted MRI of the hips. Normal adult bone marrow is high signal due to fat; note also low signal from urine in the bladder.
Courtesy of Norwich Radiology Department

Advantages MRI's great bonus is that it does not involve ionizing radiation. It has no known long-term adverse effects. It is *excellent for imaging soft tissues* (water- and hence proton-dense) and is preferred over CT for musculoskeletal disorders and for many intracranial, head, and neck pathologies (figs 16.18–16.20). Multiplanar acquisition of images can provide multiple views and 3D reconstruction from one scan. MR angiography is also excellent for reconstructing vascular anatomy. This avoids the need for invasive angiography with femoral puncture or CT contrast in patients with renal impairment.

Disadvantages Long acquisition times. Poor imaging of lung parenchyma. Claustrophobic. Incompatible with some metal implants. High cost and specialized interpretation (= limited availability).

Contraindications Absolute •Certain pacemakers; other implanted electrical devices. •Metallic foreign bodies, eg intra-ocular (consider orbital x-ray to exclude). •Noncompatible surgical clips/coils/heart valves. **Relative** •If unable to complete the pre-scan questionnaire. •Cochlear implants. NB: orthopaedic prostheses and extracranial metallic clips are generally safe. ▶If uncertain, ask a radiologist. **Contrast** •Risk of nephrogenic system fibrosis with use of gadolinium in advanced CKD. •Allergy. •Pregnancy.

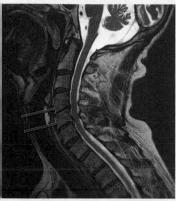

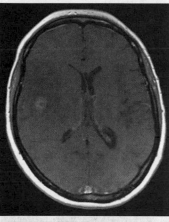

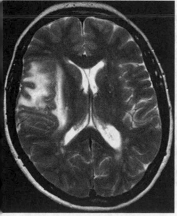

Fig 16.18 T2-weighted sagittal MRI of the cervical spine. There is impingement of the spinal cord at the C4/5 and C5/6 levels caused by degenerative disease. C2 (axis) is identifiable from the odontoid peg, which is embryologically derived from the body of C1 (atlas).

Courtesy of Norwich Radiology Department.

Fig 16.19 Axial T1-weighted MRI of the brain post IV gadolinium. In the right temporoparietal region there is a small area of high signal enhancement with a more central area of low signal, surrounded by a region of low signal (presumably vasogenic cerebral oedema) in comparison to the normal brain tissue. This is all causing mass effect with effacement of the sulci and adjacent right frontal horn of the lateral ventricle. There is a very subtle midline shift.

Courtesy of Norwich Radiology Department.

Fig 16.20 Axial T2-weighted MRI of the same patient at the same level as fig 16.19. The high signal in the temporoparietal region is the oedema causing mass effect. The diagnosis was of a solitary metastasis. In this T2-weighted image the oedema and the cerebrospinal fluid are of high signal due to their water content.

Courtesy of Norwich Radiology Department.

Ultrasound (us)

Unlike the other methods of imaging, us doesn't use electromagnetic radiation. Instead, it relies on properties of longitudinal sound waves. This has made it a popular and safe form of imaging with increasingly widespread applications. High-frequency sound waves (3–15MHz) are generated in the transducer (transmitter and receiver) by the vibrations of a piezo-electric quartz crystal as a voltage is applied. Passage of sound waves through tissue is affected by *attenuation* and *reflection*. Attenuation disperses waves out of the receiver's range, but it is the waves reflected back to the transducer that determine the image. Its quality depends on the difference in *acoustic impedance* between adjacent soft tissues.

Processing With the help of software a real-time 2D image is made. During processing, an average attenuation value is assumed throughout the tissue examined, so if a higher-than-average attenuation structure is in the superficial tissues (eg fibrous tissue, calcification, or gas), then everything deep to it will be in a low-intensity (black) acoustic shadow. If a lower-than-average attenuation object (eg fluid-filled/cystic structure) is in the superficial tissues then everything deep to it will be high intensity (white) or enhanced. If a tissue interface is strongly disparate, eg gas in the intestine, then all the waves are reflected back, making it impossible to image beyond it. See also figs 16.21–16.24.

Modes B (Brightness) is the most common, giving 2D slices that map the different magnitudes of echo in greyscale. M (Movement) traces the movement of structures within the line of the sound beam. It is used in imaging, eg heart valves (p102).

Duplex ultrasonography (flow and morphology) By combining Doppler effects (shifts in wavelength caused by movement of a source or reflecting surface) with B-mode ultrasound technology, flow characteristics of blood can be inferred (fig 16.21). This is extremely useful in arterial and venous studies, and echocardiography.

Advantages Portable; fast; non-ionizing; cheap; real-time; can be used with intervention; can enter organs, eg rectum, vagina, bowel. *Endoscopic* us can be used to stage and biopsy lung and GI tract cancers, eg stomach, pancreas, and also image the heart = transoesophageal echocardiogram (TOE), p102.

Disadvantages Operator dependent—interoperator variability high; poor quality if patient is obese; interference from bone, bowel gas, calculi, or superimposed organs can limit depth and quality of imaging.

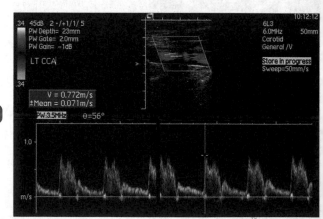

Fig 16.21 A normal Duplex US of the right common carotid artery with a flow rate = 77cm/s. The Doppler trace (orange) is displayed below the main image.

Courtesy of Norwich Radiology Department.

16 Radiology

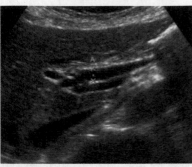

Fig 16.22 Ultrasound of the liver shows the common bile duct (CBD) to be dilated. Distal obstruction of the CBD causes proximal dilatation of the duct. It is important to correlate the width of the CBD with the ALP, as the normal diameter varies with age and previous interventions. Also check that the distal CBD tapers as it enters the duodenum. NB: the portal vein lies posterior to the duct (along with the hepatic artery) in the free edge of the lesser omentum. Next, ask 'What is causing the obstruction?' and 'Where can I get that information?'
Courtesy of Norwich Radiology Department.

16 Radiology

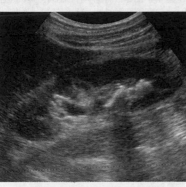

Fig 16.23 Ultrasound of the kidney. At first the image may seem normal but there is a wedge of posterior acoustic shadow cast by the object which is causing increased echogenicity in the lower pole calyces. Acoustic shadows in the kidney suggest stones—as here—or nephrocalcinosis.
Courtesy of Norwich Radiology Department.

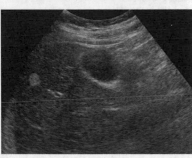

Fig 16.24 Longitudinal ultrasound of the right lobe of the liver showing a well-defined small area of echogenicity. This is the typical appearance of a liver haemangioma, a common benign liver lesion.
Courtesy of Norwich Radiology Department.

Searching for the bat signal

The first time someone started exploring the use of waves in spatial orientation was in 1794 when Lazzaro Spallanzani, an Italian physiologist, conducted experiments to explain how bats were able to fly at night. He noticed that even if the bat was blinded, it was still able to fly confidently through space. However, if the bat was deaf (even in one ear), it could not fly safely. In 1938, Griffin and Galambos coined the word 'echolocation' to explain how bats generate high-frequency clicks that bounce off surfaces and then receive and use the returned echoes to calculate the exact location of objects. However, it wasn't until 1956 that ultrasound was introduced as a medical diagnostic tool, when Ian Donald used the one-dimensional A-mode (amplitude mode) to measure the parietal diameter of the fetal head.

The majority of medical imaging is concerned with passing external waves (eg radiation) through the patient to a detector, and measuring scatter, slowing, or other alterations by various tissues. Nuclear medicine is the opposite; it measures emitted radiation from an internal source, introduced into the patient via injection, inhalation, or ingestion. It can be diagnostic (eg PET scanning) or therapeutic (eg radio-iodine (^{131}I) ablation in thyrotoxicosis).

Because molecules labelled with radioisotopes are introduced into the patient, there is exposure to ionizing radiation, though doses are usually less than those from CT (see table 16.1, p703). The selection of molecule for labelling depends on the tissue of interest, as it should be something that will be readily taken up by that tissue, eg bisphosphonates for bone, glucose for fast-turnover tissue. Examples include:

Positron emission tomography (PET) One of the key investigations in malignancy, but also has a wide range of other uses. The most commonly administered PET tracer is ^{18}F-fluorodeoxyglucose (FDG). FDG is a glucose analogue with a short half-life which becomes concentrated in metabolically active tissues. It is an unstable isotope which decays rapidly to release a positron which, after travelling a small distance, combines with an electron to produce a gamma ray, which can be detected and used to create an image. Normal high uptake of FDG occurs in brain, liver, kidney, bladder, larynx, and lymphoid tissue of pharynx and must be considered when assessing images. *Neoplasms* have high uptake of FDG with hotspots suggesting primary disease or metastases. Since inflammatory lesions will also show high uptake, there is a risk of false-positive results (eg sarcoid, TB); diagnosis must be confirmed with histology of suspicious lesions. PET allows *staging* of many solid organ malignancies (lung, melanoma, oesophageal) as well as lymphomas, and is particularly useful for *planning* of radiotherapy and surgery for both primary disease and metastases. PET can also be used to image occult sources of infection. PET can be combined with CT or MRI to provide high-quality images combining anatomy with physiology (fig 16.29). A range of alternative tracers are now entering clinical use with radiotracers conjugated to other tissue-specific substrates (eg ^{11}C-labelled metomidate to detect tumours of adrenocortical origin, somatostatin tracers in neuroendocrine tumours, and amyloid tracers in Alzheimer's disease). As the field of precision medicine expands, optimized PET probes for specific malignancies are being increasingly incorporated into clinical practice, such as prostate-specific membrane antigen (PSMA) PET imaging of prostate cancer

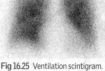

Fig 16.25 Ventilation scintigram.
Courtesy of Norwich Radiology Department.

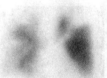

Fig 16.26 Perfusion scintigram showing mismatches with fig 16.25.
Courtesy of Norwich Radiology Department.

Ventilation/perfusion (V/Q) scan Uses inhaled technetium (Tc) or, less commonly, xenon-133 (^{133}Xe) plus injected ^{99m}Tc macro-aggregates, which lodge in lung capillaries. Normal perfusion excludes PE but ventilation component requires a normal CXR for comparison (figs 16.25, 16.26). Due to the large number of 'indeterminate' scans V/Q is considered inferior to CTPA for the investigation of PE except in pregnancy (p186).

Bone scintigraphy ^{99m}Tc-labelled bisphosphonates are readily taken up by bone, and concentrate in areas of pathology, eg tumours, fractures. It is much more sensitive in identifying metastases than X-ray, where lesions may not appear until >50% of bone matrix has been destroyed (fig 16.27).

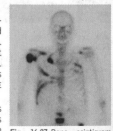

Fig 16.27 Bone scintigram showing metastases.
Courtesy of Norwich Radiology Department.

Thyroid disease TcO_4 is used for differentiating Graves', toxic multinodular goitre, and subacute thyroiditis (fig 13.21, p593) as well as identifying ectopic tissue, functioning nodules, and residual/recurrent thyroid tissue after surgery. ~15% of cold (non-functioning) nodules are malignant. Hot nodules are often toxic adenomas.

Phaeochromocytoma Iodine-123 (^{123}I) meta-iodobenzylguanidine (MIBG) is taken up by sympathetic tissues, and indicates functioning, ectopic, and metastatic adrenal medullary (+ other neural crest) tumours. ^{131}I-MIBG is also used for treatment.

Hyperparathyroidism ^{99m}Tc-methoxyisobutyl isonitrile (MIBI) scans can detect parathyroid adenomas.

Haemorrhage Red cells are removed from the patient and labelled with ^{99m}Tc, then re-injected to allow identification of a bleeding point. Used in both acute (after endoscopy and CT) and chronic GI bleeding, red cell scans are more sensitive than CT angiography and useful in intermittent bleeding, although localization can be challenging.

Kidney function Chromium-51 (^{51}Cr) EDTA or DTPA (^{99m}Tc, p661) are used to formally measure GFR, often in potential living kidney transplant donors. ^{99m}Tc-mercapto-acetyltriglycine (MAG3) technique assesses relative (left–right) renal function and renal transit time (eg in renovascular disease or to differentiate between obstructive and non-obstructive hydronephrosis in infants and children). ^{99m}Tc-dimercaptosuccinic acid (DMSA) scanning (fig 16.28) is the gold standard for evaluation of renal scarring that occurs, eg in reflux nephropathy.

Relative kidney uptake :

Left 45 %

Right 55 %

Fig 16.28 DMSA showing relative renal function of each kidney.
Courtesy of Norwich Radiology Department.

Single photon emission computed tomography (SPECT) Similar to PET but rather than using positron emission, it uses a radioisotope-labelled molecule as per conventional nuclear imaging, but with two gamma cameras for detection. The images produced are of lower resolution than PET but the isotopes used are longer lived and more easily available. Examples include myocardial perfusion scanning (p725). PET and SPECT also play an increasingly important role in the evaluation of patients with medically refractory epilepsy. They are employed to better localize epileptogenic onset zones, to identify MRI-occult lesions, and to map neurological functions as part of surgical planning.

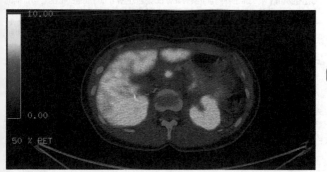

Fig 16.29 Gallium-68 DOTATATE scan in a 30-year-old woman with a history of a previous phaeochromocytoma, showing enhanced uptake in a new paraganglioma (arrow).

CT Cardiac CT Modern CT scanners can acquire images with sufficient speed and resolution to image coronary arteries and exclude significant disease with a negative predictive value of 97–99%. It can also visualize CABG patency, provide coronary artery Ca^{2+} scoring (a risk factor for coronary artery disease, p113), demonstrate cardiac anatomy including congenital anomalies, and estimate ventricular function. **Vascular CT** Has become routine in emergency assessment of suspected dissections, ruptured aneurysms, and arterial and venous thromboses (fig 16.30). CT angiography has overtaken invasive angiography in the assessment of many conditions such as stable angina and renal artery stenosis.

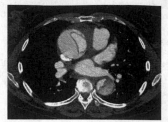

Fig 16.30 CT angiogram showing type A (ascending) aortic dissection with haemopericardium.
Courtesy of Dr C Cousins.

Catheter angiography Wherever intervention may be required, contrast studies such as angiography provide both image clarity and the possibility of proceeding to intervention, eg angioplasty or stenting of vessels, endovascular repair of aneurysms, clipping/coiling of aneurysms (p730). Remember that these have a high burden of both radiation and contrast medium, so check kidney function before requesting. *Complications* include those of arterial puncture (bleeding, infection, thrombosis, dissection, pseudoaneurysm formation) plus cholesterol emboli, thromboemboli, and vasospasm.

Cardiac MRI Using ECG-gating to acquire the imaging data and relate it to the position in the cardiac cycle (best when the patient is in sinus rhythm) can reduce movement artefact and lead to excellent resolution images for functional assessment. This, coupled with a lack of radiation, makes it ideal for the assessment of a wide range of structural and functional heart diseases. Flow velocities can be measured and, because the flow is proportional to the pressure differences, degrees of stenosis and regurgitation across heart valves can be calculated. Myocardial infarction, perfusion, and viability can also be imaged with the use of IV gadolinium contrast (p732). **Vascular MRI** is used to limit radiation exposure where multiple investigations may be required over a long time period, eg follow-up of intracranial aneurysm coiling, aortic root size in a young patient with Marfan's syndrome, or Takayasu's arteritis (p554).

Ultrasound Non-invasive, relatively low cost, and with no radiation, US is excellent for assessing the heart and vasculature particularly in acute settings where the test can be performed at the bedside. **Cardiac US** (= echocardiography) evaluates myocardial and valvular anatomy and function (p102). The use of exercise or pharmacological agents for 'stress echocardiography' can permit more detailed functional assessment. **Vascular US** Doppler ultrasonography is widely used for detection of thrombotic disease (eg DVT, p578; portal vein thrombosis, p272) and carotid atherosclerosis (p466).

Multiple-gated acquisition (MUGA) scanning is a non-invasive way to measure left ventricular ejection fraction (LVEF). After injection of ^{99m}Tc-labelled RBCs, a dynamic image of the left ventricle is obtained for a few hundred heartbeats by gamma camera. Since estimates of LVEF show less interoperator variation than with echocardiography, uses include the detailed serial assessment of LVEF in patients undergoing cardiotoxic chemotherapy (eg anthracyclines, trastuzumab).

Myocardial perfusion imaging A non-invasive method of assessing regional myocardial blood flow and the cellular integrity of myocytes. The technique uses radionuclide tracers which cross the myocyte membrane and are trapped intracellularly. Thallium-201 (^{201}Tl), a K^+ analogue, is distributed via regional myocardial blood flow and requires cellular integrity for uptake. Newer technetium-99 (^{99}Tc)-based agents are similar to ^{201}Tl but have improved imaging characteristics, and can be used to assess myocardial perfusion and LV performance in the same study (fig 16.31). Myocardial territories supplied by unobstructed coronary vessels have normal perfusion whereas regions supplied by stenosed coronary vessels have poorer relative perfusion, a difference that is accentuated by exercise. For this reason, exercise tests are used in conjunction with radionuclide imaging to identify areas at risk of ischaemia/infarction. Exercise scans are compared with resting views: *reversible* (ischaemia) or *fixed defects* (infarct) can be seen and the coronary artery involved reliably predicted. Drugs (eg adenosine, dobutamine, and dipyridamole) can also be used to induce perfusion differences between normal and underperfused tissues.

Myocardial perfusion imaging adds information in patients presenting with acute MI (to determine the amount of myocardium salvaged by thrombolysis) and in diagnosing acute chest pain in those without classical ECG changes (to define the presence of significant perfusion defects).

16 Radiology

Stress

Rest

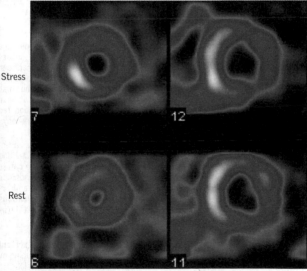

Fig 16.31 ^{99}Tc perfusion study showing perfusion defect in the left ventricle anterior and lateral walls at stress which is partially reversible (difference between stress and rest images). This study is good for small vessel disease such as in diabetes; CT and coronary angiography do not show small vessel disease well.

Courtesy of Dr C Cousins.

Ultrasound
Widely used for imaging all intra-abdominal organs, including an emerging role in small bowel imaging (though overlying bowel gas can cast acoustic shadows). US is the 1st-line imaging choice for abnormal LFTs, jaundice, hepatomegaly, renal dysfunction, and abdominal masses. Ensure the patient is 'nil by mouth' for 4 hours beforehand (aids gallbladder filling). Pelvic US needs a full bladder (consider clamping the catheter if appropriate). US may also guide diagnostic biopsy and therapeutic aspiration of cysts or collections.

CT
Plays an important role in the investigation of acute abdominal pain (pp714–17). It is unparalleled in the detection of free gas and intra-abdominal collections, and allows good visualization of the colon and retroperitoneal areas. Oral or IV contrast medium enhances definition (p714). The big disadvantage is the radiation dose. *CT colonography* (CTC; fig 16.32) uses rectal air or CO_2 insufflation, usually coupled with an oral 'stool tagging' agent to visualize the colonic mucosa in those unfit for endoscopic evaluation or in whom endoscopic evaluation has failed (eg in a stenosing tumour, where it can be used to assess the proximal colon and allow assessment of liver and nodal metastases at the same time). A negative test can be regarded as definitive but if polyps or masses are seen then patients will usually require a colonoscopy.

Wireless capsule endoscopy See p244.

Magnetic resonance imaging (MRI)
This gives excellent soft tissue imaging, giving it an important role in imaging the liver, biliary system, pancreas, and pancreatic duct (MRCP—magnetic resonance cholangiopancreatography; fig 16.33). As well as assessing potential malignant disease, MRCP is the imaging modality of choice for detection of common bile duct stones that can be missed on US. MRI performed after fluid loading of the small bowel (fluid delivered orally = MRI enterography; fluid delivered via nasoduodenal tube = MRI enteroclysis) permits assessment of small bowel inflammation (eg Crohn's) and lesions that can be challenging to reach with conventional endoscopy.

Endoscopic retrograde cholangiopancreatography (ERCP)
(See fig 16.34.) **Indications** No longer routinely used for diagnosis, it still has a significant therapeutic role: sphincterotomy for common bile duct stones; stenting of benign or malignant strictures and obtaining brushings to diagnose the nature of a stricture. **Method** A catheter is advanced from a side-viewing duodenoscope via the ampulla into the common bile duct. Contrast medium is injected and images taken to show lesions in the biliary tree and pancreatic ducts. **Complications** Pancreatitis; bleeding; cholangitis; perforation. Mortality <0.2% overall; 0.4% if performing stone removal.

Endoscopic ultrasound (EUS)
(See p720.) Commonly used in diagnosis of upper GI abnormalities, and is excellent for diagnosis of oesophageal, gastric, and pancreatic cancers. It allows staging by assessing depth of invasion, as well as histological diagnosis by biopsy of lesions.

Contrast studies
(See fig 16.35.) These can help in dysphagia (p246) and assessing integrity of anastomoses post-op. Real-time fluoroscopic imaging studies assess swallowing function. Barium gives better contrast but iodine-based water-soluble contrast medium is used if there is a concern of perforation. *Contrast enemas* are increasingly obsolete and now used to exclude a leak following a low anterior resection, for proctograms, and not much else.

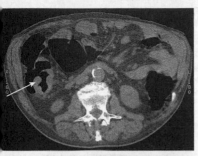

Fig 16.32 Axial CT colonogram: mural thickening (?ascending colon tumour).

Courtesy of Norwich Radiology Department.

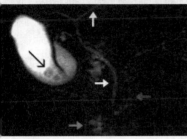

Fig 16.33 MRCP of the biliary system showing: left hepatic duct (yellow arrow); multiple gallstones in the gallbladder (black arrow); common bile duct (white arrow); pancreatic duct (red arrow); duodenum (green arrow).

Courtesy of Norwich Radiology Department.

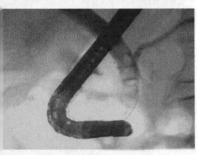

Fig 16.34 The ERCP shows a dilated common bile duct. The multiple filling defects are calculi within and obstructing the duct.

Courtesy of Norwich Radiology Department.

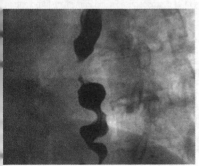

Fig 16.35 Barium swallow: note 'corkscrew' appearance of the oesophagus found in some motility disorders.

Courtesy of Norwich Radiology Department.

Ultrasound

Imaging modality of choice for genitourinary problems. Can be used to assess:

Kidneys

• Kidney size—small in chronic kidney disease, large if mass(es) present, cysts, hypertrophy if other kidney missing, polycystic kidney disease (fig 16.36), and rarities (eg amyloidosis, p364). Asymmetrical kidney size can indicate underlying renal artery stenosis.
• Hydronephrosis, which may indicate ureteric obstruction or reflux (fig 13.49, p633).
• Perinephric collections (trauma, post-biopsy).
• Kidney perfusion (assessment of renovascular disease: Doppler US of renal arteries).
• Transplanted kidneys (collections, obstruction, perfusion).

Lower urinary tract

• Bladder volume: useful in assessment of the need to catheterize (p632) or for assessment of adequacy of bladder emptying (post-micturition residual volume).
• Prostate: transrectal ultrasound enables US-guided biopsy of focal lesions. NB: prostate size does not correlate with symptoms.

Other

• Ovarian cysts, size, infections (pyosalpinx), uterine fibroids and other masses.
• Testicular masses, hydrocele, varicocele.

Advantages Fast; cheap; independent of renal function; no IV contrast or radiation risk.

Disadvantages Intraluminal masses (eg transitional cell cancer) in the upper tracts may not be seen; not a functional study; only suggests obstruction if there is dilatation of the collecting system (95% of obstructed kidneys) and so can miss obstruction from, eg retroperitoneal fibrosis.

CT

(See fig 16.37.) First choice in renal colic. Performed without IV contrast so safe in renal impairment; such unenhanced images miss <2% of stones, but can show other pathologies. With IV contrast, CT can delineate masses (cystic or solid, contrast enhancement, calcification, local/distant extension, renal vein involvement); assess renal trauma (presence of two kidneys; haemorrhage; devascularization; laceration; urine leak); and show retroperitoneal lesions. CT urogram has all but replaced IV urography and the radiation dose is similar.

Plain abdominal x-ray

Can be used to look at the kidneys, the paths of the ureters, and bladder. However, in practice it is only useful for monitoring known renal calculi.

Contrast studies

Retrograde pyelography/ureterograms are good at showing pelvicalyceal, ureteric anatomy, and transitional cell carcinomas (TCCs). Contrast medium is injected via a ureteric catheter. With the advent of cystoscopy, allowing immediate intervention, these are rarely done in isolation. However, contrast medium is routinely used in cystoscopic placement of retrograde stents for obstruction.

Percutaneous nephrostomy is used in obstruction to decompress the renal pelvis, which is punctured under local anaesthetic with imaging guidance. Images are obtained following contrast injection (antegrade pyelogram). A nephrostomy tube is then placed to allow decompression, sometimes followed by an antegrade stent depending on the cause of obstruction.

Renal arteriography (See fig 16.38.) Therapeutic indications: angioplasty; stenting; embolization (bleeding tumour, trauma, AV malformation).

Magnetic resonance imaging (MRI) Soft tissue resolution can help clarify equivocal CT findings. Magnetic resonance angiography (MRA) helps image renal artery anatomy/stenosis (fig 16.39) and is also used in the assessment of potential live donors for kidney transplant, as well as to monitor patients following embolization of tumours, arteriovenous malformations, and aneurysms.

Radionuclide imaging

See p722.

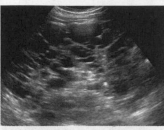

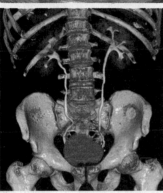

Fig 16.36 Ultrasound of the kidney showing multiple simple cysts.

Fig 16.37 3D reconstruction of CT urogram showing normal appearances of kidneys, ureters, and bladder.

Courtesy of Dr Edmund Godfrey.

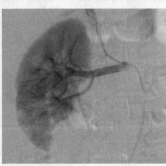

Fig 16.38 Renal artery digital subtraction angiogram (DSA; DSA is the final arbiter of renal artery stenosis). It is possible to tell that this is a DSA as no other structure has any definition or contrast in the image. There is, however, some interference from overlying bowel gas, which is not an uncommon problem. GI tract peristalsis can be diminished during the examination by using IV Buscopan®.

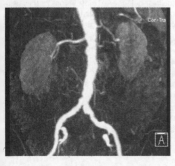

Fig 16.39 Coronal 3D MRA of the kidneys showing two renal arteries supplying the left kidney. This is important information pre-transplant. Anomalous renal arteries are common and, like the normal renal arteries, are end arteries, hence the consequence of infarction if tied at surgery.

16 Radiology

CT

(See **fig 16.40**.) Imaging modality of choice for patients presenting with acute neurological symptoms suggestive of a stroke. It is better than MRI at showing *acute haemorrhage* and *fractures*, and is much easier to do in ill or anaesthetized patients, and so is useful in emergencies. The attenuation of biological soft tissues is in a narrow range from about +80 for blood and muscle, to 0 for CSF, and down to −100 for fat (Hounsfield units, p714). IV contrast medium initially gives an angiographic effect, whitening the vessels. Later, if there is a defect in the blood–brain barrier (eg tumours or infection), contrast medium will opacify a lesion's margins, enhancing white areas.

* Some CNS areas, eg pituitary gland, choroid plexus, have no blood–brain barrier and enhance normally.
* Fresh blood is of higher attenuation (ie whiter) than brain tissue.
* In old haematomas, Hb breaks down and loses attenuation, so a subacute subdural haematoma at 2wks may be of the same attenuation as adjacent brain.
* A chronic subdural haematoma will be of relatively low attenuation.

CT is often used in *acute stroke* to exclude haemorrhage (eg pre-antiplatelets) and with perfusion scanning (**fig 16.14**, p715) to aid management decisions regarding thrombolysis. ▶If the patient is a potential candidate for thrombectomy, perform imaging with CT contrast angiography following initial non-enhanced CT. CT perfusion imaging (or MR equivalent) to assess for irreversible ischaemic brain injury and brain perfusion status is now a standard part of the CT stroke protocol to help guide suitability for tPA/thrombectomy.

Tumours and abscesses appear similar, eg a ring-enhancing mass, surrounding vasogenic oedema, and mass effect. Vasogenic oedema (from leaky capillaries) is extracellular and spreads through the white matter (grey matter spared). Mass effect causes compression of the sulci and ipsilateral ventricles, and may also cause herniation (subfalcine, transtentorial, or tonsillar). ▶See p477 (and also **fig 16.41**).

Another indication for CT is acute, *severe headache*, eg suggestive of subarachnoid haemorrhage (p474). The sensitivity of CT for subarachnoid haemorrhage approaches 100% within 6 hours of headache/symptom onset. An unenhanced CT may show fresh blood, hydrocephalus, or ↑ICP, any of which could make LP unsafe.

CT angiography gives excellent mapping of the cerebral circulation (**fig 16.42**), and can be done directly after unenhanced CT, looking for an aneurysm if the unenhanced CT shows subarachnoid haemorrhage.

MRI

(MRI in stroke: **fig 10.22**, p477) The chief image sequences are:

* **T1-weighted images** Give good anatomical detail to which the T2 image can be compared. Fat is brightest (↑signal intensity); other tissues are darker to varying degrees. Flowing blood is low signal. Gadolinium contrast (p732) usually results in an increase in signal intensity. See **table 16.4**.
* **T2-weighted images** These provide the best detection of most lesions as they usually contain some oedema or fluid and therefore appear white (eg **fig 16.20**, p719). Fat and fluid appear brightest. Flowing blood is again low signal.

Magnetic resonance angiography maps carotid, vertebrobasilar, and cerebral arterial circulations (and sinuses, veins). Functional MRI can image local blood flow.

Catheter angiography (See **fig 16.43**.) Facilitates endovascular intervention in cases of acute stroke (see above). Less commonly used since the advent of MRA and CT angiography and perfusion techniques, though it has the advantage of allowing immediate therapy—eg coil embolization of saccular aneurysms.

Radionuclide imaging (See p722.) PET is mostly used as a research tool in dementia, but perfusion scintigraphy can be used in the assessment of Alzheimer's disease, other dementias, and localizing epileptogenic foci. SPECT to visualize uptake of ^{123}I-FP-CIT (DaTscan™) can be used to assess reduced striatal dopaminergic transport in Parkinson's disease.

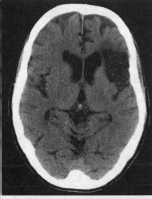

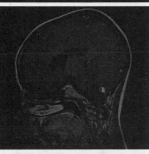

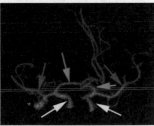

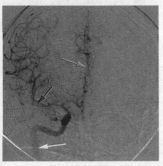

Fig 16.40 Unenhanced axial CT head: note the old infarct in the left middle cerebral artery territory.

Courtesy of Norwich Radiology Department.

Fig 16.41 T1-weighted MRI of the brain showing a haemangioblastoma in a patient with von Hippel–Lindau syndrome (p698). Note enhancement with contrast medium.

Courtesy of Dr Edmund Godfrey.

Fig 16.42 A 3D reconstruction of a CT angiogram of the paired internal carotid arteries (yellow arrows) and their branches (anterior cerebral arteries—green arrows; middle cerebral arteries—red arrows), seen from the front and slightly to the right. There is an aneurysm of the right middle cerebral artery (*).

Courtesy of Norwich Radiology Department.

Fig 16.43 Digital subtraction angiogram (DSA). The right internal carotid artery (yellow arrow), anterior cerebral artery (green arrow), and middle cerebral artery (red arrow) are shown.

Courtesy of Norwich Radiology Department.

The use of a contrast medium can alter the electron density of two previously similar tissues, thus allowing them to be distinguished. Contrast medium is usually administered by the following routes:

- *PO:* barium- or iodine-based agents for, eg swallow or enhancing visualization of bowel lumen on CT.
- *Inhaled:* technetium or xenon used in ventilation scintigraphy.
- *IV:* (most widespread clinical application.) Iodine or gadolinium.
- *PR:* air or CO_2 can be introduced to the colon for CT colonography, iodinated contrast medium is used for water-soluble enemas.

Iodine-based contrast agents Iodine is used because of its relatively high electron density and good physiological tolerance. When used with CT, the examination is said to be contrast enhanced—look for '+ c' amongst the scan details. *Exercise caution in:* advanced CKD (though the importance of contrast-induced or contrast-associated nephropathy is now highly disputed). ►Avoid iodine-based agents in active hyperthyroidism.

►Have renal function to hand in these patients. Patients who have eGFR <30mL/min/1.73m^2 and have proteinuria and diabetes or other comorbidities (ie heart failure, liver failure, or multiple myeloma) should be considered theoretically at higher risk of contrast-induced acute kidney injury (see p315 for prevention and treatment). Optimization of volume and haemodynamic status as well as avoidance of other nephrotoxins where possible in this context is reasonable. However, the guidelines would dictate that if the contrast-enhanced scan is clinically indicated and no other imaging modality suitable/available, that the contrast should not be withheld or delayed in this context, particularly if the patient is critically ill or the imaging time-sensitive, eg in the setting of stroke.

►Minor reactions include nausea, vomiting, and a sensation of warmth. More severe reactions include urticaria, bronchospasm, angioedema, and low BP (1:250); theoretical risk of death for 1:150 000.

Barium sulfate Used in examination of the GI tract. Water-insoluble particles of 0.6–1.4μm diameter are mixed with large organic molecules such as pectin and gum to promote good flow, mucosal adherence, and high density in thin layers. **Complications** Chemical pneumonitis or peritonitis. Never administer if you suspect perforated viscus.

Water-soluble, non-ionic, iodine-based contrast agents Used instead of barium where there is a risk of peritoneal contamination (eg fistula, megacolon, ulceration, diverticulitis, bowel anastomosis, acute intestinal haemorrhage). Gastrografin* should not be used.

►Contains iodine so establish allergy history and thyroid status.

Air In CT colonography, air (or CO_2) is insufflated as a negative contrast medium after barium administration to enhance mucosal definition. Water can also be used PO and PR to outline the lumen of the gut.

Gadolinium A lanthanide series element with paramagnetic qualities that is administered intravenously (as gadolinium-DTPA) to enhance the contrast of certain structures in MRI. It works by reducing the time to relaxation (TR) of hydrogen nuclei in its proximity and appears as high signal on T1-weighted scans. It does not cross the blood–brain barrier so is useful in enhancing isointense extra-axial tumours such as meningiomas. It can highlight areas where the blood–brain barrier has broken down secondary to inflammatory or neoplastic processes. It is renally excreted: ►check eGFR: if <30mL/min/1.73m^2, gadolinium is contraindicated (or at least should only be used in emergencies when no other imaging options possible) as there is a risk of a chronic, unremitting, and progressive condition known as nephrogenic systemic fibrosis. It is characterized by thickening and hardening of the skin overlying the extremities and trunk with eventual organ involvement with increased mortality. Group II gadolinium-based contrast agents (eg gadobutrol, gadoteridol) appear to be associated with lower risk. Seek nephrology advice if in doubt. Other adverse reactions include headache, nausea, and local irritation at the site of injection, with idiosyncratic reaction reported in less than 1%.

Imaging the acutely unwell patient

Asking yourself *'Does this investigation need to be done right now?'* will often yield the answer *'No!'*, yet there are a few occasions when early imaging can provide vital diagnostic information and influence the prognosis for a patient:

- Acute cauda equina syndrome (p462): ►►MRI lumbar spine.
- Suspected thoracic aorta dissection (p647): ►►CT aorta + IV contrast, MRI or transoesophageal echo (TOE). The mediastinum is rarely widened on CXR.
- Suspected leaking abdominal aortic aneurysm (p646): ►►CT aorta.
- Acute kidney injury (p294): ►►US of renal tract to exclude obstruction.
- Acute pulmonary oedema: ►►portable CXR: don't delay to get an ideal film.
- Acute abdomen with signs of peritonism: ►►erect CXR to find intraperitoneal free gas (fig 13.25, p599; ≈ GI perforation). Remember: post-op there will be detectable gas (air/CO_2) in the abdomen for ~10 days. ►►CT if suspicion of intra-abdominal source for sepsis or pathology requiring prompt surgery (eg appendicitis). US for ectopic pregnancy.
- Any patient with post-traumatic midline cervical spine tenderness—not just for the emergency department! ►►Collar and spinal precautions followed by a CT. All the vertebrae down to the top of T1 must be visualized and cleared before it is safe to take the collar off.
- Sudden-onset focal neurology, worst-ever headache, deteriorating GCS: ►►CT head, then LP if no evidence of ↑ICP.

Remember that imaging—or re-imaging for a poor-quality film—should never delay the definitive treatment of an emergency condition, eg:
- Tension pneumothorax (p799 and fig 16.44): ►►decompression *not* CXR.
- Intra-abdominal haemorrhage or viscus rupture (p598): ►►laparotomy.
- High clinical suspicion of torsion of testis (p644): ►►surgery *not* Doppler US.

Prior to the advent of interventional radiology, a collapsed, shocked patient with an acute abdomen would have skipped CT and gone straight for a laparotomy. However, you should bear in mind that ruptured aneurysms are increasingly being managed by endovascular repair under fluoroscopic guidance (p646) so this is one area where rapid imaging may be preferable to immediate intervention.

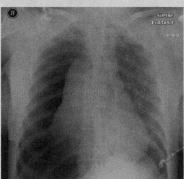

Fig 16.44 This is a great educational image from ICU. The inexperienced doctor could be distracted by the poor-quality image, missing the lung bases: technicians do their best under difficult conditions. To ask for a new CXR here would be a mistake: ►►note the large right-sided tension pneumothorax needing immediate decompression! *Lungs:* the right lung field is too black compared to the left, the right hemidiaphragm is depressed, and the right lung is seen collapsed against the mediastinum. *Mediastinum:* left-shifted, obstructing venous return—so ↓cardiac output, and a threat to life. Is it being pushed or pulled? Check hila, bones, and soft tissues. Since the right lung is collapsed and mediastinum shifted to left this suggests ►►right tension pneumothorax. Needle thoracocentesis decompression and a chest drain are needed now.

Courtesy of Dr Edmund Godfrey.

16 Radiology

17 Reference intervals, etc.

Contents

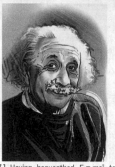

Fig 17.1 Having bequeathed $E = mc^2$ to the world, there is an informal agreement that Albert Einstein sits above the 97.5th centile (upper limit of the 95% reference range) for human intelligence. Despite his pre-expressed wish that his remains be cremated after his death and ashes scattered 'in order to discourage idolaters', his brain was surreptitiously removed within 8 hours of death, carved into 240 pieces, preserved, and stashed in a cider box underneath a beer cooler for many years. Studies later performed with unclear retrospective consent, compared the brain of Einstein (n = 1, unblinded) with 'brain of not-Einstein' (unmatched, uncontrolled, unimpressive numbers). A smaller neuron-to-glia ratio, more densely packed neurons within the 1mm² of brain examined, and a different folding pattern in a 15% wider, more symmetrical parietal lobe are tenuous surrogate markers of intelligence, driven by a need to quantify the extraordinary brain of Albert Einstein. If only Einstein had written the commonly misattributed quote: 'Not everything that counts can be counted, and not everything that can be counted counts', for it would have proven the perfect eulogy. Instead, hats off to sociologist William Bruce Cameron who, though unable to compete with the provenance of Einstein, was indeed correct.

Artwork by Gillian Turner.

- **The normal (Gaussian) distribution curve** This bell-shaped curve (fig 17.2) forms the theoretical basis of reference intervals, and explains 'lab error'—why repeated tests reveal slightly different values. Hb, for example, has a lab error of ~5g/L. This emphasizes the importance of *clinical picture* rather than treating numbers alone: don't subject patients with anaemia to transfusions unless clinical need, and transfuse bleeding patients before the haemoglobin decreases. See p324.
- **Range** The difference between the lowest and highest observation values.
- **Arithmetic mean** The sum of all observations ÷ by the number of observations.
- **Geometric mean** The nth root of the product of all observations—multiply all observations together and take the nth root (square root for two values, cube root for three values, etc.). Extreme values have less effect on the geometric mean compared to the arithmetic mean, although all values must be greater than zero.
- **Median** The middle value. In a normal distribution the median coincides with the mean.
- **Standard deviation (SD)** A measure of the spread of data away from the mean. It is calculated as the square root of the variance (where variance is the average of the square of the distance of each data point from the mean). When the distribution is normal, 95% of observations are within 1.96 SD of the mean.
- **Standard error (SE)** A measure of sample precision, measures the uncertainty of the sample mean compared to the mean of the population from which the sample was taken. It is the SD of the sample ÷ by the square root of the number of observations in the sample. Thus, the larger the sample size, the smaller the standard error, and the better the precision of the sample. SE is used to calculate confidence intervals and p-values in many circumstances.
- **Reference interval** Provides a reference point by which to interpret an individual's result. This is most commonly derived from a population of healthy individuals, with the pragmatic decision to include 95% (mean ±1.96 SD) of values. 5% of 'healthy' individuals will have results outside the reference interval (some above and some below). Do not interchange the terms 'reference interval' and 'normal range'. *A reference interval is not normal and it is not a range.* It is a fictitious dichotomy which proffers the illusion of a cliff-edge between health and disease. Do not let a reference interval obtund your inquiring mind. Form a multidisciplinary team with philosophers and social scientists to determine what is normal.

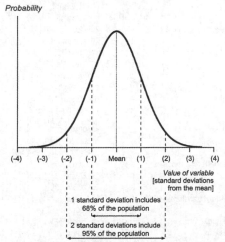

Fig 17.2 Normal (Gaussian) distribution curve.

Reproduced from Bhopal, *Concepts of Epidemiology*, 2008, with permission from Oxford University Press.

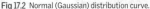

Biochemistry reference intervals

Refer to local reference intervals in preference to those listed here (tables 17.1, 17.2, 17.3, 17.4). Tests may have been re-validated for your local population.

The following factors may affect reference interval and/or assay:
- Age (see *OHCS* p314 for *children*).
- Pregnancy (see *OHCS* p9).
- Medication.

Table 17.1

Substance	Sample	Reference interval	Your hospital
Adrenocorticotrophic hormone	P	<46ng/L	
Alanine aminotransferase (ALT)	S	♂ 4–59IU/L	
		♀ 4–45IU/L	
Albumin	S	35–50g/L	
Aldosterone[1]	P	Upright 100–800pmol/L	
		Supine 100–450pmol/L	
Aldosterone:renin ratio	P	<80 (>200 suspect Conn's)	
Alkaline phosphatase	S	35–129IU/L	
α₁-antitrypsin	P/LI	0.9–2.0g/L	
α-fetoprotein	S	0–5.8kIU/L	
Ammonia	LI	12–50µmol/L	
Amylase	S	<100IU/dL	
Angiotensin-converting enzyme	S	8–52IU/L	
Aspartate transaminase	S	10–50IU/L	
β-HCG	S	<2IU/L	
Bicarbonate	S	22–30mmol/L	
Bile acids	S	<14µmol/L	
Bilirubin	S	3–20µmol/L	
NT proBNP (see p135)	S	<400pg/mL heart failure unlikely	
C-reactive protein	S	0–4mg/L	
Calcitonin[1]	PL	♂ <11.8pg/mL	
		♀ <4.8pg/mL	
Calcium (corrected, see p668)	S	2.15–2.55mmol/L	
Chloride	S	90–110mmol/L	
Cholesterol (see p682)	S	<5.0mmol/L	
LDL	S	<2.0mmol/L	
HDL	S	>1.0mmol/L	
Complement C3	P	0.70–1.65g/L	
Complement C4	P	0.16–0.54g/L	
Cortisol	S	7–10AM 171–536nmol/L	
		4–8PM 64–327nmol/L	
Creatine kinase (CK)	S	<150IU/L	
Creatinine	S	♂ 50–100µmol/L (eGFR >59)	
		♀ 45–90µmol/L (eGFR >59)	
Double-stranded DNA antibodies	S	<10IU/mL	
Ferritin	S	22–275mcg/L	
Folate	S	3.1–20.5mcg/L	
Gamma-glutamyl transferase (GGT)	S	♂ 4–72IU/L	
		♀ 4–60IU/L	
Glucose (fasting)	FL	3.5–5.5mmol/L	
Glucose (random)	FL	<11.0mmol/L	
HbA1c	P	20–41mmol/mol	
		>48mmol/mol = diabetes	

Iron	S	♂ 14–25µmol/L
		♀ 11–29µmol/L
Lactate (venous)	P/FL	0.7–2.0mmol/L
Lactate dehydrogenase (LDH)	S	240–480IU/L
Lead	B	<0.5µmol/L
Lipase	S	5–65IU/L
Magnesium	S	0.65–1.05mmol/L
Parathyroid hormone (PTH)	S/P	1.0–7.0pmol/L (10–65ng/L)
Phosphate	S	0.9–1.4mmol/L
Potassium	S	3.5–5.0mmol/L
Prolactin	S	♂ 86–324mIU/L
		♀ 102–496mIU/L
Prostate-specific antigen (PSA)	S	0.5–4.0mcg/L (see p526)
Protein (total)	S	64–86g/L
Red cell folate	B	135–750mcg/L
Renin[1]	P	Upright 5.4–60.0mU/L
		Supine 5.4–30mU/L
Rheumatoid factor	S	<12IU/mL
Sodium	S	135–145mmol/L
Thyroid-stimulating hormone (TSH)	S	0.25–4.0mU/L
Thyroxine (free T_4)	S	12–22pmol/L
Total iron-binding capacity	S	41–77µmol/L
Transferrin saturation	S/LI	<20% suggests iron deficiency
		>50% suggests iron overload
Triglycerides (fasting)	S	0.5–2.0mmol/L
Triiodothyronine (T_3)	S	3.1–6.8pmol/L
Troponin	S	See local reference interval
Urate	S	♂ 0.20–0.42mmol/L
		♀ 0.14–0.34mmol/L
Urea	S	1.7–7.0mmol/L
Vitamin B_{12}	S	187–883ng/L
Vitamin D	S	<25nmol/L = deficiency
		25–50nmol/L = insufficiency
		>50nmol/L = treatment target

B = whole blood.
FL = fluoride oxalate (plasma).
LI = lithium heparin (plasma).
P = plasma (EDTA).
PL = plain tube.
S = serum.
[1] The sample requires special handling: contact the laboratory.

Table 17.2

Arterial blood gas reference intervals	
pH	7.35–7.45
P_aO_2	12.0–15.0kPa
P_aCO_2	4.7–6.0kPa
Bicarbonate	22–30mmol/L
Lactate (arterial)	0.5–1.6mmol/L
Base excess	±2mmol/L
Fractional carboxyhaemoglobin (FCOHb)	0.2–2.4%
Fractional methaemoglobin (FMETHb)	0.2–1.2%

Note: 7.6mmHg = 1kPa.

17 Reference intervals, etc.

Table 17.3 (For B₁₂, folate, and iron studies see pp736–7.)

Cell/parameter		Reference interval	Your hospital
Haemoglobin	♂	130–180g/L	
	♀	115–165g/L	
White cell count (wcc)		4.0–11.0 × 10⁹/L	
Platelet count		150–450 × 10⁹/L	
Red cell count	♂	4.5–6.5 × 10¹²/L	
	♀	3.8–5.8 × 10¹²/L	
Packed red cell volume (PCV) (haematocrit)	♂	0.40–0.52L/L	
	♀	0.37–0.47L/L	
Mean cell volume (MCV)		80–100fL	
Mean cell haemoglobin (MCH)		27–32pg	
Mean cell haemoglobin concentration (MCHC)		320–360g/L	
Red cell distribution width (RCDW, RDW)		39–46fL 11.6–14.6% (p368)	
Neutrophils		2.0–7.5 × 10⁹/L 40–75% wcc	
Lymphocytes		1.5–4.5 × 10⁹/L 20–45% wcc	
Monocytes		0.2–0.8 × 10⁹/L 2–10% wcc	
Eosinophils		0.0–0.4 × 10⁹/L 1–6% wcc	
Basophils		0.0–0.1 × 10⁹/L 0–1% wcc	
Reticulocyte count		0.2–2.0%¹ 25–100 × 10⁹/L	
Erythrocyte sedimentation rate		1–12mm/h (p347)	
Prothrombin time (factors I, II, VII, X)		10–14 seconds	
International normalized ratio (INR)		0.8–1.2 (p351)	
Activated partial thromboplastin time (APTT) (factors VIII, IX, XI, XII)		23–30 seconds	
APTT ratio (APTTR)		0.8–1.2	
Fibrinogen		1.5–4.5g/L	
D-dimers		<500ng/mL FEU	
Fibrin degradation products (FDPs)		<10mcg/mL	

FEU = fibrinogen equivalent units.
¹ Only use percentages as reference interval if red cell count is normal; otherwise, use the absolute value.

Table 17.4

Urine reference intervals	Reference interval	Your hospital
Calcium[1]	2.5–2.5mmol/24h, 100–300mg/24h	
Cortisol (free)	<200nmol/24h	
5-Hydroxyindoleacetic acid (5-HIAA)	0–40µmol/24h	
Metanephrine	<2.0µmol/24h	
Normetanephrine	<4.4µmol/24h	
Osmolality[1]	50–1200mosmol/kg	
Potassium[1]	25–125mmol/24h >10mmol/L may suggest renal loss	
Protein	<150mg/24h (p290)	
Sodium[1]	100–250mmol/24h	

[1] Interpret based upon plasma values.

What value a test?

The diagnostic capacity of a medical test is apocryphal. It cannot define normality, which is a nebulous construct at best. Normality and health are not the same. A sore throat is normal, but it is not healthy. And if a person is only normal when healthy, then those with disease are abnormal by default, and the consequences for society are bleak and terrible. Hence the term 'reference range' rather than 'normal range'. Consider also how a reference range is derived. Are military recruits, blood donors, and medical students a good reference? If they are not representative of population bravery, civic duty, or a tendency to last-minute revision, then why for serum rhubarb? A reference cohort is like the utopia of a mirror image, a reality that does not exist, yet upon which judgements are made. And even within the limitations of such ontological ambiguity, a presumed Gaussian distribution means that 5% of normal and healthy individuals sit outside reference intervals. The temptation to tick additional boxes on a pathology form is strong. But the more tests sent, the more abnormality thrives. If 10 analytes are requested there is a 23% of chance of finding abnormality when none exists. Beware of tests that you do not need: they may bite.

Serial numbers

If you accept the premise that the result of a test is important for health, then effective treatments change that result for the better. So when cholesterol, creatinine, and CRP fall, you pat yourself on the back for a job well done. Yet a single reported figure may be a false icon of precision, particularly when reported to an overly reassuring but needless number of decimal places. Uncertainty is the reprobate cousin of diagnostic accuracy, disinherited and no longer invited to the family party of blood results. But the legal claim to inaccuracy is valid. Unavoidable variability is inherent in medical measurement.[1] There is frustrating diversity in physiology, with random fluctuation about the 'true' concentrations of salts, acids, chemicals, and proteins of which we are made. Sometimes this is a hum, sometimes a cacophony, depending on what is being measured. Regression to the mean is the statistical phenomenon in which natural variation leads to the mirage of real change. In reality, any excessive value is statistically more likely to be closer to the mean when repeated. A difference between measurements must be outside that of analytical and biological variation for it to be clinically significant: haemoglobin needs to change by greater than 20%, urea by 40%, TSH by 50%, and lactate by more than 50%. You can enter your serial results at https://www.bmj.com/content/368/bmj.m149/infographic and discover whether to pat yourself on the back after all.

►Reference intervals provide a guide to treatment. A drug may have utility even in low concentrations, and high concentrations may not equate with toxicity.

►The time since the last dose should be confirmed and documented.

Aminoglycosides All have a narrow therapeutic index with wide variability between prescribed dose and resulting serum concentrations. Toxicity includes nephrotoxicity, ototoxicity, and neuromuscular block, and is related to both dose and length of exposure: use the minimum effective dose for the shortest effective time. *Signs of toxicity:* tinnitus, deafness, nystagmus, vertigo, AKI. Monitor kidney function daily. The evidence base for dosing is limited. Most common dosing in the UK is once daily. For once-daily dosing, peak levels are presumed to be in the therapeutic range and monitoring trough (pre-dose) levels is undertaken to reduce the risk of toxicity. If trough concentration is high, withhold next dose and repeat test 12–24 hours later. Repeat trough levels every 3 days, or more if change in kidney function or clinical concern. Consider peak levels (1 hour after administration) where the volume of distribution is unpredictable: eg septic shock, burns, liver failure/ascites.
Amikacin Once-daily dose: 15mg/kg (maximum 1.5g). Trough: <5mg/L.
Gentamicin Once-daily dose: 5mg/kg. Trough: <1mg/L.
Tobramycin Once-daily dose: 3–5mg/kg. Trough <1mg/L.

Anti-epileptic medication The therapeutic concentration range for an individual patient is the range that achieves the optimum clinical response, determined according to symptoms and associated risk. Monitoring is used for initial dose optimization, uncontrolled seizures, suspected toxicity, pregnancy, pharmacokinetic interactions, and comorbidities that affect levels.

Carbamazepine Steady state 20 days after commencement due to auto-induction, 2–4 days after change in dose. Target concentration: 4–12mg/L.

Phenytoin Steady state at 6–21 days. Target concentration: 10–20mg/L. Assay measures bound phenytoin, but it is free phenytoin that is pharmacologically important. Consider use of free phenytoin concentrations if hypoalbuminaemia (free concentration = measured total concentration ÷ [((0.9 × albumin in g/L) ÷ 42) + 0.1]). *Signs of toxicity:* ataxia, diplopia, nystagmus, sedation, dysarthria, confusion, hallucinations, tremor, irritability.

Lamotrigine Concentrations decrease with oestrogen-containing contraceptives (use alternative) and pregnancy (monitor concentrations). Titrate dose slowly due to possible severe skin reactions including Steven–Johnson syndrome. Target concentration: 2.5–15mg/L.

Calcineurin inhibitors Ciclosporin and tacrolimus. Monitor trough levels. Target depends on indication and time after transplantation. Contact the patient's transplant unit for individual target. Do not stop treatment in transplant recipients unless instructed by the transplant team—provide NG/IV if oral route not possible. Enzyme inhibitors (erythromycin/clarithromycin) will increase concentrations so use alternatives where possible.

Digoxin Monitor trough concentrations (>6h after dose). Target is ventricular rate or 0.5–0.8ng/mL in heart failure. *Signs of toxicity:* CVS: arrhythmias, heart block. CNS: confusion, insomnia, agitation, xanthopsia, delirium. GI: nausea. Consider monitoring if AKI, ↓K⁺, ↓Mg²⁺.

Lithium Check levels at 12h post dose, 5–7 days after dose increase and every 6–12 months. Target: 0.8–1.2mmol/L. Signs of toxicity (>1.5mmol/L): tremor, slurred speech, lethargy, spasm, coma, seizure, arrhythmias, kidney failure.

Theophylline Target peak concentration: 10–15mg/L (avoid >20mg/L). (►See p794.) Take sample 4–6h after starting an infusion (stop for ~15min just before specimen taken). *Signs of toxicity:* arrhythmias, anxiety, tremor, convulsions.

Vancomycin Dosing guided by age and kidney function but typically 1g/12h. Check trough levels prior to 4th dose. Target: 10–15mg/L (possible higher target for deep-seated infection). Check kidney function daily and trough concentrations every 3 days.

▶ See p681 for a list of cytochrome P450 inducers and inhibitors.

▶ See *BNF* (https://bnf.nice.org.uk/interaction/).

▶ See https://reference.medscape.com/drug-interactionchecker.

▶ For HIV medication see https://www.hiv-druginteractions.org.

▶ For hepatitis medication see https://www.hep-druginteractions.org.

▶ For cancer medications see https://cancer-druginteractions.org.

Adverse drug events lead to 6.5% of unplanned hospital admissions in the UK. Fatal interactions are most commonly due to bleeding and kidney failure.

The following drugs are important for interactions. Monitoring for interactions is clinical, or using concentrations if these are routinely measured. This is not an exhaustive list; if in doubt, check:

• **Warfarin**

Beware an increased INR with erythromycin, clarithromycin, fluconazole, amiodarone, and tramadol.

• **Statins**

Particularly simvastatin, less with pravastatin.

Increase in concentrations with erythromycin/clarithromycin (avoid), diltiazem (monitor), verapamil (monitor), itraconazole (avoid), fluconazole (monitor), amiodarone (monitor), grapefruit juice (avoid). Decrease in statin concentrations with carbamazepine, phenytoin, rifampicin.

• **Macrolide antibiotics**

Particularly erythromycin and clarithromycin, minimal with azithromycin.

Increase in calcineurin inhibitor (ciclosporin, tacrolimus) concentrations (avoid), increase in statin concentrations (monitor), increase in calcium channel blocker concentrations (monitor), increase in INR on warfarin (monitor), increase in digoxin concentrations (monitor).

• **Calcium channel blockers**

Particularly diltiazem and verapamil.

Increase in calcineurin inhibitor (ciclosporin, tacrolimus) concentrations (monitor), increase in statin concentrations (monitor), increase in digoxin concentrations (monitor).

• **-azole antifungals**

Increase statin concentrations (avoid simvastatin, monitor others), increase in calcineurin inhibitor (ciclosporin, tacrolimus) concentrations (monitor), increase in digoxin concentrations (monitor), increased INR with warfarin (monitor).

• **SSRI**

Increased concentrations with tricyclic antidepressants (monitor: serotonin syndrome, seizures).

• **Amiodarone**

Increase in statin concentrations (monitor), increase in calcineurin inhibitor (ciclosporin, tacrolimus) concentrations (monitor), increase in digoxin concentrations (monitor), increased INR with warfarin (monitor).

• **Digoxin**

Increase in concentrations with erythromycin (avoid), clarithromycin (avoid), diltiazem (monitor), verapamil (monitor), -azole antifungals (monitor), amiodarone (monitor), rifampicin (monitor).

• **Calcineurin inhibitors (ciclosporin, tacrolimus)**

Increase in concentrations with erythromycin/clarithromycin (avoid), diltiazem/verapamil (monitor), -azole antifungals (monitor), amiodarone (monitor), grapefruit juice (avoid). Decrease in concentrations with rifampicin, phenytoin, and carbamazepine (monitor) and St John's wort (avoid).

• **Lithium**

Increased concentrations with ACE-i, ARA, diuretics, NSAIDs (monitor).

Others to remember:

• ACE-i/ARA ± diuretic ± NSAID ± intercurrent illness = AKI.

• Allopurinol: increased azathioprine/6-mercaptopurine concentrations and pancytopenia.

18 Practical procedures

Contents

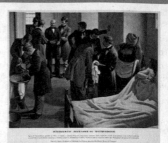

Fig 18.1 *Semmelweis: Defender of Motherhood.* Hungarian obstetrician Ignaz Semmelweis demonstrated the benefits of handwashing in the 1840s: he observed that maternal mortality was nearly three times as high on a doctor-run maternity ward compared to a midwife-run ward. The explanation remained elusive until Semmelweis' friend Jakob Kolletschka died after receiving an accidental scalpel cut from a student during a postmortem demonstration. Semmelweis recognized in Kolletschka's death many of the features of the dying mothers. The explanation: the maternity ward doctors' day started with postmortem examinations, from which they would proceed to perform vaginal examinations on the living without washing their hands. Noticing this, Semmelweis introduced the practice of washing hands with chloride of lime and cut death rates to that of the midwives' patients. Despite the evidence he amassed, Semmelweis' theory was rejected by his contemporaries, a rejection which undoubtedly contributed to his psychiatric distress, eventual commitment to an asylum, and ultimate death from the blows of his guards. It would take another 20 years and countless deaths before Lister published his landmark work on the use of carbolic acid in surgery. Take a minute to wash your hands thoroughly before undertaking any procedure. This prerequisite will not only reduce infection risk for your patients, but give you a moment for mindfulness: focus on the hot water running over your hands, breathe deeply, and for a while forget about your list of jobs. Perhaps spare Dr Kolletschka a thought. You may find that the subsequent procedure goes more smoothly than anticipated...

Robert Thom, 'Semmelweis-Defender of Motherhood', ca. 1952. From the collection of Michigan Medicine, University of Michigan, Gift of Pfizer, Inc., UMHS.26

Training and the business of medicine

As medical training has evolved in an environment where patient safety is paramount, the old adage of 'see one, do one, teach one' is no longer relevant. 'Just having a go' when you aren't confident can have devastating consequences for the patient, and also for you and your future. This creates tensions for training, but these are not insurmountable. Seek out opportunities to learn practical procedures, ideally in a controlled, elective setting, so that your first attempt isn't a life-or-death emergency attempt—time spent in theatres or ICU will pay dividends in this regard. Many seniors will be happy to make time to teach if you contact them in advance—let them know you are interested and leave your bleep. ▶Even in an emergency setting, it is still wiser to seek help rather than attempting an urgent procedure for the first time.

Nasogastric tubes

These tubes are passed into the stomach via the nose. Large (eg 16F) are good for drainage but can be uncomfortable for patients. Small (eg 10F) are more comfortable for feeding but can be difficult to aspirate and are poor for drainage. Used:
* To decompress the stomach/gastrointestinal tract especially when there is obstruction, eg gastric outflow obstruction, ileus, intestinal obstruction.
* For gastric lavage.
* To administer feed/drugs, especially in critically ill patients or those with dysphagia, eg motor neuron disease, post CVA.

Passing the tube Nurses are experts and will ask you (who may never have passed one) to do so only when they fail—so the first question to ask is: 'Have you asked the charge-nurse from the ward next door?'
* Wear non-sterile gloves and an apron to protect both you and the patient.
* Explain the procedure. Take a new, cool (hence less flexible) tube. Have a cup of water to hand. Lubricate well with aqueous gel.
* Use the tube, by holding it against the patient's head, to estimate the length required to get from the nostril to the back of the throat.
* Place lubricated tube in nostril with its natural curve promoting passage down, rather than up. The right nostril is often easier than the left but, if feasible, ask the patient for their preference. Advance directly backwards (not upwards).
* When the tip is estimated to be entering the throat, rotate the tube by ~180° to discourage passage into the mouth.
* Ask the patient to swallow a sip of water, and advance as they do, timing each push with a swallow. **If this fails** Try the other nostril.
* The tube has distance markings along it: the stomach is at ~35–40cm in adults, so advance > this distance, preferably 10–20cm beyond. Tape securely to the nose.

Confirming position This is vital prior to commencing any treatment through the tube. Misplaced nasogastric tubes have led to a number of preventable deaths, and feeding via a misplaced tube is considered an NHS Never Event (a serious, largely preventable patient safety incident that should *never* occur if the available preventative measures have been implemented).
* Use pH paper to test that you are in the stomach: aspirated gastric contents are acid (pH ≤5.5) although antacids or PPIs may increase the pH. Small tubes can be difficult to aspirate, try withdrawing or advancing a few cm or turning the patient on the left side to help dip the tube in gastric contents. Aspirates should be >0.5mL and tested directly on unhandled pH paper. Allow 10s for colour change to occur.
* If the pH is >5.5 and the NGT is needed for drug or feed administration then the position must be checked radiologically. Request a CXR/abdo x-ray (tell the radiologist why you need it). Look for the radio-opaque line/tip (this can be hard to see, look below the diaphragm, but if in doubt, ask for help from the radiologist).
* *The 'whoosh' test is NOT an accepted method of testing for tube position.*
* Either spigot the tube, or allow to drain into a dependent catheter bag secured to clothing (zinc oxide tape around tube to form a flap, safety pin through flap).
▶Do not pass a tube nasally if there is any suspicion of a facial fracture.
▶Get senior help if the patient has recently had upper GI surgery—it is not good practice to push the tube through a fresh anastomosis.

Complications •Pain, or, rarely: •loss of electrolytes •oesophagitis •tracheal or duodenal intubation •necrosis: retro- or nasopharyngeal •stomach perforation.

Weaning When planning removal of an NGT *in situ* for decompression or relief of obstruction, it is wise to wean it so that the patient manages well without it. Drainage should be <750mL/24 hours for successful weaning.
* First it should be on free drainage with, eg 4hrly aspirations.
* Then spigot with 4hrly aspirations.
* Then spigot only. If this is tolerated along with oral intake then it is probably safe to remove the tube; if not, then take a step backwards.

▶Much of what we do is not evidence based; however, in more recent years, particularly in intensive care units, the rise of hospital-acquired infections and multidrug-resistant organisms has prompted a review of standard practice and a series of evidence-based interventions put together as a 'care bundle' to reduce hospital-acquired infections. The technique for placing a cannula is best shown at the bedside by an expert, but following these simple rules will significantly reduce the risk of infection from the cannula.

Preparation is key, remember the following before you start

1 **Equipment** Set up a tray with cleaning swabs, gauze, cannulae (swallow your pride and take at least three of different sizes, see table 18.1), dressings, 0.9% saline, 10mL syringe, needle-free adaptor (eg octopus with Bionector®), blood tubes if required, portable sharps bin → needlestick injuries do happen.

2 **Patient** Have them lying down, explain procedure, obtain verbal consent, place tourniquet around arm, rest the arm below the heart to aid venous filling.

3 **Site** Look for the best vein—it should be palpable; some of the best veins are not easily visible, some of the most visible collapse on insertion. Tapping gently helps. ▶ **Never cannulate** AV fistulae arms, limbs with lymphoedema. ▶**Avoid** Sites crossing a joint (if possible), the cephalic vein in a renal patient.

4 **Consider** EMLA® cream, cold spray, or 1% lidocaine for children or those with needle phobia. EMLA® takes 45min to work, but can save you hassle later.

Insertion care bundle

1 Aseptic technique. 2 Hand hygiene. 3 Apron + non-sterile gloves. 4 Skin preparation—2% chlorhexidine in 70% isopropyl alcohol (allow to dry for 30 seconds). Do not re-palpate vein after cleaning unless wearing sterile gloves. 5 Dressing—sterile and transparent so that insertion site can be observed.

After insertion

1 Take blood with syringe or adaptor. 2 Remove tourniquet. 3 Attach needle-free device (if appropriate) and flush with 10mL 0.9% saline. 4 Apply dressing. 5 Let nursing staff know that cannula is in place and ready for use. 6 Document insertion according to local policy. 7 Write up appropriate fluids or parenteral medication.

When seeing your patient on the daily ward round (and to avoid being called to review or replace cannulae at 6pm) do a **RAID**[1] assessment: consider if the drip is:

Required—can the patient manage with oral medication/fluids?

Appropriate—should you consider a PICC, central line, long-term line, etc?

Infected—any signs of inflammation or infection? Remove if yes. Peripheral cannulae should be replaced every 72–96 hours.

Dressed properly—many drips are replaced early because they have 'fallen out', or are kinked from poor dressings.

Tissued or infected cannulae need replacing, either with another peripheral cannula, or with a longer-term access device, such as a PICC line.

If you fail after three attempts ▶Shocked patients need fluid quickly: if you are having trouble putting in a drip, call your senior. The following advice assumes that the drip is not immediately life-saving. ▶▶If it is, see BOX.

• Ask for help—from colleagues or seniors—do not be ashamed, everyone has to learn and even senior doctors have bad days; a fresh pair of eyes can be all it takes. As a house officer, one of us was asked to place a drip when a very shame-faced consultant had 'had a go' to prove he still could, and found out that he couldn't!

• Help yourself—try putting the hand in warm water, using a small amount of GTN paste over the vein, or using ultrasound if available to help you identify the vein.

• If there is no one else to help, take a break and come back in half an hour. Veins come and go, and coming back with fresh eyes can make all the difference.

Table 18.1 Intravenous cannulae sizes and UK colour conventions

Gauge	Colour	Diameter (mm)	Length (mm)	Flow rate (mL/min)
14G	ORANGE/**BROWN**	2.0	45	250
16G	GREY	1.7	42	170
18G	GREEN	1.2	40	90
20G	PINK	1.0	32	55
22G	BLUE	0.28	25	25
24G	YELLOW	0.07	19	24

Flow rate is given as maximum flow rate under gravity; faster rates may be achievable with rapid infusion devices.

According to Poiseuille's law[1] the flow rate (Q) of a fluid through a tubular structure is inversely proportional to viscosity (η) and length (l) and proportional to the pressure difference across it ($P_i - P_o$) and the radius *to the power of 4*(r^4). Hence:

$$Q \propto \frac{(P_i - P_o)\, r^4}{\eta l}$$

A last throw of the dice

Just once it may come down to you. For some, this is one of the challenges and thrills in medicine. There may be no one else available to help when there is an absolute and urgent indication for IV drugs/fluids/blood—and all of the previously discussed measures have been tried, and have failed. Think of lonesome night shifts, over-run emergency departments, a disaster scene, war, or medicine in the field. The following measures are not recommended for non-life-threatening scenarios:

▶▶Don't worry. Have a good look again. Feet (avoid in diabetics)? Inside of the forearm? Upper arm?

▶▶Have you really exhausted all of your options for help from a colleague? Maybe the anaesthetist or ICU registrar is approachable—they do have remarkable skills.

▶▶Is the patient familiar with his/her own veins (eg previous IV drug abuser)?

▶▶If there is only a small amount of IV medication required and a small, short vein, you may be able to gain access with a carefully placed butterfly needle that is taped down. Some drugs cannot be passed this way (eg amiodarone, K+).

▶▶The external jugular vein may become prominent when the patient is head down (Trendelenburg) by 5–10° (▶not in situations of fluid overload, LVF, ↑ICP). Only attempt cannulation of this vein if you are not going to jeopardize future central line insertion, and if you can clearly determine the surrounding anatomy.

▶▶In an arrest situation, the 2015 Advanced Life Support Guidelines recommend the intraosseous route in both adults and children if venous access is not possible; access devices should be available within resuscitation settings (eg emergency department).

Only do the following if you have had the appropriate training/experience

▶▶In children, consider cannulating a scalp vein.

▶▶Central venous catheterization (p759). This may be just as hard in a profoundly hypovolaemic arrest patient, and a good knowledge of local anatomy and of the procedure (± ultrasound guidance) will be invaluable.

If you don't have an intraosseous access device, a cut down to the long saphenous vein may be attempted, *in extremis*, even if you have no prior experience (at this site you won't kill by being ham-fisted). ▶▶Make a transverse incision 1–2cm anterior and superior to the medial malleolus. ▶▶Free vein with forceps. ▶▶Cannulate it under direct vision. ▶Here, 'first do no harm' is trumped by 'nothing ventured, nothing gained'.

Hopefully, it shouldn't ever have to come to these measures, but one day …

---

1 Poiseuille's law is a neat piece of physiology and worth remembering—it is applicable in some form to almost every system in the body. Note that it is a 4th-power law: a small change in the radius makes a huge difference to flow.

Urinary tract infections are the second commonest healthcare-associated infection, and urinary catheters are frequently to blame. Think, does the patient really need a catheter? If so, use the smallest you can and take out as soon as possible.

Size (In French gauge): 12 = small; 16 = large; 20 = very large (eg 3-way). **Material** Coated latex catheters are soft and a good short-term option ▶but unsuitable in true latex allergy. Silastic (silicone) catheters may be used long term, but cost more. Silver alloy coating reduces infections. **Shape** Foley is typical (fig 18.2); coudé (elbow) catheters have an angled tip to ease around prostates but are more risky; 3-way catheters are used in clot or debris retention and have an extra lumen for irrigation fluid, attached to the irrigation set via an extra port on the distal end (fig 18.3). Get urology advice before starting irrigation. Condom catheters are often preferred by patients (less discomfort) even though they may leak and fall off.

Catheter problems • Infection ~5% develop bacteraemia (most will have bacterial colonization, antibiotics may not be required unless systemically unwell—discuss with microbiology). A stat dose of, eg gentamicin 80mg is sometimes given pre-insertion despite a lack of evidence for benefit. Check your local policy. • **Bladder spasm** May be painful—try reducing the water in the balloon or an anticholinergic drug, eg oxybutynin.

Per urethram Aseptic technique required.

Indications • Relieve urinary retention. • Monitor urine output in critically ill patients. • Collect uncontaminated urine for diagnosis. ▶It is contraindicated in urethral injury (eg pelvic fracture) and acute prostatitis.

• Explain the procedure, and obtain verbal consent. Prepare a catheterization trolley: gloves, catheter, lidocaine jelly, cleaning solution, drape, kidney dish, gauze swabs, drainage bag, 10mL water and syringe, specimen container.

• Lie the patient supine: women with knees flexed and hips abducted with heels together. Use a gloved hand to clean urethral meatus in a pubis-to-anus direction, holding the labia apart with the other hand. With uncircumcised men, retract the foreskin to clean the glans; use a gloved hand to hold the penis still. The hand used to hold the penis or labia should not touch the catheter. Place a sterile drape with a hole in the middle to help you maintain asepsis. Remember: left hand dirty, right hand clean.

• Put sterile lidocaine 1–2% gel on the catheter tip and ≤10mL into the urethra (≤5mL if ♀). In men, lift and gently stretch the penis upwards to eliminate any urethral folds that may lead to false passage formation.

• Use steady gentle pressure to advance the catheter, rotating slightly can help it slide in. ▶Never force the catheter. Tilting the penis up towards the umbilicus while inserting may help negotiate the prostate. Insert to the hilt; wait until urine emerges before inflating the balloon. Remember to check the balloon's capacity before inflation (written on the outer end). Collect a sterile specimen and attach a drainage bag. Pull the catheter back so that the balloon comes to rest at the bladder neck.

• If you are having trouble getting past the prostate, try: more lubrication, a gentle twisting motion; a larger catheter; or call the urologists, who may use a guidewire.

▶Remember to reposition the foreskin in uncircumcised men after the catheter is inserted to prevent oedema of the glans and paraphimosis.

Documentation In the notes be sure to document the indication for catheterization, size of catheter, whether insertion was difficult or straightforward, any complications, residual volume, and colour of urine. It is good practice to document that the foreskin has been replaced. Sign with your name, date, and designation.

Suprapubic catheterization Sterile technique required. ▶Absolutely contraindicated unless there is a large bladder palpable or visible on ultrasound, because of the risk of bowel perforation. Be wary, particularly if there is a history of abdominal or pelvic surgery. Suprapubic catheter insertion is high risk and you should be trained before attempting it, speak to the urologists first.

Self-catheterization

This is a good, safe way of managing chronic retention from a neuropathic bladder (eg in multiple sclerosis, diabetic neuropathy, spinal tumour, or trauma). Never consider a patient in difficulties from a big residual volume to be too old, young, or disabled to learn. 5yr-old children can learn the technique, and can have their lives transformed—so motivation may be excellent. There may be fewer UTIs as there is no residual urine—and less reflux obstructive uropathy. Assessing suitability entails testing sacral dermatomes: a 'numb bum' implies ↓sensation of a full bladder; higher sensory loss may mean catheterization will be painless. Get help from your continence adviser who will be in a position to teach the patient or carer that catheterizations must be gentle (the catheter is of a much smaller calibre), particularly if sensation is lacking, and must number >4/d ('always keep your catheter with you; don't wait for an urge before catheterizing'). See fig 18.4.

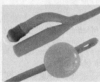

Fig 18.2 A size 14F latex Foley catheter with the balloon inflated via the topmost port of the outer end (green).
© Dr Tom Turmezei (not to scale).

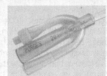

Fig 18.3 The external end of a size 20F 3-way catheter. The lowest port is for the bladder irrigation fluid and the uppermost port (yellow) is for balloon inflation.
© Dr Tom Turmezei (not to scale).

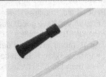

Fig 18.4 A size 10F catheter for self-catheterization. They are usually smaller than indwelling catheters, eg 10F compared to 14F. Note that this catheter also has no balloon.
© Dr Tom Turmezei (not to scale).

'The catheter is not draining ...'

You will be asked to check catheters that are not draining. Check the fluid chart and the patient:

• **Previously good output, now anuric** Blocked catheter until proven otherwise. Was the urine clear previously or bloodstained? Consider flushing the catheter: with aseptic technique flush and withdraw 20mL of sterile 0.9% saline with a bladder syringe. This may get the flow going again. A 3-way catheter may be needed if there is clot or debris retention. If it blocks again, replace it. Repeated flushes lead to infection.
• **Slow decline in urine output over several hours** In a dehydrated/post-op patient a fluid challenge of 500mL STAT (250mL if cardiac comorbidity) may help, come back and check the response in 30min. Check all other parameters (eg pulse, BP, CVP) and increase rate of background IV fluids if appropriate. ▶▶Acute kidney injury (p294): if urine output has tailed off and now stopped, the cause is often renal hypoperfusion (ie pre-renal failure), but consider other factors, eg nephrotoxic drugs.
• **Catheter is bypassing** A condom catheter may be more appropriate.
• **Catheter has dislodged into the proximal (prostatic) urethra** Possible even if the balloon is fully inflated. Consider this if a flush enters but cannot be withdrawn. If the patient still needs a catheter then replace it, consider a larger size.
• **The catheter has perforated the lower urinary tract on insertion and is not lying in the bladder or urethra** ▶▶If suspected, call the urologists immediately.

Remember: urine output should be >400mL in 24h or >0.5mL/kg/h (p574).

Trial without catheter (TWOC)

When it is time to remove a catheter, the possibility of urinary retention must be considered. Remove the catheter first thing one morning. If retention does occur, insert a long-term catheter (eg silicone), consider an α-blocker (p634), and arrange urology TWOC clinic follow-up.

Draining ascites

For patients with refractory or recurrent ascites that is symptomatic, it is possible to drain the ascites using a long pig-tail catheter. Paracentesis in such patients even in the presence of spontaneous bacterial peritonitis may be safe. Learn at the bedside from an expert.

Contraindications (these are relative, not absolute) End-stage cirrhosis; coagulopathy; hyponatraemia ($\leq$126mmol/L); sepsis. The main complication of the procedure is severe hypovolaemia secondary to re-accumulation of the ascites, so intravascular replenishment with a plasma expander is required. For smaller volumes, eg less than 5L, 500mL of 5% human albumin or Gelofusine® would be sufficient. For volumes over 5L, reasonable replacement would be 100mL 20% human albumin IV for each 1–3L of ascites drained (check your local policy). You may need to call the haematology lab to request this in advance.

Procedure Requires sterile technique.
- Ensure you have good IV access—eg 18G cannula in the antecubital fossa.
- Explain the procedure including the risks of infection, bleeding, hyponatraemia, renal impairment, and damage to surrounding structures (such as liver, spleen, and bowel), and obtain consent from the patient. Serious complications occur in less than 1 in 1000 patients. Ask the patient to empty their bladder.
- Examine the abdomen carefully, evaluating the ascites and checking for organomegaly. Mark where you are going to enter. If in doubt, ask the radiology department to ultrasound the abdomen and mark a spot for drainage. Approach from the left side unless previous local surgery/stoma prevents this—call a senior for support and advice if this is the case.
- Prepare a tray with 2% chlorhexidine solution, sterile drapes, 1% lidocaine, syringes, needles, sample bottles, and your drain. Clean the abdomen thoroughly and place sterile drapes, ensure you maintain sterile technique throughout. Infiltrate the local anaesthetic.
- Perform an ascitic tap (p749) first so that you know you are in the correct place: remove 20mL fluid for MC&S.
- Away from the patient, carefully thread the catheter over the (large and long) needle using the guide so that the pig-tail has been straightened out. Remove the guide.
- With the left hand hold the needle ~2.5cm (1 inch) from the tip—this will stop it from advancing too far (and from performing an aortic biopsy). With the right hand, hold the other end.
- Gently insert the needle perpendicular to the skin at the site of the ascitic tap up to your hold with your left hand—ascites should now drain easily. If necessary, advance the needle and catheter a short distance until good flow is achieved.
- Advance the catheter over the needle with your left hand, keeping the needle in exactly the same place with your right hand. ▶Do not re-advance the needle because it will go through the curled pig-tail and do not withdraw it because you won't be able to thread in the catheter.
- When fully inserted, remove the needle, connect the catheter to a drainage bag (keep it below the level of the abdomen), and tape it down securely to the skin.
- The patient should stay in bed as the ascites drains.
- Document clearly in the notes the indication for the procedure, that consent was obtained, clotting and U&E checked pre-procedure, how much lidocaine was required, how much fluid was removed for investigations, and whether there were any complications to the procedure.
- Replenish intravascular volume with human albumin (see 'Contraindications' earlier in topic).
- Ask the nursing staff to remove the catheter after 6h or after a predetermined volume has been drained (up to 20L can come off in 6h) and document this clearly in the medical notes. Drains are removed after 4–6h to prevent infection.
- Check U&E after the procedure and re-examine the patient.

Diagnostic taps

If you are unsure whether a drain is needed, a diagnostic tap can be helpful. Whatever fluid you are sampling, a green needle carries far less risk than a formal drain. It also allows you to decide whether a drain is required.

Ascites may be sampled to give a cytological or bacterial diagnosis, eg to exclude spontaneous bacterial peritonitis (SBP; p272). Before starting, know the patient's platelets + clotting times. If they are abnormal, seek help before proceeding.

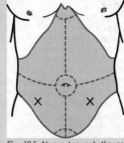

- Place the patient flat and tap out the ascites, marking a point where fluid has been identified, avoiding vessels, stomas, and scars (adhesions to the anterior abdominal wall). The left side may be safer—less chance of nicking liver (fig 18.5).

Fig 18.5 Always tap out the ascites, but aim approximately for 5cm medial to and superior to the anterior superior iliac spine. If in doubt, ask for an ultrasound to mark the spot.

- Clean the skin. Infiltrate some local anaesthetic, eg 1% lidocaine (p571).
- Insert a 21G needle on a 20mL syringe into the skin and advance while aspirating until fluid is withdrawn, try to obtain 60mL of fluid.
- Remove the needle, apply a sterile dressing.
- Send fluid to microbiology (15mL) for microscopy and culture, biochemistry (5mL for protein, see p176), and cytology (40mL). Call microbiology to forewarn them if urgent analysis of the specimen is required.

Diagnostic aspiration of a pleural effusion

- If not yet done, a CXR may help evaluate the side and size of the effusion.
- Ideally use US guidance at the bedside (↑chance of successful aspirate and ↓chance of organ puncture). If this is unavailable, ask an ultrasonographer to mark a spot, or percuss the upper border of the pleural effusion and choose a site 1 or 2 intercostal spaces below it (usually posteriorly or laterally).
- Clean the area around the marked spot with 2% chlorhexidine solution.
- Infiltrate down to the pleura with 5–10mL of 1% lidocaine.
- Attach a 21G needle to a syringe and insert it just above the upper border of the rib below the mark to avoid the neurovascular bundle (fig 18.6). Aspirate whilst advancing the needle. Draw off 10–30mL of pleural fluid. Send fluid to the lab for chemistry (protein, glucose, pH, LDH); bacteriology (microscopy and culture, auramine stain, TB culture); cytology, and, if indicated, amylase and immunology (rheumatoid factor, antinuclear antibodies, complement).
- ►►If you cannot obtain fluid with a 21G needle, seek help.
- If any cause for concern, arrange a repeat CXR.

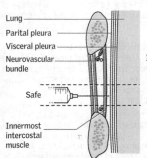
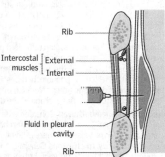

Lung
Parital pleura
Visceral pleura
Neurovascular bundle
Safe
Innermost intercostal muscle

Rib
Intercostal muscles { External / Internal }
Fluid in pleural cavity
Rib

Fig 18.6 Safe approach to entering the pleura by the intercostal route.

18 Practical procedures

Indications

- Pneumothorax (p798): ventilated; tension; persistent/recurrent despite aspiration (eg <24h after 1st aspiration); large 2nd spontaneous pneumothorax if >50yrs old.
- Malignant pleural effusion, empyema, or complicated parapneumonic effusion.
- Pleural effusion compromising ventilation, eg in ICU patients.
- Traumatic haemopneumothorax.
- Post-operatively: eg thoracotomy; oesophagectomy; cardiothoracic surgery.

▶Pleural effusions are best drained under US guidance using a Seldinger technique. This technique is also used for pneumothoraces (except in traumatic or post-operative situations) without US guidance; for this reason it is detailed here.

Sterile procedure

- Identify the point for drainage. In effusions, this should be done with US, ideally under direct guidance or with a marked spot. For pneumothoraces, check the drainage point from CXR/CT/examination.
- Preparation: trolley with dressing pack; 2% chlorhexidine; needles; 10mL syringes; 1% lidocaine; scalpel; suture; Seldinger chest drain kit; underwater drainage bottle; connection tubes; sterile H_2O; dressings. Incontinence pad under patient.
- Choose insertion site: 4th–6th intercostal space, anterior- to mid-axillary line—the 'safe triangle' (see BOX 'The "safe triangle" for insertion' and fig 18.7). A more posterior approach, eg the 7th space posteriorly, may be required to drain a loculated effusion (under direct US visualization) and occasionally the 2nd intercostal space in the mid-clavicular line may be used for apical pneumothoraces—however, both approaches tend to be less comfortable.
- Maintain sterile technique—clean and place sterile drapes. Scrub for insertion.
- Prepare your underwater drain by filling the bottle to the marked line with sterile water. Ensure this is kept sterile until you need it.
- Infiltrate down to pleura with 10mL of 1% lidocaine and a 21G needle. Check that air/fluid can be aspirated from the proposed insertion site; if not, do not proceed.
- Attach the Seldinger needle to the syringe containing 1–2mL of sterile saline. The needle is bevelled and will direct the guidewire; in general, advance bevel up for pneumothoraces, bevel down for effusions.
- Insert the needle gently, aspirating constantly. When fluid/air is obtained in the syringe, stop, note insertion depth from the markings on the Seldinger needle. Remove syringe, thread the guidewire through the needle. Remove the needle and clamp the guidewire to the sterile drapes to ensure it does not move. Using the markings on the Seldinger needle, move the rubber stops on the dilators to the depth noted earlier, to prevent the dilator slipping in further than intended.
- Make a nick in the skin where the wire enters, and slide the dilators over the wire sequentially from smallest to largest to enlarge the hole, keep gauze on hand. Slide the Seldinger drain over the wire into the pleural cavity. Remove the wire and attach a 3-way tap to the drain, then connect to the underwater drainage bottle.
- Suture the drain in place using a drain stitch—make a stitch in the skin close to the drain site, tie this fairly loosely with a double knot. Then tie the suture to the drain. It is usually best to be shown this before attempting it for yourself. Dress the drain, and ensure it is well taped down.
- Check that the drain is swinging (effusion) or bubbling (pneumothorax) and ensure the water bottle remains below the level of the patient at all times. If the drain needs to be lifted above the patient, clamp it briefly. ▶You should never clamp chest drains inserted for pneumothoraces. Clamping for pleural effusions can control the rate of drainage and prevent expansion pulmonary oedema.
- Request a CXR to check the position of the drain.

Removal In pneumothorax Consider when drain is no longer bubbling and CXR shows re-inflation. Give analgesia beforehand, eg morphine. Smartly withdraw during expiration or Valsalva. There is no need to clamp the drain beforehand as re-insertion is unlikely. **In effusions** Generally the drain can be removed when drainage is <200mL/24h, but for cirrhotic hydrothoraces the chest drain is treated similarly to the ascitic drain (p748) with HAS supplementation and removal at 4–6h.

The 'safe triangle' for insertion of a chest drain

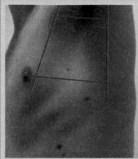

Fig 18.7 The safe 'triangle' is not really a triangle, as the axilla cuts off the point of the triangle. Draw a line along the lateral border of pectoralis major, a line along the anterior border of latissimus dorsi, and a line superior to the horizontal level of the nipple. The apex of the triangle is the axilla. Often chest drains are inserted directly under ultrasound guidance, or with a pre-marked spot; however, in an emergency or for aspiration, the landmarks of the safe triangle are important to know.

Complications
- Thoracic or abdominal organ injury. • Lymphatic damage ∴ chylothorax.
- Damage to long thoracic nerve of Bell ∴ wing scapula. • Rarely, arrhythmia.

Watch out for
- Retrograde flow back into the chest.
- Persistent bubbling—there may be a continual leak from the lung.
- Blockage of the tube from clots or kinking—no swinging or bubbling.
- Malposition—check position with CXR.

Relieving a tension pneumothorax

Symptoms Acute respiratory distress, chest pain, ►► respiratory arrest.

Signs Hypotension; distended neck veins; asymmetrical lung expansion; trachea and apex deviated away from side of reduced air entry and hyperresonance to percussion. ►► There is no time for a CXR (but see fig 16.44, p733).

Aim To release air from the pleural space. In a tension pneumothorax, air is drawn into the intrapleural space with each breath, but cannot escape due to a valve-like effect of the tiny flap in the parietal pleura. The increasing pressure progressively embarrasses the heart and the other lung.

►►100% oxygen

Procedure
- Insert a large-bore IV cannula (eg Venflon®) usually through the 2nd intercostal space in the midclavicular line or the 'safe triangle' for chest drain insertion (see BOX 'The "safe triangle" for insertion'). Remove the stylet, allowing the trapped air to escape, usually with an audible hiss. This converts the tension pneumothorax to an open pneumothorax. Tape securely. • Don't recover the cannula as tensioning will recur.
- Proceed to formal chest drain insertion (p750).

Aspiration of a pneumothorax

Identify the 2nd intercostal space in the midclavicular line (or 4th–6th intercostal space in the midaxillary line) and infiltrate with 1% lidocaine down to the pleura overlying the pneumothorax.
- Insert a 16G cannula into the pleural space. Remove the needle and connect the cannula to a 3-way tap and a 50mL syringe. Aspirate up to 2.5L of air (50mL × 50). Stop if resistance is felt, or if the patient coughs excessively.
- Request a CXR to confirm resolution of the pneumothorax. If successful, consider discharging the patient and repeating the CXR after 24h to exclude recurrence, and again after 7–10d. Advise to avoid air travel for 6 weeks after a normal CXR. Diving should be permanently avoided.
- If aspiration is unsuccessful (in a significant, symptomatic pneumothorax), insert an intercostal drain (p750).

18 Practical procedures

Contraindications • Bleeding diathesis. • Cardiorespiratory compromise. • Infection at site of needle insertion. Most importantly: ▶▶↑ICP (suspect if very severe headache, ↓level of consciousness with falling pulse, rising BP, vomiting, focal neurology, or papilloedema)—LP in these patients will cause coning, so unless it is a routine procedure, eg for known idiopathic intracranial hypertension, obtain a CT prior to LP. CT is not infallible, so be sure your indication for LP is strong.

Method Explain to the patient what sampling CSF entails, why it is needed, that co-operation is vital, and that they can communicate with you at all stages.
• Place the patient on their left side, with the back on the edge of the bed, fully flexed (knees to chin). A pillow under the head and another between the knees may keep them more stable.
• Landmarks: plane of iliac crests through the level of L3/4 (fig 18.8). In adults, the spinal cord ends at the L1/2 disc (fig 18.9). Mark L3/4 intervertebral space (or one space below, L4/5), eg by a gentle indentation of a needle cap on the overlying skin (better than a ballpoint pen mark, which might be erased by the sterilizing fluid).
• Use aseptic technique (mask, gloves, gown) and 2% chlorhexidine in 70% alcohol to clean the skin, allow to dry, and then place sterile drapes.
• Open the spinal pack. Assemble the manometer and 3-way tap. Have three plain sterile tubes and one fluoride tube (for glucose) ready.
• Using a 25G (orange) needle, raise a bleb of local anaesthetic, then use a 21G (green) needle to infiltrate deeper.
• Wait 1min, then insert spinal needle (22G, stilette in place) perpendicular to the body, through your mark, *aiming slightly up towards the umbilicus*. Feel resistance of spinal ligaments, and then the dura, then a 'give' as the needle enters the subarachnoid space. NB: keep the bevel of the needle facing up, parallel with dural fibres.
• Withdraw stilette. Check CSF fills needle and attach manometer (3-way tap turned off towards you) to measure 'opening' pressure.
• Catch fluid in numbered bottles (to volume required, mark tubes in advance).
• Remove needle and apply dressing. Document the procedure clearly in the notes including CSF appearance and opening pressure (in cmH$_2$O).
• Send CSF promptly for *microscopy*, *culture*, *protein*, *lactate*, and *glucose* (do plasma glucose too)—call the lab to let them know. If applicable, also send for: cytology, fungal studies, TB culture, virology (± herpes and other PCR), syphilis serology, oligoclonal bands (+ serum sample for comparison) if multiple sclerosis suspected. Is there xanthochromia (p474)?
• If you fail; ask for help—try with the patient sitting (but opening pressure is unreliable) or with radiological guidance.

CSF composition Normal values Lymphocytes <5/mm³; no polymorphs; protein <0.4g/L; glucose >2.2mmol/L (or ≥50% plasma level); pressure <200mm CSF. **In meningitis** See p806. **In multiple sclerosis** See p492.

Bloody tap This is an artefact due to piercing a blood vessel, which is indicated (unreliably) by fewer red cells in successive bottles, and no yellowing of CSF (xanthochromia). To estimate how many white cells (*W*) were in the CSF before the blood was added, use the following:

$$W = CSF\ WCC - [(blood\ WCC \times CSF\ RBC) \div blood\ RBC].$$

If the blood count is normal, the rule of thumb is to subtract from the total CSF WCC (per µL) one white cell for every 1000 RBCs. To estimate the true protein level, subtract 10mg/L for every 1000 RBCs/mm³ (be sure to do the count and protein estimation on the same bottle). NB: high protein levels in CSF make it appear yellow. **Subarachnoid haemorrhage** Xanthochromia (yellow supernatant on spun CSF). Red cells in equal numbers in all bottles (unreliable). RBCs will excite an inflammatory response (eg CSF WCC raised), but not marked after 48h. **Raised protein** Meningitis; MS; Guillain–Barré syndrome. **Very raised CSF protein** Spinal block; TB; or severe bacterial meningitis.

Complications

• Postdural puncture headache. • Infection. • Bleeding. • Cerebral herniation (rare, check for signs of ↑ICP before proceeding). • Minor/transient neurological symptoms, eg paraesthesia, radiculopathy.

Any change in lower body neurology after an LP (pain, weakness, sensory changes, bladder/bowel disturbance) should be treated as cauda equina compression (haematoma/abscess) until proven otherwise. Obtain an urgent MRI spine.

Post-LP brain MRI scans often show diffuse meningeal enhancement with gadolinium. This is thought to be a reflection of increased blood flow secondary to intracranial hypotension. Interpret these scans with caution and in the context of the patient's clinical situation. Ensure the reason for the scan and current neurological examination are discussed with the radiologist pre-procedure.

Post-LP headache

Risk 10–30%, typically occurring within 24h of LP, resolution over hours to 2wks (mean: 3–4d). Patients describe a constant, dull ache, more frontal than occipital. The most characteristic symptom is of positional exacerbation—worse when upright. There may be mild meningism or nausea. The pathology is thought to be continued leakage of CSF from the puncture site and intracranial *hypo*tension, though there may be other mechanisms involved.

Prevention Use the smallest spinal needle that is practical (22G) and keep the bevel aligned as described on p752. Blunt needles (more expensive) can reduce risk and are recommended (ask an anaesthetist about supply); however, collection of CSF takes too long (>6min) if needles smaller than 22G are used. Before withdrawing the needle, reinsert the stilette.

Treatment Despite years of anecdotal advice to the contrary, none of the following has ever been shown to be a risk factor: position during or after the procedure; hydration status before, during, or after; amount of CSF removed; immediate activity or rest post-LP. Time is a consistent healer. For severe or prolonged headaches, ask an anaesthetist about a blood patch. This is a careful injection of 20mL of autologous venous blood into the adjacent epidural space (said to 'clog up the hole'). Immediate relief occurs in 95%.

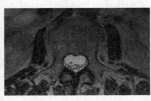

Fig 18.8 Defining the 3rd–4th lumbar vertebral interspace.
Adapted with permission from Vakil *et al., Diagnosis and Management of Medical Emergencies*, 1977. Oxford University Press.

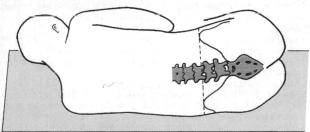

Fig 18.9 Axial T2-weighted MRI of the lumbar spine. The conus ends at the L1/L2 level with continuation of the cauda equina. Lumbar puncture below the L2 level will not damage the cauda equina as the nerve roots will part around an LP needle.

Image courtesy of Norwich Radiology Dept.

18 Practical procedures

▶Do not wait for a crisis before familiarizing yourself with the defibrillator, as there are several types. All hospitals should include this information in your induction but check how the machine on your ward works.

Indications To restore sinus rhythm if VF/VT; AF, flutter, or supraventricular tachycardias if other treatments (p122) have failed, or there is haemodynamic compromise (p126 & p790). This may be done as an emergency, eg VF/VT, or electively, eg AF.

Aim To completely depolarize the heart using a direct current.

Procedure ▶▶*For VF/pulseless VT follow the ALS algorithm on p878 and call the arrest team!*
- Unless critically unwell, conscious patients require a general anaesthetic or monitored heavy sedation.
- If elective cardioversion of AF, ensure adequate anticoagulation beforehand.

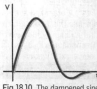
Fig 18.10 The dampened sine monophasic waveform.

- Almost all defibrillators are now paddle-free and use 'hands-free' pads instead (less chance of skin arc than jelly). Place the pads on chest, one over apex (p39) and one below right clavicle. The positions are often given by a diagram on the reverse of the pad.

Cardioversion Synchronize the shock with the rhythm by pressing the 'SYNC' button on the machine. This ensures the shock does not initiate a ventricular arrhythmia. However, this only works for cardioversion; if the sync mode is engaged in VF, the defibrillator will not discharge.

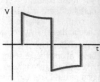
Fig 18.11 Rectilinear biphasic waveform with truncated exponential decay. Most new external defibrillators use this waveform.

- **Monophasic defibrillators** (fig 18.10) Set the energy level at 360J for VF/VT (▶▶arrest situation); 200J for AF; 50J for atrial flutter.
- **Biphasic defibrillators** (fig 18.11) Impedance is less with a biphasic shock and 120–200J is used for shocks for VF/VT. They use less energy and are just as effective as monophasic defibs in cardioversion. 120–200J will cardiovert most arrhythmias.
- **Automatic external defibrillators** (AEDs) Can be used by anyone who can turn them on and apply the pads. Follow the instructions given by the AED.

Shocking
1 Consider anticoagulation in AF (see p126).
2 Clearly state that you are charging the defibrillator.
3 Make sure no one else is touching the patient, the bed, or anything is in turn touching these.
4 Clearly state that you are about to shock the patient.
5 Give the shock. If there is a change in rhythm before you shock and the shock is no longer required, turn the dial to 'discharge'. Do not allow anyone to approach until the reading has dropped to 0J.
6 After a shock: ▶▶in resuscitation, resume CPR immediately and do not reassess rhythm until the end of the cycle (see p878, fig A3); in cardioversion, watch ECG; consider need to repeat the shock. Up to three are usual for AF/flutter.
7 Get an up-to-date 12-lead ECG.
▶In children, use 4J/kg in VF/VT; see *OHCS* p181.

Taking arterial blood gas (ABG) samples

Having an artery sampled is more unpleasant for the patient than venepuncture: explain that it is going to feel different and is for a different purpose (p154 for indications and analysis). The usual site is the radial artery at the wrist. ►*Check with the patient that they do not have an arteriovenous fistula for haemodialysis. Never, ever sample from a fistula.*

Procedure
* Get kit ready; include: portable sharps bin; pre-heparinized syringe; needle (blue size (23G) is good, although many syringes now come pre-made with needle); gloves; 2% chlorhexidine/70% alcohol swab; gauze; tape.
* Feel thoroughly for the best site. Look at both sides.
* Wipe with cleaning swab. Let the area dry. Get yourself comfortable.
* If the patient is drowsy or unconscious, ask an assistant to hold the hand and arm with the wrist slightly extended (fig 18.12).

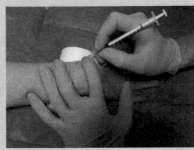

Fig 18.12 The ideal position for the wrist, slightly hyperextended, resting on an unopened litre bag of fluid or a bandage is ideal. In an unconscious patient or for arterial line insertion, taping the thumb to the bed can hold the wrist in the perfect position if you do not have an assistant.

* Before sampling, expel any excess heparin in the syringe. Infiltration over the artery with a small amount of 1% lidocaine (p571) through a 25G (orange) needle makes the procedure painless.
* Hold the syringe like a pen, with the needle bevel up. Let the patient know you are about to take the sample. Feel for the pulse with your other hand and enter at 45°, aiming beneath the finger you are feeling with.
* In most syringes, the plunger will move up on its own in a pulsatile manner if you are in the artery; rarely, entry into a vein next to the artery will give a similar result. Colour of the blood is little guide to its source.
* Allow the syringe to fill with 1–2mL, then remove the needle and apply firm pressure for 5 minutes (10 minutes if anticoagulated).
* Expel any air from the syringe as this will alter the oxygenation of the blood. Cap and label the sample, check the patient's temperature and FiO₂ (0.21 if on air). Take the sample to the nearest analysis machine or send it by express delivery to the lab (which may be by your own feet, get someone else to apply pressure) as it should be analysed within 15 minutes of sampling.
* Syringes and analysis machines differ, so get familiar with the local nuances.

The other site that is amenable to ABG sampling is the femoral artery (fig 18.13). Surprisingly this may be less uncomfortable as it is a relatively less sensitive area and because, when supine, the patient cannot see the needle and thus may feel less apprehensive. The brachial artery can also be used, but be aware that the median nerve sits closely on its medial side and it is an end-artery. Normal values: p737.

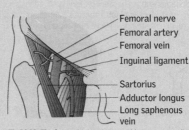

Femoral nerve
Femoral artery
Femoral vein
Inguinal ligament

Sartorius
Adductor longus
Long saphenous vein

Fig 18.13 The femoral artery is amenable to ABG sampling.

Cricothyroidotomy This is an emergency procedure to overcome airway obstruction above the level of the larynx. It should only be done in absolute 'can't intubate, can't ventilate' situations, ie where ventilation is impossible with a bag and mask (± airway adjuncts) and where there is an immediate threat to life. If not, call anaesthetics or ENT for immediate help.

Indications Upper airway obstruction when endotracheal intubation not possible, eg irretrievable foreign body; facial oedema (burns, angioedema); maxillofacial trauma; infection (epiglottitis).

Procedure Lie the patient supine with neck extended (eg pillow under shoulders) unless there is suspected cervical spine instability. Run your index finger down the neck anteriorly in the midline to find the notch in the upper border of the thyroid cartilage (the Adam's apple): just below this, between the thyroid and cricoid cartilages, is a depression—the cricothyroid membrane (fig 18.14). If you cannot feel the depression and it is an emergency, you can access the trachea directly approximately halfway between the cricoid cartilage and the suprasternal notch.

Ideally use a purpose-designed kit (eg QuickTrach®, MiniTrach®), all hospitals will stock one version. If no kit is available then a

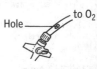

Thyroid cartilage

Cricothyroid membrane

Cricoid cartilage

Fig 18.14 The cricothyroid membrane.

cannula (needle cricothyroidotomy) can buy time, and in out-of-hospital situations a blade and empty biro case have saved lives. ▶▶Needle and kit cricothyroidotomies are temporary measures pending formal tracheostomy.

1 **Needle cricothyroidotomy** Pierce the membrane perpendicular to the skin with a large-bore cannula (14G) attached to a syringe: withdrawal of air confirms position; lidocaine may or may not be required. Slide cannula over needle at 45° to the skin superiorly in the sagittal plane. Use a Y-connector (fig 18.15) or improvise connection to O_2 supply at 15L/min: use thumb on Y-connector to allow O_2 in over 1s and CO_2 out over 4s ('transtracheal jet insufflation'). This is the preferred method in children <12yrs. This will only sustain life for 30–45min before CO_2 builds up. However, if the patient has a completely obstructed airway then they will not be able to exhale through this, and it will lead to cardiovascular compromise and pneumothoraces.

2 **Cricothyroidotomy kit** Most contain a guarded blade, and a large (4–6mm) shaped cannula (cuffed or uncuffed depending on brand) over an introducer, plus a connector and binding tape. The patient will have to be ventilated via a bag, as the resistance is too high to breathe spontaneously. This will sustain for 30–45min.

3 **Surgical cricothyroidotomy** Smallest tube for prolonged ventilation is 6mm. Introduce high-volume, low-pressure cuff tracheostomy tube through a horizontal incision in membrane. Take care not to cut the thyroid or cricoid cartilages.

Complications Local haemorrhage ± aspiration; posterior perforation of trachea ± oesophagus; subglottic stenosis; laryngeal stenosis if membrane over-incised in childhood; tube blockage; subcutaneous tunnelling; vocal cord paralysis or hoarseness (the recurrent laryngeal nerve runs superiorly in the tracheo-oesophageal groove).

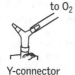

to O_2

Hole — to O_2

Hole — to O_2

Y-connector

2mL syringe

Intravenous
giving-set

Fig 18.15 Methods of providing oxygen.

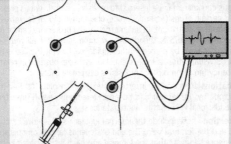

Fig 18.16 Emergency needle pericardiocentesis.

- Get your senior's help (for whom this page may serve as an *aide-memoire*).
- Equipment: 20mL syringe, long 18G cannula, 3-way tap, ECG monitor, skin cleanser. Use echo guidance if there is time.
- If time allows, use full aseptic technique, at a minimum clean skin with 2% chlorhexidine in 70% alcohol and wear sterile gloves, and, if conscious, use local anaesthesia and sedation, eg with slow IV midazolam: titrate up to 3.5–5mg—start with 2mg over 1min, 0.5–1mg in elderly (in whom the maximum dose is 3.5mg; inject at the rate of 2mg/min)—antidote: flumazenil 0.2mg IV over 15s, then 0.1mg every 60s, up to 1mg in total.
  ►*Ensure you have IV access and full resuscitation equipment to hand.*
- Introduce needle at 45° to skin just below and to left of xiphisternum, aiming for tip of left scapula (fig 18.16). Aspirate continuously and watch ECG. Frequent ventricular ectopics or an injury pattern (↓ST segment) on ECG imply that the myocardium has been breached—withdraw slightly. As soon as fluid is obtained through the needle, slide the cannula into place.
- Evacuate pericardial contents through the syringe and 3-way tap. Removal of only a small amount of fluid (eg 20mL) can produce marked clinical improvement. If you are not sure whether the fluid you are aspirating is pure blood (eg on entering a ventricle), see if it clots (heavily bloodstained pericardial fluid does not clot), or measure its PCV (though this may be difficult in the acute setting but some blood gas analysers may give this).
- You can leave the cannula *in situ* temporarily, for repeated aspiration. If there is re-accumulation, insert a drain but pericardiectomy may be needed.
- Send fluid for microscopy and culture, as needed, including tests for TB.

Complications Laceration of ventricle or coronary artery (± subsequent haemopericardium); aspiration of ventricular blood; arrhythmias (ventricular fibrillation); pneumothorax; puncture of aorta, oesophagus (± mediastinitis), or peritoneum (± peritonitis).

18 Practical procedures

Central venous cannulae may be inserted to measure central venous pressure (CVP), to administer certain drugs (eg amiodarone, chemotherapy), or for intravenous access (fluid, parenteral nutrition). In an emergency, the procedure can be done using the landmark method (p759), though NICE recommends that all routine internal jugular catheters should be placed with US guidance. Even if the line is not placed under direct US visualization, a look to check vessel size, position in relation to artery, and patency (no thrombus or stenosis) is extremely useful.

Contraindications Infection at insertion site is an absolute CI. Relative CIs include: coagulopathy; ipsilateral carotid endarterectomy; newly inserted cardiac pacemaker leads; local venous thrombosis/stenosis.

Sites of insertion These include the internal jugular vein (see p759 and p41), subclavian vein, and the femoral vein. The choice depends largely on operator experience, but evidence suggests that the femoral approach is associated with a higher rate of line infection and thrombosis. Overall, the internal jugular approach (with ultrasound guidance) is most commonly used and risks fewer complications than the subclavian. If possible, get written consent (p566). Check clotting and platelets.

Complications (~20%.) ▸Bleeding; arterial puncture/cannulation; AV fistula formation; air embolism; pneumothorax; haemothorax; chylothorax (lymph); phrenic nerve palsy (the right phrenic nerve passes over the brachiocephalic artery, posterior to the subclavian vein (fig 18.18)—hiccups may be a sign of injury); phlebitis; thrombus formation on tip or in vein (if high risk for thromboembolism, eg malignancy, consider anticoagulation, eg LMWH); bacterial colonization; cellulitis; sepsis (can be reduced by adherence to a strict aseptic technique; if taking blood cultures in a febrile patient with a central venous line, remember to take samples from the central line and from a peripheral vein).

Peripherally inserted central cannulas (PICC lines)
These are a good alternative to central lines, as they can stay *in situ* for up to 6 months, and provide access for blood sampling, fluids, antibiotics (allowing home IV therapy). They are placed using a Seldinger technique, puncturing the brachial or basilic vein then threading the line into the subclavian or superior vena cava. Because of the insertion site there is a much lower risk of pneumo- or haemothorax, but they are tricky to insert in an emergency.

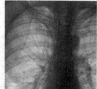

Removing central lines Should be done carefully with aseptic technique. Position the patient slightly head down, remove dressings, clean and drape the area, remove sutures. Ask the patient to inhale and hold their breath, then ▸breathe out smoothly while you are pulling the line out. This helps to prevent air emboli. Ask the patient to rehearse this sequence with you to ensure they have understood their role. Apply pressure for 5 minutes (longer if coagulopathic).

Fig 18.17 Right arm PICC with a wire still in the lumen. The tip lies in the SVC—ie good positioning for TPN or long-term antibiotic therapy. The tip of a Hickman line, for cytotoxic administration, is better in the right atrium, to avoid possible irritation of the SVC and consequent thrombosis or stenosis.
Image courtesy of Prof. Peter Scally.

The venous system at the thoracic outlet

When trying to judge the position of a central venous line tip on CXR (fig 18.17) it helps to know the anatomical landmarks of the venous system (fig 18.18). The subclavian veins join the internal jugular veins behind the sternoclavicular joints to form the brachiocephalic veins. These come together behind the right 1st sternocostal joint to form the superior vena cava (SVC), which runs from this point to the right 3rd sternocostal joint. The right atrium starts here.

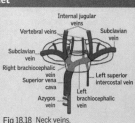

Fig 18.18 Neck veins.

Internal jugular Should be the approach of choice in a non-emergency situation. Ideally the right side as it offers a direct route to the heart and there is less chance of misplacement of the line compared to the left. The subclavian approach is trickier and best taught by an expert. Use US guidance if at all possible, ideally to insert the line under direct vision, but at least to define the anatomy. If possible, have the patient attached to a cardiac monitor in case of arrhythmias.

• Position the patient slightly head down to avoid air embolism and fill the veins to improve your chances of success. ▶This can compromise cardiac function and precipitate acute LVF so check if your patient has a cardiac history. Minimize the time the patient is head down; if they are unable to lie flat, consider a femoral approach. Turn their head slightly to the left.

• This should be a sterile procedure so use full aseptic technique (hat, mask, gloves, gown) and clean with 2% chlorhexidine in 70% isopropyl alcohol before draping. Ensure your equipment is prepared, flush the catheter lumens with saline.

• If US is unavailable, the *landmark procedure* can be used to identify insertion point—approximately at the junction of the two heads of sternocleidomastoid at about the level of the thyroid cartilage (fig 18.19). Feel gently for the carotid pulse, then infiltrate with 1% lidocaine just lateral to this. The vein is usually superficial (fig 18.20).

• Insert the introducer needle with a 5mL syringe attached, advance gently at a 45° angle, aiming for the ipsilateral nipple and aspirating continuously. If you are using US, watch the needle tip enter the vein, if the landmark approach keep your fingers on the carotid pulse.

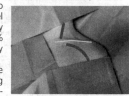
Fig 18.19 Position of internal jugular and subclavian veins (red) compared to the clavicle (yellow).

• As soon as blood is aspirated, lay down the US probe and hold the introducer needle in position, remove the syringe, and thread the guidewire through the needle. It should pass easily; if there is resistance try lowering the angle of the needle and gently advancing the wire. If the wire will not pass do not remove it alone, the tip can shear off and embolize; remove the needle with the wire, apply pressure, and attempt a second puncture.

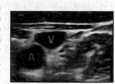
Fig 18.20 Vessels seen on ultrasound. The compressible vein is above the artery.

• If the wire threads easily, insert to 30cm (see markings on the wire), remove the needle keeping hold of the wire at all times. Make a nick in the skin with a scalpel at the insertion point, and gently thread the dilator over the wire. You do not need to insert the dilator far, only as far as the vein (you often feel a loss of resistance as the dilator enters the vein, so insert gently: a pneumothorax can result from enthusiastic dilating).

• Remove the dilator, keeping hold of the wire, thread the flushed catheter over the wire, then remove the wire. The line should sit at about 13cm on the right side (17cm on the left). Check you can aspirate blood from each lumen, then flush them.

• Suture the catheter in place (many have little 'wings' for suturing) and dress. Request a CXR to confirm position and exclude pneumothorax. The tip of the catheter should sit vertically in the SVC.

Femoral vein In an emergency situation where ultrasound is not easily accessible, if the patient is unable to lie flat, or where speed is of the essence, the femoral approach is often the safest, as there is no risk of pneumothorax or haemothorax and a much reduced risk of arrhythmia. The technique is similar to internal jugular, except the insertion point is just medial to the femoral artery at the groin crease.

Subclavian vein Should be taught by an expert and should ideally be carried out under US guidance. Some physicians prefer this approach, but even in experienced hands there is an ↑risk of complications compared to US-guided internal jugular lines.

Often it is wiser to liaise with a specialist pacing centre to arrange prompt, definitive pacing than to try temporary transvenous pacing, which often has complications (see later in topic) and therefore may delay a definitive procedure.

Possible indications in the acute phase of myocardial infarction
- **Complete AV block**
  - With inferior MI (right coronary artery occlusion) pacing may only be needed if symptomatic; spontaneous recovery may occur.
  - With anterior MI (representing massive septal infarction).
- **Second-degree block**
  - Wenckebach (p91; implies decremental AV node conduction; may respond to atropine in an inferior MI; pace if anterior MI).
  - Mobitz type 2 block is usually associated with distal fascicular disease and carries high risk of complete heart block, so pace in both types of MI.
- **First-degree block** Observe carefully: 40% develop higher degrees of block.
- **Bundle branch block** Pace prophylactically if evidence of trifascicular disease (p92) or non-adjacent bifascicular disease.
- **Sino-atrial disease + serious symptoms** Pace unless responds to atropine.

Other indications where temporary pacing may be needed
- Pre-op: if surgery is required in patients with type 2 or complete heart block (whether or not MI has occurred); do 24h ECG; liaise with the anaesthetist.
- Drug poisoning, eg with β-blockers, digoxin, or verapamil.
- Symptomatic bradycardia, uncontrolled by atropine or isoprenaline.
- Suppression of drug-resistant VT and SVT (overdrive pacing; do on ICU).
- Asystolic cardiac arrest with P-wave activity (ventricular standstill).
- During or after cardiac surgery—eg around the AV node or bundle of His.

Technique for temporary transvenous pacing Learn from an expert.
- **Preparation** Monitor ECG; have a defibrillator to hand, ensure the patient has peripheral access; check that a radiographer with screening equipment is present. If you are screening, wear a protective lead apron.
- **Insertion** Using an aseptic technique, place the introducer into the (ideally right) internal jugular vein (p759) or subclavian. If this is difficult, access to the right atrium can be achieved via the femoral vein. Pass the pacing wire through the introducer into the right atrium, ideally under radiological screening. It will either pass easily through the tricuspid valve or loop within the atrium. If the latter occurs, it is usually possible to flip the wire across the valve with a combined twisting and withdrawing movement (fig 18.21). Advance the wire slightly. At this stage the wire may try to exit the ventricle through the pulmonary outflow tract. A further withdrawing and rotation of the wire will aim the tip at the apex of the right ventricle. Advance slightly again to place the wire in contact with the endocardium. Remove any slack to ↓ risk of subsequent displacement.
- **Checking the threshold** Connect the wire to the pacing box and set the 'demand' rate slightly higher than the patient's own heart rate and the output to 3V. A paced rhythm should be seen. Find the pacing threshold by slowly reducing the voltage until the pacemaker fails to stimulate the tissue (pacing spikes are no longer followed by paced beats). The threshold should be less than 1V, but a slightly higher value may be acceptable if it is stable—eg after a large infarction.
- **Setting the pacemaker** Set the output to 3V or over 3 times the threshold value (whichever is higher) in 'demand' mode. Set the rate as required. Suture the wire to the skin, and fix with a sterile dressing.
- Check the position of the wire (and exclude pneumothorax) with a CXR.
- Recurrent checks of the pacing threshold are required over the next few days. The formation of endocardial oedema can raise the threshold by a factor of 2–3.

Complications Pneumothorax; sepsis; cardiac perforation; pacing failure: from loss of capture, loss of electrical continuity in pacing circuit, or electrode displacement.

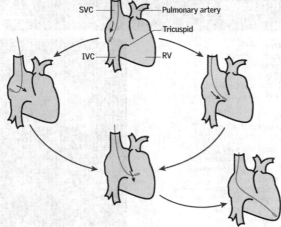

Fig 18.21 Siting a temporary cardiac pacemaker.

Non-invasive transcutaneous cardiac pacing

This method (performed through a defibrillator with external pacing facility) has the advantages of being quicker, less risky than the transvenous route, and easier to perform. Its main disadvantage is the pain caused by skeletal muscle contraction in the non-sedated patient. Indications for pacing via the transcutaneous route are as p760, *plus* if transvenous pacing (or someone able to perform it) is unavailable or will be delayed in an emergency situation.

- Give sedation and analgesia, eg midazolam + morphine IV titrated to effect.
- Clipping chest hair may help improve electrical contact; ▶don't shave the skin, as nicks can predispose to electrical burns. Ensure the skin is dry.
- Almost all modern transcutaneous devices can function through defibrillation 'hands-free' pads, and so these can be applied as for defibrillation (p754). If necessary, the pads can be placed in an AP position: anteriorly over the V_2–V_3 electrode position and posteriorly at the same level, just below the scapula.
- Select 'demand' mode, (which synchronizes the stimulus with the R wave, so avoiding pacing on the T wave—which can provoke VF or VT) and adjust the ECG gain so that QRS complexes can be seen.
- Select an appropriate pacing rate: eg 60–90bpm in an adult.
- Set the pacing current at the lowest setting and turn on the pacemaker.
- Increase the pacing current until electrical capture occurs (normally from 50–100mA), which can be confirmed by seeing a wide QRS complex and a T wave on the trace (ventricular electrical capture).
- There will be some interference from skeletal muscle contraction on the ECG trace, as well as possible artefact, which could be mistaken for a QRS complex. The absence of a T wave in the former is an important discriminator between the two.
- CPR can continue with the pads in place, though only when the pacing unit is *off*.
- Once adequate cardiac output has been maintained, seek expert help, and arrange transvenous pacing.

19 Emergencies

Contents

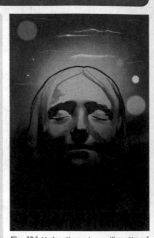

Fig 19.1 Under the unique silhouette of lattice work girders destined to become the Eiffel Tower, an unknown woman's body was pulled from the River Seine. The mortuarist was so struck by the serene face of *l'inconnue de la Seine* (the unknown woman of the Seine) that he preserved her image as a plaster mask. This mask's beauty went on to inspire artwork, poetry, and literature throughout late 19th-century France. The mask was also mass-produced, bringing her tranquil allure into homes across the world. And so *l'inconnue de la Seine* looked over the lives of Norwegian toy-maker Asmund Laerdal and his family. And her gaze remained timelessly untroubled even when it witnessed the near-drowning of Laerdal's son. Inspired by this near-tragedy, Laerdal worked with pioneers of CPR to produce a mannikin for resuscitation training, giving his Resusci-Anne the face that had witnessed the return of his son's life from death. Although too late to save her own life, her face would look upon millions of others as they gained the skills needed to save lives. But why does her mask remain with us? Do we continue to be damsels in distress seeking heroism against the grain of contemporary society? Or is this peaceful face simply what we need death to look like, even in simulation? For her serenity belies the brutal reality of many resuscitation scenarios. But rather than directing us to shield behind our own masks when facing the reality of death, her face should better serve to remind us of the patient's story behind theirs.

Artwork by Gillian Turner.

We thank Paul Cacciottolo, Simon Campbell, Marc Edwards, Thomas Hughes, Michael Matheou, Rustam Rea, Nicola Ronan, and Helen Turner, our Specialist Readers for this chapter.

Introduction to emergencies

SBAR facilitates clear communication between professionals, offering useful focus in emergent situations:

Situation Your first shift in a new hospital (a night-shift, of course).

Background Some people thrive in the adrenaline bath of acuity and unexpected presentations within the emergency department, seeing a patient recover (or not) from the brink of death. Others find the perpetual storm of severe disease nauseating, anxious about risk and error when time, rather than cerebration, is of the essence. Recognize where you sit on this spectrum and try to develop the skills you need to act and think. Or make sure you know where to find them in your team.

Assessment Though expectations of medicine may dictate otherwise, it is disease that kills patients, not doctors (for those that cause deliberate harm are not doctors). Reflect and learn. Ask: what could you do differently next time? Were there any useful predictors before the emergency? When did you ask for help? When should you have asked for help? Such questions do not need to be written down as part of formal learning and appraisal (though they can be); rather ask and answer them honestly of yourself, for yourself, and for your patients, in every emergency.

Recommendation Use your team. Observe senior clinicians in emergency situations. Often, the best leaders are those who have learned to stand back and maintain an overview of the whole situation. Look after yourself. We are not superheroes and capes do not comply with infection control policies. Make the patient central to the process. Communicate. What do they want? What are their priorities? Be honest about prognosis. Do not offer futile treatments including resuscitation. Electricity will not treat a heart that has failed due to an irreversible disease. Recognizing dying may be a challenge (for both doctor and patient); providing comfort, honesty, and a listening ear is not.

The ABCDE approach to an emergency

Airway *Assessment:* protect the cervical spine if injury is possible. Look for obstruction. No breath sounds at the mouth/nose = complete obstruction. Diminished/noisy air entry = partial obstruction. Paradoxical chest and abdominal movements may be present ('see-saw' respiration). Depressed consciousness can lead to airway obstruction. *Management:* establish a patent airway: airway opening manoeuvres, suction, oropharyngeal or nasopharyngeal airway. Tracheal intubation if these fail.

Breathing *Assessment:* accessory muscle use, cyanosis, tracheal position, respiratory rate, oxygen saturation (will not detect hypercapnia), bilateral and symmetrical chest expansion, percussion, auscultation. Abdominal distension may worsen respiratory distress. *Management:* if no respiratory effort, treat as cardiac arrest (see p878, fig A3). High-concentration O_2 to keep O_2 saturation 94–98% (88–92% if COPD). If breathing inadequate: ventilate (bag-mask, non-invasive/invasive). Treat cause: eg asthma, tension pneumothorax, pulmonary oedema.

Circulation *Assessment:* peripheral perfusion: colour, temperature, capillary refill time (normal <2s). Heart rate, peripheral and central pulse, BP, cardiac auscultation, oliguria (if catheterized). Any haemorrhage? *Management:* if no cardiac output, treat as cardiac arrest (see p878, fig A3). Replace lost fluid or blood, and stop further loss. Treat cause, eg sepsis, ACS, tamponade, arrhythmia.

Disability *Assessment:* AVPU score: **A**lert? responds to **V**oice? to **P**ain? **U**nresponsive? GCS if time allows. Pupils: size, symmetry, reactions. Blood glucose. *Management:* protect airway. Treat cause, eg hypoxia, hypercapnia, hypotension, hypoglycaemia, sepsis, stop sedative medication.

Exposure Look for cause, eg bleeding, melaena, rash, injury. Maintain dignity and temperature.

Exclude any potentially life-threatening causes. Then consider other potential causes (**fig 19.2**). Chest pain warrants a diagnosis, not just the exclusion of ACS and PE. A dull/heavy pain, radiation to the jaw, arm, or epigastrium, and pain associated with exertion suggest cardiac pain, thought it rarely comes as neatly packaged as this. For the full assessment of cardiac pain, see p94 and p118.

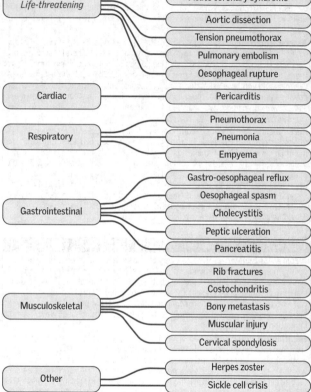

Fig 19.2 Differential diagnosis for chest pain.

Key investigations
- Troponin (p114), ECG, CXR.
- D-dimer only if low probability of venous thromboembolism. See modified Wells score for PE, p187.

Beware
- Atypical presentations are common.
- Chest wall tenderness does not always exclude heart/lung pathology.
- Advise patients to return or seek further advice if pain changes/worsens/fails to settle.

There may not be time to ask, or the patient may not be able to give you a history in acute breathlessness. This in itself is an assessment of severity:
• Inability to complete sentences in one breath = severe breathlessness.
• Inability to speak/impaired conscious level = life-threatening.
• Collateral history of respiratory disease and anaphylaxis can be helpful but do not delay. Examination findings help determine cause (fig 19.3).

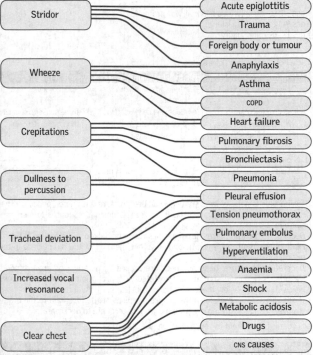

Fig 19.3 Emergency presentations of breathlessness and their potential differentials.

Key investigations
• ABG if O₂ saturations <94%.
• ECG: right heart strain, LVH, ACS?
• CXR.
• Bloods determined by likely cause: FBC, D-dimer (only if low probability of venous thromboembolism, see p187), sepsis screen, glucose, pH, lactate, drug screen.

This gives a reliable, objective way of recording the conscious state of a person. It was initially developed for use after head injury, but is now widely used in all patients with impaired consciousness for initial and continuing assessment. It also has prognostic value. Three types of response are assessed: motor, verbal, and eye (table 19.1). The best response in each category (or best of any limb) is recorded. An overall score is made by summing the score in the three areas assessed.
• GCS 3: the lowest possible score possible; no motor and verbal responses and no eye opening.
• GCS ≤8: severe injury, consider airway protection.
• GCS 9–12: moderate injury.
• GCS 13–15: minor injury.

Table 19.1 The Glasgow Coma Scale

Best motor response		Best verbal response		Eye opening	
6	Obeying commands	5	Oriented (time, place, person)	4	Spontaneous
5	Localizing to pain	4	Confused conversation	3	In response to speech
4	Withdrawing to pain	3	Inappropriate speech	2	In response to pain
3	Flexor response to pain	2	Incomprehensible sounds	1	None
2	Extensor response to pain	1	None		
1	No response to pain				

Adapted from 'Assessment of coma and impaired consciousness: a practical scale', Graham Teasdale and Bryan Jennett, *The Lancet*, Vol 304, No. 7872, 81–84 (1974), Elsevier.

Causing pain is not pleasant: try fingernail bed pressure with a pen/pencil, sternal pressure (not a rub), or suprascapular squeeze. Abnormal responses to pain may help to localize pathology:
• *Decorticate posture:* arms flexed on chest, thumbs tucked in a clenched fist, legs rigid in extension. CNS lesion/damage is above the level of the red nucleus in the midbrain.
• *Decerebrate posture:* head and neck are arched, arms and legs are extended, shoulder is adducted and internally rotated with pronation of the forearm. CNS lesion/damage is below the level of the red nucleus in the midbrain.[1]
• If CNS disease/compression advances from regions of the forebrain to the brainstem, abnormal posturing can progress from decorticate to decerebrate.

GCS scoring is different in young children; see *OHCS* p200.

AVPU

AVPU is a brief and easy tool used to rapidly assess conscious level, which is graded as A, V, P or U:
    A = **A**lert.
    V = responds to **V**ocal stimuli.
    P = responds to **P**ain.
    U = **U**nresponsive.

---

1 Red nucleus output reinforces upper limb antigravity flexion. When its output is damaged, the unregulated reticulospinal and vestibulospinal tracts reinforce extension tone of upper and lower limbs and a decerebrate posture results.

Assessment of awareness (the ability to perceive stimuli) and arousal (overall level or consciousness) helps to define the underlying CNS pathology:

1 Loss of awareness with normal arousal = diffuse, bilateral, cortical dysfunction.
2 Loss of arousal (which means awareness cannot be assessed) = damage to the ascending reticular activating system (ARAS) located throughout the brainstem from the medulla to the thalami. The brainstem can be affected directly (eg pontine haemorrhage) or indirectly (eg compression from transtentorial or cerebellar herniation secondary to a mass effect or oedema).

Systematic examination
- Level of consciousness: described objectively with GCS/AVPU.
- Respiratory pattern:
  - Cheyne-Stokes (periods of fast, shallow breathing followed by slow, heavier breathing and apnoea): brainstem lesion/compression.
  - Hyperventilation: hypoxia, acidosis, neurogenic (rare).
  - Apneustic breathing (deep inspiration, a pause in inspiration, then inadequate expiration): brainstem damage with poor prognosis.
- Eyes: almost all patients with ARAS pathology will have eye signs.
  1 *Visual fields:* in light coma, test fields with visual threat. No blink in one field suggests hemianopia and contralateral hemisphere lesion.
  2 *Pupils:*
  - Normal direct and consensual reflexes = intact midbrain.
  - Non-reactive (at midposition, 3–5mm) or irregular = midbrain lesion.
  - 'Fixed' = dilated and unreactive = IIIrd nerve compression/damage.
  - Small, reactive = pontine lesion ('pin-point pontine pupils'), or drugs, eg opioids.
  - Horner's syndrome (p48, fig 2.18) = ipsilateral lateral medulla or hypothalamus lesion, may precede uncal herniation.
  - Beware false signs: prosthetic eyes, glaucoma treatment.
  3 *Eye movements:*
  - Note resting position and spontaneous movement.
  - Vestibulo-ocular reflex (VOR). Test with *doll's-head manoeuvre* (normal if the eyes keep looking at the same point in space when the head is quickly moved laterally or vertically) or *ice water calorics* (normal if eyes deviate towards the cold ear with nystagmus to the other side). If present, the VOR exonerates most of the brainstem from the VIIth nerve nucleus (medulla) to the IIIrd (midbrain). *Do not move the head unless the cervical spine has been cleared.*
  4 *Fundi:* papilloedema, subhyaloid haemorrhage, hypertensive retinopathy, signs of other disease (eg diabetic retinopathy).
- Examine for CNS asymmetry (tone, spontaneous movements, reflexes). One way to test for hemiplegia in coma is to raise both arms together and compare how they fall under gravity. If one descends fast, like a lead weight, but the other descends more gracefully, you have found a valuable focal sign of cortical dysfunction. The same applies to the legs. Neurological exam should always be correlated to the clinical context.

19 Emergencies

Definition Unrousable unresponsiveness. Measure using *Glasgow Coma Scale (GCS)* or *AVPU* (p766).

Causes of impaired conscious level/coma
Metabolic
* Drugs, poisoning, eg carbon monoxide (p826), alcohol, tricyclic antidepressants.
* Hypoglycaemia (p818), hyperglycaemia, eg ketoacidosis (p816), or HHS (p818).
* Hypoxia, CO_2 narcosis, eg in COPD (p796).
* Sepsis (p772).
* Hypothermia (p830).
* Endocrine: hypothyroidism (p820), Addisonian crisis (p819).
* Hepatic/uraemic encephalopathy (p271, p294).

Central nervous system pathology
* Trauma (p812).
* Infection: meningitis (p806); encephalitis (p400, p808). *Tropical*: malaria (p412), typhoid, typhus, rabies, trypanosomiasis.
* Tumour: 1° or 2° (p524).
* Vascular: stroke (p466), subdural (p476), subarachnoid (p474), hypertensive encephalopathy (p110).
* Epilepsy: non-convulsive status (p488, p810), post-ictal.

Focused history
From family, ambulance staff, bystanders:
* Onset: abrupt (?seizure activity) or gradual onset.
* Surroundings: drug use, possible injury (stabilize cervical spine, *OHCS* p642), suicide note.
* Recent symptoms: headache, fever, vertigo, depression, vomiting, infection.
* Medical history: epilepsy, diabetes, hypertension, cancer, psychiatric, ENT (sinusitis, otitis), CNS disease/neurosurgery.
* Drug or toxin exposure (including alcohol and recreational drugs).
* Recent travel.

Examination
►Glasgow Coma Scale or AVPU (p766).
* Signs of trauma: haematoma, laceration, bruising, CSF/blood in nose or ears, fracture 'step' deformity of skull, subcutaneous emphysema, 'panda eyes'.
* Temperature.
* Skin: cyanosis, pallor, rash (meningitis, typhus), needle marks.
* Mouth/breath: tongue-biting, alcohol, hepatic fetor, ketosis, uraemia.
* Stigmata of other disease: jaundice, spider naevi, clubbing, cyanosis, myxoedema.
* Neurological features:
  * Opisthotonus (fig 9.47, p432): meningitis, tetanus.
  * Decerebrate/decorticate posture (p766).
  * Pupils (p767): size, reactivity, gaze.
  * Meningism (p452, p806): neck stiffness (►do *not* move neck unless cervical spine is cleared), rash.
  * Focal neurological signs.
* Cardiovascular examination: heart rate and rhythm, BP, murmurs.
* Respiratory examination: trachea, air entry and symmetry, wheeze, signs of consolidation or collapse.
* Abdomen/rectal examination: organomegaly, ascites, bruising, peritonism, melaena.
* Are there any other foci of infection: abscess, bite, middle ear infection?

Immediate management See fig 19.4.

If the diagnosis is unclear
* Review any treatable causes: eg hypoglycaemia, ↑pCO_2, sepsis.
* Biochemistry, haematology, thick films, blood cultures, blood ethanol, drug screen.
* Urgent CT head. If normal, and no CI, proceed to LP.

▲ **Coma: immediate management**

If suspected or possible trauma, stabilize the cervical spine

Airway
Consider airway adjunct and/or intubation if GCS ≤8

Breathing
• Breathing pattern: Cheynes–Stokes, apneustic (p767)
• Oxygen saturation, respiratory rate, trachea, bilateral/symmetrical expansion
• Oxygen to target saturation 94-98% (88-92% if COPD)

Circulation
• Peripheral perfusion, heart rate and rhythm, BP, heart sounds
• IV access: circulatory support if indicated, eg volume depletion, sepsis

Disability
• AVPU (p766), GCS (p766)
• Pupils: size, symmetry, reactions
• Check blood glucose

Exposure
Full inspection and examination for possible cause: trauma, tongue-biting, incontinence, bleeding, skin changes/rash, neurological signs, foci of infection, drug/toxin

Treat
• Hypoglycaemia (<4.0mmol/L): 50–250mL 10% glucose IV
• Small pupils, RR <8, or possible opioid toxicity: naloxone 400mcg IV (or IM/SC)
• Non-convulsive seizures (p810)
• Possible Wernicke's encephalopathy (alcohol dependency, liver disease, head injury, trauma, acute illness): IV thiamine (Pabrinex®) (p700)

Investigations
• ABG, FBC, U&E, LFT, CRP, ethanol, toxin screen, drug concentrations
• Blood cultures, urine culture, consider malaria
• ECG, CXR, CT head

Reassess with collateral history, investigation results, and clinical response/change

Fig 19.4 The immediate management of coma.

The eyes have it
• Check the pupils every few minutes during assessment of the comatose patient.
• This is a quick way of finding a localizing sign (but remember that false localizing signs do occur).
• Pupil changes (eg the development of fixed and dilated pupils) might be the quickest way of finding out just how bad things are.

Definition

Circulatory failure resulting in inadequate organ perfusion.

Circulatory failure
* Systolic BP (SBP) <90mmHg.
* Mean arterial pressure (MAP) <65mmHg.

Hypoperfusion
* Serum lactate >2mmol/L.
* Oliguria: urine output <0.5mL/kg/h.

Signs

↓GCS/agitation, pallor, cool peripheries/mottled skin, tachycardia, hypotension, slow capillary refill, tachypnoea, oliguria.

Aetiology

MAP = cardiac output (CO) × systemic vascular resistance (SVR) ► ∴ shock can result from inadequate CO, or a loss of SVR, or both.

Inadequate CO
* *Hypovolaemia:*
    * Haemorrhage: trauma, ruptured aortic aneurysm, GI/postpartum bleed.
    * Fluid loss: vomiting, burns, 'third-space' losses, eg pancreatitis.
* *Pump failure:*
    * Cardiogenic shock: ACS, arrhythmia, acute valve failure.
    * Due to obstructed CO, eg PE, tension pneumothorax, cardiac tamponade.

Loss of *SVR* = distributive shock
* *Sepsis* (p772): a dysregulated immune response to infection leads to vasodilatation. Classically, patients are warm & vasodilated, but may be cold & shut down. Not all sepsis has classical signs of infection (fever, ↑ WCC) especially if immunosuppressed. Other diseases, eg pancreatitis, can give a similar picture due to activation of the inflammatory cascade.
* *Anaphylactic shock:* see p776.
* *Neurogenic:* eg spinal cord injury, epidural/spinal anaesthesia.
* *Endocrine failure:* adrenal insufficiency (p819), hypothyroidism (p820).
* *Other:* drugs, eg anaesthetics, antihypertensives, cyanide poisoning (p826).

Assessment

►►ABCDE (p763).

►Focus on 'C'. Large-bore IV access ×2 as soon as possible.

►Grade shock according to class (table 19.2).

* **General** Cold and clammy suggests cardiogenic shock or fluid/blood loss. Look for signs of volume loss, eg skin turgor, postural hypotension. Warm and well perfused with bounding pulse points to septic shock. Check for features of anaphylaxis: history, urticaria, angioedema, wheeze?
* **CVS** Usually tachycardic (unless on β-blocker, or in spinal shock, see *OHCS* p563) and hypotensive. ►If young and fit, including pregnant women, the systolic BP may remain normal until there is sudden decompensation so check for a narrow pulse pressure and measure the respiratory rate (table 19.2). ECG for rate, rhythm, and signs of ischaemia. Difference in BP between arms (>20mmHg) may indicate aortic dissection (p647).
* **JVP** If raised, cardiogenic shock is likely.
* **Abdomen** Trauma, aneurysm, GI bleed?

Management
▶If BP is unrecordable, call the cardiac arrest team.
• **Septic shock** See p772.
• **Anaphylactic shock** See p776.
• **Cardiogenic shock** See p786.
• **Hypovolaemic shock**
  • Identify and treat underlying cause. Raise the legs.
  • Fluid bolus 10–15mL/kg crystalloid via large peripheral line. If shock improves, titrate ongoing fluid replacement to HR (aim <100), BP (aim SBP >90mmHg), and urinary output (aim >0.5mL/kg/h).
  • If no improvement after 2 boluses, get expert help. Consider critical care referral for vasopressor support.
• **Haemorrhagic shock**
  • Stop bleeding if possible.
  • Replace significant blood loss with blood whenever possible. If class III/IV shock (table 19.2) then red cell transfusion with cross-matched blood is usually necessary (or 0 Rh–ve, p344).
  • Replacement of blood requires more than red cells: platelets and clotting factors/proteins are also required. Additional products can be given according to investigation results (haemoglobin, platelet count, prothrombin time, fibrinogen) but provision should be anticipated while results are awaited, eg in major bleeding due to trauma, give red blood cells, plasma, and platelets in a 1:1:1 ratio, or follow local major haemorrhage protocol. Discuss with haematology early.
  • Consider tranexamic acid 1–2g IV.
• **Heatstroke (heat exhaustion)**
  • Tepid sponging, fanning. Avoid ice and immersion.
  • Resuscitate: eg 0.9% saline ± hydrocortisone 100mg IV.
  • Stop cooling when core temperature <39°C.
  • Lorazepam 1–2mg IV may be used to stop shivering.

Table 19.2 Categorizing shock

⚠ Class of shock	1	2	3	4
Blood loss (mL)	<750	750–1500	1500–2000	>2000
Circulating volume loss (%)	<15	15–30	31–40	>40
Heart rate (bpm)	<100	>100	>120	>140
Systolic BP	Normal	Normal	<90mmHg	<90mmHg/ unrecordable
Pulse pressure	Normal	Narrow	Narrow	Narrow/ absent
Capillary refill (seconds)	<2	>2	>2	Absent
Respiratory rate (per min)	14–20	>20	>30	>35
Urine output (mL/h)	>30	<30	<20	<5
Cerebral function	Normal/ anxious	Anxious/ hostile	Anxious/ confused	Confused/ unresponsive

Sepsis is a major killer. There are >150 000 cases of sepsis in the UK each year resulting in >44 000 deaths, and much morbidity.

Definitions
Sepsis: life-threatening organ dysfunction caused by a dysregulated response to infection. (Fever is part of a regulated response to infection and so fever alone is not sepsis.)

Septic shock: sepsis in combination with either:
• Lactate >2mmol/L despite adequate fluid resuscitation.
• Vasopressors to maintain MAP ≥65mmHg.

Recognition
Early treatment saves lives. Failure to recognize sepsis causes harm, including death. Early warning scores (p876, fig A1) help to identify sepsis.

Have a low threshold for assessment and treatment of sepsis if:
• Barriers to communication: language, cognition.
• Immunosuppression, on chemotherapy, or injects drugs.
• Recent surgery or pregnant/postpartum.
• Indwelling lines or other foreign material.

Risk

▶Criteria (table 19.3) are used to assess risk of death or serious illness in sepsis:

• **High-risk** One or more high-risk criterion *or* two or more moderate-high-risk criteria with AKI or lactate >2.
• **Moderate-to-high risk** One or more moderate-to-high risk criterion.
• **Low-risk** No moderate- or high-risk criteria.

Table 19.3 Risk criteria in sepsis

Category	Moderate-to-high risk	High-risk
History	History of change in mental or functional state, immunosuppression, surgery/trauma <6 weeks ago	Objective evidence of altered mental state
Respiratory	Respiratory rate 21–24/min	Respiratory rate >24/min *or* new >40% O_2 requirement to keep sats >92% (>88% in COPD)
Systolic BP	91–100mmHg	<90mmHg (or >40 below baseline)
Heart rate	91–130bpm or new arrhythmia	>130bpm
Urine output	Nil for 12–18h if not catheterized 0.5–1.0mL/kg/h if catheterized	Nil for 18h if not catheterized <0.5mL/kg/h if catheterized
Skin	Local infection: red, swelling, or discharge	Mottled, ashen, or cyanotic skin Non-blanching rash (p806)
Temp	Rigors, or temperature <36°C	

Management See fig 19.5.[1]

Antibiotics Broad-spectrum antibiotics without delay, and always within 1h. Consider non-bacterial infection, eg give aciclovir if HSV encephalitis is suspected (p808).

Fluids Within 1h if systolic BP <90, AKI, or lactate >2mmol/L (consider if <2mmol/L).
• 500mL IV crystalloid (containing Na^+ 130–154mmol/L, eg Hartmann's, Plasma-Lyte®, 0.9% saline) over 15min, then review. Caution in heart failure.
• Senior/expert review if no improvement after two boluses.

Oxygen As required to achieve O_2 saturations 94–98% (88–92% if risk of CO_2 retention, eg COPD, p796).

Critical care review Ask for help early if higher level care (eg invasive monitoring, vasopressor/inotropes, ventilation, haemofiltration) is anticipated.

Surgery For source, eg wound debridement.

Manage complications Shock (p770), AKI (p294), DIC (p350), ARDS (p178).

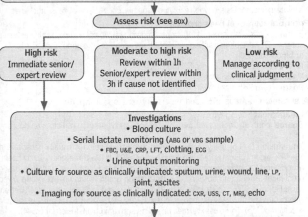

▲ Acute management of sepsis in adults

Recognize
• Consider sepsis in any patient with signs or symptoms of infection
• Consider non-specific signs: patient/carer concern, mental and functional status
• Consider risk factors for sepsis: >75 years, immunosuppression, surgery, pregnancy/postpartum, persons who inject drugs, skin breach, lines, catheters

Clinical assessment
History Infective symptoms, time course, immunosuppression, surgery, travel
Examination
• *General* Conscious level, capillary refill time, mottled/ashen skin, rash
• *Observations* Temperature, HR, BP, RR, O₂ saturation, urine output

Assess risk (see BOX)

High risk
Immediate senior/expert review

Moderate to high risk
Review within 1h
Senior/expert review within 3h if cause not identified

Low risk
Manage according to clinical judgment

Investigations
• Blood culture
• Serial lactate monitoring (ABG or VBG sample)
• FBC, U&E, CRP, LFT, clotting, ECG
• Urine output monitoring
• Culture for source as clinically indicated: sputum, urine, wound, line, LP, joint, ascites
• Imaging for source as clinically indicated: CXR, USS, CT, MRI, echo

Treatment
• Antibiotics (and other antimicrobials if clinically indicated)
• Oxygen to achieve O₂ saturation 94–98% (88–92% if COPD)
• Fluid: 500mL bolus of crystalloid and review
• Liaise with other teams: critical care, surgery, medical speciality
• Manage acute complications: shock (p770), AKI (p294), DIC (p350), ARDS (p178)

Review
Senior/expert review if 1h antibiotics and fluid resuscitation:
• SBP <90 • RR >30 • Reduced GCS • High lactate not reduced by >20%
►► Consider critical care referral

Fig 19.5 Management of sepsis in adults.

►The clinical priorities in sepsis are recognition and the timely administration of antibiotics. This often requires deviation from the usual clinical approach of history, examination, investigation, then treatment.

►Consider the six most important actions—3 'in' and 3 'out':

'IN'	'OUT'
1 Antibiotics	1 Blood culture
2 Fluid	2 Lactate
3 Oxygen.	3 Urine output.

Massive blood loss has variable definitions:
• Loss of one blood volume within a 24h period.
• 50% blood volume loss (2500mL for a 70kg adult) within 3h.
• Blood loss of 150mL/min.
But these definitions are arbitrary and difficult to apply in an acute situation.

A more useful definition may be bleeding which leads to:
• Heart rate 120bpm or more, and/or sbp <90mmHg.
▶Remember: up to 30% of blood volume can be lost before BP drops (table 19.2, p771).
▶Recognize blood loss early and trigger the local major haemorrhage protocol.

Goals of management
• Find the bleeding, stop the bleeding.
• Rapid and effective restoration of blood volume.
• Maintain haemostasis, oxygen carrying capacity, oncotic pressure, & biochemistry.

Potential sources of haemorrhage
• **Trauma** Chest, abdomen, long bones, pelvis, retroperitoneum, scalp, external sources. Beware of distracting injuries: always consider bleeding from >1 site.
• **GI bleed** See p804.
• **Respiratory** Eg haemoptysis, haemothorax.
• **Vascular** Eg ruptured AAA.
• **Postpartum** See OHCS p96.

Assessment ▶▶ABCDE (p763) and as per approach to shock (p770).

Management See fig 19.6.
• **Source control** Contact surgery/obstetrics/interventional radiology/endoscopy early.
• **Transfusion** Do not delay transfusion. Red cell transfusion is usually necessary if 30–40% blood volume is lost, and rapid loss of >40% is life-threatening. Early haematocrit and FBC may be misleading after major acute blood loss: transfuse based on clinical criteria and observations. Until blood group is known, use group O red cells. Females <50yrs should receive RhD-negative red cells to avoid sensitization. Use group-specific RBCs as soon as possible (usually within 10 minutes of sample received by lab). Try to use warmed products and rapid transfusion kit (p344).
• **Balanced transfusion** Resuscitate with blood components resembling whole blood = RBCs + plasma + platelets. If major bleeding due to trauma give red blood cells, plasma, and platelets in a 1:1:1 ratio. If other contexts, follow your local major haemorrhage protocol.
• **Minimize resuscitation with crystalloids** Use only in hypotensive patients until blood products available. Risk of oedema, worsening anaemia and thrombocytopenia, and dilutional coagulopathy.
• **Tranexamic acid** 1g over 10 minutes followed by an infusion of 1g over 8 hours reduces death in bleeding due to trauma. Good safety profile, easy administration, and low cost mean increasing use for all major haemorrhage.
• **Prevent/treat hypothermia** Monitor temperature. Transfuse warmed products (eg level 1 fluid warmer), Bair Hugger™/warm blankets, minimize exposure.
• **Imaging** CTs are quick and may help plan intervention. Consider safety including anaesthetic/critical care support. Speak to your interventional radiologist.
• **Anticoagulant reversal** See p346.
• **Desmopressin (DDAVP)** Robust evidence for desmopressin is not available and further studies in major bleeding are required.
▶Beware paradoxical bradycardia due to β-blockade.
▶Coagulopathy, acidosis, & hypothermia are a lethal triad contributing coagulopathy and adverse outcome from major haemorrhage.

⚠ **Acute management of major haemorrhage**

ABCDE (p763)
- Recognize blood loss, seek expert/senior help
- Trigger major blood haemorrhage protocol including haematology

↓

IV access
- Wide-bore cannula: 18G (green) as minimum, 16G (grey)/14G (brown) preferable
- Large vein
- Pressure bag with a pressure bag

↓

Investigations
- Full blood count
- Blood group and cross-match
- Clotting screen including fibrinogen
- Point-of-care thromboelastography, eg TEG®, ROTEM®

↓

Control haemorrhage
- Contact surgery/obstetrics/interventional radiology/endoscopy
- Initial measures, if applicable:
  - Direct pressure and elevation, adrenaline-soaked gauze, haemostatic dressing
  - Reduce/splint factures
  - Tourniquet
- Invasive measures: suture, tamponade (eg packing, balloon tamponade), cautery, injection, embolization by interventional radiology, surgery
- Correct coagulopathy and reverse anticoagulants
- *Tranexamic acid* if trauma and <3h from injury: 1g bolus over 10 minutes followed by 1g over 8h IV. Consider 1g bolus over 10 minutes in non-traumatic bleeding

Blood products
Until laboratory results available follow your local major haemorrhage protocol:
eg RBCS, FFP, and platelets in a ratio of 1:1:1

When laboratory results available:
- Falling Hb: red cells
- APPT or PT ratio >1.5: FFP 15–20mL/kg
- Fibrinogen <1.5g/L: cryoprecipitate (2 pools)
- Platelet <50×10⁹/L: 1 pool of platelets

Review thromboelastography results if available:
=Real-time kinetics of clot formation
- *How fast?* ↑Clotting time: give FFP/prothrombin complex concentrate
- *How strong?* ↓Clot strength:
  - Abnormal functional fibrinogen test: give cryoprecipitate
  - Normal functional fibrinogen test: give platelets
- *How long?* ↑Clot lysis: give anti-fibrinolytic, eg tranexamic acid
►► Defer to your local protocol for values and interpretation

⚠

↓

Cycles of monitoring and appropriate blood components until bleeding ceases

Fig 19.6 Management of major haemorrhage in adults.

Anaphylactic shock

Type I *IgE-mediated* hypersensitivity reaction to an allergen.

Release of histamine and other agents causes:
- Urticaria.
- Capillary leak and oedema, eg eyelids, lids, tongue, lips.
- Laryngeal oedema → hoarse voice, stridor.
- Hypotension.
- Wheeze.
- Hypoxia and cyanosis.

More common in atopic individuals.

In contrast, an *anaphylactoid reaction* results from direct release of mediators from inflammatory cells, without antibodies, usually in response to a drug.

Precipitants
- Drugs, eg antibiotics, NSAIDs, opiates, anaesthetic agents, contrast media.
- Latex.
- Insect venom.
- Foods: milk, eggs, fish, nuts.

Assessment
▶▶Suspect anaphylaxis in any sudden-onset ABC (DE) problem.
- Airway: stridor, airway oedema.
- Breathing: wheeze, cyanosis.
- Circulation: tachycardia, hypotension.
- Disability: confusion.
- Exposure: urticarial rash, oedema.

Management ▶ See fig 19.7.

Atypical presentations: anaphylaxis mimics
- Acute asthma (p794).
- Hereditary angioedema.
- Carcinoid syndrome (p266).
- Foreign body inhalation.
- Systemic mastocytosis.

▲ Emergency management of anaphylaxis

Suspect: sudden ABC problem, often with rash
If unresponsive: manage as cardiac arrest

↓

• Remove the trigger (ie stop infusion)
• Call for help: resuscitation team/ambulance
• Lie flat (if pregnant use left tilt), consider raising legs

↓

▶▶ *Adrenaline IM 0.5mg (0.5mL of 1:1000)*
Anterolateral aspect of the thigh
Repeat after 5 minutes if no improvement: monitor HR, BP, O₂ saturation

↓

Airway
Secure airway
Resuscitation team for intubation if airway obstruction

↓

Breathing
O₂ to achieve saturations 94–98%
If wheeze: bronchodilator, eg salbutamol (p794)

↓

Circulation
500–1000mL IV crystalloid
May require repeat

↓

If no improvement after 2 doses IM adrenaline:
Get expert help: critical care review
Treatment for refractory anaphylaxis: IV adrenaline infusion, fluid
resuscitation, additional vasopressors, glucagon if on β-blockers (p826)

↓

Further management
• Admit to ward (biphasic response possible In hours after anaphylaxis)
• Monitor HR, BP, O₂ saturation, ECG
• Measure serum tryptase 1–6h if suspected anaphylaxis
• Antihistamine for persistent skin symptoms only. Do not use to treat
  respiratory or cardiovascular symptoms
• 'MedicAlert' bracelet naming the culprit allergen
• Teach about self-injected adrenaline

Fig 19.7 Management of anaphylaxis.

▶▶Adrenaline (= epinephrine) is given IM and not IV unless the patient is in cardiac arrest or is being managed with an infusion for refractory anaphylaxis.

▶Steroids are not advised for the emergency treatment of anaphylaxis: there is little evidence that they shorten symptoms or prevent a biphasic reaction. Steroids should be given if acute asthma is contributing to the symptoms of anaphylaxis.

Severe hypertension is often defined as BP ≥200/120mmHg, but there is no specific threshold. Lower BPs may also be concerning, eg if end-organ damage, in pregnancy.

►Most severe hypertension is not associated with target organ damage/dysfunction. This is sometimes termed hypertensive 'urgency' and is not an emergency.

►Hypertensive emergencies occur when severe hypertension is associated with new or progressive target organ dysfunction:
• Hypertensive encephalopathy.
• Hypertensive retinopathy.
• Hypertensive kidney damage.
• Hypertensive heart failure.
• Aortic dissection.

Hypertensive emergencies can develop with or without chronic hypertension.

Assessment

Context Precipitants include pre-eclampsia, head trauma (►Cushing reflex: ↑BP to ↑ICP, with associated bradycardia), inadequate pain control, drug use (heroin, cocaine, amphetamines).

History
• Symptoms: headache, confusion, visual disturbance, seizures, focal neurological deficits, nausea and vomiting (due to ↑ICP), back/chest pain (dissection/MI), breathlessness (pulmonary oedema).
• Chronic hypertension: treatment, control, adherence.
• Other comorbidity, eg kidney disease, vascular disease.
• Other substances: over-the-counter (eg NSAIDs, sympathomimetics), recent steroid use, illegal drug use.

Examination BP in both arms, radiofemoral delay, signs of heart failure (gallop rhythm, ↑JVP, bibasal crepitations), pregnant abdomen, focal neurological deficits, skin changes of scleroderma. ►Fundoscopy for papilloedema/haemorrhage.

Investigation
• Blood: FBC & film (evidence of (MAHA)?), kidney function, troponin, TSH, β-HCG, glucose.
• Urinalysis: proteinuria/haematuria, pregnancy test, toxicology.
• ECG: ischaemic changes, LVH.
• As clinically indicated: CXR (pulmonary oedema), brain CT/MRI, TTE, CT aorta.
• Secondary hypertension work-up later (p112) as secondary activation of RAS occurs in hypertensive emergencies due to pressure natriuresis and volume depletion.

Management

►Severe hypertension *without* hypertensive emergency: *slow* reduction in BP. Aim <200/110mmHg over 24h using oral therapy, eg nifedipine LA 20–30mg, atenolol 25mg. IV therapy and short-acting/immediate-release preparations confer a risk of precipitous fall in BP, and MI or stroke, due to loss of autoregulation.

►Hypertensive emergencies: see fig 19.8. Patients should be closely monitored, and an arterial line considered. The choice of antihypertensive agent and BP goal depends on the specific emergency. Generally, BP should be reduced by no more than 10–25% over the first few hours, before more gradual reduction over hours to days. Aortic dissection is the exception, when BP control needs to be quicker and lower.

Pre-eclampsia/eclampsia

Occurs after 20 weeks' gestation. Severe maternal hypertension is >160/110mmHg. Treat with oral labetalol 100mg, or nifedipine MR 10mg and review. IV antihypertensives (labetalol or hydralazine) may be needed if refractory to oral therapy. If pre-eclampsia with severe features or eclampsia, give magnesium sulfate (4g over 5–15min IV, followed by 1g/hour IVI). Monitor in an enhanced care setting and plan delivery.

Hyperadrenergic state
• Phaeochromocytoma: seek expert advice. See p820.
• Sympathomimetics, eg cocaine, amphetamines. Treat with benzodiazepine, eg lorazepam (1mg IV, repeated every 10–15min, max 8mg) or diazepam (5mg IV, repeated every 5–10min, max 50mg). Monitor for sedation. Also labetalol, phentolamine 5–15mg IV, GTN.

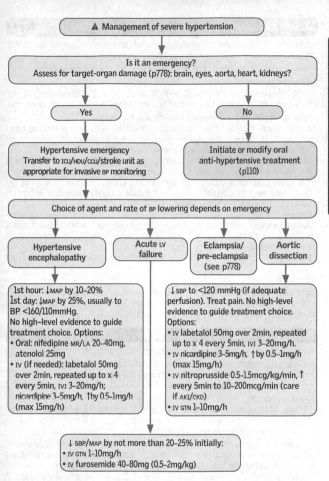

Fig 19.8 Management of hypertensive emergencies.

Acute coronary syndrome (ACS) includes unstable angina, STEMI, and NSTEMI (p782). STEMI is a common medical emergency. Prompt treatment saves lives.

▶Females may present later, and with atypical symptoms compared to males.

Initial treatment

See fig 19.9.² History, examination, 12-lead ECG, U&E, troponin, glucose, cholesterol, FBC, CXR. Monitor heart rate/rhythm via cardiac monitor/telemetry as risk of arrhythmia.

▶**Assess eligibility for coronary reperfusion** (see BOX).

• **Antiplatelets** Aspirin 300mg PO. Use in combination with prasugrel 60mg PO (if not high bleeding risk), or ticagrelor 180mg PO (if high bleeding risk), or clopidogrel 300–600mg PO (if already taking an oral anticoagulant).

• **Morphine** 2.5–5mg IV, repeated according to pain. Give anti-emetic with 1st dose of morphine: metoclopramide 10mg IV (1st line), or cyclizine 50mg IV (2nd line).

• **GTN** Sublingual (spray/tablet) if persistent chest discomfort/pain. IV if persistent symptoms, hypertension (p779) or LV dysfunction. Care if hypotension or concurrent use of phosphodiesterase inhibitors.

• **Oxygen** If SaO₂ <90%.

• **Anticoagulation** Fondaparinux, unless undergoing immediate PCI. If radial access for PCI: unfractionated heparin. If femoral access: bivalirudin. GP-IIb/IIIa blocker if angiographically indicated.

• **β-blockers** Start early, eg bisoprolol 2.5mg PO OD if no cardiogenic shock, or heart block. Care if asthma/COPD.

• **ACE-i/ARB** When stable.

Right ventricular infarction: consider if inferior MI, ST elevation in RV3/4 (p92), ↓BP with clear lung fields and ↑JVP, or echo findings. Treat hypotension by optimizing pre-load with fluid. Caution with nitrates and diuretics.

Reperfusion therapy

Coronary reperfusion saves lives. Assess eligibility if symptoms plus ECG criteria:

• ST elevation >1mm in ≥2 adjacent limb leads or >2mm in ≥2 adjacent chest leads.
• LBBB (unless prior LBBB). RBBB if ischaemic symptoms are present.
• Posterior changes: ST depression and tall R waves in leads V₁ to V₃.

Therapy may be:

1 Percutaneous intervention (PCI): angiographic identification of blockage(s) and revascularization via stenting.
2 Fibrinolysis with systemically administered clot-dissolving enzymes.

Primary PCI ▶▶Offer to all patients presenting with STEMI within 12h of symptom onset at (or after transfer to) a primary PCI centre within 120min. If this is not possible, patients should receive thrombolysis and be transferred to a primary PCI centre for either rescue PCI (if residual ST elevation) or angiography. Seek specialist advice for use beyond 12h if evidence of ongoing ischaemia or in patients presenting at 12–24h.

Fibrinolysis ▶▶Benefit reduces steadily from onset of pain, target time is <10min from diagnosis if PCI is not available. Use >12h from symptom onset requires specialist advice. ▶Do not use for isolated ST depression/T-wave inversion, or normal ECG. Thrombolysis is best achieved with tissue plasminogen activators (eg tenecteplase as a single IV bolus). Contraindications:

• Previous intracranial haemorrhage
• Cerebral malignancy/AVM
• Major trauma/surgery/head injury <3 weeks
• Non-compressible puncture <24h, eg biopsy, LP

• Ischaemic stroke <6 months
• GI bleed <1 month
• Known bleeding disorder
• Aortic dissection

Relative contraindications: TIA <6 months, anticoagulant therapy, <1wk postpartum, refractory BP >180/110mmHg, advanced liver disease, infective endocarditis, active peptic ulcer disease, prolonged/traumatic resuscitation.

▶Anticoagulation, eg LMWH is recommended in patients treated with thrombolysis until revascularization (if performed), or during hospital stay up to 8 days.

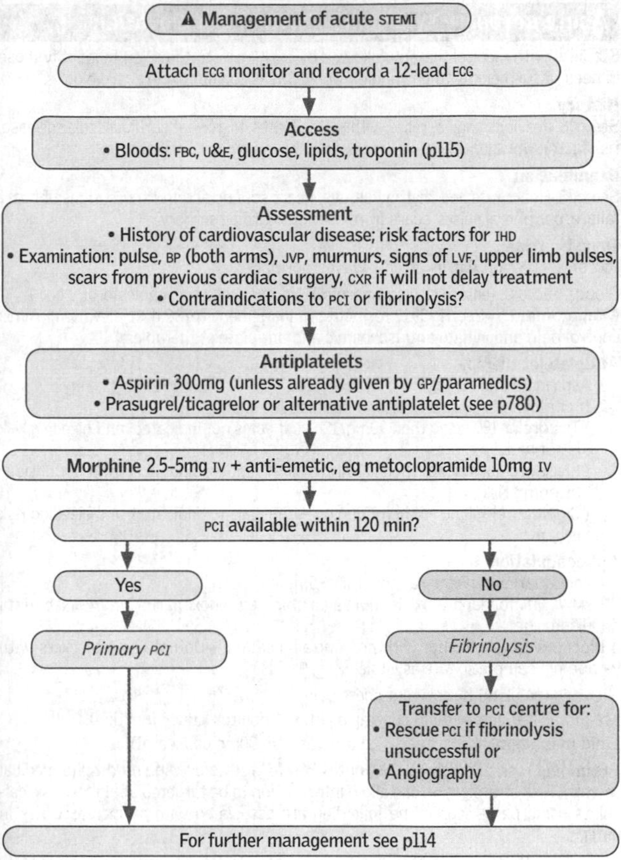

▲ **Management of acute STEMI**

Attach ECG monitor and record a 12-lead ECG

↓

Access
• Bloods: FBC, U&E, glucose, lipids, troponin (p115)

↓

Assessment
• History of cardiovascular disease; risk factors for IHD
• Examination: pulse, BP (both arms), JVP, murmurs, signs of LVF, upper limb pulses, scars from previous cardiac surgery, CXR if will not delay treatment
• Contraindications to PCI or fibrinolysis?

↓

Antiplatelets
• Aspirin 300mg (unless already given by GP/paramedics)
• Prasugrel/ticagrelor or alternative antiplatelet (see p780)

↓

Morphine 2.5–5mg IV + anti-emetic, eg metoclopramide 10mg IV

↓

PCI available within 120 min?

↓ Yes   ↓ No

Primary PCI   *Fibrinolysis*

↓   Transfer to PCI centre for:
                                            • Rescue PCI if fibrinolysis unsuccessful or
                                            • Angiography

↓

For further management see p114

Fig 19.9 Management of an acute STEMI.

Stabilize with medical therapy followed by early risk stratification to identify those in need of further treatment/angiography. Speak to your expert cardiologist.

History
See p36. Previous angina, relief with rest/nitrates, history of cardiovascular disease, risk factors for IHD. ≥75yrs/DM/female may have atypical presentation.

Examination
See p38. Heart rate and rhythm, BP, JVP, heart sounds and murmurs, signs of heart failure, peripheral pulses, scars from previous cardiac surgery.

Investigations
ECG: ST depression, flat/inverted T-waves, normal ECG.

Bloods: FBC, U&E (ensure K⁺/Mg²⁺ normal), troponin, glucose, cholesterol. CXR.

Management ►See fig 19.10 for acute management (p780 if ST elevation). Aims: control pain and initiate anti-ischaemic and antiplatelet therapies.

Antiplatelet therapy
1 Aspirin 300mg PO, followed by 75mg OD.
2 If confirmed ACS give a second antiplatelet agent:
  • Ticagrelor 180mg PO then 90mg/12h PO if PCI is not indicated, and bleeding risk is not high.
  • Prasugrel 60mg PO then 10mg/d PO if undergoing PCI (p780). Consider bleeding risk.
  • Clopidogrel 300mg PO then 75mg OD PO, if PCI is not indicated, and bleeding risk is high.

Anticoagulation
1 Fondaparinux (factor Xa inhibitor) 2.5mg OD.
2 LMWH if fondaparinux is not available, eg enoxaparin 1mg/kg/12h until discharge.

β-blockers In all patients with no contraindication. ►Do not use β-blockers with verapamil: can precipitate asystole.

Nitrates (PO or IV) If recurrent chest pain.

ACE-i In all patients with no contraindication (monitor kidney function).

Lipid management Start early, eg atorvastatin 80mg OD (see p116).

Prognosis Risk of death ~1–2%, but ~15% for refractory angina despite medical therapy. Risk stratification can allow intervention to be targeted at highest risk: calculate using GRACE score.[2] The following are associated with an increased risk in NSTEMI:
• History of unstable angina.
• ST depression or widespread T-wave inversion.
• Raised troponin.
• Age >70 years.
• Comorbidity, previous MI, poor LV function, DM.

►High-risk patients should be considered for inpatient coronary angiography. Symptomatic lesions may be addressed by coronary stenting or CABG (see p119).

Further measures
• Serial ECGs, and troponin >12h after pain.
• Observe on cardiac monitor/telemetry in case of arrhythmia.
• Wean off *glyceryl trinitrate* (GTN) infusion when stabilized on oral medication.
• Continue fondaparinux (or LMWH) until discharge.
• Address modifiable risk factors: smoking, hypertension, hyperlipidaemia, diabetes.
• Ensure optimum management: dual antiplatelets, β-blocker, ACE-i/ARB, statin.

►*If symptoms recur, refer for angiography & PCI, or CABG.*

2 GRACE = Global Registry of Acute Coronary Events. A risk score based on age, heart rate, BP, kidney function, Killip class of heart failure, and other events, eg raised troponin. Use an online calculator, eg http://www.outcomes-umassmed.org/grace/

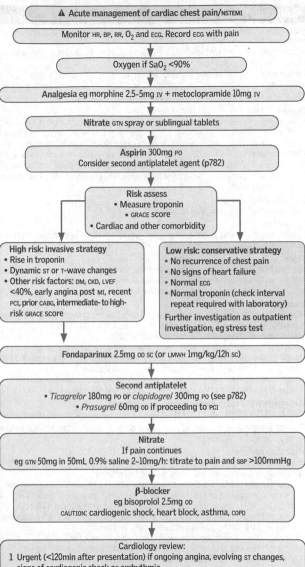

⚠ Acute management of cardiac chest pain/NSTEMI

Monitor HR, BP, RR, O₂ and ECG. Record ECG with pain

Oxygen if SaO₂ <90%

Analgesia eg morphine 2.5–5mg IV + metoclopramide 10mg IV

Nitrate GTN spray or sublingual tablets

Aspirin 300mg PO
Consider second antiplatelet agent (p782)

Risk assess
• Measure troponin
• GRACE score
• Cardiac and other comorbidity

High risk: invasive strategy
• Rise in troponin
• Dynamic ST or T-wave changes
• Other risk factors: DM, CKD, LVEF <40%, early angina post MI, recent PCI, prior CABG, intermediate- to high-risk GRACE score

Low risk: conservative strategy
• No recurrence of chest pain
• No signs of heart failure
• Normal ECG
• Normal troponin (check interval repeat required with laboratory)

Further investigation as outpatient investigation, eg stress test

Fondaparinux 2.5mg OD SC (or LMWH 1mg/kg/12h SC)

Second antiplatelet
• *Ticagrelor* 180mg PO or *clopidogrel* 300mg PO (see p782)
• *Prasugrel* 60mg OD if proceeding to PCI

Nitrate
If pain continues
eg GTN 50mg in 50mL 0.9% saline 2–10mg/h: titrate to pain and SBP >100mmHg

β-blocker
eg bisoprolol 2.5mg OD
CAUTION: cardiogenic shock, heart block, asthma, COPD

Cardiology review:
1 Urgent (<120min after presentation) if ongoing angina, evolving ST changes, signs of cardiogenic shock or arrhythmia
2 Early (<24h) if GRACE score >140 and high-risk patient
3 Within 72h if lower-risk patient

Fig 19.10 Acute management of chest pain and ACS without ST-segment elevation.

Pulmonary oedema is due to excess fluid in the alveoli as a result of change in one or more of Starling's forces:
- Cardiogenic pulmonary oedema: increased capillary hydrostatic pressure secondary to elevated pulmonary venous pressure.
- Non-cardiogenic pulmonary oedema: altered capillary permeability as a result of a direct or an indirect pathological insult, eg sepsis. Or reduced capillary oncotic pressure, eg nephrotic syndrome (pp308–9).

Causes
- Cardiogenic. Usually left ventricular failure due to ischaemic heart disease, cardiomyopathy, myocarditis, acute valve syndromes (eg IE or chordae/papillary muscle rupture), arrhythmia, hypertensive emergency (pp778–9). Severe mitral stenosis.
- Non-cardiogenic: ARDS (p178) from any cause, eg sepsis, trauma. Neurogenic pulmonary oedema (eg head injury, subarachnoid/intracerebral haemorrhage). Re-expansion pulmonary oedema (after pneumothorax). High altitude (rapid ascension to >3600m).

Differential diagnosis
Asthma/COPD, pneumonia. May coexist.

Symptoms
Dyspnoea, orthopnoea (paroxysmal), pink frothy sputum. Symptoms of precipitant: MI, infection.

Signs
↑HR, ↑RR, pink frothy sputum, pulsus alternans, ↑JVP, fine lung crackles, triple/gallop rhythm (p42), wheeze. If significant hypoxia: sitting up, leaning forward, distressed, pale, sweaty. Also signs of cause/precipitants.

Investigations
- CXR (p135, p706–8): cardiomegaly, bilateral airspace shadowing, effusions (check costophrenic angles), fluid in lung fissures, Kerley B lines (septal linear opacities).
- ECG: ischaemic changes/MI, tachycardia, arrhythmia.
- U&E (AKI), troponin (raised in ACS), ABG (hypoxia, raised lactate in cardiogenic shock).
- BNP/NT-proBNP (p135): useful −ve predictive value if BNP <100ng/L or NT-proBNP <300ng/L.
- Echo (early if cardiogenic shock): LV function, valve disease.
- Lung US: multiple B lines per intercostal space (non-specific, user dependent).
- If due to ACS (including new RBBB): urgent PCI/coronary angiography.

Management of cardiogenic pulmonary oedema
►See fig 19.11. ►►Treat before investigations if hypoxia/haemodynamic compromise.

Monitor progress HR, BP, RR, SaO₂, JVP, urine output, ABG. Cardiac monitor or telemetry in case of arrhythmia.

After stabilization
- Salt and fluid restrict <1.5L/day.
- Weigh daily, aim reduction of 0.5kg/day until euvolaemic.
- Convert to oral diuretics once fluid state optimized: eg furosemide, bumetanide.
- Consider combination of loop plus thiazide diuretic if inadequate diuresis on loop diuretic alone, eg metolazone 2.5–5mg daily PO, chlortalidone 25mg daily PO.
- Angiotensin receptor neprilysin inhibitor (ARNI): better outcomes than ACE-i/ARB alone.
- β-blocker: once stable, ie IV diuretics no longer required.
- Mineralocorticoid receptor antagonist (MRA), eg spironolactone.
- SGLT2 inhibitor: add to optimized care with ARNI/ACE-i/ARB, β-blocker, and MRA.
- Consider suitability for biventricular pacing or cardiac transplantation.
- Arrhythmias: manage if present (AF, pp120–7); consider anticoagulation.
- VTE prophylaxis.

Refractory disease
- Opiates are not recommended due to risk of cardiorespiratory depression. They will relieve dyspnoea and anxiety if no reversibility.
- Discuss care with the patient, their advocates, and senior clinicians. Mechanical ventilation may be futile without a reversible underlying cause.

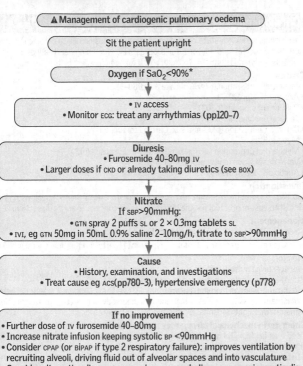

Fig 19.11 Management of cardiogenic pulmonary oedema.

* Avoid supplemental oxygen if not hypoxaemic as it causes vasoconstriction and may reduce cardiac output. If known COPD monitor for CO_2 retention with serial ABGs and reduce O_2 as soon as possible (see pp796–7).

Loop diuretic dosing

- If diuretic naïve, the usual initial IV bolus dose of furosemide is 40–80mg (0.5–2mg/kg).
- If taking regular oral diuretics, up to 2–3 times the previously ineffective oral dose may be needed.
- In CKD higher doses of diuretic are needed for tubular delivery to be sufficient to cause diuresis (2–5 times depending on CKD stage).
- Furosemide has a short duration of action (except in CKD) and post-diuretic sodium retention can occur. Although there is no measurable difference in all-cause mortality, length of hospital stay, or electrolyte disturbance with bolus versus continuous infusion, a continuous infusion may be superior in initial measured diuretic effect and reduction in BNP.

Cardiogenic shock

Cardiogenic shock is a state of inadequate tissue perfusion due to cardiac dysfunction. It may occur suddenly, or after progressively worsening heart failure. It has a high mortality and is difficult to treat. ► Ask for senior/expert help.

Causes
- Myocardial infarction (~80% of cases) (pp780–3).
- Arrhythmia (pp120–7).
- Pulmonary embolus (p802).
- Tension pneumothorax (p799).
- Cardiac tamponade (p132 and BOX 'Cardiac tamponade').
- Myocarditis.
- Myocardial depression (drugs, hypoxia, acidosis, sepsis) (p130).
- Valve destruction (endocarditis—p144).
- Aortic dissection (p647).

Investigation
ECG, FBC, U&E, lactate, troponin, ABG, echocardiogram, CXR. CT thorax: speak with radiologist to ensure protocol for the differential(s) of concern, ie aortic dissection/PE.

Management
► See fig 19.12. Manage in coronary or critical care unit.

►► If the cause is myocardial infarction prompt reperfusion therapy is vital (p780).

Monitor:
- BP, ECG, urine output, lactate.
- Cardiac monitor/telemetry and serial 12-lead ECG.
- Real-time haemodynamics, eg arterial line, CVP line, pulmonary artery catheter. Minimally invasive devices which monitor haemodynamics (eg via transduction, pneumatics, light transmission, thermodilution) may be available.

Short-term mechanical circulatory support devices
Used as a bridging therapy to recovery (where possible) or definitive treatment (eg transplant). Include:
- **Intra-aortic balloon pump** A balloon is inflated during diastole to increase coronary perfusion and then deflated during systole to decrease afterload. Increases myocardial oxygenation, CO, and organ perfusion, with decrease in LV workload.
- **Left ventricular assist device** (LVAD) Pumps blood from the LV to the aorta.
- **Extracorporeal membrane oxygenation** (ECMO) A prolonged mechanical cardiopulmonary support system indicated for potentially reversible acute respiratory or cardiac failure that is unresponsive to other therapies.

Cardiac tamponade

Compression of the heart by an accumulation of fluid in the pericardial sac.

Causes
Trauma, primary malignancy (cardiac/pericardial), metastatic disease (eg lung, breast, lymphoma), pericarditis, autoimmune, infection (viral, bacterial, fungal, parasitic, don't forget TB), coronary artery dissection (after PCI), ruptured ventricle. *Rarely:* ↑urea, radiation, myxoedema.

Signs
↓BP, ↑JVP, muffled heart sounds (= Beck's triad). ↑JVP on inspiration (Kussmaul's sign), pulsus paradoxus (↓BP on inspiration). CXR: globular heart, left heart border convex or straight, right cardiophrenic angle <90°. ECG: electrical alternans (p132).

Echocardiography is diagnostic.

Management
►► If haemodynamic compromise request expert support for pericardiocentesis (p757). Prepare: O₂, monitor ECG, set up IVI, take blood for group & save.

Contact cardiothoracic surgery for definitive solution, eg CABG, ventricular repair, pericardial window.

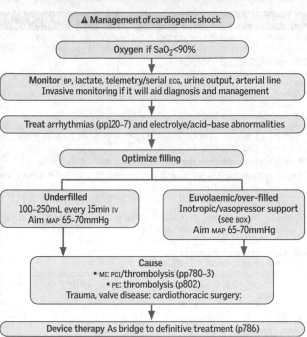

Fig 19.12 Management of cardiogenic shock.

Inotropes and vasopressors

- Inotropes: increase cardiac contractility (inotropy), eg phenylephrine.
- Vasopressors: induce vasoconstriction, elevating MAP by increasing systemic vascular resistance, eg norepinephrine.
- Drugs are classified by their predominant function—pure inotropes and vasopressors are rare, eg norepinephrine is classified as a vasopressor due to its potent vasoconstrictive effects, though it also confers some inotropy (which helps the heart manage the increase in afterload it has just caused).
- A third class of drug is the inodilator, which increases cardiac contractility with arterial vasodilatation, eg levosimendan, milrinone.
- There is limited randomized trial evidence to guide the choice of inotropes and vasopressors in cardiogenic shock.
- If SBP <90mmHg and evidence of shock (eg cool extremities, narrow pulse pressure, low urine output, confusion) despite an adequate preload, an inotrope (or even inodilator) may be useful, though a vasopressor may be needed to maintain BP.

ECG shows HR >100bpm and QRS complexes >120ms (>3 small squares on ECG at the standard UK rate of 25mm/s). Identify the underlying rhythm and treat accordingly.[3]

Differential diagnosis (See p124.)
• *Ventricular tachycardia (VT):* consider the pre-ECG probability of VT: older age, LV dysfunction, and known IHD increase the likelihood of VT. >30s = sustained VT.
• *Torsades de pointes:* a form of VT with a constantly varying axis, often in the setting of long QT.
• *SVT with aberrant conduction:* SVT with bundle branch block (p790).
• *Pre-excited tachycardia:* atrial arrhythmia conducted down an accessory pathway, eg pre-excited AF. Consider if irregularly irregular, varying QRS duration, delta wave (not always seen).

Identifying the underlying rhythm See p124. ▸▸If in doubt, treat as VT.

General management ▸See fig 19.13. Connect patient to a cardiac monitor and ensure a defibrillator is available.
• Monitor O_2 sats and give supplemental oxygen if <90%.
• Obtain IV access.
• Check for adverse signs: HR >150, SBP <90mmHg, ↓consciousness, chest pain, breathlessness (pulmonary oedema), oliguria.
• Correct electrolyte abnormalities: K^+ and Mg^{2+}.

Haemodynamically unstable VT
▸▸Synchronized DC shock (see p878, fig A3).
• Correct K^+ <3.5mmol/L: 20mmol/h IV (20mmol/20min if imminent arrest).
• Correct Mg^{2+} <0.6mmol/L: 4mL 50% magnesium sulfate (=2g=8mmol) IV over 10min.
• Amiodarone 300mg IV over 10–20min (peripherally in an emergency).
• If refractory, consider lidocaine 1mg/kg IV.

Haemodynamically stable VT
• Correct hypokalaemia and hypomagnesaemia as above.
• Amiodarone 300mg IV over 20–60min via central line/wide-bore cannula.
• Consider synchronized DC shock—a heart may not cope with VT for long.

After correction of VT
• Establish the cause.
• If VT occurs after MI: IV amiodarone infusion for 12–24h.
• A maintenance oral anti-arrhythmic may be required/indicated, eg β-blocker in IHD.
• Recurrent VT: electrophysiology study (EPS)-guided ablation of the arrhythmogenic area.

▸▸All patients with VT should be assessed for an implantable cardiac defibrillator (ICD).

Torsade de pointes
ECG, p125, fig 3.36.

Cause Congenital. Acquired is usually secondary to medication, eg antiarrhythmic, tricyclic, antimalarial, antipsychotic. See p697.

Treatment 4mL 50% magnesium sulfate (=2g=8mmol) IV over 10min. Correct hypokalaemia. If bradycardia and prolonged QT, an increase in HR can shorten QT: overdrive pacing (pace at a faster rate, then slowly reduce), or isoprenaline IVI.

Prevent Congenital long-QT syndrome: β-blocker. Acquired: stop predisposing drugs.

SVT with aberrant conduction
Manage as SVT, eg adenosine (see p790).

Ventricular extrasystoles (ectopics)
Found in 1–4% of population. Can be frequent, eg up to >60/h. If no underlying heart disease they are considered benign, with no role for treatment. If IHD, a β-blocker is indicated and effective.

Ventricular fibrillation
ECG, p125, fig 3.34. Manage as cardiac arrest. Use *non-synchronized* DC shock (there is no R wave which can trigger fibrillation, p754). See p878, fig A3.

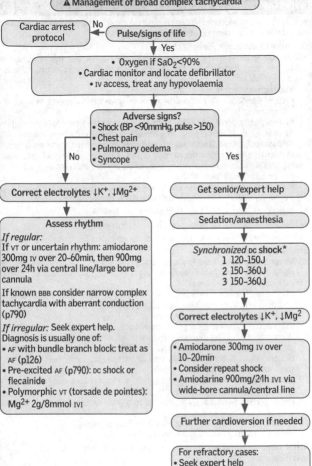

▲ Management of broad complex tachycardia

Pulse/signs of life
— No → Cardiac arrest protocol
— Yes ↓

• Oxygen if SaO₂<90%
• Cardiac monitor and locate defibrillator
• IV access, treat any hypovolaemia

↓

Adverse signs?
• Shock (BP <90mmHg, pulse >150)
• Chest pain
• Pulmonary oedema
• Syncope

No → (left branch)   Yes → (right branch)

Left branch (No):

Correct electrolytes ↓K⁺, ↓Mg²⁺

↓

Assess rhythm

If regular:
If VT or uncertain rhythm: amiodarone 300mg IV over 20–60min, then 900mg over 24h via central line/large bore cannula

If known BBB consider narrow complex tachycardia with aberrant conduction (p790)

If irregular: Seek expert help.
Diagnosis is usually one of:
• AF with bundle branch block: treat as AF (p126)
• Pre-excited AF (p790): DC shock or flecainide
• Polymorphic VT (torsade de pointes): Mg²⁺ 2g/8mmol IVI

Right branch (Yes):

Get senior/expert help

↓

Sedation/anaesthesia

↓

Synchronized DC shock*
1   120–150J
2   150–360J
3   150–360J

↓

Correct electrolytes ↓K⁺, ↓Mg²

↓

• Amiodarone 300mg IV over 10–20min
• Consider repeat shock
• Amiodarine 900mg/24h IVI via wide-bore cannula/central line

↓

Further cardioversion if needed

↓

For refractory cases:
• Seek expert help
• Consider lidocaine

*Check your defibrillator: energies given are for a typical biphasic defibrillator (preferred). If a monophasic device is used, higher energies will be required.

Fig 19.13 Management of broad complex tachycardia.

ECG shows rate of >100bpm and QRS complex duration of <120ms (<3 small squares on ECG done at the standard UK rate of 25mm/s).

Differential diagnosis (See p122.)

- **Sinus tachycardia** Normal P wave followed by normal QRS. This is not an arrhythmia. Look for and treat the underlying cause, eg hypovolaemia, PE, sepsis, hyperthyroidism.
- **Atrial tachyarrhythmias**
  - *Atrial fibrillation (AF):* absent P wave, irregular QRS complexes. If rhythm is irregular, AF is likely.
  - *Atrial flutter:* atrial rate ~260–340bpm. Saw-tooth baseline, due to a re-entrant circuit usually in the right atrium. Ventricular rate often ~150bpm (ie 2:1 block).
  - *Atrial tachycardia:* abnormally shaped P waves, which may outnumber QRS.
- **Supraventricular tachycardia** AV node is part of the arrhythmogenic pathway. P wave may be either buried in QRS complex or occur after QRS complex.
  - AV nodal re-entry tachycardia.
  - AV re-entry tachycardia via an accessory pathway. Can occur with pre-excitation, eg WPW (p129), or without pre-excitation if only retrograde conduction.

Management ▶Be guided by patient status. See fig 19.14.

▶▶Identify the underlying rhythm and treat accordingly.

▶▶Prepare for DC cardioversion if patient is compromised due to arrhythmia.

Supraventricular tachycardia

1 *Vagal manoeuvres:* carotid sinus massage, modified Valsalva manoeuvre (see p126). Transient increase in AV block may unmask underlying atrial arrhythmia.
2 *Adenosine:* short half-life (10–15s).
   - Give 6mg IV bolus into a large vein, followed by 0.9% saline flush, while recording a rhythm strip (or 12-lead ECG if possible).
   - If unsuccessful after 2min, give 12mg IV.
   - If unsuccessful after 2min, give 18mg IV bolus.
   Warn about SE: chest tightness, dyspnoea, headache, flushing. Do not use in pre-excited AF as can precipitate VT, see p788. Will not work in cardiac transplant as heart is denervated. Caution in asthma (but remember adenosine is short-acting and effective).
3 *Review rhythm strip* after adenosine. If adenosine does not cardiovert, AV block may reveal an alternative atrial arrhythmia.
4 Recurrent SVT: β-blocker, eg metoprolol 5mg IV or atenolol 2.5mg IV; verapamil 5mg IV.
5 *DC cardioversion* if other measures fail or if compromised.
6 Refer for specialist electrophysiology review.

Atrial fibrillation/flutter See BOX: irregular narrow complex tachycardia. Seek help if resistant (p126).

Atrial tachycardia Rare. Manage with rate control. Seek expert help.

Wolff–Parkinson–White (WPW) syndrome (*ECG*, p129, fig 3.42.)

Congenital accessory conduction pathway between atria and ventricles. Resting ECG shows short PR interval, widened QRS complex due to slurred upstroke (= 'delta wave'). Presents with SVT which may be:

- AVRT (p122).
- pre-excited AF/atrial flutter with risk of degeneration to VF and sudden death. Consider if irregularly irregular, varying QRS duration, delta wave, variable rate up to 300bpm (ie too high to be conducted via AV node). Do not use medications which block the AV node as this increases the risk of VF via the accessory pathway. Treat with cardioversion or flecainide.

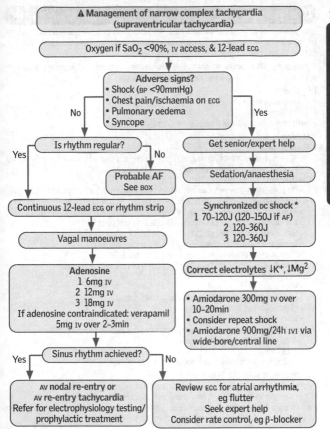

⚠ Management of narrow complex tachycardia
(supraventricular tachycardia)

Oxygen if SaO_2 <90%, IV access, & 12-lead ECG

Adverse signs?
• Shock (BP <90mmHg)
• Chest pain/ischaemia on ECG
• Pulmonary oedema
• Syncope

No ——— Yes

Is rhythm regular?

Yes

No ——— **Probable AF**
See BOX

Continuous 12-lead ECG or rhythm strip

Vagal manoeuvres

Adenosine
1 6mg IV
2 12mg IV
3 18mg IV
If adenosine contraindicated: verapamil
5mg IV over 2–3min

Get senior/expert help

Sedation/anaesthesia

Synchronized DC shock *
1 70–120J (120–150J if AF)
2 120–360J
3 120–360J

Correct electrolytes ↓K⁺, ↓Mg²

• Amiodarone 300mg IV over
10–20min
• Consider repeat shock
• Amiodarone 900mg/24h IVI via
wide-bore/central line

Sinus rhythm achieved?

Yes ——— No

AV nodal re-entry or
AV re-entry tachycardia
Refer for electrophysiology testing/
prophylactic treatment

Review ECG for atrial arrhythmia,
eg flutter
Seek expert help
Consider rate control, eg β-blocker

*Check your defibrillator: energies given are for a typical biphasic defibrillator (preferred). If a monophasic device is used, higher energies will be required.

Fig 19.14 Management of narrow complex tachycardia.

⚠ Irregular narrow complex tachycardia

• AF is the most likely diagnosis.
• The need for emergency rate control is uncommon. Treat precipitants, eg hypovolaemia, sepsis. Consider:
  • β-blocker: eg metoprolol 5mg IV if rapid rate control needed. Otherwise oral β-blocker. Caution if LVF.
  • Rate limiting calcium-channel blocker: eg diltiazem, verapamil.
  • Digoxin. Load (eg 500mcg PO every 8h for 3 doses), then maintenance (eg 125–250mcg PO daily).
• LMWH or DOAC based on persistence beyond 48h, and stroke/bleeding risk.
• Rhythm control. Cardioversion. Risk of thromboembolism unless clear onset <48h, or effectively anticoagulated for >3wk.
  • Electrical cardioversion: synchronized DC cardioversion under sedation.
  • Chemical cardioversion: flecainide (normal heart structure and no IHD), amiodarone.

Bradycardia is defined as a heart rate <60bpm. This may be normal and asymptomatic in fit individuals as large stroke volumes will maintain adequate cardiac output at low heart rates.

Symptoms Often asymptomatic. Fatigue, nausea, dizziness. The presence of syncope, chest pain, or breathlessness are adverse signs.

Rhythm
- Sinus bradycardia.
- Heart block (p90).
- AF/flutter with a slow ventricular response.

Aetiology
- **Physiological**
  - Sinus rhythm of <40bpm can occur in the absence of pathology in athletes and at night. If asymptomatic, this needs no treatment.
- **Cardiac**
  - Degenerative changes causing fibrosis of conduction pathways. May have previous ECG showing bundle branch block or 1st- or 2nd-degree heart block.
  - Post-MI. Particularly after an inferior MI as the right coronary artery supplies the sinoatrial and atrioventricular nodes in most people.
  - Sick-sinus syndrome (p121).
  - Iatrogenic: anti-arrhythmic drugs, post-cardiac surgery.
  - Myocarditis, cardiomyopathy, amyloid, sarcoid.
  - Infective endocarditis (p144) with erosion of conduction tissue.
- **Non-cardiac**
  - Vasovagal: common (p456).
  - Endocrine: hypothyroidism, adrenal insufficiency.
  - Metabolic: hyperkalaemia, hypoxia.
  - Infective: Lyme disease.
  - Other: hypothermia, ↑ICP (hypertension with a widening pulse pressure, bradycardia, and abnormal respiration).
- **Drug induced**
  - β-blockers, amiodarone, verapamil, diltiazem, digoxin.

Management ►See fig 19.15
- Perform a 12-lead ECG, ensure cardiac monitor/telemetry.
- Check electrolytes (K^+, Ca^{2+}, Mg^{2+}), digoxin concentration.
- Address the cause: correct metabolic defects. Reverse toxicity, eg glucagon in β-blocker overdose, digoxin-specific antibody, see p826.

Atropine
Use if adverse signs or risk of asystole (►ineffective if heart transplant as it is denervated).

If atropine is insufficient and adverse signs persist, consider transcutaneous pacing (p761). Remember electrical 'capture' with transcutaneous pacing does not guarantee mechanical 'capture'. Once pacing is established, check the patient's pulse.

If pacing cannot be initiated immediately (eg delay for sedation/anaesthesia), consider isoprenaline/adrenaline.

►It is possible to have two patients sat next to each other with identical bradycardic ECG tracings, one of whom is peri-arrest, the other is sat comfortably and cannot understand your concern. The clinical state is more important than the numbers on the screen.

►►Anticipate the need for an anaesthetist to sedate the patient for transcutaneous pacing, or a cardiologist for transvenous pacing. Contact them early.

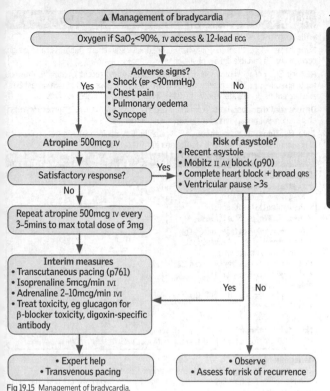

Fig 19.15 Management of bradycardia.

Acute severe asthma

►The severity of an attack is easily underestimated. See BOX.

Symptoms More than one of wheeze, breathlessness, chest tightness, and cough, occurring with variable airflow obstruction.

History See p46. Symptoms and progression. Usual and recent treatment. Previous acute episodes and their severity including critical care admission. Best (within last 2yrs) and current peak expiratory flow rate (PEF). Triggers: infection, allergy, reflux.

Differential diagnosis COPD, pulmonary oedema, anaphylaxis, upper respiratory tract obstruction, pulmonary embolus, pneumonia/pneumonitis.

Investigations PEF, ABG if saturations <92% or life-threatening features, CXR (if suspicion of pneumothorax, infection, or if life-threatening attack), FBC, U&E.

Asthma severity

Severe attack Any one of:
- Unable to complete sentences in one breath.
- Respiratory rate ≥25/min.
- Pulse rate ≥110 beats/min.
- PEF 33–50% of predicted or best.

Life-threatening attack Any one of:
- Altered conscious level, exhaustion.
- Arrhythmia or hypotension.
- Silent chest, cyanosis, feeble respiratory effort.
- PEF <33% of predicted or best.
- Arterial blood gas:
  - Inappropriately 'normal' P_aCO_2 >4.6kPa.
  - P_aO_2 <8kPa.
  - S_aO_2 <92%.

Near-fatal asthma
High P_aCO_2 and/or requiring mechanical ventilation with raised inflation pressures.

Management
►Recognition, rapid treatment and reassessment are key,[4] see fig 19.16.
►Monitor oxygen saturation, heart rate, respiratory rate, and PEF before and after nebulized treatment.
- Supplementary oxygen to maintain saturations 94–98%.
- Nebulized β_2 agonist (eg salbutamol 5mg, terbutaline 10mg), driven by oxygen (usually 6L/min). Repeat doses every 15–30min. Continuous nebulizer therapy (5–10mg/h) if inadequate response. SE: tachycardia, arrhythmias, tremor, ↓K⁺. IV β_2-agonists only if inhaled therapy not reliable/possible.
- Prednisolone 40–50mg PO for minimum 5d. Continue inhaled corticosteroids. Hydrocortisone 100mg every 6h only if parenteral route not available.
- Nebulized ipratropium bromide 500mcg every 4–6h if severe asthma, or poor response to β_2 agonists alone.
- Consider magnesium sulfate 1.2–2g IV over 20min in severe disease. Use a single dose as toxicity leads to muscle weakness and possible respiratory fatigue.
- Antibiotics are not given routinely: look for evidence of bacterial infection including procalcitonin.
- Aminophylline is not recommended. It does not provide any additional bronchodilation compared to inhaled β_2-agonists alone, and adverse effects include ↓BP, arrhythmias, and seizures.

Discharge
- Increased risk of relapse/readmission if PEF <75% predicted/best with diurnal variability >25%.
- Education on inhaler technique and PEF monitoring prior to discharge. Provide a written PEF and symptom-based plan for patient-led adjustment of therapy. These interventions reduce morbidity and relapse.
- Follow-up: GP/asthma nurse (ideally within 2d of discharge), respiratory specialist.

Management of acute asthma

Assess
- Ability to speak, O_2 saturation, PEF, RR, HR
- Expert/senior help
- Critical care if severe or life-threatening attack (p794)

↓

Treat
- O_2 to maintain sats 94–98%
- Salbutamol 5mg nebulized with O_2
- Prednisolone 40–50mg PO
- If severe disease: ipratropium bromide 0.5mg/4–6h nebulized with O_2

↓

Reassess every 15 min
- Monitor: ability to speak, O_2 saturation, PEF, RR, HR, ECG
- Salbutamol 5mg nebulized with O_2 every 15–30min, or 10mg/h continuously
- Ipratropium bromide 500mcg/4–6h nebulized with O_2, if poor clinical response and not already given
- Consider $MgSO_4$ 1.2–2g IV over 20min in severe/life-threatening disease

↓

►► If not improving
Refer to critical care for consideration of ventilatory support if:
- Deteriorating PEF
- Persistent/worsening hypoxia
- Exhaustion, feeble respiration
- Hypercapnia
- Acidosis: respiratory or lactic
- Drowsiness, confusion, altered conscious level
- Respiratory arrest
- Other clinical concern

Fig 19.16 Management of acute asthma.

19 Emergencies

Risk factors for asthma-related death

- Difficulty with adherence to asthma monitoring/medications/self-escalation.
- β_2-agonist monotherapy with no inhaled corticosteroid use.
- Current or recent use of oral steroids.
- History of poorly controlled asthma including:
  - near-fatal asthma requiring intubation and mechanical ventilation
  - hospitalization or ED visit for asthma in the past year.
- Coexisting psychiatric disease.
- Social deprivation.

Acute exacerbation of COPD

An acute-onset, sustained worsening of symptoms compared to usual symptoms that is beyond normal day-to-day variation. Common, especially in winter.

Presentation Increase in dyspnoea, worsening of chronic cough, increase in volume/purulence of sputum.

History Breathlessness, cough, sputum production. Exercise tolerance (distance on flat, number of stairs) now and recent best. Usual/recent treatment. Haemoptysis. Weight loss. Smoking status. Independence in activities of daily living. Quality of life from the patient's perspective. Comorbidity, eg IHD, CKD. Complicating symptoms, eg chest pain, palpitations. See p46.

Differential diagnosis Asthma, pulmonary oedema, upper respiratory tract obstruction, pulmonary embolus, anaphylaxis.

Investigations
- ABG (p755).
- CXR: airspace shadowing, pneumothorax, pulmonary oedema, malignancy.
- Blood tests: FBC, U&E, CRP. Theophylline concentration.
- Microbiology: sputum culture, viral swab (including SARS-COV-2), blood culture.

Management ▶ Ensure oxygenation and treat the reversible.[5,6] See fig 19.17.
- Location of care depends on community expertise (eg hospital-at-home) and patient preference. Hospital admission usually indicated if severe dyspnoea, deteriorating condition, cyanosis, worsening peripheral oedema, confusion/impaired consciousness, significant comorbidity, worsening hypoxia/acidosis.
- Assess symptom burden/severity: eg COPD Assessment Test (CAT) score, **DECAF** (**D**yspnoea, **E**osinopenia, **C**onsolidation, **A**cidaemia, atrial **F**ibrillation).
- Treat hypoxia: O_2 to target saturation 94–98% for most acutely unwell patients, or 88–92% or individualized target range if risk of hypercapnic respiratory failure (see BOX). Prescribe O_2 like a drug and monitor P_aO_2 and P_aCO_2.
- β_2 agonist: nebulized (eg salbutamol 5mg) or hand-held inhaler. If hypercapnic or acidotic, drive nebulizer with compressed air, with additional oxygen guided by O_2 saturation and P_aO_2 and P_aCO_2.
- Ipratropium bromide: 500mcg/4–6h, driven with compressed air.
- Corticosteroids: 30–40mg prednisolone PO daily for 5 days (may be less effective if blood eosinophil count <300 cells/microlitre).
- IV theophylline has significant side effects (↓BP, arrhythmia, seizures) with no high-quality evidence of efficacy and is not recommended.
- Treat trigger(s): infection, pneumothorax.
- Treat/prevent complications: sepsis, haemodynamic instability, fluid balance, heart failure, arrhythmia, VTE prophylaxis, nutrition.

Ceiling of care Ventilation may be futile if no reversibility. Ventilation also confers risk of infection, pneumothorax, & VTE. Can the patient survive critical care admission? Consider comorbidity, lung function, functional status, home oxygen, and patient's wishes. Talk to the patient, their family/advocates, and expert physicians early.

Oxygen therapy

▶▶ Prescribe O_2 as if it were a drug.

▶▶ Hypoxia is more dangerous than hypercapnia. *Use high-flow oxygen for all who are critically unwell and then adjust.*

▶▶ Monitor ABG within 60min of initiation or change of oxygen therapy.
- Some patients have a hypoxic drive to breathe. Excess oxygen leads to ↓respiratory drive, hypercapnia, respiratory acidosis, and ↓consciousness.
- If risk factors for hypercapnia (moderate/severe COPD, previous hypercapnic respiratory failure, long-term oxygen, chest wall/spinal disease, bronchiectasis, obesity) and not critically unwell:
  - Start with 24–28% humidified O_2 via venturi mask, aim O_2 saturations 88–92%.
  - P_aO_2 <8.0kPa and P_aCO_2 ≤6.0kPa: aim O_2 saturations 94–98%.
  - P_aO_2 <8.0kPa and P_aCO_2 >6.0kPa consider non-invasive ventilation/critical-care.

19 Emergencies

▲ **Management of acute exacerbation of COPD**

Treat hypoxia
If hypoxic and critically unwell/peri-arrest treat with high-flow O_2

Risk of hypercapnia

- Moderate or severe COPD
- Previous hypercapnic respiratory failure
- Long-term oxygen
- Chest wall/spinal disease
- Bronchiectasis
- Obesity

Yes

- 24–28% O_2 via Venturi mask
- Aim O_2 saturations 88–92%
- Monitor ABG at 30–60min:
  1 P_aO_2 ≥8.0kPa and P_aCO_2 ≤6.0kPa: no change
  2 P_aO_2 <8.0kPa and P_aCO_2 ≤6.0kPa: aim O_2 saturations 94–98%
  3 P_aO_2 <8.0kPa and P_aCO_2 >6.0kPa: NIPPV/critical care

No

- Aim O_2 saturations 94–98%
- Monitor ABG at 30–60 min
  1 P_aO_2 ≥8.0kPa and P_aCO_2 ≤6.0kPa: no change
  2 P_aO_2 ≥8.0kPa and P_aCO_2 >6.0kPa: aim O_2 saturations 88–92%
  3 P_aO_2 <8.0kPa and P_aCO_2 >6.0kPa: NIPPV/critical care

Bronchodilators
- Salbutamol 5mg/4h driven with air
- Ipratropium bromide 500mcg/6h driven with air

Corticosteroids
eg prednisolone 30–40mg OD for 5d
Consider eosinophil count. Monitor blood glucose and fluid balance

Adjuncts
- Antibiotics: if symptoms/evidence of infection, according to local sensitivities
- Physiotherapy to aid sputum expectoration

Ventilatory support (see BOX)
- Consider if no response/deterioration: RR >23, pH <7.35, P_aCO_2 >6.5kPa
- Review ceiling of care (p796)

Fig 19.17 Management of acute COPD.

Ventilatory support: non-invasive ventilation (NIV)

- Bilevel positive airways pressure (BiPAP): a tight-fitting face mask delivers two different airway pressures: inspiratory (IPAP) and expiratory (EPAP) pressures.
- Consider in modest respiratory acidosis to try to prevent deterioration to invasive ventilation, or as highest level of support if invasive ventilation not suitable.
- Prior to start: ABG, CXR (but do not delay start), treat reversible causes, agree measures if NIV fails. Explain treatment to patient.
- Start: IPAP 10–15cmH$_2$O, EPAP 4cmH$_2$O, FiO$_2$ to saturations 88–92%. Other settings with guidance: eg backup rate 10–16/min, I:E 1:2–3, inspiratory time 0.8–1.2s.
- Escalate: IPAP over 10–30 minutes to 20–30cmH$_2$O, as tolerated.
- Adjust: ABG 1 hour after a settings change, or if clinically indicated.
  - ↑P_aCO_2: ↑tidal volume by ↑IPAP (expert review for IPAP >30cmH$_2$O).
  - ↓P_aO_2: ↑FiO$_2$ (consider ↑IPAP to prevent ↑P_aCO_2) or ↑EPAP (expert review for EPAP >8cmH$_2$O).
- Maximize NIV use for as much time as possible in first 24h. Wean over 48–72h depending on self-ventilating P_aCO_2 and clinical review.

Aetiology
- **Primary spontaneous**
  - Occurs in the absence of trauma, usually due to rupture of a subpleural bulla.
- **Secondary spontaneous**
  - Chronic lung disease: asthma, COPD, cystic fibrosis, lung fibrosis, sarcoidosis.
  - Infection: TB, pneumonia, SARS-COV-2, *Pneumocystis jirovecii*, lung abscess.
  - Lung cancer.
  - Connective tissue disorder: Marfan's syndrome, Ehlers–Danlos syndrome.
  - Suspected lung disease: aged >50yrs and significant smoking history.
- **Traumatic**
  - Includes iatrogenic, eg CVP line insertion, pleural aspiration/biopsy, percutaneous liver biopsy, positive pressure ventilation.

Clinical features
Symptoms

Asymptomatic (especially if small pneumothorax) or sudden onset of dyspnoea and/or pleuritic chest pain. Patients with asthma or COPD may present with a sudden deterioration. Sudden hypoxia or an increase in ventilation pressures in mechanically ventilated patients.

Signs

Reduced expansion, hyperresonance to percussion, and diminished breath sounds on the affected side. With a *tension pneumothorax*, the trachea will be deviated away from the affected side (see BOX).

Tests

▶*A CXR should not be performed if a tension pneumothorax is suspected, as it will delay immediate necessary treatment.*
- If no tension pneumothorax, request an expiratory film, and look for an area devoid of lung markings peripheral to a visible edge of the collapsed lung (see p709). Measured from the visible lung margin to chest wall at level of the hilum.
- Oxygen saturation and ABG in dyspnoeic patients and those with chronic lung disease.
- CT thorax can differentiate emphysematous bulla from pneumothorax. May be warranted to investigate underlying lung disease.

Management
Analgesia and oxygen as required.

Management depends on the degree of compromise and the likelihood of spontaneous resolution. Response to needle aspiration may be different if there is underlying lung disease. See fig 19.18. Management includes:
- Oxygen if hypoxic.
- Aspiration of a pneumothorax with 16–18G cannula, see p751.
- Chest drain insertion see p750. Use a small tube (10–14F) unless blood/pus is also present. Negative pressure suction may be required. Tubes may be removed 24h after the lung has re-expanded and air leak has stopped (ie the drain stops bubbling). Remove during expiration or Valsalva manoeuvre. Pneumothorax in mechanical ventilation usually requires a chest drain.

Cardiothoracic input
If:
- Bilateral pneumothoraces.
- Lung fails to expand within 48h of drain insertion.
- Persistent air leak.
- Two or more previous pneumothoraces on the same side, or history of pneumothorax on the opposite side.
- Tension pneumothorax.
- High-risk occupation (eg pilot, diver).

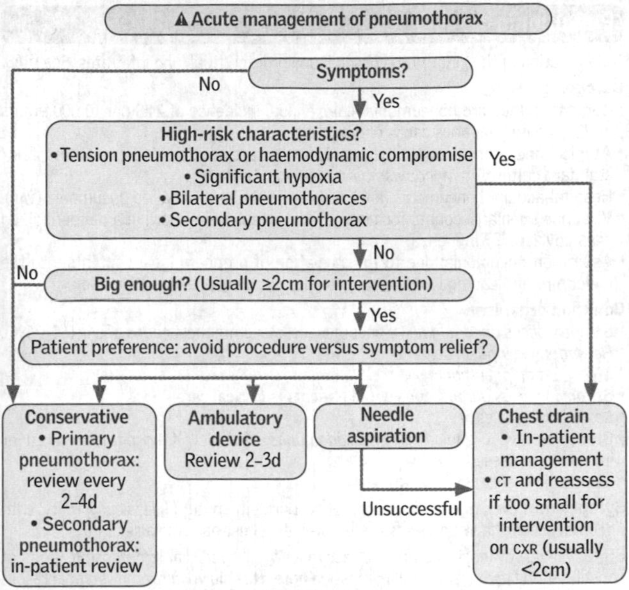

Fig 19.18 Acute management of pneumothorax.

Tension pneumothorax

This is a medical emergency. See fig 16.44, p733.

Aetiology

Air drawn into the pleural space with each inspiration has no route of escape during expiration. The mediastinum is pushed over into the contralateral hemithorax, compressing the great veins. Unless the air is rapidly removed, cardiorespiratory arrest will occur.

Signs

Respiratory distress, tachycardia, hypotension, distended neck veins, tracheal deviation away from side of pneumothorax, increased percussion note, reduced air entry/breath sounds on the affected side.

Treatment

▶▶Do not delay treatment in order to get a CXR.

1 Insert a large-bore (14-16G) needle connected to a syringe partially filled with 0.9% saline, into the 2nd intercostal interspace in the midclavicular line on the side of the pneumothorax. Remove plunger to allow the trapped air to bubble through the syringe (with saline as a water seal) until a chest tube can be placed. Alternatively, insert a large-bore Venflon in the same location.

2 Insert a chest drain. See p750.

Inflammation of the lungs with consolidation or interstitial lung infiltrates. See p168.

Categories

- Community-acquired pneumonia (CAP): annual incidence of 24.8 per 10 000 adults and a leading infectious cause of death.
- Atypical pneumonia: caused by organisms that are not detectable on Gram stain/ standard culture, eg *Mycoplasma pneumoniae*, *Legionella*.
- Hospital-acquired pneumonia (HAP), including ventilator-acquired pneumonia (VAP).
- Viral pneumonia: accounts for up to 15% of pneumonia (more in a pandemic), eg SARS-COV-2 (p172), influenza.
- Aspiration pneumonia: due to the inhalation of oropharyngeal contents into the lower airways leading to chemical pneumonitis, lung injury, and infection.

Common organisms

- *Streptococcus pneumoniae* (= pneumococcus): commonest cause of CAP (60–75%).
- *Haemophilus influenzae*.
- *Mycoplasma pneumoniae*.
- *Staphylococcus aureus:* consider in patients in critical care.
- *Legionella* species.
- Gram-negative organisms, eg *Pseudomonas*: consider if hospital acquired or immunosuppressed.
- Viruses: influenza, SARS-COV-2.

Symptoms Fever, rigors, dyspnoea, cough, purulent sputum (classically 'rusty' with pneumococcus), haemoptysis (see BOX), pleuritic chest pain, malaise.

Signs Fever, cyanosis, confusion, tachypnoea, tachycardia, hypotension, signs of consolidation (↓expansion, dull percussion note, ↑tactile vocal fremitus/vocal resonance, bronchial breathing), pleural rub.

Severity 'CURB-65' score

- **C**onfusion (abbreviated mental test score ≤8).
- **U**rea >7mmol/L.
- **R**espiratory rate ≥30/min.
- **B**P <90/60mmHg.
- Age ≥**65**.

Score: 0–1: home treatment if possible; ≥2: hospital treatment; ≥3: severe pneumonia with high risk of mortality.

Mortality is also increased in: coexisting disease, bilateral/multilobar involvement P_aO_2 <8kPa or S_aO_2 <92%.

Investigations

- Oxygen saturation, ABG if S_aO_2 <92% or severe pneumonia.
- FBC, U&E, LFT, CRP.
- CXR (fig 16.4, p709). CT may be helpful to identify complications (eg in immunosuppression) or if CXR non-diagnostic.
- Culture: sputum, blood, pleural fluid.
- Viral throat swabs including influenza, parainfluenza, and SARS-COV-2.
- Urine pneumococcal antigen, *Legionella* antigen, *Mycoplasma* PCR/serology.
- Consider bronchoscopy and bronchoalveolar lavage if immunocompromised, critical illness or not responding to treatment.

Management

▶Ensure oxygenation. See fig 19.19.

- Antibiotics: as soon as possible and within 1h if sepsis (p772–3, fig 19.5). See antibiotic guidance in table 4.6, p169. Use of IV antibiotics should be reviewed daily and switched to PO therapy as soon as clinically improved and able to take oral medication. Narrow spectrum to target specific organism if identified. Antibiotics can be stopped after 5d depending on fever in last 48h, BP, HR, RR, and oxygen saturation.

Complications Pleural effusion, empyema, lung abscess, AKI. See p168.

Prevention Smoking cessation. Influenza, pneumococcal, and SARS-COV-2 vaccination (p169).

▲ Management of pneumonia

Sepsis
If signs/risk of sepsis: manage as sepsis with chest source (fig 19.5, p773)

↓

Assess (p800)
• Symptoms and signs
• Investigation
• Risk assessment, eg CURB-65 score

↓

Treat
• Oxygen if hypoxia
• Controlled O_2 therapy if hypercapnia/risk of hypercapnia (fig 19.17, p797)
• Treat hypotension: IV crystalloid if volume deplete
• Antibiotics (p169)

↓

Adjuncts
• VTE prophylaxis
• Steroids if asthma (fig 19.16, p795)/COPD (fig 19.7, p797)/SARS-COV-2 pneumonitis (pp172–3)
• Analgesia for pleuritic chest pain, eg paracetamol 1g/6h or NSAID
• Physiotherapy
• Nutrition

↓

Response
Ventilatory support/critical care if fails to respond to treatment

Fig 19.19 Management of pneumonia.

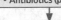

19 Emergencies

Life-threatening haemoptysis

Definition

=Any amount of haemoptysis that causes significant haemodynamic decompensation or respiratory distress, which may lead to death if left untreated.

Definitions using volume of haemoptysis are variable, difficult to measure, and less clinically useful, eg up to 1L/24h, bleeding ≥100mL/h.

Causes

Lung cancer, bronchiectasis, TB, lung abscess, pulmonary AVM, autoimmune (eg ANCA vasculitis, anti-GBM disease), cryptogenic (↑ in smokers), post-biopsy.

Investigations

FBC, PT/APTT/INR, blood type and cross-match, kidney function and urine dip, autoimmune screen, infection screen, CT thorax ± aortogram.

Management

▶Ensure adequate oxygenation and ventilation.
• Secure the airway, eg with a endotracheal tube. If available, a double lumen tube can isolate the lungs, but do not delay intubation of non-bleeding side.
• Turn patient bleeding side down so blood localizes in affected lung due to gravity.
• Treat haemodynamic instability: blood product replacement ± vasopressors.
• Correct any coagulopathy.
• Diagnostic and therapeutic bronchoscopy: clears airway of blood, locates bleeding site, bronchial balloon/blockade, thermal ablation.
• Radiological bronchial artery embolization.
• Surgery (typically a lobectomy) if bronchoscopic/angiographic interventions fail.
• Specific treatments, eg immunosuppression in pulmonary–renal syndromes: ANCA vasculitis (p310), anti-GBM disease (p307).

Pulmonary embolism (PE)

Mechanism Venous thrombi migrate to the pulmonary arterial tree and cause obstruction. The source may be occult.

▶Suspect a PE in sudden collapse in anyone with risk factors for VTE.

Types
- *High risk (massive):* haemodynamically unstable, SBP <90mmHg or drop ≥40mmHg (not due to hypovolaemia/arrhythmia/sepsis), tissue hypoperfusion. ↑Risk of death: up to 50% within 30min. Thrombolysis is indicated.
- *Intermediate risk (submassive):* haemodynamically stable but evidence of RV strain (hypokinesis, dilatation, pulmonary hypertension). Risk/benefit of thrombolysis less clear and thrombolysis is not routine.
- *Low risk (non-massive):* haemodynamically stable with no right heart strain.

Risk factors
- Malignancy, myeloproliferative disorder.
- Immobility, including surgery (especially pelvic/lower limb), hospital admission.
- Active inflammation: eg infection, SARS-COV-2, IBD.
- Oestrogens: pregnancy, combined OCP, HRT.
- Previous VTE, inherited thrombophilia (p370), antiphospholipid syndrome (APLS).

Signs and symptoms
- Acute dyspnoea, pleuritic chest pain, haemoptysis, syncope, cardiac arrest.
- Hypotension, tachycardia, gallop rhythm, ↑JVP, loud P₂, right ventricular heave, pleural rub, tachypnoea, cyanosis, AF.

Investigations
▶A clinical decision tool that predicts pre-test probability of PE helps determine necessary investigations. Use 2-level Wells score for PE (p187).
- *D-dimer:* in a low-probability patient, a negative result effectively excludes PE (not in pregnancy).[7] Low specificity: also ↑ in inflammation/infection, post-op, infection, pregnancy ∴ check only in patients with low pre-test probability (p187).
- *Other bloods:* FBC, U&E, clotting, troponin (marker of RV dysfunction).
- *ECG:* normal, sinus tachycardia, right ventricular strain pattern V₁–V₃ (p90), right axis deviation, RBBB, AF. 'SI QIII TIII' = S wave in I, Q wave in III, inverted T in III.
- *CXR:* normal, decreased vascular markings, small pleural effusion, wedge-shaped area of infarction, atelectasis.
- *ABG:* hypoxia despite hyperventilation: ↓P_aO_2, ↓P_aCO_2, ↑pH.
- *CT pulmonary angiography (CTPA):* sensitive and specific in high-risk patients and low-risk patients with a +ve D-dimer. A *ventilation·perfusion (V/Q) scan* can aid diagnosis but may be inconclusive, and will not exclude other differentials.
- **P**ulmonary **E**mbolism **S**everity **I**ndex (PESI) (or simplified SPESI) assesses risk of mortality and complications. Close monitoring of intermediate-risk PE with ↑ scores may allow early detection of instability and need for rescue reperfusion.

Management ▶Treat[7] (fig 19.20) before definitive investigations if convincing presentation: most PE deaths occur <1h.
- Commence LMWH or DOAC (eg apixaban, rivaroxaban). Consider haemodynamic stability, kidney function, pregnancy status, and aetiology, eg malignancy, APLS, when choosing agent/dose.
- If high-risk (massive) PE with haemodynamic instability: thrombolyse, eg alteplase 10mg IV over 1min, then 90mg IVI over 2h (max 1.5mg/kg). Catheter-directed thrombolysis, or catheter/surgical embolectomy if thrombolysis is contraindicated or fails.
- Long-term anticoagulation: DOAC (p346, switch directly from LMWH) or warfarin (continue LMWH until INR >2).
- Is there an underlying cause, eg thrombophilia (p370), SLE, polycythaemia? Consider malignancy: history and physical examination, CXR, FBC, LFT, Ca^{2+}; urinalysis, consider CT abdomen/pelvis and mammogram.
- If clear temporary/reversible precipitant, 3 months of anticoagulation (p347) may be enough, otherwise, continue for ≥3–6 months. Long-term anticoagulation for recurrent emboli, or ongoing risk, eg malignancy, APLS.

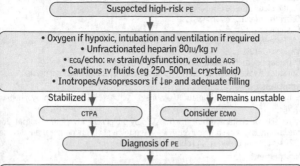

△ Management of high-risk (massive) pulmonary embolism

Suspected high-risk PE

• Oxygen if hypoxic, intubation and ventilation if required
• Unfractionated heparin 80IU/kg IV
• ECG/echo: RV strain/dysfunction, exclude ACS
• Cautious IV fluids (eg 250–500mL crystalloid)
• Inotropes/vasopressors if ↓BP and adequate filling

Stabilized → CTPA

Remains unstable → Consider ECMO

Diagnosis of PE

Reperfusion therapy
Thrombolysis: eg IV alteplase 10mg in 1min, then 90mg over 2h (max 1.5mg/kg)
If contraindications to thrombolysis: *surgical/catheter embolectomy*

Fig 19.20 Management of high-risk pulmonary embolism.[7]

Thrombolysis therapy in PE

Indication for thrombolysis
• High-risk (massive) PE.

Review risk versus benefit of thrombolysis
• Intermediate-risk PE with high risk of mortality/complications (eg PESI score).
• Patients with acute PE who appear to be decompensating but are not yet hypotensive.
• Patients with extensive clot burden.

Absolute contraindications
• Active bleeding or bleeding diathesis (eg severe thrombocytopenia).
• Recent (<2 months) intracranial or spinal surgery or trauma.
• Intracranial neoplasm.
• History of intracerebral haemorrhage, or ischaemic stroke within the previous 3 months.

Relative contraindications
• Severe uncontrolled hypertension (ie systolic BP >200mmHg or diastolic BP >110mmHg).
• Ischaemic stroke >3 months.
• Surgery within previous 10 days.
• Pregnancy (can be given and may be life-saving).
• Recent invasive procedure.
• Non-compressible vascular punctures.
• Active peptic ulcer disease.

Causes
• Peptic ulcer disease (35–50%).
• Gastroduodenal erosions (8–15%).
• Oesophagitis (5–15%).
• Mallory–Weiss tear (15%).
• Varices (5–10%).
• Other: upper GI malignancy, vascular malformation.
• Consider swallowed blood due to facial trauma, epistaxis, or haemoptysis.

Symptoms
Haematemesis, melaena, (postural) dizziness, fainting, abdominal pain, dysphagia.

Signs
↓BP (check for postural drop), ↑HR (masked by β-blocker), ↓JVP, ↓urine output, cool and clammy, signs of chronic liver disease (eg telangiectasia, purpura, jaundice, see p272). Ask about previous GI problems, drug use, alcohol.

Management
►Focus on circulation,[8] see fig 19.21.
• Assess for shock:
    • Peripherally cool/clammy, capillary refill time >2s, urine output <0.5mL/kg/h.
    • Tachycardic (HR >100bpm).
    • Systolic BP <90mmHg or postural drop >20mmHg.
• If shock or ↓GCS/encephalopathy (p271), seek expert/senior advice and refer to critical care.
• Risk stratify, eg Glasgow–Blatchford score (GBS). If low score (GBS 0–1), consider outpatient management. A higher score means ↑risk of needing transfusion/endoscopy/surgery (GBS score ≥6 = risk of needing intervention >50%).
• Monitor HR, BP, RR, oxygen saturation, temperature, consciousness, urine output.
• Insert two large-bore (14–16G) IV cannulae and take blood for FBC, U&E, LFT, clotting, lactate, glucose, blood group ± cross-match. Consider ABG, ECG, CXR.
• IV fluid if haemodynamically unstable (fig 19.21). Avoid saline if cirrhotic. CVP may facilitate monitoring and/or guide fluid replacement.
• Transfuse if significant Hb drop (<70g/L), aim Hb 70–100g/L.
• Correct clotting abnormalities (vitamin K (p270), FFP, platelets).
• Continue aspirin but stop other antiplatelets/anticoagulants.
• If suspicion of varices (eg known history of liver disease or alcohol excess): terlipressin 2mg IV/6h and initiate broad-spectrum IV antibiotics (according to local guidance, eg piperacillin/tazobactam IV 4.5g/8h).
• Nil by mouth for urgent *endoscopy* (p244).
• If endoscopic control fails, mesenteric angiography/embolization or surgery may be needed. For uncontrolled oesophageal variceal bleeding, a Sengstaken–Blakemore tube may compress the varices.

Acute drug therapy There is no role for routine proton pump inhibitor (PPI) treatment pre-endoscopy (provided endoscopy can be arranged in a timely manner). If endoscopic evidence/treatment of bleeding give PPI (eg omeprazole 40mg/12h IV/PO or intermittent IV or high-dose PO). Treat if positive for *Helicobacter pylori* (p249).

Re-bleeds Serious event: mortality up to 40%. Maintain a high index of suspicion. Seek expert/senior advice regarding repeat endoscopy or radiological/surgical intervention.

Signs of a (re)bleed

• ↑Heart rate.
• ↓BP.
• ↓JVP.
• ↓Urine output.
• Haematemesis or 'fresh' rectal bleeding (NB: it is normal to pass decreasing amounts of melaena after haemostasis, as blood makes its way through the GI tract).
• ↓Conscious level.

Fig 19.21 Management of an upper GI bleed.

⚠ Management of GI bleed

Protect airway and keep NBM
► If major haemorrhage, manage with major haemorrhage protocol (p774)

• Insert two large-bore cannulae (14–16G)
• Urgent: FBC, U&E, LFT, glucose, clotting screen, lactate, cross-match 4–6 units

Monitor
• Monitor HR, BP, RR, oxygen saturation, temperature, conscious level
• Monitor urine output. Aim for >30mL/h

Circulation
• IV crystalloid if unstable: 500mL in <15min
• Transfuse if Hb <70g/L, aim Hb 70–100g/L

Coagulation
• Correct clotting abnormalities
• Platelet tranfusion if ≤50 x 10⁹/L
• Continue low dose aspirin, stop/reverse other antiplatelets/anticoagulants

Liver disease
If suspected cirrhosis/variceal bleed (eg known liver disease, alcohol excess):
• Terlipressin IV 2mg/6h (care in IHD/PVD, check ECG)
• Broad-spectrum IV antibiotics according to local guidance

Endoscopy
• Haemodynamic instability: urgent endoscopy
• Haemodynamically stable: within 24h

Proton pump inhibitor
If ulcer with evidence of recent bleed
eg IV omeprazole 80mg then 8mg/h for 72h or intermittent IV or high dose oral

Other expertise
• Gastroenterology follow-up if endoscopic therapy given, or if varices
• Radiological/surgical intervention for failed endoscopic therapy
• Post-haemostasis plan for antiplatelets/anticoagulants

Meningitis

Primary care ► Prompt actions save lives.
►► *If meningitis suspected: urgent transfer to secondary care.*
►► *If non-blanching rash: benzylpenicillin 1.2g IM/IV before transfer.*

Organisms Meningococcus, pneumococcus. Less common: *Haemophilus influenzae*; *Listeria monocytogenes*, HSV, VZV, enteroviruses. If immunocompromised, consider CMV, cryptococcus (p396), TB (p389).

Differential diagnosis Malaria, encephalitis, subarachnoid haemorrhage, dengue,
tetanus.

Features

Early Headache, fever, cold peripheries, abnormal skin colour.

Late
• Meningism: neck stiffness, photophobia,
Kernig's sign (pain + resistance on passive
knee extension with hip fully flexed).
• Non-blanching petechial rash (fig 19.22).
Inspect carefully: may only be 1 or 2 spots.

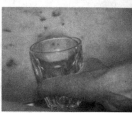
Fig 19.22 Glass test for petechiae.
Courtesy of Meningitis Research Foundation.

• ↓GCS, coma.
• Seizures (~20%), focal CNS signs (~20%), opisthotonus (p432, fig 9.47).
• Septic shock. See pp772–3.

Signs of infective cause VZV: zoster rash. HSV: cold sore/genital vesicles. HIV: lymphadenopathy, dermatitis, candidiasis, uveitis. Leptospirosis: bleeding ± red eye.
Mumps: parotid swelling. EBV (p401): sore throat, jaundice, lymphadenopathy.

Management ► See fig 19.23. Treat and investigate in parallel.
• *Early antibiotics:* blood culture out, antibiotics in. LP prior to antibiotics only if no
septic shock, petechial rash, or ↑ICP, and if able to obtain LP within 1h (table 19.4).
Antibiotics according to local guidance, eg ceftriaxone 2g/12h IV. Cover listeria if
immunocompromised, >50 years, or pregnant, eg amoxicillin 2g/4h IV. If suspect
encephalitis see p808.
• *↑ICP:* signs include papilloedema, seizures, focal neurology, reduced conscious level.
Seek expert help and transfer to critical care.
• *Meningism:* dexamethasone (after antibiotics given) 10mg/6h IV for 12h (4d if
pneumococcal meningitis).
• *Other investigation:* FBC (get help if neutropenia), U&E, LFT, glucose, clotting
studies. Throat swabs (bacterial and viral). CXR. Consider HIV, TB.
• *Prophylaxis:* according to public health/expert advice. Give to contacts in droplet
range, eg 1 dose ciprofloxacin 500mg PO, or rifampicin 600mg BD PO for 2d.

Differential diagnosis for petechial rash

► Considering other causes should not delay treatment if meningitis suspected.

Other causes of petechial rash may also be urgent:
• Acute leukaemia.
• Vasculitis.
• Thrombocytopenia (eg ITP, p343).
• Dengue.
• Severe vitamin deficiency (B₁₂, folate).
• Drugs (eg carbamazepine, valproate).

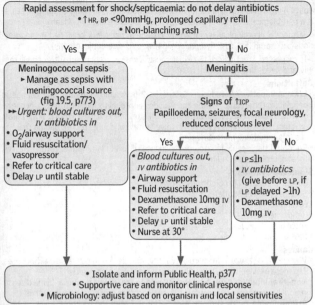

Fig 19.23 Management of suspected bacterial meningitis and meningococcal sepsis in immuno-competent adults.

Lumbar puncture in meningitis

LP (p752) before CT except if ↓GCS, focal neurology, papilloedema, seizure. Wait for clotting screen only if coagulopathy suspected. Send CSF for MC&S, protein, lactate, glucose, virology/PCR. See table 19.4.

Table 19.4 CSF analysis in meningitis

CSF	Normal	Bacterial	TB (p389)	Viral	Fungal
Pressure	<25cmH$_2$O	>30cmH$_2$O	Variable	Variable	>30cmH$_2$O
Appearance	Clear	Turbid	Turbid	Clear	Fibrin web
wcc/mm^3	≤5	>500	100–500	50–1000	Up to 1000
Dominant cell	Lymphocyte	Neutrophil	Lymphocyte	Lymphocyte	Lymphocyte
Glucose	⅔ plasma	<½ plasma	<½ plasma	>½ plasma	<½ plasma
Protein (g/L)	0.18–0.45	>1.5	1–5	<1	0.1–0.5

Encephalitis is inflammation of the brain. This leads to brain dysfunction (encephalopathy) with evidence of inflammation measured in CSF, or using imaging or EEG. It is a neurological emergency which can result in severe disability/death.

▶Suspect if neurological symptoms or change in behaviour preceded by an infectious prodrome (↑T°, rash, lymphadenopathy, cold sore, conjunctivitis).

▶If suspected, treat before the exact cause is known: HSV encephalitis can kill rapidly and needs urgent antiviral treatment.

Definitions
- **Encephalopathy** Altered consciousness >24h including lethargy and change in behaviour. Differential is wide and includes encephalitis, but also sepsis, hypoglycaemia, hepatic encephalopathy, diabetic ketoacidosis, drugs, hypoxic brain injury, uraemia, SLE, vasculitis, Wernicke's (give vit B₁ if in doubt (p700)), glioma (mimics CNS inflammation), metastases.
- **Encephalitis** Encephalopathy *and* evidence of CNS inflammation: fever, seizures, focal neurology, CSF findings, EEG, neuroimaging.

Signs and symptoms
- Confusion, change in personality, drowsiness.
- Seizures (may be subtle).
- Fever.
- Headache.
- Focal neurological signs.
- ↓GCS or coma.

Causes
- **Viral** HSV-1 & 2, VZV, adenovirus, CMV, HIV, measles, mumps, rabies, arboviruses, Japanese B encephalitis, West Nile virus, tick-borne encephalitis.
- **Non-viral infections** Any bacterial meningitis, TB, malaria, listeria, Lyme disease, legionella, leptospirosis, aspergillosis, cryptococcus, schistosomiasis, typhus.
- **Auto-immune (with tumour associations)** Anti-NMDA receptor (ovarian teratoma), anti-LGI-1 (thymoma), anti-Hu (small cell lung), anti-Ma (testicular tumour) anti-GAD, acute disseminated, Bickerstaff's encephalitis.
▶Ask about travel history and risk factors for immunocompromise.

Investigations
- **LP** Imaging is not needed prior if no focal neurological signs, no papilloedema, no seizures, and GCS >12. Moderate ↑CSF protein, ↑lymphocytes (table 19.4, p807), glucose often normal. Viral PCR including HSV (high sensitivity and specificity, though may be negative early in disease course so consider repeat). ▶Do not delay treatment if encephalitis is suspected and LP is delayed. CSF will remain PCR positive for a few days so can be done after treatment is given.
- **Bloods** HIV, blood culture, serum for viral PCR, throat swab, toxoplasma IgM titre, malaria film. Consider autoantibody testing.
- **MRI** Abnormal in 90% of HSV encephalitis. Normal or subtle abnormalities in autoimmune encephalitis.
- **CT, CT-PET** If paraneoplastic cause suspected.
- **EEG** Diffuse abnormalities are non-specific and can be abnormal in encephalopathy due to other causes.

Management
▶Mortality in untreated viral encephalitis is >70%.

▶▶Aciclovir 10mg/kg/8h IV for 14d. Consider repeat CSF HSV PCR at 14 days to confirm discontinuation. May need longer (eg 21d) if immunosuppressed.
- Supportive therapy in high-dependency unit or critical care may be needed.
- Monitor kidney function with IV aciclovir (small risk of crystal nephropathy).
- CMV encephalitis: ganciclovir, foscarnet.
- Toxoplasmosis: see p421.
Symptomatic treatment: eg anticonvulsant medication for seizures (p810).

►Suspect in any patient with ↑ICP and signs of infection, eg fever, ↑WCC.

►Can occur in the absence of systemic signs of inflammation especially if immunosuppressed.

►Consider risk:
• Recent ear, sinus, dental, or periodontal infection.
• Skull fracture.
• Congenital heart disease, endocarditis.
• Bronchiectasis.
• Immunosuppression.

Signs
• Fever.
• Focal neurological signs.
• Seizure.
• Signs of ↑ICP: papilloedema, seizures, focal neurology, reduced conscious level.
• Signs of infection elsewhere, eg teeth, ears, lungs, endocarditis.

Investigations
↑WCC, ↑ESR, blood culture, HIV, CT/MRI (see p730), drainage and culture.

Treatment ►►Urgent neurosurgical referral for evacuation.
• Treat ↑ICP (p814).
• Antimicrobial therapy depends on likely source, (eg *Streptococcus milleri* or oropharyngeal anaerobes from frontal sinuses or teeth, *Bacteroides fragilis* or anaerobes from ear), immunosuppression (risk of toxoplasmosis), and local sensitivities. Seek expert advice from microbiology/infectious disease physicians.

19 Emergencies

Definition Clinical or electroencephalographic (EEG) seizure activity for 5 minutes or more, or recurrent seizures without recovery in between. (The historical definition of seizure activity for >30min is not practical or appropriate given the urgent need for treatment.)

Usually occurs in patients with known epilepsy. Diagnosis of tonic–clonic status is usually clear. Non-convulsive status (eg absence or continuous partial seizures with preserved consciousness) may be more difficult: look for subtle eye or lid movement. For other signs, see p480, pp486–9. An EEG can be very helpful.

▶Could the patient be *pregnant*? If so, manage as eclampsia (occurs after 20 weeks' gestation so a pelvic mass is palpable): obstetric help, IV magnesium, and delivery when stable (*OHCS* p90).

Investigations
• Capillary glucose.
• Other tests after treatment: FBC, U&E, Ca^{2+}, ABG, ECG.
• MRI (if first presentation of seizure).
• Consider: anticonvulsant concentrations, toxicology screen, LP, blood and urine culture, EEG, carbon monoxide concentration.

Management
▶See fig 19.24.[9]
• Basic life support. Treat hypoglycaemia.
• If the patient has an individualized emergency management plan that is immediately available, administer medication as detailed in the plan.
• If no individualized emergency management plan:
  1 **Benzodiazepine**
    • *IV lorazepam:* 4mg, repeat after 5–10min. Use if no delay to IV access and resuscitation facilities available. Beware respiratory depression.
    • *Buccal midazolam:* 10mg, repeat after 5–10min.
    • *Rectal diazepam:* 10–20mg, repeat after 5–10min.
  2 **Second-line IV anticonvulsant** If ongoing seizure activity. Follow local guidance. For example:
    • *Levetiracetam:* 60mg/kg (max 4500mg) IV over 10min. Can use in patients already on levetiracetam. Avoid if known advanced CKD.
    • *Phenytoin:* 20mg/kg (max 2000mg) IV at max rate of 50mg/min. ECG and blood pressure monitoring due to risk of hypotension and bradycardia. Use with caution in elderly and in cardiac disease (consider ↓rate, eg ≤25mg/min).
    • *Sodium valproate:* 40mg/kg (max 3000mg) IV over 10min. Avoid in pregnancy, advanced liver disease, mitochondrial disease.
    • Continue medication given as a loading dose as a maintenance treatment according to expert neurology advice. Give maintenance dose of levetiracetam or sodium valproate 12h after loading, or phenytoin 6–8h after loading.
  3 Refer to critical care for general anaesthesia if above measures fail.
• Adjuncts:
    • Dexamethasone 10mg IV if vasculitis/cerebral oedema (tumour) possible.
    • IV thiamine in malnutrition/alcohol withdrawal.

What was the cause?

• Consider precipitants, eg hypoglycaemia, pregnancy, alcohol, drugs, CNS lesion or infection, hypertensive encephalopathy, inadequate anticonvulsant dose, non-adherence (p486).
• Consider non-epileptic seizures (p460) if atypical features: pelvic thrusts, resisting eye-lid opening or passive movements, flailing rather than clonic movements of limbs.

△ Management of status epilepticus

Immediate life support
- Secure airway
- Give oxygen
- Assess cardiac and respiratory function
- Secure IV access
- If hypoglycaemia treat, eg 100mL 20% glucose IV, buccal glucose gel

Benzodiazepine
- IV lorazepam 4mg
OR
- Buccal midazolam 10mg
OR
- Rectal diazepam 10–20mg

If indicated: thiamine, toxin-reversal, treat acidosis, treat infection, steroids

↓ If ongoing seizure activity

Repeat benzodiazepine after 5–10 minutes

↓ If ongoing seizure activity

Second-line IV anticonvulsant (p810)
Follow local guidance. For example:
- Levetiracetam: 60mg/kg (max 4500mg) IV over 10 minutes
OR
- Phenytoin: 20mg/kg (max 2000mg) IV at max rate of 50mg/min
OR
- Sodium valproate 40mg/kg (max 3000mg) IV over 10 minutes

↓ If ongoing seizure activity

General anaesthesia
If 30 minutes since seizure onset do not delay anaesthesia
Ongoing critical and expert neurology care

Fig 19.24 Management of status epilepticus.

△

Initial management ►See fig 19.25.[10]

►►Do not presume ↓GCS is due to intoxication unless a head injury has been excluded.

►►Stabilize airway, breathing, and circulation. If GCS ≤8 seek anaesthetic or critical care expertise in order to protect the airway.

• If GCS ≤12 without active extracranial bleeding, give tranexamic acid 2g IV.

• Involve neurosurgeons early if ↓GCS, falling GCS, persistent confusion, ↑ICP suspected, abnormal intracranial imaging, CSF leak, penetrating injury.

• Monitor HR, BP, T°, RR, pupil size/symmetry every 15min.

• Complete neurological examination is needed. Assess amnesia. Distinguish anterograde (from time of injury, post-traumatic) and retrograde (events prior to injury).

• There is no risk to cervical spine if low-risk features: rear-end motor collision, comfortable sitting, ambulatory, no cervical spine tenderness, delayed-onset pain, and able to actively rotate neck 45° to the left and right.

• Nurse semi-prone if no spinal injury.

CT head
• Within 1h if:
    • GCS ≤12 on initial assessment, or GCS <15 at 2h following injury.
    • Focal neurological deficit.
    • Suspected open or depressed skull fracture, or signs of basal skull fracture (periorbital ecchymoses ('panda' eyes/racoon sign), postauricular ecchymosis (Battle's sign), CSF leak through nose/ears, haemotympanum).
    • Post-traumatic seizure.
    • Vomiting more than once.
• Within 8h if loss of consciousness or amnesia since the injury and any of:
    • Age ≥65yrs.
    • Bleeding/clotting disorder or on anticoagulant treatment.
    • Dangerous mechanism of injury: pedestrian/cyclist struck by motor vehicle, ejection from motor vehicle, fall >1m or 5 stairs.
    • Retrograde amnesia (events before head injury) of >30min.

CT cervical spine
Within 1h if any of the following:
• GCS ≤12 on initial assessment.
• The patient has been intubated.
• Definitive diagnosis of cervical spine injury is needed urgently (eg before surgery).
• The patient is having other body areas scanned, eg due to polytrauma.
• Clinical suspicion of cervical spine injury *and* increased risk due to any of:
    • Age ≥65yrs.
    • High-impact injury.
    • Focal neurological deficit or limb paraesthesia.
• Unsafe to assess the range of movement in the neck.
• Person cannot actively rotate neck 45° to left and right in safe assessment.
• Condition predisposing to higher risk of injury, eg axial spondyloarthritis.

MRI cervical spine
If neurological signs or symptoms of cervical spine injury or if needed to clarify CT findings. MRA if suspicion of vascular injury.

Admission and observation
• New, clinically important abnormalities on CT (consider anticoagulant treatment in assessing significance).
• GCS has not recovered to pre-injury baseline.
• Ongoing symptoms, eg persistent vomiting, seizures, severe headache, meningism.
• Other injuries or safe-guarding concerns.

Complications Extradural/subdural haemorrhage (p476), seizures (pp810–11), hypopituitarism (p819), Parkinsonism, dementia.

Poor prognostic indicators: decerebrate rigidity, extensor spasms, prolonged coma, ↑BP, ↓P_aO_2, T° >39°C.

⚠ Immediate management of head injury

ABCDE assessment
- Protect airway and c-spine: anaesthetic review for intubation if GCS ≤8
- Oxygen if hypoxic
- Support circulation, treat shock (p770)
- Clinical clearance of cervical spine if low-risk features (p812)
- Neurological examination and assess amnesia
- Evaluate facial lacerations, check for step-deformity
- Signs of base-of-skull fracture (p812)

↓

Tranexamic acid
2g IV if GCS ≤12 without active extracranial bleeding

↓

CT head
Within 1h or 8h according to risk (p812)

↓

CT cervical spine
- Within 1h according to risk (p812)
- MRI if neurological signs/symptoms
- MRA if suspicion for vascular injury

↓

Neurosurgical expertise for
- ↓GCS
- Abnormality on imaging
- Falling GCS
- ↑ICP
- CSF leak
- Penetrating injury

►►Ensure safe (airway, bleeding, seizures) if transfer to neurosurgical unit

↓

Ongoing management
- Monitor: HR, BP, T°, RR, pupil size and symmetry, GCS
- Analgesia
- Tetanus vaccine if indicated for penetrating injuries
- Ongoing circulatory support as required
- Correct coagulopathy
- Good communication and information
- Specialist rehabilitation

Fig 19.25 Immediate management of head injury.

Raised intracranial pressure (ICP)

The volume inside the cranium is fixed, so any increase in the contents can lead to raised ICP. This can be mass effect, oedema, or obstruction to fluid outflow. ↑ICP leads to secondary brain injury and death, so needs urgent treatment. Normal ICP in adults is <15mmHg. A measurement >20mmHg suggests ↑ICP.

Causes
- Primary or metastatic tumours.
- Head injury (pp812–13).
- Haemorrhage: subdural, extradural, subarachnoid, intracerebral, intraventricular.
- Infection: meningitis (pp806–7), encephalitis (p808), brain abscess (p809).
- Hydrocephalus.
- Cerebral oedema.
- Status epilepticus (pp810–11).
- Idiopathic.

Signs and symptoms
- History of trauma.
- Headache (worse on coughing, leaning forwards), vomiting.
- Altered GCS: drowsiness, listlessness, irritability, coma.
- ↓HR and ↑BP (Cushing's response).
- Irregular/Cheyne–Stokes respiration.
- Pupil changes: constriction first, later dilation (do not mask these signs by using agents such as tropicamide to dilate the pupil for fundoscopy).
- ↓Visual acuity, peripheral visual field loss.
- Papilloedema has low sensitivity for ↑ICP. Loss of venous pulsation at the optic disc is more sensitive but difficult to detect and may be absent in ~10% of population.

Investigations
- U&E, FBC, LFT, glucose, serum osmolality, clotting, blood culture.
- Consider toxicology screen.
- CXR, and other source of infection that might indicate abscess.
- CT head.
- LP if papilloedema with normal imaging: measure the opening pressure.

Management ►See fig 19.26. The goal is to ↓ICP and avert secondary injury. Urgent neurosurgery may be required for definitive treatment of ↑ICP from focal causes. This can be achieved via evacuation, or temporized with burr hole/craniotomy. An ICP monitor (or bolt) can be placed to monitor pressure and guide neurosurgical critical care.

Herniation syndromes
Uncal herniation
A supratentorial mass pushes the inferomedial temporal lobe (uncus) through the tentorial notch (the opening between supratentorial and infratentorial regions of the brain), to compress the midbrain. The IIIrd nerve, travelling in this space, gets compressed, causing a dilated ipsilateral pupil, then ophthalmoplegia (a fixed pupil does not localize the lesion: it is due to compression, not the lesion itself, but does indicate the side of the lesion). This may be followed (quickly) by contralateral hemiparesis due to pressure on the cerebral peduncle. Coma then occurs due to pressure on the ascending reticular activating system in the midbrain.

Cerebellar tonsil herniation
↑Pressure in the posterior fossa forces the cerebellar tonsils through the foramen magnum. Ataxia, VIth nerve palsy, and up-going plantar reflexes occur first, then loss of consciousness, irregular breathing, and apnoea. May proceed very rapidly given the small size and poor compliance of the posterior fossa.

Subfalcian (cingulate) herniation
A frontal mass forces the cingulate gyrus (medial frontal lobe) under the rigid falx cerebri. May be silent unless the anterior cerebral artery is compressed and causes a stroke: contralateral leg weakness ± abulia (lack of decision-making).

▲ Management of raised intracranial pressure

Airway and breathing
- Oxygen if hypoxic: hypoxia can ↑ICP due to vasodilatation and cerebral oedema
- Consider sedation for laryngoscopy if needed to secure airway: coughing/resistance can ↑ICP
- Normocapnia: CO_2 is a vasodilator causing ↑cerebral blood flow and ↑ICP

Circulation
- SBP >100–110mmHg: hypotension will ↓cerebral perfusion when cerebral autoregulation is impaired
- Hypertension needs expert/specialist advice. It may be a compensatory response to ↓cerebral perfusion and BP targets may need to be higher. Avoid cerebral vasodilators
- Fluids: only if indicated for volume depletion, avoid hypo-osmolar fluids as ↓Na^+ will increase cerebral oedema

Adjuncts
- Head of bed elevated to 15–30°. Tracheostomy/endotracheal ties positioned to prevent internal jugular vein compression
- Treat seizures (pp810–11)
- Sedation/analgesia: to prevent coughing, bucking, agitation, and pain contributing to ↑ICP. Needs expert/critical care
- Fever control: fever increases metabolic rate and causes vasodilatation
- Steroids: only to reduce oedema due to space–occupying tumour, or if indicated to treat meningitis (pp822–3). ↑Risk of death in ↑ICP due to haemorrhage
- In select cases under expert guidance only: osmotic agents (eg mannitol), hypertonic saline (benefit may be transient, risks of haemodilution and ↑BP), hypothermia (conflicting evidence)

Diagnosis and definitive treatment
- History, examination, and imaging
- Treat meningitis (pp806–7), encephalitis (p808) and cerebral abscess (p809), and idiopathic intercranial hypertension (p494)
- Neurosurgical management of ↑ICP and definitive treatment of cause where possible

Fig 19.26 Immediate management of raised intracranial pressure.

Diabetic ketoacidosis (DKA)

Mechanism
Insulin deficiency and an increase in counter-regulatory hormones (glucagon, catecholamines, cortisol) lead to metabolism of triglycerides and amino acids instead of glucose for energy. Overproduction of β-hydroxybutyric acid, acetoacetic acid, and acetone ('fruity' breath) leads to acidosis.

▶Early recognition and treatment are important. The combination of acidosis and hyperglycaemia can be fatal.

Presentation
Unexplained weight loss, vomiting, abdominal pain, polyuria, polydipsia, lethargy, anorexia, dehydration, rapid/deep breathing (= 'Kussmaul' hyperventilation, consider if ↑RR without hypoxia), drowsiness, coma.

▶Check glucose in all patients with diabetes who are unwell. Triggers for DKA include infection, surgery, MI, pancreatitis, medication (eg corticosteroids, calcineurin inhibitors, thiazides, antipsychotics, SGLT2 inhibitors (see BOX)), wrong insulin dose/non-adherence.

Diagnosis
1 Acidaemia (pH <7.3 or HCO_3^- <15.0mmol/L).
2 Hyperglycaemia (blood glucose >11.0mmol/L) or known DM.
3 Ketonaemia (≥3.0mmol/L) or significant ketonuria (more than 2+ on dipstick).

Blood Capillary and lab glucose, ketones, venous pH (ABG if ↓GCS or hypoxia), U&E, HCO_3^-, osmolality, FBC, blood culture. **Urine** Dipstick and MSU. **Other** ECG, CXR.

Severe DKA Get senior/critical care help. Includes one or more of the following:
- Blood ketones >6mmol/L.
- Venous bicarbonate <10mmol/L.
- Venous/arterial pH <7.0.
- Anion gap >16.
- K^+ <3.5mmol/L on admission.
- GCS <12.
- O_2 sats <92% on air (no respiratory disease).
- Systolic BP <90mmHg.
- Pulse >100bpm or <60bpm.

Management ▶Provide insulin, correct volume/metabolic abnormalities (fig 19.27).[11]

Pitfalls in diabetic ketoacidosis
- **Plasma glucose** Consider DKA at lower concentrations of glucose if some insulin therapy ongoing, SGLT2 inhibitors (see BOX), pregnancy.
- **WCC** May be elevated in the absence of infection.
- **Infection** Often there is no fever. Check MSU, blood cultures, and CXR. Broad-spectrum antibiotics (eg co-amoxiclav) if infection suspected.
- **Ketones** Ketonuria does not always mean ketoacidosis. It can occur after a normal overnight fast. ▶Check blood/capillary ketones. Not all ketones are due to diabetes: consider alcohol, starvation, vomiting.
- **Recurrent ketoacidosis** Blood glucose may normalize before ketosis is corrected. Premature termination of insulin infusion may lead to recurrent DKA. Continue insulin infusion by supplementing with IV glucose until blood ketones <0.6mmol/L and pH >7.3.
- **Acidosis** May occur without gross elevation of glucose. Consider also lactic acidosis (eg sepsis, volume depletion).
- **Serum amylase** This may be raised (up to ×10) and non-specific abdominal pain is common, even in the absence of pancreatitis.

Complications ▶Cerebral oedema (get help if sudden CNS decline), aspiration pneumonia, hypokalaemia, hypomagnesaemia, hypophosphataemia, thromboembolism.

Prevention ▶Talk to the patient. Evaluate adherence. Provide information about triggers, and 'sick day' rules. Ensure specialist diabetes input.

Atypical normoglycaemic DKA
Associated with SGLT2 inhibitors ('flozins') ≈ 1 in 1000. ▶Check blood ketones, even if glucose is normal. Do not use if previous DKA. Stop SGLT2 inhibitors if hospitalized for surgery or acute illness. Restart when stabilized.

△ **Management of diabetic ketoacidosis**

Airway and breathing
- Ensure safe airway (critical care review if GCS <12)
- Oxygen if hypoxic (and investigate for cause, eg infection, VTE)

Restore circulating volume
- Significant volume depletion is likely (consider also cardiac disease, sepsis)
- SBP <90mmHg: 500mL 0.9% saline over 10–15min then review. Repeat if remains volume deplete
- SBP <90mmHg after 1000mL fluid resuscitation, or if cardiac comorbidity/sepsis: get senior/critical care advice
- SBP ≥90mmHg: 1000mL 0.9% saline over 1h

Insulin
- Prepare: 50u human soluble insulin (Actrapid®, Humulin S®) in 50mL 0.9% saline
- Fixed rate insulin infusion at 0.1u/kg/h
- Continue regular long-acting insulin (glargine, detemir, degludec) at usual doses and times. Consider initiating long-acting insulin if newly diagnosed T1DM

Assess and monitor
Assess HR, BP, T°, RR, O₂ saturation, GCS, full clinical examination
Investigate Capillary and lab glucose, VBG, U&E, FBC, blood cultures, ECG, CXR, MSU
Monitor
- Capillary blood glucose and capillary ketones: every hour
- Venous bicarbonate and K⁺: at 60min, then every 2h
- Plasma electrolytes: every 4h
- Catheter if no urine output at 1h

Titrate insulin
Aims:
- ↓*blood ketones by 0.5mmol/L/h*
- ↑*venous bicarbonate by 3mmol/L/h*
- ↓*glucose 3mmol/L/h and avoid hypoglycaemia*
→ Increase insulin infusion by 1u/h until target rates achieved
→ *Consider* reduce insulin infusion to 0.05u/kg/h when glucose <14mmol/L

Ongoing fluid and K⁺ replacement
1 0.9% sodium chloride 1L with KCl over 2 hours
2 0.9% sodium chloride 1L with KCl over 2 hours
3 0.9% sodium chloride 1L with KCl over 4 hours
→ Adjust volume according to clinical review and if age <25 or elderly, IHD, or CKD
- Add 10% glucose 125mL/h if blood glucose <14mmol/L
- K⁺ replacement: plasma K⁺
Plasma K⁺<3.5mmol/L: expert/critical care advice
Plasma K⁺ 3.5–5.5mmol/L: add KCl 40mmol/L
Plasma K⁺>5.5mmol/L: no supplementary K⁺ and expert advice if >6.0mmol/L.

Further management
- *Specialist diabetes advice for ongoing management*
- Treat/manage precipitants, eg infection, adherence
- VTE prophylaxis
- IV insulin until: DKA resolved, eating and drinking, and 30min *after* SC short-acting insulin given

△

Fig 19.27 Management of diabetic ketoacidosis.

Hyperglycaemic hyperosmolar state (HHS)

Usually affects patients with type 2 DM (and may be first presentation of type 2 DM). Usually develops over several days before presenting with very high blood glucose concentration and marked volume depletion. Infection is a common precipitant, eg chest, UTI.

Characterized by:
• Marked elevation in plasma glucose, eg >30mmol/L.
• Osmolality typically >320mOsmol/kg.
• Significant volume depletion.

There is no switch to ketone metabolism, so blood ketones <3mmol/L and pH >7.3. High mortality due to:
• Vascular events (precipitant or consequence), eg MI, stroke, peripheral thrombosis.
• Risk of neurological complications, eg cerebral oedema and osmotic demyelination.
▶A mixed picture may occur with DKA.

Management

Ensure specialist diabetologist input. Principles: correct osmolality and fluid deficits, whilst avoiding complications from rapid osmotic change, eg cerebral oedema and central pontine myelinolysis (p664).[12]

• Monitor: HR, BP, T°, RR, O_2 saturation, conscious level. Airway/critical care support if indicated. Assess for cause: sepsis, adherence, vascular event.
• Measure and monitor osmolality. Calculate as $((2 \times Na^+) + glucose)$ until urea is available, then re-calculate as $((2 \times Na^+) + urea + glucose)$.
• Replace fluid deficit. Typical deficits are 110–220mL/kg, ie 8–15L for a 70kg adult. 0.9% sodium chloride should be the principal fluid used, eg 1L over 1h, then 2h, then 4h. Aim 2–3L positive balance by 6h. Caution if LV dysfunction (or risk).
• ↓Osmolality by 3–8mOsmol/kg/h. If ↓ <3mOsmol/kg/h: ↑ rate of fluid replacement. If ↓ >8mOsmol/kg/h: ↓ rate of fluid replacement (or insulin if given). If ↑osmolality or fluid overload: seek expert advice regarding use of 0.45% sodium chloride.
• Aim to ↓ blood glucose by 5mmol/L/h to reach 10–15mmol/L at 24h. Usually falls with fluid resuscitation. IV insulin if:
  • Blood ketones >3mmol/L and acidosis (pH<7.3 or bicarbonate <15mmol/L): manage as DKA (pp816–7).
  • Blood ketones >3mmol/L without acidosis: start fixed rate insulin infusion 0.05 units/kg/h and review.
  • Raised blood glucose not falling on repeat measures despite +ve fluid balance.
• K⁺ replacement according to serum K⁺ (see p817).
• LMWH prophylaxis if no contraindication.
▶Ensure management of any precipitant, eg infection, vascular event, adherence.

Hypoglycaemia

Definitions

• <4mmol/L in diabetes. Exclude hypoglycaemia if a person with diabetes is unwell, drowsy, unconscious, unable to cooperate/aggressive, or has seizures. Insulin and sulfonylurea treatment may precipitate hypoglycaemia.
• <3mmol/L plus symptoms in the absence of diabetes.

Management

• If able to swallow: fast-acting oral carbohydrate, eg glucose tablets, 40% glucose gel, pure fruit juice (not if ↓K⁺ diet), sucrose in water. Repeat up to 3 times, every 15min. Avoid biscuits/chocolate as sugar content is less and fat delays stomach emptying.
• If unresponsive to oral glucose or oral route not possible: 100mL 20% dextrose IV over 15 minutes. 1mg glucagon IM (not if starvation/alcohol excess/sulfonylurea).
• Investigate underlying causes (p817) if persistent.

Lactic acidosis and metformin

Lactic acidosis is a rare complication of metformin use (6 in 100 000). Seek expert help. Look for and treat other sources of ↑lactate: sepsis, liver disease, ischaemic bowel. Discontinue metformin in AKI. Care with metformin use in CKD: low dose if eGFR <45mL/min/1.73m², don't initiate/consider stopping if eGFR <30mL/min/1.73m².

Acute adrenal insufficiency

Presentation
- Undiagnosed adrenal insufficiency, eg autoimmune, non-classical congenital adrenal hyperplasia, bilateral adrenal haemorrhage (meningococcal sepsis). Consider if current/previous exogenous glucocorticoids within the last year (oral, intra-articular, IM, inhaled, nasal, topical).
- Known adrenal insufficiency. Existing cortisol replacement does not meet an increased need, eg intercurrent illness, vomiting/diarrhoea, pregnancy, surgery, non-adherence.

Signs and symptoms
Hypoglycaemia, ↑HR, postural hypotension/↓BP, vomiting, weakness, shock, confusion, coma.

Precipitating factors
Infection, trauma, surgery, missed medication.

Investigation
- ►If suspected, treat before biochemical results.
- Blood: paired cortisol and ACTH (direct to lab on ice, call ahead), glucose, U&Es.
- Monitor blood glucose: risk of hypoglycaemia.
- Look for infectious trigger: blood, urine, and sputum cultures, CXR.

Treatment
- Initial fluid resuscitation, eg 0.9% sodium chloride 500mL over 15min.
- Hydrocortisone 100mg IV. Followed by 200mg hydrocortisone/24h continuous IVI in 5% glucose or hydrocortisone 50mg IM/6h (100mg if BMI >40).
- Ongoing rehydration, eg 3–4L sodium chloride 0.9% solution in 24h. IV glucose may be needed if hypoglycaemic.
- ↑K⁺: ECG, cardiac monitor, and treatment (p297).
- Treat underlying infection.
- Expert endocrine input for diagnosis, conversion/tapering of oral steroids, indications for fludrocortisone, and 'sick day rules' education before hospital discharge.

Pituitary apoplexy

Rare. Usually due to pituitary haemorrhage or infarction. Often in conjunction with an (undiagnosed) pituitary adenoma, and thought to occur due to ↑metabolic demand and/or compromise of pituitary vasculature. Also head injury, subarachnoid haemorrhage, coagulopathy, surgery, postpartum (Sheehan syndrome, p228).

►Rapid glucocorticoid replacement may be life-saving.

Presentation
Mimics common neurological conditions: fever, neck stiffness, photophobia, ↓GCS/altered mental status. Consider if sudden-onset severe headache and:
- Subarachnoid haemorrhage and meningitis excluded.
- Visual disturbance: ↓ acuity, visual field defect, eg bitemporal hemianopia due to optic chiasm compression.
- Ocular palsies (CIII due to cavernous sinus involvement).

Also: nausea/vomiting, ↓BP, hypothermia, hypoglycaemia, hypopituitarism (p228).

Investigation FBC, U&E, LFT, clotting screen, cortisol, prolactin, TSH, T₄, insulin-like growth factor, growth hormone, LH, FSH, testosterone/oestradiol. Urgent MRI.

Management
- ►Get expert endocrine advice.
  1 Fluid resuscitate, eg 500mL 0.9% saline over 15min. Treat ↑K⁺ (p297).
  2 Hydrocortisone 100mg IV. Followed by 200mg hydrocortisone/24h IVI in 5% glucose or hydrocortisone 50mg IM/6h (100mg if BMI >40).
  3 Consider surgical management if severely reduced visual acuity, severe and persistent/deteriorating visual field defects, or ↓GCS.
  4 Other pituitary hormone replacement only after established on glucocorticoid.
  5 Close monitoring of pituitary and visual function by specialist endocrine/neurosurgical service.

Phaeochromocytoma emergency

Rare, life-threatening emergency due to release of high concentrations of catecholamines. Mimics other conditions, therefore difficult to diagnose if not known
to have a phaeochromocytoma/paraganglioma. Occurs spontaneously, or may be a
triggering event: trauma, surgery, medication, eg corticosteroids, β-blockers (unopposed β-blockade can ↑α effects), metoclopramide, anaesthetic agents.

Signs and symptoms
▶Emergency = symptoms of phaeochromocytoma (severe hypertension, headache,
sweating/fever, anxiety, palpitations) plus life-threatening complications:
• Haemodynamic instability: labile SBP 60–250mmHg.
• End-organ dysfunction: cardiac (LVF, IHD, arrhythmia cardiogenic shock), pulmonary (oedema, ARDS), neurological (encephalopathy, stroke, seizure), renal (AKI),
hepatic (acute liver failure), GI (paralytic ileus, intestinal ischaemia), metabolic
(lactic acidosis, DKA, rhabdomyolysis), coagulopathy.

Investigation Plasma metanephrines (metanephrine, normetanephrine, 3-meth-
oxytyramine), CT (adrenal), MRI (extra-adrenal), functional scan, eg PET-CT, genetics.

Management Aims: medical stabilization and sufficient α-blockade to block cat-
echolamine effects. ▶Get help from critical care and endocrinology.
• **α-blockade** Titrate to BP control, eg:
  • Doxazosin 4–32mg/d PO (selective, ↓tachycardia).
  • Phenoxybenzamine 10mg/12h PO, up to 1mg/kg/d (non-selective, ↑↑tachycardia).
  • Phentolamine 2–5mg IV. Short acting. Repeat if required.
• **β-blocker** Only *after* α-blockade if tachycardia, arrhythmia, myocardial ischaemia.
• **Volume** Expansion if required.
• **Supportive care** As well as management of end-organ dysfunction.
• **Surgery** For resectable disease once stable with sufficient α-blockade and appro-
priate volume expansion.

Thyroid emergencies

Hyperthyroid crisis ('thyrotoxic storm')
Signs and symptoms ↑T°, agitation, confusion, tremor, tachycardia, AF/arrhythmia,
heart failure, D&V, acute abdomen (exclude surgical causes), proptosis/exophthalmos/
ophthalmoplegia, goitre, thyroid bruit, coma. Triggers: infection, surgery.
Investigation ↓TSH, ↑free T₄, ↑free T₃, TSH-receptor antibodies (+ve in Graves' disease). Also: U&E, FBC, LFT, calcium, glucose, ECG. Look for precipitants: CXR, blood and
urine cultures.

Treatment ▶See fig 19.28. Seek endocrinology advice.

Myxoedema coma
Signs and symptoms Hypothyroid appearance (p215, fig 5.16), hypothermia, bradycardia, hypercapnic respiratory failure, hyporeflexia, hypoglycaemia, psychosis
('myxoedema madness'), seizure, coma. Triggers: infection, MI, stroke, trauma.

Investigation ↑TSH, ↓free T₄, ↓free T₃, U&E (often ↓Na⁺). Also cortisol, glucose, FBC,
ABG, infection screen: CXR, blood and urine cultures.

Treatment ▶Seek endocrinology advice.
• Secure airway, O₂ if hypoxic. Refer to critical care.
• Correct hypoglycaemia: eg 100mL 20% glucose IV over 15min.
• Assume (relative) cortisol deficiency until tests prove otherwise: hydrocortisone
100mg IV (p821).
• Thyroid hormone replacement, eg liothyronine (T₃) 5–10mcg PO/NG (↑risk of car-
diac complications if IV), repeat/titrate depending on response/cardiac status.
Thyroxine (T₄) can also be used but conversion to T₃ may be ↓ in severe illness. Dose
depends on cardiac risk, eg 25–75mcg/day PO/NG.
• IV fluids if needed for volume depletion: care due to risk of pulmonary oedema.
• Other: slow warming, treat infection. Establish on oral thyroxine before discharge.

⚠ Management of hyperthyroid crisis

- IV access
- Check: TSH, T_4, T_3, U&E, FBC, liver function, calcium, glucose
- Precipitants/sequelae: septic screen, CXR, blood and urine cultures, ECG

↓

Propranolol
- 80mg PO TDS (IV only if PO/NG not possible: 1–2mg IV over 10min, rarely required)
- β-blockade is *not* contraindicated if acute heart failure is due to thyrotoxicosis
- If contraindicated: rate-controlling calcium channel blocker, eg verapamil

↓

Thionamide
- Propylthiouracil (PTU) 200mg PO/NG/PR TDS
- PTU is preferred over carbimazole due to ↓peripheral conversion of $T_4 \rightarrow T_3$

↓

Glucocorticoid
- Benefits: ↓peripheral conversion of $T_4 \rightarrow T_3$, autoimmune effect in Graves' disease, protects if limited adrenal reserve
- eg Hydrocortisone 200mg IV or equivalent
- Then hydrocortisone 100mg TDS or prednisolone 20mg TDS

↓

Other
- Treat infection
- Monitor blood glucose and treat hypoglycaemia
- Cooling
- Risk of pulmonary oedema: IV fluids only if volume deplete
- Nutritional support
- Critical care if respiratory or cardiovascular support/monitoring needed

↓

Specialist endocrine advice
- Iodine oral solution: eg potassium iodide (100mg/mL) plus iodine (50mg/mL) 0.3mL PO TDS. Blocks T_4 and T_3 release. Give at least *1 hour after* thionamide to prevent utilization as a substrate for more thyroid hormone production
- Cholestyramine 3–4g PO TDS/QDS: ↓enterohepatic circulation of thyroid hormone
- Monitoring and titration of thionamide (liver function and neutrophil count)
- Monitoring and tapering of glucocorticoid treatment

Fig 19.28 Management of hyperthyroid crisis.

The patient may or may not be able to tell you what they have taken. If there are any tablets with the patient use *MIMS Colour Index*, *EMIMS* images, *BNF* descriptions, or online drug identification services, eg *TICTAC visual ID system*.

Examination and investigations

May offer a clue as to the toxin taken:
- **Fast/irregular pulse** Salbutamol, tricyclic, quinine, phenothiazine (p827).
- **Respiratory depression** Opiate (p826), benzodiazepine (p826).
- **Hypothermia** Phenothiazine (p827), barbiturate.
- **Hyperthermia** Amphetamine, MAOIs, cocaine, ecstasy (p827).
- **Coma** Benzodiazepine (p826), alcohol, opiate, tricyclic, barbiturate.
- **Seizures** Hypoglycaemics, tricyclic, phenothiazine (p827), theophylline, cocaine.
- **Constricted pupils** Opiates (p826), organophosphate (p827).
- **Dilated pupils** Amphetamine, cocaine, quinine, tricyclics.
- **Hyperglycaemia** Organophosphates, theophylline, MAOIs.
- **Hypoglycaemia** Insulin, sulfonylurea, alcohol, salicylate (p825).
- **Kidney injury** Salicylate (p825), paracetamol (p824), ethylene glycol.
- **Acidosis** Salicylate (p825), carbon monoxide (p826), iron (p826), alcohol, ethylene glycol.
- **↑Osmolality** Alcohol, ethylene glycol (p660).

Management

1 *ABC:* secure airway. O_2 if hypoxic.
2 *Blood:* check paracetamol and salicylate concentrations. Other drug concentrations and assessment of toxicity guided by toxin taken (or likely toxin taken).
3 *Reduce toxicity:* activated charcoal (p823) and/or specific treatment (pp826–7).
4 *Information:* ▶if in doubt how best to act, contact the National Poisons Information Service. Advice is available 24/7 via your NHS unit's login, the TOXBASE app, or UK phone information line: 0844 892 0111.
5 *Supportive care:*
   - Monitor GCS and ensure safe airway. O_2 if hypoxic. May need intubation, ventilation, critical care.
   - Monitor: according to toxin, T°, HR, BP, RR, O_2 sats, glucose, ECG, urine output.
   - Treat hypoglycaemia (p818).
   - IV fluids if volume deplete.
   - Cool/warm if hypo/hyperthermia.

Psychiatric assessment

Be kind. Aim to establish:
- *Intentions at time.* Was this a suicide attempt? If so, was the act planned? Did they take precautions against being found? Did the patient seek help afterwards? Does the patient think the method was dangerous? Any final act, eg suicide note?
- *Present intentions.* Do they still feel suicidal?
- *What problems* led to the act and do they still exist?
- Is there a *psychiatric disorder*? Is there an established diagnosis or current symptoms, eg depression, psychosis, schizophrenia, dementia, substance misuse disorder, personality disorder?
- What are the patient's *resources*, eg friends, family, work, personality?

Assess suicide risk See *OHCS* p726. There is ↑risk of death in the first year following a presentation with attempted suicide. Risk factors for future suicide include:
- Intention to die.
- Psychiatric disorder.
- Poor resources.
- Previous suicide attempts.
- Social isolation.
- Unemployed.
- Male.
- >50yrs old.

Refer for psychiatric assessment and support Seek advice about all presentations with deliberate self-poisoning. Refer for formal assessment if symptoms or known to have a psychiatric disorder, or if high suicide risk.

Toxicology
- Check blood glucose, paracetamol, and aspirin concentrations.
- Necessity of other assays and tests depends on the drug taken, the anticipated toxicity, and the index of suspicion.
- Be guided by the National Poisons Information Service (p822).
- Therapeutic monitoring is available for some poisons, eg digoxin, methanol, lithium, anti-epileptic drugs, iron, theophylline.
- Screening of urine, especially for recreational drugs, may be useful in some, but not all, cases (see BOX 'New psychoactive substances').

New psychoactive substances

New 'designer' drugs, with chemical properties similar to established illicit drugs, may cause toxicity. They were termed 'legal highs' until UK legislation banned them in 2016. These drugs pose a difficult problem for the assessing physician as the precise chemistry and mechanisms of action of both the active compound, as well as any impurities, are often unclear. They can cause life-threatening complications and death. Obtain as much detail as possible about specific agents taken in a drug history; there may be no available screening tool.

Decontamination
▶Do not induce vomiting.

Activated charcoal
- Binds toxins in GI tract to ↓ absorption. Includes: ACE-i, amphetamine, antidepressants (not lithium), antiepileptics, aspirin, benzodiazepines, β-blockers, calcium-channel blockers, digoxin, diuretics, oral hypoglycaemic drugs, opiates, paracetamol, death cap, ricin, yew, ie taxanes.
- The sooner activated charcoal is given, the more effective it is.
- It is generally effective up to 1h after ingestion, but longer if poisons are:
    - Adsorbed beyond the stomach in the distal GI tract.
    - Modified-release preparations.
    - Slowly absorbed.
    - Undergo significant enterohepatic or entero-enteric circulation which is interrupted by activated charcoal. (In entero-enteric circulation, the intestinal wall functions as a semipermeable membrane: toxins can diffuse out of the blood onto the charcoal in the intestinal lumen.)
- A multi-dose regimen is useful in poisoning due to carbamazepine, quinine, dapsone, phenobarbital, theophylline, digoxin, slow-release quetiapine, aspirin, amitriptyline, phenytoin, sotalol, oxcarbazepine, lamotrigine, citalopram, venlafaxine, eg 50g/4h (if unable to tolerate, reduce to 25g/2h or 12.5g/h though may ↓ efficacy).
- Activated charcoal does not adsorb alcohols or metals so is ineffective in poisoning due to lithium, lead, mercury, organic solvents, acids/bases, cyanide.

Gastric lavage
- Rarely used as outcome studies (in high-income countries with access to supportive care and antidotes) do not show benefit.
- Risks include pulmonary aspiration, laryngospasm and hypoxia, perforation.

Haemodialysis
May be indicated if significant toxicity from substances that can be cleared by haemodialysis, eg alcohol, ethylene glycol, methanol, aspirin, lithium, barbiturates, sodium valproate, phenytoin, carbamazepine, theophylline.

►12g (= 24 tablets) or 150mg/kg in adults may be fatal.

►If >110kg, calculate ingested dose using a weight of 110kg to avoid underestimating toxicity.

►If the patient is malnourished then 75mg/kg can kill.

Signs and symptoms None initially, or vomiting ± RUQ pain. Later, jaundice and encephalopathy from liver damage, AKI.

Management

Decontamination Activated charcoal 1g/kg (max 50g) if <4h after overdose (p823).

Investigation Blood paracetamol concentration at ≥4h post-ingestion. Plot this result on the paracetamol nomogram (**fig 19.29**). Also: glucose, U&E, LFT, INR, FBC, HCO₃⁻, lactate.

Acetylcysteine Is indicated if:
- Paracetamol concentration is above the treatment line (the 100 mg/L at 4h after ingestion line), see **fig 19.29**.
- Presentation >8h after ingestion, before paracetamol concentration available. Stop later if concentration below line (use clinical judgement, review INR and ALT).
- Unknown timing or staggered overdose.

Seek expert advice if HIV, enzyme-inducing drugs, alcohol, or nutrition affects interpretation of paracetamol nomogram, or in critical illness.

Scottish and Newcastle Acetylcysteine Protocol (SNAP) regimen:
1. Bag 1: 100mg/kg NAC in 200mL 5% glucose/0.9% sodium chloride over 2 hours.
2. Bag 2: 200mg/kg NAC in 1000mL 5% glucose/0.9% sodium chloride over 10 hours. Send LFTs, INR, venous blood gases, paracetamol concentration at 10 hours (2 hours before end). If INR ≤1.3 and ALT normal and paracetamol level <10mg/L and no symptoms suggestive of liver failure, treatment may stop after bag 2.
3. If criteria to stop are not met, repeat step 2. If INR ≤1.3 and ALT <x2 upper limit of normal and not >x2 compared to admission, treatment may stop after bag 3.
4. If criteria to stop are not met, continue to repeat step 2. ►Seek expert hepatology advice. Continue extended treatment until INR <3 and falling.

Psychiatric assessment Prior to hospital discharge.

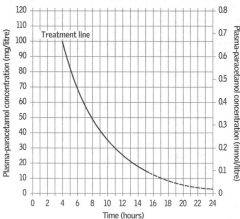

Fig 19.29 Plasma concentration of paracetamol vs time. The graph may mislead if HIV +ve (↓hepatic glutathione), long-acting paracetamol taken, pre-existing liver disease or liver enzyme induction. Do not use in staggered overdose.

Aspirin is a weak acid with poor water solubility. It is present in many over-the-counter preparations. Metabolism leads to uncoupling of oxidative phosphorylation, anaerobic metabolism, and lactic acidosis. Direct stimulation of the medulla contributes to an increase in respiratory rate. Salicylate metabolites worsen acidosis. Eventually the patient decompensates with severe metabolic acidosis, haemodynamic instability, and organ failure.

Effects are dose related (NB: salicylate concentrations correlate poorly with toxicity, especially if chronic):
• Dose 150mg/kg ≈ blood salicylate concentration >2.5mmol/L: mild toxicity.
• 250mg/kg ≈ blood salicylate concentration >4mmol/L: moderate toxicity.
• >500mg/kg ≈ blood salicylate concentration >6mmol/L: severe toxicity.

Signs and symptoms
Unlike paracetamol, there are many early features:
• Mild toxicity: tinnitus, tachypnoea, nausea, vomiting, headache, abdominal pain.
• Moderate toxicity: tachypnoea, tachycardia, orthostatic hypotension, confusion, slurred speech, hallucinations, hypoglycaemia.
• Severe toxicity: cerebral and pulmonary oedema, hypotension, arrhythmias. Hypoventilation heralds respiratory failure: prepare for intubation.

Management
1 **Activated charcoal** 1g/kg (max 50g) to all presenting within 1h of ingestion. Consider repeat doses (two further doses of 50g, 4h apart) as food in the stomach, bezoar formation, and pyloric sphincter spasm due to aspirin can all delay absorption.
2 **Investigations** Paracetamol and salicylate concentrations, U&E, bicarbonate, lactate, ABG, glucose, FBC, clotting studies, calcium, magnesium, LFT. ECG and cardiac monitor. Repeat salicylate concentrations every 2h to assess for delayed absorption/increasing toxicity.
3 **Fluid balance and urine output** Correct volume and K+ depletion. Consider catheterization to monitor output and pH.
4 **Alkalization of urine** Enhances excretion. Consider if moderate toxicity/rising concentration, eg 1L 1.2–1.4% sodium bicarbonate IV over 3–4h. Aim for urine pH 7.5–8. NB: monitor serum K+ as hypokalaemia may occur, and should be replaced, caution if AKI.
5 **Haemodialysis** For moderate and severe toxicity. Contact nephrology early.
6 **Supportive care** Correct hypoglycaemia (p818), treat seizures (pp810–11), early critical care input.
7 **Psychiatric assessment** Assess before discharge home.

Anticoagulants See pp346–7.

Benzodiazepines

Symptoms Sedation, coma, respiratory depression.

Treatment Supportive. Ensure airway. Ventilation and haemodynamic support may be needed. Risks of reversal with flumazenil outweigh benefits for most. Risk of provoking seizures, which are then treatment resistant. Use only after expert advice.

β-blocker

Symptoms Bradycardia, hypotension.

Treatment Atropine 500mcg IV, repeat up to 3mg (pp792–3). Glucagon, eg 5–10mg IV over 2min, then infusion of 50–150mcg/kg/h. Contact cardiology for temporary pacing. ↓Evidence for calcium (eg 10mL of 10% calcium chloride), IV insulin plus dextrose, Intralipid®.

Cyanide Binds iron and inhibits the cytochrome system. Leads to anaerobic respiration and lactic acidosis.

Symptoms
• Mild: dizziness, anxiety, tachycardia, nausea, confusion.
• Moderate: reduced consciousness, convulsions, cyanosis, arrhythmias.
• Severe: coma, fixed pupils, cardiorespiratory failure, death.

Treatment ►►100% O_2. If mild, supportive care is usually sufficient. ►If moderate/severe, specific treatment to bind cyanide is required, eg:
• Hydroxocobalamin (Cyanokit®) 5g over 15min, repeated once if required.
• Sodium thiosulfate: 50mL of 25% sodium thiosulfate (12.5g) IV over 10min. Repeat after 30–60min if required.

Carbon monoxide Despite hypoxaemia, skin is pink or pale (not blue), as carboxyhaemoglobin (COHb) displaces O_2 from Hb binding sites. For the same reason, O_2 saturation measured by a pulse oximeter may be normal. Check ABG in a co-oximeter (ie ensure it measures haemoglobin, SaO_2, Meth-Hb, and COHb): ↓SaO_2 and ↑COHb (normal <5%). Confirm diagnosis with an ABG quickly as concentrations soon return to normal.

Symptoms Headache, vomiting, tachycardia, tachypnoea, arrhythmias (monitor ECG). If severe toxicity (COHb >50%): seizures, coma, cardiac arrest.

Treatment ►►Remove source. Give 100% O_2 until COHb <10%. With 100% O_2 $t_{1/2}$ of COHb is reduced from 250min to 40min. Metabolic acidosis usually responds to correction of hypoxia. Consider hyperbaric O_2 if COHb >25–30%, neurological features, cardiovascular impairment, failure to respond to treatment, pregnancy.

Digoxin

Symptoms GI upset, diarrhoea, yellow-green visual halos, palpitations, ↓cognition. ECG ST 'scooping', ventricular ectopics, bidirectional VT (beat-to-beat alteration of QRS axis).

Treatment Activated charcoal, correct ↓K^+. If severe/life-threatening toxicity, eg ventricular arrhythmia, high-grade heart block, or concentration >15ng/mL: inactivate with digoxin-specific antibody fragments (DigiFab®). Dose according to amount ingested, or use concentration and weight.

Iron <20mg/kg of elemental iron is non-toxic. Moderate symptoms can occur with ingestion 20–60mg/kg. >60mg/kg causes severe toxicity and mortality.

Symptoms GI upset, shock, metabolic acidosis, coagulopathy, cardiomyopathy, AKI, liver dysfunction/failure. Healing of bowel leaves scarring and stenoses.

Treatment Desferrioxamine 15mg/kg/h IVI (max 80mg/kg/d). Whole-bowel irrigation to clear non-absorbed pills. Support circulation. Vitamin K for coagulopathy.

Opiates

Symptoms Itch, nausea, miosis, CNS and respiratory depression, apnoea.

Treatment ABC. Naloxone, eg 400mcg IM/IV every 2min until ↑RR (max 10mg). Short $t_{1/2}$, so toxicity can recur. Consider IVI. 'Take home' naloxone to prevent death if ↑risk.

Phenothiazines Includes chlorpromazine, prochlorperazine, promethazine, thioridazine.

Symptoms Hyperthermia, ↑HR, labile BP, dystonia, confusion, seizures.

Treatment ABC. Circulatory support with IV fluids. Cool. Acute dystonia: procyclidine 5–10mg IM/IV. Treat seizures (p810–11).

Neuroleptic malignant syndrome: hyperthermia, rigidity, extrapyramidal signs, autonomic dysfunction (labile BP, ↑HR, sweating, urinary incontinence), confusion, coma, ↑WCC, ↑CK. Treatment: cool, benzodiazepines can help fever and rigidity, eg lorazepam 1–2mg PO/IV every 4–6h. Also bromocriptine 2.5mg 2–3/d.

Carbon tetrachloride Present in industrial solvents. Exposure via ingestion, transdermal, or inhalation.

Symptoms Nausea, gastrointestinal irritation, headache, dizziness, dyspnoea, drowsiness, tachycardia, tachypnoea, liver and kidney toxicity.

Treatment Remove clothing, irrigate eyes. Supportive. Case reports of treatment with antioxidants, eg methionine, acetylcysteine. Hyperbaric O_2 if severe exposure (before liver dysfunction as oxidative processes may contribute to liver toxicity).

Organophosphates Insecticides and chemical warfare. Rapidly absorbed via skin, mucous membranes, inhalation. Main concern is respiratory failure from excess secretions.

Symptoms Inactivates acetylcholinesterase, leading to an increase in acetylcholine and muscarinic **SLUDGE** effects: **S**alivation, **L**acrimation, **U**rination, **D**iarrhoea, **G**I upset, **E**mesis. Also: diaphoresis, diarrhoea, miosis, bradycardia, bronchospasm, fasciculation, paralysis.

Treatment PPE. Remove soiled clothes, wash skin. Atropine 1–2mg IV every 3–5min aiming for control of respiratory secretions and oxygenation. Pralidoxime (binds to organophosphate and reactivates acetylcholinesterase) may help paralysis (but not respiratory effects so give with atropine), eg 1–2g (20–40mg/kg) IV over 15–30min, repeat in 1h, then repeat every 3–8h depending on weakness. See also p830.

Paraquat Found in weed-killers, contaminated cocaine. Diagnosis: blood/urine concentration.

Symptoms D&V, painful oral ulcers, alveolitis, kidney/liver/heart failure, coma.

Treatment Activated charcoal. Supportive. No antidote available. Excess oxygen may worsen lung toxicity.

Ecstasy = 3,4-methylenedioxymethamphetamine (MDMA).

Symptoms Nausea, muscle pain, blurred vision, amnesia, fever, confusion, ataxia, tachyarrhythmias, hyperthermia, hyper/hypotension, water intoxication, DIC, ↑K^+, AKI, hepatocellular and muscle necrosis, cardiovascular collapse, ARDS.

Treatment No antidote available. Supportive: activated charcoal, cooling, IV fluid resuscitation. Benzodiazepine for agitation/seizures (pp810–11). Treat hypoglycaemia (p818), ↑K^+ (p297), narrow complex tachycardia (p790–1), hypertension (p778). Consider dantrolene for hyperthermia, eg 2–3mg/kg, then 1mg/kg repeated if necessary (max 10mg/kg).

Snake bite (envenomation)

Symptoms ↓BP, swelling spreading proximally within 4h of bite, compartment syndrome, bleeding gums or venepuncture sites, D&V, ptosis, trismus, rhabdomyolysis, kidney failure, pulmonary oedema, shock.

20-minute whole blood clotting test if limited access to laboratory facilities: collect 2–3mL of venous blood into a clean, dry test tube, leave for 20 minutes at room temperature. Unclotted blood or a friable clot that breaks down on tipping indicates a possible clotting disorder.

Management ABC. Immobilize to reduce venom spread. Avoid tourniquet due to risk of local gangrene. Antivenom (if available) if shock, coagulopathy, neurotoxicity, AKI (black urine), rapidly progressive local swelling, bites known to cause local necrosis, or digital bites. Also tetanus toxoid (once coagulopathy corrected). Monitor for adverse reaction to antivenom (3–80% depending on dose/quality). Treat anaphylaxis (p776).

Assessment

- *Burn size* is proportional to the inflammatory response (vasodilation, increased vascular permeability) and thus fluid shift from the intravascular volume. Calculate burn as % of total body surface area using a Lund and Browder chart (fig 19.30), or the *'rule of nines'*:
  - Head and neck: 9%.
  - Arm: 9%.
  - Front of trunk: $2 \times 9\% = 18\%$.
  - Back of trunk $2 \times 9\% = 18\%$.
  - Each leg $2 \times 9\% = 18\%$.
  - Perineum 1%.
- *Burn depth* determines healing time/scarring. Assessment is hard, even with experience. Burns can also evolve, particularly over the first 48h. Distinguish:
  - Partial-thickness burns: painful, red, and blistered.
  - Full-thickness burns: insensate/painless; grey-white.

Management
Resuscitate

- *Airway:* beware of upper airway compromise if hot gases inhaled. Suspect if history of fire in enclosed space, soot in oral/nasal cavity, singed nasal hairs, or hoarse voice. Flexible laryngoscopy/bronchoscopy can be used to diagnose upper airway injury and inform intubation decision. Involve anaesthetists early. Monitor: obstruction can develop in the first 24h.
- *Breathing:* exclude life-threatening chest injuries (eg tension pneumothorax) and constricting burns. Consider escharotomy if circumferential chest burns are impairing thorax excursion (*OHCS* p598). Suspect carbon monoxide poisoning from history, cherry-red skin. If COHb >10%, treat with 100% O_2 (p826).
- *Circulation:* >15% partial-thickness burns require IV fluid resuscitation. Use 2 large-bore (14–16G) IV lines, through burned skin if needed, or intraosseous (see *OHCS* p182). Use a burns calculator or formula to determine amount of IV fluid needed, eg *Parkland formula:* $4 \times$ weight in kg $\times$ % burn = mL of crystalloid needed in first 24h, half given within 8h. Replace fluid from the time of burn, not from the time admitted. Formulae are only guides: adjust IVI according to clinical response and urine output (aim ≥0.5mL/kg/h). Beware of over-resuscitation ('fluid creep') which can lead to complications, eg abdominal compartment syndrome.
- *Disability:* assess GCS. Consider carbon monoxide toxicity (p826), cyanide toxicity (p826), and trauma.

Immediate burn management

- 'Cool the burn, warm the patient.' Remove burned/constricting/contaminated clothing unless molten/adherent. Cool the burn within 3h with cold water (not ice or iced water), or use a cooled, clean compress. Aim for 20 minutes of cooling. Cover non-burned areas, and keep these areas warm during cooling of burns.
- Cover burns with saline gauze. Specialist dressings may be available. Cling film can be a useful temporary measure and relieve pain. Do not burst blisters.
- Analgesia. Paracetamol, NSAIDs, codeine. If severe pain: Entonox®, titrate IV morphine until pain controlled.
- Surgical/plastics input. If circumferential burn of chest or limbs (above wrist/ankle) refer for escharotomy/fasciotomy.
- Ensure tetanus immunity.

Burns unit care

Burns unit specialist advice ± transfer care if:
- Total body surface area burnt >10%, or full-thickness burn >5%.
- Airway compromise/inhalation injury.
- Circumferential burns to trunk or limbs requiring escharotomy.
- Chemical/high voltage electrical burn.
- Special area burns: hands, face, neck, feet, perineum/genitalia, joint affecting mobility.

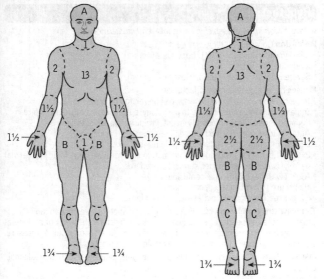

Relative percentage of body surface area affected by growth

Area	Age	0	1	5	10	15	Adult
A: half of head		9½	8½	6½	5½	4½	3½
B: half of thigh		2¾	3¼	4	4¼	4½	4¾
C: half of leg		2½	2½	2¾	3	3¼	3½

Fig 19.30 Lund and Browder chart for estimating the total body surface area affected by burns.

►*Have a high index of suspicion and a low-reading thermometer.*

Definition Core (rectal) temperature <35°C.
• Mild hypothermia: 32.2–<35°C (may see shivering).
• Moderate: 28–32.1°C.
• Severe: <28°C (shivering usually lost).

Causes Often a combination of factors:
• Impaired homeostatic mechanisms: eg age-related ↓thermoregulation.
• Impaired thermoregulation due to pathology: eg pneumonia, MI, heart failure.
• Reduced metabolism: immobility, hypothyroidism, hypoglycaemia.
• Autonomic neuropathy (p501): eg diabetes mellitus, Parkinson's.
• Low room temperature: poverty, poor housing.
• Excess heat loss: widespread dermatological disease, eg toxic epidermal necrolysis/eczema; prolonged surgical procedures.
• ↓Cold awareness: dementia, confusion.
• ↑Exposure to cold: falls, especially nocturnal.
• CNS depression: alcohol, opiates, benzodiazepines.

Temperature measurement Infrared ear thermometers give only an indirect estimate of core temperature. Sublingual or axillary T° can be checked slightly as peripheral site temperatures are often inaccurate. ►Confirm using a direct accurate measure, eg rectal temperature taken with a low-reading thermometer.

Presentation Common: after fall with long-lie, houseless patients, alcohol/drug use.
• Symptoms: confusion, agitation, ↓GCS, coma.
• Signs: bradycardia, hypotension, arrhythmias (AF, VT, VF).

There are many stories of people 'returning to life' when warmed despite absence of vital signs, see BOX. It is essential to rewarm and re-examine.

Investigation FBC, U&E, thyroid function, cortisol, plasma glucose, amylase, lactate. Screen for infection. Consider blood gas. ECG: may show J-waves (fig 19.31).

Management
• Ensure safe airway. Warm, humidified O₂. Consider ventilation if ↓GCS, ↓pO₂, ↑pCO₂.
• Re-warming depends on context.
    • *Slow rewarming* for most. Remove wet clothing. Warm IVI. Using blankets or active external warming (hot air duvets). Aim for core temperature rise of 0.5°C/h. If T° rising too quickly, stop and allow to cool slightly as rapid rewarming can lead to peripheral vasodilation and shock. Monitor temperature, HR, BP, RR. ↑HR or ↓BP can be signs of too rapid warming.
    • Rapid rewarming if hypothermia with cardiovascular instability/cardiac arrest. Consider warmed fluid lavage (eg intravesical, intraperitoneal) and intravascular warming (eg extracorporeal membrane oxygenation (ECMO)). In the event of cardiac arrest, defibrillation may be unsuccessful if T° <30°C. If VF persists after three shocks, continue resuscitation but delay further shocks until core T°>30°C (*OHCS* p579). Increase administration intervals for adrenaline to 6–10 minutes if the core temperature is <34°C.
• Monitor for arrhythmias, eg AF, VT, VF. Can occur at any time during rewarming or on stimulation.

Complications Arrhythmia, pneumonia, pancreatitis, AKI, DIC.

Prognosis Depends on age and degree of hypothermia. If age >70yrs and T° <32°C then mortality >50%.

Prevention Assess/provide support: accommodation, personal alarm/telemonitoring. Review medication, especially sedatives. Support with drug/alcohol dependency.

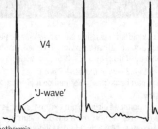

V4

'J-wave'

Fig 19.31 J-wave in hypothermia.

Courtesy of Dr R Luke and Dr E McLachlan.

'I did not die, and alive I remained not'

Remember that death is a process. In hypothermia, all processes are suspended: metabolism may slow to as much as 10% of baseline, drastically diminishing the oxygen requirements of tissues.

Perhaps this is what Dante had in mind for the last round of the 9th circle of hell, in which those betraying their benefactors are encased in ice:

> How frozen I became and powerless then.
> Ask it not, reader, for I write it not,
> because all language would be insufficient.
> I did not die, and I alive remained not.

13-month-old Canadian Erica Nordby was successfully resuscitated 2 hours after her heart stopped (core $T°$: 16°C).

Anna Bågenholm, a Swedish trainee orthopaedic surgeon, became trapped under freezing water covered by a layer of ice for 80 minutes following a skiing accident, suffering a cardiac arrest (core $T°$: 13.7°C). After resuscitation and 20 days in intensive care, she regained consciousness, suffering no permanent brain damage. She is now a radiologist.

▶No one is dead until they are warm and dead.

Definition

An incident (or series of incidents) causing casualties on a scale beyond the normal resources of emergency and healthcare services.[13] Usually caused by sudden-onset events. (Does not include casualties as a result of infectious disease/pandemics.)

►All hospitals have a detailed *Major Incident Plan*.
►Tasks of key personnel can be helpfully defined on individual *Action Cards*.

Major incident standby

A 'standby' message is announced either from external sources (eg NHS England) or internally (due to activity level or alert from another source, eg social media). This is communicated via METHANE: **M**ajor incident standby, **E**xact location of incident, **T**ype of incident, **H**azards/potential hazards, **A**ccess routes to hospital, **N**umber of casualties, which **E**mergency services are involved.

Patients at the scene undergo triage to one of:
• Adult major trauma centre.
• Adult trauma unit.
• Local hospitals/walk-in-centres.
• Comfort at scene as unlikely to survive injuries.
• Survivor reception for uninjured survivors.

Immediate wound management

• Examine all wounds, consider photographs to avoid unnecessary re-looks.
• Examine sequentially to minimize temperature and fluid loss.
• Intra-cavity and junctional (between torso and limbs) bleeding needs surgery/interventional radiology.
• Tranexamic acid if major haemorrhage (pp774–5).
• Young patients may have significant blood loss with normal physiology (until late).
• Beware of compartment syndrome/pressure effects with prolonged tourniquet use. Use pressure dressings and elevation first, record tourniquet time if they are used.
• Use saline-soaked gauze to cover exposed viscera/brain.

Ballistic injury

• Small exit and entry wounds can mask catastrophic internal damage.
• Some bullets fragment, leading to multiple wound tracts.
• CT for fragments (may contain steel and be moved by MRI field).

Crush injury

• Look for crush syndrome (rhabdomyolysis): check serum CK, urine myoglobin. Treat with crystalloid (blood products first if haemorrhagic shock).
• Monitor for cardiac arrhythmias and treat: ↑risk with reperfusion.
• Avoid suxamethonium for intubation: risk of hyperkalaemia and death.
• Surgical stabilization of flail chest.
• Cranial trauma needs expert neurosurgical review and management.

Hazardous materials (HAZMAT), chemical, biological, radiological, and nuclear (CBRN) events

• Recognize: symptoms in emergency service/hospital staff, multiple casualties with similar non-traumatic symptoms, unusual taste or smell, unexplained dead animals, unexplained symptoms (eg altered vision, eye pain, excessive secretions, non-thermal burns/blistering/necrosis), unusual investigation results.
• Assistance with management of event in UK: National Emergency Co-Ordinated Scientific Advice (ECOSA) system, 0300 303 3493.
• Clinical guidance for individual patient in UK: National Poisons Information Service (NPIS), 0344 892 0111.
• Emergency combination treatment for nerve agents is available, eg Combopen® (2mg atropine, 500mg pralidoxime, 5mg diazepam). Give 3 pens if unconscious, convulsions, respiratory paralysis/arrest, cyanosis, HR >40. Give 1 pen every 15min if not walking, excessive secretions, confusion, wheezing, incontinence. See also p827.

Domestic (eg gas explosion), industrial (eg mining), or explosive device (eg terrorist bomb). Death may occur without obvious external injury. Injury occurs in a number of ways:

1 **Blast wave** A transient (milliseconds) wave of overpressure expands rapidly producing cellular disruption, shearing forces along tissue planes (submucosal/ subserosal haemorrhage), and re-expansion of compressed trapped gas causing bowel perforation, fatal air embolism.

2 **Blast wind** This can totally disrupt a body or cause avulsive amputations. Bodies can be thrown and sustain injuries on landing.

3 **Missiles** Penetration or laceration from missiles from the bomb or secondary missiles, eg broken glass.

4 **Flash burns** Usually superficial and occur on exposed skin.

5 **Crush injuries** Beware sudden death or acute kidney injury from rhabdomyolysis after release.

6 **Contamination** Domestic and industrial blasts can scatter chemicals widely, and cause both superficial and penetrating contamination. There may be concern about the use of biological or radioactive material in man-made explosive devices. Consider the location and mechanism of the blast. Seek advice.

7 **Psychological injury** Eg post-traumatic stress disorder (*OHCS* p721).

Management
See major trauma, *OHCS* p586.
- Aggressive resuscitation in close-range survivors.
- Look for occult injury and monitor for evolving injury.
- Blast thorax: high risk of great vessel and aortic disruption. Needs early cardiothoracic review.
- Blast lung ($\downarrow pO_2$, associated rib fracture/pneumothorax/contusions): early intubation, and lung protective ventilation.
- Blast abdomen: risk of significant intra-abdominal bleeding and late bowel perforation, even if abdominal wall not breached.
- Blast pelvis: high mortality from exsanguination, especially if sacroiliac joints are open.
- Early CT.
- Use rapid transfuser for blood products.
- Crystalloid resuscitation may worsen coagulopathy.
- Prioritize damage control surgery.

19 Emergencies

20 References

Contents

1 Schneider EC, Shah A, Doty MM, *et al. Mirror, mirror 2021: reflecting poorly. health care in the U.S. compared to other high-income countries.* 2021. Available at: https://www.commonwealthfund.org/publications/fund-reports/2021/aug/mirror-mirror-2021-reflecting-poorly#rank

2 Mani N, Slevin N, Hudson A. What three wise men have to say about diagnosis. *BMJ* 2011; 343:d7769. http://www.bmj.com/content/343/bmj.d7769

3 Schulz K. *Being wrong: adventures in the margin of error.* London: Portobello Books, 2011.

4 Francis R. *Report of the Mid-Staffordshire NHS Foundation Trust Public Enquiry.* London: The Stationery Office, 2013. http://webarchive.nationalarchives.gov.uk/20150407084003/http://www.midstaffspublicinquiry.com/home

5 Cerdeña JP, Plaisime MV, Tsai J. From race-based to race-conscious medicine: how anti-racist uprisings call us to act. *Lancet* 2020; 396(10257):1125–8

6 Walker M. *Why we sleep.* Harmondsworth: Penguin Books, 2018.

7 Jewitt C. *Sexism in medicine.* British Medical Association. 2021. https://www.bma.org.uk/media/4487/sexism-in-medicine-bma-report.pdf

8 British Medical Association. *Commentary on mend the gap: the independent review into gender pay gaps in medicine in England.* https://www.bma.org.uk/media/3617/bma-commentary-on-medicine-gender-pay-gap-dec-2020.pdf

9 Ruegger J, Hodgkinson S, Field-Smith A, *et al.* Care of adults in the last days of life: summary of NICE guidance. *BMJ* 2015; 351:h6631. http://www.bmj.com/content/351/bmj.h6631

10 Academy of Royal Colleges. *A code of practice for the diagnosis and confirmation of death.* 2010. http://www.aomrc.org.uk/publications/reports-guidance/ukdec-reports-and-guidance/code-practice-diagnosis-confirmation-death

11 Sokol DK, McFadzean WA, Dickson WA, *et al.* Ethical dilemmas in the acute setting: a frame-work for clinicians. *BMJ* 2011; 343:d5528. http://www.bmj.com/content/343/bmj.d5528.long

12 NICE. *Depression: the treatment and management of depression in adults* [CG90]. 2009, updated 2016. https://www.nice.org.uk/guidance/CG90

13 NICE. *Violence and aggression: short-term management in mental health, health and community setting* [NG10]. 2015. https://www.nice.org.uk/guidance/ng10

14 Greenland S, Senn SJ, Rothman KJ, *et al.* Statistical tests, P values, confidence intervals, and power: a guide to misinterpretations. *Eur J Epidemiol* 2016; 31:337–50.

15 Greenhalgh T. *How to read a paper* (6th edn). Oxford: Wiley-Blackwell, 2019.

16 O'Mahony D, O'Sullivan D, Byrne S, *et al.* STOPP/START criteria for potentially inappropriate prescribing in older people: version 2. *Age Ageing* 2015; 44(2):213–8. https://academic.oup.com/ageing/article-lookup/doi/10.1093/ageing/afu145

17 NICE. *Falls in older people: assessing risk and prevention* [CG161]. 2013. https://www.nice.org.uk/guidance/cg161

18 Knight M, Bunch K, Tuffnell D, *et al.* on behalf of MBRRACE-UK. *Saving lives, improving mothers' care: lessons learned to inform maternity care from the UK and Ireland.* National Perinatal Epidemiology Unit, University of Oxford. Up-to-date reports available at: https://www.npeu.ox.ac.uk/mbrrace-uk/reports

Chapter 2: History and examination

No references for this chapter

20 References

1 Arnett DK, Blumenthal RS, Albert MA, *et al*. AHA guideline on the primary prevention of cardiovascular disease: a report of the American College of Cardiology/American Heart Association Task Force on Clinical Practice Guidelines. *Circulation* 2019; 140(11):e596–646. https://www.ahajournals.org/doi/full/10.1161/CIR.0000000000000678

2 Stead LF, Buitrago D, Preciado N, *et al*. Physician advice for smoking cessation. *Cochrane Database Syst Rev* 2013; 5:CD000165. https://www.cochranelibrary.com/cdsr/doi/10.1002/14651858.CD000165.pub4/full

3 NICE. *Cardiovascular disease: risk assessment and reduction, including lipid modification* [CG181]. 2014, updated 2023. https://www.nice.org.uk/guidance/cg181

4 Kidney Disease: Improving Global Outcomes (KDIGO) Blood Pressure Work Group. KDIGO 2021 Clinical Practice Guideline for the Management of Blood Pressure in Chronic Kidney Disease. *Kidney Int* 2021; Mar;99 (3S):S1–S87.

5 Smith SW, Dodd KW, Henry TD, *et al*. Diagnosis of ST-elevation myocardial infarction in the presence of left bundle branch block with the ST-elevation to S-wave ratio in a modified Sgarbossa rule. *Ann Emerg Med* 2012; 60(6):766–76. https://www.annemergmed.com/article/S0196-0644(12)01368-6/fulltext

6 Maw AM, Hassanin A, Ho PM, *et al*. Diagnostic accuracy of point-of-care lung ultrasonography and chest radiography in adults with symptoms suggestive of acute decompensated heart failure: a systematic review and meta-analysis. *JAMA Netw Open* 2019; 2(3):e190703. https://jamanetwork.com/journals/jamanetworkopen/fullarticle/2728006

7 Aspirin for primary prevention of disease. http://www.nyrdtc.nhs.uk/docs/dud/DU_65_Aspirin.pdf

8 McNeil JJ, Wolfe R, Woods RL, *et al*. Effect of aspirin on cardiovascular events and bleeding in the healthy elderly. *N Engl J Med* 2018; 379(16):1509–18. https://www.nejm.org/doi/full/10.1056/NEJMoa1805819

9 Wallentin L, Becker RC, Budaj A, *et al*. Ticagrelor versus clopidogrel in patients with acute coronary syndromes. *N Engl J Med* 2009; 361(11):1045–57. https://www.nejm.org/doi/10.1056/NEJMoa0904327

10 Eikelboom JW, Connolly SJ, Bosch J, *et al*. Rivaroxaban with or without aspirin in stable cardiovascular disease. *N Engl J Med* 2017; 377(14):1319–30. https://www.nejm.org/doi/full/10.1056/nejmoa1709118

11 Schmidt M, Mansfield KE, Bhaskaran K, *et al*. Serum creatinine elevation after renin-angiotensin system blockade and long term cardiorenal risks: cohort study. *BMJ* 2017; 356:j791. https://www.bmj.com/content/356/bmj.j791

12 McMurray JJ, Packer M, Desai AS, *et al*. Angiotensin-neprilysin inhibition versus enalapril in heart failure. *N Engl J Med* 2014; 371(11):993–1004. https://www.nejm.org/doi/10.1056/NEJMoa1409077

13 The Digitalis Investigation Group. The effect of digoxin on mortality and morbidity in patients with heart failure. *N Engl J Med* 1997; 336:525–33. http://www.nejm.org/doi/full/10.1056/NEJM199702203360801

14 Lewington S, Clarke R, Qizilbash N, *et al*. Age-specific relevance of usual blood pressure to vascular mortality: a meta-analysis of individual data for one million adults in 61 prospective studies. *Lancet* 2002; 360(9349):1903–13. https://www.thelancet.com/journals/lancet/article/PIIS0140-6736(03)12816-4/fulltext

15 NICE. *Hypertension in adults: diagnosis and management* [CG127]. 2011, updated 2016. https://www.nice.org.uk/guidance/cg127

16 Beckett NS, Peters R, Fletcher AE, *et al*. Treatment of hypertension in patients 80 years of age or older. *N Engl J Med* 2008; 58:1887–98. http://content.nejm.org/cgi/reprint/358/18/1887.pdf

17 Bakris G, Ali W, Parati G. ACC/AHA versus ESC/ESH on hypertension guidelines: JACC guideline comparison. *J Am Coll Cardiol* 2019; 73(23):3018–26. https://www.sciencedirect.com/science/article/pii/S0735109719348879

18 Cohen JB, Lotito MJ, Trivedi UK, *et al*. Cardiovascular events and mortality in white coat hypertension: a systematic review and meta-analysis. *Ann Intern Med* 2019; 170(12):853–62. https://www.acpjournals.org/doi/10.7326/M19-0223

19 NICE. *Hypertension in adults: diagnosis and management* [NG136]. 2019, updated 2022. https://www.nice.org.uk/guidance/ng136

20 Law M, Wald N, Morris J. Lowering blood pressure to prevent myocardial infarction and stroke: a new preventive strategy. *Health Technol Assess* 2003; 7(31):1–94. https://www.ncbi.nlm.nih.gov/pubmedhealth/PMH0015113/

21 ALLHAT Officers and Coordinators for the ALLHAT Collaborative Research Group. The Antihypertensive and Lipid-Lowering Treatment to Prevent Heart Attack Trial. Major outcomes in high-risk hypertensive patients randomized to angiotensin-converting enzyme inhibitor or calcium channel blocker vs diuretic. *JAMA* 2002; 288:2981–97. http://jama.ama-assn.org/content/288/23/2981.full

22 NICE. General principles for treating people with stable angina. In *Stable angina: management* [CG126], Chapter 1.3. 2011, updated 2016. https://www.nice.org.uk/guidance/cg126/chapter/1-Guidance#general-principles-for-treating-people-with-stable-angina

23 NICE. *Chest pain of recent onset: assessment and diagnosis* [CG95]. 2010, updated 2016. http://www.nice.org.uk/guidance/CG95

24 Thygesen K, Alpert JS, Jaffe AS, *et al*. Fourth universal definition of myocardial infarction (2018). *J Am Coll Cardiol* 2018; 72(18):2231–64. https://www.jacc.org/doi/10.1016/j.jacc.2018.08.1038

25 Stacy SR, Suarez-Cuervo C, Berger Z, *et al*. Role of troponin in patients with chronic kidney disease and suspected acute coronary syndrome: a systematic review. *Ann Intern Med* 2014; 161(7):502–12. https://www.acpjournals.org/doi/full/10.7326/M14-0746

26 Driver and Vehicle Licensing Agency. *Cardiovascular disorders: assessing fitness to drive*. March 2016. https://www.gov.uk/guidance/cardiovascular-disorders-assessing-fitness-to-drive

27 Lopes RD, Heizer G, Aronson R, *et al*. Antithrombotic therapy after acute coronary syndrome or PCI in atrial fibrillation. *N Engl J Med* 2019; 380(16):1509–24. https://www.nejm.org/doi/10.1056/NEJMoa1817083

28 Massimo M. Minimally invasive coronary surgery: fad or future? *BMJ* 1998; 316:88.

29 Takagi H, Matsui M, Umemoto T. Lower graft patency after off-pump than on-pump coronary artery bypass grafting: an updated meta-analysis of randomized trials. *J Thorac Cardiovasc Surg* 2010; 140(3):e45–7. https://www.jtcvs.org/article/S0022-5223(09)01543-8/fulltext

30 Brown WR, Moody DM, Venkata R, *et al*. Longer duration of cardiopulmonary bypass is associated with greater numbers of cerebral microemboli. *Stroke* 2000; 31:707–13. http://stroke.ahajournals.org/content/31/3/707

31 Corrado D, Pelliccia A, Bjørnstad HH, *et al*. Cardiovascular pre-participation screening of young competitive athletes for prevention of sudden death: proposal for a common European protocol. *Eur Heart J* 2005; 26(5):516–24. https://academic.oup.com/eurheartj/article/26/5/516/2888062

32 Appelboam A, Reuben A, Mann C, *et al*. Postural modification to the standard Valsalva manoeuvre for emergency treatment of supraventricular tachycardias (REVERT): a randomised controlled trial. *Lancet* 2015; 386(10005):1747–53. https://www.thelancet.com/journals/lancet/article/PIIS0140-6736(15)61485-4/fulltext

33 NICE. *Atrial fibrillation: management*. 2014. https://www.nice.org.uk/guidance/cg180/chapter/1-Recommendations

34 Wyse DG, Waldo AL, DiMarco JP, *et al*. A comparison of rate control and rhythm control in patients with atrial fibrillation. *N Engl J Med* 2002; 347:1825–33. http://www.nejm.org/doi/full/10.1056/NEJMoa021328

35 Mant J. Warfarin vs aspirin for stroke prevention in elderly with atrial fibrillation (the Birmingham Atrial Fibrillation Treatment of the Aged Study, BAFTA): a randomised controlled trial. *Lancet* 2007; 370:493–503. http://www.thelancet.com/journals/lancet/article/PIIS0140673607612331/abstract

36 Bristow M, Saxon L, Boehmer J, *et al*. Cardiac-resynchronization therapy with or without an implantable defibrillator in advanced chronic heart failure. *N Engl J Med* 2004; 350(21):2140–50. http://www.nejm.org/doi/full/10.1056/NEJMoa032423

37 NICE. *Implantable cardioverter defibrillators and cardiac resynchronisation therapy for arrhythmias and heart failure [TA314]*. 2014. https://www.nice.org.uk/guidance/ta314

38 Adler Y, Charron P, Imazio M, *et al*. 2015 ESC Guidelines for the diagnosis and management of pericardial diseases. *BMJ* 2002; 325(7370):915–16. https://www.ncbi.nlm.nih.gov/pmc/articles/PMC1124429/

39 Ponikowski P, Voors AA, Anker SD, *et al*. 2016 ESC Guidelines for the diagnosis and treatment of acute and chronic heart failure. *Eur J Heart Fail* 2016; 18(8):891–975. https://academic.oup.com/eurheartj/article/37/27/2129/1748921

40 McKee PA, Castelli WP, McNamara PM, *et al*. The natural history of congestive heart failure: the Framingham study. *N Engl J Med* 1971; 285(26):1441–6. http://www.nejm.org/doi/full/10.1056/NEJM197112232852601

41 NICE. *Chronic heart failure [CG108]*. 2010. https://www.nice.org.uk/guidance/cg108

42 Fonarow GC, Abraham WT, Albert NM, *et al*. Influence of beta-blocker continuation or withdrawal on outcomes in patients hospitalized with heart failure: findings from the OPTIMIZE-HF program. *J Am Coll Cardiol* 2008; 52(3):190–9.

43 Pitt B, Zannad F, Remme WJ, *et al*. The effect of spironolactone on morbidity and mortality in patients with severe heart failure. *N Engl J Med* 1999; 341:709–17. http://content.nejm.org/cgi/reprint/341/10/709.pdf

44 Taylor AL, Ziesche S, Yancy C, *et al*. Combination of isosorbide dinitrate and hydralazine in blacks with heart failure. *N Engl J Med* 2004; 351(20):2049–57. http://content.nejm.org/cgi/content/full/351/20/2049

45 McMurray JJV, Solomon SD, Inzucchi SE, *et al*. Dapagliflozin in patients with heart failure and reduced ejection fraction. *N Engl J Med* 2019; 381:1995–2008. https://www.nejm.org/doi/full/10.1056/NEJMoa1911303

46 Chopra HL, Nanda N. *Textbook of cardiology (a clinical & historical perspective)*. New Delhi: Jaypee Brothers Medical Publishers, 2012:667.

47 Soutter H. The repair of mitral stenosis. *Br Med J* 1925; 2(3379):603–6.

48 Stout KK, Daniels CJ, Aboulhosn JA, *et al*. 2018 AHA/ACC guideline for the management of adults with congenital heart disease. *Circulation* 2019; 139(14):e637–97. https://www.ahajournals.org/doi/full/10.1161/CIR.0000000000000602

49 Durack D, Lukes AS, Bright DK. New criteria for diagnosis of infective endocarditis: utilization of specific echocardiographic findings. Duke Endocarditis Service. *Am J Med* 1994; 96:200–9.

50 Habib G, Lancellotti P, Antunes MJ, *et al*. *Eur Heart J* 2015; 36:3075–128. https://academic.oup.com/eurheartj/article/36/44/3075/2293384

51 Driver and Vehicle Licensing Agency. *Assessing fitness to drive—a guide for medical professionals*. 2016. https://www.gov.uk/government/publications/assessing-fitness-to-drive-a-guide-for-medical-professionals

1 Johnson DC. Importance of adjusting carbon monoxide diffusing capacity (DLCO) and carbon monoxide transfer coefficient (KCO) for alveolar volume. *Respir Med* 2000; 94(1):28–37. http://www.resmedjournal.com/article/S0954-6111(99)90740-0/abstract

2 Spira A. Airway gene expression; a novel diagnostic test for lung cancer in smokers. *Proc Amer Assoc Cancer Res* 2006; 47:242.

3 Størdal K, Johannesdottir GB, Bentsen BS, *et al*. Acid suppression does not change respiratory symptoms in children with asthma and gastro-oesophageal reflux disease. *Arch Dis Child* 2005; 90(9):956–60. https://www.ncbi.nlm.nih.gov/pmc/articles/PMC1720585/

4 Douglas JD. If you want to cure their asthma, ask about their job. *Prim Care Respir J* 2005; 14(2):65–71. http://www.nature.com/articles/pcrj2004122

5 Global Initiative for Asthmas. *2021 GINA Report, Global Strategy for Asthma Management and Prevention.* 2020. https://ginasthma.org/wp-content/uploads/2020/04/GINA-2020-full-report_-final-_wms.pdf

6 NICE. *Omalizumab for severe persistent allergic asthma* [TA133]. 2007. https://www.nice.org.uk/guidance/TA133

7 Hensley MJ. Use of inhaled corticosteroids was associated with the development of cataracts. *Evid Based Med* 1998; 3:24. http://ebm.bmj.com/content/3/1/24.full.pdf+html

8 Lozano R, Naghavi M, Foreman K, *et al*. Global and regional mortality from 235 causes of death for 20 age groups in 1990 and 2010: a systematic analysis for the Global Burden of Disease Study 2010. *Lancet* 2012; 380(9859):2095–128.

9 Steiner M, Barton RL, Singh SJ, *et al*. Nutritional enhancement of exercise performance in chronic obstructive pulmonary disease: a randomised controlled trial. *Thorax* 200358(9):745–51. https://www.ncbi.nlm.nih.gov/pmc/articles/PMC1746806/

10 Poole PJ, Black PN. Mucolytic agents for chronic bronchitis or chronic obstructive pulmonary disease. *Cochrane Database Syst Rev* 2006; 3:CD001287. http://onlinelibrary.wiley.com/doi/10.1002/14651858.CD001287.pub2/abstract

11 Nannini L, Cates CJ, Lasserson TJ, *et al*. Combined corticosteroid and long-acting beta-agonist in one inhaler versus separate components for COPD. *Cochrane Database Syst Rev* 2007; 4:CD003794. http://www.ncbi.nlm.nih.gov/pubmed/17943798

12 BTS. *National Adult Community Acquired Pneumonia Audit 2018/19.* Available here: https://brit-thoracic.org.uk/quality-improvement/clinical-audit/national-adult-community-acquired-pneumonia-audit-201819/

13 Burk M, El-Kersh K, Saad M, *et al*. Viral infection in community-acquired pneumonia: a systematic review and meta-analysis. *Eur Respir Rev* 2016; 25(140):178–88.

14 Man SY, Lee N, Ip M, *et al*. Prospective comparison of three predictive rules for assessing severity of community-acquired pneumonia in Hong Kong. *Thorax* 2007 62:348–53. https://www.ncbi.nlm.nih.gov/pmc/articles/PMC2092476/

15 Lim WS. Severity assessment in community-acquired pneumonia: moving on. *Thorax* 2007; 62:287–8. https://www.ncbi.nlm.nih.gov/pmc/articles/PMC2092475/

16 NICE. *Summary of antimicrobial prescribing guidance–managing common infections.* March 2020. https://www.nice.org.uk/Media/Default/About/what-we-do/NICE-guidance/antimicrobial%20guidance/summary-antimicrobial-prescribing-guidance.pdf

17 Kumar S, Hammerschlag MR. Acute respiratory infection due to *Chlamydia pneumoniae*: current status of diagnostic methods. *Clin Infect Dis* 2007; 44(4):568–76. http://cid.oxfordjournals.org/content/44/4/568.long

18 Stringer JR, Beard CB, Miller RF, *et al*. A new name (Pneumocystis jiroveci) for Pneumocystis from humans. *Emerg Infect Dis* 2002; 8(9):891–6.

19 Kaplan JE, Benson C, Holmes KT, *et al*. Guidelines for prevention and treatment of opportunistic infections in HIV-infected adults and adolescents. Atlanta, GA: CDC, 2009. http://www.cdc.gov/mmwr/preview/mmwrhtml/rr5804a1.htm

20 Hui DS. Review of clinical symptoms and spectrum in humans with influenza A/H5N1 infection. *Respirology* 2008; 13(Suppl 1):S10–13. http://www.ncbi.nlm.nih.gov/pubmed/18366521

21 The Writing Committee of the World Health Organization (WHO) Consultation on Human Influenza A/H5. Avian Influenza A (H5N1) Infection in Humans. *N Engl J Med* 2005; 353:1374–85. http://content.nejm.org/cgi/content/full/353/13/1374

22 Engin A. Influenza type A (H5N1) virus infection. *Mikrobiyol Bul* 2007; 41(3):485–94. http://www.ncbi.nlm.nih.gov/pubmed/17933264

23 Public Health England. *Avian influenza: guidance and algorithms for managing human cases.* 2014. https://www.gov.uk/government/publications/avian-influenza-guidance-and-algorithms-for-managing-human-cases

24 HPA. *Avian influenza guidance and algorithms.* http://www.hpa.org.uk/web/HPAweb&HPAwebStandard/HPAweb_C/1195733851442

25 British Thoracic Society. *Guidelines on severe acute respiratory syndrome.* 2004. http://www.brit-thoracic.org.uk/guidelines/severe-acute-respiratory-syndrome-guideline.aspx

26 Hui DS. An overview on severe acute respiratory syndrome (SARS). *Monaldi Arch Chest Dis* 2005; 63(3):149–57.

27 Williamson EJ, Walker AJ, Bhaskaran K, *et al*. Factors associated with COVID-19-related death using OpenSAFELY. *Nature* 2020; 584:430–6. doi: 10.1038/s41586-020-2521-4

28 Lauer SA, Grantz KH, Bi Q, *et al*. The incubation period of coronavirus disease 2019 (COVID-19) from publicly reported confirmed cases: estimation and application. *Ann Intern Med* 2020; 172(9):577–82.

29 Horby P, Lim WS, Emberson JR, *et al*. Dexamethasone in Hospitalized Patients with Covid-19. *N Engl J Med* 2021; 384(8):693–704.

30 Agarwal R. Allergic bronchopulmonary aspergillosis. *Chest* 2009; 135:805–26. http://www.sciencedirect.com/science/article/pii/S0012369209602099

31 Graf K. Five-years surveillance of invasive aspergillosis in a university hospital. *BMC Infect Dis* 2011; 11:163. https://www.ncbi.nlm.nih.gov/pmc/articles/PMC3128051/

32 Herbrecht R, Denning DW, Patterson TF, et al. Voriconazole versus amphotericin B for primary therapy of invasive aspergillosis. *N Engl J Med* 2002; 347:408–15. http://www.nejm.org/doi/full/10.1056/NEJMoa020191

33 BTS Pleural Guideline Group. Investigation of a unilateral pleural effusion in adults: British Thoracic Society Pleural Disease Guideline 2010. *Thorax* 2010; 65(Suppl 2):ii4–17.

34 Davies C, Gleeson FV, Davies RJ, et al. BTS guidelines for the management of pleural infection. *Thorax* 2003; 58(Suppl 2):ii18–28. https://www.ncbi.nlm.nih.gov/pmc/articles/PMC1766018/

35 Wheeler AP, Bernard GR, Thompson BT, et al. Pulmonary-artery versus central venous catheter to guide treatment of acute lung injury. *N Engl J Med* 2006; 354(21):2213–24.

36 The ARDS Definition Task Force. Acute respiratory distress syndrome: the Berlin definition. *JAMA* 2012; 307(23):2526–33.

37 The Acute Respiratory Distress Syndrome Network. Ventilation with lower tidal volumes as compared with traditional tidal volumes for acute lung injury and the acute respiratory distress syndrome. *N Engl J Med* 2000; 342:1301–8.

38 Annane D, Pastores SM, Rochwerg B, et al. Guidelines for the diagnosis and management of critical illness-related corticosteroid insufficiency (CIRCI) in critically ill patients (part I): Society of Critical Care Medicine (SCCM) and European Society of Intensive Care Medicine (ESICM) 2017. *Intensive Care Med* 2017; 43(12):1751.

39 Zambon M, Vincent JL. Mortality rates for patients with acute lung injury/ARDS have decreased over time. *Chest* 2008; 133(5):1120

40 Erickson SE, Martin GS, Davis JL, et al. Recent trends in acute lung injury mortality: 1996–2005. *Crit Care Med* 2009; 37(5):1574.

41 Ramsey BW, Davies J, McElvaney NG, et al. A CFTR potentiator in patients with cystic fibrosis and the G551D mutation. *N Engl J Med* 2011; 365(18):1663–72. https://www.ncbi.nlm.nih.gov/pmc/articles/PMC3230303/

42 Middleton PG, Mall MA, Drevínek P, et al. Elexacaftor-tezacaftor-ivacaftor for cystic fibrosis with a single Phe508del allele. *N Engl J Med* 2019; 381(19):1809.

43 Alton EW, Armstrong DK, Ashby D, et al. Repeated nebulisation of non-viral CFTR gene therapy in patients with cystic fibrosis: a randomised, double-blind, placebo-controlled, phase 2b trial. *Lancet Respir Med* 2015; 3(9):684–91. https://www.ncbi.nlm.nih.gov/pmc/articles/PMC4673100/

44 Cancer Research UK. Lung cancer statistics. https://www.cancerresearchuk.org/health-professional/cancer-statistics/statistics-by-cancer-type/lung-cancer

45 NICE. *Guidance on the diagnosis and treatment of lung cancer* [CG121]. 2011. http://guidance.nice.org.uk/CG121

46 Bertazzi PA. Descriptive epidemiology of malignant mesothelioma. *Med Lav* 2005; 96(4):287–303. http://www.ncbi.nlm.nih.gov/pubmed/16457426

47 Tsiouris A, Walesby RK. Malignant pleural mesothelioma: current concepts in treatment. *Nat Clin Pract Oncol* 2007; 4(6):344–52. http://www.nature.com/nrclinonc/journal/v4/n6/full/ncponc0839.html

48 Aberle DR, Adams AM, Berg CD, et al. Reduced lung-cancer mortality with low-dose computed tomographic screening. *N Engl J Med* 2011; 365(5):395.

49 Horeweg N, Scholten ET, de Jong PA, et al. Detection of lung cancer through low-dose CT screening (NELSON): a prespecified analysis of screening test performance and interval cancers. *Lancet Oncol* 2014; 15(12):1342.

50 NICE. *Lung cancer: diagnosis and management* [CG121]. 2011. http://guidance.nice.org.uk/CG121

51 NICE. *Pulmonary embolism.* 2019. https://cks.nice.org.uk/pulmonary-embolism

52 NICE. *Continuous positive airway pressure for the treatment of obstructive sleep apnoea/hypopnoea syndrome* [TA139]. 2008. http://www.nice.org.uk/Guidance/TA139

53 Simonneau G, Montani D, Celermajer DS, et al. Haemodynamic definitions and updated clinical classification of pulmonary hypertension. *Eur Respir J* 2019; 53(1):1801913.

54 Iannuzzi MC, Rybicki BA, Teirstein AS. Sarcoidosis. *N Engl J Med* 2007; 357(21):2153–65. http://www.nejm.org/doi/full/10.1056/NEJMra071714

55 Bradley B, Branley HM, Egan JJ, et al. Interstitial lung disease guideline: the British Thoracic Society in collaboration with the Thoracic Society of Australia and New Zealand and the Irish Thoracic Society. *Thorax* 2008; 63(Suppl V):v1–v58. http://thorax.bmj.com/content/63/Suppl_5/v1.long

56 Grönhagen-Riska C. Angiotensin-converting enzyme. I. Activity and correlation with serum lysozyme in sarcoidosis, other chest or lymph node diseases and healthy persons. *Scand J Respir Dis* 1979; 60(2):83–93.

57 Iannuzzi MC, Sah BP. Sarcoidosis. In: *Merk Manual.* http://www.merckmanuals.com/professional/pulmonary_disorders/sarcoidosis/sarcoidosis.html

58 Evans M, Sharma O, LaBree L, et al. Differences in clinical findings between Caucasians and African Americans with biopsy-proven sarcoidosis. *Ophthalmology* 2007; 114(2):325–33. http://www.aaojournal.org/article/S0161-6420(06)00994-8/abstract

59 Raghu G, Remy-Jardin M, Ryerson CJ, et al. Diagnosis of hypersensitivity pneumonitis in adults. An official ATS/JRS/ALAT clinical practice guideline. *Am J Respir Crit Care Med* 2020; 202(3):e36.

60 Nathan SD, Shlobin OA, Weir N, et al. Long-term course and prognosis of idiopathic pulmonary fibrosis in the new millennium. *Chest* 2011; 140(1):221.

61 Ley B, Ryerson CJ, Vittinghoff E, et al. A multidimensional index and staging system for idiopathic pulmonary fibrosis. *Ann Intern Med* 2012; 156(10):684–91.

20 References

20 References

1 Simpson RW, Shaw JE, Zimmet PZ. The prevention of type 2 diabetes—lifestyle change or pharmacotherapy? A challenge for the 21st century. *Diabetes Res Clin Pract* 2003; 59(3):165–80. http://www.ncbi.nlm.nih.gov/m/pubmed/12590013/

2 Cartwright RD. The role of sleep in changing our minds: a psychologist's discussion of papers on memory reactivation and consolidation in sleep. *Learn Mem* 2004; 11(6):660–3. https://www.ncbi.nlm.nih.gov/pmc/articles/

3 Weetman AP. Autoimmune thyroid disease: propagation and progression. *Eur J Endocrinol* 2003; 148(1):1–9. http://www.eje-online.org/content/148/1/1.long

4 Gale E. Is there really an epidemic of type 2 diabetes? *Lancet* 2003; 362:503–4. http://www.thelancet.com/journals/lancet/article/PIIS0140-6736(03)14148-7/abstract

5 Bilous RW, Jacklin PB, Maresh MJ, *et al*. Resolving the gestational diabetes diagnosis conundrum: the need for a randomized controlled trial of treatment. *Diabetes Care* 2021; 44:858–64. 10.2337/dc20-2941

6 Inoue K, Matsumoto M, Akimoto K. Fasting plasma glucose and HbA1c as risk factors for type 2 diabetes. *Diabet Med* 2008; 25(10):1157–63. http://onlinelibrary.wiley.com/doi/10.1111/j.1464-5491.2008.02572.x/abstract

7 Westman EC, Yancy WS Jr, Mavropoulos JC, *et al*. The effect of a low-carbohydrate, ketogenic diet versus a low-glycemic index diet on glycemic control in type 2 diabetes mellitus. *Nutr Metab (Lond)* 2008; 5:36. https://www.ncbi.nlm.nih.gov/pmc/articles/PMC2633336/

8 The Diabetes Control and Complications Trial Research Group. The effect of intensive treatment of diabetes on the development and progression of long-term complications in insulin-dependent diabetes mellitus. *N Engl J Med* 1993; 329(14):977–86. http://www.nejm.org/doi/full/10.1056/NEJM199309303291401

9 Belch J. Aspirin does not help as primary prevention in DM. *BMJ* 2008; 337:a1840. http://www.bmj.com/cgi/content/full/337/a1840

10 Murad MH, Coto-Yglesias F, Wang AT, *et al*. Clinical review: drug-induced hypoglycemia: a systematic review. *J Clin Endocrinol Metab* 2009; 94(3):741–5. http://press.endocrine.org/doi/pdf/10.1210/jc.2008-1416

11 Kapoor RR, James C, Hussain K. Advances in the diagnosis and management of hyperinsulinemic hypoglycemia. *Nat Clin Pract Endocrinol Metab* 2009; 5(2):101–12. http://www.nature.com/nrendo/journal/v5/n2/full/ncpendmet1046.html

12 Geraghty M, Draman M, Moran D, *et al*. Hypoglycaemia in an adult male: a surprising finding in pursuit of insulinoma. *Surgeon* 2008; 6(1):57–60.

13 Abraham P, Avenell A, Park CM, *et al*. A systematic review of drug therapy for Graves' hyperthyroidism. *Eur J Endocrinol* 2005; 153(4):489–98. http://www.eje-online.org/content/153/4/489.long

14 Hedback G, Odén A. Recurrence of hyperparathyroidism; a long-term follow-up after surgery for primary hyperparathyroidism. *Eur J Endocrinol* 1994; 40:479–84. http://onlinelibrary.wiley.com/doi/10.1111/j.1365-2265.1994.tb02486.x/abstract

15 Hoff AO, Cote GJ, Gagel RF. Multiple endocrine neoplasias. *Annu Rev Physiol* 2000; 62:377. http://www.annualreviews.org/doi/pdf/10.1146/annurev.physiol.62.1.377

16 Renehan AG, Brennan BM. Acromegaly, growth hormone and cancer risk. *Best Pract Res Clin Endocrinol Metab* 2008; 22(4):639–57. http://pubmedhh.nlm.nih.gov/cgi-bin/abstract.cgi?id=18971124&from=cqsr

17 Etxabe J, Vazquez JA. Morbidity and mortality in Cushing's disease: an epidemiological approach. *Clin Endocrinol* 1994; 40:479–84. http://onlinelibrary.wiley.com/doi/10.1111/j.1365-2265.1994.tb02486.x/abstract

18 Brosnan CM, Gowing NF. Addison's disease. *BMJ* 1996; 312(7038):1085–7. https://www.ncbi.nlm.nih.gov/pmc/articles/PMC2350885/

19 State Coroner for Western Australia. *Failure to diagnose: Addison's disease*. 2007. http://www.racgp.org.au/afp/200710/200710bird.pdf

20 Herrmann HC, Chang G, Klugherz BD, *et al*. Hemodynamic effects of sildenafil in men with severe coronary artery disease. *N Engl J Med* 2000; 342(22):1622–6. http://www.nejm.org/doi/full/10.1056/NEJM200006013422201

21 Minniti G, Gilbert DC, Brada M. Modern techniques for pituitary radiotherapy. *Rev Endocr Metab Disord* 2009; 10(2):135–44. http://link.springer.com/article/10.1007%2Fs11154-008-9106-0

22 Chanson P. Acromegaly. *Presse Med* 2009; 38(1):92–102. https://www.ncbi.nlm.nih.gov/pubmed/19004612

Chapter 6: Gastroenterology

1 Seidelmann SB, Claggett B, Cheng S, *et al*. Dietary carbohydrate intake and mortality: a prospective co-hort study and meta-analysis. *Lancet Public Health* 2018; 3:e419–28.

2 Reynolds A, Mann J, Cummings J, *et al*. Carbohydrate quality and human health: a series of systematic reviews and meta-analyses. *Lancet* 2019; 393:434–45.

3 Batur P, Stewart WJ, Isaacson JH. Increased prevalence of aortic stenosis in patients with arteriovenous malformations of the gastrointestinal tract in Heyde syndrome. *Arch Intern Med* 2003; 163(15):1821–4. http://jamanetwork.com/journals/jamainternalmedicine/fullarticle/755859

4 Unlugenc H, Guler T, Gunes Y, *et al*. Comparative study of the antiemetic efficacy of ondansetron, propofol and midazolam in the early postoperative period. *Eur J Anaesthesiol* 2004; 21(1):60–5. http://pubmedhh.nlm.nih.gov/cgi-bin/abstract.cgi?id=14768925&from=cqsr

5 NICE. *Dyspepsia and gastro-oesophageal reflux disease* [CG184]. 2014. https://www.nice.org.uk/Guidance/cg184

6 Spechler SJ, Hunter JG, Jones KM, *et al*. Randomized trial of medical versus surgical treatment for refractory heartburn. *N Engl J Med* 2019; 381(16):1513–23. doi: 10.1056/NEJMoa1811424

7 Fitzgerald RC, di Pietro M, Ragunath K, *et al*. British Society of Gastroenterology guidelines on the diagnosis and management of Barrett's oesophagus. *Gut* 2014; 63(1):7–42. http://gut.bmj.com/content/63/1/7.long

8 Odutayo A, Desborough MJ, Trivella M, *et al*. Restrictive versus liberal blood transfusion for gastrointestinal bleeding: a systematic review and meta-analysis of randomised controlled trials. *Lancet Gastroenterol Hepatol* 2017; 2(5):354. doi: 10.1016/S2468-1253(17)30054-7

9 NICE. *Suspected cancer: recognition and referral* [NG12]. 2015. https://www.nice.org.uk/Guidance/ng12

10 Ludvigsson JF, Bai JC, Biagi F, *et al*. Diagnosis and management of adult coeliac disease: guidelines from the British Society of Gastroenterology. *Gut* 2014; 63(8):1210–28. https://www.ncbi.nlm.nih.gov/pmc/articles/PMC4112432/

11 Marth T, Raoult D. Whipple's disease. *Lancet* 2003; 361(9353):239–46. http://www.thelancet.com/journals/lancet/article/PIIS0140-6736(03)12274-X/abstract

12 Lacy BE, Mearin F, Chang L, *et al*. Bowel disorders. *Gastroenterology* 2016; 150:1393–407.e5. https://doi.org/10.1053/j.gastro.2016.02.031

13 Auernhammer CJ, Göke B. Medical treatment of gastrinomas. *Wien Klin Wochenschr* 2007; 119(19–20):609–15. https://www.ncbi.nlm.nih.gov/pubmed/17985097

14 Hillbom M, Pieninkeroinen I, Leone M. Seizures in alcohol-dependent patients: epidemiology, pathophysiology and management. *CNS Drugs* 2003; 17(14):1013–30. https://www.ncbi.nlm.nih.gov/pubmed/14594442

15 European Association for the Study of the Liver (EASL). EASL–EASD–EASO Clinical Practice Guidelines for the management of non-alcoholic fatty liver disease. *J Hepatol* 2016; 64(6):1388–402. http://www.journal-of-hepatology.eu/article/S0168-8278(15)00734-5/fulltext

16 Galle PR, Forner A, Llovet JM, *et al*. EASL clinical practice guidelines: management of hepatocellular carcinoma. *J Hepatol* 2018; 69:182–236.

17 Snook J, Bhala N, Beales ILP, *et al*. British Society of Gastroenterology guidelines for the management of iron deficiency anaemia in adults. *Gut* 2021; 70(11):2030–51.

Chapter 7: Kidney medicine

1 Scottish Intercollegiate Guidelines Network. *Management of suspected bacterial urinary tract infection in adults: a national clinical guideline* (SIGN 88). 2012. http://www.sign.ac.uk/pdf/sign88.pdf

2 KDIGO Acute Kidney Injury Work Group. KDIGO clinical practice guideline for acute kidney injury. *Kidney Int Suppl* 2012; 2:1–138. http://kdigo.org/home/guidelines/acute-kidney-injury/

3 London AKI Network. *Guidelines and pathways*. http://www.londonaki.net/clinical/guidelines-pathways.html

4 NICE. *Algorithms for IV fluid therapy in adults*. 2013. https://www.nice.org.uk/guidance/cg174/resources/intravenous-fluid-therapy-in-adults-in-hospital-algorithm-poster-set-191627821

5 UK Renal Association. *Clinical practice guidelines: treatment of acute hyperkalaemia in adults*. March 2014. http://www.renal.org/guidelines/joint-guidelines/treatment-of-acute-hyperkalaemia-in-adults#sthash.LACGYarj.dpbs

6 KDIGO CKD Work Group. KDIGO 2012 clinical practice guideline for the evaluation and management of chronic kidney disease. *Kidney Int Suppl* 2013; 3:1–150. http://kdigo.org/home/guidelines/ckd-evaluation-management/

7 Evans PD, Taal MW. Epidemiology and causes of chronic kidney disease. *Medicine* 2015; 43:450–3. http://www.medicinejournal.co.uk/article/S1357-3039(15)00117-6/fulltext

8 KDIGO Glomerulonephritis Work Group. KDIGO clinical practice guideline for glomerulonephritis. *Kidney Int Suppl* 2012; 2:139–274. http://kdigo.org/home/glomerulonephritis-gn/

9 Molitch ME, Adler AI, Flyvbjerg A, *et al*. Diabetic kidney disease: a clinical update from Kidney Disease: Improving Global Outcomes. *Kidney Int* 2015; 87(1):20–30. http://www.kidney-international.theisn.org/article/S0085-2538(15)30004-1/abstract

Chapter 8: Haematology

1 van der Klooster JM. A medical mystery. Lead poisoning. *Singapore Med J* 2004; 45(10):497–9. http://pubmedhh.nlm.nih.gov/cgi-bin/abstract.cgi?id=15455173&from=cqsr

2 World Health Organization. *WHO global anaemia estimates, 2021 edition.* https://www.who.int/data/gho/data/themes/topics/anaemia_in_women_and_children

3 Angelucci E. A new medical therapy for anemia in thalassemia. *Blood* 2019; 133(12):1267.

4 The Joint United Kingdom (UK) Blood Transfusion and Tissue Transplantation Services Professional Advisory Committee. *Transfusion handbook* (5th edn). 2014. Available free at: http://www.transfusion-guidelines.org/transfusion-handbook

5 NICE. *Neutropenic sepsis: prevention and management in people with cancer* [CG151]. 2012. https://www.nice.org.uk/guidance/cg151

6 Kantarjian H, Kadia T, DiNardo C, *et al.* Acute myeloid leukemia: current progress and future directions. *Blood Cancer J* 2021; 11(2):41.

7 Connors JM, Jurczak W, Straus DJ, *et al.* Brentuximab vedotin with chemotherapy for stage III or IV Hodgkin's lymphoma. *N Engl J Med* 2018; 378(4):331.

8 Khorana AA, Kuderer NM, Culakova E, *et al.* Development and validation of a predictive model for chemotherapy-associated thrombosis. *Blood* 2008; 111(10):4902–7.

Chapter 9: Infectious diseases

1 Laxminarayan R, Duse A, Wattal C, *et al.* Antibiotic resistance—the need for global solutions. *Lancet Infect Dis* 2013; 13(12):1057–98. http://www.thelancet.com/journals/laninf/article/PIIS1473-3099(13)70318-9/abstract

2 NICE. *Antimicrobial stewardship: systems and processes for effective antimicrobial medicine use* [NG15]. 2015. https://www.nice.org.uk/guidance/ng15

3 NICE. *Tuberculosis* [NG33]. 2016. https://www.nice.org.uk/guidance/ng33

4 Public Health England. *PHE guidance on the use of antiviral agents for the treatment and prophylaxis of seasonal influenza.* 2019. https://assets.publishing.service.gov.uk/government/uploads/system/uploads/attachment_data/file/833572/PHE_guidance_antivirals_influenza_201920.pdf

5 Goldacre B. What the Tamiflu saga tells us about drug trials and big pharma. *Guardian* 2014; 10 April. https://www.theguardian.com/business/2014/apr/10/tamiflu-saga-drug-trials-big-pharma

6 British Association for Sexual Health and HIV. *BASHH guidelines.* https://www.bashh.org/guidelines

7 British HIV Association. *British HIV Association guidelines for the treatment of HIV-1-positive adults with antiretroviral therapy 2015 (2016 interim update).* 2016. https://www.bhiva.org/file/RVYKzFwyxpgiI/treatment-guidelines-2016-interim-update.pdf

8 Loveday HP, Wilson JA, Pratt RJ, *et al.* epic3: National evidence based guidelines for preventing healthcare-associated infections in NHS hospitals in England. *J Hosp Infect* 2014; 86s1:s1–70. https://pubmed.ncbi.nlm.nih.gov/24330862/

9 Fink D, Wani RS, Johnston V. Fever in the returning traveller. *BMJ* 2018; 360:j5773. https://pubmed.ncbi.nlm.nih.gov/29371218

10 Johnson V, Stockley JM, Dockrell D, *et al.* Fever in returned travellers presenting in the United Kingdom: recommendations for investigation and initial management. *J Infect* 2009; 59(1):1–18. https://www.ncbi.nlm.nih.gov/pubmed/19595360

11 Lalloo DG, Shingadia D, Bell DJ. UK malaria treatment guidelines 2016. *J Infect* 2016; 72(6):635–49. http://www.journalofinfection.com/article/S0163-4453(16)00047-5/abstract

12 Sinclair D, Donegan S, Iba R, *et al.* Artesunate versus quinine for severe malaria. *Cochrane Database Syst Rev* 2012; 6:CD005967. http://onlinelibrary.wiley.com/doi/10.1002/14651858.CD005967.pub4/full

13 World Health Organization. *Health topics.* http://www.who.int/topics/en/

14 Musso D, Ko A, Baud D. Virus infection—after the pandemic. *N Engl J Med* 2019; 381:1444–57. https://www.nejm.org/doi/full/10.1056/NEJMra1808246

15 Medlock JM, Leach SA. Effect of climate change on vector borne disease in the UK. *Lancet Infect Dis* 2015; 15(6):721–30. http://www.thelancet.com/journals/laninf/article/PIIS1473-3099(15)70091-5/abstract

16 Sudarshi D, Brown M. Human African trypanosomiasis in non-endemic countries. *Clin Med* 2015; 15(1):70–3. http://www.clinmed.rcpjournal.org/content/15/1/70.full.pdf

17 Lambourne JR, Brooks T. Brucella and coxiella: if you don't look, you don't find. *Clin Med* 2015; 15(1):91–2. http://www.clinmed.rcpjournal.org/content/15/1/91.abstract

18 Forbes AE, Zochowski WJ, Dubrey SW, *et al.* Leptospirosis and Weil's disease in the UK. *QJM* 2012; 105(2):1151–62. http://qjmed.oxfordjournals.org/content/105/12/1151.long

19 World Health Organization. *Notes for the record: consultation on monitored emergency use of unregistered and investigational interventions (MEURI) for Ebola virus disease (EVD).* 2018. https://www.who.int/ebola/drc-2018/notes-for-the-record-meuri-ebola.pdf

20 Barrett J, Brown M. Traveller's diarrhoea. *BMJ* 2016; 353:i1937. http://www.bmj.com/content/353/bmj.i1937.long

21 Riddle MS, DuPont HL, Connor BA. ACG clinical guideline: diagnosis, treatment, and prevention of acute diarrheal infections in adults. *Am J Gastroenterol* 2016; 111:602–22. doi:10.1038/ajg.2016.126. http://gi.org/wp-content/uploads/2016/05/ajg2016126a.pdf

22 Beeching N, Dassanayake A. Tropical liver disease. *Medicine* 2011; 39(9):556–60. http://www.medicinejournal.co.uk/article/S1357-3039(11)00154-X/abstract

23 Rodrigo C, Fernando D, Rajapakse S. Pharmacological management of tetanus: an evidence based review. *Crit Care* 2014; 18:217. https://ccforum.biomedcentral.com/articles/10.1186/cc13797

24 Varghese GM, Trowbridge P, Doherty T. Investigating and managing pyrexia of unknown origin. *BMJ* 2010; 341:c5470. http://www.bmj.com/content/341/bmj.c5470.long

Chapter 10: Neurology

1 Lipton RB, Fanning KM, Serrano D, *et al*. Ineffective acute treatment of episodic migraine is associated with new-onset chronic migraine. *Neurology* 2015; 84(7):688–95. doi: 10.1212/WNL.0000000000001256

2 Chandrasekhar SS, *et al*. Clinical practice guideline: sudden hearing loss (update) executive summary. *Otolaryngol Head Neck Surg* 2019; 161(2):195–210. doi: 10.1177/0194599819859883

3 Stone J. Functional neurological disorders: the neurological assessment as treatment. *Pract Neurol* 2016; 16(1):7–17. doi: 10.1136/practneurol-2015-001241

4 Nogueira RG, Jadhav AP, Haussen DC, *et al*. DAWN trial: thrombectomy 6 to 24 hours after stroke with a mismatch between deficit and infarct. *N Engl J Med* 2018; 378:11–21. doi: 10.1056/NEJMoa1706442

5 NICE. *Stroke and transient ischaemic attack in over 16s: diagnosis and initial management* [CG128]. 2019. https://www.nice.org.uk/guidance/ng128

6 Claiborne Johnston S, *et al*. Clopidogrel and aspirin in acute ischemic stroke and high-risk TIA. *N Engl J Med* 2018; 379:215–25. doi: 10.1056/NEJMoa1800410

7 Shah R, Nayyar M, Jovin IS, *et al*. Device closure versus medical therapy alone for patent foramen ovale in patients with cryptogenic stroke: a systematic review and meta-analysis. *Ann Intern Med* 2018; 168(5):335–42. doi: 10.7326/M17-2679

8 Stinear CM, Lang CE, Zeiler S, *et al*. Advances and challenges in stroke rehabilitation. *Lancet Neurology* 2020; 19(4):348–60. doi: 10.1016/S1474-4422(19)30415-6

9 Fong TG, Davis D, Growdon ME, *et al*. The interface between delirium and dementia in elderly adults. *Lancet Neurol* 2015; 14(8).823–32. https://www.ncbi.nlm.nih.gov/pmc/articles/PMC4535349

10 Green AJE. RT-QuIC: a new test for sporadic CJD. *Practical Neurology* 2019; 19:49–55.

11 NICE. *Multiple sclerosis in adults: management* [CG186]. 2014. https://www.nice.org.uk/guidance/cg186

Chapter 11: Oncology and palliative care

1 Cancer Research. *UK statistics*. http://www.cancerresearchuk.org/health-professional/cancer-statistics

2 National Cancer Institute. *Communication in cancer health: professional version*. http://www.cancer.gov/about-cancer/coping/adjusting-to-cancer/communication-hp-pdq#section/_9

3 Baile WF, Buckman R, Lenzi R, *et al*. SPIKES: a six-step protocol for delivering bad news: application to the patient with cancer. *Oncologist* 2000; 5(4):302–11. http://theoncologist.alphamedpress.org/content/5/4/302.long

4 NICE. *Suspected cancer: recognition and referral* [NG12]. 2015. https://www.nice.org.uk/guidance/ng12

5 Kerr DJ, Haller DG, Verweij J. Principles of chemotherapy. In Kerr DJ, Haller DG, van der Valde CJH, *et al*. (eds) *Oxford Textbook of Oncology* (3rd edn). Oxford: Oxford University Press, 2016:186–95.

6 Pérez Fidalgo JA, García Fabregat L, Cervantes A, *et al*. Management of chemotherapy extravasation: ESMO–EONS clinical practice guidelines. *Ann Oncol* 2012; 23(Suppl 7): vii167–73. https://academic.oup.com/annonc/article/23/suppl_7/vii167/145139/Management-of-chemotherapy-extravasation-ESMO-EONS

7 Ahmad SS, Duke S, Jena R, *et al*. Advances in radiotherapy. *BMJ* 2012; 345e7765. http://www.bmj.com/content/345/bmj.e7765.long

8 Loren AW, Mangu PB, Beck LN, *et al*. Fertility preservation for patients with cancer: American Society of Clinical Oncology clinical practice guideline update. *J Clin Oncol* 2013; 31(19):2500–10. http://ascopubs.org/doi/full/10.1200/JCO.2013.49.2678

9 DeAngelo D, Alyea EP. Oncologic emergencies. In: Singh AK, Loscalzo J (eds) *The Brigham Intensive Review of Internal Medicine*. Oxford: Oxford University Press; 2014:159–67.

10 Lee DLY, Anthoney A. Complications of systemic therapy—gut infections and acute diarrhoea. *Clin Med* 2014(5):528–45. http://www.clinmed.rcpjournal.org/content/14/5/528.full.pdf+html

11 Pelosof LC, Gerber DE. Paraneoplastic syndromes: an approach to diagnosis and treatment. *Mayo Clin Proc* 2010; 85(9):838–54. http://www.mayoclinicproceedings.org/article/S0025-6196(11)60214-0/abstract

12 Sturgeon CM, Lai LC, Duffy MJ. Serum tumour markers: how to order and interpret them. *BMJ* 2009; 339:b3527. http://www.bmj.com/content/339/bmj.b3527.long

13 Schröder FH, Hugosson J, Roobol MJ, *et al*. Screening and prostate cancer mortality: results of the European Randomised Study of Screening for Prostate Cancer (ERSPC) at 13 years of follow up. *Lancet* 2014; 384(9959):2027–35. http://www.thelancet.com/journals/lancet/article/PIIS0140-6736(14)60525-0/abstract

14 Temel JS, Greer JA, Muzikansky A, *et al*. Early palliative care for patients with metastatic non-small-cell lung cancer. *N Engl J Med* 2010; 363:733–42. http://www.nejm.org/doi/full/10.1056/NEJMoa1000678

15 World Health Organization. *Analgesic ladder*. http://www.who.int/cancer/palliative/painladder/en/

16 NHS England. NPSA safety alert: risk of distress and death from inappropriate doses of naloxone in patients on long-term opioid/opiate treatment. 2014. https://www.england.nhs.uk/wp-content/uploads/2014/11/psa-inappropriate-doses-naloxone.pdf

17 NHS Scotland. *Scottish palliative care guidelines*. 2014. http://www.palliativecareguidelines.scot.nhs.uk/

18 Universities of Hull, Staffordshire, and Aberdeen. *Spiritual care at the end of life: a systematic review*. 2010. https://www.gov.uk/government/system/uploads/attachment_data/file/215798/dh_123804.pdf

19 Kaye P. Spiritual pain. In: *Notes on symptom control in hospice and palliative care*. London: Hospice Education Institute, 1990:261–7.

20 Ruegger J, Hodgkinson S, Field-Smith A, *et al*. Care of adults in the last days of life. *BMJ* 2015; 351:h6631. http://www.bmj.com/content/351/bmj.h6631

21 General Medical Council. *Treatment and care towards the end of life*. 2010. http://www.gmc-uk.org/static/documents/content/Treatment_and_care_towards_the_end_of_life_-_English_1015.pdf

Chapter 12: Rheumatology

1 Doherty M, Dacre J, Dieppe P, *et al*. The 'GALS' locomotor screen. *Ann Rheum Dis* 1992; 51:1165–9. https://www.ncbi.nlm.nih.gov/pmc/articles/PMC1012427/

2 Courtney P, Doherty M. Joint aspiration and injection. *Best Pract Res Clin Rheumatol* 2005; 19:345–69. http://www.bprclinrheum.com/article/S1521-6942(05)00010-0/abstract

3 Speed C. Low back pain. *BMJ* 2004; 328:1119–21. https://www.ncbi.nlm.nih.gov/pmc/articles/PMC406328/

4 NICE. *Osteoarthritis: care and management* [NG226]. Available at: https://www.nice.org.uk/guidance/ng226

5 McGettigan P, Henry D. Cardiovascular risk with non-steroidal anti-inflammatory drugs: systematic review of population-based controlled observational studies. *PLoS Med* 2011; 8(9):e1001098. https://www.ncbi.nlm.nih.gov/pmc/articles/PMC3181230/

6 Chan F, Wong VW, Suen BY, *et al*. Combination of COX-2 and PPI for prevention of recurrent ulcer bleeding in patients at very high risk. *Lancet* 2007; 369:1621–6. http://www.thelancet.com/journals/lancet/article/PIIS0140-6736(07)60749-1/abstract

7 Brown AK, Wakefield RJ, Conaghan PG, *et al*. New approaches to imaging early inflammatory arthritis. *Clin Exp Rheumatol* 2004; 22(5 Suppl 35): S18–25. http://www.clinexprheumatol.org/article.asp?a=2432

8 Szekanecz Z, Kerekes G, Dér H, *et al*. Accelerated atherosclerosis in rheumatoid arthritis. *Ann N Y Acad Sci* 2007; 1108:349–58. http://onlinelibrary.wiley.com/doi/10.1196/annals.1422.036/abstract

9 Aletaha D, Neogi T, Silman AJ, *et al*. 2010 Rheumatoid arthritis classification criteria: an American College of Rheumatology/European League Against Rheumatism collaborative initiative. *Arthritis Rheum* 2010; 62(9):2569–81. http://onlinelibrary.wiley.com/doi/10.1002/art.27584/abstract

10 Ramiro S, Gaujoux-Viala C, Nam JL, *et al*. Safety of synthetic and biological DMARDs: a systematic literature review informing the 2013 update of the EULAR recommendations for management of rheumatoid arthritis. *Ann Rheum Dis* 2014; 73(3):529–35.

11 Thompson A, Gandhi KK, Hochberg MC, *et al*. Incidence of malignancy in adult patients with rheumatoid arthritis: a meta-analysis. *Arthritis Res Ther* 2015; 17(1):212. https://www.ncbi.nlm.nih.gov/pmc/articles/PMC4536786/

12 Charles-Schoeman C, Buch MH, Dougados M, *et al*. Risk of major adverse cardiovascular events with tofacitinib versus tumour necrosis factor inhibitors in patients with rheumatoid arthritis with or without a history of atherosclerotic cardiovascular disease: a post hoc analysis from ORAL Surveillance. *Ann Rheum Dis* 2023; 82(1):119–29. doi: 10.1136/ard-2022-222259

13 Gross WL, Reinhold-Keller E. [ANCA-associated vasculitis (Wegener's granulomatosis, Churg-Strauss syndrome, microscopic polyangiitis). 1. Systemic aspects, pathogenesis and clinical aspects.] *Z Rheumatol* 1995; 54(5):279–90. https://www.ncbi.nlm.nih.gov/pubmed/8578884

14 Petri M, Orbai AM, Alarcón GS, *et al*. Derivation and validation of the Systemic Lupus International Collaborating Clinics classification criteria for systemic lupus erythematosus. *Arthritis Rheum* 2012; 64(8):2677–86. https://www.ncbi.nlm.nih.gov/pmc/articles/PMC3409311

15 Jennette JC, Falk RJ, Bacon PA, *et al*. 2012 Revised International Chapel Hill Consensus Conference nomenclature of vasculitides. *Arthritis Rheum* 2012; 65(1):1–11. doi: 10.1002/art.37715

16 New Zealand Guidelines Group. *New Zealand acute low back pain guide*. 2004. http://www.acc.co.nz/PRD_EXT_CSMP/groups/external_communications/documents/guide/prd_ctrb112930.pdf

17 Reichrath J, Bens G, Bonowitz A, *et al*. Treatment recommendations for pyoderma gangrenosum: an evidence-based review of the literature based on more than 350 patients. *J Am Acad Dermatol* 2005; 53(2):273–83. https://www.ncbi.nlm.nih.gov/pubmed/16021123

Chapter 13: Surgery

1 Rogozov V, Bermel N. Auto-appendectomy in the Antarctic: case report. *BMJ* 2009; 339:b4965. doi: 10.1136/bmj.b4965

2 NICE. *Plus Sutures for preventing surgical site infection* [MTG59]. 2021. https://www.nice.org.uk/guidance/mtg59/chapter/1-Recommendations

3 Wolchok JD, Chiarion-Sileni V, Gonzalez R, *et al*. Long-term outcomes with nivolumab plus ipilimumab or nivolumab alone versus ipilimumab in patients with advanced melanoma. *J Clin Oncol* 2022; 40(2):127–37. doi: 10.1200/JCO.21.02229

4 Jávor P, Hanák L, Hegyi P, *et al*. Predictive value of tachycardia for mortality in trauma-related haemorrhagic shock: a systematic review and meta-regression. *BMJ Open* 2022; 12:e059271. doi: 10.1136/bmjopen-2021-059271

5 Juturi JV, Maghfoor I, Doll DC, *et al*. A case of biliary carcinoid presenting with pancreatitis and obstructive jaundice. *Am J Gastroenterol* 2000; 95(10):2973–4. http://www.nature.com/ajg/journal/v95/n10/full/ajg20001463a.html

6 NICE. *Obesity: identification, assessment and management* [CG189]. 2014. https://www.nice.org.uk/guidance/cg189

1 NICE. *Intravenous fluid therapy in adults in hospital* [CG174]. 2013. https://www.nice.org.uk/Guidance/cg174

2 Semler MW, Self WH, Wanderer JP, *et al*. Balanced crystalloids versus saline in critically ill adults. *N Engl J Med* 2018; 378(9):829–39. doi: 10.1056/NEJMoa1711584

3 Finfer S, Bellomo R, Boyce N, *et al*. A comparison of albumin and saline for fluid resuscitation in the intensive care unit. *N Engl J Med* 2004; 350(22):2247–56.

4 Delgado C, Baweja M, Crews DC, *et al*. A unifying approach for GFR estimation: recommendations of the NKF-ASN Task Force on reassessing the inclusion of race in diagnosing kidney disease. *Am J Kidney Dis* 2022; 79(2):268–88.e1. doi: 10.1053/j.ajkd.2021.08.003

5 Kelly YP, Waikar SS, Mendu ML. When to stop renal replacement therapy in anticipation of renal recovery in AKI: the need for consensus guidelines. *Semin Dial* 2019; 32(3):205–9.

6 Renneboog B, Musch W, Vandemergel X, *et al*. Mild chronic hyponatremia is associated with falls, unsteadiness, and attention deficits. *Am J Med* 2006; 119:71.e1–8. https://www.ncbi.nlm.nih.gov/pubmed/16431193

7 Robertson GL. Vaptan for the treatment of hyponatraemia. *Nat Rev Endocrinol* 2011; 7:151–61. http://www.nature.com/nrendo/journal/v7/n3/full/nrendo.2010.229.html

8 Smellie S. Spurious hypokalaemia. *BMJ* 2007; 334:693. http://www.bmj.com/content/334/7595/693

9 Kosiborod M, Rasmussen HS, Lavin P, *et al*. Effect of sodium zirconium cyclosilicate on potassium lowering for 28 days among outpatients with hyperkalemia: the HARMONIZE randomized clinical trial. *JAMA* 2014; 312(21):2223–33.

10 Thomas J, Doherty SM. HIV infection—a risk factor for osteoporosis. *J Acquir Immune Defic Syndr* 2003; 33(3):281–91. https://www.ncbi.nlm.nih.gov/pubmed/12843738

11 Fitzpatrick LA. The hypocalcemic states. In: Favus M (ed) *Disorders of bone and mineral metabolism*. Philadelphia, PA: Lippincott Williams & Wilkins, 2002:568–88.

12 Jones GL, Will A, Jackson GH, *et al*. Guidelines for the management of tumour lysis syndrome in adults and children with haematological malignancies on behalf of the British Committee for Standards in Haematology. *Br J Haematol* 2015; 169:661–71.

13 Kramer HJ, Choi HK, Atkinson K, *et al*. The association between gout and nephrolithiasis in men: the Health Professionals' Follow-Up Study. *Kidney Int* 2003; 64:1022–6. https://www.ncbi.nlm.nih.gov/pubmed/12911552

14 Sarafrazi N, Wambogo EA, Shepherd JA. Osteoporosis or low bone mass in older adults: United States, 2017–2018. *NCHS Data Brief, no 405*. Hyattsville, MD: National Center for Health Statistics, 2021. doi: https://dx.doi.org/10.15620/cdc:103477

15 Howe TE, Shea B, Dawson LJ, *et al*. Exercise for preventing and treating osteoporosis in postmenopausal women. *Cochrane Database Syst Rev* 2011; 7:CD000333. http://onlinelibrary.wiley.com/doi/10.1002/14651858.CD000333.pub2/abstract

16 National Osteoporosis Foundation. *2013 Clinician's Guide to Prevention and Treatment of Osteoporosis*. http://nof.public/content/resource/913/files/580.pdf

17 Vollbrecht J, Rao DS. Tumor-induced osteomalacia. *N Engl J Med* 2008; 358:1282. http://www.nejm.org/doi/full/10.1056/NEJMicm066066#t=article

18 Wermers RA, Tiegs RD, Atkinson EJ, *et al*. Morbidity and mortality associated with Paget's disease of bone: a population study. *J Bone Miner Res* 2008; 23:819–25. https://www.ncbi.nlm.nih.gov/pmc/articles/PMC2515478/

19 NICE. *Chronic kidney disease: assessment and management* [CG203]. 2021. https://www.nice.org.uk/guidance/cg203

20 Anon. Randomised trial of cholesterol lowering in 4444 patients with coronary heart disease: the Scandinavian Simvastatin Survival Study (4S). *Lancet* 1994; 344:1383–9. https://www.ncbi.nlm.nih.gov/pubmed/7968073

21 Shepherd J, Cobbe SM, Ford I, *et al*. Prevention of coronary heart disease with pravastatin in men with hypercholesterolemia. West of Scotland Coronary Prevention Study Group. *N Engl J Med* 1995; 333:1301–8. http://www.nejm.org/doi/full/10.1056/NEJM199511163332001#t=article

22 Sacks FM, Pfeffer MA, Moye LA, *et al*. The effect of pravastatin on coronary events after myocardial infarction in patients with average cholesterol levels. Cholesterol and Recurrent Events Trial investigators. *N Engl J Med* 1996; 335:1001–9. http://www.nejm.org/doi/full/10.1056/NEJM199610033351401#t=article

23 Heart Protection Study Collaborative Group. MRC/BHF Heart Protection Study of cholesterol lowering with simvastatin in 20,536 high-risk individuals: a randomised placebo-controlled trial. *Lancet* 2002; 360:7–22. http://www.thelancet.com/journals/lancet/article/PIIS0140-6736(02)09327-3/abstract

24 Libby P. Inflammation in atherosclerosis. *Nature* 2002; 420:868–74. http://www.nature.com/nature/journal/v420/n6917/full/nature01323.html

25 Mach F, Baigent C, Catapano AL, *et al*. ESC/EAS Guidelines for the management of dyslipidaemias: lipid modification to reduce cardiovascular risk: the Task Force for the management of dyslipidaemias of the European Society of Cardiology (ESC) and European Atherosclerosis Society (EAS). *Eur Heart J* 2020; 41:111–88. https://doi.org/10.1093/eurheartj/ehz455

26 Versmissen J, Oosterveer DM, Yazdanpanah M, *et al*. Efficacy of statins in familial hypercholesterolaemia: a long term cohort study. *BMJ* 2008; 337:a2423 https://www.ncbi.nlm.nih.gov/pmc/articles/PMC2583391/

27 McKenney JM, Davidson MH, Jacobson TA, *et al*. Final conclusions and recommendations of the National Lipid Association Statin Safety Assessment Task Force. *Am J Cardiol* 2006; 8A:89C–94C. https://www.ncbi.nlm.nih.gov/pubmed/16581336

1 Todd J. The syndrome of Alice in Wonderland. *Can Med Assoc J* 1955; 73(9):701–4. https://www.ncbi.nlm.nih.gov/pmc/articles/PMC1826192/

2 Cau C. The Alice in Wonderland syndrome. *Minerva Med* 1999; 90(10):397–401. https://www.ncbi.nlm.nih.gov/pubmed/10767914

3 Fritschy D, Fasel J, Imbert JC, *et al*. The popliteal cyst. *Knee Surg Sports Traumatol Arthrosc* 2006; 14(7):623–8. https://www.ncbi.nlm.nih.gov/pubmed/16362357

4 Scheinfeld NS. Erythema induratum (nodular vasculitis). *Medscape*. 2016. http://emedicine.medscape.com/article/1083213-overview

5 Wakerley BR, Uncini A, Yuki N, *et al*. Guillain-Barré and Miller Fisher syndromes—new diagnostic classification. *Nat Rev Neurol* 2014; 10:537–44. https://www.nature.com/articles/nrneurol.2014.138

6 Brugada J, Campuzano O, Arbelo E, *et al*. Present status of Brugada syndrome: JACC state-of-the-art review. *J Am Coll Cardiol* 2018; 72:1046–59. https://www.sciencedirect.com/science/article/pii/S0735109718353622

7 Vaglio A, Moosig F, Zwerina J. Churg–Strauss syndrome: update on pathophysiology and treatment. *Curr Opin Rheumatol* 2012; 24(1):24–30. https://www.ncbi.nlm.nih.gov/pubmed/22089097

8 Bliss M. *Harvey Cushing: a life in surgery*. Toronto: University of Toronto Press, 2005.

9 Lepur D, Peterković V, Kalabrić-Lepur N. Neuromyelitis optica with CSF examination mimicking bacterial meningomyelitis. *Neurol Sci* 2009; 30(1):51–4. https://www.ncbi.nlm.nih.gov/pubmed/19145403

10 Kim SH, Kim W, Li XF, *et al*. Repeated treatment with rituximab based on the assessment of peripheral circulating memory B cells in patients with relapsing neuromyelitis optica over 2 years. *Arch Neurol* 2011; 68(11):1412–20. http://jamanetwork.com/journals/jamaneurology/fullarticle/1107915

11 Trauner M, Meier PJ, Boyer JL. Molecular pathogenesis of cholestasis. *N Engl J Med* 1998; 339:1217–27. http://www.nejm.org/doi/full/10.1056/NEJM199810223391707

12 Badalamente MA, Hurst LC. Efficacy and safety of injectable mixed collagenase subtypes in the treatment of Dupuytren's contracture. *J Hand Surg Am* 2007; 32(6):767–74. https://www.ncbi.nlm.nih.gov/pubmed/17606053

13 Schaefer RM, Tylki-Szymańska A, Hilz MJ. Enzyme replacement therapy for Fabry disease: a systematic review of available evidence. *Drugs* 2009; 69(16):2179–205. https://www.ncbi.nlm.nih.gov/pubmed/19852524

14 Weinshenker BG. Neuromyelitis optica: what it is and what it might be. *Lancet* 2003; 361(9361):889–90. http://www.thelancet.com/journals/lancet/article/PIIS0140-6736(03)12784-5/abstract

15 Losacco T, Punzo C, Santacroce L. Gardner syndrome: clinical and epidemiologic up to date. *Clin Ter* 2005; 156(6):267–71. https://www.ncbi.nlm.nih.gov/pubmed/16463563

16 Okai T, Yamaguchi Y, Sakai J, *et al*. Case report: complete regression of colonic adenomas after treatment with sulindac in Gardner's syndrome: a 4-year follow-up. *J Gastroenterol* 2001; 36:778–82. https://www.ncbi.nlm.nih.gov/pubmed/11757751

17 Mignot E. Narcolepsy and the HLA system. *N Engl J Med* 2001; 344:692. http://www.nejm.org/doi/full/10.1056/NEJM200103013440918#t=article

18 Freeman RD, Zinner SH, Müller-Vahl KR, *et al*. Coprophenomena in Tourette syndrome. *Dev Med Child Neurol* 2009; 51(3):218–27. https://www.ncbi.nlm.nih.gov/pubmed/19183216

19 Turtle L, Robertson MM. Tics, twitches, tales: the experiences of Gilles de la Tourette's syndrome. *Am J Orthopsychiatry* 2008; 78(4):449–55. https://www.ncbi.nlm.nih.gov/pubmed/19123766

20 Himle MB, Woods DW, Piacentini JC, *et al*. Brief review of habit reversal training for Tourette syndrome. *J Child Neurol* 2006; 21(8):719–25. https://www.ncbi.nlm.nih.gov/pubmed/16970874

21 Bersudsky M, Rosenberg P, Rudensky B, *et al*. Lipopolysaccharides of a Campylobacter coli isolate from a patient with Guillain-Barré syndrome display ganglioside mimicry. *Neuromuscul Disord* 2000; 10:182–6. https://www.ncbi.nlm.nih.gov/pubmed/10734265

22 Janniger CK. Klippel–Trenaunay–Weber syndrome. *Medscape*. 2016. http://reference.medscape.com/article/1084257-overview

23 Vassalo R, Ryu JH, Colby TV, *et al*. Pulmonary Langerhans cell histiocytosis. *N Engl J Med* 2000 342:1969–78. http://www.nejm.org/doi/full/10.1056/NEJM200006293422607

24 Beyerbach DM. Lown–Ganong–Levine syndrome. *Medscape*. 2015. http://emedicine.medscape.com/article/160097-overview

25 Quinlivan R, Vissing J, Hilton-Jones D, *et al*. Physical training for McArdle disease. *Cochrane Database Syst Rev* 2011; 12:CD007931. http://onlinelibrary.wiley.com/doi/10.1002/14651858.CD007931.pub2/abstract

26 Quinlivan R, Martinuzzi A, Schoser B. Pharmacological and nutritional treatment for McArdle disease (glycogen storage disease type V). *Cochrane Database Syst Rev* 2010; 12:CD003458. http://onlinelibrary.wiley.com/doi/10.1002/14651858.CD003458.pub4/abstract

27 Ault J. Marchiafava-Bignami disease. *Medscape*. 2016. http://emedicine.medscape.com/article/1146086-overview

28 Lambrecht NW. Ménétrier's disease of the stomach: a clinical challenge. *Curr Gastroenterol Rep* 2011; 13(6):513–17. https://www.ncbi.nlm.nih.gov/pubmed/21931998

29 Yamamoto M, Harada S, Ohara M, *et al*. Clinical and pathological differences between Mikulicz's disease and Sjögren's syndrome. *Rheumatology (Oxford)* 2005; 44(2):227–34. http://rheumatology.oxfordjournals.org/content/44/2/227.long

30 Asher RAJ. Munchausen's syndrome. *Lancet* 1951; 257:339–41. https://www.ncbi.nlm.nih.gov/pubmed/14805062

31 Ponec RJ, Saunders MD, Kimmey MB. Neostigmine for the treatment of acute colonic pseudo-obstruction. *N Engl J Med* 1999; 341:137–41. http://www.nejm.org/doi/full/10.1056/NEJM199907153410301#t=article

32 Hatzimouratidis K, Eardley I, Giuliano F, *et al*. EAU guidelines on penile curvature. *Eur Urol* 2012; 62(3):543–52. https://www.ncbi.nlm.nih.gov/pubmed/22658761

33 Kim ED. Local therapies to heal the penis: fact or fiction? *J Androl* 2008; 30(4):384–90. https://www.ncbi.nlm.nih.gov/pubmed/19023141

34 Wanders RJA, Waterham HR, Leroy BP. Refsum disease. *GeneReviews®* 2006; 20 March [updated 11 June 2015]. https://www.ncbi.nlm.nih.gov/books/NBK1353/

35 Worswick S, Cotliar J. Stevens–Johnson syndrome and toxic epidermal necrolysis: a review of treatment options. *Dermatol Ther* 2011; 24(2):207–18. https://www.ncbi.nlm.nih.gov/pubmed/21410610

36 Shirley MD, Tang H, Gallione CJ, *et al*. Sturge–Weber Syndrome and port-wine stains caused by somatic mutation. *N Eng J Med* 2013; 368(21):1971–9. doi:10.1056/NEJMoa1213507

37 Aomar Millán IF, Candel Erenas JM, *et al*. Up-date of the diagnosis and treatment of vasospastic angina. *Rev Clin Esp* 2008; 208(2):94–6. https://www.ncbi.nlm.nih.gov/pubmed/18261397

38 Keller KB, Lemberg L. Prinzmetal's angina. *Am J Crit Care* 2004; 13(4):350–4. https://www.ncbi.nlm.nih.gov/pubmed/15293589

39 Jayne DRW. Conventional treatment and outcome of Wegener's granulomatosis and microscopic polyangiitis. *CCJM* 2002; 69(Suppl 2):SII110–5. http://www.ccjm.org/supplements/single-view/conventional-treatment-and-outcome-of-wegener-s-granulomatosis-and-microscopic-polyangiitis/0d8061df0951aa4829194e88a0a1ba6b.html

40 Kuo SH, Debnam JM, Fuller GN, *et al*. Wernicke's encephalopathy: an underrecognized and reversible cause of confusional state in cancer patients. *J Oncology* 2009; 76(1):10–18. https://www.karger.com/Article/Abstract/174951

41 Anon. Listening to patients with rare diseases. *Lancet* 2009; 373:868. http://www.thelancet.com/pdfs/journals/lancet/PIIS0140-6736(09)60519-5.pdf

20 References

Chapter 16: Radiology

No references for this chapter

Chapter 17: Reference intervals, etc.

No references for this chapter

Chapter 18: Practical procedures

1 Johnston AJ, Streater CT, Noorani R, *et al*. The effect of peripherally inserted central catheter (PICC) valve technology on catheter occlusion rates—The 'ELeCTRiC study. *J Vasc Access* 2012; 13(4):421–5. https://www.ncbi.nlm.nih.gov/pubmed/22505280

Chapter 19: Emergencies

1 NICE. *Sepsis: recognition, diagnosis and early management* [NG51]. 2016, updated September 2017. https://www.nice.org.uk/guidance/ng51

2 NICE. *Acute coronary syndromes* [NG185]. November 2020. https://www.nice.org.uk/guidance/ng185

3 Resuscitation Council (UK). *Advanced life support* (8th edn). London: Resuscitation Council (UK), 2021.

4 Scottish Intercollegiate Guidelines Network. *British guideline on the management of asthma* (SIGN 158). Revised July 2019. https://www.brit-thoracic.org.uk/quality-improvement/guidelines/asthma

5 NICE. Management of exacerbations of COPD. In: *Chronic obstructive pulmonary disease in over 16s* [NG115]. Updated 2019. https://www.nice.org.uk/guidance/ng115

6 Agustí A, Celli BR, Criner GJ, *et al*. Global Initiative for chronic obstructive lung disease 2023 report. *Eur Respir J* 2023; 61(4):2300239.

7 NICE. *Venous thromboembolic diseases: diagnosis, management and thrombophilia testing* [NG158]. March 2020. https://www.nice.org.uk/guidance/ng158

8 Siau K, Hearnshaw S, Stanley AJ, *et al*. British Society of Gastroenterology (BSG)-led multisociety consensus care bundle for the early clinical management of acute upper gastrointestinal bleeding. *Frontline Gastroenterol* 2020; 11(4):311–23.

9 NICE. *Epilepsies in children, young people and adults* [NG217]. 2022. https://www.nice.org.uk/guidance/ng217

10 NICE. *Head injury: assessment and early management* [NG232]. 2023. https://www.nice.org.uk/guidance/ng232

11 Joint British Diabetes Societies for In-patient Care. *The management of diabetic ketoacidosis in adults*. Update 2023. https://abcd.care/sites/abcd.care/files/site_uploads/JBDS_Guidelines_Current/JBDS_02_DKA_Guideline_with_QR_code_March_2023.pdf

12 Joint British Diabetes Societies Inpatient Care Group. *Hyperosmolar hyperglycaemic state (HHS) care pathway in adults*. 2022. https://abcd.care/sites/abcd.care/files/site_uploads/JBDS_Guidelines_Current/JBDS_06_HHS_care_pathway_in_adults_2022.pdf

13 NHS England. *Clinical guidelines for major incidents and mass casualty events*. Version 2, 2020. https://www.england.nhs.uk/publication/clinical-guidelines-for-major-incidents-and-mass-casualty-events

Abbreviations: **F** indicates a notable figure or image; dis = disease; syn = syndrome.

Early warning scores are scoring systems based on physiological parameters. The magnitude of the given score reflects how far the parameter varies from normal.

The collated score from different parameters is used in:
• the assessment of acute illness
• the detection of a clinical deterioration
• the initiation of a timely and competent clinical response.

A standardized National Early Warning Score (NEWS) is recommended for use across the NHS.[1] The components of the NEWS are detailed in **fig A1**. An appropriate clinical response to the aggregate score from fig A1 is outlined in **fig A2**.

Physiological parameter	Score						
	3	2	1	0	1	2	3
Respiration rate (per minute)	≤8		9–11	12–20		21–24	≥25
SpO$_2$ Scale 1(%)*	≤91	92–93	94–95	≥96			
SpO$_2$ Scale 2(%)*	≤83	84–85	86–87	88–92 ≥93 on air	93–94 on oxygen	95–96 on oxygen	≥97 on oxygen
Air or oxygen?		Oxygen		Air			
Systolic blood pressure (mmHg)	≤90	91–100	101–110	111–219			≥220
Pulse (per minute)	≤40		41–50	51–90	91–110	111–130	≥131
Consciousness				Alert			CVPU
Temperature (°C)	≤35.0		35.1–36.0	36.1–38.0	38.1–39.0	≥39.1	

Fig A1 National Early Warning Score for adult patients. * Scale 1 is recommended for most patients including patients with COPD without hypercapnic respiratory failure. Scale 2 is recommended for patients with hypercapnic respiratory failure, whose target saturations are set lower (ie, 88–92%).

Reproduced from: Royal College of Physicians. *National Early Warning Score (NEWS) 2: Standardising the assessment of acute-illness severity in the NHS. Updated report of a working party*. London: RCP, 2017.

1 Royal College of Physicians. *National Early Warning Scores (NEWS) 2: Standardising the assessment of acute-illness severity in the NHS*. London: RCP, 2017.

NEW score	Frequency of monitoring	Clinical response
0	Minimum 12 hourly	• Continue routine NEWS monitoring
Total 1-4	Minimum 4-6 hourly	• Inform registered nurse, who must assess the patient • Registered nurse decides whether increased frequency of monitoring and/or escalation of care is required
3 in single parameter	Minimum 1 hourly	• Registered nurse to inform medical team caring for the patient, who will review and decide whether escalation of care is necessary
Total 5 or more Urgent response threshold	Minimum 1 hourly	• Registered nurse to immediately inform the medical team caring for the patient • Registered nurse to request urgent assessment by a clinician or team with core competencies in the care of acutely ill patients • Provide clinical care in an environment with monitoring facilities
Total 7 or more Emergency response threshold	Continuous monitoring of vital signs	• Registered nurse to immediately inform the medical team caring for the patient – this should be at least at specialist registrar level • Emergency assessment by a team with critical care competencies, including practitioner(s) with advanced airway management skills • Consider transfer of care to a level 2 or 3 clinical care facility, ie higher-dependency unit or ICU • Clinical care in an environment with monitoring facilities

Fig A2 Clinical response to NEWS triggers.
Reproduced from: Royal College of Physicians. *National Early Warning Score (NEWS) 2: Standardising the assessment of acute-illness severity in the NHS. Updated report of a working party.* London: RCP, 2017.

► Early warning scores are tools to aid assessment. They do not replace clinical judgment: use yours and respect the clinical opinion of others.
► Refer to local early warning scores where available.

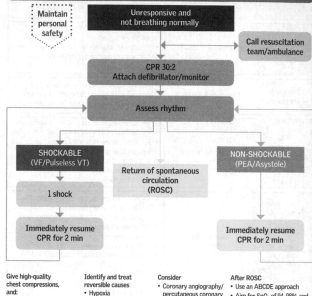

Fig A3 Cardiac arrest: advanced life support algorithm 2021.

Reproduced with the kind permission of the Resuscitation Council (UK), © 2021.

►►Ensure the safety of the patient and yourself.

►►Confirm diagnosis: a patient who is unresponsive and not breathing properly is in cardiac arrest (a manual pulse check is inaccurate and not recommended).

Basic life support Shout for help. Ask someone to call the arrest team and bring the defibrillator. Note the time. ABC:

►►*Airway:* head tilt (if no spine injury) and chin lift/jaw thrust.

►►*Breathing:* look, listen, and feel for breathing for no more than 10 seconds. If there is any doubt whether breathing is normal, proceed to chest compressions.

►►*Chest compressions:* place the heel of one hand on the centre of the chest (lower half of the sternum). Place your second hand on top and interlock fingers. Use straight arms. Give compressions at a rate of 100–120/min. Aim to compress the sternum 5–6cm. After 30 compressions give 2 rescue breaths. Do not interrupt compressions >10s. Continue with a ratio of 30:2 until defibrillator is available.

Advanced life support See algorithm fig A3.
• Continue chest compressions while adhesive defibrillation/monitoring pads are put in place. Plan all actions before pausing chest compressions.
• Stop chest compression for <5s to assess rhythm. Determine whether the rhythm is shockable (VF/pulseless VT) or non-shockable (asystole, pulseless electrical activity).

Shockable rhythm: VF/pulseless VT

►►A single person performs uninterrupted chest compressions while everyone else prepares for defibrillation: stand clear, move oxygen delivery device 1m away.

►►Select the appropriate energy on the defibrillator (150J or manufacturer's guidelines). When defibrillator is charged and safety check complete, the rescuer performing chest compressions stands clear and the shock is delivered.

►►CPR is resumed immediately (30:2). Reassess pulse/rhythm only after 2 minutes of CPR.

►►Repeat if shockable rhythm remains. Give drugs after 3 shocks (see Drugs, this topic).

Non-shockable rhythm: asystole/pulseless electrical activity (PEA)

►►Continue CPR 30:2. Obtain IV access and secure airway. Once airway secure switch to continuous compressions and ventilation. Give adrenaline 1mg IV.

►► Check rhythm every 2 minutes.

►►Consider reversible causes (4HS and 4TS: hypoxia, hypovolaemia, hyper/hypokalaemia/other metabolic derangement, hypothermia, thrombosis, tension pneumothorax, tamponade, toxins).

Drugs
• Give adrenaline 1mg IV every 3–5 mins for both shockable (from 3rd shock) and non-shockable rhythms. In practice this means at every other rhythm check or shock.[1]
• In shockable rhythms give amiodarone 300mg IV after 3 defibrillation attempts. Consider a further 150mg IV after 5 shocks. Lidocaine is an alternative.

Discontinuing resuscitation Needs clinical judgement: what is the likelihood of achieving a successful return of spontaneous circulation? If there is a shockable rhythm or a reversible cause then attempts are usually continued. It is reasonable to discontinue if asystole >20min without a reversible cause. Ask for the opinion of others in the resuscitation team.

Resuscitation decisions Consider, discuss, and record CPR decisions:
• at the request of a patient with capacity
• as part of end of life care (p12, p532)
• in deteriorating, severe illness.

►Your patient should be involved in decisions about CPR (unless it would cause physical or psychological harm). Explain your clinical decision to them, including futility.

►Do not make judgements about the quality of life of others based on your own perception.

1 The PARAMEDIC2 trial in the UK demonstrated a small increase in 30-day survival in those receiving adrenaline compared to placebo, but a higher rate of severe neurological impairment (PMID 30021076).

Useful doses for the new doctor

▶These pages outline the typical adult doses of drugs that a foundation doctor will be called upon to prescribe. Refer to local guidelines first. If in any doubt, consult a drug formulary (eg *British National Formulary*: www.bnf.org) especially if ↓eGFR or weight <50kg. Always check allergies before prescribing.

Drug	Dose and frequency	Notes
Analgesics		
Paracetamol	1g/6h PO/PR/IV, max 4g/24h	Avoid if hepatic impairment.
Ibuprofen	400mg/8h PO, max 2.4g/24h	SE: gastritis; broncho-spasm; AKI; fluid retention; hypersensitivity. CI: peptic ulcer; NSAID-induced asthma; coagulopathy; advanced CKD; heart failure.
Diclofenac sodium	50mg/8h PO/PR	
Codeine phosphate	30–60mg/4h PO/IM, max 240mg/24h	Chronic pain, eg malignancy, may require higher doses (see p532). Reduce dose if ↓eGFR. Care in head injury, as may hinder neurological assessment. SE: N&V; constipation; drowsiness; hypotension; respiratory depression, dependence. CI: respiratory depression.
Dihydrocodeine tartrate	30mg/4–6h PO, or 50mg/4–6h IM/SC	
Morphine	5–10mg/4h PO/IM	
Oxycodone	2.5–5mg/4h PO	
Tramadol	50–100mg/4h PO/IM/IV	
Antibiotics (refer to local guidelines)		
Phenoxymeth-ylpenicillin	500mg/6h PO (max 4g/24h)	SE: rash; hypersensitivity and anaphylaxis; diarrhoea. CI: history of allergy.
Benzylpenicillin	0.6–1.2g/6h IV/IM	
Flucloxacillin	250–500mg/6h PO/IM 1g/6h IV	
Erythromycin	250–500mg/6h PO	IV only if oral treatment not possible. Beware of cyto-chrome P450 interactions (not azithromycin). SE: N&V; diarrhoea; cholestasis; QT prolongation; pancreatitis.
Clarithromycin	250–500mg/6h PO	
Azithromycin	500mg/24h PO	
Doxycycline	200mg/24h PO as a single dose then 100mg/24h	SE: hypersensitivity; hepatotox-icity; may exacerbate myas-thenia gravis and SLE. CI: pregnancy; age <12yrs.
Metronidazole	400mg/8h PO, or 500mg/8h IV, or 1g/8h PR	IV only if oral treatment not possible.
Gentamicin	5mg/kg/24h IV adjusted to serum concentration	Adjust dose for renal function. SE: nephrotoxicity (correct volume depletion); electrolyte disturbance; ototoxicity.
Trimethoprim	200mg/12h PO	CI: 1st trimester (folate antagonist).
Anti-emetics		
Cyclizine	50mg/8h PO/IM/IV	SE: drowsiness.
Metoclopramide	10mg/8h PO/IM/IV	SE: extrapyramidal SE, espe-cially in young adults.
Ondansetron	4–8mg/8–12h PO/IV	SE: constipation; headache. CI: long QT syndrome.